Surgical Anatomy & Techniques to the Spine

Surgical Anatomy & Techniques to the Spine

Daniel H. Kim
Director, Spinal Neurosurgery and
Reconstructive Peripheral Nerve
Surgery
Department of Neurosurgery
Stanford University Medical Center
Stanford, CA

Alexander R. Vaccaro
Professor of Orthopaedic Surgery
Thomas Jefferson University
The Rothman Institute
Philadelphia, PA

Jeffrey S. Henn
Department of Neurosurgery
Lee Memorial Hospital
Fort Myers, FL

Curtis A. Dickman
Associate Chief, Spine Section
Director of Spinal Research
Division of Neurological Surgery
Barrow Neurological Institute
St. Joseph's Hospital and Medical Center
Phoenix, AZ

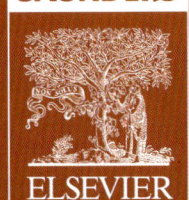

SAUNDERS
ELSEVIER

SAUNDERS
ELSEVIER

1600 John F. Kennedy Boulevard
Suite 1800
Philadelphia, PA 19103-2899

SURGICAL ANATOMY AND TECHNIQUES TO THE SPINE

Copyright © 2006, Elsevier Inc. All rights reserved.

No part of this publication may be reproduced or transmitted in any form or by any means, electronic or mechanical, including photocopying, recording, or any information storage and retrieval system, without permission in writing from the publisher. Permissions may be sought directly from Elsevier's Health Sciences Rights Department in Philadelphia, PA, USA: phone: (+1) 215 239 3804, fax: (+1) 215 239 3805, e-mail: healthpermissions@elsevier.com. You may also complete your request on-line via the Elsevier homepage (http://www.elsevier.com), by selecting 'Customer Support' and then 'Obtaining Permissions'.

NOTICE

Knowledge and best practice in this field are constantly changing. As new research and experience broaden our knowledge, changes in practice, treatment and drug therapy may become necessary or appropriate. Readers are advised to check the most current information provided (i) on procedures featured or (ii) by the manufacturer of each product to be administered, to verify the recommended dose or formula, the method and duration of administration, and contraindications. It is the responsibility of the practitioner, relying on their own experience and knowledge of the patient, to make diagnoses, to determine dosages and the best treatment for each individual patient, and to take all appropriate safety precautions. To the fullest extent of the law, neither the Publisher nor the Editors assume any liability for any injury and/or damage to persons or property arising out or related to any use of the material contained in this book.

Library of Congress Cataloging-in-Publication Data
Surgical anatomy and techniques to the spine / Daniel H. Kim . . . [et al.].
  p. ; cm.
   ISBN-13: 978-1-4160-0313-7   ISBN-10: 1-4160-0313-4
    1. Spine—Surgery. 2. Spine—Anatomy. 3. Anatomy, Surgical and topographical.   I. Kim, Daniel H.
    [DNLM: 1. Spinal Diseases—surgery. 2. Neurosurgical Procedures—methods. 3. Spinal Cord Injuries—surgery. 4. Spine—surgery. WE 725 S96185 2006]
RD533.S888 2006
617.5'6059—dc22

2005046536

ISBN-13: 978-1-4160-0313-7
ISBN-10: 1-4160-0313-4

Acquisitions Editor: Rebecca Schmidt Gaertner
Editorial Assistant: Suzanne Flint
Project Manager: David Saltzberg

Printed in China

Last digit is the print number: 9   8   7   6   5   4   3

Dedications

Daniel H. Kim:
I dedicate this book to all of the residents and fellows that I have had the privilege and honor to work with over the years at the Stanford University Medical Center.

Jeffrey S. Henn:
I would like to dedicate this book to my wife, Deana, my inspiration and support.

Alexander R. Vaccaro:
I wish to dedicate this book to my wife, Midge, and three children, Max, Alex, and Juliana. Without their love and support my contributions to this project would not have been possible.

Curtis A. Dickman:
I would like to dedicate this book to my wife, Celeste; my children, Alexander, Rachel, and Jacob; and my entire family. Thank you for enriching my life, for teaching me, and for your love.

Acknowledgments

Daniel H. Kim:
I would like to acknowledge the following individuals whose combined hard work, long hours, and dedicated resolve made this book possible: Max C. Lee, Karen M. Shibata, Thelma M. Prescott, and medical illustrators Christine M. Field, Justin Greene, and Curtis Mothershed.

Jeffrey S. Henn:
I would like to acknowledge my parents, Don and Eileen, for their support throughout my education and career.

Preface

The fundamentals of spine surgery revolve around a thorough understanding of anatomy and surgical technique. With new instrumentation and minimally invasive techniques, spinal surgery has become complex in the 21st century. From occipital cervical fusions to sacroiliac fixation, the spine surgeon of today is confronted with an extensive array of surgical options. The rapid pace of technological change in this field has left many spine surgeons and colleagues struggling to keep up. The increasing variety of options for surgical treatments of spinal injury and disease renders the decision-making process regarding the use of any particular approach, procedure, or technology more and more difficult.

In addition to instrumentation, minimally invasive spine (MIS) techniques are becoming common. With smaller and smaller incisions, spine surgeons find themselves working with a smaller aperture and, subsequently, a limited view. Without exposure of the adjacent anatomical structures, these MIS techniques can create a challenge. This challenge occurs not only with decompressions but also with percutaneous instrumentation placement.

This instrumentation and these techniques are being used for an increasing patient base. Spinal instrumentation is used not only for trauma and degenerative disease, but also, with new techniques, increasingly in cases of tumor and infection.

In light of the myriad advancements, we sought to cover the topics of occipital cervical fusion—including cervical plating techniques along with atlantoaxial fixation devices. In addition, we provide a review of fusions of the cervicothoracic and thoracolumbar regions, as these transition zones have led to a new level of complexity. Last, longer fusion constructs have led to sacroiliac fixation.

Whether confronted with new instrumentation or minimally invasive techniques, the spine surgeon has to rely on the fundamentals of anatomy and technique. Thus, we wished to review these essential items to provide the spinal surgeon with an armamentarium to approach increasingly complex issues facing medicine today.

Max C. Lee

Contributors

Frank Acosta, Jr., MD
Department of Neurosurgery
University of California, San Francisco Spine Center
San Francisco, CA
Secondary Metastatic Tumors of the Spine

Christopher J. Aho, MD
Resident
Department of Neurological Surgery
University of Southern California Keck School of Medicine
Los Angeles, CA
Lateral Lumbar Interbody Fusion

Todd J. Albert, MD
Vice Chairman and Professor
Department of Orthopaedic Surgery
Jefferson Medical College of Thomas Jefferson University
Co-Director of Reconstructive Surgery and Spine Fellowship Program
Thomas Jefferson University
The Rothman Institute
Philadelphia, PA
Anterior Retroperitoneal Approach

Howard S. An, MD
The Morton International Professor of Orthopaedic Surgery
Director
Division of Spine Surgery and Spine Fellowship Program
Department of Orthopaedic Surgery
Rush University Medical Center
Chicago, IL
Laminoplasty Techniques

D. Greg Anderson, MD
Associate Professor
Jefferson Medical College
The Rothman Institute
Philadelphia, PA
Transperitoneal Approaches to the Lumbosacral Junction

Todd Applegate, DO
Senior Assistant Resident
Department of Orthopaedic Surgery
Boston University Medical Center
Boston, MA
Posterior Approaches to the Sacrum

Ashok Biyani, MD
Assistant Professor
Department of Orthopaedic Surgery
Medical College of Ohio
Toledo, OH
Laminoplasty Techniques

Christopher M. Bono, MD
Assistant Professor
Department of Orthopaedic Surgery
Boston University Medical Center
Boston, MA
Posterior Approaches to the Sacrum

Ungkyu Chang, MD
Research Fellow
Department of Neurosurgery
Stanford University Medical Center
Stanford, CA
High Cervical Retropharyngeal Approach to the Craniocervical Junction; Anterior Approach to the Midcervical Spine; Posterior Approach to the Midcervical Spine; Anterior Corpectomy and Fusion

Fady T. Charbel, MD
Professor and Head
Chief of Neurovascular Section
Department of Neurological Surgery
University of Illinois at Chicago
Chicago, IL
Vascular Lesions of the Spinal Cord

Won-Ho Choo, MD
Visiting Assistant Professor
Department of Neurosurgery
Stanford University Medical Center
Stanford, CA
Posterior and Far-Lateral Approaches to the Craniovertebral Junction

Dean Chou, MD
Assistant Clinical Professor
Department of Neurological Surgery
University of California, San Francisco
San Francisco, CA
Primary Malignant and Benign Tumors of the Vertebral Column; Secondary Metastatic Tumors of the Spine

Andrew Dailey, MD
Associate Professor
Department of Neurological Surgery
University of Washington School of Medicine
Seattle, WA
Ossification of the Posterior Longitudinal Ligament

Matthew D. Eichenbaum, MD
Spine Research Fellow
Department of Orthopaedic Surgery
Thomas Jefferson University
The Rothman Institute
Philadelphia, PA
Ankylosing Spondylitis—Posterior Approaches (Osteotomy) to the Cervical and Lumbar Spine in the Management of a Fixed Sagittal Plane Deformity

Ron El-Hawary, MD, MSc
Fellow
Department of Orthopaedics
Texas Scottish Rite Hospital for Children
Dallas, TX
Anterior Treatment for Thoracolumbar/Lumbar Scoliosis

Azadeh Farin, MD
Resident Physician
Department of Neurological Surgery
University of Southern California Keck School of Medicine
Los Angeles, CA
Posterior Keyhole Cervical Foraminotomy; The Transoral Approach for Ventral Cervicomedullary Decompression in Rheumatoid Arthritis

Farrokh R. Farrokhi, MD
Chief Resident
Department of Neurological Surgery
University of Washington Medical Center
Seattle, WA
Ossification of the Posterior Longitudinal Ligament

Amir H. Fayyazi, MD
Assistant Professor
Division of Spine Surgery
Department of Orthopedic Surgery
State University of New York Upstate Medical University
Syracuse, NY
Laminoplasty Techniques

Iman Feiz-Erfan, MD
Neurosurgical Resident
Division of Neurological Surgery
Barrow Neurological Institute
St. Joseph's Hospital and Medical Center
Phoenix, AZ
Surgical Therapy for Fractures and Dislocations of the Craniocervical Junction and Upper Cervical Spine

Maurice L. Goins, MD
Department of Orthopaedic Surgery
Balboa Naval Medical Center
San Diego, CA
Ankylosing Spondylitis—Posterior Approaches (Osteotomy) to the Cervical and Lumbar Spine in the Management of a Fixed Sagittal Plane Deformity

L. Fernando Gonzalez, MD
Research Fellow
Surgical Neuroanatomy Laboratory
Division of Neurological Surgery
Barrow Neurological Institute
St. Joseph's Hospital and Medical Center
Phoenix, AZ
Surgical Technique for Resection of Intradural Tumors

Nitin Goyal, MD
Jefferson Medical College
Thomas Jefferson University
Philadelphia, PA
Minimal Access Exposure for Posterior Lumbar Instrumented Fusions

Alan S. Hilibrand, MD
Assistant Professor and Director of Medical Education
Department of Orthopaedic Surgery
Thomas Jefferson University
The Rothman Institute
Philadelphia, PA
Ankylosing Spondylitis—Posterior Approaches (Osteotomy) to the Cervical and Lumbar Spine in the Management of a Fixed Sagittal Plane Deformity

Langston Holly, MD
Assistant Professor and Co-Director
UCLA Comprehensive Spine Center
Division of Neurosurgery
Department of Orthopedic Surgery
University of California, Los Angeles Medical Center
Los Angeles, CA
Anterior Retroperitoneal Approach to the Lumbar Spine; Posterior and Posterolateral Approaches to the Thoracic and Lumbar Spine

Jin-Woo Hur, MD
Staff Neurosurgeon
Cheongju St. Mary's Hospital
Chungbuk, Korea
Surgical Anatomy and Operative Techniques of Lumbar Stenosis

Dean G. Karahalios, MD
Chicago Institute of Neurosurgery and Neuroresearch (CINN)
Neurologic and Orthopedic Institute of Chicago
Chicago, IL
Thoracic Diskectomy

Larry T. Khoo, MD
Assistant Professor and Co-Director
UCLA Comprehensive Spine Center
Division of Neurosurgery
Department of Orthopedic Surgery
University of California, Los Angeles Medical Center
Los Angeles, CA
Anterior Retroperitoneal Approach to the Lumbar Spine

Jeffrey D. Klopfenstein, MD
Neurosurgical Resident
Division of Neurological Surgery
Barrow Neurological Institute
St. Joseph's Hospital and Medical Center;
Phoenix, AZ
Surgical Therapy for Fractures and Dislocations of the Craniocervical Junction and Upper Cervical Spine

Timothy R. Kuklo, MD
Department of Orthopaedic Surgery
Walter Reed Army Medical Center
Washington, DC
Surgical Management of Flatback Syndrome

Carl Lauryssen, MD
Medical Director of Research and Education
Cedars-Sinai Institute for Spinal Disorders
Department of Neurological Surgery
Cedars-Sinai Medical Center
Los Angeles, CA
Anterior Lumbar Interbody Fusion

Hoang N. Le, MD
Department of Neurosurgery
Stanford University Medical Center
Stanford, CA
Anterior Approaches to the Cervicothoracic Junction (Low Cervical-Supraclavicular, Transclavicular-Transmanubrial, Trans-sternal-Transthoracic); Anterolateral Transthoracic Approaches to the Cervicothoracic Junction (Transaxillary Approach, Transpleural Transthoracic Third Rib Resection Approach); Posterolateral Approaches to the Cervicothoracic Junction (Transpedicular, Costotransversectomy, Lateral Extracavitary, and Parascapular Extrapleural Approaches); Thoracoabdominal Approach; Cervicothoracic Junction Fractures; Thoracic and Thoracolumbar Fractures

Max C. Lee, MD
Clinical Instructor
Department of Neurosurgery
Stanford University Medical Center
Stanford, CA
Transoral Approach to the Craniocervical Junction and Upper Cervical Spine; Transmaxillary Approach to the Clivus and Upper Cervical Spine; High Cervical Retropharyngeal Approach to the Craniocervical Junction; Posterior and Far-Lateral Approaches to Craniovertebral Junction; Anterior Approach to the Midcervical Spine; Posterior Approach to the Midcervical Spine; Anterior Corpectomy and Fusion; Burst Fractures of the Cervical Spine; Subaxial Cervical Spinal Injuries and Facet Dislocation Injuries

G. Michael Lemole, Jr., MD
Assistant Professor
Department of Neurosurgery
University of Illinois at Chicago
Neuropsychiatric Unit
Chicago, IL
Vascular Lesions of the Spinal Cord

Lawrence G. Lenke, MD
The Jerome S. Gilden Professor of Orthopaedic Surgery
Washington University of St. Louis
Co-Chief, Pediatric and Adult Scoliosis and Spinal Reconstruction
Department of Orthopaedic Surgery
Barnes-Jewish Hospital
St. Louis, MO
Surgical Treatment of Adolescent Idiopathic Scoliosis: Lenke Curve Types 1 to 6

Brian M. Leo, MD
Resident
Department of Orthopaedic Surgery
University of Virginia Health System
Charlottesville, VA
Transperitoneal Approaches to the Lumbosacral Junction

K. Charles Y. Liu, MD, PhD
Assistant Professor
Department of Neurological Surgery
University of Southern California Keck School of Medicine
Los Angeles, CA
The Transoral Approach for Ventral Cervicomedullary Decompression in Rheumatoid Arthritis

Amir A. Mehbod, MD
Twin Cities Spine Center
Minneapolis, MN
Spondylolisthesis Reduction

Ronnie I. Mimran, MD
Staff Physician
Pacific Brain and Spine Medical Group
Eden Medical Center
Castro Valley, CA
Minimally Invasive Lumbar Decompression

Sergey Neckrysh, MD
Resident
Department of Neurological Surgery
University of Illinois at Chicago
Chicago, IL
Vascular Lesions of the Spinal Cord

Bryan C. Oh, MD
Resident
Department of Neurological Surgery
University of Southern California Keck School of Medicine
Los Angeles, CA
Lateral Lumbar Interbody Fusion

Adebukola Onibokun, MD
Senior Resident
Division of Neurological Surgery
University of California, Los Angeles Medical Center
Los Angeles, CA
Anterior Retroperitoneal Approach to the Lumbar Spine; Posterior and Posterolateral Approaches to the Thoracic and Lumbar Spine

Michael A. Pahl, MD
Orthopaedic Spine Research Fellow
Thomas Jefferson University
The Rothman Institute
Philadelphia, PA
Minimal Access Exposure for Posterior Lumbar Instrumented Fusions

Jon Park, MD, FRCSC
Assistant Professor
Department of Neurosurgery
Stanford University Medical Center
Stanford, CA
Thoracoabdominal Approach; Thoracic and Thoracolumbar Fractures

David A. Peace, MS
Medical Illustrator
Department of Neurosurgery
University of Florida
Gainesville, FL
Lumbar Microdiskectomy: Midline Open and Far-Lateral Techniques; Percutaneous and Endoscopic Diskectomy

Randall W. Porter, MD
Chief, Intradisciplinary Skull Base Section
Division of Neurological Surgery
Barrow Neurological Institute
St. Joseph's Hospital and Medical Center
Phoenix, AZ
Surgical Technique for Resection of Intradural Tumors

Benjamin K. Potter, MD
Resident
Department of Orthopaedics and Rehabilitation
Walter Reed Army Medical Center
Washington, DC
Surgical Management of Flatback Syndrome

Eric A. Potts, MD
Indianapolis Neurosurgical Group
Indianapolis, IN
Thoracic Diskectomy

Kian Raiszadeh, MD
Resident
Department of Orthopaedic Surgery
University of Medicine and Dentistry of New Jersey—
New Jersey Medical School
Newark, NJ
Bacterial, Fungal, and Tuberculosis Diskitis and Osteomyelitis of the Cervical, Thoracic, and Lumbar Spine

Albert L. Rhoton, Jr., MD
R.D. Keene Family Professor and Chairman Emeritus
Department of Neurosurgery
University of Florida
McKnight Brain Institute
Gainesville, FL
Transoral Approach to the Craniocervical Junction and Upper Cervical Spine; Transmaxillary Approach to the Clivus and Upper Cervical Spine; High Cervical Retropharyngeal Approach to the Craniocervical Junction

Erich O. Richter, MD
Resident
Department of Neurological Surgery
University of Florida
Gainesville, FL
Lumbar Microdiskectomy: Midline Open and Far-Lateral Techniques; Percutaneous and Endoscopic Diskectomy

Stephen I. Ryu, MD
Resident
Department of Neurosurgery
Stanford University Medical Center
Stanford, CA
Transmaxillary Approach to the Clivus and Upper Cervical Spine

Darren B. Schneider, MD
Assistant Professor of Surgery and Radiology
Division of Vascular Surgery
University of California, San Francisco
San Francisco, CA
Secondary Metastatic Tumors of the Spine

Fernando E. Silva, MD
Visiting Spinal Fellow
Department of Orthopaedics
Pediatric and Adult Spinal, Scoliosis and Reconstructive Surgery
Washington University Medical Center
St. Louis, MO
Surgical Treatment of Adolescent Idiopathic Scoliosis: Lenke Curve Types 1 to 6

Carl Spivak, MD, FRCSC
Clinical Instructor
Department of Neurological Surgery
Jackson-Madison County General Hospital
Jackson, TN
Laminotomy and Laminectomy for Cervical Stenosis

Daniel J. Sucato, MD
Assistant Professor
Department of Orthopaedic Surgery
University of Texas Southwestern Medical Center at Dallas
Department of Orthopedics
Texas Scottish Rite Hospital for Children
Dallas, TX
Anterior Release and Fusion Techniques for Thoracic Scoliosis; Anterior Treatment for Thoracolumbar/Lumbar Scoliosis

Issada Thongtrangan, MD
Fellow
Department of Orthopaedic Surgery
Virginia Commonwealth University Medical Center
Richmond, VA
Thoracoabdominal Approach; Thoracic and Thoracolumbar Fractures

Ensor E. Transfeldt, MD
Associate Professor
Cervical Spine Disorders, Scoliosis, and Spondylolisthesis
University of Minnesota, Twin Cities
Twin Cities Spine Center
Minneapolis, MN
Spondylolisthesis Reduction

Arthur J. Ulm, III, MD
Resident
Department of Neurosurgery
University of Florida
Gainesville, FL
Lumbar Microdiskectomy: Midline Open and Far-Lateral Techniques; Percutaneous and Endoscopic Diskectomy

Michael J. Vives, MD
Assistant Professor
Department of Orthopaedic Surgery
University of Medicine and Dentistry of New Jersey—New Jersey Medical School
Newark, NJ
Bacterial, Fungal, and Tuberculosis Diskitis and Osteomyelitis of the Cervical, Thoracic, and Lumbar Spine

Vassilios I. Vougioukas, MD
Department of Neurosurgery
Neurocenter
Albert Ludwigs University of Freiburg
Freiburg, Germany
Surgical Therapy for Fractures and Dislocations of the Craniocervical Junction and Upper Cervical Spine

Michael Y. Wang, MD
Assistant Professor
Department of Neurological Surgery
University of Southern California Keck School of Medicine
Los Angeles, California
Posterior Keyhole Cervical Foraminotomy; Anterior Lumbar Interbody Fusion; Lateral Lumbar Interbody Fusion; The Transoral Approach for Ventral Cervicomedullary Decompression in Rheumatoid Arthritis

Kirkham B. Wood, MD
Chief of Orthopaedic Spine Service
Department of Orthopaedic Surgery
Massachusetts General Hospital
Orthopaedic Associates
Boston, MA
The Surgical Management of Scheuermann's Kyphosis

Steven C. Zeiller, MD
Resident
Department of Orthopaedic Surgery
Thomas Jefferson University
Philadelphia, PA
Anterior Retroperitoneal Approach

Ho-Yeol Zhang, MD, PhD
Clinical Associate Professor
Chief, Department of Neurosurgery
National Health Insurance Corporation
Ilsan Hospital
Yonsei University College of Medicine
Kyonggi-do, Korea
Anterior Cervical Diskectomy and Fusion; Anterior Cervical Microforaminotomy; Anterior Cervical Fusion and Instrumentation Techniques; Transpedicular Screw Fixations; Posterior Lumbar Interbody Fusion; Unilateral Transforaminal Lumbar Interbody Fusion; Lumbar and Sacral Fractures

Table of Contents

Section I
Surgical Anatomy and Approaches

Section A Craniovertebral Junction and Upper Cervical Spine

Chapter 1 Transoral Approach to Craniocervical Junction and Upper Cervical Spine **3**
Jeffrey S. Henn, Max C. Lee, Albert L. Rhoton, Jr.

Chapter 2 Transmaxillary Approach to the Clivus and Upper Cervical Spine **13**
Max C. Lee, Stephen I. Ryu, Albert L. Rhoton, Jr., Daniel H. Kim

Chapter 3 High Cervical Retropharyngeal Approach to the Craniocervical Junction **22**
Ungkyu Chang, Jeffrey S. Henn, Max C. Lee, Albert L. Rhoton, Jr.

Chapter 4 Posterior and Far-Lateral Approaches to the Craniovertebral Junction **33**
Won-Ho Choo, Max C. Lee, Daniel H. Kim

Section B Mid and Lower Cervical Spine

Chapter 5 Anterior Approach to the Midcervical Spine **45**
Ungkyu Chang, Max C. Lee, Daniel H. Kim

Chapter 6 Posterior Approach to the Midcervical Spine **57**
Ungkyu Chang, Max C. Lee, Daniel H. Kim

Section C Cervicothoracic Junction and Thoracic Spine

Chapter 7 Anterior Approaches to the Cervicothoracic Junction (Low Cervical-Supraclavicular, Transclavicular-Transmanubrial, Trans-sternal-Transthoracic) **65**
Hoang N. Le, Daniel H. Kim

Chapter 8 Anterolateral Transthoracic Approaches to the Cervicothoracic Junction (Transaxillary Approach, Transpleural Transthoracic Third Rib Resection Approach) **71**
Hoang N. Le, Daniel H. Kim

Chapter 9 Posterolateral Approaches to the Cervicothoracic Junction (Transpedicular, Costotransversectomy, Lateral Extracavitary, and Parascapular Extrapleural Approaches) **78**
Hoang N. Le, Daniel H. Kim

Section D Thoracolumbar and Lumbar Spines

Chapter 10 Thoracoabdominal Approach **89**
Issada Thongtrangan, Hoang N. Le, Jon Park, Daniel H. Kim

Chapter 11 Anterior Retroperitoneal Approach to the Lumbar Spine **101**
Adebukola Onibokun, Larry T. Khoo, Langston Holly

Chapter 12 Posterior and Posterolateral Approaches to the Thoracic and Lumbar Spine **106**
Adebukola Onibokun, Langston Holly

Section E Lumbar Sacral Junction

Chapter 13 Transperitoneal Approaches to the Lumbosacral Junction **113**
Brian M. Leo, D. Greg Anderson

Chapter 14 Anterior Retroperitoneal Approach **126**
Steven C. Zeiller, Todd J. Albert

Chapter 15 Posterior Approaches to the Sacrum **133**
Todd Applegate, Christopher M. Bono

Section II
Degenerative Disease of the Spine

Section A Cervical Disk Herniation

- Chapter 16 Anterior Cervical Diskectomy and Fusion **141**
  Ho-Yeol Zhang, Daniel H. Kim
- Chapter 17 Anterior Cervical Microforaminotomy **150**
  Ho-Yeol Zhang, Daniel H. Kim
- Chapter 18 Anterior Cervical Fusion and Instrumentation Techniques **157**
  Ho-Yeol Zhang, Daniel H. Kim
- Chapter 19 Posterior Keyhole Cervical Foraminotomy **164**
  Azadeh Farin, Michael Y. Wang

Section B Cervical Stenosis

- Chapter 20 Anterior Corpectomy and Fusion **169**
  Ungkyu Chang, Max C. Lee, Daniel H. Kim
- Chapter 21 Laminotomy and Laminectomy for Cervical Stenosis **174**
  Carl Spivak, Daniel H. Kim
- Chapter 22 Laminoplasty Techniques **180**
  Howard S. An, Amir H. Fayyazi, Ashok Biyani
- Chapter 23 Ossification of the Posterior Longitudinal Ligament **191**
  Farrokh R. Farrokhi, Andrew Dailey

Section C Thoracic Disk Herniation

- Chapter 24 Thoracic Diskectomy **201**
  Dean G. Karahalios, Eric A. Potts

Section D Lumbar Disk Herniation

- Chapter 25 Lumbar Microdiskectomy: Midline Open and Far-Lateral Techniques **213**
  Arthur J. Ulm, III, Erich O. Richter, David A. Peace, Jeffrey S. Henn
- Chapter 26 Percutaneous and Endoscopic Diskectomy **219**
  Erich O. Richter, Arthur J. Ulm, III, David A. Peace, Jeffrey S. Henn

Section E Lumbar Stenosis

- Chapter 27 Surgical Anatomy and Operative Techniques of Lumbar Stenosis **227**
  Jin-Woo Hur, Daniel H. Kim
- Chapter 28 Minimally Invasive Lumbar Decompression **231**
  Ronnie I. Mimran, Jeffrey S. Henn

Section F Lumbar Fusion and Instrumentation Techniques

- Chapter 29 Transpedicular Screw Fixations **239**
  Ho-Yeol Zhang, Daniel H. Kim
- Chapter 30 Posterior Lumbar Interbody Fusion **246**
  Ho-Yeol Zhang, Daniel H. Kim
- Chapter 31 Unilateral Transforaminal Lumbar Interbody Fusion **255**
  Ho-Yeol Zhang, Daniel H. Kim
- Chapter 32 Anterior Lumbar Interbody Fusion **263**
  Michael Y. Wang, Carl Lauryssen

Chapter 33 Lateral Lumbar Interbody Fusion **272**
Michael Y. Wang, Bryan C. Oh, Christopher J. Aho

Chapter 34 Spondylolisthesis Reduction **280**
Ensor E. Transfeldt, Amir A. Mehbod

Chapter 35 Minimal Access Exposure for Posterior Lumbar Instrumented Fusions **287**
Nitin Goyal, Alexander R. Vaccaro, Michael A. Pahl

Section III
Inflammatory Disease

Chapter 36 The Transoral Approach for Ventral Cervicomedullary Decompression in Rheumatoid Arthritis **297**
Azadeh Farin, K. Charles Y. Liu, Michael Y. Wang

Chapter 37 Ankylosing Spondylitis—Posterior Approaches (Osteotomy) to the Cervical and Lumbar Spine in the Management of a Fixed Sagittal Plane Deformity **305**
Maurice L. Goins, Matthew D. Eichenbaum, Alan S. Hilibrand

Section IV
Spinal Trauma

Section A Craniovertebral and Cervical Spine

Chapter 38 Surgical Therapy for Fractures and Dislocations of the Craniocervical Junction and Upper Cervical Spine **317**
Iman Feiz-Erfan, Jeffrey D. Klopfenstein, Vassilios I. Vougioukas, Curtis A. Dickman

Chapter 39 Burst Fractures of the Cervical Spine **331**
Max C. Lee, Daniel H. Kim

Chapter 40 Subaxial Cervical Spinal Injuries and Facet Dislocation Injuries **337**
Max C. Lee, Daniel H. Kim

Section B Thoracic Spine

Chapter 41 Cervicothoracic Junction Fractures **344**
Hoang N. Le, Daniel H. Kim

Chapter 42 Thoracic and Thoracolumbar Fractures **352**
Issada Thongtrangan, Hoang N. Le, Jon Park, Daniel H. Kim

Section C Lumbar and Sacral Spine

Chapter 43 Lumbar and Sacral Fractures **365**
Ho-Yeol Zhang, Daniel H. Kim

Section V
Spinal Deformity

Chapter 44 Anterior Release and Fusion Techniques for Thoracic Scoliosis **379**
Daniel J. Sucato

Chapter 45 Anterior Treatment for Thoracolumbar/Lumbar Scoliosis **392**
Ron El-Hawary, Daniel J. Sucato

Chapter 46 Surgical Treatment of Adolescent Idiopathic Scoliosis: Lenke Curve Types 1 to 6 **406**
Fernando E. Silva, Lawrence G. Lenke

Chapter 47 Surgical Management of Flatback Syndrome **421**
Timothy R. Kuklo, Benjamin K. Potter

Chapter 48 The Surgical Management of Scheuermann's Kyphosis **432**
Kirkham B. Wood

Section VI
Spinal Tumor

Chapter 49 Primary Malignant and Benign Tumors of the Vertebral Column **441**
Dean Chou, Curtis A. Dickman

Chapter 50 Secondary Metastatic Tumors of the Spine **449**
Dean Chou, Frank Acosta, Jr., Darren B. Schneider, Curtis A. Dickman

Chapter 51 Surgical Technique for Resection of Intradural Tumors **462**
L. Fernando Gonzalez, Randall W. Porter

Chapter 52 Vascular Lesions of the Spinal Cord **474**
Sergey Neckrysh, Fady T. Charbel, G. Michael Lemole, Jr.

Section VII
Spinal Infection

Chapter 53 Bacterial, Fungal, and Tuberculosis Diskitis and Osteomyelitis of the Cervical, Thoracic, and Lumbar Spine **489**
Michael J. Vives, Kian Raiszadeh

Section VIII
Miscellaneous

Chapter 54 Bone Graft Harvesting Techniques **505**
Jeffrey S. Henn, Curtis A. Dickman

Index **513**

SECTION I

SURGICAL ANATOMY AND APPROACHES

SECTION A
Craniovertebral Junction and Upper Cervical Spine

CHAPTER 1

JEFFREY S. HENN
MAX C. LEE
ALBERT L. RHOTON, JR.

Transoral Approach to the Craniocervical Junction and Upper Cervical Spine

INTRODUCTION

Lesions of the craniocervical junction have intrigued spine surgeons for centuries. Pathology at this location was first described in literature written by physicians in the nineteenth century. These lesions have presented with a multitude of signs and symptoms. In addition, treatment has varied. In the past, posterior decompression and fixation offered the only solution, and the outcomes were poor. Currently, newer techniques have included an anterior decompression and posterior fixation.

The transoral approach was initially described by Fang and Ong in 1962. Because of complications (which included cerebrospinal fluid leak, infections, and vertebral artery injury), this procedure did not gain popularity until the 1980s. Approaches to the craniocervical junction include transoral, transfacial, high cervical retropharyngeal, posterior, and far-lateral approaches.

A standard transoral approach will expose the caudal clivus with the anterior arch of the atlas and the C2-C3 disk space. Thus, the transoral approach has been used to reach tumors of the atlas, axis, and clivus for resection and fixation of the odontoid process after ligamentous and osseous injury, and for decompressing bony malformations of the craniovertebral junction, such as basilar invagination, which compress the medulla or spinal cord anteriorly. Historically, the transoral approach has also been used for intradural lesions, such as aneurysms of the vertebrobasilar junction or foramen magnum meningiomas. However, significant inherent risks have resulted in general abandonment of this strategy.

The transoral approach may be modified to include a transpalatine (approach in which the soft palate or both the soft and hard palates are opened) and a labiomandibular or labioglossomandibular approach in which the lip, mandible, and possibly the tongue and floor of the mouth are split to increase the exposure. In addition, a median glossotomy may be incorporated into a mandibular spit, in order to incorporate more caudal levels. Lastly, a transoral approach may also incorporate a transpalatal or transmaxillary approach for increased rostral exposure. The transmaxillary approach will be discussed in Chapter 2.

This chapter will focus on transoral approaches. This approach is used to reach lesions of the anterior craniovertebral junction and is best suited for midline, irreducible extradural lesions. This approach has been used for the diagnosis and débridement of infection and resection of tumors and compressive masses within this region. The main advantage of the anterior approach is the direct route to the lesion, avoiding the potential need to work around or to manipulate neural structures. The major disadvantages include a contaminated field and a limited working field, especially for lesions extending off-midline. When exposing intradural lesions, or in cases of inadvertent duratomy, other risks include cerebrospinal fluid fistula, pseudomeningocele, and meningitis. Although the depth of the operative field is a potential disadvantage, the use of the operating microscope has reduced the importance of this factor.

The stability of the craniocervical junction has to be accounted for at all times, with the understanding that an anterior decompression may necessitate posterior fixation. Reconstruction, as it is elsewhere within the spinal axis, is paramount. In addition, contraindications to transoral surgery include active nasopharyngeal infection and anomalous vascular anatomy resulting in vessels within or ventral to the lesion. Relative contraindications include posterior pathology, which may guide one toward a posterior decompression and fusion. In addition, reducible ventral lesions may be taken care of via strict posterior stabilization. In other words, decompression of the cervicomedullary junction may be obtained via posterior reduction. Lastly, intradural work via a transfacial, transoral approach has been fraught with complications of cerebrospinal fluid leakage and meningitis. Thus, intradural work may be considered a relative contraindication.

SURGICAL ANATOMY

Transoral exposure is generally limited by the amount of mouth opening and degree of neck extension.

- Opening of the mouth permits exposure to the clivus. The hard palate limits access to the upper clivus (Fig. 1-1).
- The soft palate and posterior pharyngeal wall are visualized. The soft palate extends backward from the hard palate and blocks the view of the upper clivus. An incision through the midline soft palate is outlined (Fig. 1-2).
- After the soft palate has been opened, the lower clivus may be exposed by opening the posterior pharyngeal wall in a single layer and retracting the soft tissue laterally (Fig. 1-3).
- For access to the upper anterior spine, the soft palate may be retracted and the posterior pharyngeal wall, including the mucosa and muscles, are opened in a single layer and retracted laterally (Fig. 1-4).
- Lesions involving the clivus and upper spine can be approached by opening the soft palate and extending the opening of the posterior pharyngeal wall (Fig. 1-5).
- Cadaveric dissection in Figure 1-6 shows extent of exposure. The right-sided longus colli and longus capitis muscles are shown for reference.
- If further cranial exposure is needed, laterally based mucoperiosteal flaps are elevated from the surface of the hard palate (interrupted lines). The posterior aspect of the hard palate may then be removed (oblique lines). The posterior pharyngeal opening is extended up through the vault of the nasopharynx to the posterior border of the vomer (Fig. 1-7).
- The transmandibular extension of the transoral approach requires a midline skin incision through the lip and chin. The mandibular osteotomy is performed in a step-like fashion to maximize postoperative stability. Spreading the mandibular halves laterally allows the tongue to be depressed downward. If necessary, the tongue can also be split in the midline to gain further exposure inferiorly (Fig. 1-8).

OPERATIVE TECHNIQUES

PREPARATION AND POSITIONING

The patient should be given a broad-spectrum antibiotic with gram-positive and gram-negative coverage prior to surgery. The patient is positioned supine, ideally with the head somewhat extended (proper positioning should be carefully performed with fluoroscopic guidance if appropriate). The skull is rigidly fixated using a Mayfield head holder (or a halo brace if spinal instability is a consideration). The surgeon is positioned at the top of the patient's head and uses an operating microscope for illumination, magnification, and binocular visualization. Image guidance can be helpful, and cranial image guidance techniques are often applicable based on the fixed relationships of the clivus and C1 vertebra to the rest of the skull.

SURGICAL PROCEDURE

Custom-designed self-retaining retractor systems are used to facilitate the transoral approach. Others have used a modified Dingman self-retaining mouth retractor. The patient's tongue and the endotracheal tube are retracted caudally with a rigid adjustable wide retractor blade. Teeth guards attached to the retractor frame help protect the patient's dentition. After the retractor is positioned, the patient's tongue should be inspected in order to ensure that it is not compressed by the teeth. Such compression can result in severe swelling. In addition, during a lengthy case, intermittent relaxation of this retraction may be accomplished.

For access to the upper spine, the soft palate may be retracted using the table-mounted retractor system. Alternatively, catheters may be passed through the nasal passages and brought out the mouth for retraction (see Fig. 1-3). If the lesion involves the clivus, it may be necessary to split the soft palate in the midline. Although typically well tolerated, this split may result in nasal regurgitation, dysphagia, and a nasal tone of voice. If even more cranial exposure is needed, it may become necessary to remove the posterior part of the hard palate, which can be replaced at the completion of the procedure using miniplates. A transpalatal approach includes an incision along the hard palate in the midline. The vomer is identified and removed in order to allow exposure of the basisphenoid region. Menezes describes an alternative incision paralleling the upper dentition and en bloc removal of the hard palate.

Prior to incision, the oropharynx and retractors are sterilized with betadine solution after the retractors have been positioned. In addition, packing the pharynx will occlude the laryngopharynx and the esophagus. Injection may be carried out with local anesthetic and epinephrine. Depending on the extent of exposure, the soft palate is opened in a midline fashion, and, if necessary, laterally based mucoperiosteal flaps may be elevated from the lower surface of the hard palate. The mucosa covering the upper surface of the hard palate should be retracted and not opened.

The posterior pharyngeal wall is incised longitudinally in the midline. The mucosa and prevertebral muscles are elevated as a single mucoperiosteal layer, using subperiosteal dissection, and are retracted laterally. The longus coli and the longus capitis muscles are dissected free. By not dissecting the layers separately, a single thick layer of tissue allows a strong closure. Adjustable soft tissue retractors are used to retract the pharyngeal tissue flaps laterally. If the mucoperiosteal layer is elevated from the clivus, the lateral margins slope dorsally

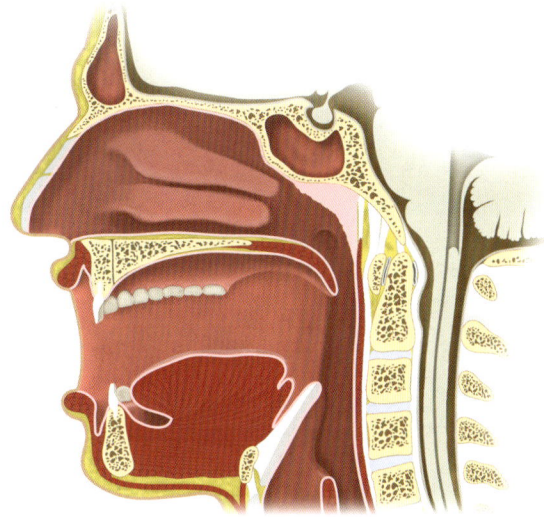

CHAPTER 1 Transoral Approach to the Craniocervical Junction and Upper Cervical Spine

Fig. 1-1 Opening of the mouth permits exposure to the clivus and upper cervical spine. *A*, Artist's rendering. *B*, Lateral view of the skull with mouth opened. *C*, Anteroposterior view of the skull with the mouth opened. (*B* and *C* from Rhoton AL Jr: The foramen magnum. The posterior cranial fossa: Microsurgical anatomy and surgical approaches. Neurosurgery 2000; 47(Suppl 3):S155–S193.)

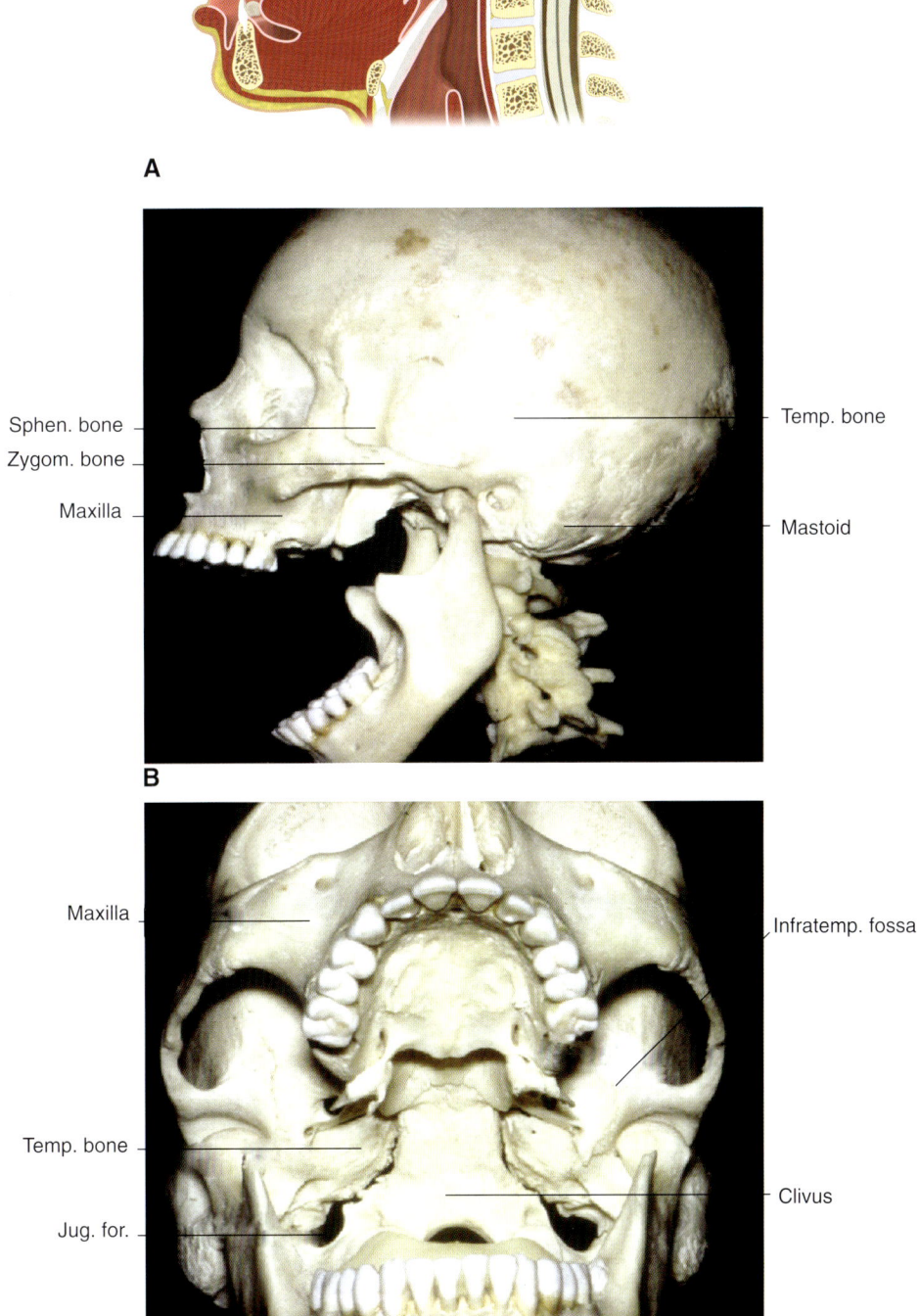

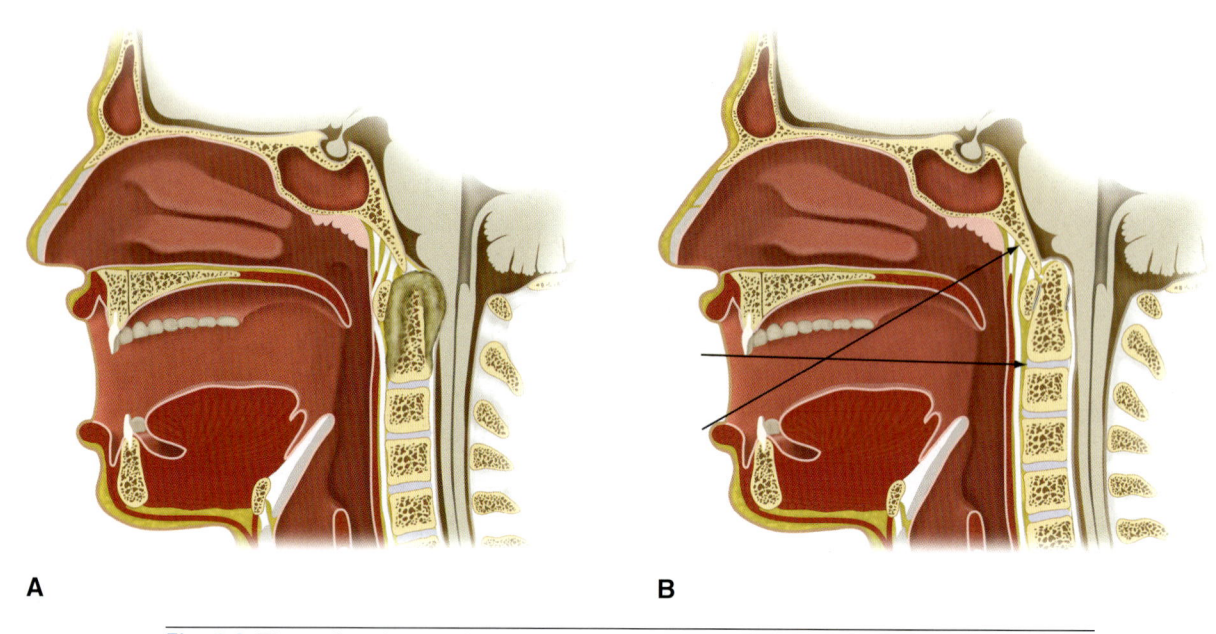

Fig. 1-2 The soft palate and posterior pharyngeal wall. The soft palate extends backward from the hard palate and blocks the view of the upper clivus. *A*, Tumor invading the odontoid process. *B*, Basilar invagination.

into "gutter-like" depressions in which the tissue becomes thicker and more adherent.

Depending on the lesion, the clivus, the anterior arch of the atlas, the dens, and the bodies of C2 and C3 vertebrae may be removed with a drill and rongeurs. The clival exposure between the occipital condyles is 2 to 2.5 cm wide and 2.5 to 3.0 cm long. Care must be taken to avoid the sixth through the twelfth cranial nerves, the internal carotid arteries, the internal jugular veins, and the inferior petrosal sinuses that are on the periphery of the exposure. Lateral dissection is limited to 1.5 cm from the midline because of the proximity of the vertebral arteries and eustachian tubes.

In the case of a transoral odontoidectomy, curettes are used to define the boundaries of the arch of C1, the body of C2, the dens, and the clivus. The inferior rim of the C1 arch is resected to expose the base of the dens. If possible, the continuity of the anterior arch of C1 should be maintained to preserve the structural integrity of the C1 ring. The base of the dens is partially transected using a drill with cutting bit, followed by either a diamond bit or a 1-mm Kerrison rongeur. The dens is grasped with a toothed rongeur and pulled ventrally and caudally after the alar and apical ligaments are sharply detached with curved curettes. Typically, the soft tissue pathology must also be removed to achieve adequate decompression. However, this removal must be done with extreme care to avoid inadvertent durotomy.

After completion of the procedure, hemostasis is obtained and the wound is irrigated with antibiotic solution. The pharyngeal incision is closed in a single layer with running or interrupted 2-0 vicryl suture. A small-diameter needle is useful for closing in this deep working space. If opened, the palatal incisions are then similarly closed. Immediately after the incision is closed, a nasogastric feeding tube is placed under direct vision of the wound to avoid dangerous malplacement. Orders are written that the tube is not to be replaced if inadvertently pulled out. The endotracheal tube should be maintained until the patient's tongue swelling subsides, usually within 24 to 36 hours. Some surgeons apply topical steroids to the tongue to minimize swelling. Tube feedings are begun on the first postoperative day, after tube position is verified. After 1 week the patient is started on clear liquids, and then advanced to a soft diet as tolerated.

Occasionally, it is necessary to further extend the inferior exposure and reduce operative depth. In this case a transmandibular extension of the transoral approach may be used. In this situation, a tracheostomy is required. The lip and chin may be incised vertically or in a zigzag fashion to conform to the tension lines in this region. A mandibular osteotomy is accomplished in the midline. If possible, a wide interdental space is used, or alternatively a central incisor tooth is removed. Generally, however, this process can be accomplished without a tooth removal.

The osteotomy is performed in a step-like fashion to provide a more stable reconstruction. After the future osteotomy has been outlined, miniplates are contoured and drill holes are created. This maximizes the likelihood of normal postoperative dental occlusion. Then, the osteotomy is accomplished. After the osteotomy, the mandibular edges are spread laterally, without splitting the tongue, to permit the tongue to be depressed downward between the mandibular halves. Spreading the mandibular-lingual halves exposes the pharyngeal wall down to the level of the arytenoid cartilages.

Text continued on p. 12

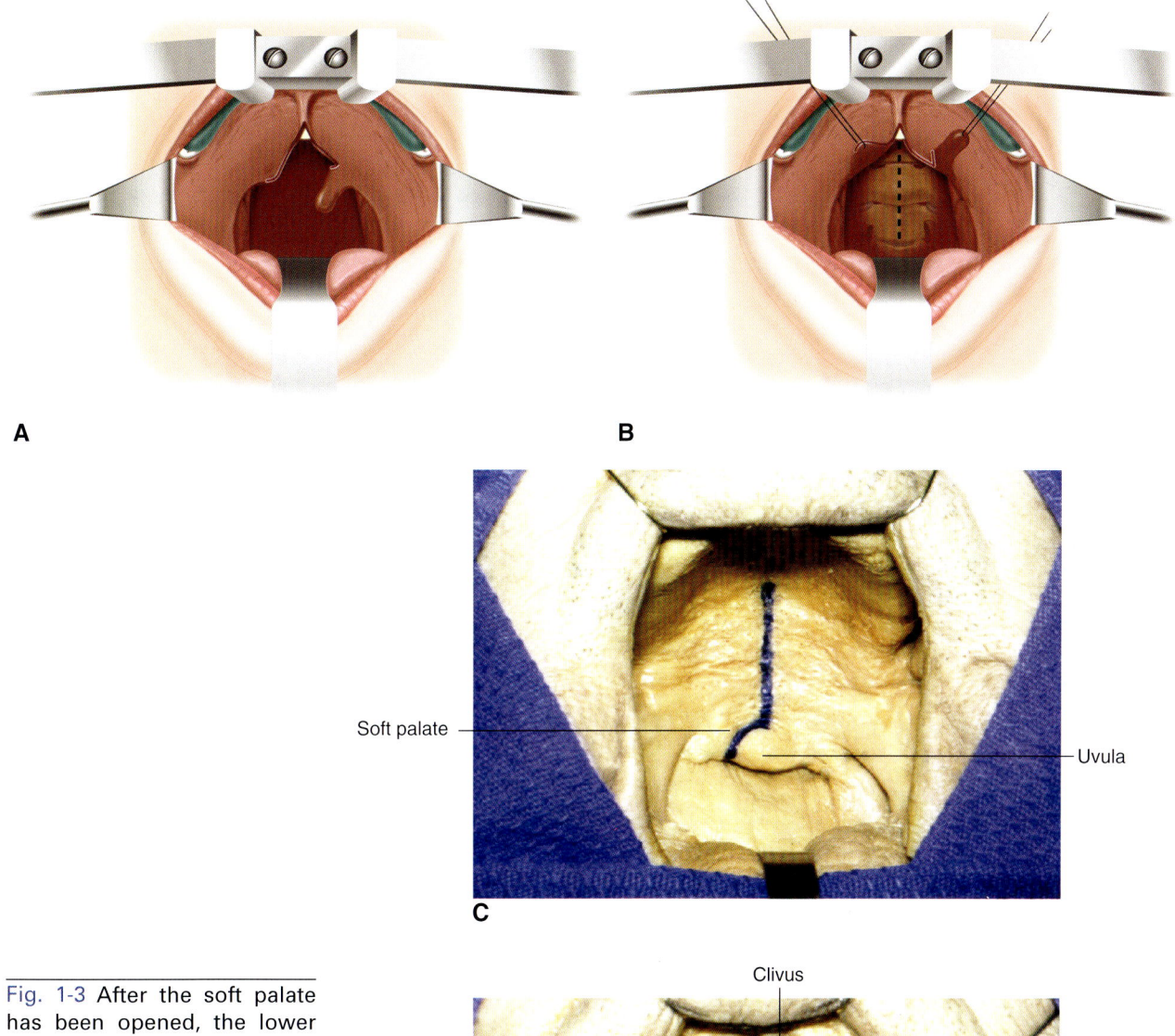

CHAPTER 1 Transoral Approach to the Craniocervical Junction and Upper Cervical Spine   7

Fig. 1-3 After the soft palate has been opened, the lower clivus may be exposed by opening the posterior pharyngeal wall in a single layer and retracting the soft tissue laterally. *A*, Artist's rendering of the incision in the soft palate. *B*, Artist's rendering of the linear incision in the posterior pharyngeal wall. *C*, Cadaveric incision of the soft palate. *D*, Retraction of the incised soft palate. (*C* and *D* from Rhoton AL Jr: The foramen magnum. The posterior cranial fossa: Microsurgical anatomy and surgical approaches. Neurosurgery 2000;47(Suppl 3):S155–S193.)

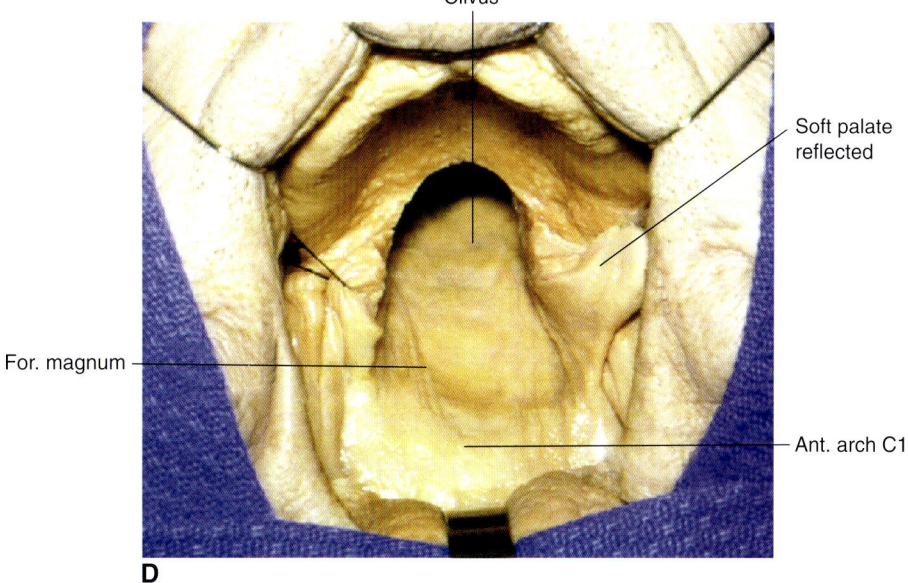

8   SECTION I   SURGICAL ANATOMY AND APPROACHES

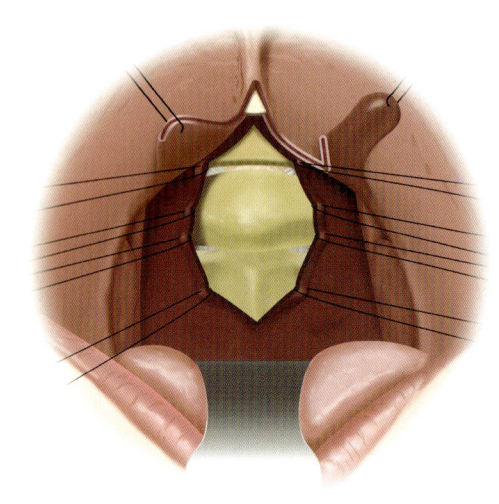

Fig. 1-4 For access to the upper anterior spine, the soft palate may be retracted and the posterior pharyngeal wall, including the mucosa and muscles, are opened in a single layer and retracted laterally.

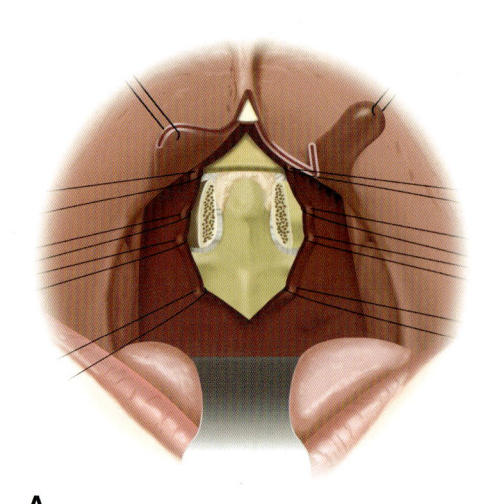

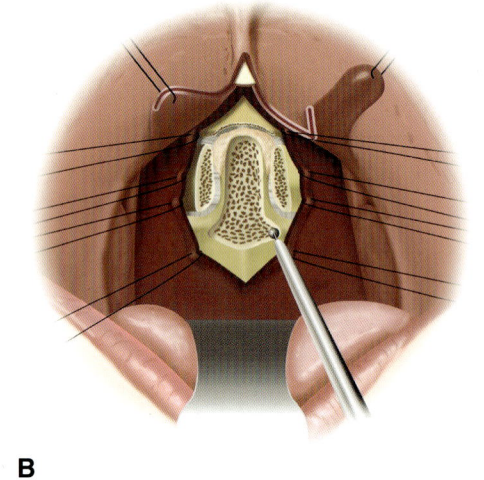

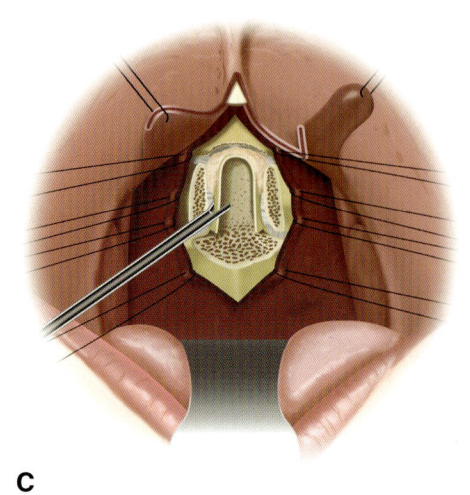

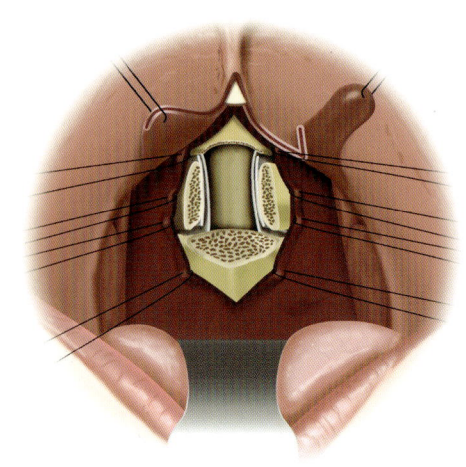

Fig. 1-5 Lesions involving the odontoid process. *A*, The anterior arch of the atlas is removed to gain access to the odontoid process. *B*, The odontoid process is drilled from rostral to caudal. *C*, Cortical rim of the odontoid process is removed. *D*, This gains exposure to the ventral aspect of the thecal sac.

A

B

C

D

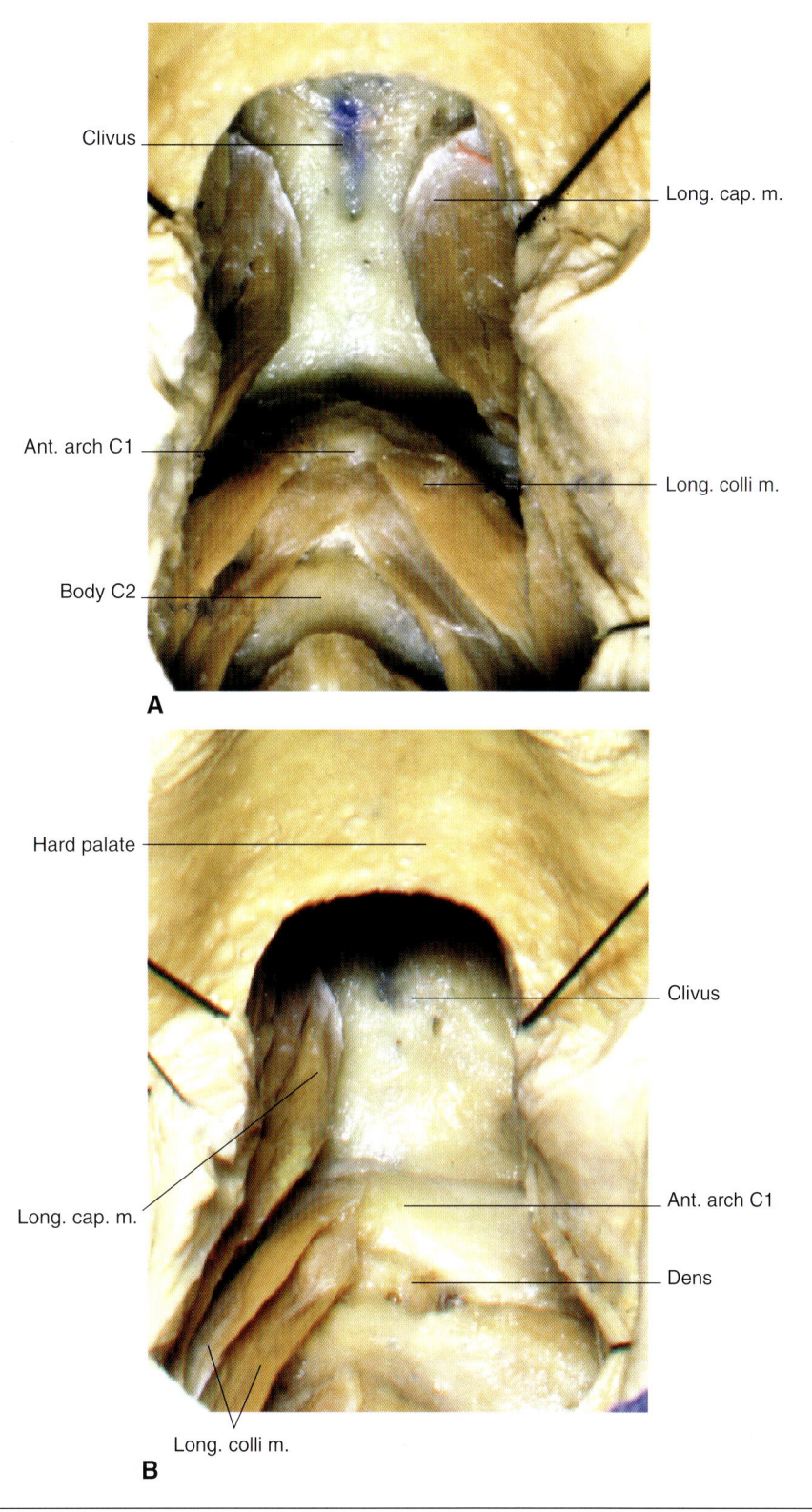

CHAPTER 1 Transoral Approach to the Craniocervical Junction and Upper Cervical Spine

Fig. 1-6 Cadaveric dissection showing extent of exposure. *A,* Longus colli and longus capitis muscles are shown here, with the anterior arch of the atlas. *B,* Further dissection demonstrating the odontoid process posterior to the anterior arch of C1. (From Rhoton AL Jr: The foramen magnum. The posterior cranial fossa: Microsurgical anatomy and surgical approaches. Neurosurgery 2000;47(Suppl 3):S155–S193.)

SECTION I SURGICAL ANATOMY AND APPROACHES

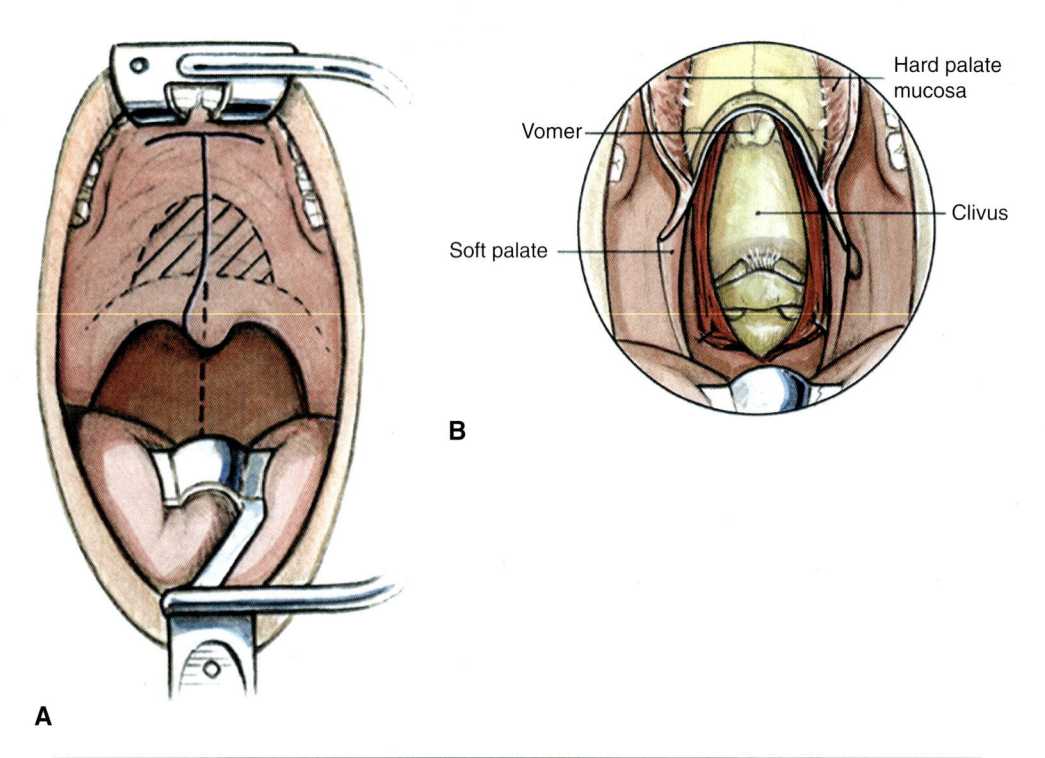

Fig. 1-7 If further cranial exposure is needed, *A*, laterally based mucoperiosteal flaps are elevated from the surface of the hard palate (*interrupted lines*). The posterior aspect of the hard palate may then be removed (*oblique lines*). *B*, The posterior pharyngeal opening is extended upward, through the vault of the nasopharynx to the posterior border of the vomer. (From Rhoton AL Jr: The foramen magnum. The posterior cranial fossa: Microsurgical anatomy and surgical approaches. Neurosurgery 2000;47(Suppl 3):S155–S193.)

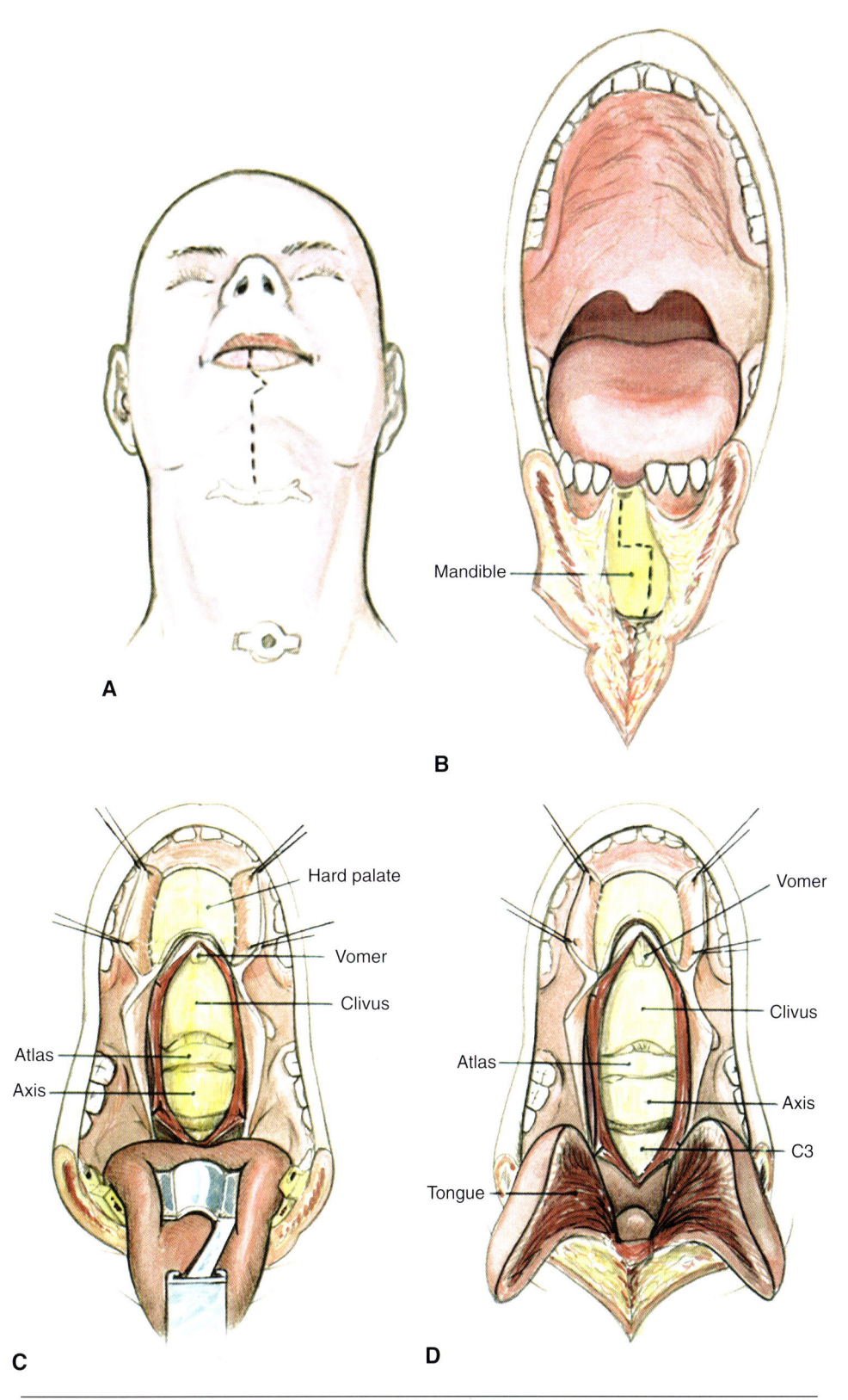

CHAPTER 1 Transoral Approach to the Craniocervical Junction and Upper Cervical Spine   11

Fig. 1-8 *A*, The transmandibular extension of the transoral approach requires a midline skin incision through the lip and chin. *B*, The mandibular osteotomy is performed in a step-like fashion to maximize postoperative stability. *C*, Spreading the mandibular halves laterally allows the tongue to be depressed downward. *D*, If necessary, the tongue can also be split in the midline to gain further exposure inferiorly. (From Rhoton AL Jr: The foramen magnum. The posterior cranial fossa: Microsurgical anatomy and surgical approaches. Neurosurgery 2000;47(Suppl 3):S155–S193.)

If the exposure is still inadequate, the tongue and floor of the mouth may be split in the midline. A midline glossotomy may be done with the placement of retention sutures on the tip of the tongue. With elevation of the tongue, cautery can assist in incising the median raphe to the midline epiglottic fold. The halves of the tongue can then be retracted laterally with a self-retaining retractor. With soft tissue depression, this glossotomy may lead to exposure down to the C5 vertebra.

After dealing with the lesion, the mucosa and musculature of the tongue and floor of the mouth are reapproximated. This may be easily accomplished by approximating the dorsal aspect of the tongue first. Second, approximate the intrinsic muscles of the tongue. Last, approximate the ventral aspect. The osteotomy is repositioned with miniplates (prefitted). Then, the lip, chin, and submandibular region are carefully closed.

COMPLICATIONS

If a dural opening occurs in surgery, a patch is placed directly over the dura and is secured with fibrin glue. A lumbar drain is placed in the operating room, and lumbar drainage and antibiotics are continued for at least 1 week.

If the transoral procedure results in destabilization of the spine, extreme care must be used until definitive fixation is accomplished. Patients undergoing a transoral odontoidectomy are typically extremely unstable and will require a posterior stabilization procedure. This percedure may be performed immediately after the transoral procedure. Some surgeons prefer to wait several days to minimize the risk of a posterior cervical wound infection. Extreme care must be exercised during positioning of these patients.

DISCUSSION

The transoral approach is well suited for anterior extradural lesions of the craniovertebral junction. The approach includes several variations, the choice of which depends on the region of interest and needed exposure.

CHAPTER 2

MAX C. LEE

STEPHEN I. RYU

ALBERT L. RHOTON, JR.

DANIEL H. KIM

Transmaxillary Approach to the Clivus and Upper Cervical Spine

INTRODUCTION

The craniovertebral junction includes the clivus, foramen magnum, and upper cervical spine. Neural elements encompassed by these bones include the pons, medulla, and upper cervical spinal cord. Pathology of this area includes structural defects, acquired and congenital mechanical dysfunction, tumors, inflammatory lesions, and intrinsic neural lesions. Collectively, lesions in this location can be difficult to diagnose and difficult to treat surgically.

Surgical approaches to the craniovertebral junction include anterior, anterolateral, lateral, posterolateral, and posterior approaches. The direct anterior approaches include the transoral approach and its variations.

The transoral approach was discussed in Chapter 1. Initially described by Fang and Ong in 1962, the transoral approach has evolved over the ensuing 40 years.[1-6] The transoral, transpharyngeal approach, also known as the buccopharyngeal approach, can allow access of the inferior third of the clivus down to the C2 vertebral body. On the other hand, lateral exposure is limited to 1.5 cm lateral to midline because of the vertebral artery anatomy and the eustachian tubes.

The transmaxillary approach may extend the upper limit of the transoral approach.[7-9] With maxillotomies, the transoral approach can expose the majority of the clivus and upper cervical spine. This method, however, does carry a greater wound infection and complication risk. Swallowing and speech difficulties are frequent, especially with soft palate division. The LeFort I followed by en bloc fracturing can obscure the lower operative field and result in greater oropalatal morbidity and dental malocclusion. The unilateral LeFort I results in more rapid recovery of oropalatal function as it preserves the soft palate and one half of the maxilla.

Three types of maxillotomies have been described[10]:
1. LeFort I osteotomy followed by fracturing the maxilla and hard palate en bloc inferiorly into the oral cavity
2. LeFort I osteotomy combined with a midline osteotomy and division of the hard and soft palate followed by swinging both maxilla halves down and out
3. Unilateral LeFort I osteotomy combined with a midline osteotomy of the hard palate followed by swinging the single maxilla half down and out attached with an intact soft palate

ANATOMY

In a supine position, with the neck slightly extended, and the mouth open, the rostral aspect of the transoral approach is limited by the soft palate. This limitation is demonstrated in a skull model (Fig. 2-1). Removal of the soft palate allows for visualization of the mucosa lining the lower clivus. Opening the pharyngeal mucosa along the midline allows for greater rostral exposure, compared to a strictly transoral approach. In addition to the anterior arch of C1 and body of C2, the clivus is appreciated (Fig. 2-1C and D).

Muscular anatomy demonstrates the longus coli muscle as seen with the previous exposure. In addition, with more rostral exposure, the longus capitus muscles are exposed. With these muscles reflected laterally, the lower clivus can be exposed (Fig. 2-1E and F).

With the transmaxillary exposure, a subperiosteal dissection exposes the maxilla and the lower part of the anterior pyriform aperture (Fig. 2-2A). LeFort I osteotomy extends throughout the maxillary sinus above the teeth and below the infraorbital canals (Fig. 2-2B). With bilateral osteotomies performed, the nasal septum and both maxillary sinuses are appreciated (Fig. 2-2C and D).

Further anatomy is appreciated via a Weber-Ferguson incision, as the masseter muscle is attached along the lower margin of the zygoma (Fig. 2-3A). With a maxillotomy,

SECTION I SURGICAL ANATOMY AND APPROACHES

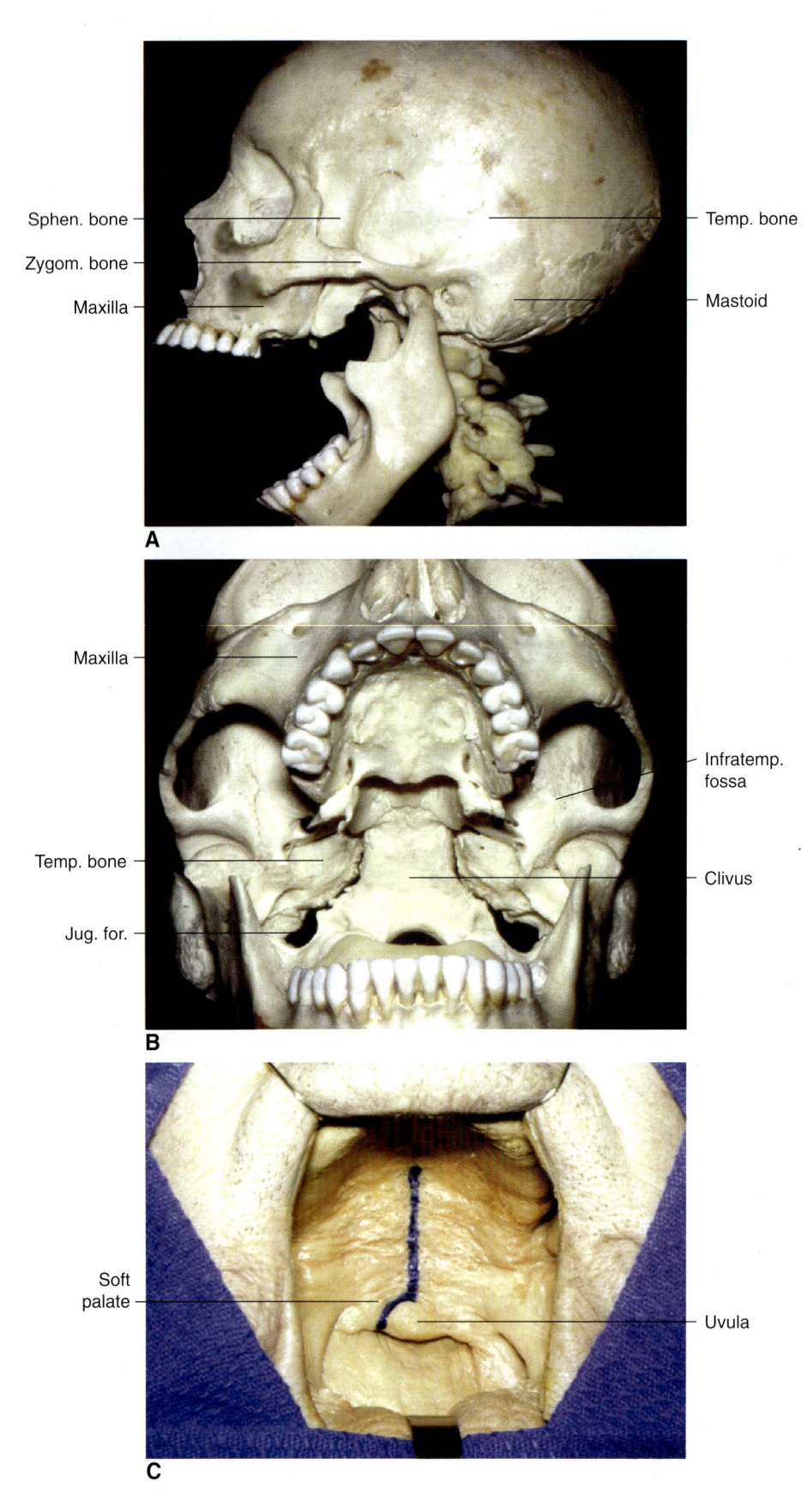

Fig. 2-1 *A* and *B*, The rostral aspect of the transoral approach is limited by the soft palate. This is demonstrated in a skull model. *C* and *D*, Removal of the soft palate allows visualization of the mucosa lining the lower clivus. In addition to the anterior arch of C1 and body of C2, the clivus is appreciated. (From Rhoton AL Jr: The foramen magnum. The posterior cranial fossa: Microsurgical anatomy and surgical approaches. Neurosurgery 2000;47(Suppl 3): S155–S193.)

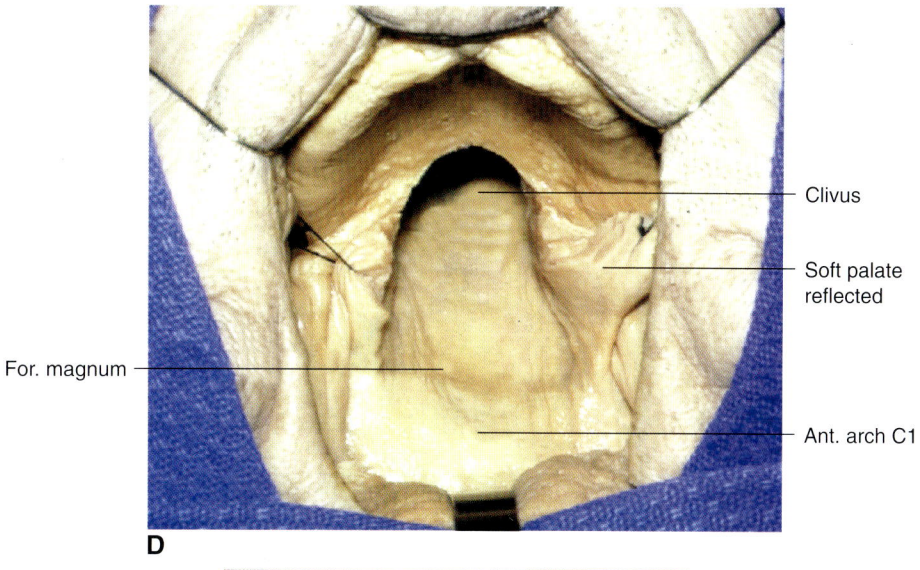

Fig. 2-1, cont'd. *E* and *F*, The longus capitis muscles are exposed with more rostral exposure. With these muscles reflected laterally, the lower clivus can be exposed. (From Rhoton AL Jr: The foramen magnum. The posterior cranial fossa: Microsurgical anatomy and surgical approaches. Neurosurgery 2000;47(suppl 3): S155–S193.)

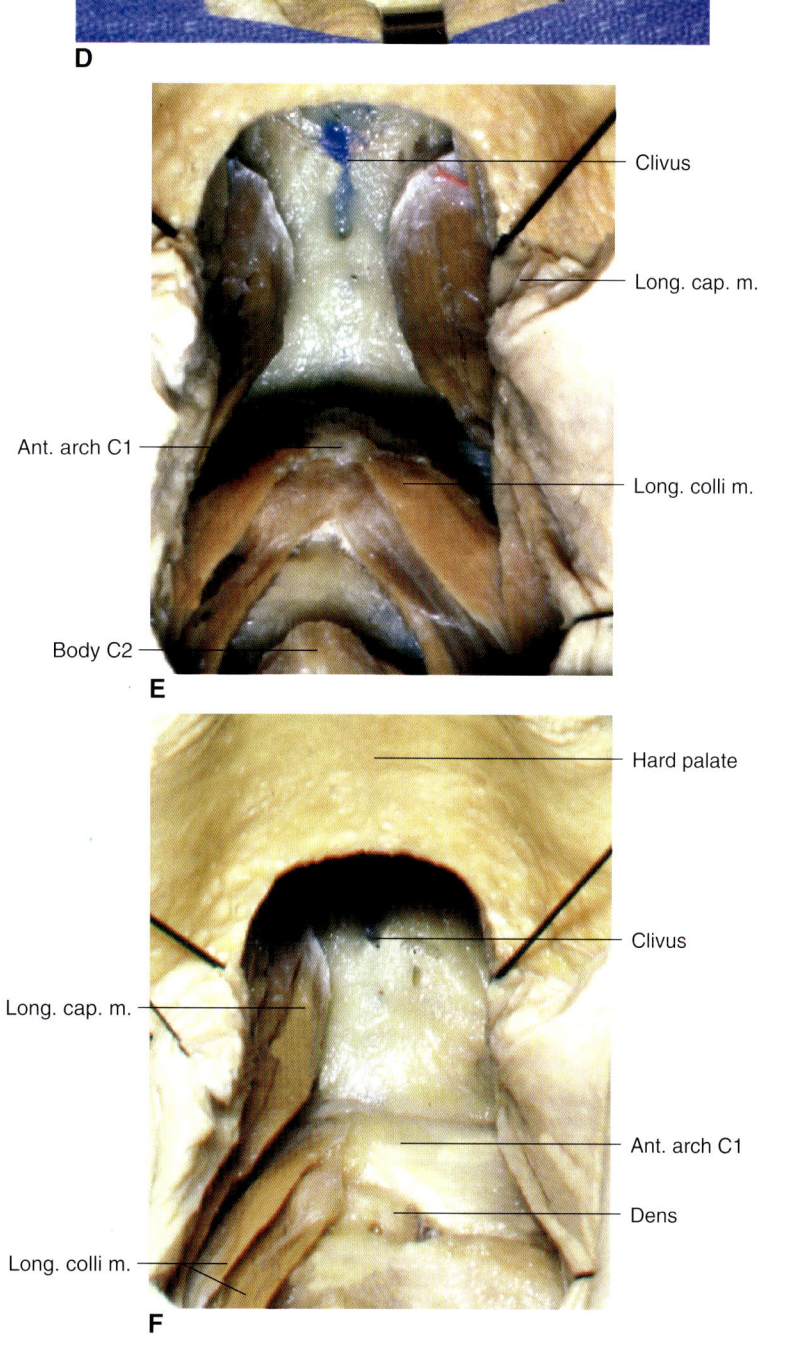

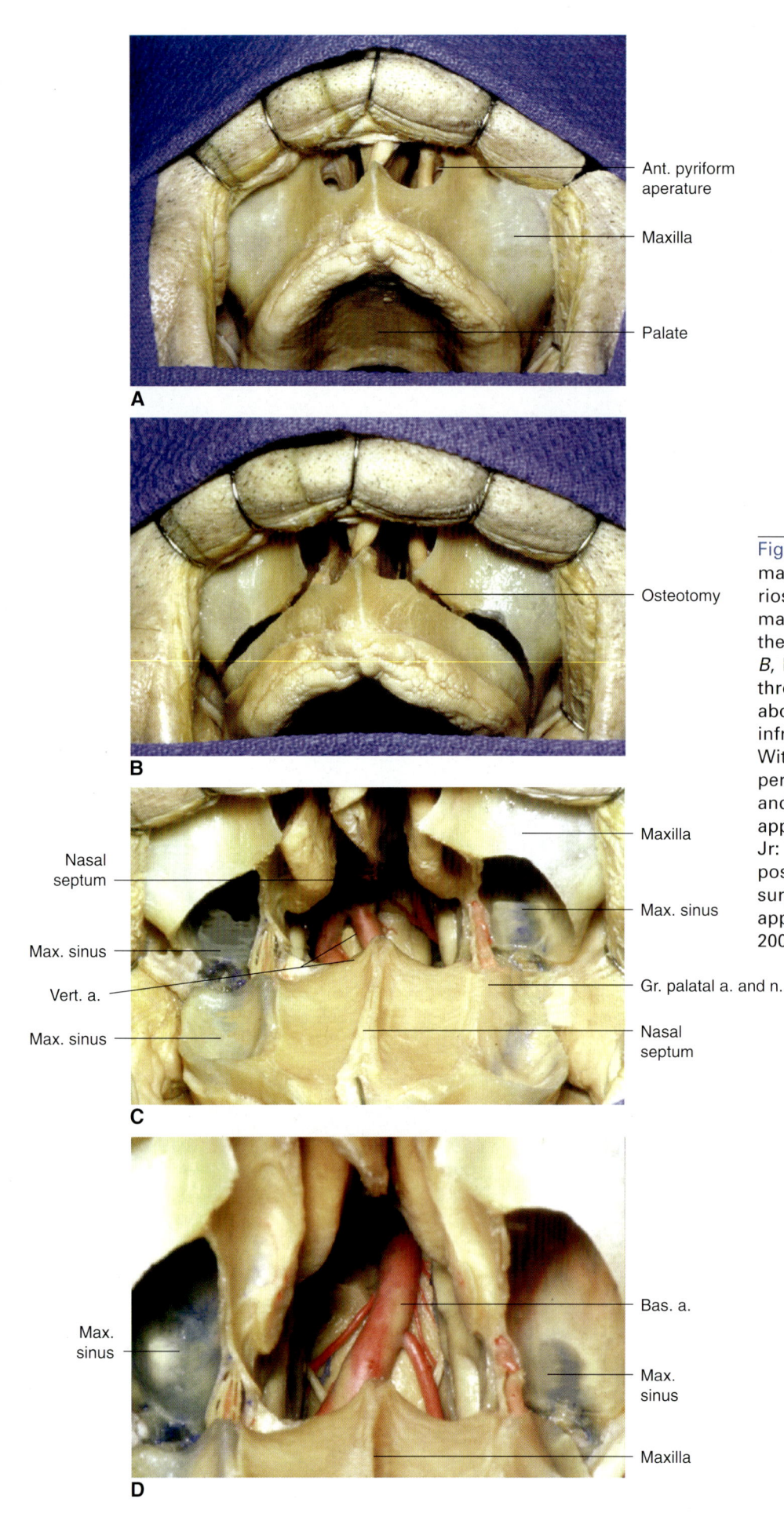

Fig. 2-2 *A*, With the transmaxillary exposure, a subperiosteal dissection exposes the maxilla and the lower part of the anterior pyriform aperture. *B*, LeFort I osteotomy extends throughout the maxillary sinus above the teeth and below the infraorbital canals. *C* and *D*, With bilateral osteotomies performed, the nasal septum and both maxillary sinuses are appreciated. (From Rhoton AL Jr: The foramen magnum. The posterior cranial fossa: Microsurgical anatomy and surgical approaches. Neurosurgery 2000;47(Suppl 3):S155–S193.)

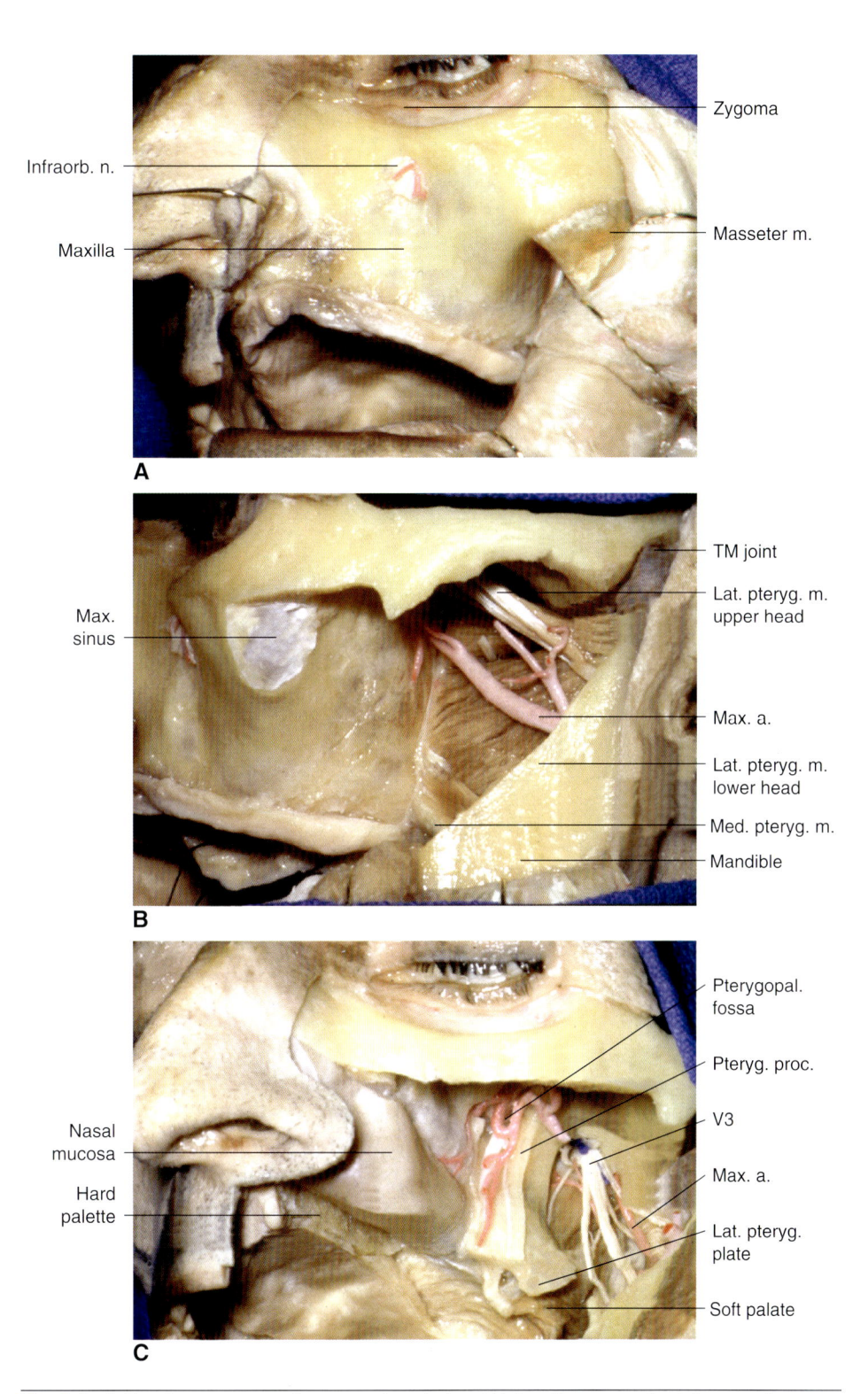

CHAPTER 2 Transmaxillary Approach to the Clivus and Upper Cervical Spine   17

Fig. 2-3 *A*, Further anatomy is appreciated via a Weber-Ferguson incision, as the masseter muscle is attached along the lower margin of the zygoma. *B* and *C*, Laterally, the maxillary artery traversing to the pterygopalatine fossa and lateral pterygoid muscle (*B*) overlie the mandibular branch of the trigeminal nerve and the tensor veli palatine (*C*). (From Rhoton AL Jr: The foramen magnum. The posterior cranial fossa: Microsurgical anatomy and surgical approaches. Neurosurgery 2000;47(Suppl 3):S155–S193.)

the maxillary sinus is appreciated. Laterally, the maxillary artery traversing to the pterygopalatine fossa and lateral pterygoid muscle (Fig. 2-3B) overlie the mandibular branch of the trigeminal nerve and the tensor veli palatine (Fig. 2-3C).

With soft tissue retraction laterally, the proximity of this dissection to the eustacian tube and carotid artery must be appreciated (Fig. 2-4A). As with the transoral approach, exposure of the upper cervical spine is easily accomplished (Fig. 2-4B).

Removal of the clivus demonstrates bilateral vertebral arteries, the basilar artery, the anterior inferior cerebellar artery, and posterior inferior cerebellar arteries. In addition, lower cranial nerves are appreciated, including cranial nerves VI and XII (CN VI, CN XII) (Fig. 2-5). More rostral dissection demonstrates the proximity of this dissection to the cavernous sinus.

Variations of the transmaxillary approach include a LeFort I osteotomy (Fig. 2-6) with a midline incision of the hard and soft palates (Fig. 2-7). In addition, a unilateral maxillotomy may be performed (Fig. 2-8). With a unilateral approach, half of the maxilla is mobilized after a midline osteotomy is performed between the two front incisors. The benefit to a unilateral approach may be appreciated by maintaining the integrity of the soft palate. In addition, the nasal septum is left undisturbed except for the posterior part, which is removed with the posterior turbinates and wall of the sinuses to allow for bilateral exposure of the clivus.

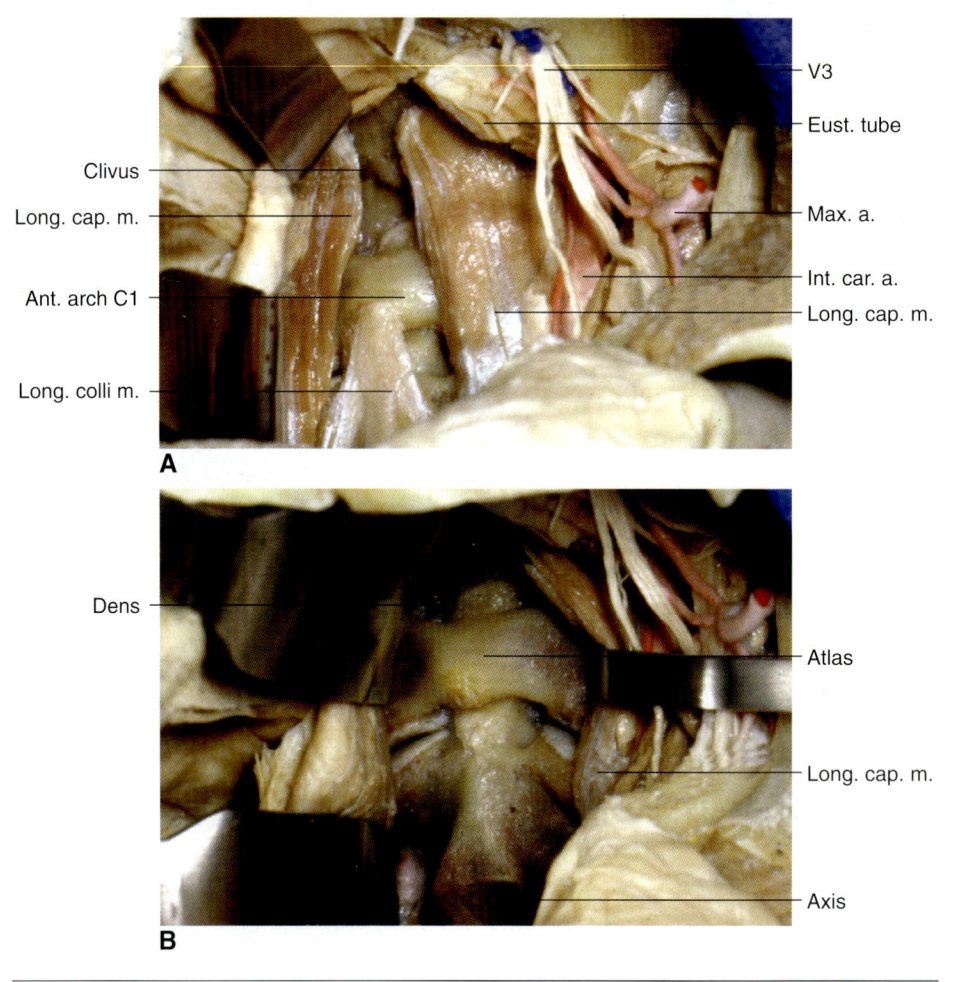

Fig. 2-4 A, With soft tissue retraction laterally, the proximity of this dissection to the eustacian tube and carotid artery must be appreciated. B, Exposure of the upper cervical spine via a transoral approach. (From Rhoton AL Jr: The foramen magnum. The posterior cranial fossa: Microsurgical anatomy and surgical approaches. Neurosurgery 2000;47(Suppl 3):S155–S193.)

Fig. 2-5 *A* and *B*, Lower cranial nerves VI and XII (CN VI, CN XII), vertebral artery, basilar artery, and anterior and posterior inferior cerebellar arteries (AICA, PICA) dissected with removal of the clivus. (From Rhoton AL Jr: The foramen magnum. The posterior cranial fossa: Microsurgical anatomy and surgical approaches. Neurosurgery 2000;47(Suppl 3):S155–S193.)

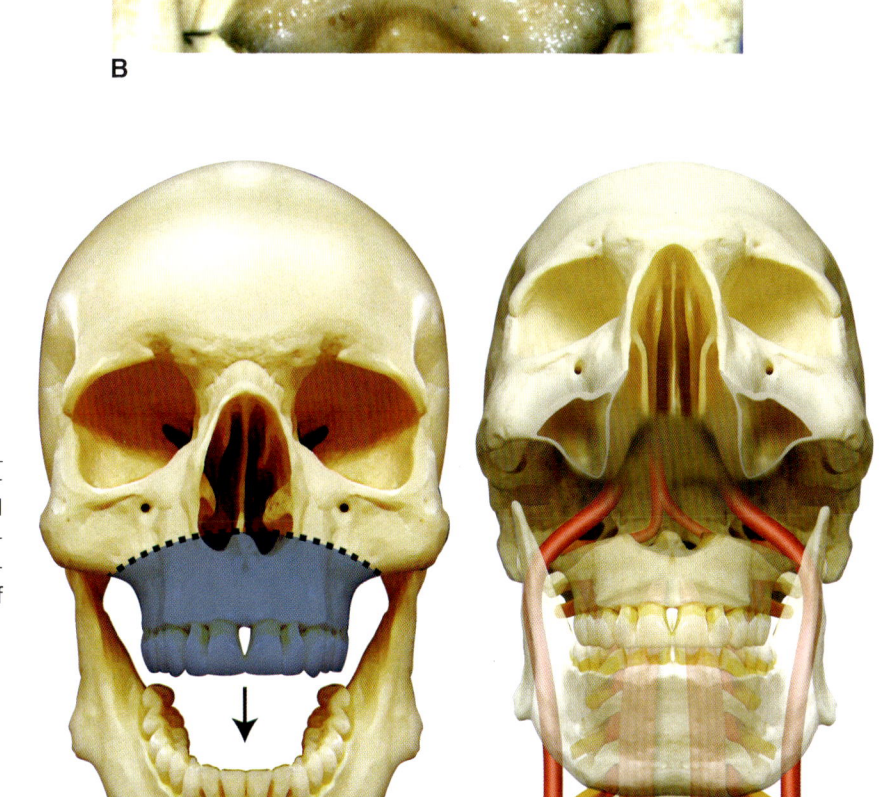

Fig. 2-6 The transmaxillary approach with a LeFort I. *A*, Skull model with a dotted line demonstrating the location of the maxillotomy. *B*, Graphic representation of the arterial system after a LeFort I.

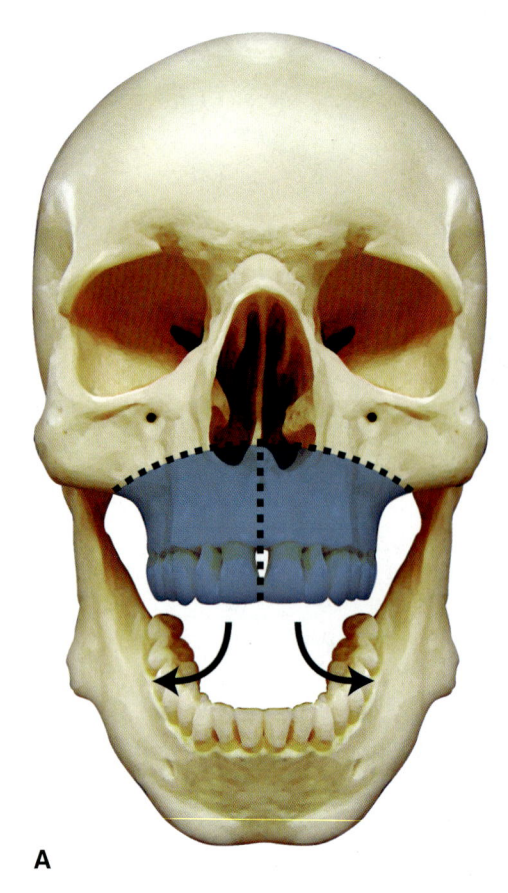

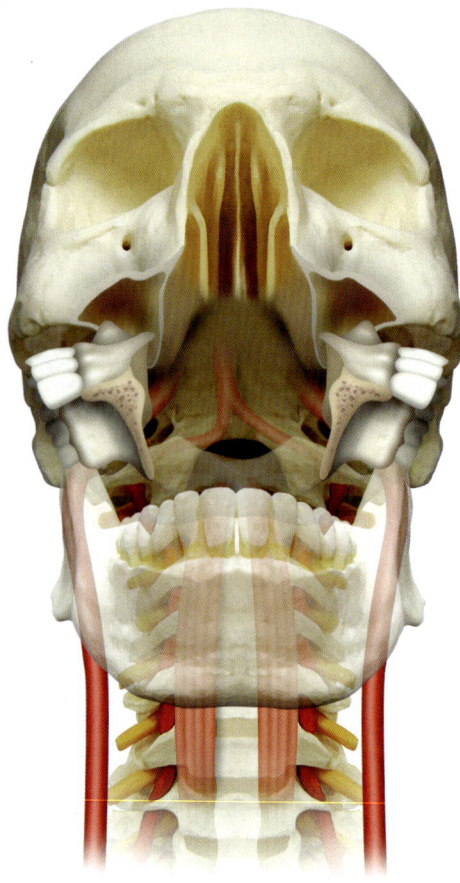

Fig. 2-7 *A*, LeFort I osteotomy with a midline incision of the hard and soft palate. *B*, Graphic representation of the arterial system after a midline split.

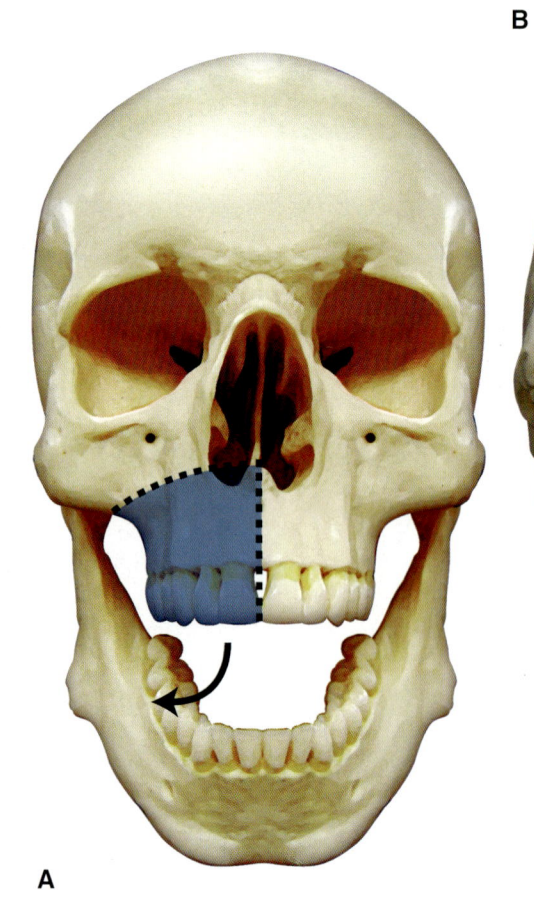

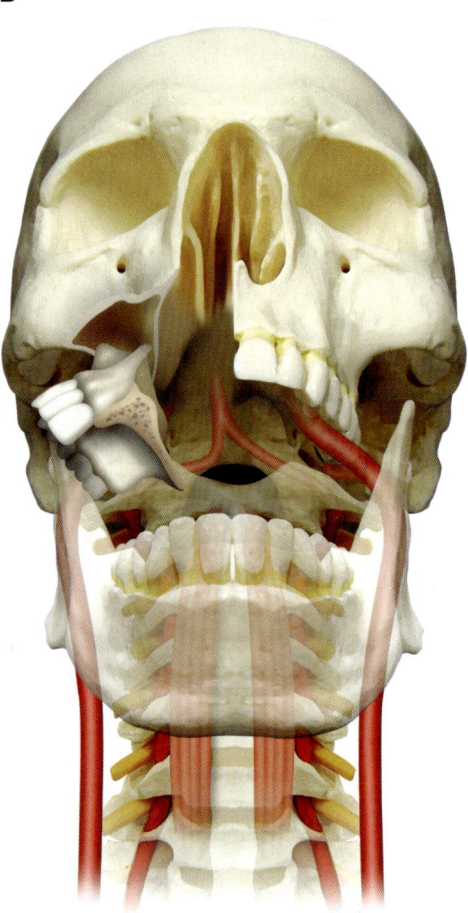

Fig. 2-8 *A*, A unilateral maxillotomy. *B*, Graphic representation of the arterial system after a unilateral maxillotomy.

SURGICAL TECHNIQUE

The general considerations mentioned in Chapter 1 for transoral surgery apply. Preoperative dental evaluation is strongly recommended. Here we describe the technique for the unilateral maxillotomy variation.

After general anesthesia is induced, a feeding tube is placed. The patient is placed supine with the neck in slight extension. The face, jaw, upper neck, and oropharynx are prepared and exposed. The mucosa is elevated off the upper alveolar margin by local anesthetic injection. A mucosal incision is made under the upper lip along the alveolar margin around the maxillary tuberosity. This alveolar tissue is elevated to the level of the nasal opening. This subperiosteal elevation can be facilitated with similar instruments as those mentioned in Chapter 1. The mucosa over the hard palate is also incised in the midline and elevated.

Miniplates are prebent and fitted along the maxilla, and screw holes are predrilled to ensure proper alignment on the conclusion of this endeavor. A unilateral LeFort I osteotomy and midline parasagittal osteotomy are cut between the front two incisors through the hard palate. The mobile maxilla half is separated from the pterygoid process and swung down and out laterally while still attached to the intact soft palate. The mobile bone is retracted out of the field, exposing the posterior nasopharynx. The posterior nasal septum is removed as needed. The posterior pharyngeal wall is opened.

The mucoperiosteal layers are spread with a self-retaining retractor. The longus and capitis muscles and the anterior longitudinal ligament are dissected free. This dissection exposes the clivus and anterior arch of C1. A high-speed pneumatic drill is used to remove the necessary bone. Careful attention to the vital structures mentioned earlier is essential, thus minimizing injury to the lower cranial nerves, carotid artery, and jugular vein.

After the posterior pharyngeal wall is closed, the mobilized maxilla is replaced and plated into its original position. The hard palate mucosa is closed with absorbable suture. The nares are packed to reset the nasal septum to the midline. The sublabial mucosa is then closed with interrupted absorbable sutures. Postoperatively, care is taken to allow for the nasal and oral mucosa to heal. Enteral nutrition is provided. Airway management is also critical. A tracheostomy may be required until pharyngeal swelling subsides. Posterior stabilization is performed as soon as possible.

SUMMARY

With the advancement of surgical techniques, a transoral approach allows for exposure of the clivus and upper cervical spine. The upper limit of this exposure is improved with a maxillotomy. With a unilateral or bilateral LeFort I, exposure of upper clivus may be accomplished, thus allowing for access to the pons and the posterior circulation arteries in addition to the atlas and the body of the axis. Involving the oropharyngeal mucosa, the transmaxillary approach may have a greater infection rate compared to the various high cervical and craniotomy exposures. In addition, this approach may lead to malocclusion. Lastly, soft tissue edema may necessitate tracheostomy and gastrostomy placement.

REFERENCES

1. Fang HSY, Ong GB: Direct anterior approach to the upper cervical spine. J Bone Joint Surg Am 1962;44:1588–1604.
2. Hall JE, Denis F, Murray J: Exposure of the upper cervical spine for spinal decompression by a mandible and tongue-splitting approach. J Bone Joint Surg Am 1977;59:121–123.
3. Crockard HA, Pozo JL, Ransford AO, et al: Transoral decompression and posterior fusion for rheumatoid atlanto-axial subluxation. J Bone Joint Surg Br 1986;68:350–356.
4. Krespi YP, Har-El G: Surgery of the clivus and anterior cervical spine. Arch Otolaryngol Head Neck Surg 1988;114(1):73–78.
5. Honma G, Murota K, Shiba R, Kondo H: Mandible and tongue-splitting approach for giant cell tumor of axis. Spine 1989;14(11):1204–1210.
6. Enepekides DJ, Donald PJ: Transoral approaches to the clivus and nasopharynx. Otolaryngol Clin North Am 2001;34(6):1105–1121, ix.
7. Archer DJ, Young S, Uttley D: Basilar aneurysms: A new transclival approach via maxillotomy. J Neurosurg 1987;67(1):54–58.
8. Cocke EW, Robertson JH, Robertson JT, et al: The extended maxillotomy and subtotal maxillectomy for excision of skull base tumours. Arch Otolaryngol Head Neck Surg 1990;116:92–104.
9. Menezes AH, Traynelis VC, Gantz BJ: Surgical approaches to the craniovertebral junction. Clin Neurosurg 1994;41:187–203.
10. Bhangoo RS, Crockard HA: Transmaxillary anterior decompressions in patients with severe basilar impression. Clin Orthop 1999;(359):115–125.

CHAPTER 3

UNGKYU CHANG
JEFFREY S. HENN
MAX C. LEE
ALBERT L. RHOTON, JR.

High Cervical Retropharyngeal Approach to the Craniocervical Junction

INTRODUCTION

The transcervical approach to the craniovertebral junction, also known as the high cervical retropharyngeal approach, is an anterior approach directed through the fascial planes of the neck. The main advantage of the anterior approaches is the direct route to the lesion, avoiding the potential need to work around or manipulate neural structures. The transcervical approach can provide access to the C2 vertebral body and odontoid process, the anterior arch of C1, and the lower clivus. Similar to the transoral approach, the transcervical approach is considered an option for anterior lesions of the craniovertebral junction. However, unlike the transoral approach, the transcervical approach avoids opening the oropharyngeal mucosa and the potential associated risks. In spite of this advantage, the transcervical approach is selected infrequently because of the relatively awkward trajectory, depth of the exposure, and long exposure time, and because it is not a direct midline exposure to the craniovertebral junction. Furthermore, this approach often requires a tracheostomy.[1,2]

SURGICAL ANATOMY

POSITION AND SKIN INCISION

On the anterolateral surface of the neck are several triangles between the prominent neck muscles (Fig. 3-1). The posterior triangle is formed by the sternocleidomastoid muscle, the clavicle, and the trapezius muscle. The omohyoid muscle divides it into the supraclavicular and the occipital triangles. The anterior triangle is made by the midline of the neck anteriorly, the lower border of the mandible superiorly, and the sternocleidomastoid muscle posteriorly. The anterior triangle is subdivided by the submental triangle, the inferior carotid triangle, the superior carotid triangle, and the submandibular triangle.[3] The target of this approach is via a submandibular and superior carotid triangle.

The patient is positioned with the head slightly extended in order to raise the mandible up and away from the surgeon's line of view and rotated 30 degrees contralateral to the surgical approach[4] (Fig. 3-2).

The four methods of skin incisions are transverse, oblique-vertical, hockey-stick, and T-shape. For the C1 and C2 bodies to be exposed, the transverse incision is enough. For the additional exposure of midcervical levels, a vertical line of incision should be combined with the transverse. Regardless of the incision, the important point is a wide dissection of the cervical fascia planes. The transverse incision is made 2 cm inferior and parallel to the lower margin of the mandible, and extends from the angle of the mandible posteriorly to the base of the mental protuberance beyond the midline anteriorly (see Fig. 3-2). The side of approach is decided by the laterality of the lesion and surgeon's preference. If the lower cranial nerve impairment is already present, the approach should be performed from the side of impairment.[4]

- The T-shaped skin incision includes a submandibular incision extending from the mastoid tip to the symphysis menti and an inferior extension carried down along the border of the sternocleidomastoid muscle. A tracheostomy allows the jaws to be closed tightly and facilitates the exposure.
- The trajectory and resectable areas are shown. The high cervical retropharyngeal approach provides access to the C2 body and odontoid process, the anterior arch of C1, and the lower clivus.[4]
- A plane is directed along the anterior border of the sternocleidomastoid muscle, between the carotid sheath laterally and the esophagus and trachea medially. Struc-

CHAPTER 3   High Cervical Retropharyngeal Approach to the Craniocervical Junction

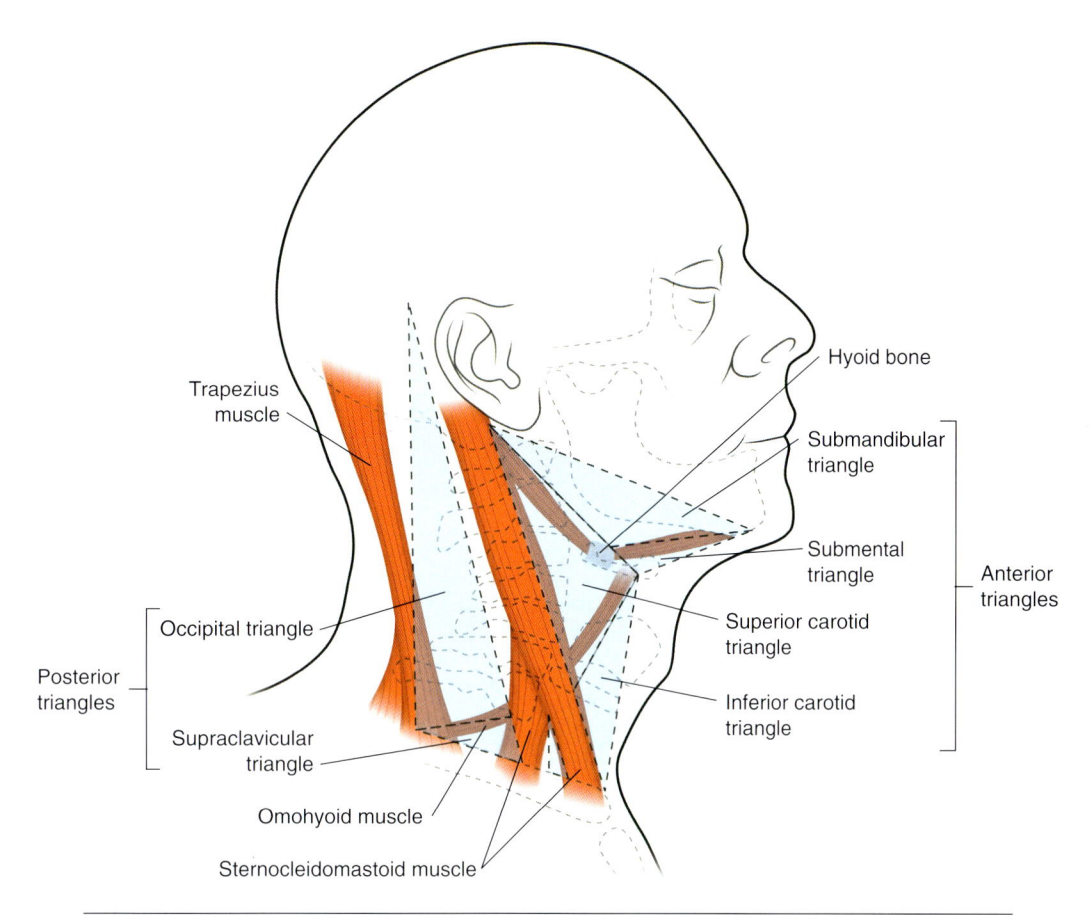

Fig. 3-1 There are several triangles on the anterolateral surface of the neck. The posterior triangle is formed by the sternocleidomastoid muscle, the clavicle, and the trapezius muscle. The omohyoid muscle divides it into the supraclavicular and the occipital triangles. The anterior triangle is made by the midline of the neck anteriorly, the lower border of the mandible superiorly, and the sternocleidomastoid muscle posteriorly. The anterior triangle is subdivided by the submental triangle, the inferior carotid triangle, the superior carotid triangle, and the submandibular triangle. The digastric muscle divides it into the submental triangle and submandibular triangle. The omohyoid muscle divides it into the superior and inferior carotid triangle.

tures that may be divided to increase the exposure include the ascending pharyngeal artery, superior thyroid artery, external laryngeal nerve, ansa hypoglossi, internal laryngeal nerve, lingual artery, stylohyoid muscle, anterior belly of the digastric muscle, stylohyoid ligament, stylopharyngeus muscle, and styloglossus muscle. Although rarely necessary, the hypoglossal and glossopharyngeal nerves may be divided if required for additional exposure. The tagged ends may be reapproximated at the conclusion of the procedure. The spinal accessory nerve passes behind the sternocleidomastoid muscle.[5]

- The prevertebral fascia along with the longus colli and longus capitis muscles are separated in the midline and retracted laterally using subperiosteal dissection. In this manner, exposure of the clivus, atlas, and axis is obtained.[4]

OPERATIVE TECHNIQUES

PREPARATION AND POSITIONING

The patient should be given a broad-spectrum antibiotic with gram-positive and gram-negative coverage prior to surgery, particularly because a tracheostomy is typically performed as part of the procedure. The patient is positioned supine; ideally with the head extended (this positioning should be carefully performed with fluoroscopic guidance if appropriate). The head may be supported on a doughnut, or the skull can be rigidly fixated using a Mayfield head holder (or a halo brace if spinal instability is a consideration). As with a standard anterior cervical approach, the surgeon works from the side of the patient and an operating microscope is employed for illumination, magnification, and binocular visualization.

24 SECTION I SURGICAL ANATOMY AND APPROACHES

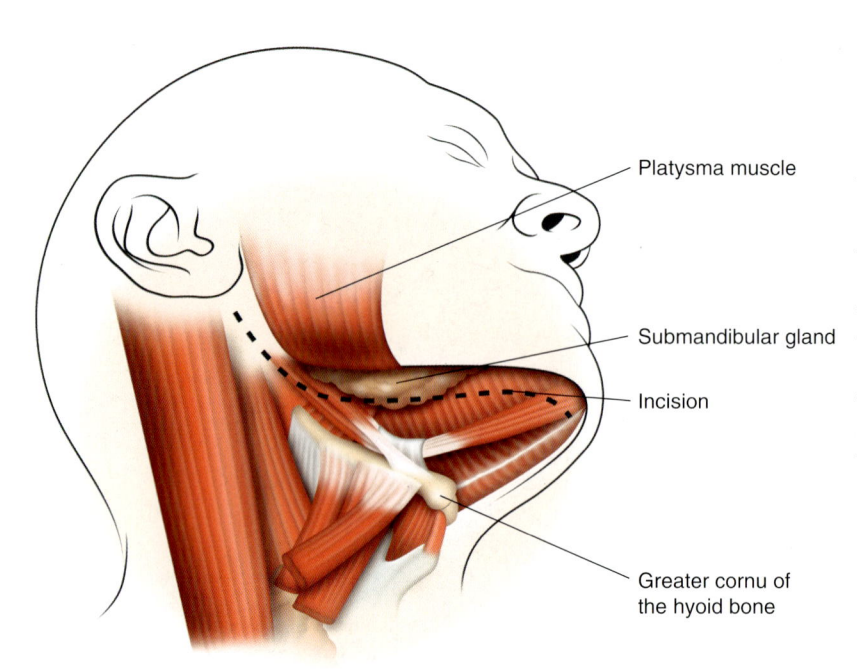

Fig. 3-2 Operative position and incision. The patient is positioned with the head slightly extended and rotated 30 degrees contralateral to the surgical approach. The transverse incision is made 2 cm inferior and parallel to the lower margin of the mandible, and extends from the angle of the mandible posteriorly to the base of the mental protuberance beyond the midline anteriorly.

A tracheostomy, which allows the jaws to be closed tightly, is placed to facilitate the exposure. The T-shaped skin incision is marked out to include a submandibular incision from the mastoid tip to the symphysis menti and an inferior extension carried from the midpoint of the submandibular incision along the anterior border of the sternocleidomastoid muscle. The entire cervical region and lower face are prepped and draped in sterile fashion, similar to an extended anterior cervical approach. Injection may be carried out with local anesthetic and epinephrine.

SURGICAL PROCEDURE

The skin incision is performed. Wide subcutaneous flap on each side of the incision superficial to the platysma muscle should be prepared. The medial edge of the platysma muscle is grasped in the midline. Vertical incision of platysma is made from the mental symphysis to the superior notch of the thyroid cartilage. Next, the platysma muscle is undermined and freed. Then the platysma can be transected across its fibers parallel to the direction of the primary incision for the full length of the exposure[5] (Fig. 3-3).

The fascial plane between the pharynx and the prevertebral muscles is reached through an exposure directed along the anterior border of the sternocleidomastoid muscle and between the carotid sheath laterally and the esophagus and trachea medially. By performing the initial exposure inferiorly, the approach can be considered an extension of the familiar anterior cervical approach.

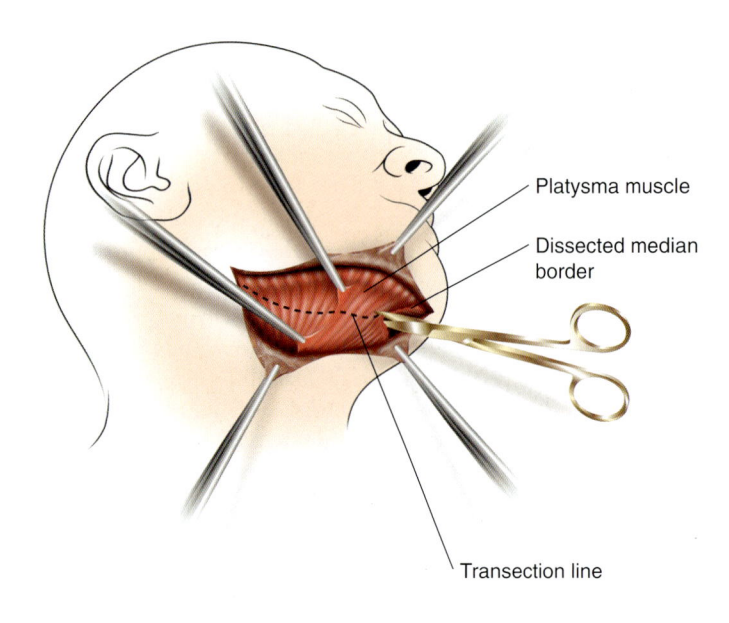

Fig. 3-3 Platysma muscle incision. The platysma muscle is transected across its fibers parallel to the direction of the primary incision for the full length of the exposure.

Fig. 3-4 Underneath the superficial cervical fascia layer, the marginal branch of the facial nerve (the ramus mandibularis nerve) is found. This nerve runs anteriorly below the angle of the mandible and lies in the upper part of the submandibular gland.

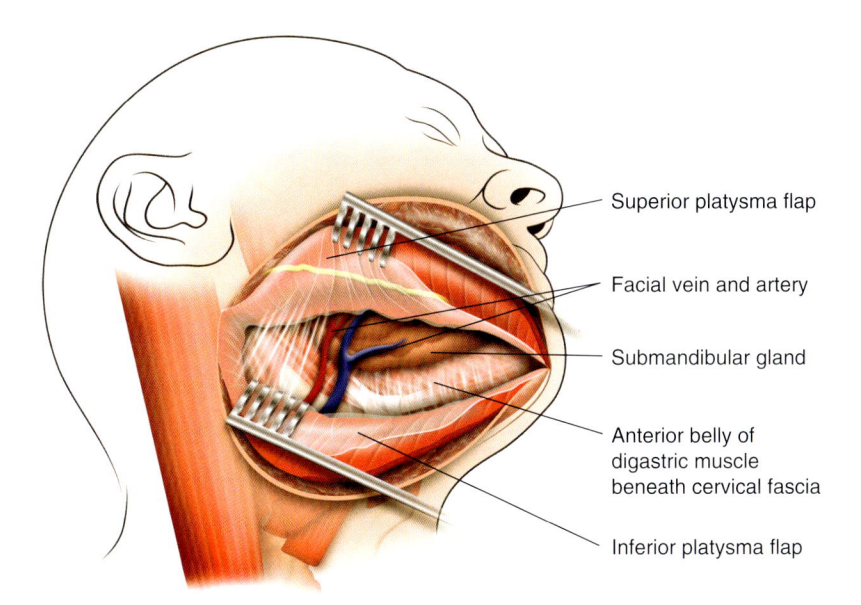

In order to expose the craniovertebral junction, additional superior exposure is needed. Structures that may be divided to increase the exposure include the ascending pharyngeal and superior thyroid arteries, external laryngeal nerve, ansa hypoglossi, internal laryngeal nerve, lingual artery, stylohyoid muscle, anterior belly of the digastric muscle, stylohyoid ligament, and the stylopharyngeus and styloglossus muscles.

SUBMANDIBULAR GLAND DISSECTION AND RETRACTION

The retraction of the divided platysma muscle will show that the next fascial layer overlies the submandibular gland and facial artery and vein. When dealing with the superficial cervical fascia layer, the marginal branch of the facial nerve (the ramus mandibularis nerve) is found[4] (Fig. 3-4). Inadvertent injury to it will result in the paresis of the orbicularis muscle, which causes the drooping at the mouth angle.

This nerve runs anteriorly, below the angle of the mandible, and lies in the upper part of the submandibular gland. So the superficial fascia should be incised below the nerve and raised over the submandibular gland. It is important to remember that the facial artery runs posterior to the submandibular gland and appears lateral to the facial vein in the mandibular notch.

The inferior edge of the gland is grasped and elevated, and the fascia is opened, undermined, and dissected. The facial vein is ligated and transected. The facial artery is dissected and preserved. When the facial artery is dissected, it can be fully retracted[5] (Fig. 3-5).

The retraction of the submandibular gland will show the next fascial layer investing the digastric muscle. The transec-

Fig. 3-5 After the retraction of the submandibular gland, the next fascial layer investing the digastric muscle is seen. The removal of the fascia exposes the digastric muscle, digastric tendon, fascial sling, and stylohyoid muscle.

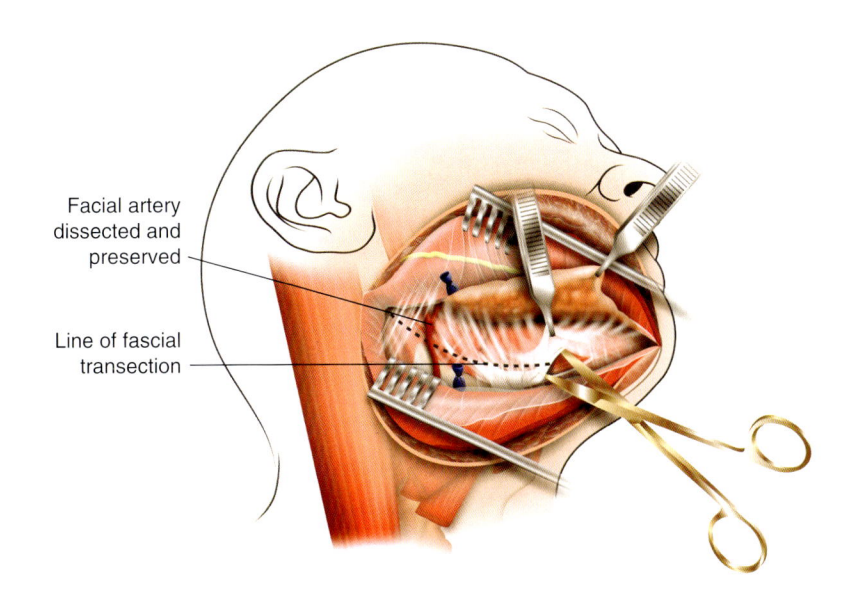

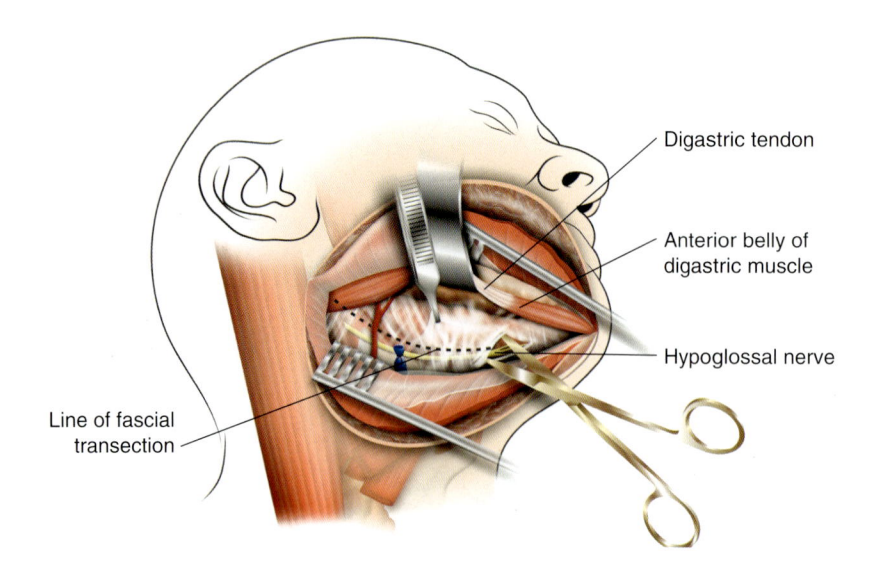

Fig. 3-6 Hypoglossal nerve identification. The digastric muscle and stylohyoid muscle are retracted toward the mandible, which exposes the next fascial layer. The hypoglossal nerve is located just deep, slightly inferior, and parallel to the digastric tendon.

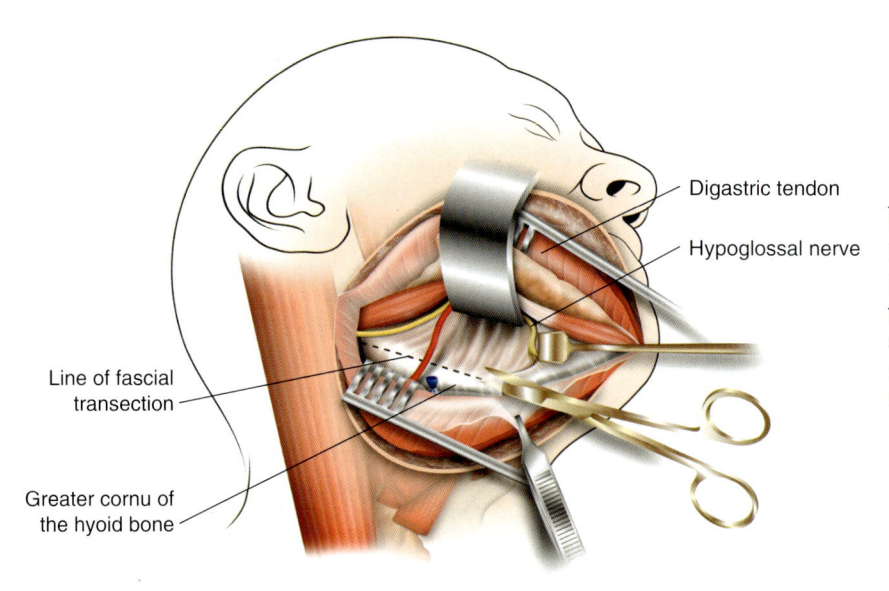

Fig. 3-7 After the hypoglossal nerve is retracted superiorly, fascia overlying the hyoid bone is incised along the course laterally to the carotid sheath, and the carotid artery is retracted laterally to open the retropharyngeal space.

tion of this fascial investment exposes the digastric muscle, digastric tendon, fascial sling, and stylohyoid muscle. The fascial sling attaches the digastric tendon to the great wing of the hyoid bone. After the transection of the fascial sling, the digastric muscle and stylohyoid muscle are retracted toward the mandible, and the next fascial layer is shown. The hypoglossal nerve is located just deep, slightly inferior, and parallel to the digastric tendon[5] (Fig. 3-6).

HYPOGLOSSAL NERVE

The hypoglossal nerve exits the skull in close proximity to the vagus nerve and courses between the internal carotid artery and internal jugular vein, becoming superficial at the angle of the mandible. After its point of identification over the arteries, it passes deep to the tendon of the digastric muscle for the distribution to the muscles of the tongue.

The hypoglossal nerve is gently dissected along its course and carefully preserved (Fig. 3-7). Posterolaterally, the dissection is done along the nerve trunk toward the descending hypoglossal ramus. After the dissection is done, the hypoglossal nerve is retracted superiorly, exposing the hypoglossus muscle.[5]

HYOID BONE AND OPENING OF THE RETROPHARYNGEAL SPACE

Fascia overlying the hyoid bone is incised along the course laterally to the carotid sheath, and carotid artery is retracted laterally to open the retropharyngeal space. The superior constrictor muscle of the pharynx is retracted medially by a deep right-angled retractor. The retropharyngeal areolar tissue is opened with scissors. The fat pad in the retropharyngeal space confirms the location. The prominent anterior tuber-

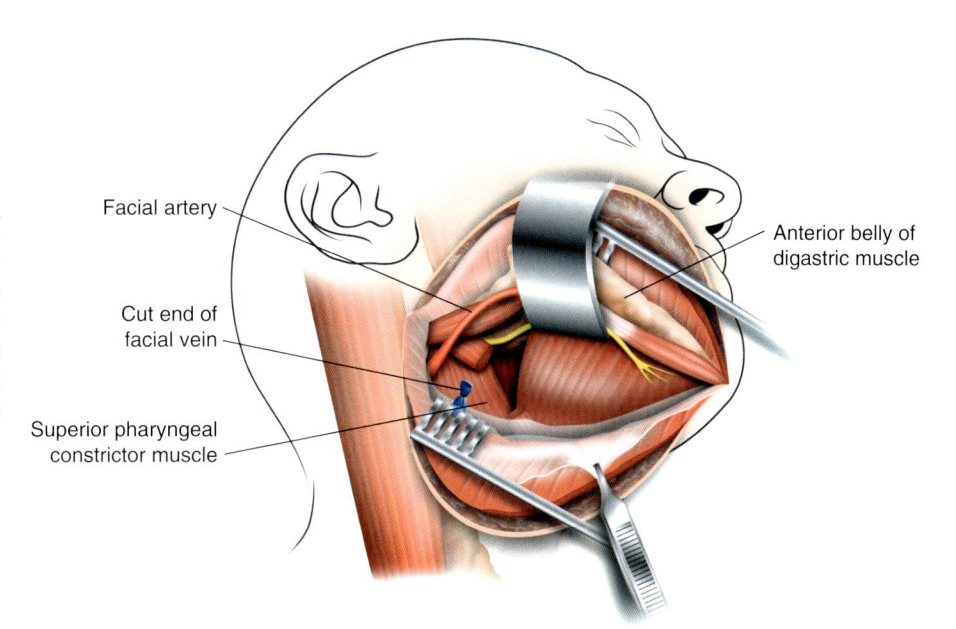

CHAPTER 3 High Cervical Retropharyngeal Approach to the Craniocervical Junction

Fig. 3-8 Opening of the retropharyngeal space. The superior constrictor muscle of the pharynx is retracted medially and the carotid artery is retracted laterally. The fat pad in the retropharyngeal space confirms the location.

cle of C1 can be palpated, and the prevertebral fascia and longus colli muscles are seen (Fig. 3-8). Entrance to the retropharyngeal space by this route is along the greater cornu of the hyoid bone and adjacent to the superior pharyngeal constrictor muscle.[6]

Be careful not to injure the superior laryngeal nerve in opening the retropharyngeal space. The superior laryngeal nerve is running deep to the internal carotid artery along the middle pharyngeal constrictor muscle, toward the superior wing of the hyoid bone and adjacent to the superior pharyngeal constrictor muscle. The superior laryngeal nerve is vulnerable to stretch injury from retraction. Wide dissection of the fascial planes will help reduce the risk of causing nerve injury. If the deep cervical fascia is opened vertically in the lateral exposure to gain access to C4 or lower cervical levels, the superior laryngeal nerve must be identified and preserved[7] (Fig. 3-9). Sometimes it is necessary to sacrifice the branches of the carotid artery and internal jugular vein for lateral mobilization of the carotid sheath[8] (Fig. 3-10). These branches are the superior thyroidal artery and vein, the lingual artery and vein, the ascending pharyngeal artery and vein and facial vein.

Although rarely necessary, the hypoglossal and glossopharyngeal nerves may be divided if required for additional exposure. The tagged ends may be reapproximated at the conclusion of the procedure. Deviation laterally may damage the internal jugular vein, internal carotid artery, eustachian tube, and the ninth through the twelfth cranial nerves.

DISSECTION OF LONGUS COLLI MUSCLE AND LONGUS CAPITIS MUSCLE

After the retropharyngel space is opened, the precervical fascia and longus colli muscle are seen. It is important to identify the midline of the cervical spine. The midline is assumed with the imaginary line between bilateral longus colli muscles, and the anterior tubercle of C1 is considered to be the midpoint. The longus colli muscle converges at the midline at the upper cervical level, so it should be elevated by sharp dissection from the anterolateral surface of C2 and C3 (Fig. 3-11). Muscle dissection should be done up to the pharyngeal tubercle of the basiocciput including the anterior arch and the lateral mass articulation of C1. The anterior rim of the foramen magnum is palpated just above the anterior arch of C1. The pharyngeal tubercle is the most rostral landmark and limit to this approach.[9]

At the anterior arch of the atlas and the odontoid process, a 2-cm width of clivus extending from the foramen magnum to the spheno-occipital synchondrosis may be removed. If necessary, the dura may be opened, providing access to the vertebrobasilar junction and anterior cervicomedullary junction. The ability to approach ventral intradural lesions represents a key advantage of this approach over the transoral approach, in which dural entry carries a high risk of meningitis and cerebrospinal fluid fistula.

APPROACH, LATERAL TO CAROTID SHEATH

This approach is medial to the sternocleidomastoid muscle and lateral to the carotid sheath. The patient is placed in the supine position, with the head extended and turned about 30 degrees. The ear lobe is temporarily reflected and sutured to the skin in front of the ear. A hockey stick–shaped incision is made transversely over the proximal sternocleidomastoid muscle, then distally along the anterior border of this muscle and posteriorly curving across the mastoid process (Fig. 3-12). Following the skin incision, the subcutaneous

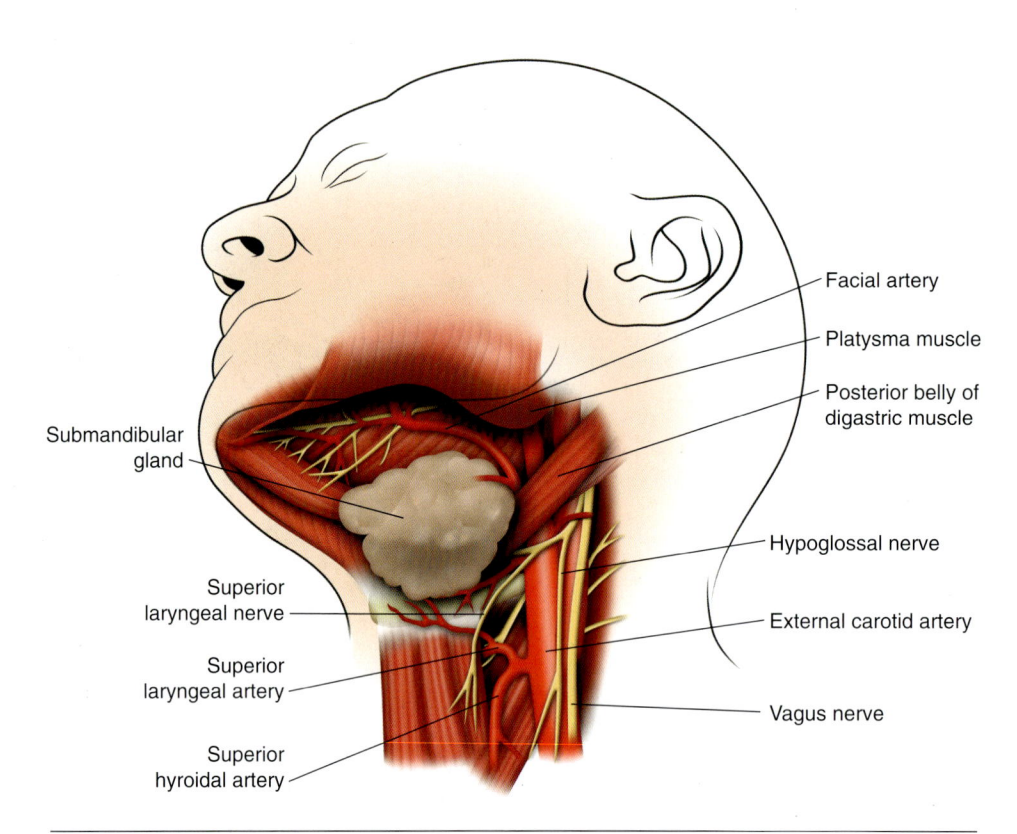

Fig. 3-9 Superior laryngeal nerve. The superior laryngeal nerve is running deep to the internal carotid artery along the middle pharyngeal constrictor muscle, toward the superior wing of the hyoid bone and adjacent to the superior pharyngeal constrictor muscle.

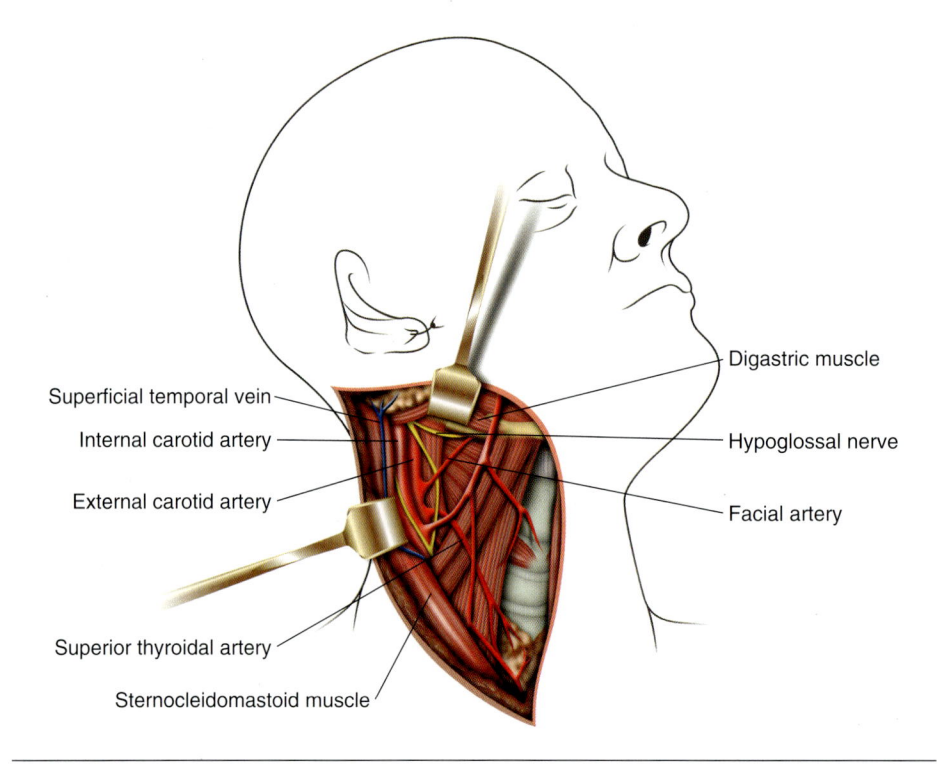

Fig. 3-10 The superior thyroidal artery and vein, the lingual artery and vein, the ascending pharyngeal artery and vein, and the facial vein are sometimes ligated for extensive exposure.

CHAPTER 3 High Cervical Retropharyngeal Approach to the Craniocervical Junction

layer and platysma muscle are divided along the skin incision line. Underneath the platysma muscle, the greater auricular nerve is dissected for mobilization. The external jugular vein is seen to overlie the sternocleidomastoid muscle. It can be ligated if necessary. The posterior portion of the parotid gland is shown on the anterior border of the sternocleidomastoid muscle and should be protected. The sternocleidomastoid muscle is divided in its tendinous portion partially along perpendicular direction to its anterior border (Fig. 3-13). Sufficient tendon tissue should be left for easy repair of the muscle. Underneath the divided sternocleidomastoid muscle, the spinal accessory nerve, common carotid artery, internal jugular vein, posterior belly of digastric muscle, and multiple lymph nodes are seen (Fig. 3-14). The spinal accessory nerve runs downward and enters the sternocleidomastoid muscle about 3 cm below the mastoid process. Usually, the nerve is retracted medially with the carotid sheath.[10]

After the division of the sternocleidomastoid muscle, the C1 transverse process is palpated. Several lymph nodes are found around the spinal accessory nerve and can be excised. The retropharyngeal space can be reached by dissecting between the internal jugular vein and the longus capitis muscle. This space can be extended in the areolar plane by blunt or sharp dissection[10] (Fig. 3-15). The C1 and C2 midline structures are easily identified with the retraction of overlying structures. To expose bony surface, it is necessary to elevate the longus colli muscle and longus capitis muscle from the transverse process of C1 and C2 from lateral to medial direction. The peeling off the muscles is completed, and the lateral mass and anterior arch of atlantoaxial complex can be visualized. The frontal view of atlantoaxial complex can be obtained by fitting the malleable retractor on the contralateral transverse process. Cephalad retraction should be cautious, taking care not to injure the facial nerve. The

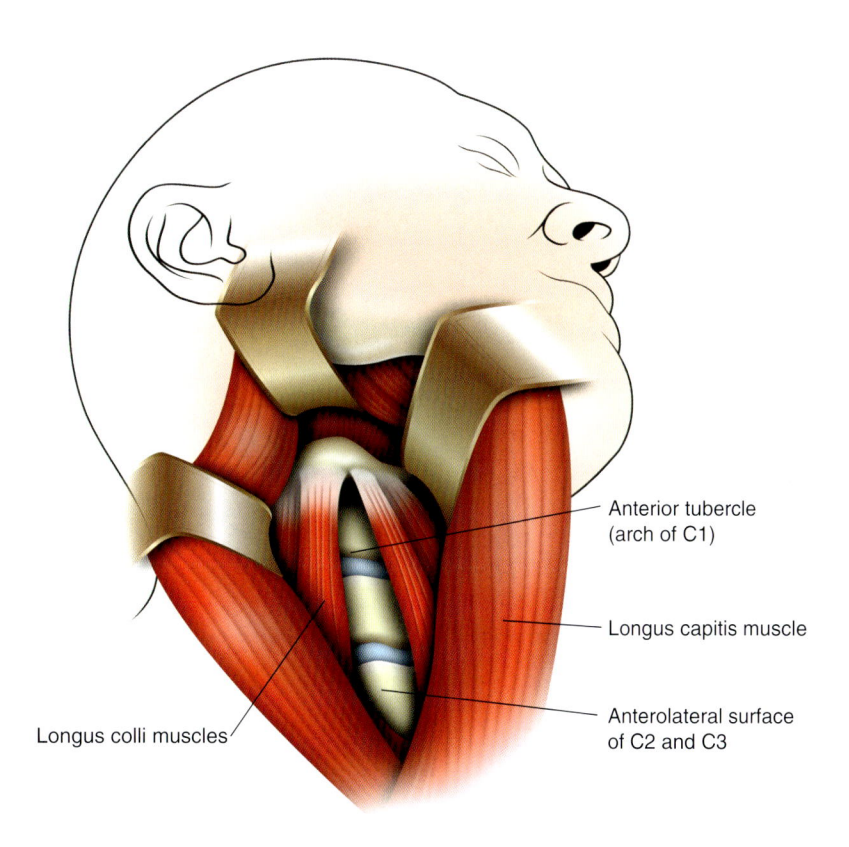

Fig. 3-11 After the retropharyngeal space is opened, the precervical fascia and longus colli muscle can be seen. The midline is identified with bilateral longus colli muscles and anterior tubercle of C1. The longus colli muscle converges at the midline at the upper cervical level, so it should be elevated by sharp dissection from the anterolateral surface of C2 and C3.

30 SECTION I SURGICAL ANATOMY AND APPROACHES

Fig. 3-12 Position and skin incision in lateral approach. The patient is placed on supine position with the head extended and turned away. A hockey stick–shaped incision is made transversely over the proximal sternocleidomastoid muscle, then distally along the anterior border of this muscle and posteriorly curving across the mastoid process.

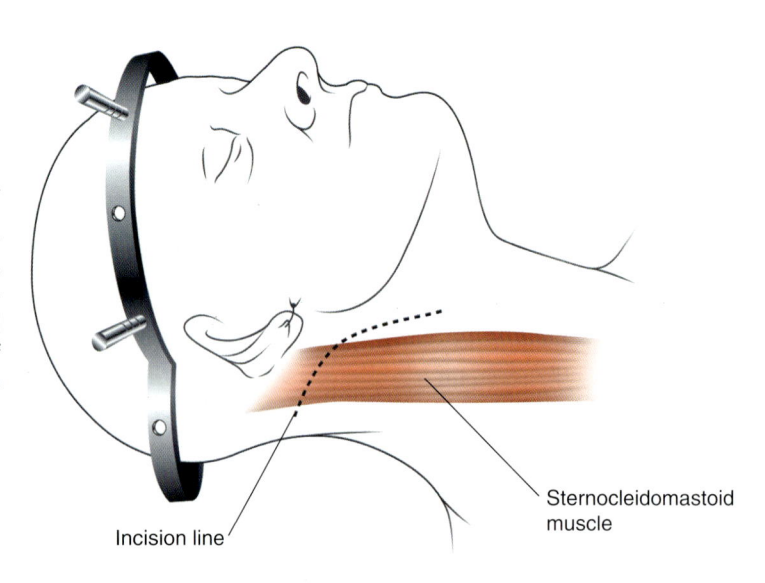

Fig. 3-13 Following the skin incision, the greater auricular nerve is dissected and mobilized. The external jugular vein can be ligated if necessary. The sternocleidomastoid muscle is divided in its tendinous portion partially along its anterior border in a perpendicular direction.

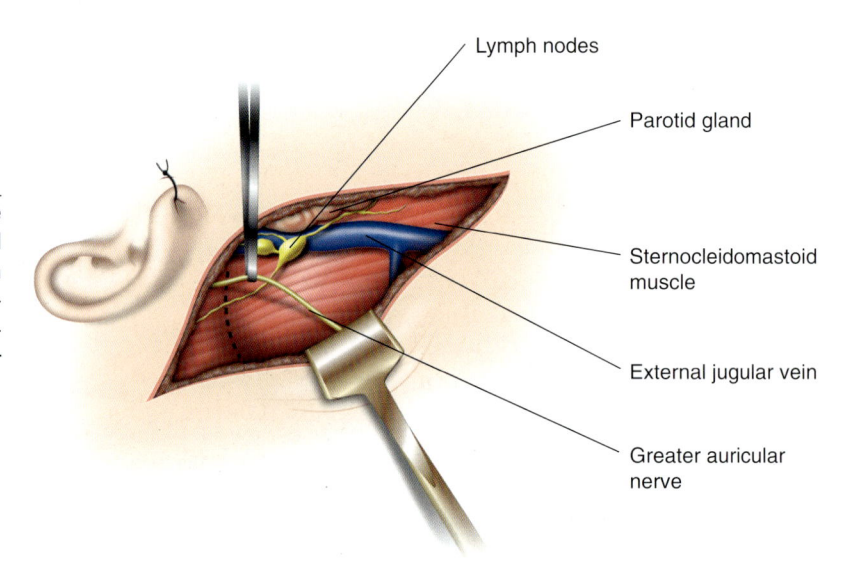

posterior belly of the digastric muscle forms the superior limit of the exposure.

After dealing with the pathology, closure is performed. After completion of the procedure, hemostasis is obtained and the wound is irrigated with antibiotic solution. The dura is closed in a watertight fashion, and a combination of muscle, fat, and fibrin glue are used to assist with the dural closure. The prevertebral fascia and muscles may also be sutured in the midline to further assist with prevention of cerebrospinal fluid fistula. The platysma and skin are then closed in a routine fashion. The tracheostomy is typically left in place until postoperative swelling has subsided and swallowing function has been assessed.

COMPLICATIONS

If the procedure results in destabilization of the spine, extreme care must be used until definitive fixation is accomplished. Patients undergoing an odontoidectomy are typically extremely unstable and will require a posterior stabilization procedure. This procedure may be performed immediately after the transcervical approach. Extreme care must be exercised during positioning of these patients.

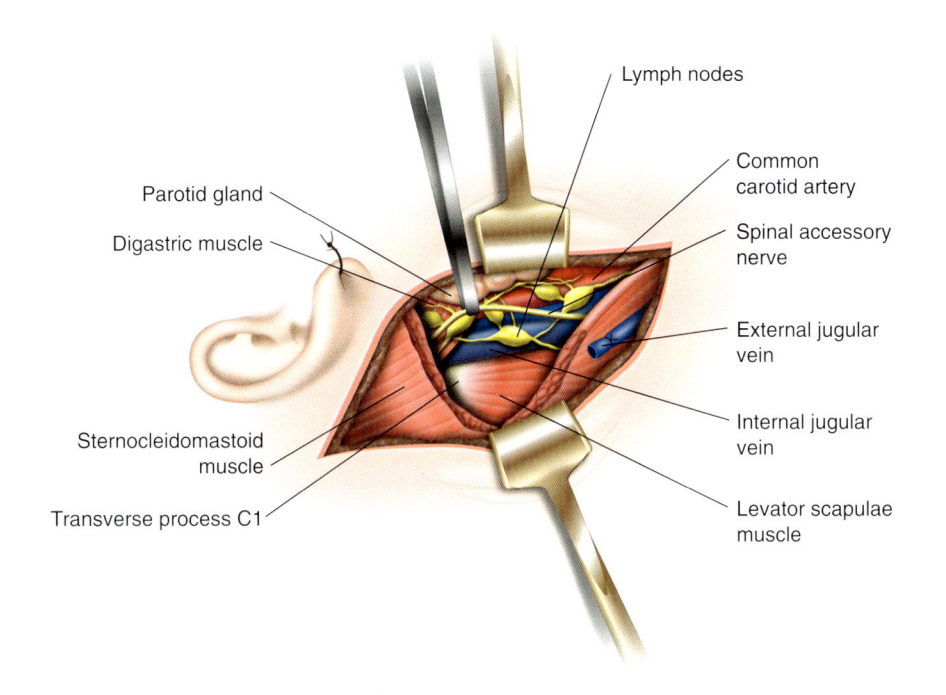

CHAPTER 3 High Cervical Retropharyngeal Approach to the Craniocervical Junction

Fig. 3-14 After the division of the sternocleidomastoid muscle, the C1 transverse process is palpated. The common carotid artery, internal jugular vein, spinal accessory nerve, and posterior belly of digastric muscle can now be seen.

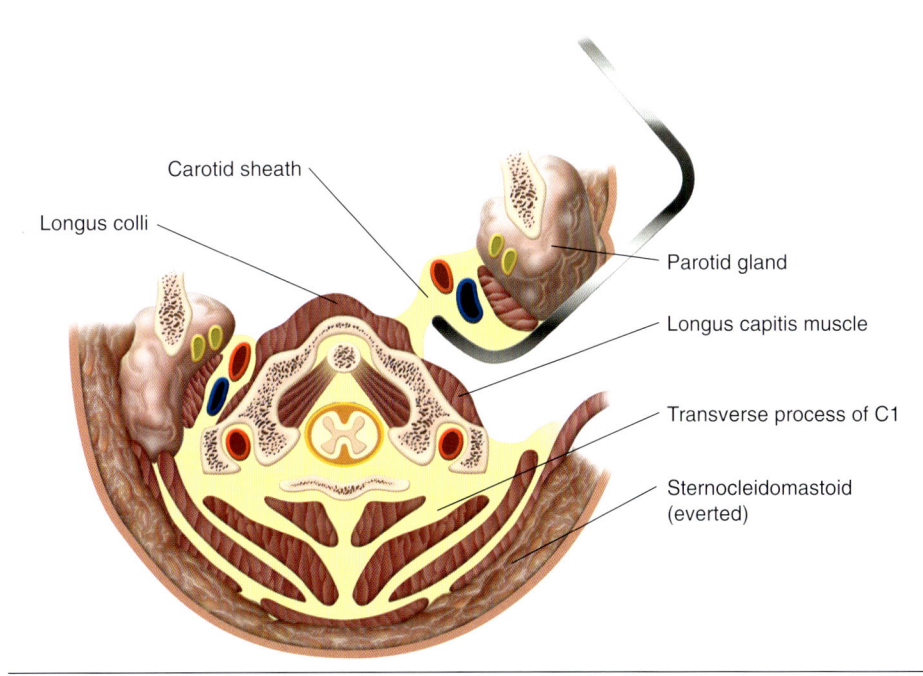

Fig. 3-15 The retropharyngeal space can be reached by dissecting between the internal jugular vein and longus capitis muscle. This space can be extended in the areolar plane by blunt or sharp dissection. To expose bony surface, it is necessary to elevate the longus colli and longus capitis muscle from the transverse process of C1 and C2 from lateral to medial direction.

SUMMARY

The transcervical approach to the craniovertebral junction is an option for anterior lesions of the craniovertebral junction. This approach has one key advantage over the transoral approach in that it does not involve opening the oropharyngeal mucosa. As a result, it is better suited to treating transdural or intradural lesions.

REFERENCES

1. Bauer R, Kerschbaumer F, Poisel S, et al: Approaches, anterior approaches, cervical spine and cervicothoracic junction. In Bauer R (ed): Atlas of Spinal Operations. New York, Thieme, 1993, pp 1–12.
2. Watkins RG: Anterior medial approach to C1, C2 and C3. In Watkins RG: Surgical Approaches to the Spine, 2nd ed. New York, Springer, 2004, pp 34–47.
3. Janfaza P, Fabian RL: The back and posterior region of the neck. In Janfaza P, Nadol JB, Galla FJ, et al (eds): Surgical Anatomy of the Head and Neck. Philadelphia, Lippincott Williams & Wilkins, 2001, pp 715–745.
4. German J, Benzel EC, Alexander JT: Anatomy and surgical approaches and exposure of the vertebral column, the cervical spine. In Benzel EC (ed): Spine Surgery, Technique, Complication Avoidance and Management. New York, Churchill Livingstone, 1999, pp 145–156.
5. McDonnell DE: Anterolateral cervical approach to the craniovertebral junction. In Rengachary SS, Wilkins RH (eds): Neurosurgical Operative Atlas, Vol 3. New York, Thieme, 1991, pp 147–164.
6. Vender JR, Harrison SJ, McDonnell DE: Fusion and instrumentation at C1-3 via the high anterior cervical approach. J Neurosurg 2000;92(1):24–29.
7. Clemente CD: Anatomy: A Regional Atlas of the Human Body, 3rd ed. Baltimore-Munich, Urban & Schwartzenberg, 1987.
8. An HS: Anatomy and the cervical spine. In An HS, Simpson JM (eds): Surgery of the Cervical Spine. Baltimore, Williams & Wilkins, 1994, pp 1–40.
9. McDonnell DE, Harrison S: Transcervical approach to the upper cervical spine. In Menezes AH (ed): Principles of Spinal Surgery. New York, McGraw-Hill, 1996, pp 1307–1324.
10. Zdeblick TA (ed): Anterior Approaches to the Spine. St. Louis, Quality Medical Publishing, 1999.

CHAPTER 4

WON-HO CHOO

MAX C. LEE

DANIEL H. KIM

Posterior and Far-Lateral Approaches to the Craniovertebral Junction

PRINCIPAL INDICATIONS

The principal indications for the posterior and far-lateral surgical approaches to the craniovertebral junction can be grouped into four types[1-4]:
1. *Occipitocervical instability*: inflammatory/infectious and iatrogenic processes, common complications of odontoid fracture, os odontoideum, rheumatoid arthritis, Chiari malformation, basilar information, achondroplasia
2. *Degenerative changes*: spondylosis, facet arthropathy, intervertebral disk degeneration
3. *Trauma*: (a) fractures (articular facet fractures, fractures of the laminae or pedicles, and vertebral body fractures) and (b) ligamentous injuries (unilateral or bilateral articular facet dislocation, posterior ligamentous incompetence, and anterior ligamentous incompetence)
4. *Tumors*: benign/malignant, congenital/acquired, primary/secondary, and intradural/extradural

OCCIPITOCERVICAL JUNCTION OPERATIVE METHODS

1. Atlantoaxial wiring
2. Posterior atlantoaxial screw fixation
3. Halifax interlaminar clamp fixation
4. Occipitocervical fusion

POSTERIOR APPROACHES TO THE CRANIOVERTEBRAL JUNCTION

POSITIONING AND INCISION

The operation is performed with the patient in the prone position with a Wilson frame under the chest. With few exceptions, throughout the positioning process it is essential to maintain the neutral cervical alignment and proper stabilization of the head. The sitting position is occasionally used for posterior stabilization procedures. This posture is particularly advantageous for obese or pregnant patients in order to minimize abdominopelvic compression and subsequent venous obstruction. Precautions must be taken to reduce the risk of venous air embolization throughout the operative procedure. Depending on the personal preference of the surgeon, the Concorde and lateral decubitus or park bench position is utilized.

Adjustments to the skeletal fixation or skeletal traction may be necessary to provide perfect alignment. A fiberoptic oral endotracheal intubation may be desirable with the spinal cord being monitored by somatosensory evoked potentials, motor evoked potential, and stimulus-evoked electromyography (EMG).

Extensive shaving of the back of the neck and head is required. The dermis and subcutaneous tissues may be infiltrated with an epinephrine-containing solution to effect vasoconstriction, thus facilitating hemostasis. The midline skin incision is made from two fingerbreadths above the external occipital protuberance and is continued as far as the tip of the spinous process of the C7 (prominent vertebra), depending on the case (Fig. 4-1).

After splitting of the subcutis, self-retaining retractors are applied and hemostasis is accomplished. Using a diathermy knife, the nuchal ligament is now approached via a midline incision of the cervical fascia. Self-retaining retractors are then inserted. The muscles are divided in the midline until the spinous process of C7 is identified and the occipital bone is found.[5-8]

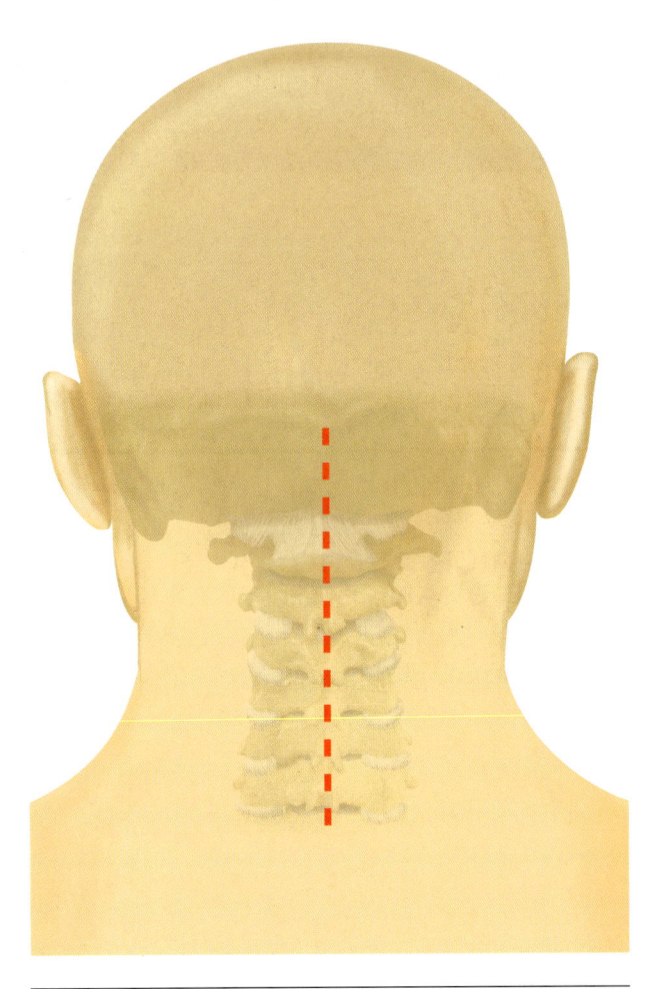

Fig. 4-1 The midline skin incision is made from two fingerbreadths above the external occipital protuberance and continued as far as the tip of the spinous process of the C7 (prominent vertebra), depending on the case.

EXPOSURE OF THE SPINE

The nuchal ligament is divided in the midline and incision as far as the tips of the spinous processes. The muscle layer that has been divided in the midline is retracted to the side. The trapezius muscle adherent to the fascia can then be mobilized bilaterally and a retractor placed in the next deeper plane.[9–14]

After this, beginning at the spinous process of the second cervical vertebra, the deep muscle layer is stripped off the spinous processes close to the bone with the electrocautery or No. 15 blade, going from cranial to caudal. The ligamentous attachment to C2 are very prominent. Insert the Cobb elevator, first facing up to elevate the tip subperiosteally, then facing down to complete the subperiosteal elevation medial to lateral approximately 1.5 cm at each level. If necessary (as with occipitocervical fusion), the musculature origination from, or attached to, the occiput (trapezius muscle, semispinalis capitis muscle) may be separated using a T-shaped dissection.

Beginning at the second spinous process (Fig. 4-2) and proceeding caudally, a sharp elevator is now used to strip the short rotator and multifidus muscles from the spinous process and articular processes. A subperiosteal dissection extending to the lateral boundary of the vertebral joints is carried out. The muscles of C1 and C2 are then dissected, with care taken not to extend too far laterally in the region of the vertebral artery. The large venous plexuses at C1 and C2 are far lateral. It is wise to carry the dissection out to the limits of the zygapophyseal joints, but not beyond and not between, to avoid these veins. This invariably leads to bleeding from the suboccipital venous plexus, which can be stopped by eletrocautery. Hemostasis may be accomplished by insertion of Gelfoam and thrombin.

Subsequently, the part of the occipital squama that lies caudal to the external occipital protuberance is exposed subperiosteally with a sharp rasp. The posterior tubercle of the atlas is now palpated with a fingertip on its deep midline location. The musculature arising from it is detached on both sides, and with an elevator, the arch of the atlas is subperiosteally dissected for about 1.5 cm bilaterally.

After passing through the foramen of the transverse process of the atlas, the vertebral artery travels medially in the sulcus of the vertebral artery, the edge of which is visible and palpable after careful dissection. Thus, the tip of the rasp must remain in constant contact with the bone to avoid damage to the vertebral artery.

In addition, between the first and second cervical vertebrae, the posterior branch of the second spinal nerve arises, the main branch of which is the greater occipital nerve. The second cervical ganglion is an important landmark on the ring of C1 laterally, which lies approximately in the area of the groove for the vertebral artery.

This nerve should likewise be spared. The retractors are inserted into the deepest muscle layer and opened further. The vertebral arches, the yellow ligaments, and the atlanto-occipital membrane are exposed with curettes and small dissectors (Fig. 4-3). The interspinal ligaments are generally removed if posterior fusion is to be performed. Bleeding from the bone is controlled with bone wax. In rheumatoid arthritis, the posterior arch of the atlas is very thin, and it can be injured by excessive dissector pressure.

With exposure of the ring of C1 and exposure to bone of the posterior occiput, different operative procedures require exposure of the dura under the edge of the foramen magnum. No attempt should be made to decompress the posterior fossa under the edge of the foramen magnum without sufficient visualization of the area cephalad to the foramen. Periosteum of the skull at this point is often conjoined with the dura of the spinal cord. There is a median venous sinus in the midline, and the fascial attachment of the periosteum of the skull to the dura often contains a transverse sinus as well.

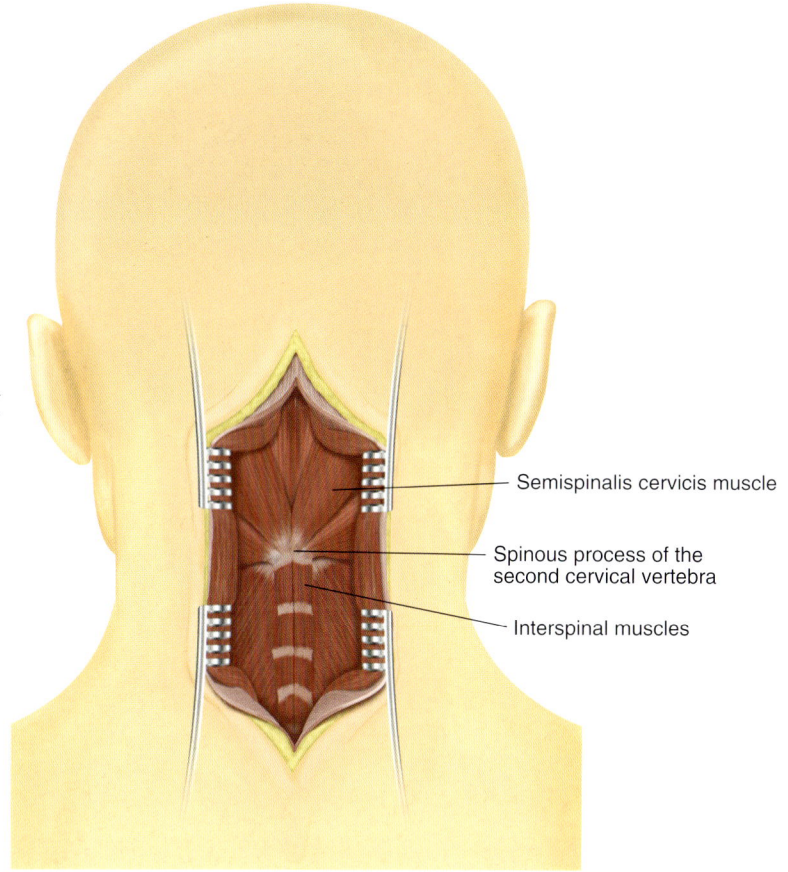

CHAPTER 4 Posterior and Far-Lateral Approaches to the Craniovertebral Junction 35

Fig. 4-2 Spinous process of the second cervical vertebra.

- Semispinalis cervicis muscle
- Spinous process of the second cervical vertebra
- Interspinal muscles

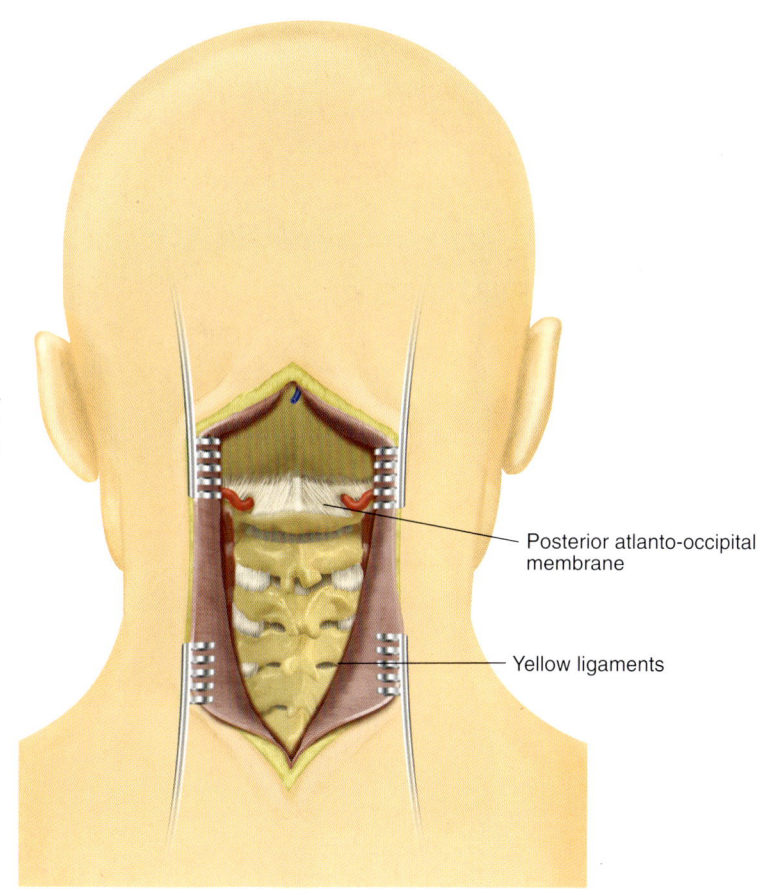

Fig. 4-3 The vertebral arches, the yellow ligaments, and the atlanto-occipital membrane are exposed with curettes and small dissectors.

- Posterior atlanto-occipital membrane
- Yellow ligaments

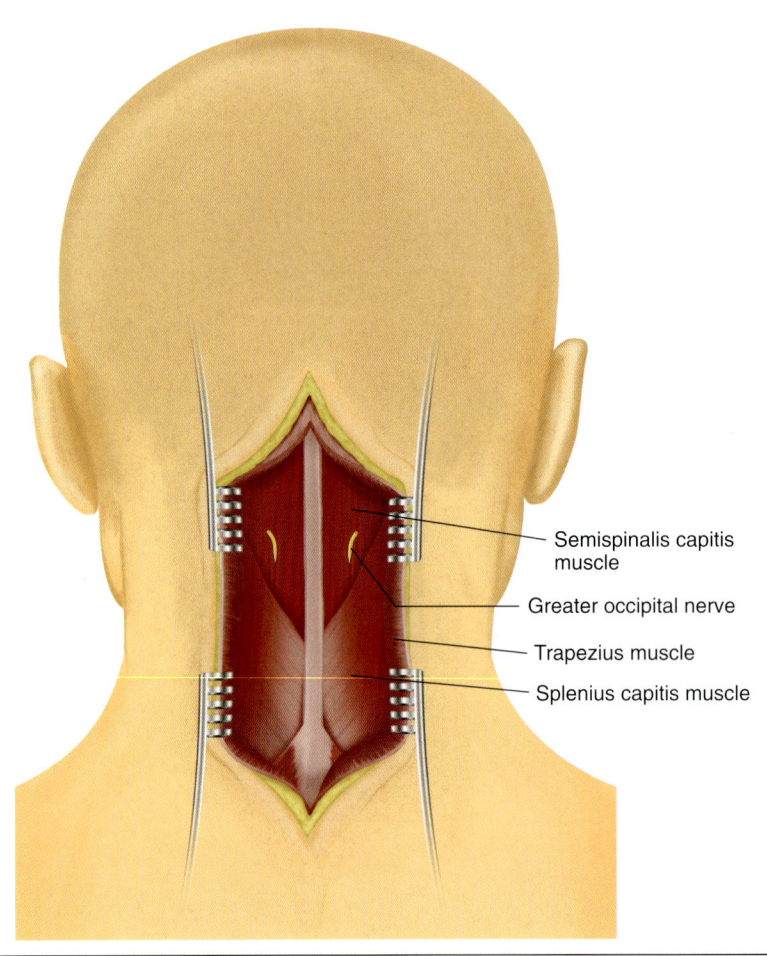

Fig. 4-4 The musculature of the neck.

To close the wound, remove the retractors, allow the muscles to fall together, and close the fascia, subcutaneous tissue, and skin.

THE MUSCULATURE OF THE NECK

The musculature of the neck is subdivided as follows (Fig. 4-4)[9-14]:
- Superficial layer: trapezius muscle—a diamond-shaped or oval aponeurosis forms
- Middle layer: lesser rhomboid muscle
- Intrinsic muscles of the neck:
  - Splenius capitis and cervicis muscles
  - Semispinalis capitis and cervicis muscles
  - Multifidus muscles
  - Rotator muscles (variable); interspinal muscles
- Short nuchal muscles:
  - Rectus capitis posterior major and minor muscles
  - Superior and inferior oblique capitis muscles of the head

Clinical tip: The rectus capitis posterior major and the superior and inferior oblique capitis muscles form the suboccipital triangle. The vertebral artery can be located here, lying along the posterior arch of the atlas. Located between the artery and the posterior arch of the atlas is the first cervical nerve, whose dorsal ramus, the suboccipital nerve, innervates these muscles.

The posterior branch of the second spinal nerve (main branch: greater occipital nerve) lies in a posterior direction between the first and second cervical vertebrae. It runs subcutaneously, one fingerbreadth distal to the tendinous arch between the trapezius and the sternocleidomastoid muscles, supplying the skin of the occiput. The posterior branch of the third spinal nerve runs posteriorly between the second and third cervical vertebrae. Its main branch, the third occipital nerve, is variable, and also supplies the skin of the occiput. The vertebral artery travels in a medial direction from the foramen of the transverse process of the atlas behind the atlanto-occipital articulation; then it runs through the posterior atlanto-occipital membrane into the great foramen and into the cranial cavity.

For a more lateral approach to the C1-C2 facet joint, the vertebral artery between C1 and C2 must be identified. In rotatory dislocations of C1-C2, the artery, which should be handled carefully because it can be damaged easily, is stretched tightly across the joint on the side where C1 is anterior to C2.

CHAPTER 4 Posterior and Far-Lateral Approaches to the Craniovertebral Junction

LATERAL APPROACH TO THE CRANIOVERTEBRAL JUNCTION

SURGICAL METHODS

In designing lateral approaches to the craniocervical junction, several surgical limitations and considerations must be given attention. These are discussed in Chapter 5.[1-3]

INDICATION AND EVALUATION

In the upper cervical spine (from the midpoint of C3 cephalad), the major uses of the lateral approach are for intradural lesions such as meningiomas or neurofibromas that are primarily ventral or ventrolateral to the spinal cord; abnormalities involving the vertebral artery; and, occasionally, fusions of C1 to C2 when posterior approaches are not feasible.[15-17]

The lateral approach to the cervical spine below C3 is best used for lesions involving the vertebral artery; lesions of the bony spine or canal in that area are more easily approached from the anterior or posterior aspect.

Evaluation of the patient for spinal problems is accomplished with plain x-rays, including dynamic views, magnetic resonance imaging (MRI), or cervical myelography followed by high-resolution computed tomography (CT). Imaging of lesions within the spinal canal is best done with MRI, which provides images in several planes. Three-dimensional CT reconstructions are often helpful in evaluating bony lesions.

MRI with flow-sensitive sequences can be useful in evaluating tumor vascularity and displacement of blood vessels, although vertebral angiography is essential for defining lesions of the vertebral arteries. If a lesion is vascular or has a rich blood supply, endovascular intervention can facilitate surgery or, in some cases, may be curative (e.g., vertebral venous plexus fistulas).

SURGICAL TECHNIQUE

Upper Cervical Spine

Prior to removing the laminae, the technique for the lateral approach is essentially the same when dealing with any lesion. The operating microscope is essential for the intraspinal portions of the operation and is very helpful in the operation after the large muscles have been reflected. The Cavitron and laser can facilitate tumor removal, and bipolar cautery is preferable throughout the procedure.[1-3,15-17]

Procedure

Nasotracheal intubation is used, as it allows the mouth to be nearly closed, keeping the angle of the mandible forward so that it does not compromise the operative field. Anterior displacement of the mandible can be increased by pulling it forward with adhesive tape. A suture is placed through the skin of the back of the ear to pull it forward. The patient is placed in the true lateral position with the neck extended and the chin turned 10 degrees toward the down side.

The skin incision is made anteriorly 1 cm below the level of the cricoid cartilage and is extended up to the base of the mastoid process (Fig. 4-5). It is then curved back across the base of the skull for 6 to 8 cm. The platysma muscle and the deep fascia are divided in the neck, and the insertions of the sternocleidomastoid muscle and part of the splenius capitis muscle are divided at the base of the skull, leaving enough bony attachment to allow reapproximation (Figs. 4-6 and 4-7).

These muscles are mobilized inferiorly and posteriorly until the spinal accessory nerve is identified entering the deep surface of the sternocleidomastoid muscle, usually 3 or 4 cm below the mastoid tip. At this point, the tip of the transverse process of C1 can be identified by palpating 1 cm below and 1 cm in front of the mastoid tip. The transverse process of C2 is shorter and more difficult to palpate and can easily be confused with the C2-C3 facet joint, which lies slightly posterior and inferior.

The deep fascia is incised from the tip of the C1 transverse process obliquely downward, parallel to the course of the spinal accessory nerve. The attachments of the thick

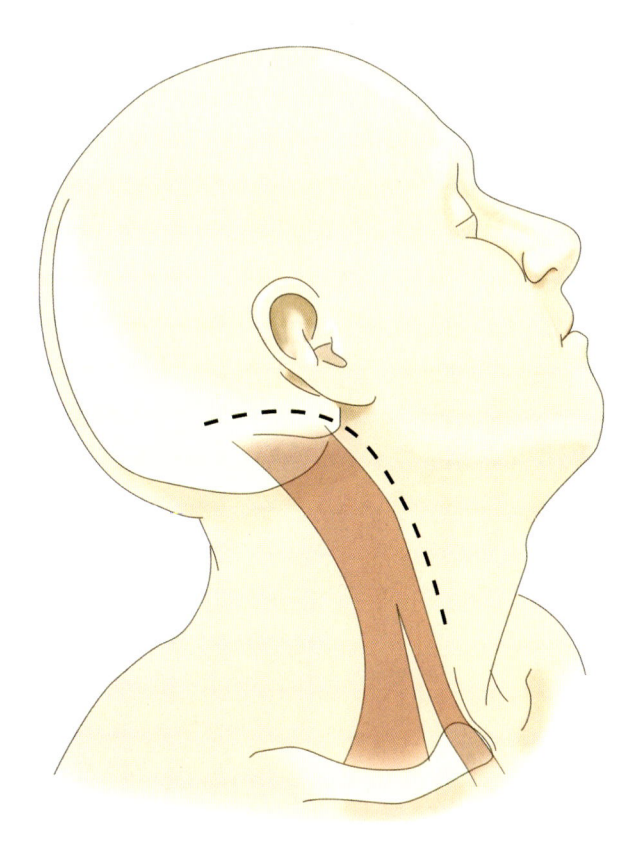

Fig. 4-5 The skin incision is made anteriorly 1 cm below the level of the cricoid cartilage and extended up to the base of the mastoid process.

38 SECTION I SURGICAL ANATOMY AND APPROACHES

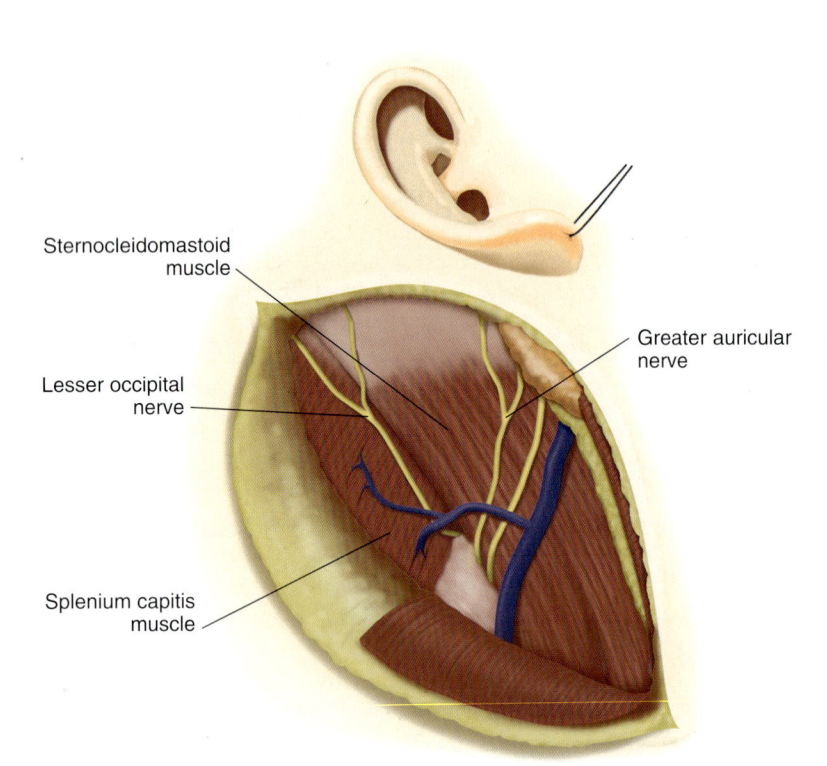

Fig. 4-6 The transverse process of C2 is shorter and more difficult to palpate and can easily be confused with the C2-C3 facet joint, which lies slightly posterior and inferior.

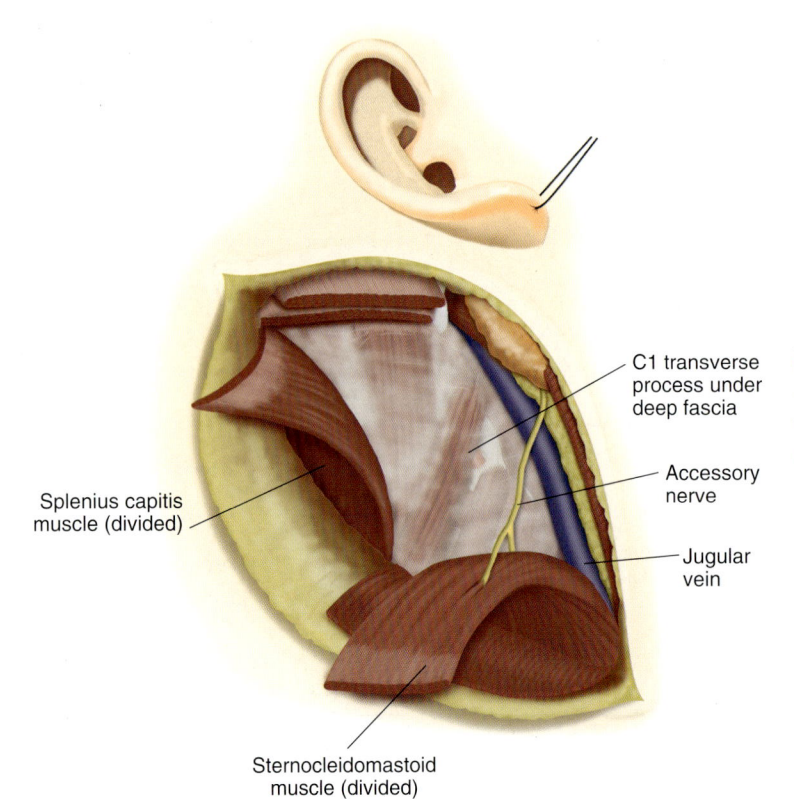

Fig. 4-7 The vertebral artery then comes clearly into view, and the remaining muscle fibers running between the transverse processes of C1 and C2 are divided.

levator scapulae muscle and the slender splenius cervicis muscle to the C1 transverse process can now be seen. These are picked up and divided, keeping in mind that the vertebral artery is located beneath them. The vertebral artery then comes clearly into view, and the remaining muscle fibers running between the transverse processes of C1 and C2 are divided (Fig. 4-8).

Next, the muscle attachments to the tip of the transverse process of C2 are divided. The lateral aspect of the arch of C1 and the C2 lamina can then be palpated and partially seen (Fig. 4-9).

Curettes are used to reflect the muscle attachments from the lamina of C2 and the inferior portion of C1. The muscle attachments to the superior portion of the C1 arch can be removed using an angled curette, keeping the plane of dissection subperiosteal to avoid injuring the vertebral artery. The muscle attachments are removed almost to the posterior midline.

With the use of a high-speed drill with diamond burrs, the exposed arch of C1 and the lamina of C2 are removed (Fig. 4-10). The lamina of C2 is removed to within a few millimeters of the foramen transversarium, but the C2-C3 facet joint and a portion of the pedicle are spared. The arch of C1 is removed to the point where the vertebral artery is on the superior surface. From that point laterally to the transverse foramen, the bone is undercut but not removed totally.

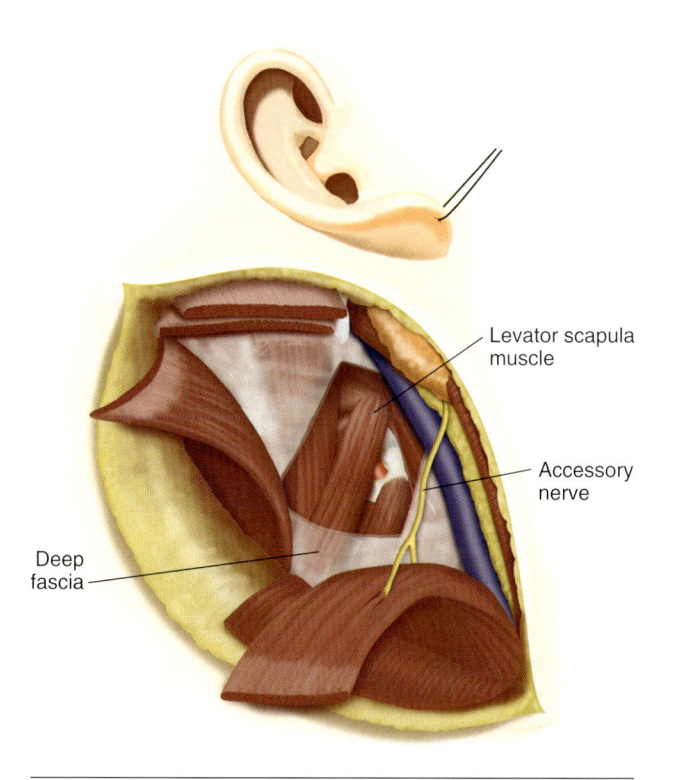

Fig. 4-8 The muscle attachments are removed almost to the posterior midline.

Usually, little epidural fat is present, and the dura is easily exposed from the foramen magnum to the superior portion of C3. The dura is best opened using a curved incision, beginning at the anterosuperior portion of the exposed dura and creating a convex backward incision that ends by coming back to the anteroinferior portion of the exposed dura (see Fig. 4-10).

This incision allows the dura to be flapped anteriorly. For tumors that are ventral to the spinal cord, this opening will expose both the compressed cord and the tumor. For ventrolateral tumors, this opening should expose at least a small portion of the normal cord in its posterior extent (Fig. 4-11).

Tumors in this area are best removed in a piecemeal fashion with minimal manipulation of the spinal cord. The Cavitron can be helpful in debulking the central portion of the lesion if standard suction and gentle curetting are not effective. The variety of curettes and forceps used for transsphenoidal pituitary surgery are particularly appropriate for this part of the operation. The laser and bipolar cautery are both helpful for shrinking the tumor. If the tumor is a meningioma, involved dura should be removed, and in some cases, the dura is patched with a fascial graft. If the dural defect is purely ventral, no graft is placed and the lateral dural incision is closed.

With this exposure, ventrally situated tumors that have displaced the spinal cord posteriorly are readily seen, and more laterally situated tumors lie just beneath the dural incision. After the tumor removal and standard dural closure, the muscles are reapproximated with 2-0 sutures and the remaining incision is closed in the usual fashion. A cervical collar helps to lessen the patient's discomfort during the first few postoperative weeks.

Potential complications include injury to the spinal accessory nerve and the vertebral artery. The landmarks for locating the vertebral artery before it is seen are so prominent that untoward injury is unlikely. Once the artery is identified, it is easy to avoid, and it remains at the periphery of the surgical area. The spinal accessory nerve is seen early in the procedure and is more likely to be injured during retraction by excessive stretching, than by division of the nerve.

The jugular vein lies anterior to the tips of the transverse processes of C1 and C2, well removed from the operative area. The risks of spine instability and spinal cord injury seem lessened with this approach than with others.

Leakage of cerebrospinal fluid is not usually a problem, as the dura can usually be closed primarily or grafted. In addition, there are several soft tissue layers between the dura and the skin.

LATERAL RETROPHARYNGEAL APPROACH

This exposure has been useful for the simultaneous exposure of the right and left lateral C1 and C2 articulations through

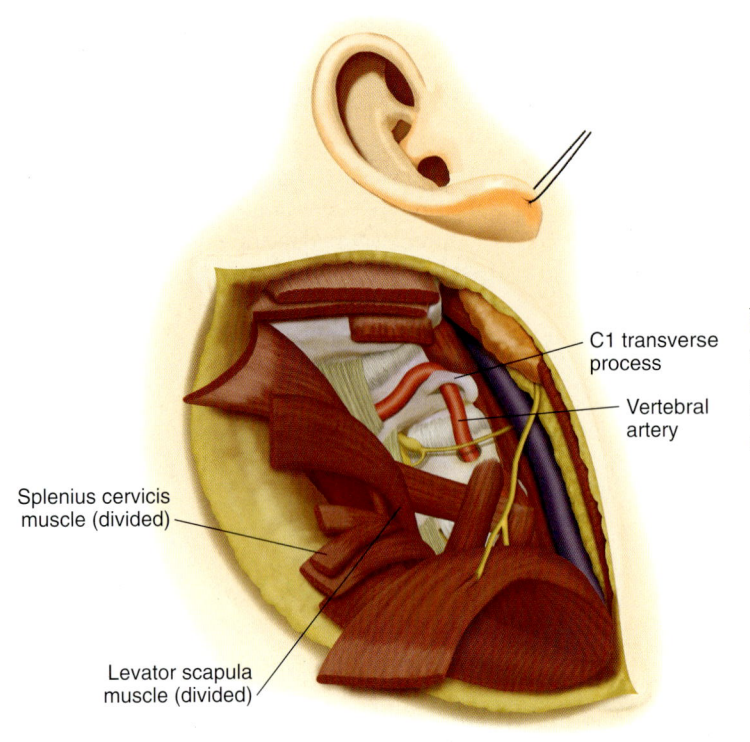

Fig. 4-9 The arch of C1 is removed to the point where the vertebral artery is on the superior surface. From that point laterally to the transverse foramen, the bone is undercut but not removed totally.

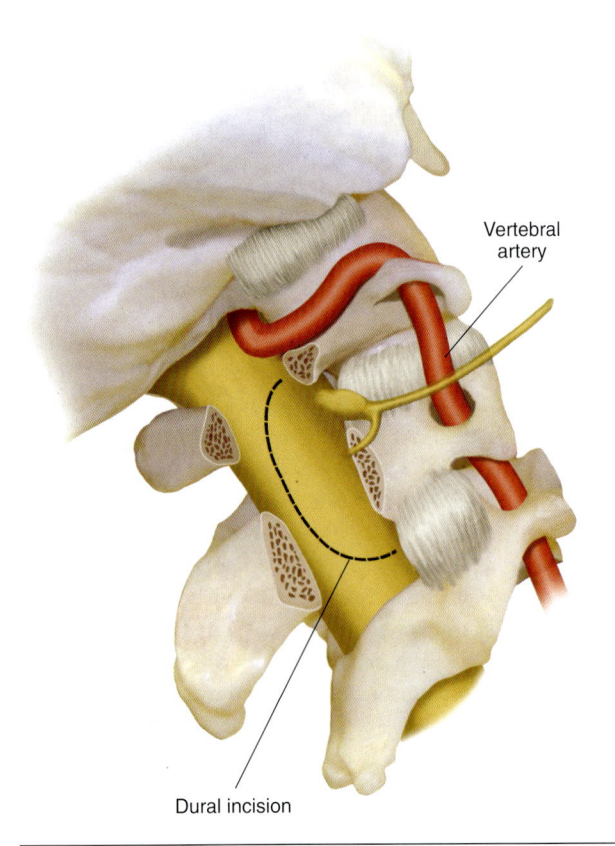

Fig. 4-10 The dura is best opened using a curved incision, beginning at the anterosuperior portion of the exposed dura and creating a convex backward incision that ends by coming back to the anteroinferior portion of the exposed dura.

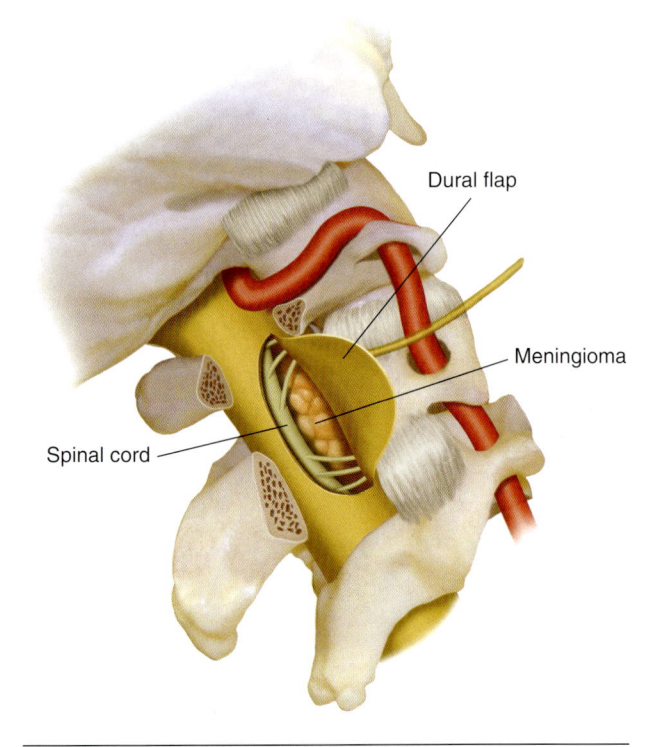

Fig. 4-11 For ventrolateral tumors, this opening should expose at least a small portion of the normal cord in its posterior extent.

a unilateral approach for removal of vertebral bodies and the odontoid for various diseases; for biopsy of lesions of all areas of the anterior spine in this region; for fusion of C1 to T1; and to expose a small amount of the basiocciput for fusion to that area when needed. This procedure is generally performed with a halo ring. Nasotracheal intubation on the side opposite the approach is recommended. The neck is extended and rotated to the opposite side as much as is possible. The inside and outside of the ear area is prepared and the ear lobe is sewn anteriorly to the cheek to facilitate exposure of the operative incision. A "hockey stick" incision is made transversely across the tip of the mastoid process and is carried distally along the anterior border of the sternocleidomastoid muscle.[1-3,18]

The greater auricular nerve is identified and dissected in both directions. The spinal accessory nerve is then identified at its entrance into the sternocleidomastoid muscle approximately 3 cm from the mastoid tip. If only the C1-C2 area needs to be approached, the nerve is retracted anteriorly with the contents of the carotid sheath. If a more extensive approach is needed, the nerve is dissected from the jugular vein up to an area near the jugular foramen and then retracted laterally and posteriorly as the sternocleidomastoid muscle is everted.

The transverse processes of the cervical vertebrae, especially C1, are easily palpable. The vertebral artery can be safely avoided by identifying the internal jugular vein and delineating it well. After identifying the transverse processes of C1 and C2, fibrous attachments directed anteriorly are divided, which allows access to the retropharyngeal space along the anterior arch of C1 and anterior body of C2. Exposure of the appropriate vertebral bodies is now possible with subperiosteal stripping and, if needed, removal of the anterior cervical muscles that cover the lateral articulations of C1 and C2. The C1-C2 lateral masses can be accessed and fused bilaterally by an extension of the lateral approach to the upper cervical spine.

This approach allows resection of bony lesions involving the lateral mass of C1-C2, the anterior arch of C1, and the body and odontoid process of C2. Transarticular screw fixation of C1-C2 is accomplished after preparation of the articular surfaces and decortication of the end plates with a small straight curette. Under fluoroscopic visualization, a screw is directed from the superolateral aspect of the lateral mass of C1 across the articular surface in an inferomedial direction into C2. Bilateral fixation requires a bilateral approach. When performing a resection of an instability, titanium plate fixation of the occiput to C3 or C4 may be needed to accompany bony fusion.

The true lateral exposure to the craniocervical junction demands resection of a portion of the lateral atlantal mass and the occipital condyle. The exposure of the lower clivus and ventral brainstem is quite satisfactory when combined with retrosigmoid craniectomy.

Its combination with the infratemporal fossa procedures allows for both posterior and anterior extension that overcomes the limitations of the sigmoid sinus and the hypoglossal nerve.

FAR-LATERAL APPROACH TO THE CRANIOVERTEBRAL JUNCTION

A standard lateral approach may not be adequate to achieve a radical tumor resection or safely clip an aneurysm with full visualization.

The basic far-lateral approach without drilling of the occipital condyle may be all that is required to reach some lesions located along the anterolateral margin of the foramen magnum, but this approach also provides a route through which the transcondylar, supracondylar, and paracondylar areas can be approached. Several modifications of these approaches can be completed.[19-26]

This discussion focuses primarily on the transcondylar approach.

The transcondylar approach consists of (1) dissection of the muscles along the posterolateral aspect of the craniocervical junction to permit an adequate lateral approach while reducing the depth of the surgical field; (2) early identification of the vertebral artery either above the posterior arch of the atlas or in its ascending course between the transverse processes of the atlas and axis; (3) a suboccipital craniectomy or craniotomy with removal of at least one half of the posterior arch of the atlas; and (4) removal of the posterior portion of the occipital condyle to allow a more lateral approach (Fig. 4-12).

The patient is placed in full lateral decubitus position with the head and neck neutral. Intraoperative monitoring includes bilateral somatosensory evoked potentials, bilateral brainstem auditory evoked response, and cranial nerves X, XI, and XII.

An inverted horseshoe incision is made with one of the limbs along the midline and the other limb at the side of the neck. The horizontal limb is at the level of the upper border of the ear. The incision begins in the midline, approximately 5 cm below the external occipital protuberance, and is directed upward to just above the external occipital protuberance, turning laterally just above the superior nuchal line, reaching the mastoid, and turning downward in front of the posterior border of the sternocleidomastoid muscle onto the lateral aspect of the neck to approximately 5 cm below the mastoid tip and below where the transverse process of the atlas can be palpated through the skin. Sometimes, a C-shaped incision has been recommended.

The skin flap is reflected downward and medially to expose the most superficial layer of muscles formed by the sternocleidomastoid and splenius capitis muscles laterally and the trapezius and the semispinalis capitis muscles medially. The sternocleidomastoid, the splenius capitis, the longis-

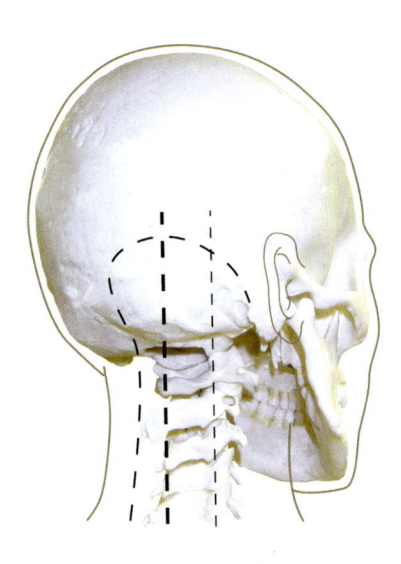

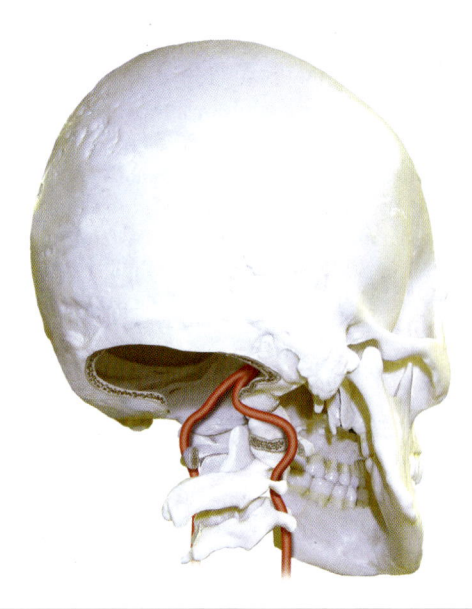

Fig. 4-12 Far-lateral approach to the craniovertebral pathology. *Left*, The incision extends from the midline to the inion, and across to the mastoid tip. The subperiosteal dissection allows the entire muscle mass to be retracted laterally. *Right*, The bony removal includes the arch of C1 from the midline to the sulcus arteriosus of the vertebral artery.

simus capitis, and the semispinalis muscles are detached from the mastoid in one layer. Muscle dissection in the posterior cervical triangle is preferably performed in anatomic layers, detaching each muscle from its cephalic attachment and reflecting it inferiorly.

At this stage, the posterior belly of the digastric muscle should be kept in place to protect the facial nerve as it exits the stylomastoid foramen. The splenius cervicis muscle, which attaches superiorly on the lateral process of C1, is kept in place to protect the jugular vein.

The deep muscular layer forms the suboccipital triangle, which is delimited by the major and minor rectus capitis muscles medially, the superior oblique muscle superiorly, and the inferior oblique muscle inferiorly. The apex of the triangle is the transverse process of C1. Inside the suboccipital triangle, the horizontal segment of the vertebral artery and C1 root can be seen.

After identification of the transverse processes of C1 and C2, the transverse segment of the vertebral artery along C1 is identified. The vertebral artery is surrounded by a plexus of veins that can be left intact if mobilization of the artery is not necessary. The artery is intimately related to the occiput-C1 joint capsule and must be carefully freed from this for circumferential control. A large craniectomy that extends up to the sigmoid and transverse sinuses is performed if the tumor in the posterior fossa is large. The sigmoid sinus is completely unroofed down to the jugular bulb.

The posterior arch of C1 is removed and a small suboccipital craniectomy is performed at the foramen magnum.

Two osseous landmarks—the asterion and the inion—are important in planning the suboccipital craniectomy. The asterion is located on the point where the transverse sinus empties into the sigmoid sinus. The inion, the site of the external occipital protuberance, is located an average of 1 cm below the apex of the internal occipital protuberance and the inferior margin of the confluence of the sagittal and transverse sinuses.

After the vertebral artery has been fully exposed as needed, the bone in front of it (the posterior part of the condyle) is carefully drilled with a diamond drill or the Midas Rex AM-8 to allow additional ventral exposure as well as access to the anterior surface of the foramen magnum. The posterior process of the occipital condyle often prevents the dural flap from being reflected anteriorly; its removal gains an additional several degrees of view.

Bone removal superiorly is limited by the hypoglossal canal, which may be partially unroofed. Areas limiting the transcondylar approach are the nasopharynx anteriorly, the spinomedullary junction posteriorly, and the jugular bulb and hypoglossal nerve superiorly. The inferior limit can be tailored to each situation: Extending the skin incision allows inferior resection to be as low as necessary.

Exposure of some lesions may be facilitated by transposition of the vertebral artery, which is accomplished by resecting the transverse processes of C1 and C2, and reflecting the vertebral artery inferiorly. At this point, the C1 nerve root may be sacrificed.

For purely intradural lesions, less than one third of the condyle typically needs to be drilled away for access. However, extradural tumors, such as chordomas and chondrosarcomas, invading the condyle may necessitate removal of the entire condyle.

The dura is opened medial to the sigmoid sinus and the jugular bulb and caudally, behind the vertebral artery entrance. The dura is incised circumferentially around the vertebral artery entrance so that the artery is completely freed to be moved anteriorly and posteriorly, facilitating its dissection from the tumor or exposure of the aneurysm.

For intradural tumors, standard microsurgical techniques are used to debulk the tumor progressively and then dissect it off the brainstem, cranial nerves, and blood vessels. Sometimes extradural tumors may invade the dura and extend inside. Removal of the extradural tumor requires drilling of the temporal bone.

Before entering the jugular bulb, the sigmoid sinus and the internal jugular vein should be ligated. All the infiltrated bone is drilled away as far as possible and the involved dura is also excised. The mastoid air cells are heavily waxed. The aditus to the middle ear, if opened, should be well sealed. The dura is closed as securely as possible. A piece of autologous fat is placed over the dural defect and the muscles are closed in layers.

Complete removal of the condyle, which sometimes includes the articular mass of C1, usually warrants an occipitocervical fusion. Several methods of occipitocervical stabilization are available and can be performed at the same sitting as the tumor removal, or at a later stage.

Thus, there are several advantages to using the lateral and far-lateral approach: (1) simultaneous lateral and posterolateral avenues of exposure are obtained on the lesion at the lower clivus, C1, and C2, allowing radical tumor resection; (2) the approach does not traverse contaminated areas such as the pharynx or the paranasal sinuses; (3) it permits excellent control and mobilization of the vertebral artery to allow its safe dissection from the tumor of elimination of the aneurysm; and (4) this operation can be combined with other approaches to enhance the completeness of tumor resection and is equally useful for intradural and extradural tumors.

DISCUSSION

The posterior approach to the spine seems to be the most natural one because the spinous processes of the neck vertebrae are easily palpable. Because of this seemingly easy accessibility, it is not surprising that posterior approaches were developed earlier than anterior approaches. The lateral and far-lateral approach to the upper cervical spine is especially suited for intradural lesions ventral and ventrolateral to the spinal cord between C1 and C2. It allows access to the ventral aspect of the spinal cord with little or no retraction. The exposure is straightforward and provides a wide, shallow field, allowing a good dural closure. The vertebral artery is identified early in the exposure and can be mobilized readily. The risk of cerebrospinal fluid leak or meningitis is low. The bony resection required for the exposure does not in itself cause spinal instability.

The lateral transcondylar approach includes removal of more of the occipital condyle and the adjacent portion of the superior facet of the atlas, with additional optimum exposure of the hypoglossal canal, and removal of the jugular tubercle in the supracondylar area, with exposure of the jugular foramen and mastoid portion of the facial nerve in the paracondylar area. This procedure can be used for lesions between the ventral or ventrolateral foramen magnum and C2, including lesions of the transverse segment of the extravertebral artery that extend from below the foramen magnum to the inferior third of the clivus.

The lateral approach is not as well suited to bony or extradural lesions. Access to the contralateral lateral mass is limited and fusion is more readily accomplished by standard posterior techniques. If C1-C2 wiring fails, or when the posterior arch of C1 or lamina of C2 is not available for fusion, bilateral transarticular screw fixation of C1 to C2 can be achieved from a posterior approach—as well as C1 lateral mass C2 pedicle screw rod fixation.

The major advantages of lateral and far-lateral approaches include the following: (1) there is no spinal instability if the joints are not disturbed, (2) the surgeon's line of vision is truly lateral, (3) little or no spinal cord retraction is necessary, and (4) the surgical exposure is wide enough and superficial enough not to be confining. The lateral approach throughout the cervical spine is excellent for dealing with vertebral artery problems.

REFERENCES

1. Menezes AH, Sonntag VKH: Principles of Spinal Surgery, Vols. 1 and 2. New York, McGraw-Hill, 1996, pp 123–139, 395–409, 539–546, 705–722, 841–854, 855–869, 871–883, 1051–1065, 1067–1079, 1081–1104, 1325–1332, 1335–1353.
2. An HS: Principles and Techniques of Spine Surgery. Baltimore, Williams & Wilkins, 1998, pp 658–674.
3. Schmidek HH: Operative Neurosurgical Techniques, Vol. 2, 4th ed. Philadelphia, WB Saunders, 2000, pp 146–149, 1923–1969.
4. Singh SK, Rickards l, Apfelbaum RI, et al: Occipitocervical reconstruction with the Ohio Medical Instruments Loop: Results of a multicenter evaluation in 30 cases. J Neurosurg (Spine 2) 2003;98:241–248.
5. Watkins RG: Approach to the Posterior Aspect of C1-C2. Surgical Approaches to the Spine, 2nd ed. New York, Springer, 2003, pp 217–223.
6. Fourney DR, York JE, Cohen ZR, et al: Management of atlanroaxial metastases with posterior occipitocervical stebilization. J Neurosurg (Spine 2) 2003;98:165–170.
7. Pait TG, Al-Mefty O, Boop FA, et al: Inside-outside technique for posterior occipitocervical spine instrumentation and stabilization: Preliminary results. J Neurosurg (Spine 2) 1999;90:1–7.
8. Amautovic KI, Al-Merfy O, Pait TG, et al: The suboccipital cavernous sinus. J Neurosurg 1997;86:252–262.
9. De Oliveira E, Rhoton AL, Peace D: Microsurgical anatomy of the region of the foramen magnum. Surg Neurol 1985;24:293–352.

10. Platzer W: Intrinsic Muscles of the Back, Locomotor System. Color Atlas and Textbook of Human Anatomy, Vol. 1. New York, Thieme Medical Publishers, 2004, pp 74–81, 346–349.
11. Long DM, McAfee PC: Atlas of Spinal Surgery. Baltimore, Williams & Wilkins, 1992, pp 158–176, 217–227, 359–368.
12. Bauer R, Kerschbaumer F, Poisel S: Atlas of Spinal Operations. New York, Thieme Medical Publishers, 1993, pp 56–59, 263–268, 347–372.
13. Netter FH: The Ciba Collection of Medical Illustrations. Ardlsey, NY, CIBA-Geigy Corp, 1986, Section I, Plate 9–13, 11–15.
14. Pait TG, Borba LA: Stabilization of the cervical spine (C3-7) with articular mass (lateral mass) plate and screws. In Rengachary SS, Wilkins RH (eds): Neurosurgical Operative Atlas, Vol. 5. Baltimore, Williams & Wilkins, 1996, pp 91–100.
15. Permeczky A: The posterolateral approach to the foramen magnum. In Samii M (ed): Surgery In and Around the Brain Stem and the Third Ventricle. Berlin, Springer-Verlag, 1986, pp 460–466.
16. Nanda A, Vincent DA, Prasad S, et al: Far-lateral approach to intradural lesions of the foramen magnum without resection of the occipital condyle. J Neurosurg 2002;96:302–309.
17. Bartolomei JC, Crockard AH: Bilateral posterolateral approach to mirror-image C-2 neurofibromas. J Neurosurg (Spine 2) 2001;94:292–298.
18. Whitesides TE: Lateral retropharyngeal approach to the upper cervical spine. In Sherk HH, Dunn EJ, Eismont FJ, et al (eds): The Cervical Spine, Vol 2. Philadelphia, Lippincott, 1989, pp 796–804.
19. Babu RP, Sekhar LN, Wright DC: Extreme lateral transcondylar approach: Technical improvements and lesions learned. J Neurosurg 1994;81:49–51.
20. Hosoda K, Fujita S, Kawaguchi T, et al: A transcondylar approach to the arteriovenous malformation at the ventral cervicomedullary junction: Report of three cases. Neurosurgery 1994;34:748–753.
21. Lang DA, Neil-Dwyer G, Iannotti F: The suboccipital transcondylar approach to the clivus and cranio-cervical junction for ventrally placed pathology at and above the foramen magnum. Acta Neurochir 1993;125:132–137.
22. Wen HT, Rhoton AL, Katsuta T, Oliveira ED: Microsurgical anatomy of the transcondylar, supracondylar, and paracondylar extensions of the far-lateral approach. J Neurosurg 1997;87:555–585.
23. Sen C, Catalano PJ: Extreme lateral transcondylar approach to the craniocervical junction. In Donald PJ (ed): Surgery of the Skull Base. Philadelphia, Lippincott-Raven, 1998, pp 491–505.
24. Al-Mefty O, Borba LA, Aoki N, et al: The trancondylar approach to extradural nonneoplastic lesions of the craniovertebral junction. J Neurosurg 1996;84:1–6.
25. Ture U, Pamir MN: Extreme lateral-transatlas approach for resection of the dens of the axis. J Neurosurg (Spine 1) 2002;96:73–82.
26. Sen C, Sekhar LN: An extreme lateral transcondylar approach to the foramen magnum and cervical spine. In Rengachary SS, Wilkins RH (eds): Neurosurgical Operative Atlas, Vol. 2. Baltimore, Williams & Wilkins, 1992, pp 163–171.

SECTION B
Mid and Lower Cervical Spine

CHAPTER 5

UNGKYU CHANG

MAX C. LEE

DANIEL H. KIM

Anterior Approach to the Midcervical Spine

ANATOMY

OSSEOUS STRUCTURE

A cervical vertebra is composed of a body, pedicle, transverse process, superior articular process, inferior articular process, lamina, and spinous process (Fig. 5-1). The lamina blends into the lateral mass, which is bone between the superior articular process and the inferior articular process. The articular processes come together to form a facet joint (Fig. 5-2A). The interfacet distances are relatively constant at different levels, with an average of 13 mm. The cervical facet joint itself is typically angled 45 degrees cephalad from the transverse plane. Important anatomic landmarks for posterior plate-screw/screw-rod instrumentation include the facet joint lines, medial and lateral margins of the lateral mass, and joint inclination. The lateral mass of C7 is more elongated in a superoinferior direction and thinner in an anteroposterior direction. Bony anatomy of the lower cervical spine from C3 to C6 is similar. They have bifid spinous processes and project posteriorly and inferiorly. But the spinous process of C7 is not bifid and large.[1]

The body is relatively small and oval in shape, with the mediolateral direction more than an anteroposterior direction. In the coronal plane, the superior surface of the vertebral body is concave, and the inferior surface of the body is convex, the anteroinferior edge of the vertebral body is lipped inferiorly and the lateral surfaces of the superior vertebral body projects upward (uncinate process), conforming to small grooves in the inferolateral borders of the cephalad vertebra, forming the uncovertebral joint or joints of Luschka (see Fig. 5-2B). The location of the uncinate process in a motion segment predisposes to uncovertebral joint hypertrophy, which, in turn, produces intervertebral foraminal stenosis and neural compression. The uncinate process is located posterolaterally on C6 and C7 levels and laterally on C3-C5 levels, and the distance between the uncinate processes increases gradually from C3-C7.

The vertebral artery and venous system pass through the transverse foramen, which is located medial to the tubercles of the transverse process and lateral to the vertebral body. The pedicles of the cervical spine measure a height of 7 mm and a width of 5 to 6 mm. The pedicle angle in the sagittal plane decreases from 45 degrees to 30 degrees for C3 down to C7.

The intervertebral foramina are bounded anteriorly by the vertebral bodies and disks, posteriorly by the facets, and cephalad and caudad by the pedicles (see Fig. 5-2C). The cervical foramina are aligned in a 45-degree oblique direction in the sagittal plane.

INTERVERTEBRAL DISKS AND LIGAMENTS

Intervertebral disks are present between vertebral bodies and comprise an inner nucleus pulposus, an outer annulus fibrosus, and the cartilaginous end plates adjacent to the vertebral surfaces. The disks are shaped to conform to the surface of the vertebral bodies, so the superior surface of the disk is concave and the inferior surface of the disk is convex in the coronal plane. The outmost fibers of the annulus fibrosus are contiguous with the anterior and posterior longitudinal ligaments. The anterior longitudinal ligament is a strong band that attaches from the skull as the anterior occipital membrane and continues caudally over the entire length of the spine down to the sacrum. The posterior longitudinal ligament is wider in the upper cervical spine than in the lower cervical spine and wider over the intervertebral disks than over the vertebral bodies. It is double-layered, with the deep layer sending fibers into the annulus fibrosis and continuing laterally to the region of the intervertebral foramina (Fig. 5-3A and B).[2,3]

SECTION I SURGICAL ANATOMY AND APPROACHES

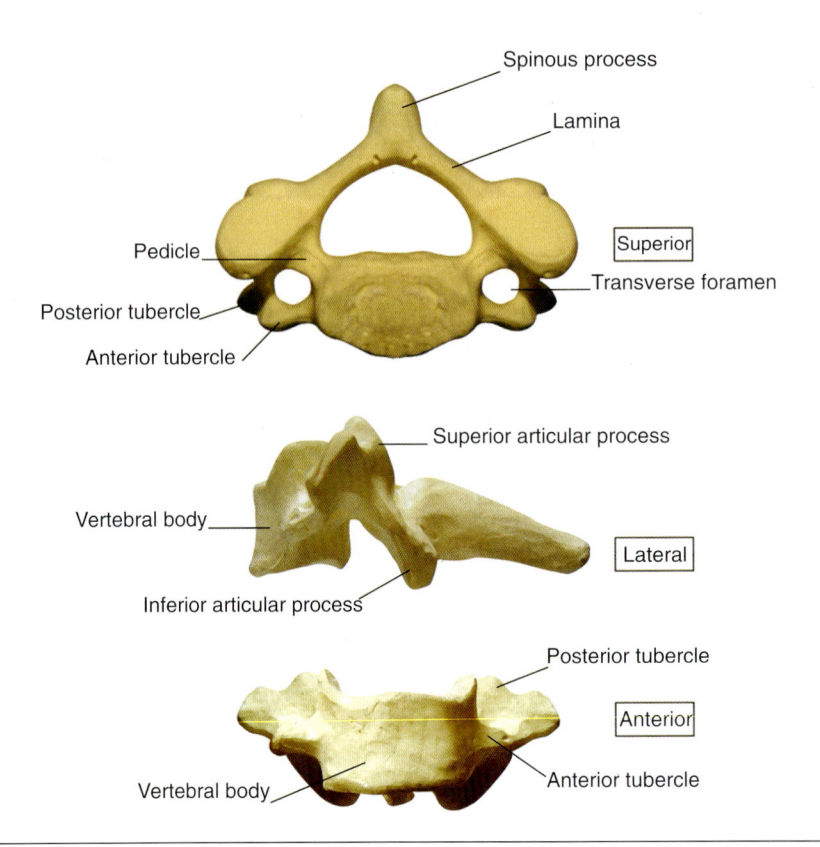

Fig. 5-1 Superior, lateral, and anterior views of a middle cervical vertebra.

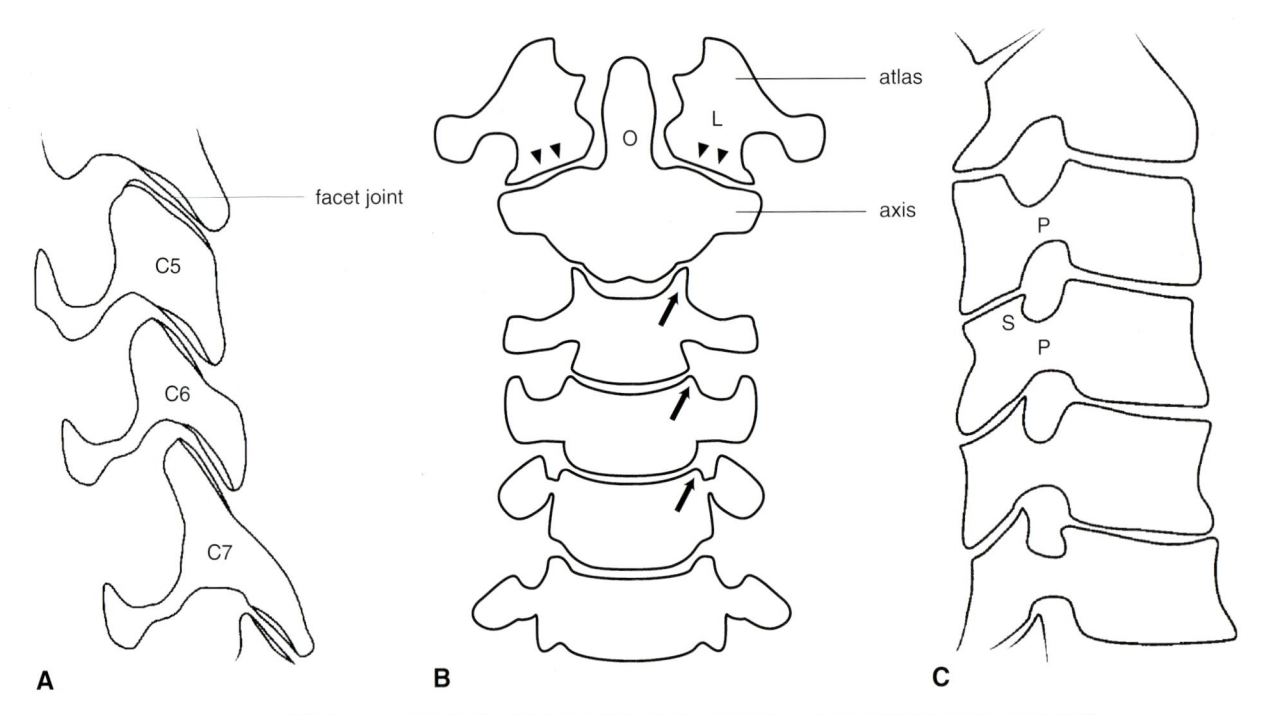

Fig. 5-2 *A*, A parasagittal microtome section of the facet joint. The angle of facet joint to transverse plane is about 45 degrees at the midcervical level and shows an increase in the lower cervical region. *B*, Coronal section of the occiput-C7 region. Lateral projections of the uncinate process of the lower cervical spine are well shown. The inferior articular facets *(arrowheads)* are facing downward laterally to articulate with the axis. Arrows, uncovertebral joints; L, lateral mass of Atlas; O, odontoid. *C*, Oblique section of cervical spine. Intervertebral foramina are shown. They are bounded anteriorly by the vertebral bodies and intervertebral disks, posteriorly by the facets and superior articular process. P, pedicle; S, superior articulating facet.

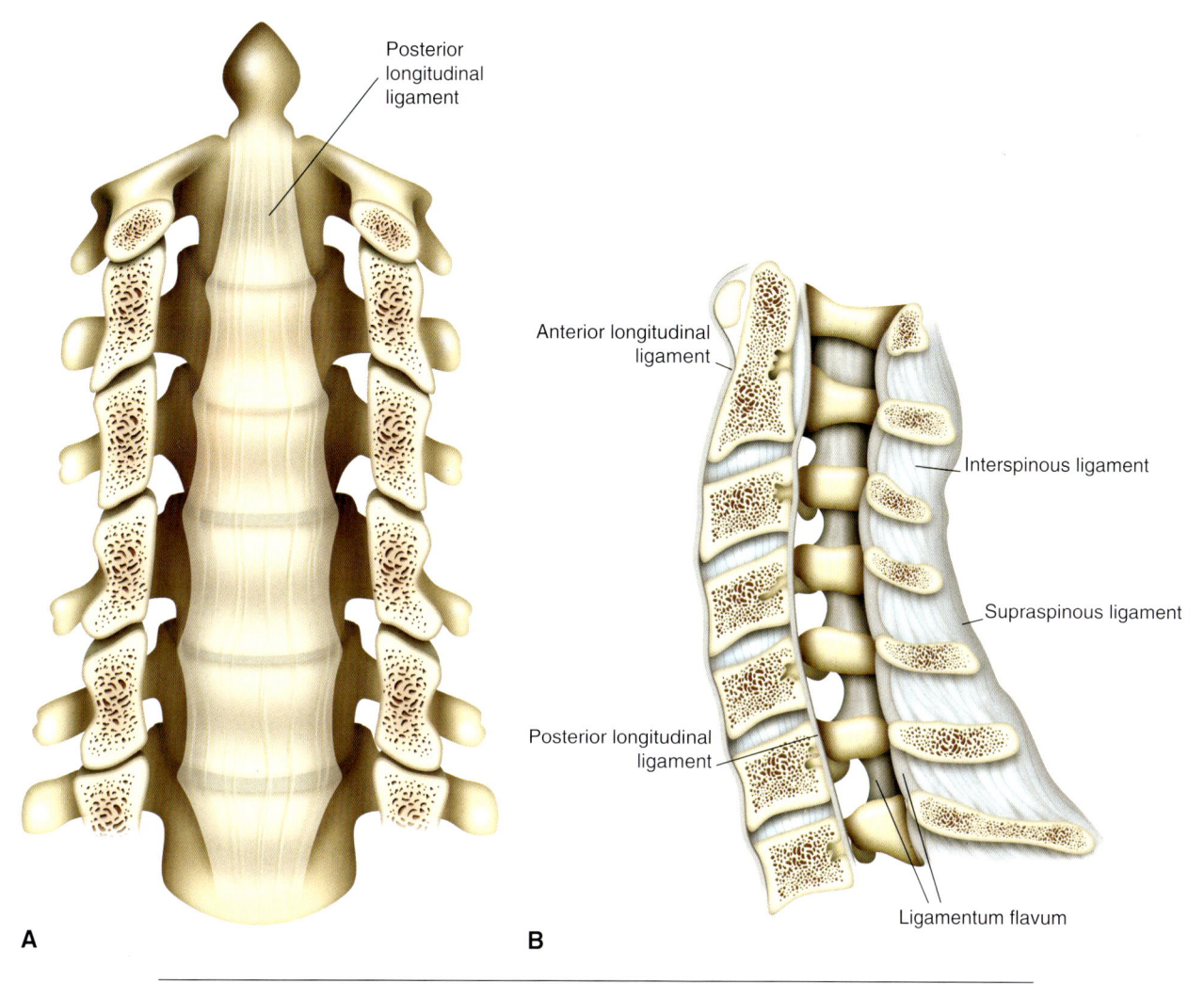

Fig. 5-3 *A* and *B*, Ligamentous structures around the spinal canal. The anterior longitudinal ligament attaches to the ventral surface of the vertebral bodies. The posterior longitudinal ligament attaches to the dorsal surface of the vertebral bodies. It is wider at the upper cervical level than at the lower cervical level and wider at the disk level than at the vertebral body level.

MUSCLE AND FASCIA

The anterolateral muscles of the neck include the platysma, sternocleidomastoid, suprahyoid muscles, strap muscles of the larynx, scalenes, longus colli, and longus capitis (Fig. 5-4). The platysma is a thin muscle just beneath the subcutaneous tissues; it spans the deltoid to the upper pectoral fascia, crosses over the clavicle, and passes obliquely upward and medially to insert onto the mandible. The sternocleidomastoid muscle (SCM) originates from the sternum and the medial clavicle and attaches to the mastoid process and the lateral half of the superior nuchal line of the occipital bone. Suprahyoid muscles that attach to the hyoid bone include the digastric, stylohyoid, mylohyoid, and geniohyoid muscles. The strap muscles of the larynx include the sternohyoid, sternothyroid, thyrohyoid, and omohyoid muscles. They cover the larynx, the thyroid gland, and the trachea. Anterior vertebral muscles are the longus colli muscle, the longus capitis muscle, the rectus capitis anterior muscle, and the rectus capitis lateralis muscle (Fig. 5-5).[4,5]

The longus colli is a wide muscle with tapered ends that spans from C1 to T3 and extends laterally to attach to the anterior tubercles of the transverse processes of C3, C4, C5, and C6. The longus capitis originates on the anterior tubercles of the transverse processes of C3, C4, C5, and C6 and attaches to the inferior surface of the basilar part of the occipital bone.

Lateral vertebral muscles include the scalenes and levator scapulae muscle. The scalenus anterior originates from the anterior tubercles of the transverse processes of C3 to C6 and inserts on the first rib. The scalenus medius originates from the posterior tubercles of the transverse processes of C2 to

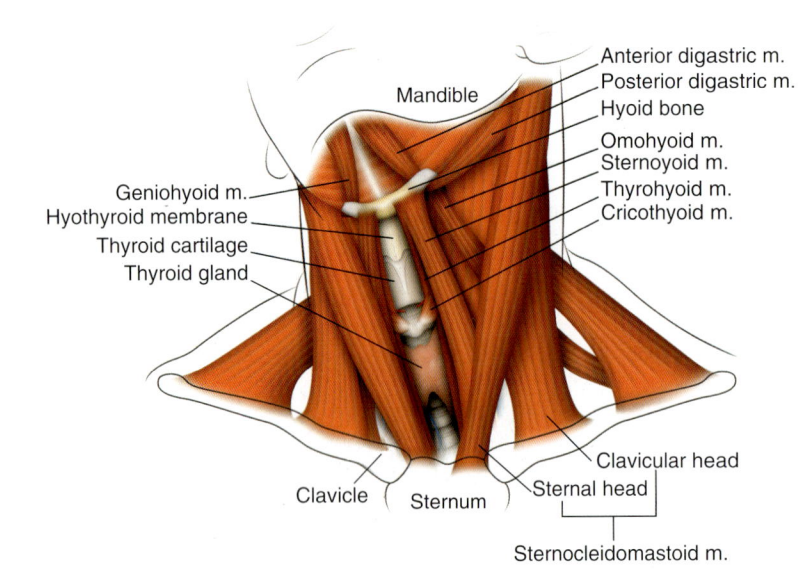

Fig. 5-4 Superficial muscles of anterior neck. Anterior neck muscles are the sternocleidomastoid muscle, suprahyoid muscles, and strap muscles. Hyoid bone represents the natural division between the muscles of the digastric triangle and the infrahyoid or strap muscles.

C7 and inserts on the first rib. The subclavian artery and inferior portion of the brachial plexus are located where the anterior and middle scalene muscles fuse at the insertion site. The scalenus posterior originates from the posterior tubercles of the transverse processes of C4 to C6 and inserts on the second rib.

The levator scapula muscle is another component of lateral neck muscles and originates from the lateral mass of the atlas and the transverse processes of the subsequent three cervical vertebrae and inserts at the cranial corner of the medial margin of the scapula.

The fascial layers of the anterior neck invest the muscles and viscera of this region to form separate compartments, and generally facilitate surgical exposure. The fascia of the neck are composed of two large layers: superficial and deep. The superficial cervical fascia is a continuous sheet of fatty subcutaneous tissue extending from the head and neck into the thorax and the shoulder. It invests the platysma muscle, the external jugular vein, and the cutaneous sensory nerve and comprises two layers—supraplatysmal and infraplatysmal (Fig. 5-6).

Deep cervical fascia includes superficial deep layer, middle deep layer, and deepest layer. The superficial layer of deep cervical fascia is a continuous layer of fibrous tissue arising from the vertebral spinous process and the nuchal ligament and completely encircling the neck (Fig. 5-7). It envelops

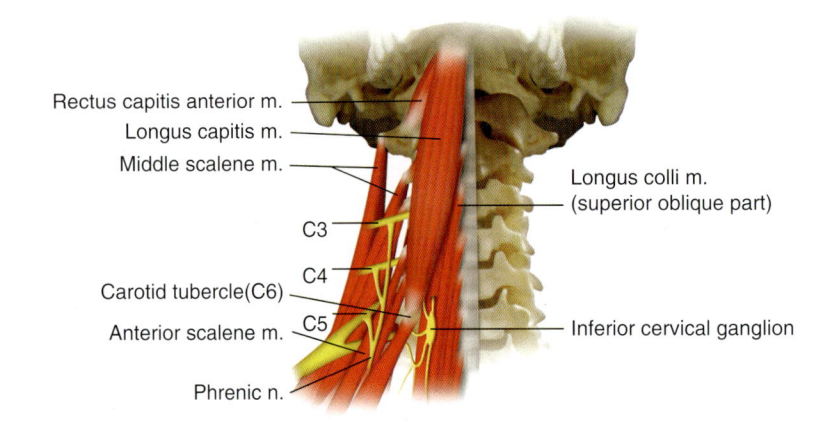

Fig. 5-5 Deep muscles of the anterior neck are the longus capitis and longus colli muscles, scalene muscles, rectus capitis anterior and lateralis muscles, and levator scapulae muscle.

CHAPTER 5 Anterior Approach to the Midcervical Spine

the scapula. A deeper position of the middle layer is the visceral fascia, which surrounds the thyroid gland, larynx, trachea, pharynx, and esophagus. The deepest layer of the deep cervical fascia is the prevertebral fascia, which covers the scalenus muscles, the longus colli muscles, and the anterior longitudinal ligament. It arises from the cervical spine and nuchal ligament, extends laterally over the muscles of the back of the neck, and crosses the midline to insert on these same structures.

NEUROVASCULAR STRUCTURES

Neurovascular structures of the cervical spine include the spinal cord, nerve roots, carotid artery, vertebral artery, laryngeal nerves, sympathetic chain, and epidural vessels. Cervical nerve roots forming from the ventral and dorsal nerve rootlet complex then extend anterolaterally at a 45-degree angle to the coronal plane and inferiorly at 10 degrees to the axial plane. The nerve roots enter the intervertebral foramen by passing directly in a lateral direction from the spinal canal adjacent to the corresponding disk and over the top of the corresponding pedicle. Each cervical spinal nerve root exits over the pedicle bearing the same number, except for the C8 nerve, which lies between the C7 and T1 pedicles. The spinal nerve divides into dorsal primary rami and ventral primary rami branches (Fig. 5-8). The gray rami connect the sympathetic cervical ganglion to the ventral primary rami. The anterior primary rami of C1 to C4 form the cervical plexus and of C5 to T1 form the brachial plexus. The sinuvertebral nerve, which innervates the posterior part of the annulus and the ventral portion of the dura, is connected to the dorsal root ganglion.[3,4]

The vertebral artery is located lateral to the uncinate process and in line with the middle one third of the

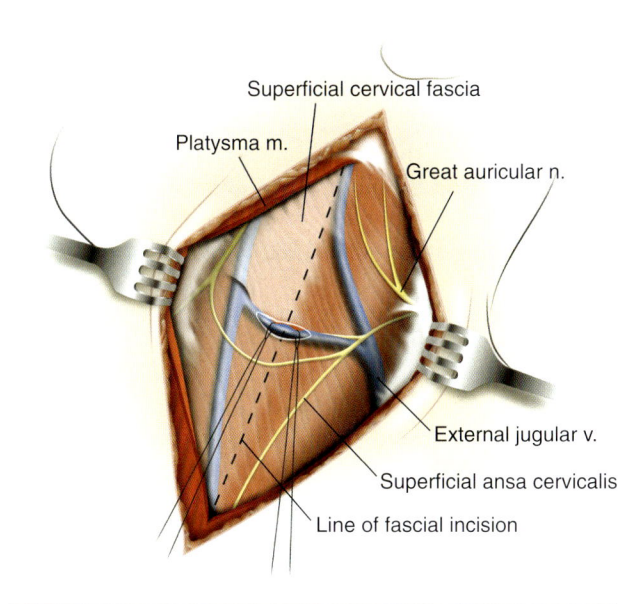

Fig. 5-6 The superficial cervical fascia is continuous sheet of fatty subcutaneous tissue extending from the head and neck into the thorax and the shoulder. It invests the platysma muscle, the external jugular vein, and the cutaneous sensory nerve and comprises two layers—supraplatysmal and infraplatysmal.

the trapezius muscle over the posterior triangle, and then splits to enclose the SCM muscle. In the mandibular triangle, it encloses the submaxillary and parotid glands.

The middle layer of the deep cervical fascia encloses the strap muscles and omohyoid, and extends as far laterally as

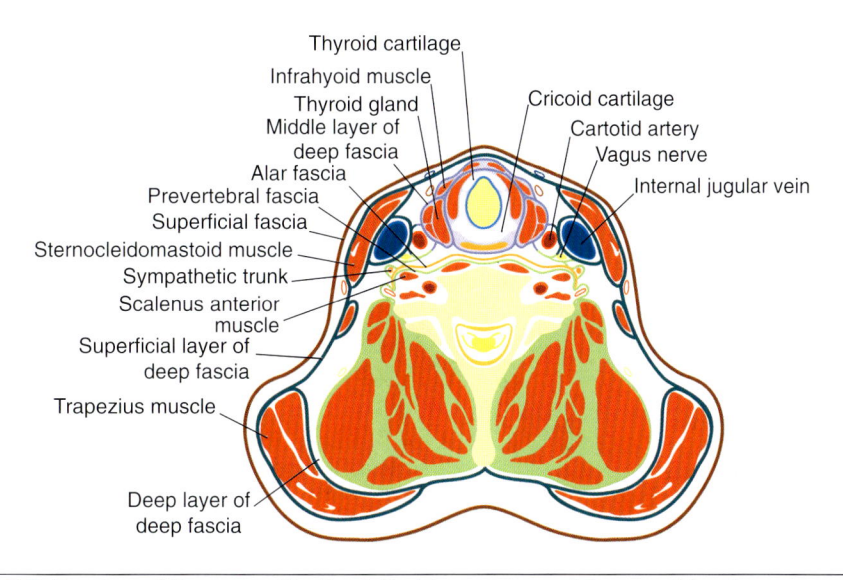

Fig. 5-7 Fasciae of the neck. On the left side are several layers of fascia.

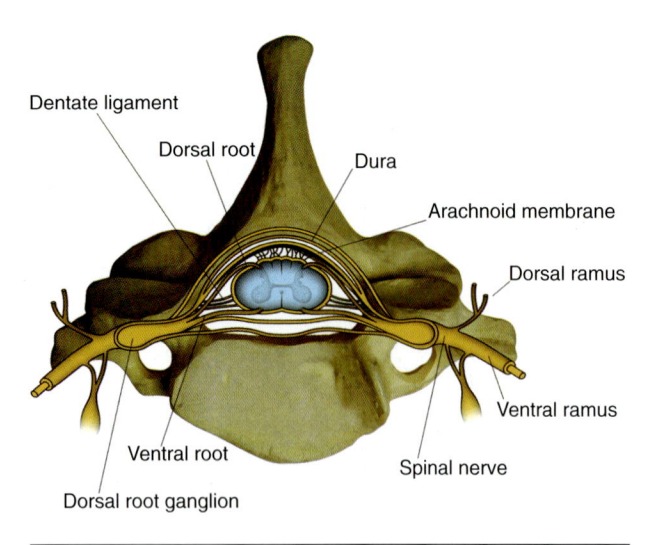

Fig. 5-8 Cross-sectional diagram showing spinal cord, dorsal root ganglion, and spinal nerve. The spinal nerve divides into dorsal primary rami and ventral primary rami branches.

vertebral body just anterior to the nerve root. It originates from the subclavian artery and enters the transverse foramen at C6 in most cases. The carotid sheath is an investment of the internal and common carotid arteries, the internal jugular vein, and the vagus nerve (Fig. 5-9). The ansa cervicalis is on the surface of the carotid sheath and the cervical sympathetic trunk in the dorsomedial aspect (Fig. 5-10). During the left side approach, the thoracic duct may be encountered. The thoracic duct runs ventral to subclavian artery, behind the carotid sheath, and terminates at the junction of the left internal jugular vein and subclavian vein (Fig. 5-11). The phrenic nerve lies on the ventral surface of the anterior scalene muscle (Fig. 5-12).

The superior laryngeal nerve (SLN) is a branch of the inferior ganglion of the vagus nerve, and travels along with the superior thyroid artery. As it descends medially toward the thyrohyoid membrane, the SLN lies in the fascia covering the longus colli muscle. The SLN divides into two branches, external branch and internal branch, immediately deep to the origin of the superior thyroidal artery from the external carotid artery (ECA) (Fig. 5-13).

The inferior laryngeal nerve is a recurrent branch of the vagus nerve. On the right side, the recurrent laryngeal nerve loops around the subclavian artery, passing dorsomedial to the side of the trachea and esophagus. It is vulnerable as it passes from the subclavian artery to the right tracheoesophageal groove because it is not protected by the tracheoesophageal groove for much of its course. The best guideline to its location is the inferior thyroidal artery. On the left side, the recurrent laryngeal nerve (RLN) travels under the arch of the aorta. The left RLN is much less vulnerable than the right RLN because it is protected by the tracheoesophageal groove and its course is lengthy and redundant.

The cervical sympathetic system consists of three ganglia with intervening cords. The sympathetic trunk is located ventral to the transverse process and is embedded in the dorsal aspect of the carotid sheath. The superior cervical ganglion is located on the level of C2-C3, the middle cervical

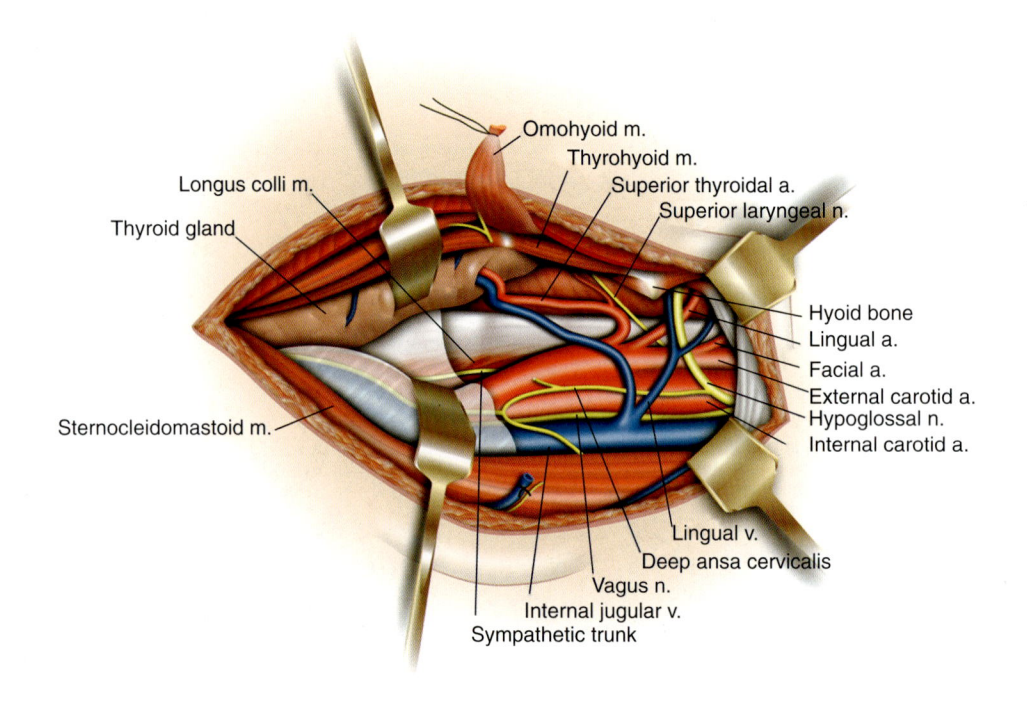

Fig. 5-9 Neurovascular structures after removing fascia, as seen from the left.

CHAPTER 5 Anterior Approach to the Midcervical Spine

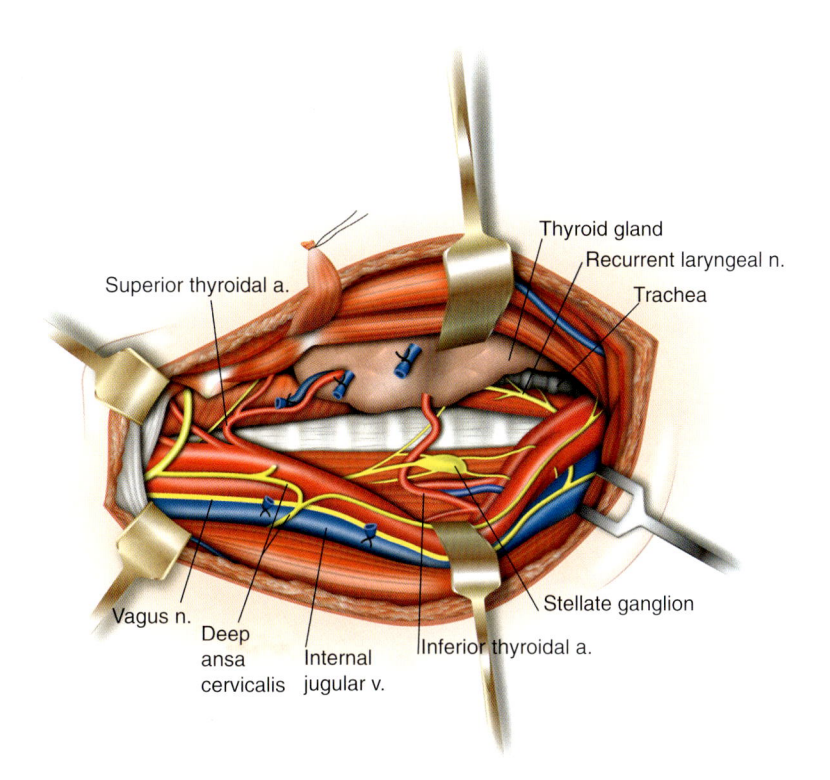

Fig. 5-10 Neurovascular structures seen from the right side. The recurrent laryngeal nerve is shown to run below the subclavian artery and then pass obliquely over the anterior side of the vertebra toward the groove between the trachea and esophagus.

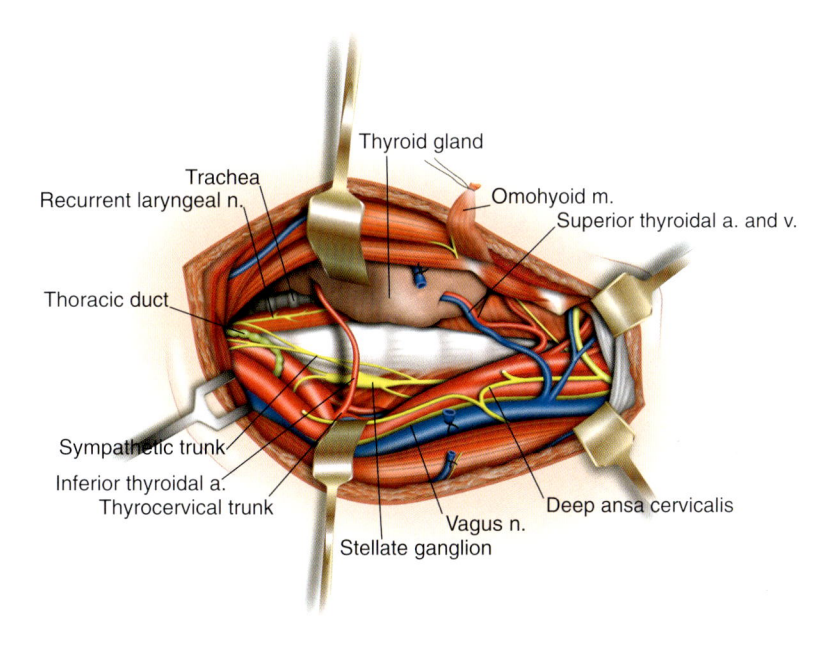

Fig. 5-11 Neurovascular structures seen from the left side. The thoracic duct runs ventral to the subclavian artery, behind the carotid sheath, and terminates at the junction of the left internal jugular vein and subclavian vein. The recurrent laryngeal nerve courses behind the aortic arch and ascends further toward the larynx between the trachea and esophagus.

52 SECTION I SURGICAL ANATOMY AND APPROACHES

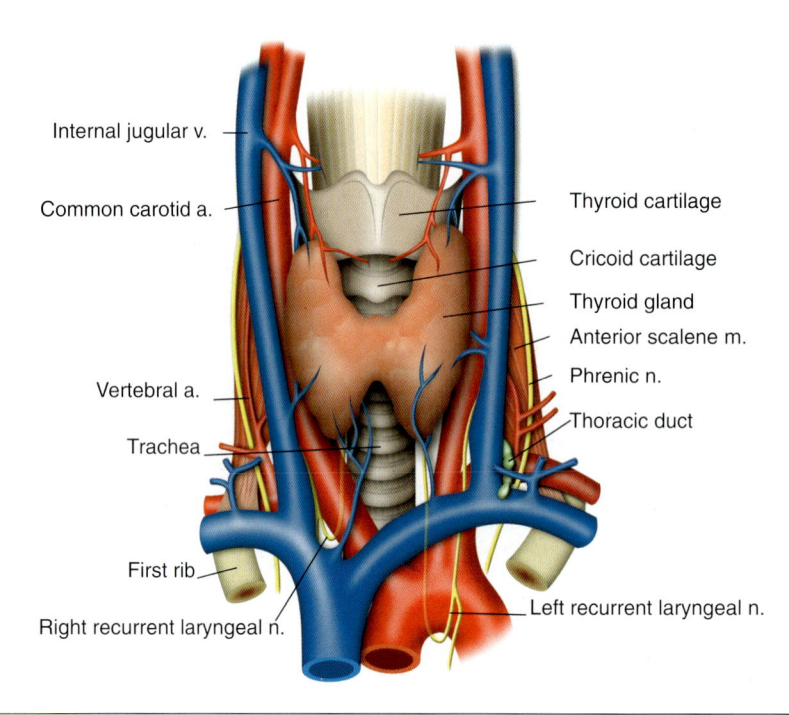

Fig. 5-12 The location of the phrenic nerve and recurrent laryngeal nerve.

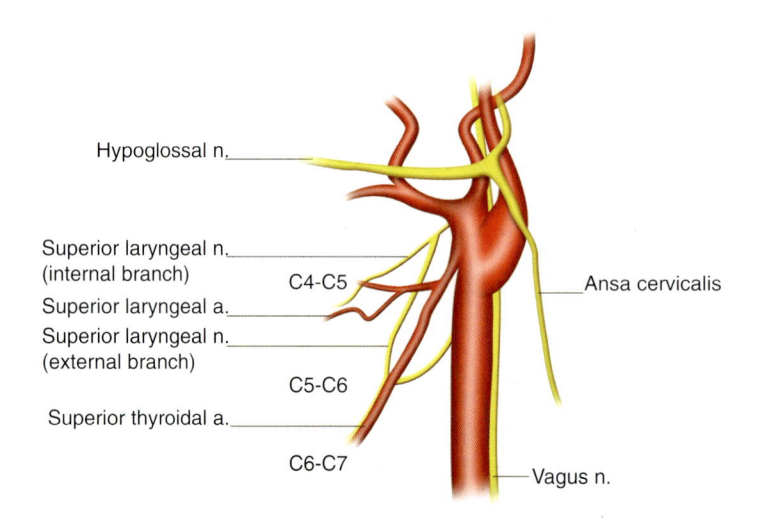

Fig. 5-13 Lateral view of the left anterior neck. The superior laryngeal nerve is divided into two branches, external and internal. Branches of the external carotid artery are observed in relation to the nerves and other structures of the anterior neck.

ganglion is at C6-C7, and the inferior ganglion lies between the transverse process of C7 and the neck of the first rib.

SURGICAL APPROACH

MEDIAL (VENTRAL APPROACH)

The ventral approach to the cervical spine is performed through a plane between the sternocleidomastoid muscle and the carotid sheath laterally and the strap muscles and tracheoesophageal viscera medially. This approach is suitable for a ventral cervical diskectomy, vertebrectomy, fusion, and instrumentation.[6–8]

The patient is placed in a supine position with a pad under the shoulder to induce slight extension. The choice of incision depends on the level to be operated (Fig. 5-14).

For the exposure of one or two segments, the transverse incision is enough. But longitudinal incision is preferred for

CHAPTER 5 Anterior Approach to the Midcervical Spine

the exposure of several segments. The transverse incision levels are determined according to the external landmarks. For the C3 operation, the incision is done overlying hyoid bone. The thyroid cartilage is the landmark for the C5 body. And the cricoid cartilage is selected for the operation of C6 vertebral bodies. The supraclavicular level is matched for C7-T1 segments (see Fig. 5-14).

After the appropriate incision for skin and subcutaneous tissue is made, platysma muscle is exposed. The platysma is divided in the same direction, and then the superficial cervical fascia is shown. This fascia is divided in a longitudinal direction along the anterior border of the sternocleidomastoid muscle. The sternocleidomastoid muscle is retracted laterally. The superior belly of omohyoid muscle is seen to run transversely across the operative field. It can be undermined and divided. Under the omohyoid muscle, the middle layer of the cervical fascia is shown and opened with blunt dissection. In the middle cervical fascia, the middle thyroid vein and transverse branch of the deep ansa cervicalis are found and can be sacrificed. After opening the middle cervical fascia, the cervical vertebrae can be palpated (Fig. 5-15). The carotid sheath is retracted laterally, whereas the visceral structures and sternohyoid and sternothyroid muscles are retracted contralaterally.

When the exposure of the cervical vertebrae above C4 is required, it is necessary to be aware of the superior thyroidal artery, the lingual artery, the facial artery, and the hypoglossal nerve (Fig. 5-16). The superior laryngeal nerve originates from the vagus nerve and runs beneath the lingual and facial arteries to pass into the larynx. The distal portions of both SLN branches are prone to injury, especially during the placement of self-retaining retractor blades. The branches of the

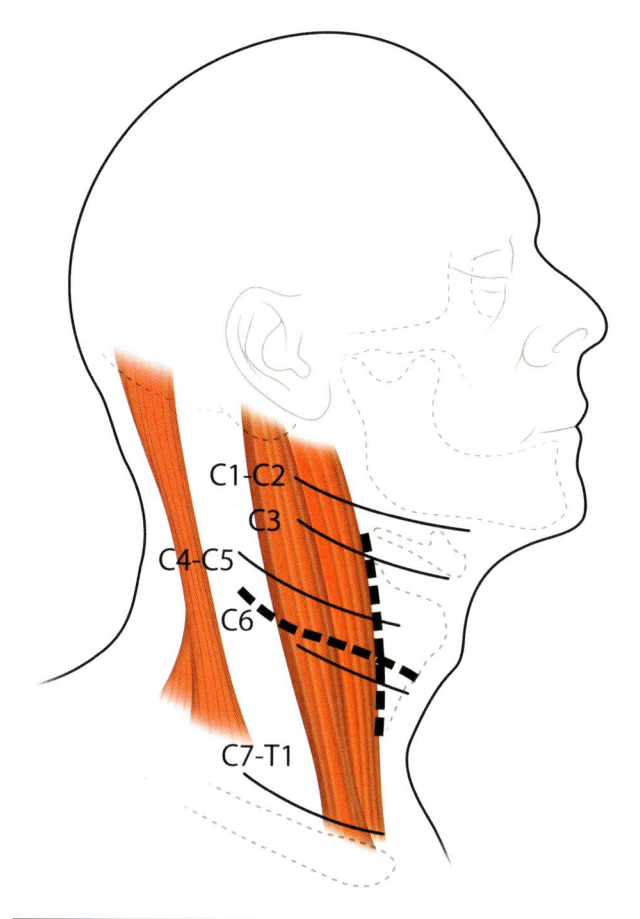

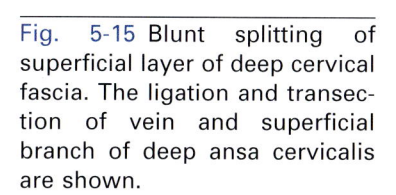

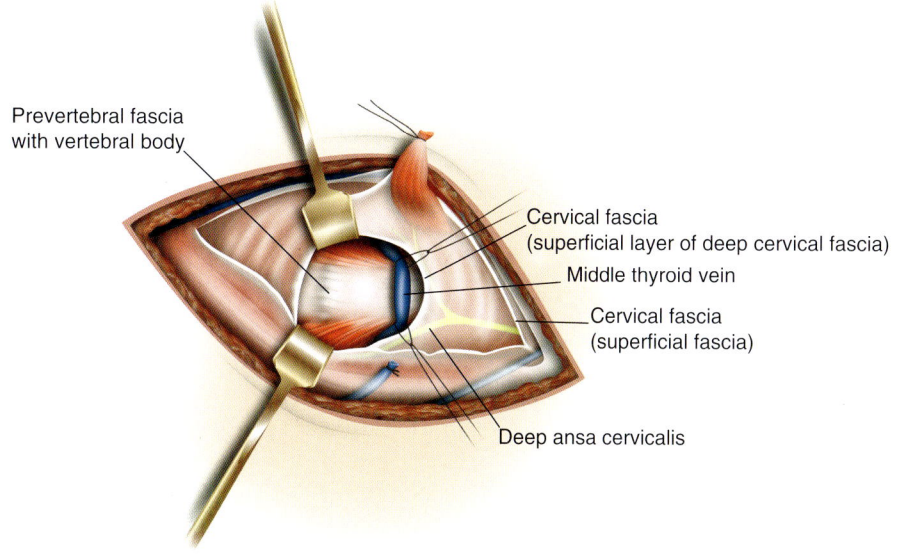

Fig. 5-14 The incision lines related to anatomic structures. The hyoid bone overlies at C3, the thyroid cartilage at C5, the cricoid ring at C6, and supraviclular level for C7-T1 region.

Fig. 5-15 Blunt splitting of superficial layer of deep cervical fascia. The ligation and transection of vein and superficial branch of deep ansa cervicalis are shown.

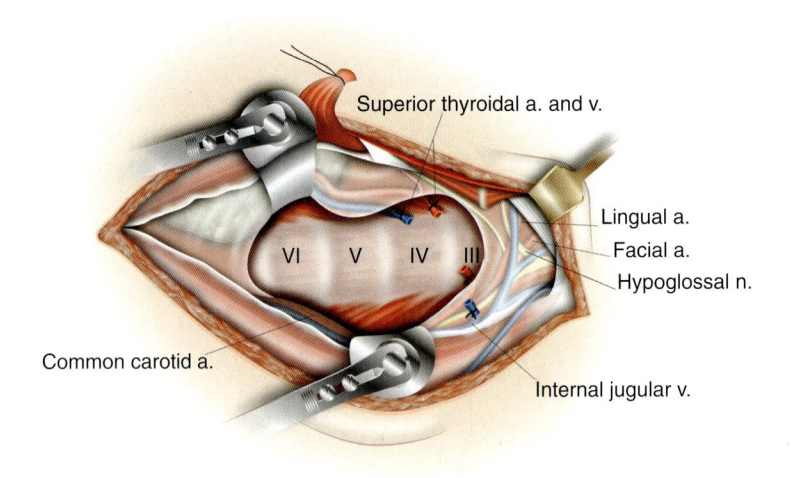

Fig. 5-16 After the superficial layer of the deep cervical fascia is opened, the deep layer of the deep cervical fascia is seen. The superior thyroidal artery and vein are ligated.

SLN cross the surgical field from the carotid bifurcation laterally toward the larynx and then lie discretely on the paratracheal fascia, covering the longus colli muscles.

The midportion of the recurrent laryngeal nerve and the superior laryngeal nerve are encountered in the anterior approach to the lower cervical spine. The recurrent laryngeal nerve is vulnerable to injury on the right side, especially if ligation of inferior thyroid vessels is performed without paying sufficient attention to the course and position of the nerve, and the external branch of the superior laryngeal nerve is vulnerable to injury during ligature and division of the superior thyroid artery.

The deep prevertebral cervical fascia has to be divided in the midline and dissected laterally to the medial margin of the longus colli muscle. With a freer, the longus colli muscles are elevated on the anterior longitudinal ligament (ALL) and retracted laterally as far as the base of the transverse process. During exposure of the transverse foramen or uncovertebral joint at the lower cervical levels, the sympathetic trunk may be injured. The sympathetic trunk is situated in close proximity to the medial border of the longus colli at the C6 level (the longus colli muscles diverge laterally, whereas the sympathetic trunk converges medially).

LATERAL APPROACH

Lateral approaches are described by Henry, Hodgson, and Verbiest (Fig. 5-17).[9-11]

Verbiest's approach is made through the same plane as is the ventral approach. However, further exposure is performed lateral to the longus colli muscle on the ipsilateral side (Fig. 5-18). Verbiest's lateral approach is a direct approach to the vertebral artery and the spinal nerves in the intervertebral foramen. After the same incision and dissection of the middle cervical fascia as in the anterior approach, a handheld Cloward retractor is used to retract the medial structures. The anterior tubercle of the transverse process is the key to this dissection. The muscular insertions on the anterior tubercle, including the longus colli, longus capitis, and anterior scalene, are dissected sharply to the bone. After the anterior tubercle is cleared up, it is removed with a narrow-tip rongeur, exposing the vertebral artery.

Hodgson's approach is posterior to the sternocleidomastoid muscle and carotid sheath. These structures are retracted medially, including the longus colli muscle (Fig. 5-19A and B). The posterior border of the sternocleidomastoid muscle is identified, and blunt dissection is done through the fat pad of the posterior triangle of the cervical spine. The dissection

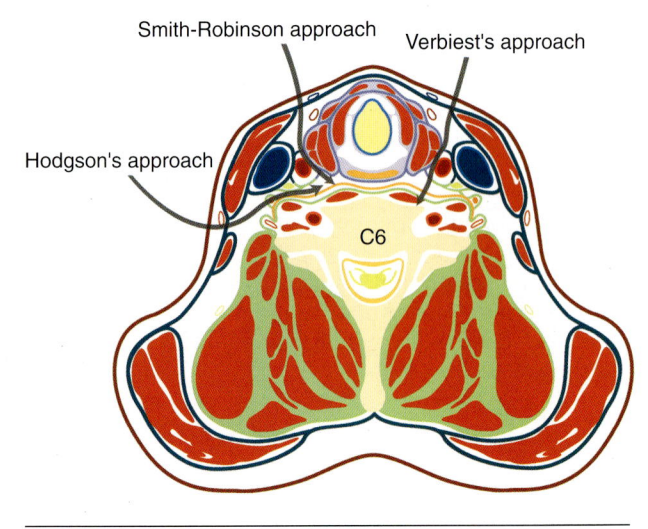

Fig. 5-17 Lateral approaches by Smith-Robinson, Hodgson, and Verbiest.

CHAPTER 5 Anterior Approach to the Midcervical Spine

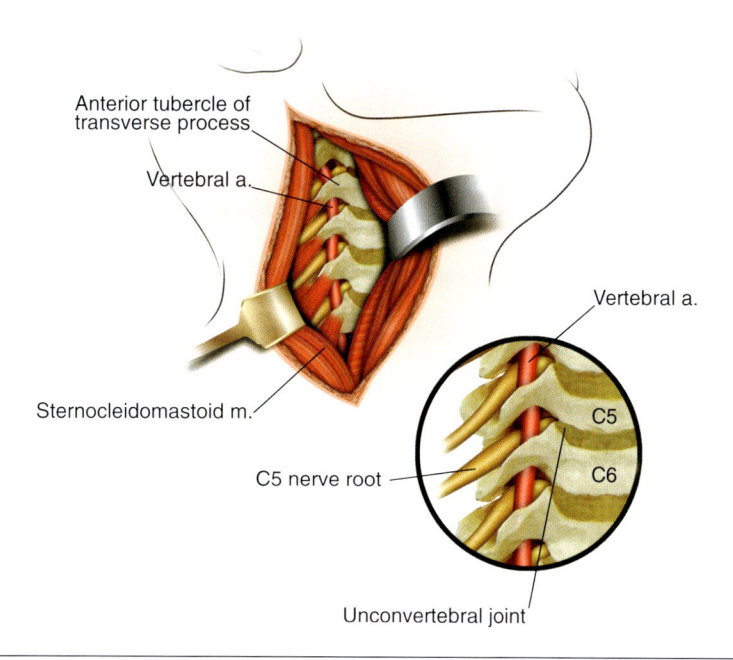

Fig. 5-18 Verbiest lateral approach. The sternocleidomastoid muscle and the carotid sheath are identified and retracted laterally. The visceral structures are retracted medially. The anterior tubercle of the transverse process, which is the key to this dissection, is identified by palpation.

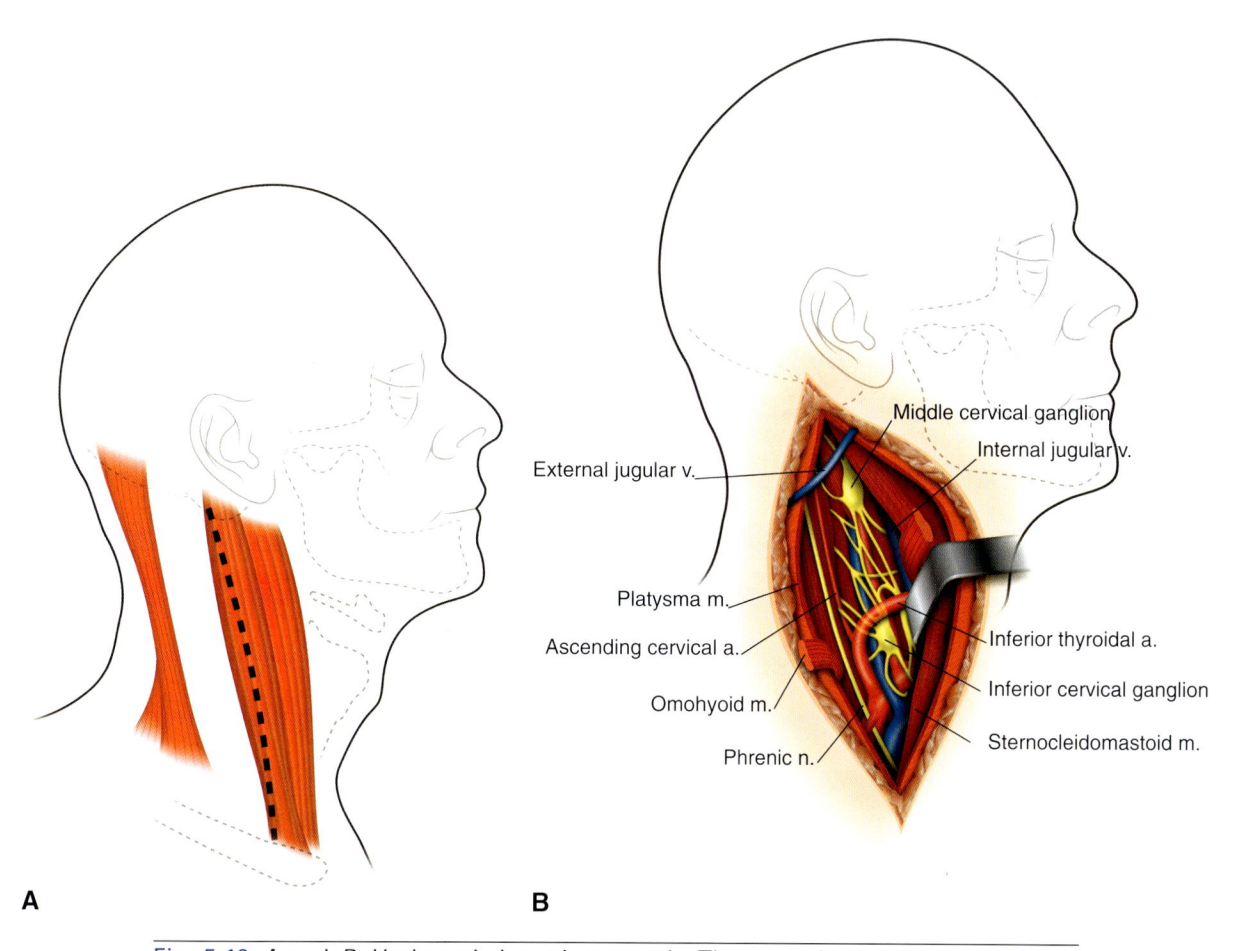

Fig. 5-19 *A* and *B*, Hodgson's lateral approach. The posterior border of the sternocleidomastoid muscle is identified, and the posterior triangle of the cervical spine is explored. The dissection should stay anterior to the anterior scalene muscle and anterior tubercle of the transverse process.

should stay anterior to the scalene muscle and the anterior tubercle of the transverse process to avoid injuries to the vertebral artery and nerve roots. The prevertebral fascia is incised in the midline, and subperiosteal dissection is achieved for the exposure of the cervical spine.

References

1. Yilmazlar S, Kocaeli H, Uz A, Tekdemir I: Clinical importance of ligamentous and osseous structures in the cervical uncovertebral foraminal region. Clin Anat 2003;16:404–410.
2. Hayashi K, Yabuki T, Kurokawa T, et al: The anterior and the posterior longitudinal ligaments of the lower cervical spine. J Anat 1977;124:633–636.
3. Lang J: Skeletal system of the cervical spine. In Lang J (ed): Clinical Anatomy of the Cervical Spine. New York, Thieme, 1993, pp 51–78.
4. An HS: Anatomy and the cervical spine. In An HS, Simpson JM (eds): Surgery of the Cervical Spine. Baltimore, Williams & Wilkins, 1994, pp 1–40.
5. Monfared A, Kim D, Jaikumar S, et al: Microsurgical anatomy of the superior and recurrent laryngeal nerves. Neurosurgery 2001;49(4):925–932.
6. Bauer R, Kerschbaumer F, Poisel S, et al: Approaches, anterior approaches, cervical spine and cervicothoracic junction. In Bauer R, Kerschbaumer F, Poisel S, et al (eds): Atlas of Spinal Operations. New York, Thieme, 1993, pp 1–12.
7. German J, Benzel EC, Alexander JT: Anatomy and surgical approaches and exposure of the vertebral column, the cervical spine. In Benzel EC (ed): Spine Surgery: Technique, Complication Avoidance and Management. New York, Churchill Livingstone, 1999, pp 145–156.
8. Johnson RM, Murphy MJ, Southwick WO: Surgical approaches to the spine. In Herkowitz HN, Garfin SR, Balderston RA, et al (eds): Rothman-Simeone's The Spine, 4th ed. Philadelphia, WB Saunders, 1999, pp 1463–1572.
9. Verbiest H: A lateral approach to the cervical spine: Technique and indications. J Neurosurg 1968;28:191–203.
10. Hodgson AR: Approach to the cervical spine C3-C7. Clin Orthop 1965;39:129–134.
11. An HS: Anatomy of the spine. In An HS (ed): Principles and Techniques of Spinal Surgery. Baltimore, Williams & Wilkins, 1998, pp 1–62.

CHAPTER 6

UNGKYU CHANG

MAX C. LEE

DANIEL H. KIM

Posterior Approach to the Midcervical Spine

ANATOMY

MUSCLE AND FASCIA

The most superficial muscle is the trapezius, which originates from the external occipital protuberance, the medial nuchal line, and the (C7 to T12) spinous processes. The trapezius muscle inserts onto the upper body of the scapula, acromion, and the lateral aspect of the clavicle.

The intermediate muscles beneath the trapezius muscle include the splenius capitis and splenius cervicis, which originate from the spinous processes of the lower cervical and upper thoracic spine, and insert on the transverse processes of the upper cervical spine and the mastoid process (Figs. 6-1 and 6-2).

In the deep layer are the sacrospinalis muscle group and transversospinalis muscle group. Sacrospinalis (the erector spinae muscles) consist of a group of muscles running from the lumbosacral spine into the cervical region. These muscles include iliocostalis laterally; longissimus cervicis and longissimus capitis centrally; and spinalis cervicis, semispinalis capitis, and semispinalis cervicis medially (see Figs. 6-1 and 6-2). The other group of deep muscle is the transversospinalis muscle group, which consists of the semispinalis muscle, multifidus muscle, and rotator muscle.

The semispinalis muscles are a part of the transverse spinal system of the erector muscles of the spine. They originate from the transverse processes of the lower cervical and upper thoracic spine and insert at the spinous processes of C2 to C5, nuchal portion of occipital squama (see Fig. 6-1). Beneath the semispinalis muscles lie the multifidus muscles and rotator muscles. The multifidus muscles are also parts of the transversus spinal system and originate at transverse processes from C4 downward to the sacrum and insert at all cervical vertebrae up to the spinous process of C2. They cover the laminae of the vertebrae and are covered by the semispinalis muscle. The rotators cross only one segment of the spine and extend from the transverse process to the spinous process of the vertebrae directly above.

Most posterior muscles are involved in producing extension of the neck and head, whereas some produce rotation and lateral flexion.[1-3]

LIGAMENTOUS STRUCTURES

Nuchal Ligament

The supraspinous ligament of the thoracolumbar spine extends into the cervical region as the ligamentum nuchae, which spans from the external occipital protuberance to the seventh cervical vertebra (Fig. 6-3). There is no separate supraspinous ligament in the cervical region. The ligamentum nuchae is a fibroelastic septum for the attachment of adjacent muscles.

Ligamentum Flavum

The ligamentum flavum of the cervical spine attaches to the anterior surface of the lamina above, and to the superior margin of the lamina below. The ligamentum flavum extends laterally to the articular processes and is connected with the facet capsular ligament (see Fig. 6-3).

Interspinous Ligament

The interspinous ligament attaches in an oblique orientation from the posterosuperior aspect to the anteroinferior aspect of the spinous process below.

FACET JOINT

The facet joint is composed of articular processes, facet capusular ligament, and intervening fibrocarilage. Approximately 80% to 90% of joint surface is covered by cartilage. The coverage surface is wider in the upper cervical spine than in the lower cervical spine. The facet width is 10 to 12 mm

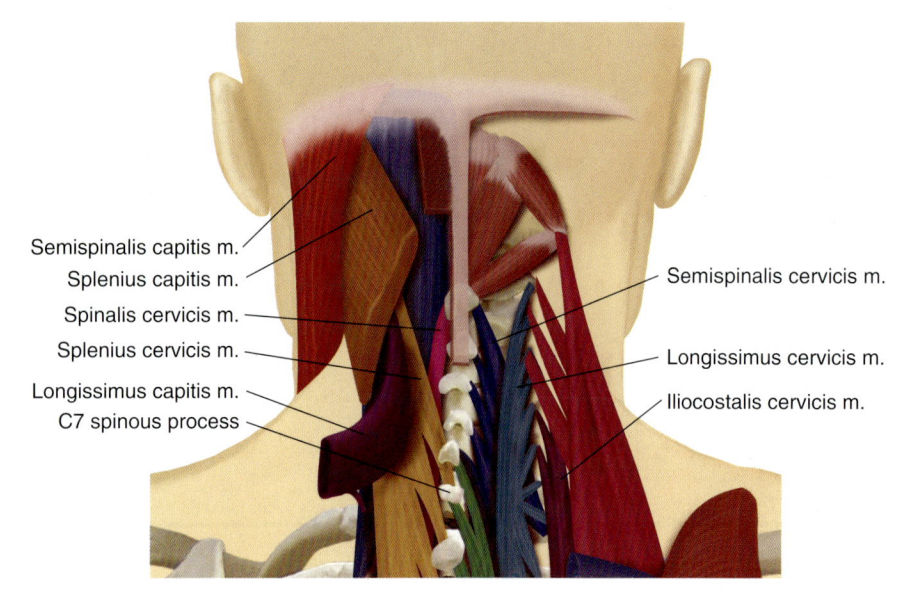

Fig. 6-1 Intermediate and deep muscles of the posterior neck. The splenius capitis and splenius cervicis muscles are included in an intermediate group. In the deep layer is the sacrospinalis muscle group (iliocostalis laterally, longissimus cervicis, and longissimus capitis centrally, and spinalis cervicis, semispinalis capitis, and semispinalis cervicis medially) and the transversospinalis muscle group (semispinalis muscle, multifidus muscle, and rotator muscle).

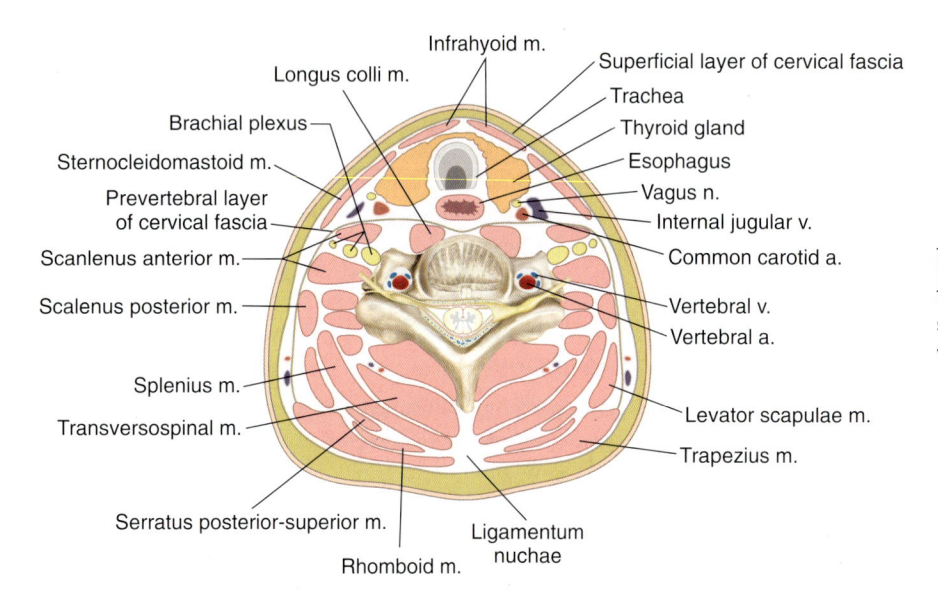

Fig. 6-2 Cross-sectional view of the middle cervical spine showing surrounding neck muscles and vascular structures.

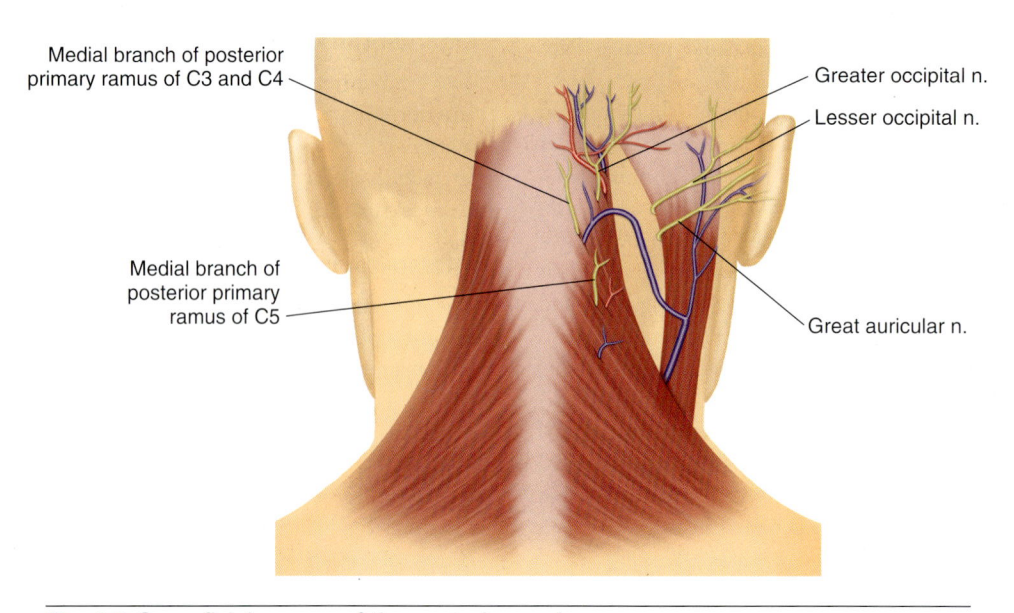

Fig. 6-3 Superficial nerves of the posterior neck.

CHAPTER 6　Posterior Approach to the Midcervical Spine

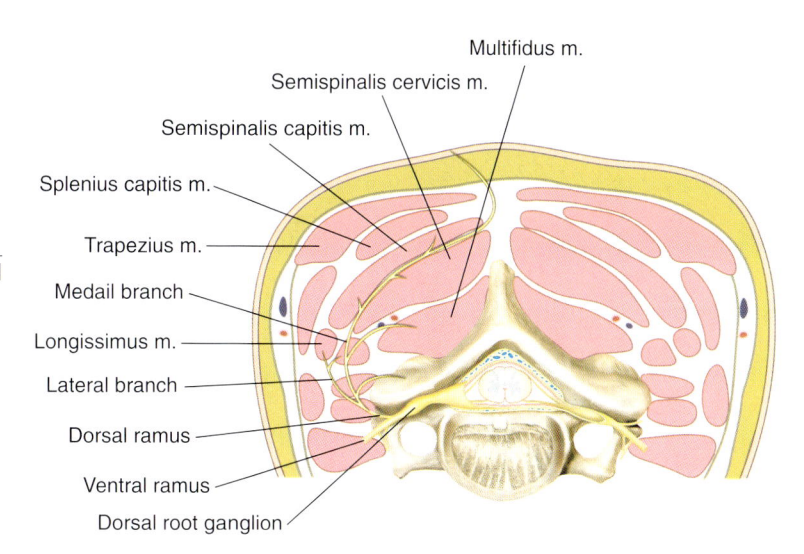

Fig. 6-4 Course of dorsal ramus of the spinal nerve root.

in the lower cervical level and 16 to 18 mm in the upper cervical spine. This suggests that the protective action of the facet joint to the segmental anatomy is more predominant in the upper cervical spine.

The orientation of the superior articular facet in relation to the transverse plane changes from posteromedial (C3, C4 level) to posterolateral (C6, C7). The shape of the superior articular facet is circular to oval at C3, C4, and C5 and gradually changes to a transversely elongated surface at C7 and T1.[4,5]

NEURAL ANATOMY

SUPERFICIAL NERVES OF THE POSTERIOR NECK

Cutaneous branches of the posterior primary rami are found adjacent to every spinous process below the C2 spinous process. The largest one is the greater occipital nerve. The lesser occipital nerve is lateral to the greater occipital nerve and is in the retroauricular area (see Fig. 6-3).

The dorsal root ganglion is located between the vertebral artery and superior articular process. The spinal nerves divide into dorsal primary rami and ventral primary rami branches.

The posterior primary rami of cervical nerves send motor fibers to the deep muscles and sensory fibers to facet joint, deep muscles, and soft tissue (Fig. 6-4). At the anterior aspect of the facet joint, the dorsal ramus curves dorsolaterally along the superior articular process. Then, the dorsal ramus branches medial and lateral, giving another small branch to the facet joint. The lateral branch crosses the transverse process and reaches to the anterior surface of the longissimus capitis. The medial branch runs dorsomedially through the tunnel between the facet capsule and the tendon of semispinalis capitis. Then, this medial branch traverses to the lateral edge of the multifidus muscle. After passing the lateral edge of the multifidus muscle, the medial branch divides into superficial and deep branches. The deep branch goes into the space between the multifidus muscle and semispinalis cervicis muscle. The superficial branch runs between semispinalis capitis and semispinalis cervicis muscles and terminates as cutaneous branches (see Fig. 6-4).

The anterior primary rami of C1 to C4 form the cervical plexus. The anterior rami of C5 to T1 form the brachial plexus (Fig. 6-5).[6]

APPROACH

MIDLINE POSTERIOR APPROACH

The position of the patient for posterior cervical spine surgery is as follows: the patient's face rests on a well-padded horseshoe-shaped headrest. Five-point fixation may also be accomplished with a Mayfield head holder. The patient is placed prone on chest holsters or a Wilson frame and the operating table is placed in reverse Trendelenburg position such that the cervical spine is parallel to the floor.

The direct posterior approach involves a midline incision centered over the palpable spinous processes. The incision is performed to the ligamentum nuchae in the midline. It is important to keep the dissection within the midline; failure to do so will cause profuse muscle bleeding. With sharp dissection, the incision is carried down to the level of the spinous process. Then, gentle subperiosteal elevation of the muscles is performed to the level of the lateral aspects of the facet joints (Fig. 6-6).

In an approach to the lateral area of the facet joint, trunks of medial branches from the dorsal ramus are likely to be injured. The nerve trunk can be visible after the complete detachment of multifidus muscle from the lateral mass.

The attachments of the cervical muscles to the spine are then cut away. It is easier to begin at the bottom because the

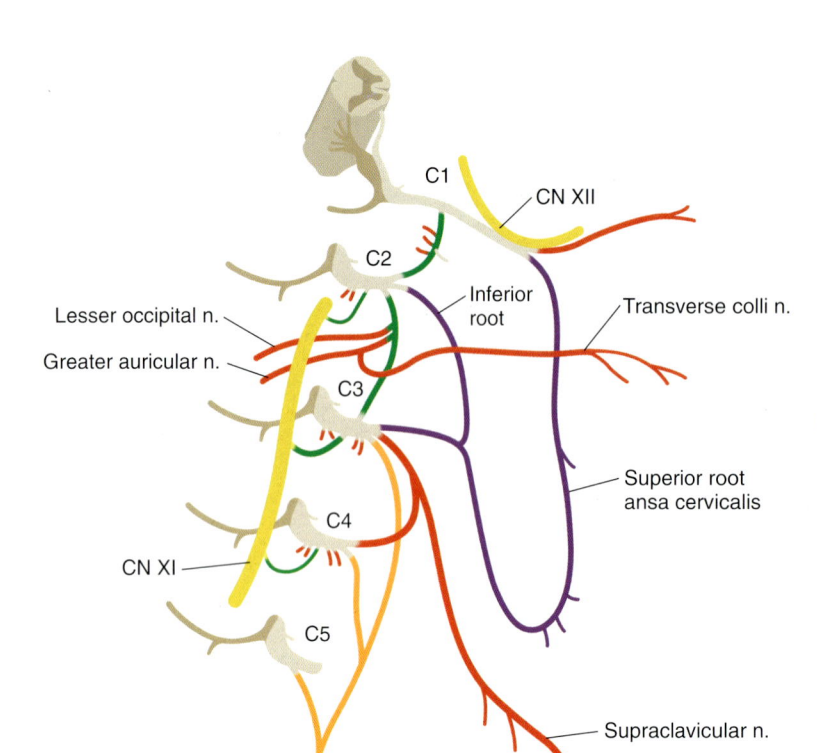

Fig. 6-5 Upper cervical roots.

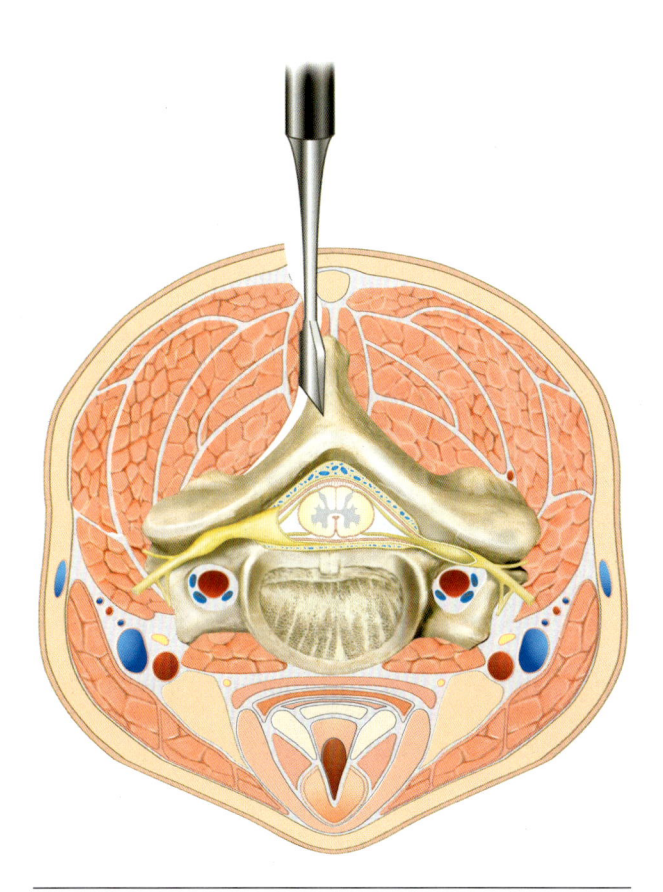

Fig. 6-6 Manipulation of osteotome for subperiosteal dissection of the paravertebral muscle.

bleeding will be less troublesome. Gauze sponges should be packed in the surgical space created to obliterate it and absorb the minor bleeding that occurs. The identification of the exposed level is accomplished by counting from the large bifid spinous process of C2 or with fluoroscopy.

After sufficient bony exposure is achieved, bony decompression is begun. The extent of the posterior decompression is determined according to the structures to be removed (Fig. 6-7).[7,8]

LATERAL MASS PLATING

After retraction of the posterior neck muscles, the lamina and facet joint are exposed. Viewed posteriorly, the facet joint appears horizontal and curves slightly inferior (Fig. 6-8). The interfacetal distance averages 13 mm, ranging from 9 to 16 mm. The medial border of the facet is identified where the lamina joins the lateral mass to form a small valley (Fig. 6-9A). The vertebral artery and exiting nerve root are directly anterior to this valley.

For posterior fixation of the cervical spine, lateral mass plating or a lateral mass screw/rod system can be useful. Lateral mass screws must be lateral to this landmark and angled outward from this point. The entry point of the screw is just lateral to the midpoint. The targeting angle is 25 to 30 degrees lateral and 25 to 30 degrees cephalad (see Fig. 6-9A and B).

If the lateral mass screw is used at the C7 level, a preoperative computed tomography (CT) scan of the level and a

CHAPTER 6 Posterior Approach to the Midcervical Spine

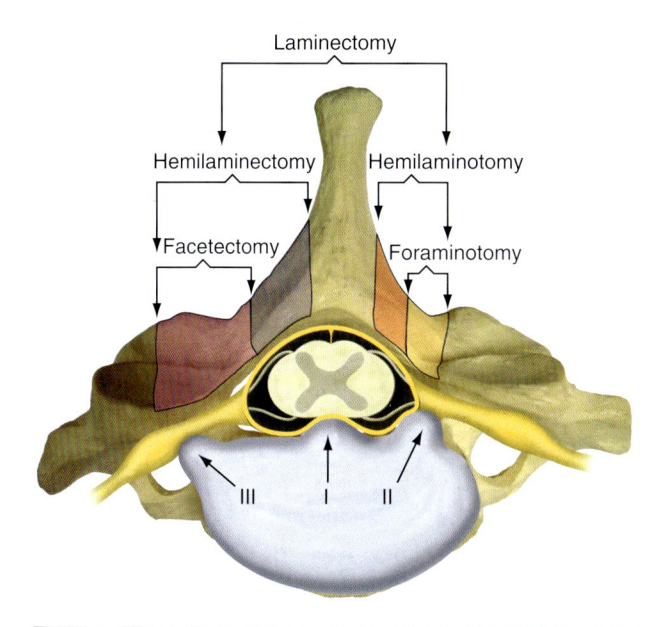

Fig. 6-7 Posterior decompression nomenclature: total laminectomy, hemilaminectomy, facetectomy, foraminotomy. I, Central disk herniation; II, lateral disk herniation; III, foraminal disk herniation.

more cephalad and lateral drilling point may be necessary (see Fig. 6-9C).[7,9,10]

CERVICAL PEDICLE SCREWING

For the cervicothoracic junction (C7-T2) fixation, the pedicle screws are stronger because the lateral masses become thinner at the C7 level. The average thickness of lateral mass is about 9 mm. This figure does not offer a sufficient length of bone purchase for lateral mass screws. The average pedicular width is about 3.5 to 6.5 mm, and the average height is 5 to 8 mm in cervical spines. The pedicular angulation in the transverse plane ranges from 35 to 45 degrees and the pedicle angulation in the sagittal plane is 3 to 5 degrees downward with reference to the lower end plate of C7. The entry point of C7 transpedicular screwing is located at the junction of two lines—the vertical line passing by the middle of the C6-C7 facet joint and the horizontal line passing just (1 mm) under the middle of C7 transverse process (Fig. 6-10A) Direction of screwing is 30 to 35 degrees medially and 5 degrees downward with reference to the C7 lower end plate (see Fig. 6-10B and C).[7,10-12]

INTERSPINOUS WIRING FOR SUBAXIAL FUSION

As in atlantoaxial fusion, the triple-wire technique can be used for all subaxial posterior cervical spine fusions with intact laminae and spinous processes. Drill holes are placed in the base of the spinous process of levels to be fused. A single cable is then passed from near to far through the drill hole in the caudad spinous process. The advancing leader is then looped around the inferior edge of the spinous process and again is passed through the drill hole. The advancing leader is then passed from far to near through the drill hole in the cephalad spinous process, looped around the cephalad edge of the spinous process, and again passed from far to near through the drill hole (Fig. 6-11A). After that, two additional cables are passed into the drill hole on the spinous process, then passed into bone grafts. The grafts are positioned on the laminae to be fused (see Fig. 6-11B).[13,14]

Fig. 6-8 Posterior view of spinal cord and nerve roots. Laminae and left side facet joints are removed.

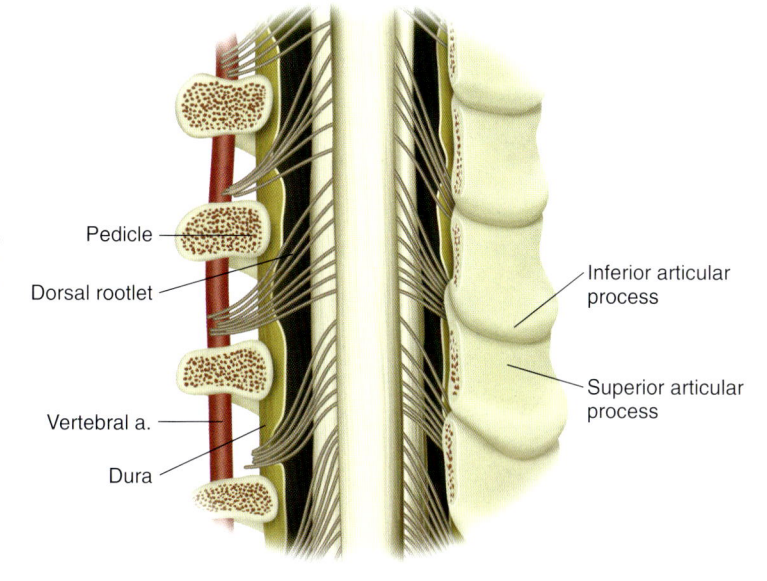

SECTION I SURGICAL ANATOMY AND APPROACHES

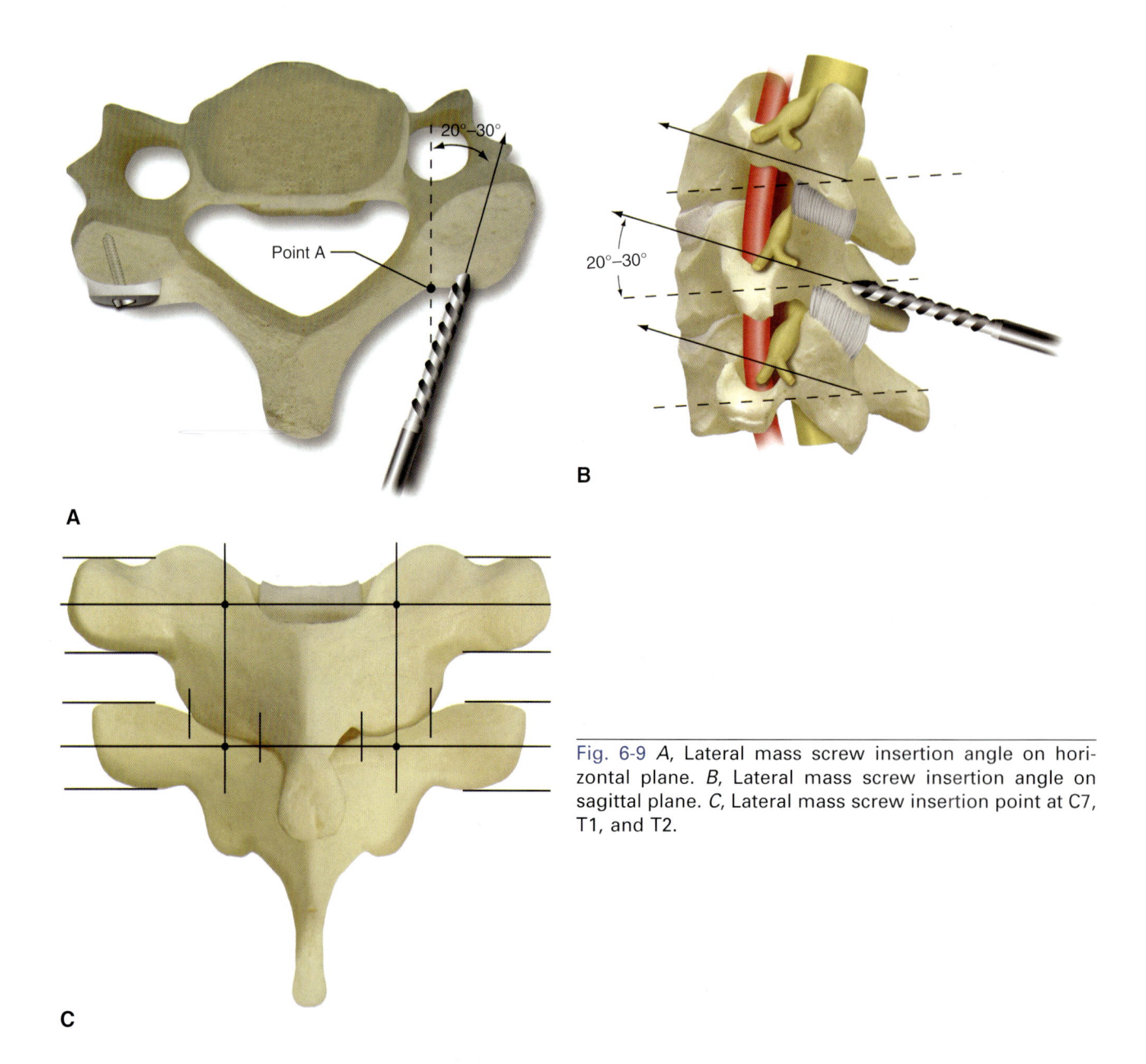

Fig. 6-9 *A,* Lateral mass screw insertion angle on horizontal plane. *B,* Lateral mass screw insertion angle on sagittal plane. *C,* Lateral mass screw insertion point at C7, T1, and T2.

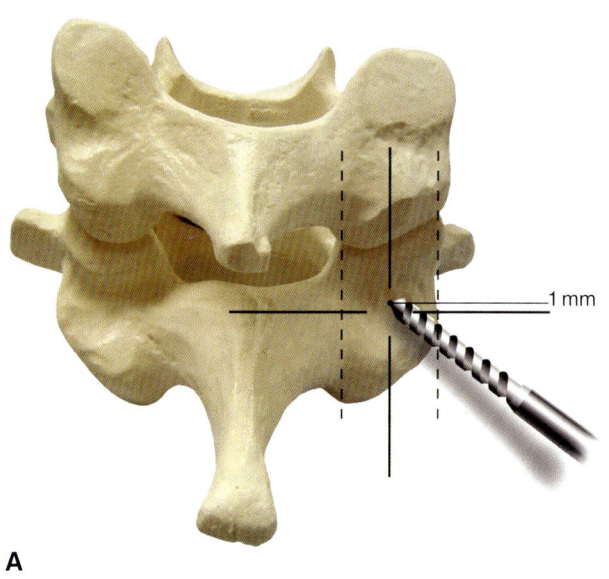

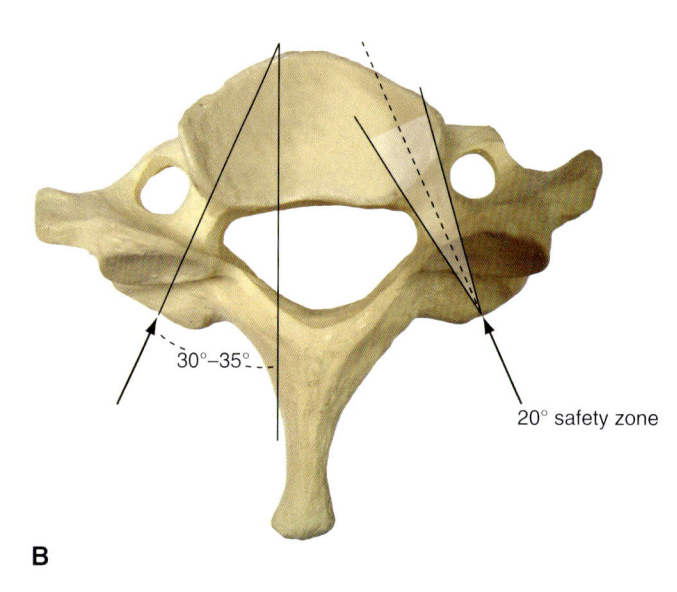

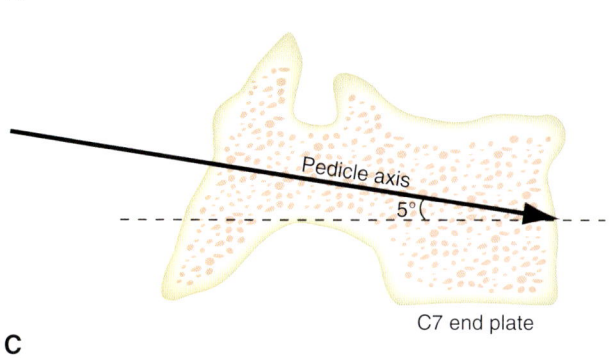

CHAPTER 6 Posterior Approach to the Midcervical Spine   63

Fig. 6-10 *A*, Pedicle screw insertion point at C7. *B*, Pedicle screw insertion angle on sagittal plane with reference to lower end plate of C7. Screws have to be pointed 5 degrees downward. *C*, Pedicle screw insertion angle on axial plane at C7 level. Transverse angulation of the pedicle with reference to the sagittal plane is between 30 and 35 degrees. Transverse angulation of the transpedicluar screwing safety zone is greater than 20 degrees.

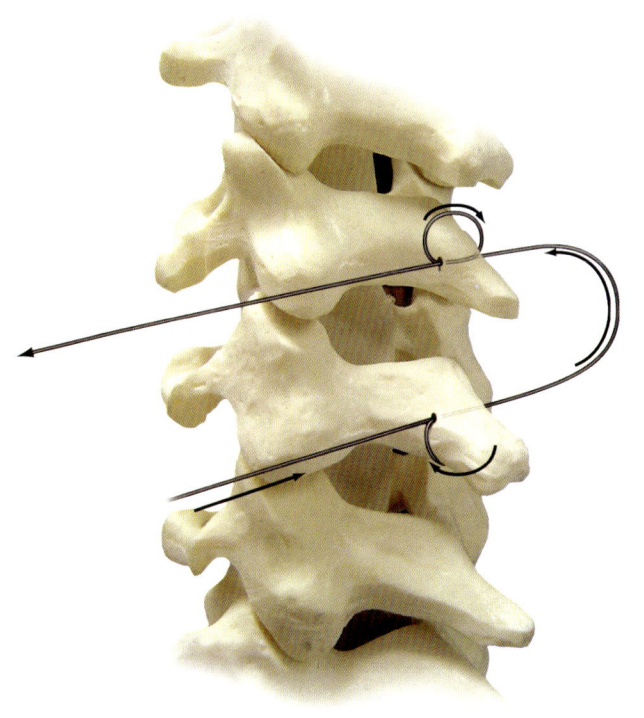

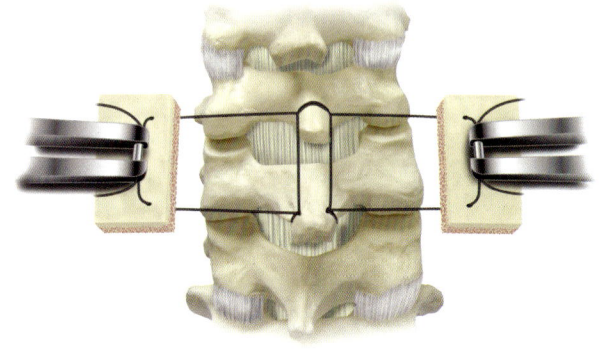

Fig. 6-11 *A*, Interspinous wiring method. The cable is passed through the C5 hole and then looped around the inferior edge of the C5 spinous process, re-entering through the C5 hole. Then, the cable is passed through the C4 hole and looped around the superior edge of the C4 spinous process. *B*, Bone graft attachment on C4 and C5 laminae. Bone grafts are cinched simultaneously onto C4 and C5.

References

1. Rauschning W: Anatomy and pathology of the cervical spine. In Frymoyer JW (ed): The Adult Spine. New York, Raven Press, 1991, pp 907–929.
2. An HS: Anatomy and the cervical spine. In An HS, Simpson JM (eds): Surgery of the Cervical Spine. Baltimore, Williams & Wilkins, 1994, pp 1–40.
3. Zhang J, Tsuzuki N, Hirabayashi H, et al: Surgical anatomy of the nerves and muscles in the posterior cervical spine. Spine 2003;28(13):1379–1384.
4. Yoganandan N, Knowles SA, Mainman DJ, Pintar FA: Anatomic study of the morphology of human cervical facet joint. Spine 2003;28(20):2317–2323.
5. Pal GP, Routal RV, Saggu SK: The orientation of the articular facet of the zygapophyseal joints at the cervical and upper thoracic region. J Anat 2001;198:431–441.
6. Janfaza P, Fabian RL: The back and posterior region of the neck. In Janfaza P, Nadol JB, Galla J, et al (eds): Surgical Anatomy of the Head and Neck. Philadelphia, Lippincott Williams & Wilkins, 2001, pp 715–745.
7. An HS, Gordin R, Renner K: Anatomical considerations for plate-screw fixation to the cervical spine. Spine 1988;13:813–816.
8. Ugur HC, Attar A, Uz A, et al: Surgical anatomic evaluation of the cervical pedicle and adjacent neural structures. Neurosurgery 2000;47(5):1162–1169.
9. Coppes MA, Howard A: Posterior cervical lateral mass plating. In Dillin WH, Simeone FA (eds): Posterior Cervical Spine Surgery. Philadelphia, Lippincott-Raven, 1998, pp 81–89.
10. Cooper PR, Cohen A, Rosiello A, Kosiow M: Posterior stabilization of cervical spine fractures and subluxations using plates and screws. Neurosurgery 1988;23:300–306.
11. Kim HS, Heller JG, Hudgins PA, Fountain JA: The accuracy of computed tomography in assessing cervical pedicle screw placement. Spine 2003;28:2441–2446.
12. Barrey C, Cotton F, Jund J, et al: Transpedicular screwing of the seventh cervical vertebra: Anatomical considerations and surgical technique. Surg Radiol Anat 2003;25:354–360.
13. Parker LM, McAfee PC: Atlantoaxial and subaxial arthrodesis with triple-wire technique. In Dillin WH, Simeone FA (eds): Posterior Cervical Spine Surgery. Philadelphia, Lippincott-Raven, 1998, pp 101–106.
14. McAfee PC, Bohlman HH, Wilson WL: The triple wire fixation technique for stabilization of acute fracture-dislocations: A biomechanical analysis. Orthop Trans 1985;9:142.

SECTION C
Cervicothoracic Junction and Thoracic Spine

CHAPTER 7

HOANG N. LE
DANIEL H. KIM

Anterior Approaches to the Cervicothoracic Junction (Low Cervical-Supraclavicular, Transclavicular-Transmanubrial, Trans-sternal-Transthoracic)

INTRODUCTION

The anterior approach to the cervicothoracic spine can be technically challenging and requires precise knowledge of cervicothoracic regional anatomy as well as careful preoperative planning. A standard low cervical approach can often expose to T1 level in most patients. In patients with long necks, it is possible to expose down to T2 with a standard low cervical approach. However, for usual anterior exposure of T2 to T4, more extensile approaches such as the transmanubrial or transsternal approaches will be necessary. The transsternal approach offers the best exposure of T3 and T4; however, it carries the highest morbidity rate of all the anterior approaches. Caudally, the aortic arch and its branches will limit access to the T3 and T4 vertebrae.

ANATOMY

THORACIC INLET

- Superior mediastinum is defined anteriorly by the manubrium (Fig. 7-1).
- T2-T3 level is at the suprasternal notch.
- T4-T5 level is at the sternal angle.
- Sternohyoid muscle, from the ventrocaudal hyoid bone to the dorsal surface of the manubrium, attaches to the sternoclavicular joint capsule.
- Sternothyroid muscle attaches along the dorsal midline of the manubrium.
- Sternocleidomastoid muscle arises on the mastoid process and superior nuchal line and attaches to the manubrioclavicular joint. Its nervous supply is from the accessory nerve. Arterial supply branches come from the superior thyroid artery.
- Removal of the manubrium and medial third of the clavicle reveals the pleural apices, which are covered by an extension of the transthoracic fascia, called *Sibson's fascia*.

VASCULAR AND VISCERAL COMPARTMENTS OF THE SUPERIOR MEDIASTINUM
Fascial Layers

- Visceral fascia circumscribes the trachea, esophagus, and thyroid gland, defining a visceral compartment.
- Carotid sheath circumscribes the carotid arterial system, internal jugular vein, and vagus nerve, defining a neurovascular compartment.
- These adjacent compartments create a potential space (the viscerocarotid space), which extends from the base of the skull to C7 to T4, depending on the location of fusion between the visceral and alar fascia.
- Blunt dissection of the viscerocarotid space exposes the alar fascia and the retropharyngeal space (Fig. 7-2).
- The visceral compartment continues down to the bronchi, where the fascia fuses with the parietal and visceral pleurae.
- Carotid sheath extends down to the subclavian vessels, where it fuses into the axillary sheath.

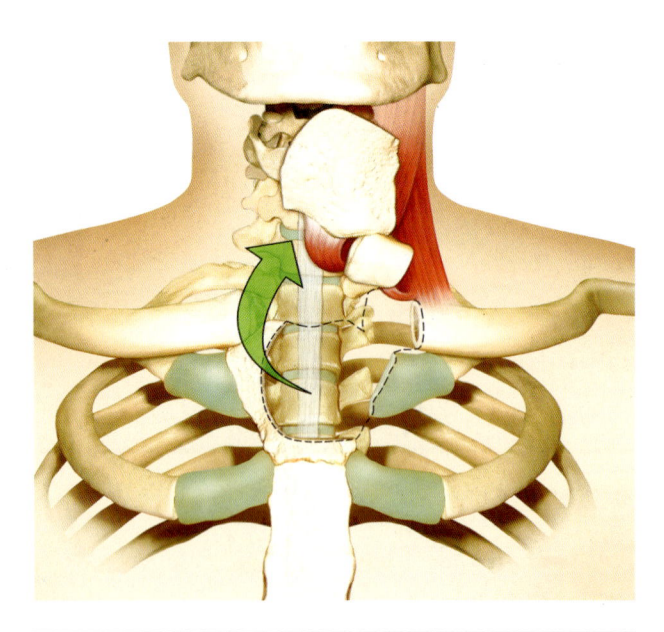

Fig. 7-1 Surgical approach will depend on the desired level of exposure. The suprasternal notch approximates the T2-T3 level and the sternal angle approximates the T4-T5 level.

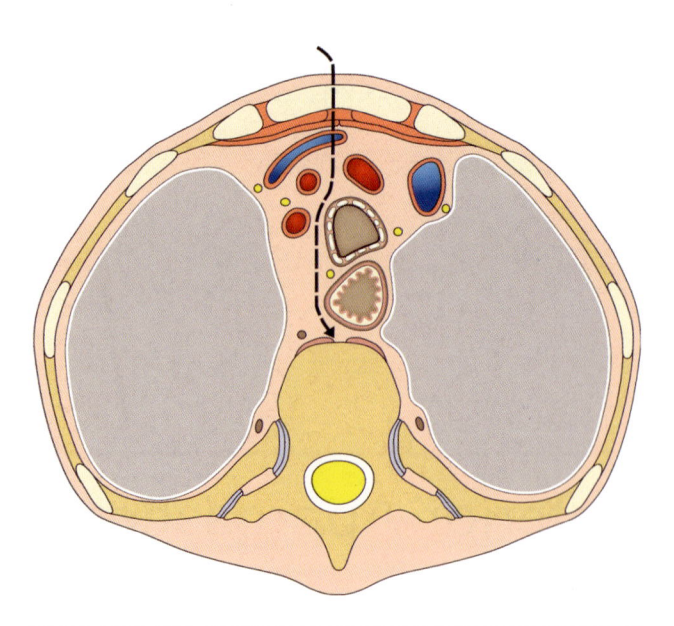

Fig. 7-2 Dissection plane through the viscerocarotid space needed to reach the upper thoracic prevertebral space.

- In the superior mediastinum, the vascular compartment is not circumscribed by its own well-defined fascial sheath but is defined secondarily by independent surrounding fascia.
  - Ventrally is the prevertebral fascial extension, the transthoracic fascia.
  - Caudally is the visceral fascia.
  - Laterally are the parietal pleurae.
  - Inferiorly is the pericardium.

Venous Structures

- Brachiocephalic veins with their branches descend from the neck into the superior mediastinum just posterior to the thymus gland.
  - Right brachiocephalic vein is formed just posterior to the medial end of the right clavicle and descends vertically into the superior mediastinum.
  - Left brachiocephalic vein is formed just posterior to the medial end of the left clavicle and descends diagonally to join the right brachiocephalic vein just posterior to the right first costal cartilage to form the superior vena cava.
  - In the superior mediastinum, the left brachiocephalic vein runs obliquely from left inferior to right superior.
- Tributaries draining into the brachiocephalic veins:
  - The vertebral and first, posterior, intercostal veins are in the neck.
  - Internal thoracic, thymic, and inferior thyroid veins are in the superior mediastinum.
  - On the left, the superior intercostal vein (which drains the second and third intercostal spaces) also drains into the left brachiocephalic vein.

Arterial Structures

- Aortic arch initially ascends posteriorly to the superior vena cava but also turns diagonally posterior, then inferior just anterior and to the left of the vertebral column.
- A second concave turn occurs as the arch curves around the anterolateral visceral compartment to reach the vertebral column.
- Brachiocephalic artery is the first branch off the aortic arch and ascends vertically and slightly rightward to branch into the right common carotid and subclavian arteries posterior to the right sternoclavicular joint.
- The left common carotid artery arises next off the arch and ascends essentially vertically into the carotid sheath without branching in the superior mediastinum.
- The left subclavian artery is the third branch and ascends superiorly and leftward to curve around the thoracic inlet and into the axillary sheath without branches in the superior mediastinum.

RETROPHARYNGEAL AND RETROMEDIASTINAL SPACES

- By incising the alar and mediastinal fascia, the median compartment of the retromediastinal space is entered.
- The prevertebral fascia covers the vertebral bodies and envelops the longus colli muscles.
- Autonomic branches to the cardiopulmonary plexi may be seen in this region and can be sacrificed if necessary.
- Structures potentially crossing the retropharyngeal and retromediastinal spaces:
  - Right recurrent laryngeal nerve can cross the retropharyngeal or retromediastinal space anywhere from C7 to T3.

- Left recurrent laryngeal nerve loops around the ligamentum arteriosum, and ascends within the visceral fascia between the esophagus and trachea.
- Lymphatics terminating in the thoracic duct (on the left side):
  - Run dorsal and to the left of the esophagus between the visceral and alar fascia in the superior mediastinum and ascend to the C7 level.
  - Lie laterally in a plane dorsal to the carotid sheath, then course caudally and ventrally to the branches of the thyrocervical trunk and phrenic nerve.
  - Terminate at the junction of the left internal jugular and subclavian veins.
  - A lymphatic trunk located on the right side follows a similar course to the thoracic duct.

ANTERIOR APPROACHES AND TECHNIQUES

LOW CERVICAL APPROACH

- The low cervical approach is the Smith-Robinson approach with possible caudal exposure to T1 or T2 in most patients. Technical description of this approach is similar to an approach used for anterior cervical diskectomy and fusion (ACDF) as described in Chapter 16.
- Visualization of the posterior aspect of the disk is difficult and may require a resection of the lower aspect of the cranial vertebrae.
- Vertebrectomy may be easier than diskectomy.
- Right-sided approach should identify the recurrent laryngeal nerve.
- Left-sided approach should spare the thoracic duct.
- Inferior thyroid vein and artery may be encountered and ligated as necessary.
- Inferiorly, the brachiocephalic vein is anterior to the trachea at T3.
- Retraction:
  - Trachea, esophagus medially
  - Lung apex, innominate vessels inferiorly
  - Carotid shealth laterally

SUPRACLAVICULAR APPROACH

- This approach uses an incision above the clavicle with dissection posterior to the carotid sheath.
- The clavicular head of the sternocleidomastoid muscle is divided.
- The subclavian artery and branches are exposed (thyrocervical, suprascapular, transcervical—latter two can be ligated if necessary).
- Identify phrenic nerve on anterior scalene muscle. This muscle is divided with sparing of the phrenic nerve.
- After division of the anterior scalene, expose Sibson's fascia, which covers the dome of the lung.
- Divide Sibson's fascia transversely to retract visceral pleura and lung inferiorly.
- A view into the thoracic inlet is now possible, as well as the posterior thorax, stellate ganglion, and upper thoracic vertebral bodies.
- Obese and muscular patients with short necks are poor candidates for the above two approaches but can be appropriate for the following approaches.

TRANSMANUBRIAL-TRANSCLAVICULAR APPROACH

- This approach can be combined with a left-sided low cervical approach.
- Various hockey stick incisions can be used (Fig. 7-3A to C).
- Platysma and deep cervical fascia are incised.
- Sternal and clavicular heads of sternocleidomastoid muscle are divided and retracted laterally.
- Sternohyoid and sternothyroid muscles are divided and retracted medially.
- Blunt dissection of the viscerocarotid plane is done.
- Expose the medial third of clavicle and manubrium periosteally.
- Divide the clavicle at junction of medial and middle thirds.
- Medial end of clavicle can be disarticulated from sternoclavicular joint.
- Left side of manubrium can be removed piecemeal along its posterior periosteum.
- Alternatively, the manubrium and sternoclavicular joint can be left intact and reflected with the sternal head of the sternocleidomastoid muscle (Fig. 7-4).
- Dissection is carried deeper until great vessels are identified (Fig. 7-5).
- Inferior thyroid vessels can be ligated.
- The left inominate vein should be identified and retracted caudally (Fig. 7-6).
- Identify the prevertebral fascia and incise to expose the vertebral bodies.
- Reconstruction of the clavicle and manubrium is optional but can be accomplished with wire or plating systems.

TRANS-STERNAL-TRANSTHORACIC APPROACH

- This approach affords the best exposure down to T4, especially in obese patients.
- Morbidity rate is higher than for other approaches.
- This approach can be combined with the low cervical approach.
- This approach does not affect shoulder function.
- Incision should be made medial to the anterior border of the sternocleidomastoid muscle down the middle of the sternum to the xiphoid process (Fig. 7-7).
- Sternohyoid and sternothyroid muscles are divided.

68 SECTION I SURGICAL ANATOMY AND APPROACHES

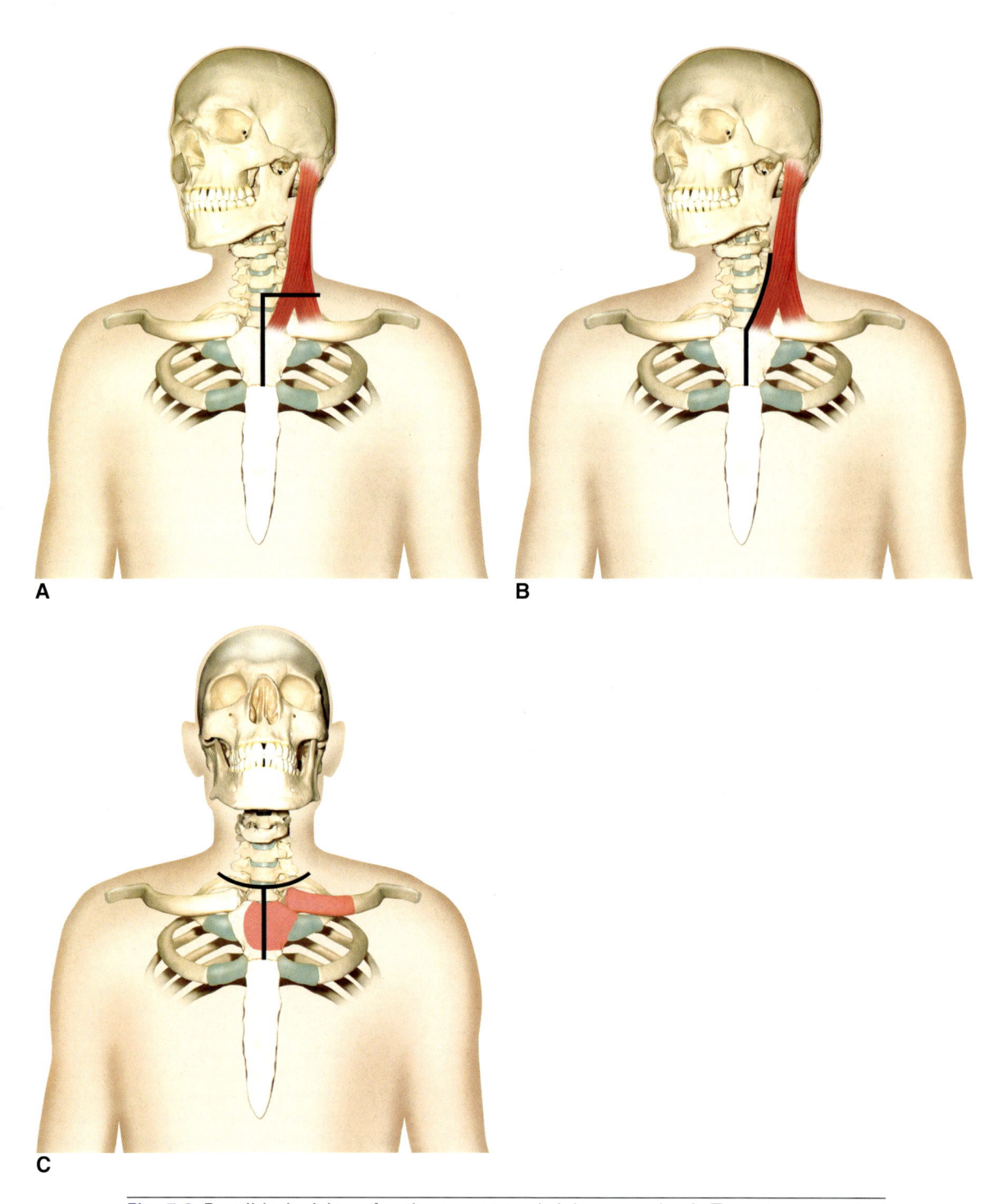

Fig. 7-3 Possible incisions for the transmanubrial approach. *A*, Transverse cervical incision combined with midline sternal incision. *B*, Oblique cervical incision along the medial border of the sternocleidomastoid muscle and a midline sternal incision. *C*, A T-shaped incision.

CHAPTER 7   Anterior Approaches to the Cervicothoracic Junction   69

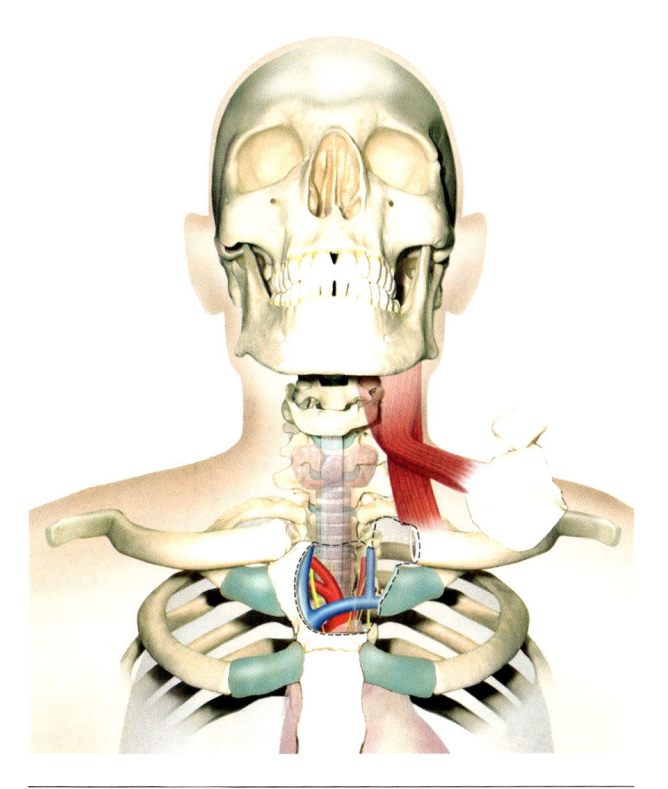

Fig. 7-4 The sternoclavicular joint can be left intact by leaving the sternal head of the sternocleidomastoid muscle attached to the manubrium and reflecting as one piece.

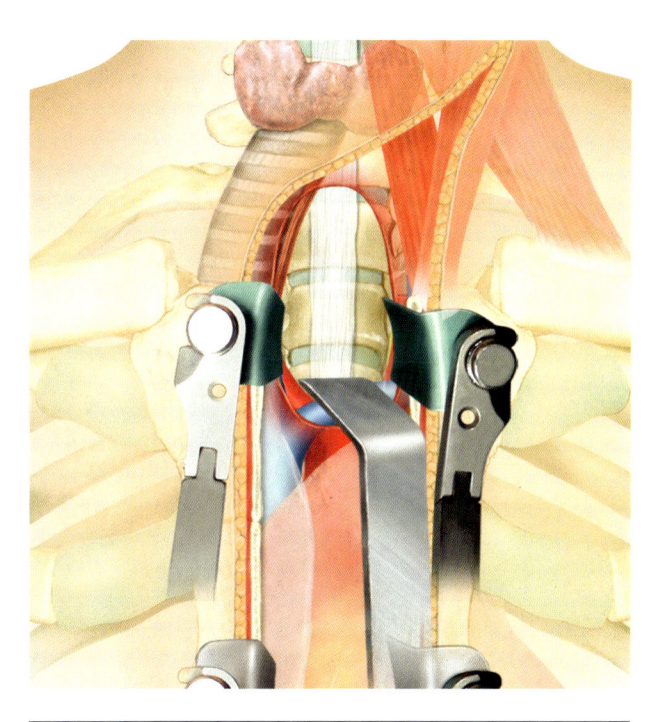

Fig. 7-6 Retraction of the great vessels caudally, visceral structures medially, and carotid shealth laterally to expose the prevertebral space.

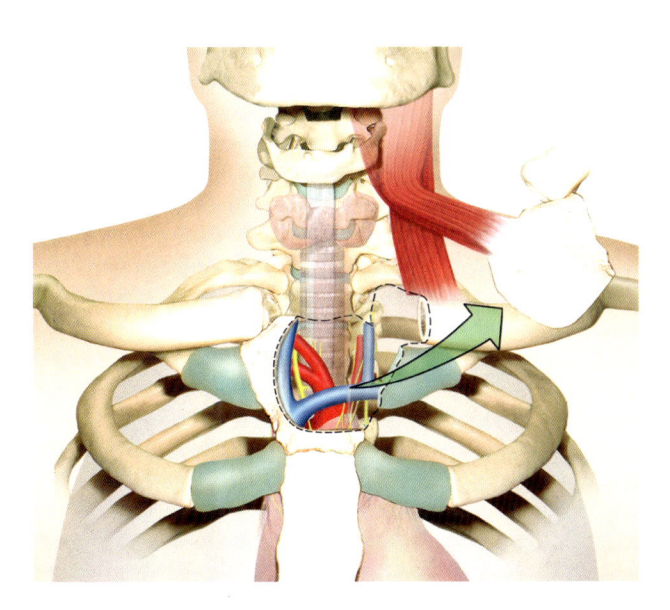

Fig. 7-5 Great vessels should be identified after reflection of the manubrium and dissection through the retrosternal fat. Inferior thyroid vessels can be ligated as needed.

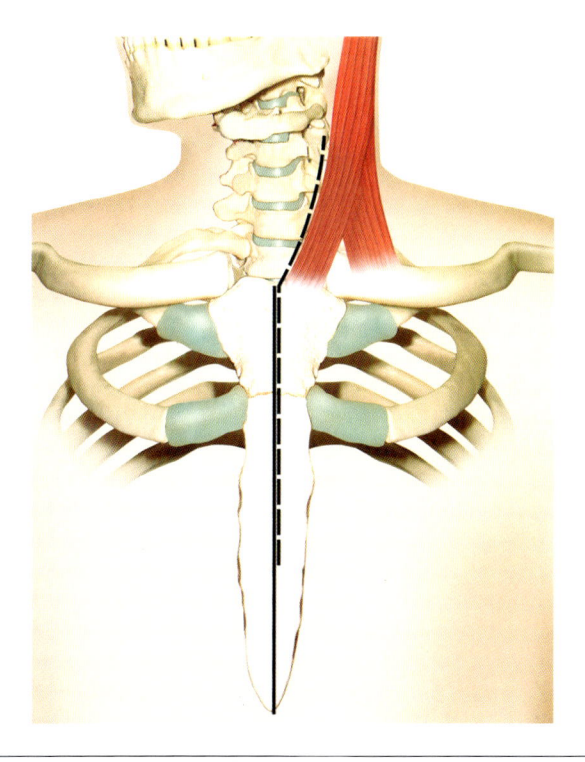

Fig. 7-7 Incision used for a combined low cervical sternotomy approach.

70 SECTION I SURGICAL ANATOMY AND APPROACHES

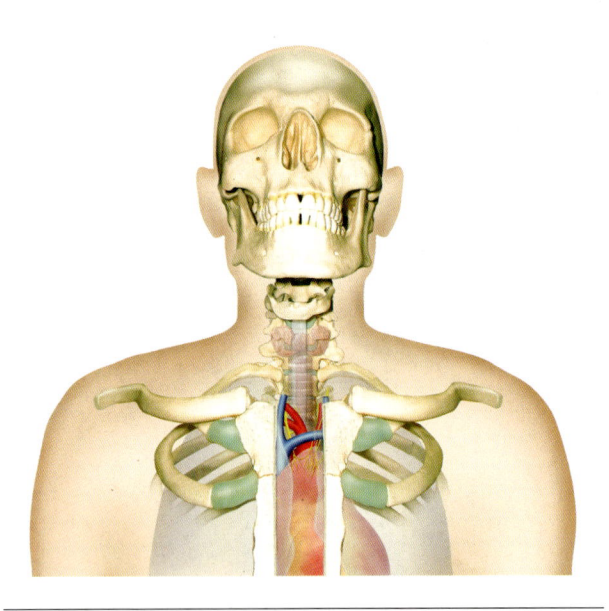

Fig. 7-8 Exposure after a midline sternotomy. Stay midline to avoid injury to the pleura. Sternotomy should be done with utmost care so that underlying vessels are not injured.

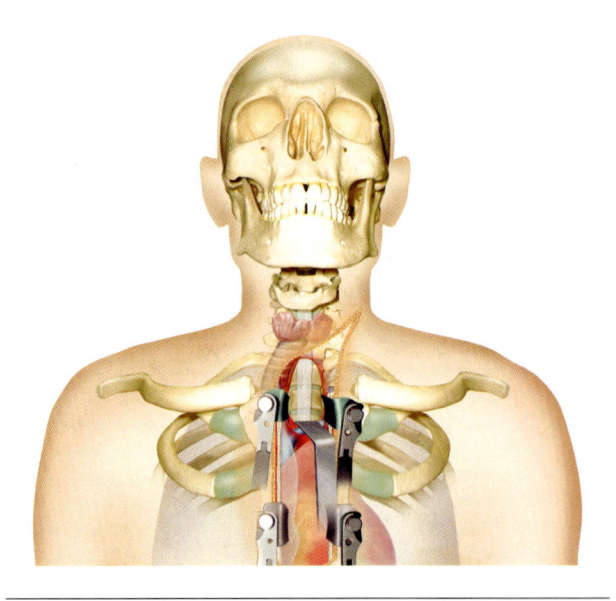

Fig. 7-10 Exposure after retractors are placed for a sternotomy approach.

- Retrosternal adipose and thymus tissues are retracted from the sternum.
- Sternum is exposed subperiosteally and divided in the middle with a sternal saw (Fig. 7-8).
- Inferior thyroid vessels can be ligated (Fig. 7-9).
- Left inominate vein is retracted caudally (or ligated if necessary), tracheoesophagus medially, carotid shealth laterally (Fig. 7-10).
- Identify the prevertebral fascia and incise to expose the vertebral bodies.
- Closure should be performed with standard wiring. Chest tube is not necessary unless there is pleural violation.

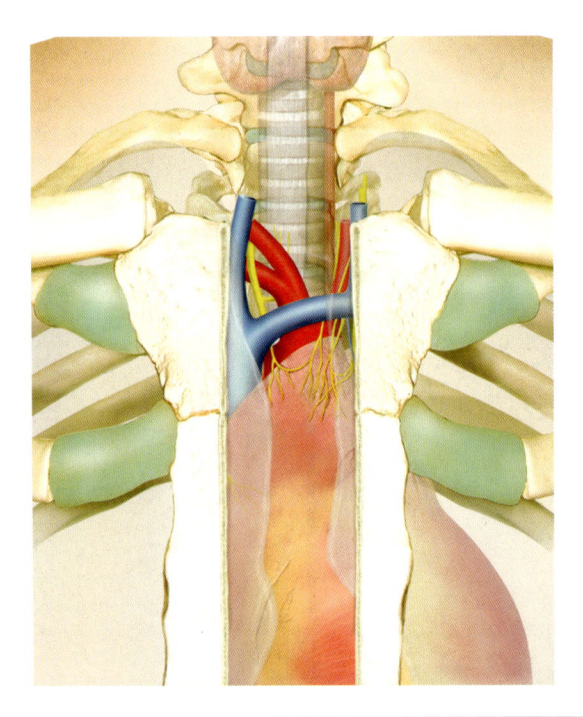

Fig. 7-9 Closeup view after median sternotomy. Recurrent laryngeal nerves can be identified with great vessels.

CHAPTER 8

HOANG N. LE

DANIEL H. KIM

Anterolateral Transthoracic Approaches to the Cervicothoracic Junction (Transaxillary Approach, Transpleural Transthoracic Third Rib Resection Approach)

INTRODUCTION

The anterolateral transthoracic approach to the cervicothoracic junction provides excellent exposure the vertebral bodies anterolaterally. T3 and T4 exposure can be easily achieved, but access to T1 and T2 can be limited by the narrowing of the thoracic inlet. Unlike in other approaches, exposure of the lower cervical vertebrae is most often not possible. Rapid exposure of the anterior spinal elements and excellent control of intercostal segmental arteries can be achieved via this approach. Lung isolation is utilized, and a small thoracotomy through the third rib bed is performed to access to the paramedian retromediastinal space of the cervicothoracic junction. Intrapleural dissection, the long depth of field, and the inability to obtain exposure of the lower cervical vertebrae may limit this exposure to a few selected cases of cervicothoracic junction pathologies.

ANATOMY

SCAPULAR AND PARASCAPULAR ANATOMY

- Mobilization of the scapular for exposure of the high thoracic region will require detachment of the posterior musculature and associated tendinous attachments to the posterior inferior medial scapular border.
- Muscles detached during exposure (Fig. 8-1):
  - Anteroinferior: serratus anterior
  - Inferomedial border of the scapula: latissimus dorsi
  - Medioposterior border: trapezius and rhomboid major and minor

SUBSCAPULAR ANATOMY

- The subscapular space is entered once the superficial muscles have been detached and the scapula is mobilized and retracted in a cephalad direction.
- The upper thoracic rib beds can be identified after division of the serratus anterior. Care should be taken to identify and preserve the long thoracic nerve.
- Once the scapula is retracted, identification of the third rib is possible. When counting ribs, the first rib is usually located inside the second rib and can be missed.
- The ribs are attached to one another through the intercostal musculature, which originates medially on each superior rib and inserts laterally on its immediately inferior rib.
- Resection of the third rib will allow for greater intercostal spreading than would a second rib resection.
- The rib bed consists of periosteum, endothoracic fascia, and parietal pleura.
- With rib resection, a strip of intercostal musculature is isolated between each rib, which contains the intercostal nerve, artery, and vein.

72 SECTION I SURGICAL ANATOMY AND APPROACHES

A

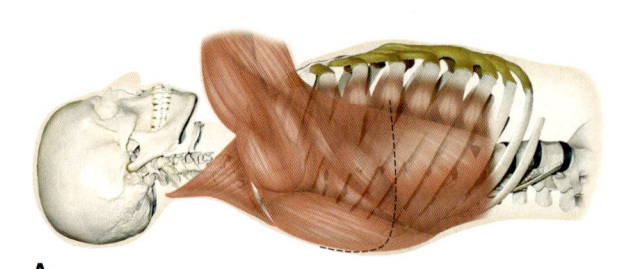

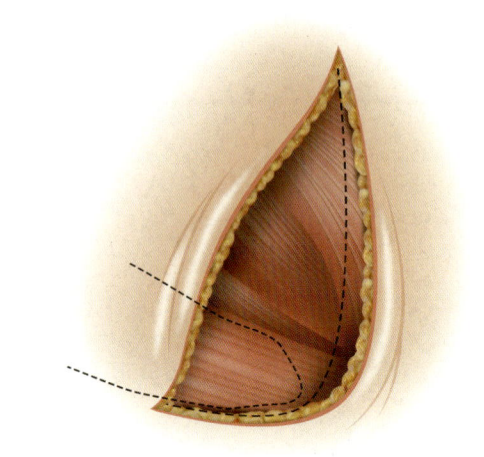

B

Fig. 8-1 Incision and underlying muscular anatomy. *A*, Incision in lateral position. Both the latissimus dorsi and trapezius muscle may be encountered superficially. *B*, Muscular view. Serratus anterior and rhomboids can also be seen with deeper exposure.

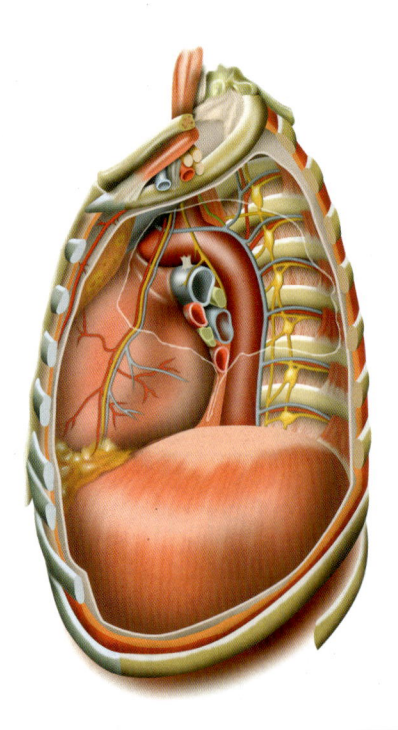

Fig. 8-2 Left lateral view of the thoracic cavity. Refer to text for anatomic description.

- Immediately ventral to the intercostal bundle lies the pleura.

SUPERIOR MEDIASTINUM PARAVERTEBRAL ANATOMY (Figs. 8-2 and 8-3)

Once the lung is deflated and retracted, important anatomic structures are as follows.

Parietal Pleura
- The parietal pleura covers the spinal column and vascular structures.
- It is removed to reveal the underlying structures.

Upper Thoracic Spine
- Disk spaces are large, white prominent surfaces.
- Intercostal vessels lie underneath the pleura and run over the midvertebral bodies.
- Ribs can be visualized and counted.

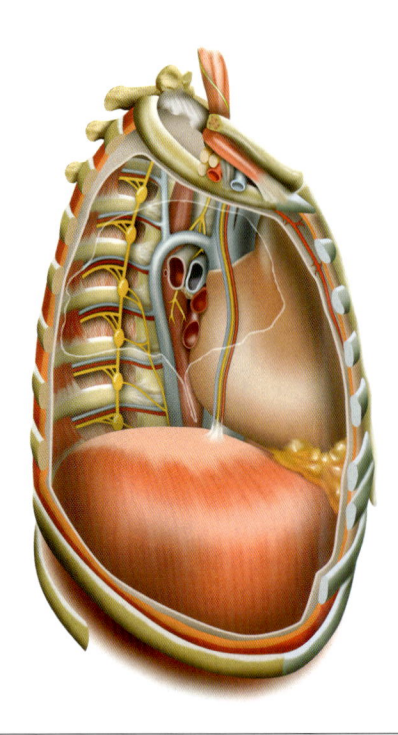

Fig. 8-3 Right lateral view of the thoracic cavity. Refer to text for anatomic description.

CHAPTER 8 Anterolateral Transthoracic Approaches to the Cervicothoracic Junction

Sympathetic Chain
- The sympathetic chain lies over the neck of the rib, close to the intervertebral disk space.
- First thoracic ganglion can combine with the lower cervical ganglion to form the satellite (cervicothoracic) ganglion.

Superior Intercostal Veins
- Drain the upper thoracic intercostal space.
- On right side, drain into the azygos venous system.
- On left side, drain above accessory hemiazygos veins.
- Drain into the left brachiocephalic vein (which also receives the thoracic duct).

Intercostal Arteries
- Superior (highest) artery supplies the first two intercostal spaces and branches off the costocervical trunk.
- Posterior (T3 to T11) artery branches off aorta and ascends obliquely to reach intercostal spaces deep to venous system.

Ascending Aorta and Arch
- Passes anterior to trachea and esophagus to remain on left side.
- Passes inferiorly on the left side of T4 vertebra.
- Three branches from the arch:
  - Brachiocephalic trunk
  - Left common carotid artery
  - Left subclavian artery

Esophagus
- Between trachea and vertebral column.
- Anterior to T1 to T4 vertebrae.
- Medial and posterior to aortic arch from left side.
- Medial and posterior to azygous vein and superior intercostal veins from right side.

Trachea
- Anterior and slightly right of the esophagus.
- Arch of aorta is at first anterior to the trachea and then is on the left side.
- Brachiocephalic trunk and left common carotid arteries ascend to straddle the trachea and separate it from the brachiocephalic veins.

APPROACHES AND TECHNIQUE

INDICATIONS AND ADVANTAGES
Transpleural Transthoracic Third Rib Resection Approach
- This approach provides the best exposure of the anterolateral region of the upper thoracic vertebrae.

Transaxillary Approach
- Ideal for thin female patients.
- Should be reserved for situations in which wide exposure of the cervicothoracic region is not necessary.
- Allows preservation of the shoulder girdle muscles.
- Violation of the pleural space is not necessary.

CONTRAINDICATIONS AND DISADVANTAGES
Transpleural Transthoracic Third Rib Resection Approach
- Requires mobilization of the scapular and muscle dissection.
- Requires violation of the pleural space and a chest tube.
- Does not expose the cervical area.
- Simultaneous posterior stabilization not possible via same exposure.

Transaxillary Approach
- Difficult in obese and muscular patients.
- Provides limited exposure as compared with the transthoracic approach.
- Places the brachial plexus at risk.
- Does not expose the cervical area.
- Simultaneous posterior stabilization is not possible via same exposure.

PATIENT POSITIONING
Transpleural Transthoracic Third Rib Resection Approach
- General endotracheal anesthesia.
- Double lumen tube with lung isolation (Fig. 8-4).
- Lateral decubitus position with the appropriate side up.

Transaxillary Approach
- Lateral decubitus position with the appropriate side up or torso of the ipsilateral side elevated beyond 60 degrees.
- Arm abducted and elbow flexed.

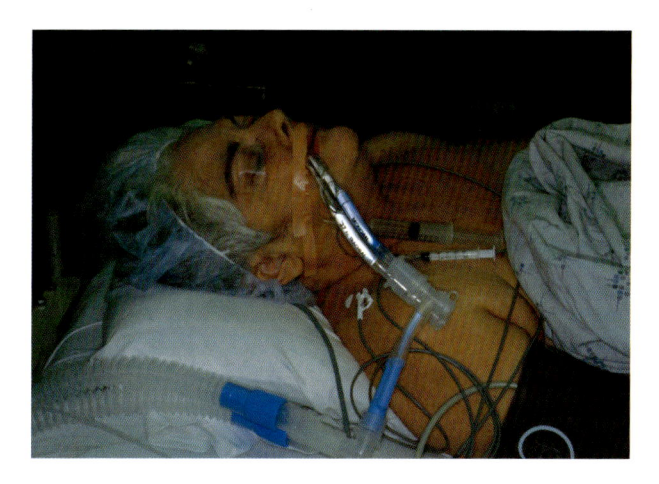

Fig. 8-4 Standard double lumen endotracheal intubation should be performed prior to positioning for the high transthoracic approach.

74　SECTION I　SURGICAL ANATOMY AND APPROACHES

Fig. 8-5 Patient is positioned in lateral on a Jackson spinal table with incision marked for a high transthoracic approach.

INCISION AND OPERATIVE PROCEDURE
Transpleural Transthoracic Third Rib Resection Approach

- Skin is incised from the paraspinous area at approximately T1 and taken distally along the medial border of the scapula to the seventh rib. This incision is continued first laterally, then anteriorly, then medially to the costal cartilage of the third rib (Fig. 8-5).
- The trapezius and latissimus dorsi (rarely, rhomboid major and serratus posterior muscles) are divided, after which the third rib is identified (Fig. 8-6A and B).
- The scapula is then retracted cephalad and medially using a scapular retractor to expose the subscapular space (Fig. 8-7).
- In identifying the third rib, it is important to recall that the first rib is located somewhat medially to the second rib.
- Lungs are isolated and deflated at this point or earlier.
- Anterior periosteal rib dissection can be done with cautery and curettes (Fig. 8-8).
- A posterior subperiosteal dissection of the third rib is performed using a doyen (Fig. 8-9).
- Third rib is resected using a rib cutter as far anteriorly and posteriorly as possible (Fig. 8-10). Resection of the third rib will allow for greater intercostal spreading than would a second rib resection and also serves as graft material, if needed.
- Third rib bed consisting of periosteum, endothoracic fascia, and parietal pleura is identified and transected to enter the thoracic cavity (Fig. 8-11).
- A chest spreader can then be inserted and opened (Fig. 8-12).
- Alternatively, an intercostal (rib preservation) approach can be performed with detachment of the intercostals superior to the third rib. This prevents injury to the neurovascular bundle located on the inferior rib border (see Fig. 8-12). Exposure, however, will be less than with rib resection.
- After deflating and retracting the lung, the spine is clearly exposed. A wet lap can be used to cover and protect the lung for retraction.
- Structures of the superior mediastinum should be identified, depending on side of approach (see Figs. 8-2 and 8-3)

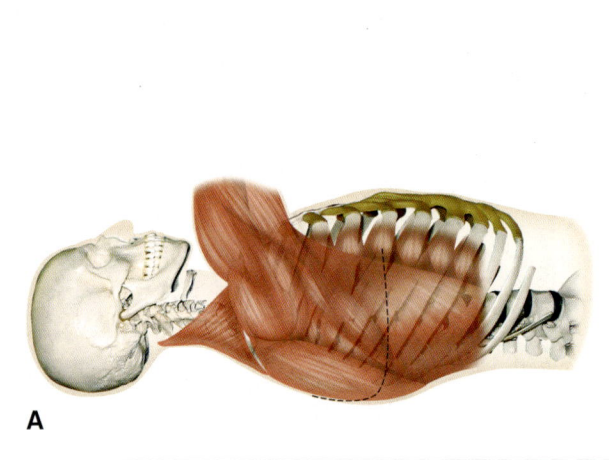

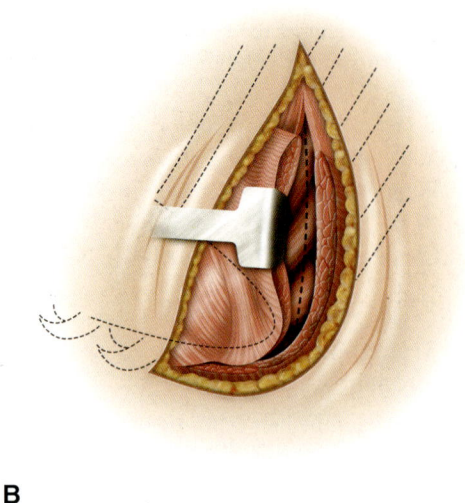

Fig. 8-6 Muscular exposure. A, Note the relationship of the periscapular muscular anatomy. B, Retracting or detaching the latissimus muscle will reveal the underlying upper thoracic ribs and the attachments of the serratus anterior muscles.

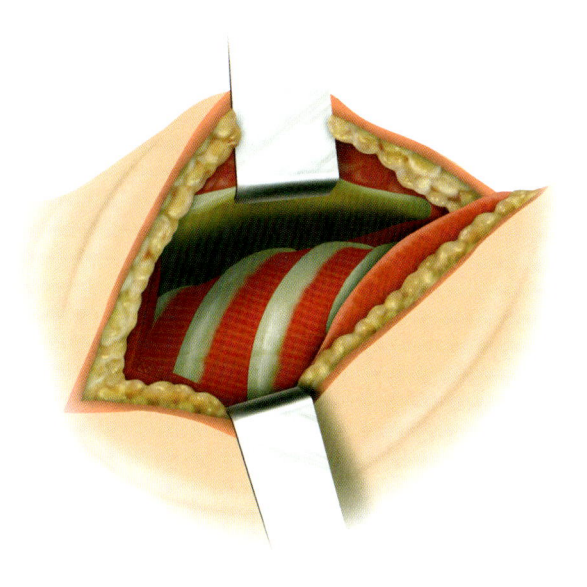

CHAPTER 8   Anterolateral Transthoracic Approaches to the Cervicothoracic Junction

Fig. 8-7 Subscapular anatomy is depicted after retraction of the scapular in a cephalad medial direction.

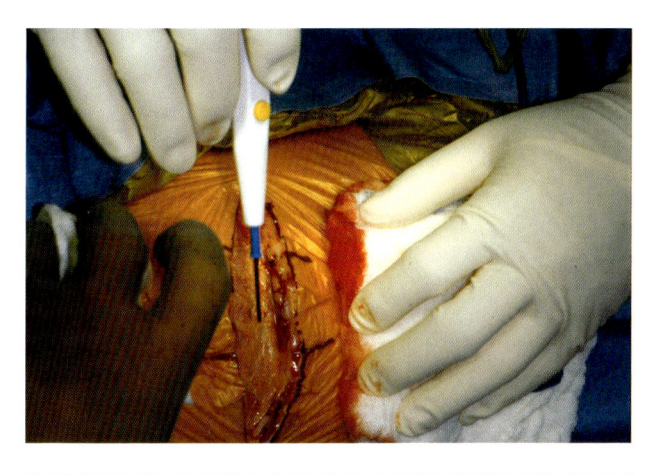

Fig. 8-8 Rib dissection can be exposed with use of cautery and subperiosteal dissection.

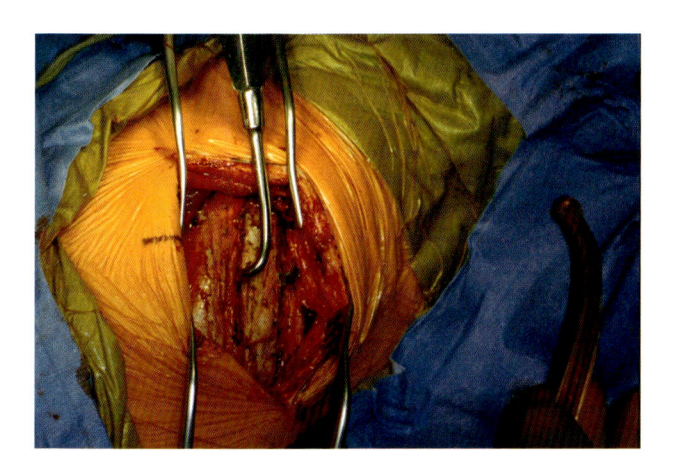

Fig. 8-9 A posterior subperiosteal dissection of the third rib is performed using a doyen.

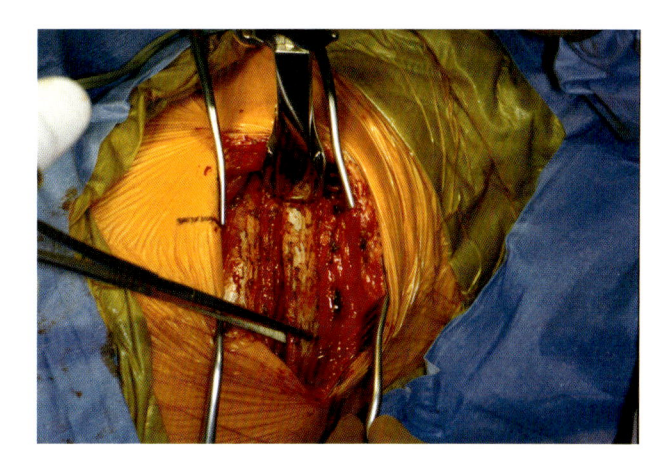

Fig. 8-10 Third rib is resected using a rib cutter as far anteriorly and posteriorly as possible.

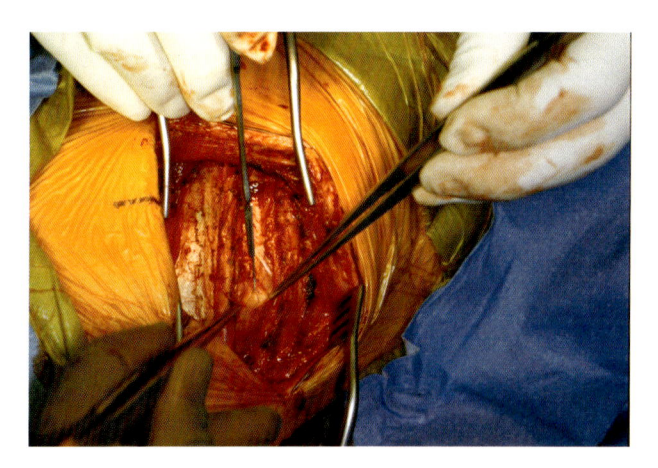

Fig. 8-11 Third rib bed consisting of periosteum, endothoracic fascia, and parietal pleura is identified and transected to enter the thoracic cavity.

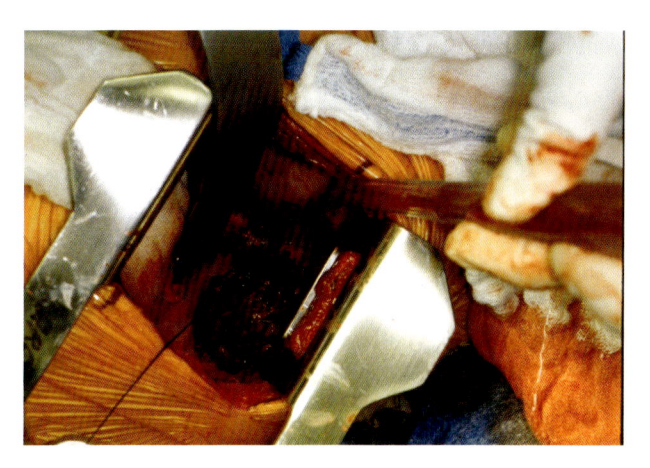

Fig. 8-12 Operative exposure. A chest spreader can then be inserted and opened after rib resection.

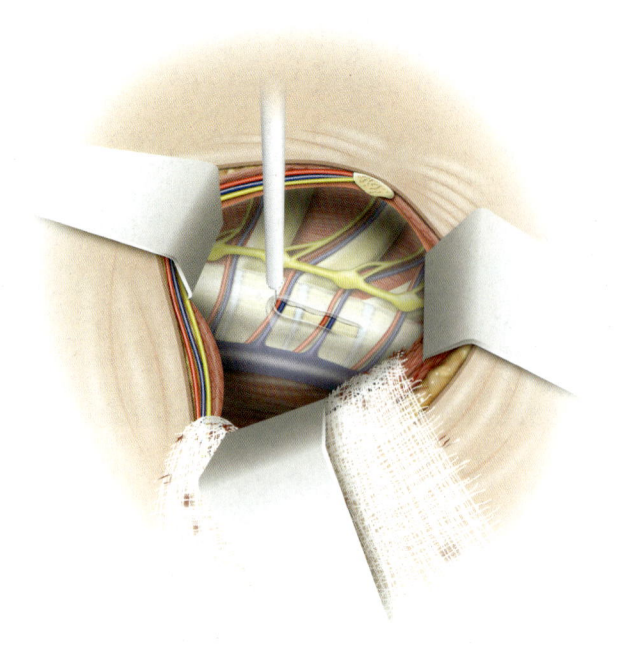

Fig. 8-13 Parietal pleura overlying the ribs and spinal column is identified and can be opened by incising from the costochondral cartilage to the midvertebral body.

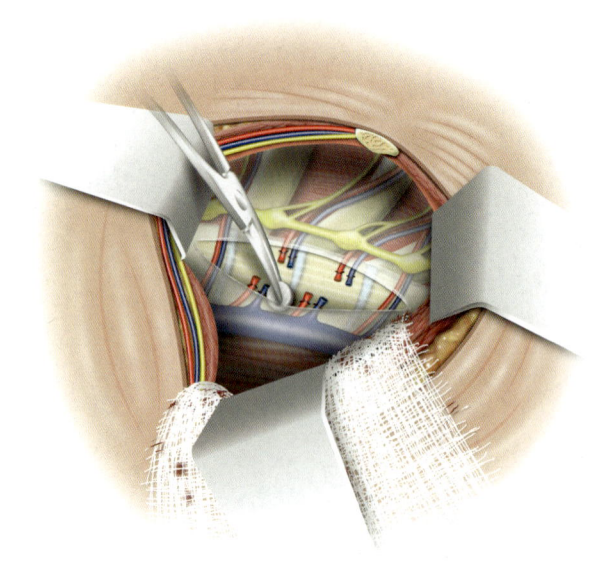

Fig. 8-14 Appropriate intercostal arteries and veins are dissected, ligated, and cut.

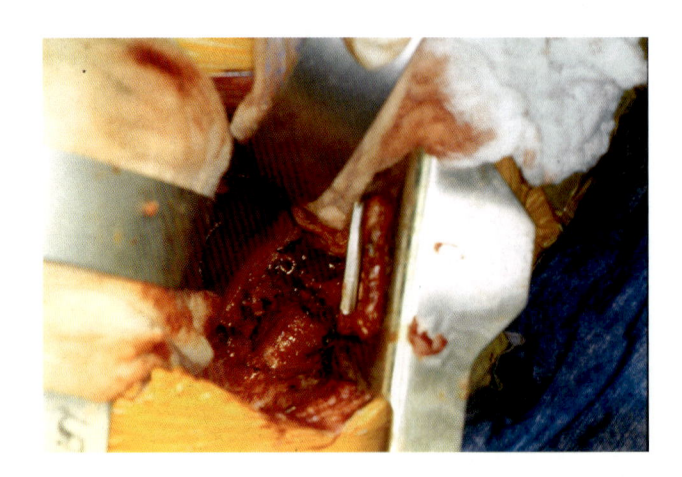

Fig. 8-15 Intraoperative photograph after vertebrectomy through a high transthoracic approach.

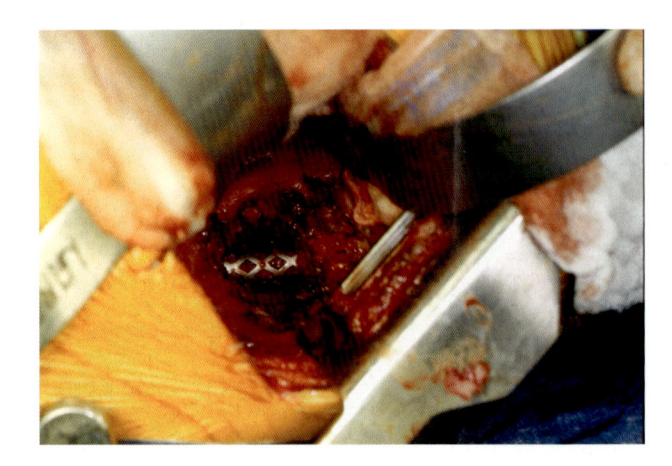

Fig. 8-16 A cage can be used to reconstruct the vertebrectomy defect.

- Parietal pleura overlying the ribs and spinal column is identified and can be opened by incising from the costochondral cartilage to the midvertebral body (Fig. 8-13).
- Opening the pleura will expose the intervertebral disks, the sympathetic chain, and the superior intercostal arteries and veins. Less bleeding will be encountered if dissection is initiated over the disk space.
- Appropriate intercostal arteries and veins are dissected, ligated, and cut (Fig. 8-14).
- Vertebrectomy can then be performed if necessary (Fig. 8-15).
- Vertebral reconstruction of the anterior column is performed if a vertebrectomy is completed (Fig. 8-16).

Transaxillary Approach

- Incision is made transversely at base of axilla from the posterior border of the pectoralis major muscle to the anterior border of the latissimus dorsi muscle.
- Identify the pectoralis major muscles anteriorly and the latissimus dorsi muscle posteriorly.
- Identify the chest wall. Some dissection of the pectoralis major may be necessary. Oblique dissection of the axillary tissues should be avoided.
- By palpation, feel the first through third ribs. The third rib will be the entry site.
- The large intercostobrachial nerve exiting from the second intercostal space may be encountered and should be sacrificed to minimize chances of postoperative neuralgia.

CHAPTER 8 Anterolateral Transthoracic Approaches to the Cervicothoracic Junction

- If dissection is carried out too far cephalad and anterior, the brachial plexus and axillary vasculature can be encountered and injured.
- The thoracodorsal nerve and artery can also be encountered during the exposure and should be preserved.
- Once the third rib is isolated, periosteal dissection should be performed as previously described.
- After rib resection, the lung apex and parietal pleura may be visible.
- At this point, either an extrapleural approach or transpleural approach is possible.
- With an extrapleural approach, the lung apex can be retracted caudally.
- For a wider caudal exposure, a transpleural approach is preferred.
- Transpleural entry is gained through the third rib bed.
- Dissection of the vertebral space is as previously described.

Closure

- Parietal pleura is closed if possible, although a small defect can be left without significant consequences.
- Lungs can be re-expanded.
- A chest tube should be placed into the wound and brought out through an inferior stab incision as low as the ninth intercostal space.
- Rib bed should be closed.
- Rib approximator is used to reapproximate the ribs for closure with wire or nylon sutures (Fig. 8-17).

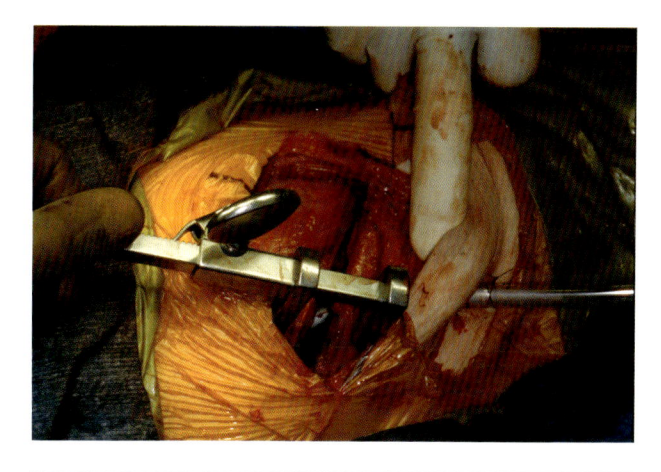

Fig. 8-17 Rib approximator is used to reapproximate the ribs for closure with wire or nylon sutures.

- Each muscle layer is independently reapproximated using 0 polyglycolic acid (Vicryl) sutures.
- Skin can be stapled and chest tube secured with a purse-string stitch.
- A subcutaneous drain should be placed (especially in the transaxillary approach because lymphatic drainage can be expected).
- Chest tube can be removed usually in 2 to 3 days once drainage is low and a persistent air leak is not demonstrated.

CHAPTER 9

HOANG N. LE

DANIEL H. KIM

Posterolateral Approaches to the Cervicothoracic Junction (Transpedicular, Costotransversectomy, Lateral Extracavitary, and Parascapular Extrapleural Approaches)

INTRODUCTION

Extended posterolateral approaches to the cervicothoracic junction allows for excellent exposure of T1 to T4 vertebral bodies but limited exposure of C7. These approaches can be subclassified based on degrees of lateral dissection and exposure of the anterior lateral spinal column. Figure 9-1 demonstrates the viewing angle and extent of lateral exposure gained from each approach. Through these approaches, decompression of neural tissue is performed under direct visualization at all times with minimal manipulation of the thecal sac. Furthermore, posterior stabilization can be performed simultaneously through the same incision. Relative disadvantages are that only the inferior aspect of C7 vertebral body is available through this approach, and that is partially obstructed by the T1 nerve root and rami communicantes to the stellate ganglion.

ANATOMY

SCAPULAR AND PARASCAPULAR ANATOMY

In order to maximize posterolateral access to the high thoracic area, mobilization of the scapula anterolaterally is necessary. This requires dissection of the posteromedial shoulder musculature and familiarity of the muscles in this area. These muscle groups can be divided into superficial, intermediate, and deep layers (Fig. 9-2).

Superficial Muscle Group

TRAPEZIUS
- Originates along the superior nuchal line and external occipital protuberance and on each spinous process (via the ligamentum nuchae) from C1 through T12.
- Functions in stabilization and abduction of the shoulder.
- Supplied by the spinal accessory nerve that arises from C1 to C5 and directly via the ventral rami of C3 and C4. The spinal accessory nerve lies deep to the trapezius muscle but superficial to the levator scapulae.
- Arterial supply is from branches of the dorsal scapular artery.

RHOMBOID MAJOR, RHOMBOID MINOR
- Immediately deep to the trapezius muscle.
- The rhomboid major originates on the ligamentum nuchae of the spinous processes T1 through T4, whereas the rhomboid minor originates similarly on the spinous processes of C6 and C7.
- Insertion into the scapular spine: rhomboid minor above and rhomboid major below.
- The nervous innervation and arterial supply: dorsal scapular nerve and artery.

LEVATOR SCAPULAE
- Immediately deep to the trapezius muscle.
- Insertion into the scapular spine above the rhomboid minor.
- Nervous supply: via branches from C3, C4, and C5.

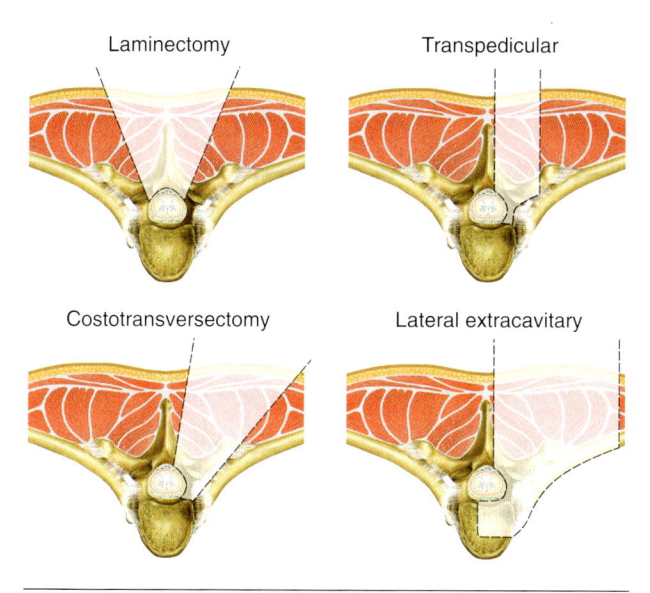

Fig. 9-1 Viewing angle and extent of lateral exposure gained from each posterior approach.

- Arterial supply: dorsal scapular artery.
- In a routine exposure, neither the dorsal scapular nerve nor the dorsal scapular artery or vein is directly exposed.

Intermediate Muscle Group

Serratus Posterior Superior Muscle
- From C6 through approximately T2.

Splenius Capitis and Splenius Cervicis
- Function in stabilization and rotation of the skull.
- Splenius capitis inserts with the sternocleidomastoid muscle on the superior nuchal line and mastoid process.
- Splenius cervicis joins the levator scapulae to insert on the transverse processes of C1 through C4.

Deep or Intrinsic Muscle Group

Erector Spinae Muscles (Spinalis, Longissimus, Iliocostalis)
- Originate as a dense aponeurotic band from the sacrum and divide into three columns below the last rib.
- Iliocostalis muscle is located most laterally and is inserted into the angles of the ribs and into the cervical transverse processes from C4 through C6.
- Longissimus muscles (thoracis, cervicis, and capitis) are inserted into lumbar and thoracic transverse processes and nearby parts of the ribs between T2 and T12. Muscle bundles arising medial to these, from T1 to T4, are relayed to the cervical transverse processes from C2 through C6 and extend to attach to the mastoid process deep to the splenius capitis and sternocleidomastoid muscles. The

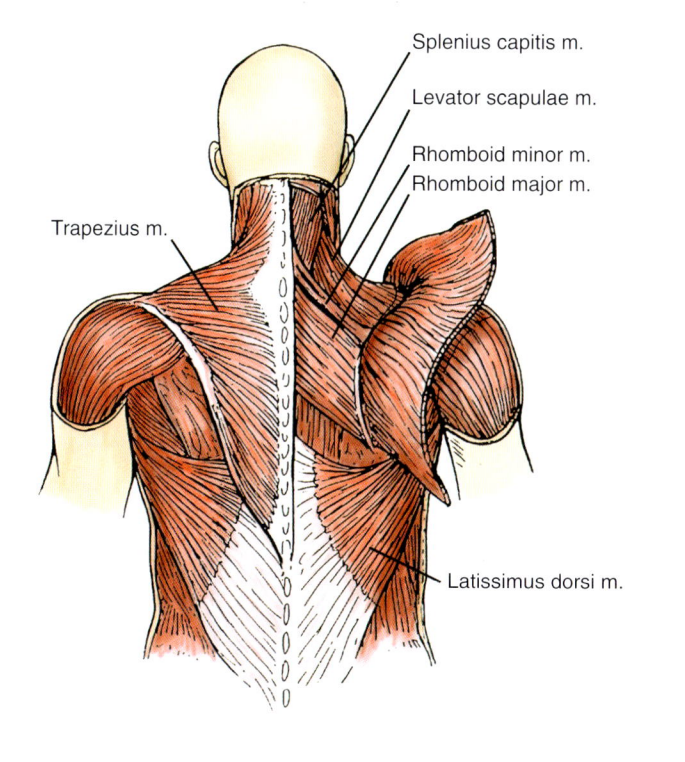

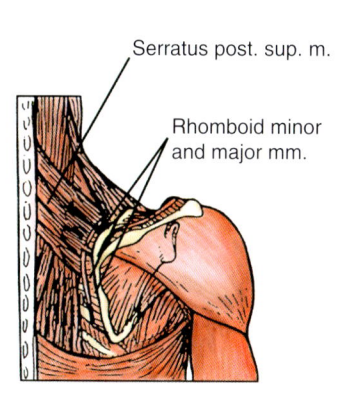

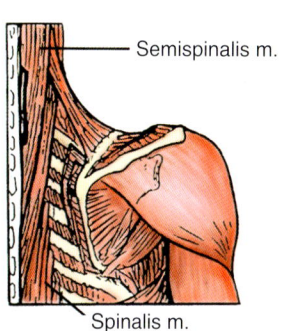

Fig. 9-2 Dissection of the posteromedial shoulder musculature. These muscle groups can be divided into superficial, intermediate, and deep layer muscles.

longissimus is the only erector spinae muscle to reach the skull.
- Spinalis muscle is largely aponeurotic and extends from the upper lumbar to the lower cervical spinous processes.

Transversospinalis Muscles (Semispinalis, Multifidus, Rotators)

- Pass obliquely cephalad from the transverse processes to the spinous processes immediately deep to the erector spinae muscles.
- Semispinalis arises near the tips of the transverse processes and inserts near the tips of the spinous processes approximately five vertebral levels cephalad. In the upper thoracic and lower cervical spine, most of this muscle is composed of the semispinalis capitis. This muscle passes from the upper thoracic transverse processes and lower cervical articular processes (C4 to T4) to the occipital bone between the superior and inferior nuchal lines.
- Multifidus arises from the dense aponeurosis of the overlying erector spinae muscle and from all transverse processes up to C4 and inserts into the lower border of each spinous process. This muscle generally spans about three levels.
- Rotatores are small muscles that bridge one interspace. They pass from the root of one transverse process to the root of the spinous process immediately above. The actions of these muscles extend the vertebral column or, when acting individually on one side, bend and rotate the vertebrae.

In the initial posterolateral dissection of the cervicothoracic junction, the spinous process insertions of the trapezius, rhomboid, serratus posterior superior, splenius capitis, and splenius cervicis are taken down as a single group for lateral retraction. As these muscles are taken down, the scapula is released from its attachments to the spinous processes and rotates anterolaterally out of the operative field. Furthermore, the entire group of erector spinae muscles and transversospinalis muscles can be dissected laterally as a single muscular mass. Control of the musculature in this way exposes all vertebral elements from the tips of the spinous processes to the tips of the transverse processes as well as the costotransverse ligaments, the joints, and the ribs. This maneuver exposes the posterior and posterior lateral rib cage for the remainder of the procedure.

Posterior Thoracic Cage

- In the thoracic spine, each rib articulates with its own vertebral body, the vertebra above, and the intervertebral disk between them. In the upper thoracic spine, the only exception to this general rule is the first rib, which articulates only with its own vertebral body.
- The tubercle of each rib also articulates with the transverse process of its own vertebra. Three important groups of ligaments articulate the rib with the corresponding vertebral body and transverse process and are disrupted for rib removal (Fig. 9-3):
  - Anterior and posterior superior costotransverse ligaments join the neck of the rib to the transverse process immediately above.
  - Lateral and medial costotransverse ligaments attach the posterior neck of the rib to the transverse process.
  - Anterior costovertebral (radiate) ligament secures head of rib to vertebral body.
- The ribs are also attached to one another through the intercostal musculature, which originates medially on each superior rib and inserts laterally on its immediately inferior rib.

After rib resection, a strip of intercostal musculature is isolated between each rib and contains the intercostal nerve, artery, and vein. Most frequently, the intercostal vein is most cephalad and the intercostal nerve most caudad. Immediately ventral to the intercostal bundle lies the pleura.

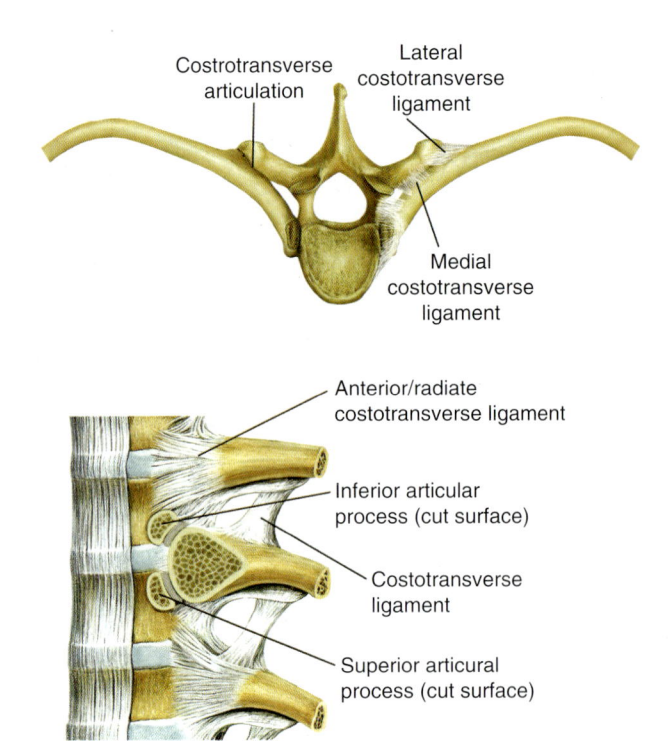

Fig. 9-3 Three groups of ligaments articulate the rib with the corresponding vertebral body and transverse process and are disrupted for rib removal: Anterior and posterior superior costotransverse ligaments, lateral and medial costotransverse ligaments, and anterior costovertebral (radiate) ligament.

Retromediastinal Space Anatomy

- Pleura can be separated from the lateral vertebral elements. A layer of retropleural fat is often apparent anteromedially and can aid in the dissection plane (Fig. 9-4).

CHAPTER 9 Posterolateral Approaches to the Cervicothoracic Junction

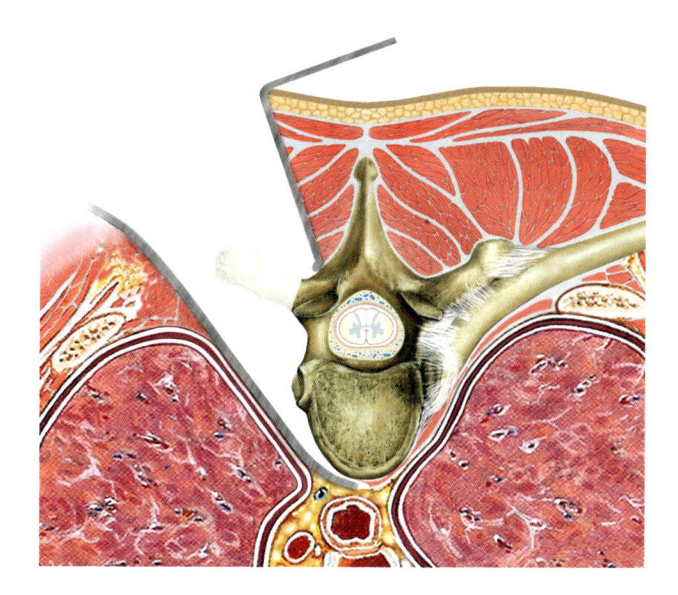

Fig. 9-4 Anatomic illustration after costotransversectomy and retractor placement. Pleura can be separated from the lateral vertebral elements. A layer of retropleural fat is often apparent anteromedially and can aid in the dissection plane.

- Tracing the intercostal bundle medially will identify the neural foramen.
- Because the aortic arch does not reach the top of the thoracic cavity, the arterial supply to the chest wall has become specialized.
  - First two intercostal spaces are supplied by branches of the costocervical trunk through the highest intercostal artery. This artery descends anteriorly to the ventral rami of the eighth cervical and first thoracic nerves on the necks of the first two ribs.
  - Remaining intercostal arteries arise from the posterior surface of the thoracic aorta. Each intercostal artery stretches obliquely across each vertebral body from caudad to cephalad close to the vertebral body periosteum and is located deep to the azygos or hemiazygos vein, the thoracic duct, and the sympathetic trunk.
- Neural structures:
  - Ventral ramus of the first thoracic nerve passes cephalad across the neck of the first rib to join the eighth cervical nerve in the brachial plexus.
  - A small intercostal branch runs across the inferior surface of the first rib to enter the first interspace close to the costal cartilage.
  - Ventral ramus of the second thoracic nerve also usually sends a small branch to the brachial plexus.
  - Although the intercostal nerves below T1 can usually be sacrificed to facilitate exposure, T1 and C7, which frequently are exposed during this procedure, cannot be sacrificed without suffering severe neurologic deficit to hand function.

POSTERIOR-POSTEROLATERAL APPROACHES AND TECHNIQUES

INDICATIONS AND ADVANTAGES
Laminectomy
- Pathology located primarily on the dorsal surface of the spinal canal (Fig. 9-5).
- Anterior and middle spinal column integrity is preserved.
- Ability to address pathologies extending the axis of the dorsal spinal column.
- When stabilization is not required.

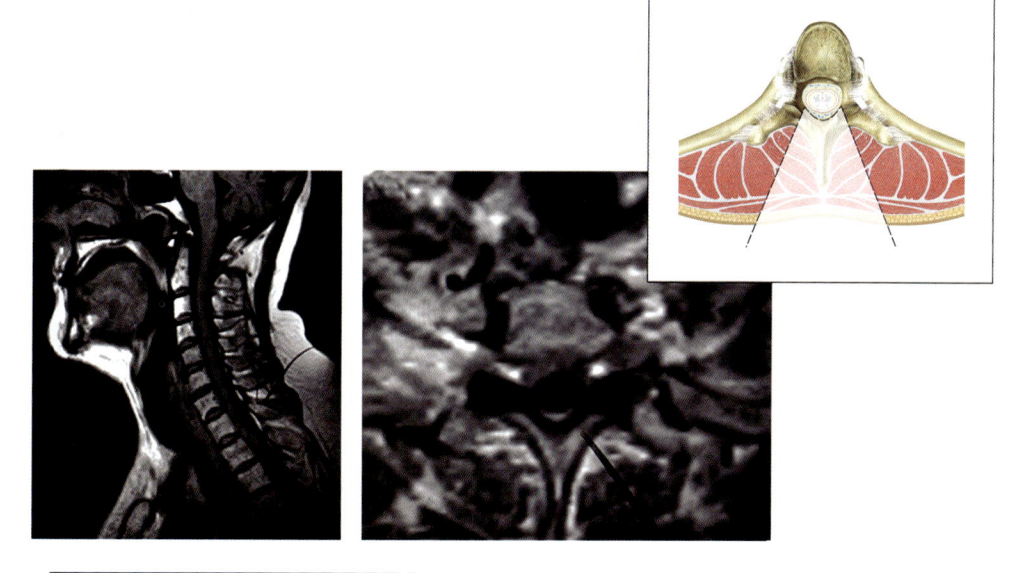

Fig. 9-5 A laminectomy approach is ideal only for pathology located dorsally.

Transpedicular Approach
- Can be used for simple biopsies of anterior column pathologies.
- Provides lateral access to the spinal cord.
- In combination with a laminectomy and ultrasound guidance, degree of spinal cord decompression can be assessed and may obviate need for extensive posterolateral dissection.
- Extensive bony-ligamentous removal not necessary, and thus, need for stabilization is minimized.

Costotransversectomy
- Provides a limited ability to address anterior column pathologies.
- Can be done bilaterally for increased vertebral body decompression.
- Possible to simultaneously reconstruct the anterior column and stabilize posteriorly.
- Pleural space violation not necessary.

Lateral Extracavitary Approach (LECA)
- Provides an opportunity for circumferential decompression and simultaneous stabilization.
- Can address midline ventral pathologies directly.
- Pleural space violation not necessary.
- Neural decompression performed under direct visualization.

Parascapular Extrapleural Approach
- Procedural modification of the LECA for the cervicothoracic junction.
- Increase mobilization of the scapula allows better exposure of the cervicothoracic junction.
- Other benefits similar to LECA.

CONTRAINDICATIONS AND DISADVANTAGES
Laminectomy
- With disruption of the anterior and middle spinal column, a stand-alone laminectomy will further destabilize the cervicothoracic region. Increasing kyphosis from increasing instability will result in progression of neurologic deficit.
- Anterior column visualization and reconstruction are not possible.
- Inability to address anterior column pathologies.
- Limited ability to address pathologies lateral to the spinal cord.

Transpedicular Approach
- Extensive anterior column decompression and reconstruction are not possible.
- Difficult to address calcified hard lesions.
- Decompression done without direct visualization.

Costotransversectomy
- Unable to address midline ventral lesions directly.
- Anterior column reconstruction possible but difficult.
- Sacrificing intercostal nerve roots may be necessary.
- Stabilization is necessary.

Lateral Extracavitary Approach
- Significant muscle dissection can lead to marked atrophy.
- Recovery time is more prolonged.
- Sacrificing intercostal nerve roots may be necessary.
- Stabilization is necessary.

Parascapular Extrapleural Approach
- Same as for LECA.

PATIENT POSITIONING (Fig. 9-6)
- General endotracheal anesthesia.
- Prone in Mayfield three-point pin fixation.
- Two padded rolls, one across under the chest and the other supporting the iliac crest.
- The abdomen should hang freely so that the inferior vena cava is not compressed and adequate ventilation can occur.
- Patient is placed in reverse Trendelenburg position with knees flexed. This will reduce the venous bleeding.
- Arms are padded and tucked to the sides.
- Shoulder tape can be placed to reduce the lordotic skinfold at the cervicothoracic area.
- Check for pressure areas (eyes, chin, ulnar, knees, genitalia, extremities).
- Prep and drape wide if stabilization is anticipated.

INCISION AND OPERATIVE PROCEDURE
For All Procedures
- Local anesthetic is given to incision site.
- We prefer a midline incision (Fig. 9-7) (length depends on need for stabilization and requirements for decompression). Other incisions may be used (hockey stick, paramedian, curvilinear, transverse).
- Midline dissection is performed down the avascular nuchal plane.
- Subperiosteal dissection is made along the spinous process and lamina.
- Paraspinal musculature should be dissected together and retracted laterally as a single bulk. Paralytics given for the initial dissection will greatly facilitate muscle dissection laterally.
- Each episode of bleeding should be controlled before proceeding:
  - Carefully coagulate any draining veins encountered during midline dissection.
  - If bleeding is not easily controlled, pack very tightly and then continue.

CHAPTER 9   Posterolateral Approaches to the Cervicothoracic Junction   83

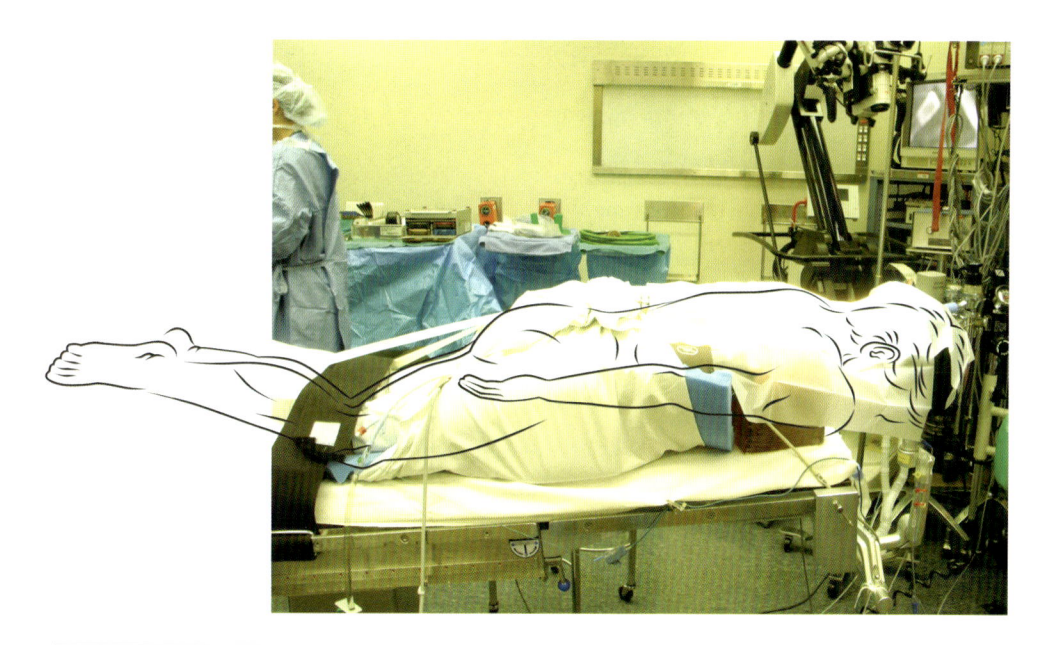

Fig. 9-6 Patient should be positioned prone in pins on chest bolsters, head elevated 15 to 30 degrees.

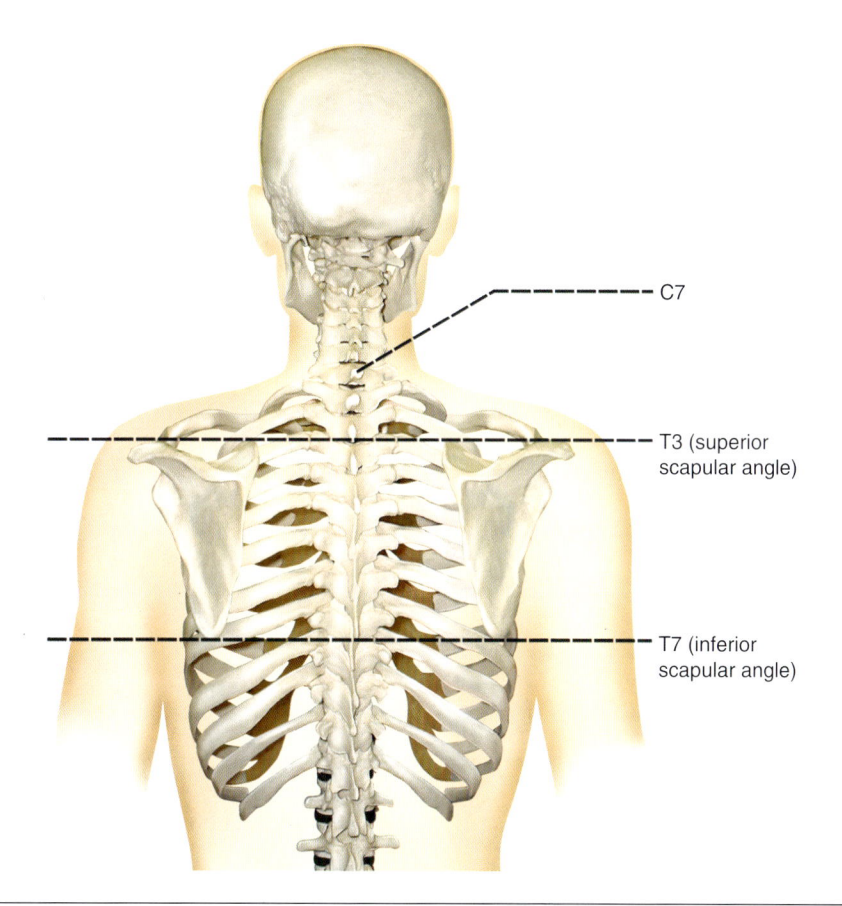

Fig. 9-7 Skeletal diagram showing approximate vertebral level with length of incision needed. T3 approximates the superior scapular angle.

- If dissection is not done in a controlled manner, significant blood loss can be encountered.
- C7-T1 junction can always be identified by the prominent transverse process of T1 and lateral mass of C7.
- In the cervical spine, the interlaminar space is wider than the thoracic area and should not be penetrated during the dissection.
- Do not dissect anterior to the lateral mass or transverse process because of the potential for injury to the nerve root and vertebral artery.
- Extent of lateral exposure will depend on the following approaches.

Transpedicular Approach

- Great variations exist at the cervicothoracic junction in regard to pedicle location.
- It is best to perform at least a laminotomy to palpate the medial wall of the pedicle.
- Pedicle is usually located toward the superior aspect of the lamina at the cervicothoracic junction.
- Cervicothoracic pedicle anatomy:
  - Medial pedicle angle decreases from 50 degrees at C5 to 10 degrees at T5.
  - Sizes of pedicles are approximately 5 mm at C5, 7.5 mm at T1, and 4.5 mm at T5.
  - Spinal nerve is closer to the superior aspect of the pedicle than the inferior aspect at the cervicothoracic junction.
  - Vertebral artery closer to C7 vertebral body than it is to T1.

Costotransversectomy

- Paraspinal muscles are dissected in bulk laterally so that exposure past the costotransverse joint is attained.
- Identify rib, costotransverse joint, and transverse process after periosteal dissection.
- Incise the costotransverse joint and remove the transverse process back toward the pedicle and lamina (Fig. 9-8).
- Rib and its costovertebral articulation can be seen.
- Neurovascular bundle can be seen on the inferior aspect of the rib and can be followed back to the neural foramen.
- Dissect off the posterior periosteum on the outer rib surface.
- Depending on the extent of lateral exposure needed, the entire costovertebral articulation complex can be removed. Care should be taken during the dissection of the anterior periosteum not to injure the pleura. Laterally, this can be separated by using a doyen (Fig. 9-9).
- Alternatively, to reduce injury to the pleura, a thin cortical shell of rib head can be left intact at the costovertebral junction with careful drilling. However, some protection can also be provided by the endothoracic fascia, periosteum, and retropleural fat. Avulsion of the rib from its costovertebral joint can cause significant bleeding. Microscopic dissection at this stage with drilling and Kerrison rongeur would be most prudent (Fig. 9-10).

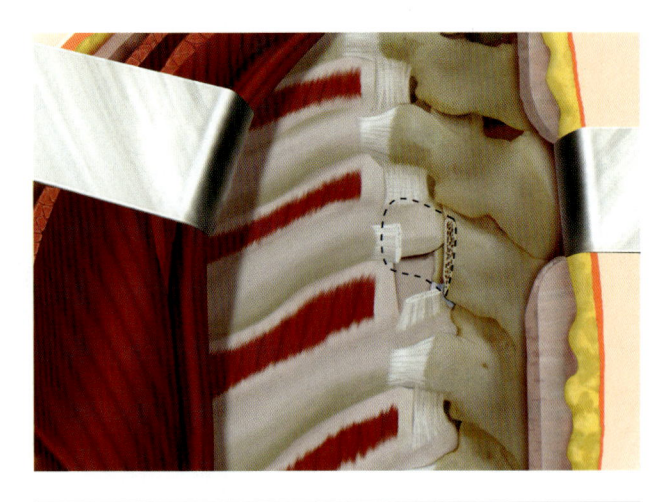

Fig. 9-8 Costotransversectomy technique. Incise the costotransverse joint and remove the transverse process back toward the pedicle and lamina.

- Also note the position of the aorta. At the lower aspect of the cervicothoracic junction the aorta is biased toward the left side of the vertebral body, making a right-sided costotransversectomy approach safer (Fig. 9-11A to C). Side of approach, however, should be dictated by side of pathology.
- With rib removal, periosteum, fascia, and pleura can be retracted anteriorly (see Fig. 9-4).
- The remainder of transverse process, pedicle, and ipsilateral lamina can be removed to identify the disk space, vertebral body, and dura (Fig. 9-12).
- Each thoracic nerve root will exit under the pedicle of its respective level. Therefore, do not sacrifice the nerve root

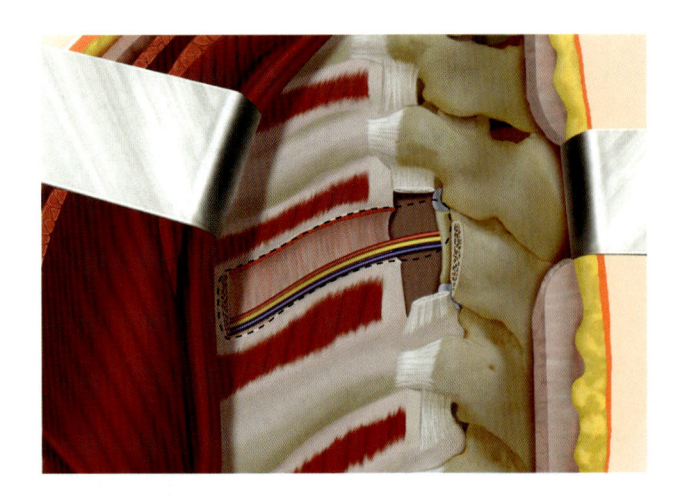

Fig. 9-9 Costotransversectomy technique. The entire costovertebral articulation complex can be removed. Care should be taken during the dissection of the anterior periosteum not to injure the pleura. Laterally, this can be separated by using a doyen.

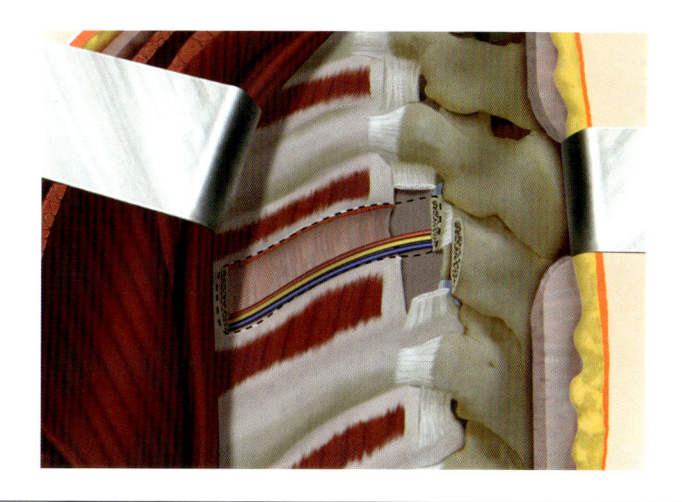

Fig. 9-10 Costotransversectomy technique. To reduce injury to the pleura, a thin cortical shell of rib head can be left intact at the costovertebral junction with careful drilling. However, some protection can also be provided by the endothoracic fascia, periosteum, and retropleural fat. Avulsion of the rib from its costovertebral joint can cause significant bleeding. Microscopic dissection at this stage with drilling and Kerrison rongeur would be most prudent.

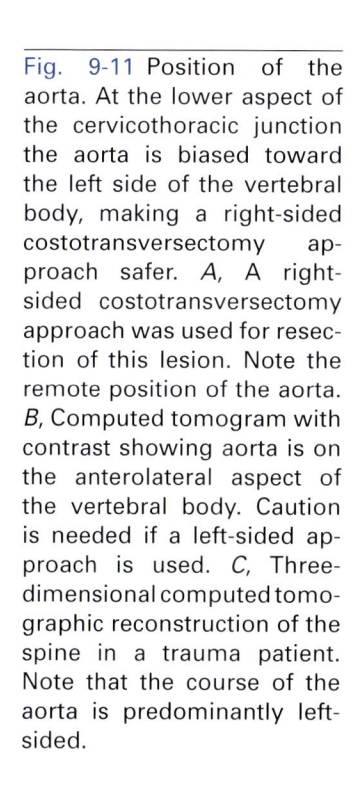

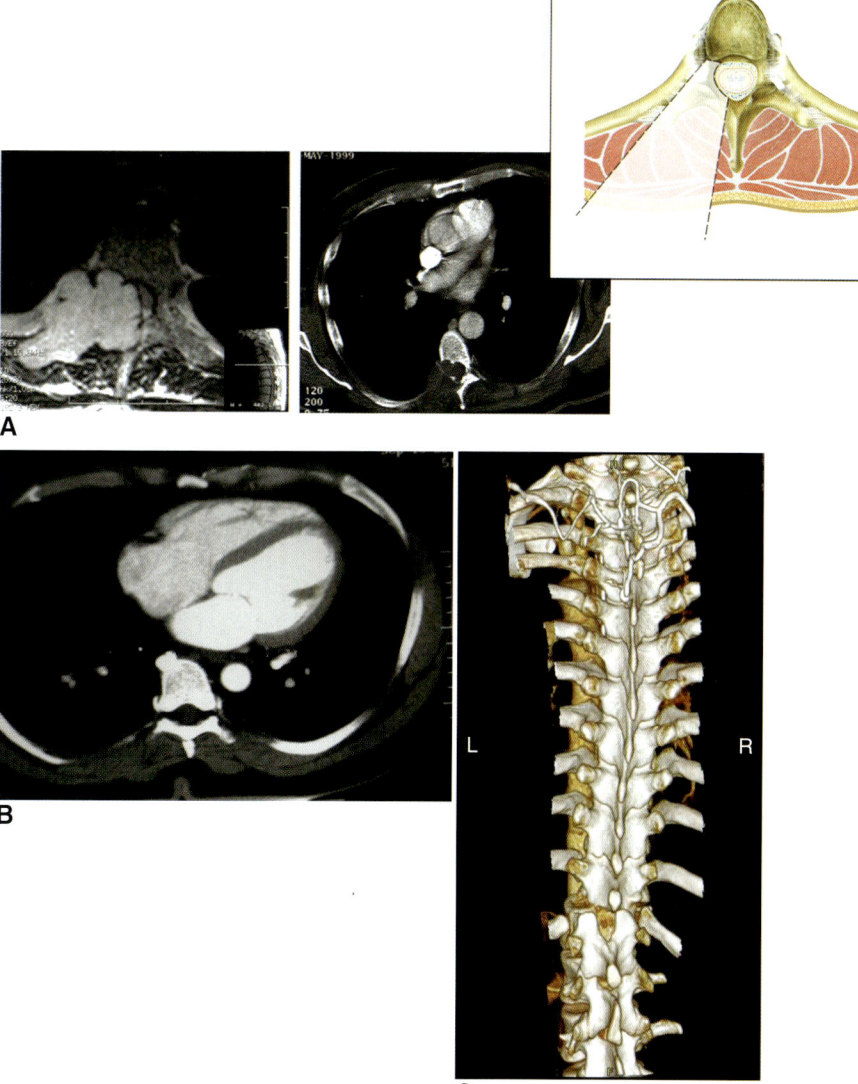

Fig. 9-11 Position of the aorta. At the lower aspect of the cervicothoracic junction the aorta is biased toward the left side of the vertebral body, making a right-sided costotransversectomy approach safer. A, A right-sided costotransversectomy approach was used for resection of this lesion. Note the remote position of the aorta. B, Computed tomogram with contrast showing aorta is on the anterolateral aspect of the vertebral body. Caution is needed if a left-sided approach is used. C, Three-dimensional computed tomographic reconstruction of the spine in a trauma patient. Note that the course of the aorta is predominantly left-sided.

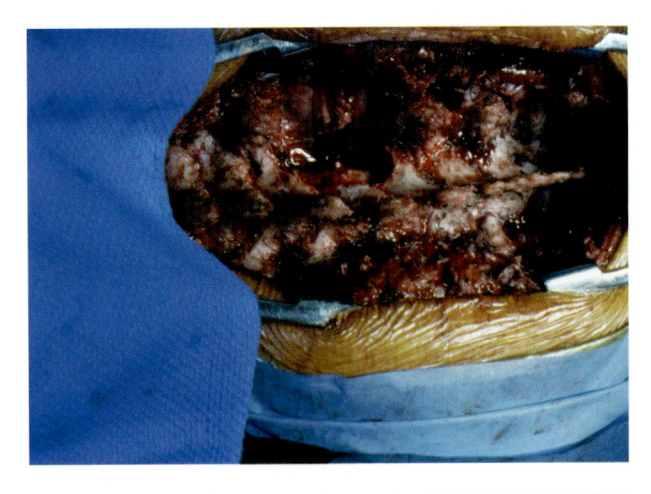

Fig. 9-12 Intraoperative photograph after a costotransvesectomy. The transverse process, pedicle, and ipsilateral lamina can be remove to identify the disk space, vertebral body, and dura.

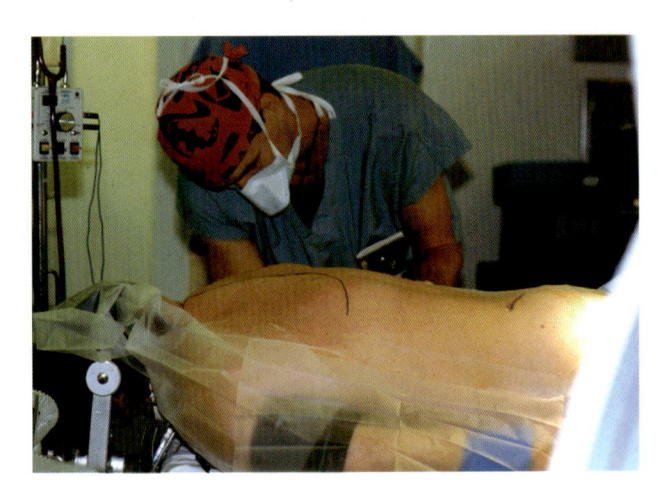

Fig. 9-13 Position and incision for the lateral extracavitary approach. Iliac crest site should also be prepped into field if autograft harvesting is expected.

under the T1 pedicle. If additional exposure is needed, a costotransversectomy procedure can be done at T2 or T3. The T2 nerve root and below can be taken without adverse effects to hand function.
- Decompression of the anterior column can be done with direct visualization of the dura.

Lateral Extracavitary (Parascapular Extrapleural) Approach

- Modification of the costotransversectomy approach.
- A hockey stick incision will facilitate reflection of a myocutaneous flap (Fig. 9-13).
- The trapezius and rhomboid are dissected off the spinous process.
- Slightly deep to the trapezius and rhomboid muscles is a loose areolar tissue plane separating the paraspinal musculature and the longissimus muscle.
- Approach will be lateral to the paraspinal musculature and medial to the longissimus muscle (Fig. 9-14).
- The inferior fibers of the trapezius will be transected in order to reflect the myocutaneous flap. A muscle cuff is left for reapproximation at the end.
- Retraction of the trapezius, rhomboid, and erector spinae muscles and medial border of the scapula laterally exposes the posterior thoracic cage (Fig. 9-15).

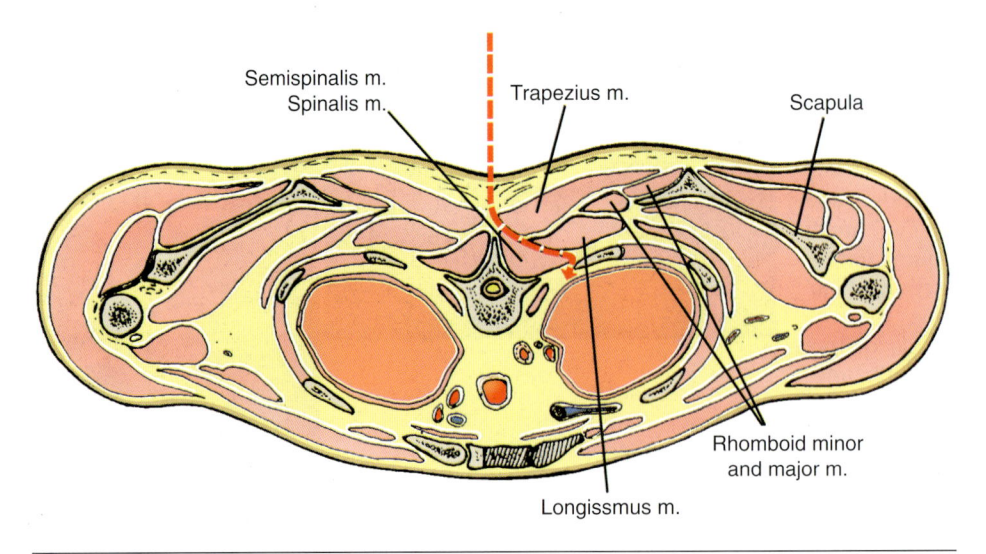

Fig. 9-14 The lateral extracavitary approach will be lateral to the paraspinal musculature and medial to the longissimus muscle.

CHAPTER 9 Posterolateral Approaches to the Cervicothoracic Junction

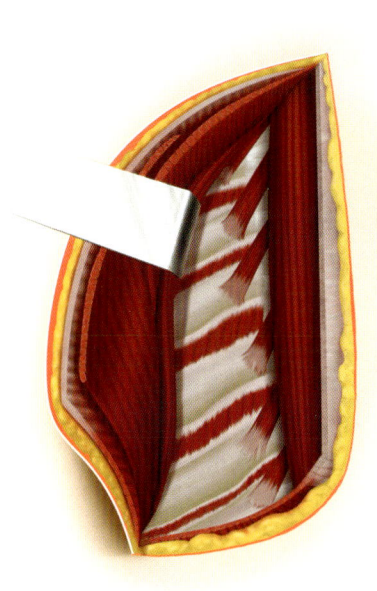

Fig. 9-15 LECA approach. Retraction of the trapezius, rhomboid, erector spinae muscles, and medial border of the scapula laterally exposes the posterior thoracic cage.

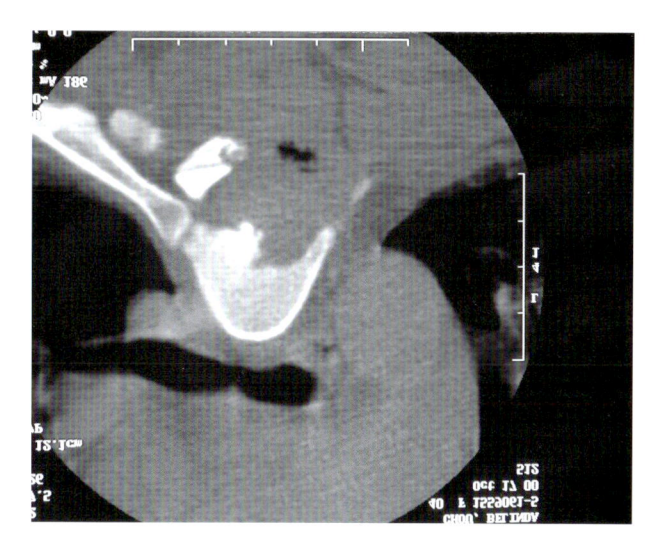

Fig. 9-17 Axial computed tomograph demonstrating the amount of rib resection required in a lateral extracavitary approach.

- Transversospinalis muscles are dissected and retracted medially (Fig. 9-16).
- Dissection of the levator scapulae muscles in the cervical region will further expose the cervicothoracic junction.
- Subperiosteal dissection and removal of the appropriate ribs can be performed as in the costotransversectomy technique except that more than an additional 3 cm of rib removal is usually required (Fig. 9-17).

- Adequate exposure of the vertebral body will often require sacrificing at least one nerve root (Fig. 9-18).
- Direct visualization of the neural elements is available during the corpectomy procedure.
- Vertebral reconstruction and posterior stabilization can be performed without an additional anterior procedure (Fig. 9-19).

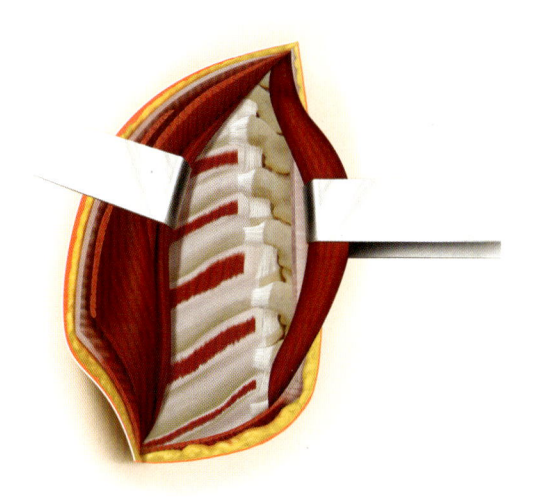

Fig. 9-16 LECA approach. Transversospinalis muscles are dissected and retracted medially.

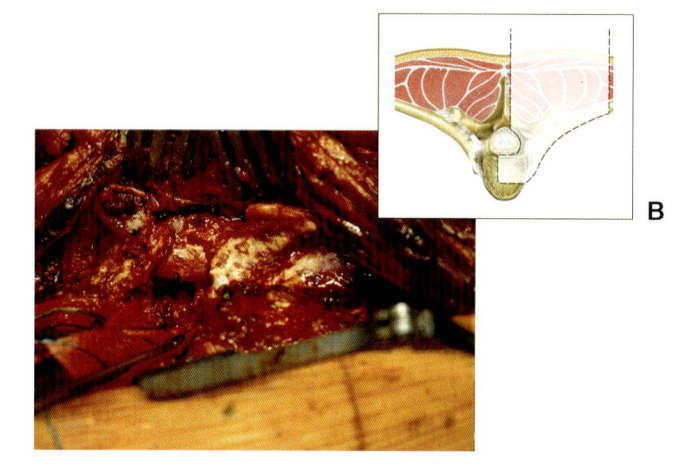

Fig. 9-18 Adequate exposure of the vertebral body will often require sacrificing at least one thoracic nerve root (T2 and below acceptable). *A*, Intraoperative view after lateral extracavitary approach. *B*, Graphic depiction of a LECA decompression.

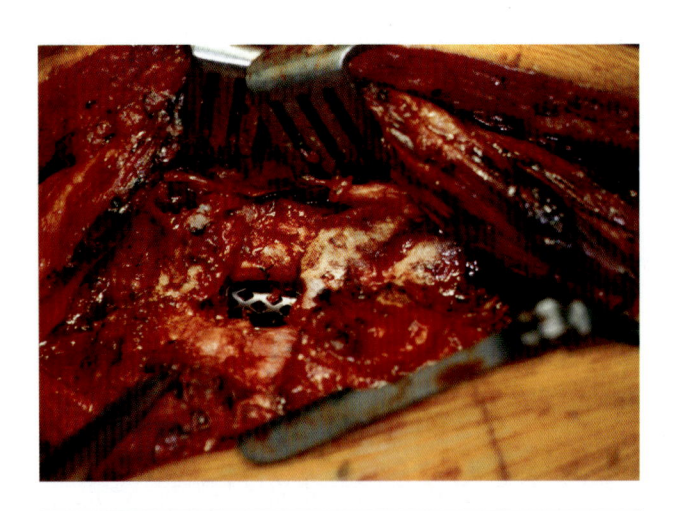

Fig. 9-19 View after cage placement. Vertebral reconstruction and posterior stabilization can be performed without an additional anterior procedure.

CLOSURE

- Before closure, wound is filled with saline to check for an air leak. If present, a 22 to 24 French chest tube should be placed into the wound and brought out through a separate stab incision.
- Any cerebrospinal fluid leak should be repaired to prevent fistula formation.
- Muscles are reapproximated.
- Tight fascia closure is performed.
- Wound is closed in multilayers.

SECTION D
Thoracolumbar and Lumbar Spines

CHAPTER 10

ISSADA THONGTRANGAN
HOANG N. LE
JON PARK
DANIEL H. KIM

Thoracoabdominal Approach

INTRODUCTION

The thoracolumbar junction is unique because it is the transitional zone from the stiff and less mobile thoracic spine to the mobile lumbar spine. It is also a transitional zone between pleural cavity and abdominal cavity. The anatomy surrounding this area is more complicated with the attachment of the diaphragm, psoas and quadratus lumborum, ribs, and major vessels. Because this is a transitional area, therefore, these structures are susceptible to trauma and deformity. The anterior approach to this area is useful; however, it appears to be difficult because of the complicated anatomy of the diaphragm.

In general, for exposure higher than T12 or lower than L2, the 10th rib can be resected and the diaphragm has to be adequately divided, and this is a traditional transpleural-transdiaphragmatic approach.[1] Technically, this exposure is difficult because of the presence of the diaphragm and increased risk involved in simultaneous exposure of the thoracic cavity and the retroperitoneal space. Dividing of the posterior insertion of diaphragm and crus of diaphragm with further retraction downward can give a very good exposure from T12 to L2, and this can be called the *transpleural-retroperitoneal approach*. The "classic" thoracoabdominal approach, made by aggressive cutting of the diaphragm, will expose the anterolateral part of the vertebral body, whereas the less aggressive approach (transpleural-retroperitoneal approach) exposes the lateral aspect of vertebral body and offers less exposure anteriorly.

RELEVANT ANATOMY

MAJOR VESSELS

- Lower in the chest, the aorta lies to the left of the midline, anterior to the vertebral bodies (Fig. 10-1A and B), and leaves the thorax at the level of the 12th thoracic vertebra, whereas the azygos vein, splanchnic nerves, and thoracic duct are to the right of the midline.
- At T10 to L2, the intercostals and lumbar arteries display an essentially horizontal segmental distribution. Arising on each side of the posterior aortic midline, they run horizontally across the middle of the corresponding vertebral bodies.
- At L2 to L4, the lumbar arteries run in a descending direction, arising on each side of the posterior aortic midline at the level of the disk just above their numerically corresponding vertebrae; they then run vertically downward behind the aorta, and they finally run horizontally toward the middle of the vertebral bodies before entering the intervertebral foramen.

DIAPHRAGM

- The diaphragm is a dome-shaped organ that is muscular in the periphery and tendinous in the center. Posteriorly, it originates from the upper lumbar vertebrae through crura, the arcuate ligaments, and the 12th ribs. Anteriorly and laterally, it attaches to the cartilaginous ends of the lower six ribs and xiphoid[2–4] (Fig. 10-2).
- The crura are musculotendinous structures that arise from the anterior longitudinal ligaments of the lumbar vertebrae and extend superiorly to surround the aorta and esophageal hiatus.[5–7]
- The medial arcuate ligaments arise from the crura on the respective sides, cross the psoas muscle as a bridge, and insert on the transverse processes of the first lumbar vertebra.[5–7]
- The lateral arcuate ligaments arise from the transverse process from the first lumbar vertebra extending over the quadratus lumborum muscles to the tips of the 12th ribs.
- The diaphragm is innervated by the phrenic nerve, which descends through the thoracic cavity on the pericardium. The phrenic nerve joins the diaphragm adjacent to the fibrous pericardium, dividing into three major branches that extend peripherally in anterolateral and posterior

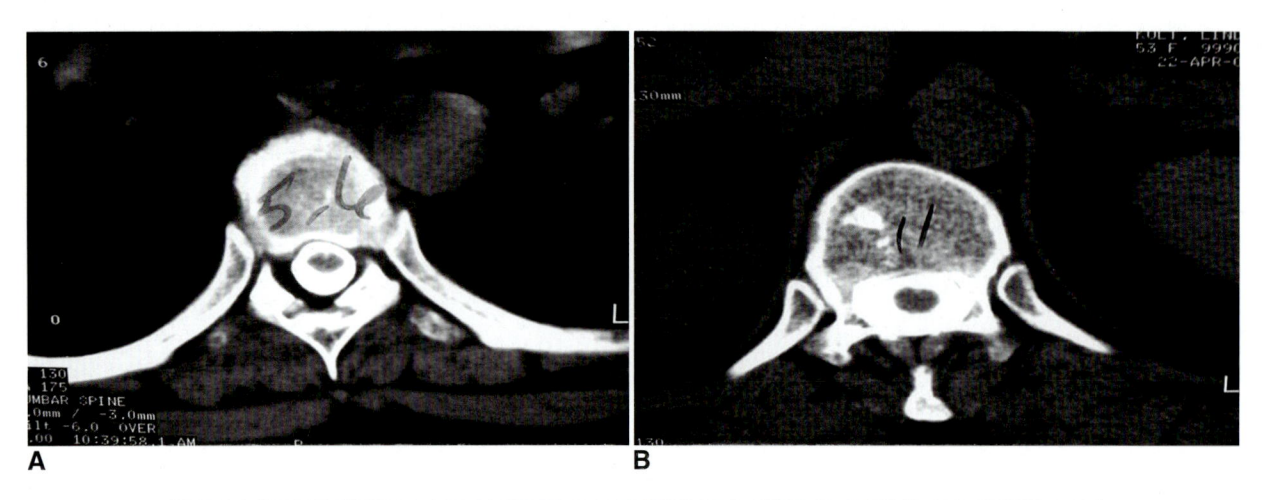

Fig. 10-1 *A,* Axial computed tomographic (CT) scan showing relationship between aortic arch and the upper thoracic vertebra. *B,* Axial CT scan showing relationship of aortic arch and the lower thoracic spine (T10).

directions. Therefore, it is best to make an incision around the periphery of the diaphragm to minimize interference with function when performing a thoracoabdominal approach to the spine.[8,9]

PSOAS MUSCLE

- It runs from the transverse processes of the lumbar vertebrae to attach to the lesser trochanter of the femur and serves to flex the thigh at the hip.

- It is located in a retroperitoneal position and is considered one of the muscles of the posterior abdominal wall muscle.
- There are major and minor components of this muscle.
- The minor component has a longer tendon and attaches to the pelvic brim instead of the lesser trochanter. The psoas minor helps the psoas major flex the hip.
- The psoas major muscle inserts at the lesser trochanter and its major function is hip flexure.[10–12]
- If tuberculosis spreads to the lumbar region, it can spread into the fascia enclosing the psoas muscles and form a psoas abscess. The pus from this abscess can spread inferiorly over the pelvic brim into the inguinal ligament. Because the muscle has important relationships with other abdominal organs such as the pancreas, cancer of the pancreas can also invade the muscle and cause spasms, leading to severe pain.

THE 12TH RIB

- The relationship of the pleural sac to the 12th rib is critical for this approach.
- In summary, if the rib is less than 6 cm long, usually it is in contact with the pleura entirely; whereas, if it is longer, only the posterior 6 cm is in contact with the pleura.[1,13]

RETROARCUATE SPACE

- This is a potential space that is very important for this exposure (Fig. 10-3).
- It is limited anteriorly by the caudal portion of the lumbar part of the diaphragm and posteriorly by the quadratus lumborum and the 12th rib.
- It is limited inferiorly by the lateral arcuate ligament and superiorly it is roofed by the pleura and medially by the transverse process of L1 and the proximal part of the psoas.

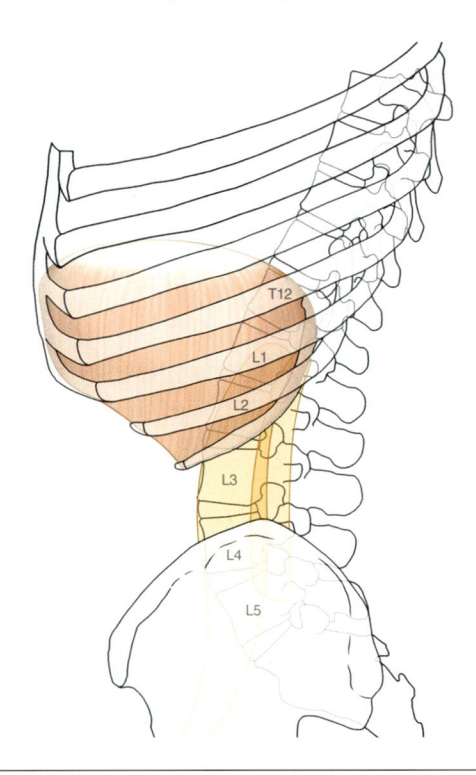

Fig. 10-2 Drawing demonstrates the relationship of diaphragm, ribs, and pleura in sagittal plane.

CHAPTER 10   Thoracoabdominal Approach   91

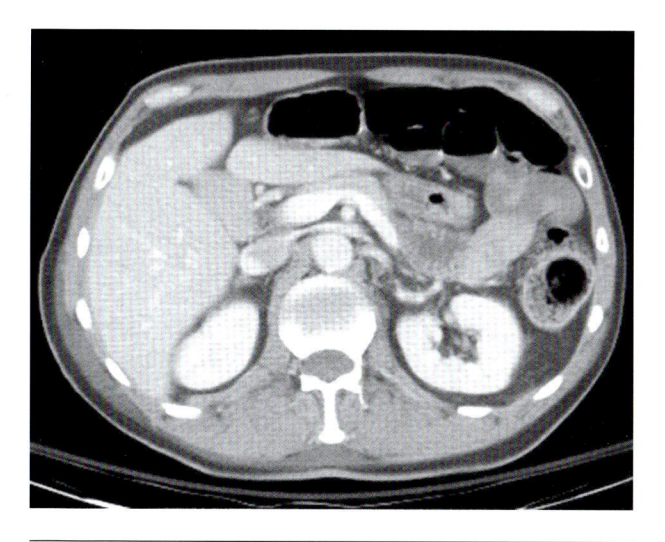

Fig. 10-3 Axial computed tomographic scan at the thoracolumbar junction showing retroperitoneal potential space and surrounding contents.

- Its apex is located laterally where the lateral arcuate ligament is attached to the 12th rib.
- The pleura is vulnerable to puncture at the point where the pleura attaches to the 12th rib.
- The space looks pyramidal in shape, with its base medial and its apex lateral. The lower thoracic vertebral bodies could be approached extrapleurally through this space.

NERVE AND PLEXUS

- The genitofemoral nerve mainly branches from the L1 and L2 nerve root, pierces through the psoas muscle toward the anterior side from the posterior side, and subsequently descends in accordance with the abdominal surface of the psoas muscle.[1,14,15]
- Recently, it was found that the level where the genitofemoral nerve passes the psoas muscle ranges from the cranial third of the L3 vertebral body to the caudal third of the L4 vertebral body.[14]
- Thus, when the psoas major muscle is split at the L3 or L4 vertebral body, there is a risk of injury to the genitofemoral nerve.
- An anatomic study by Moro and associates[14] demonstrated that above L2-L3, all parts of the lumbar plexus and nerve roots were located from the dorsal fourth of the vertebral body and dorsally. Furthermore, the genitofemoral nerve descends obliquely forward through the psoas major muscle, emerging on the abdominal surface between the cranial third of the L4 vertebra.
- Therefore, they recommended that the psoas muscle should be split more anteriorly than the dorsal fourth of lumbar vertebral body above the cranial third of the L3 vertebral body to prevent nerve injuries.

URETER

- The ureter runs between the peritoneum and the psoas fascia and is attached not to the psoas fascia but loosely to the peritoneum.
- It normally falls forward with the peritoneum and its contents, away from the operative field.

INDICATIONS

- Vertebral fracture[3,5,16,17]
- Vertebral tumor (primary, metastasis)[2,7]
- Vertebral osteomyelitis or diskitis
- Deformity includes kyphosis and scoliosis

CONTRAINDICATIONS

- No absolute contraindications; only relative contraindications
- Skin or soft tissue infection over the affected area
- Severe respiratory system conditions
- Active pleural disease or lung infection
- Severe osteoporotic bone

PATIENT POSITIONING

Overall, exposure of the thoracolumbar junction can be accessed through either left side or right side. We recommended a left-sided approach (Fig. 10-4A and B), because the vena cava on the right is less tolerant of dissection and may result in troublesome hemorrhage and the liver may be difficult to retract. Nevertheless, in cases of scoliosis, entry on the convex side of the curvature is the rule.

- Double-lumen endotracheal tube is needed to collapse the left lung during procedure.
- Intraoperative monitoring, such as somatosensory evoked potentials, is not mandatory but is recommended in deformity cases to ensure that neurologic injury is not occurring during correction.
- Place the patient in the true right lateral decubitus position with lateral attachment attached to the operating table or place the patient on the beanbag (Fig. 10-5A and B).
- The patient's right leg is flexed at the hip and knee, while the left leg is slightly flexed.
- The arms should be placed in a rest; be careful not to place the arms in the outstretched position because of risk of injury to brachial plexuses.
- All the bony prominences must be checked and padded.
- Intraoperative C-arm may bring in and position at this time.

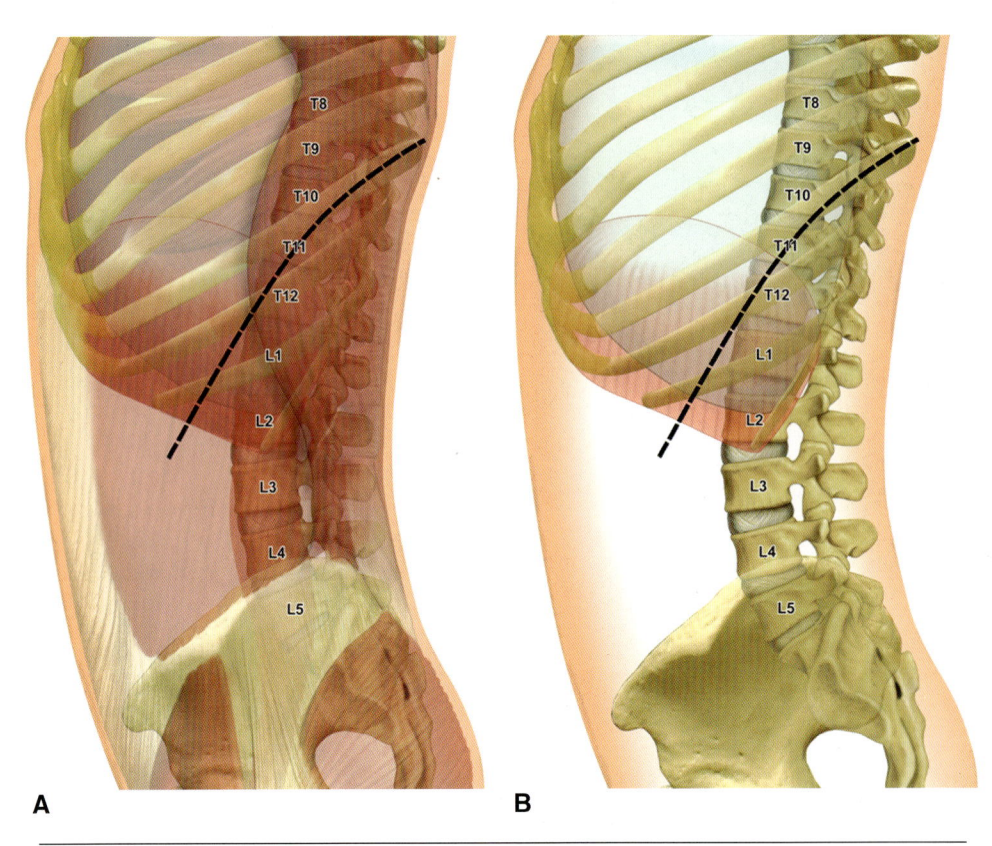

Fig. 10-4 *A* and *B*, Incision line for thoracoabdominal approach.

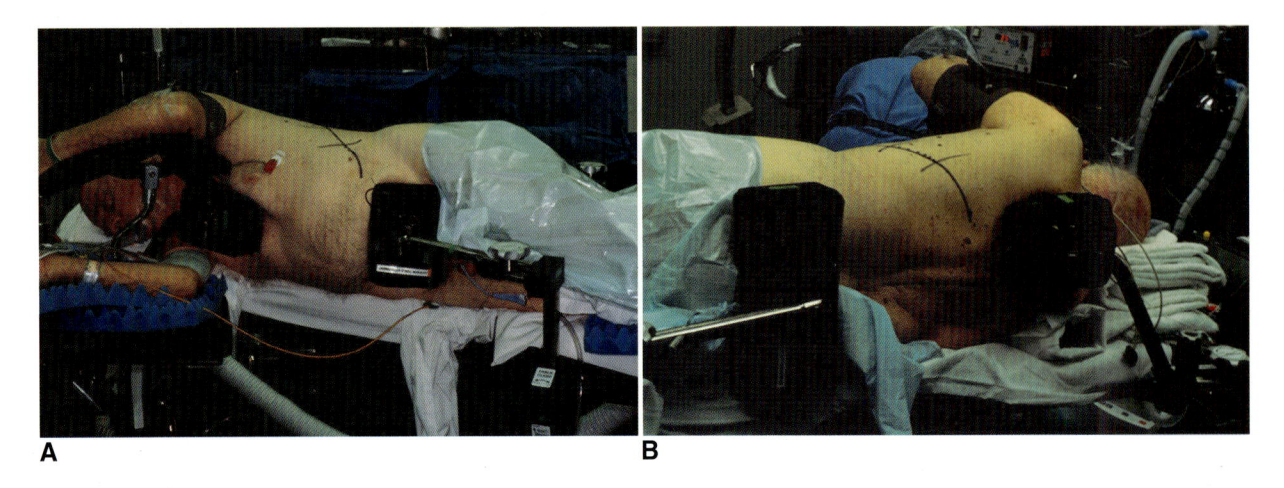

Fig. 10-5 *A* and *B*, Left-sided lateral approach positioning.

TRANSTHORACIC-TRANSDIAPHRAGMATIC APPROACH

- The 10th rib resection is almost always used and will give an access up to T10 vertebra and down to L3.[1,11–13]
- For the deformity cases, the ninth rib can be chosen and will give access up to T9 and down to L4.[1,11–13]

INCISION

- The skin incision begins posteriorly near the midline of the back, follows the course of the 10th rib as far as the costal cartilage, and then continues obliquely downward on the upper and middle abdomen. It usually ends at a level between the umbilicus and the pubic symphysis (Fig. 10-6).

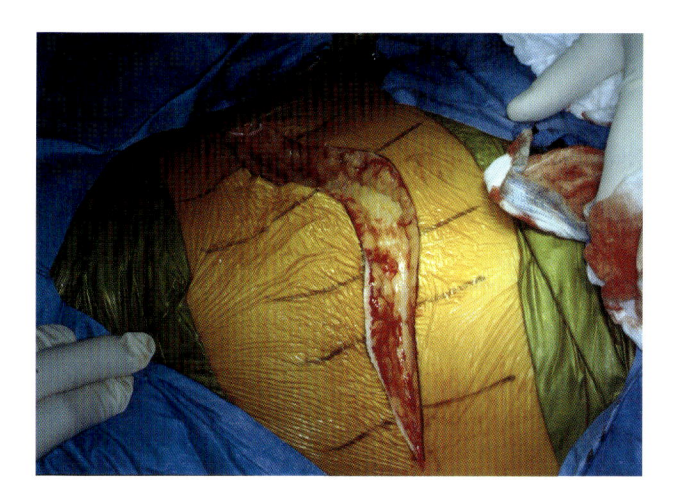

Fig. 10-6 Skin and soft tissue incision along the course of the 10th rib.

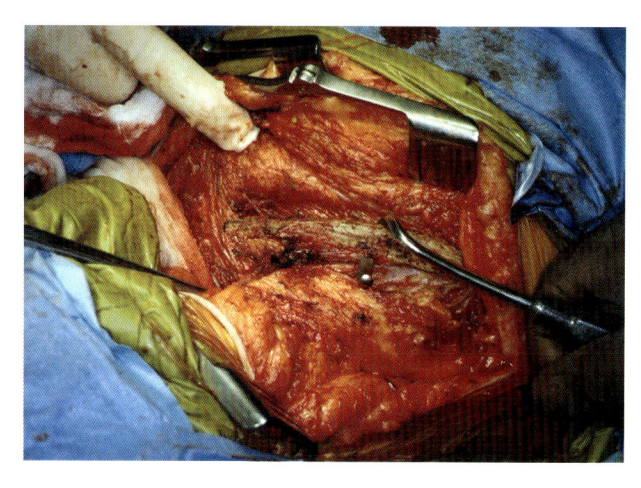

Fig. 10-8 Doyen dissector is used to isolate the rib from its bed.

- The first step is to expose the thoracic cavity, followed by exposure of the abdomen, and then to join two parts together.

Intrathoracic Dissection[8,18–20]

- After the skin incision was made, soft tissue and subcutaneous tissue were dissected along the course of the tenth rib (Fig. 10-7).
- Posteriorly, the latissimus dorsi and anterior serratus muscles are divided with electrocautery along the course of the selected rib.
- The 10th rib (or the 9th rib) was dissected subperiosteally using Alexander periosteal elevator. Intercostal neurovascular bundle was carefully dissected and protected by using Alexander periosteal elevator and doyen (Fig. 10-8).

- Then, the rib was removed using a rib cutter. The removed rib can be the best source of bone graft (Fig. 10-9).
- Before the abdominal muscles are divided, attention is directed to entering the chest. The periosteal layer of the removed rib bed is incised (Fig. 10-10).
- The chest cavity is opened. The margins of the wound are padded with moist sponges, and a rib spreader is inserted (Figs. 10-11 and 10-12).
- The costal arch at the level of rib resection is divided or, in other instances, the costal cartilage of the resected rib is split (Figs. 10-13 and 10-14), underneath which lies the preperitoneal fat, gateway to the extraperitoneal plane, and separation of the diaphragm (Figs. 10-15 and 10-16).

Diaphragm Dissection

- Attention is now directed to separation of the diaphragm peripherally according to anatomic landmarks as reviewed earlier.

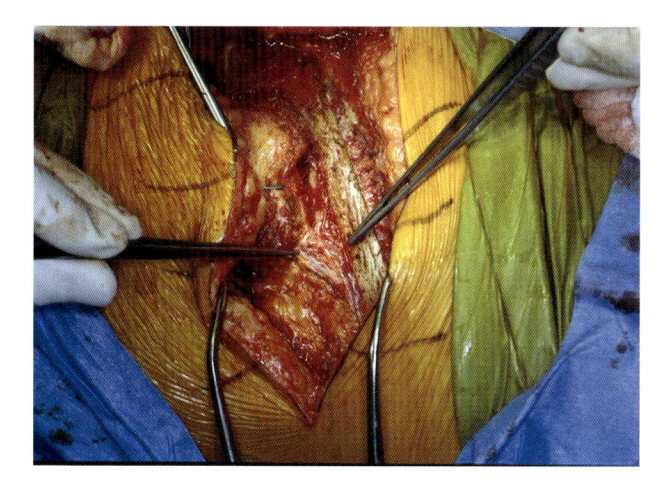

Fig. 10-7 Dissection along the course of the 10th rib, carefully preserving the neurovascular bundle.

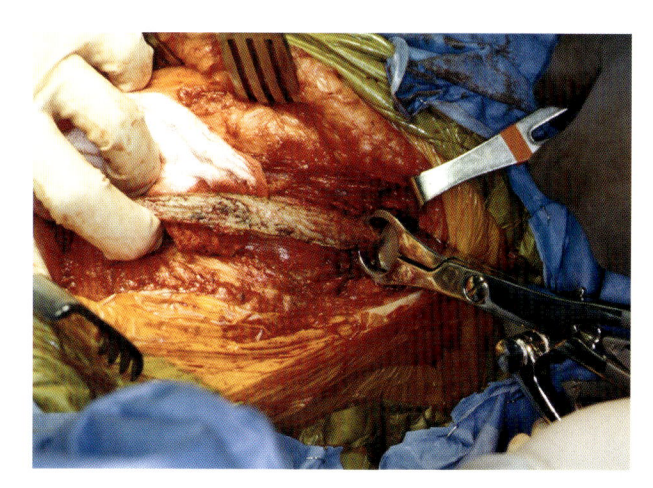

Fig. 10-9 Rib cutter is used to cut the 10th rib to expose the pleura underneath.

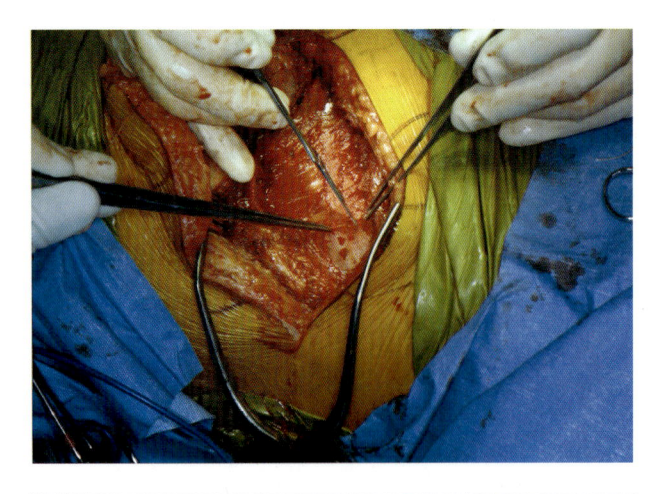

Fig. 10-10 Pleural cavity is carefully entered.

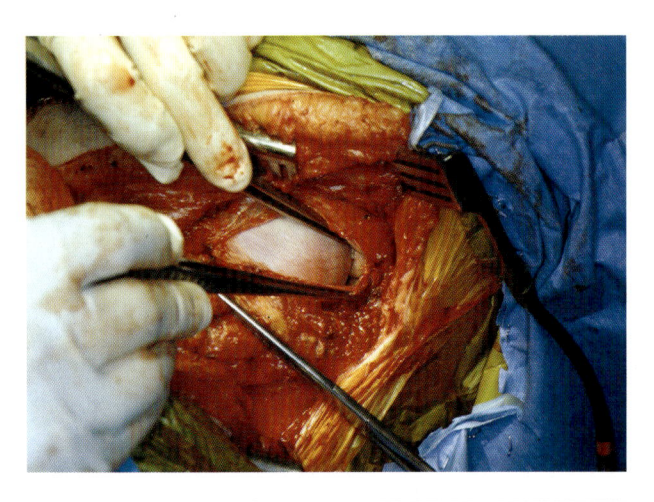

Fig. 10-11 The diaphragm is brought onto the view after pushing the lung out of the field.

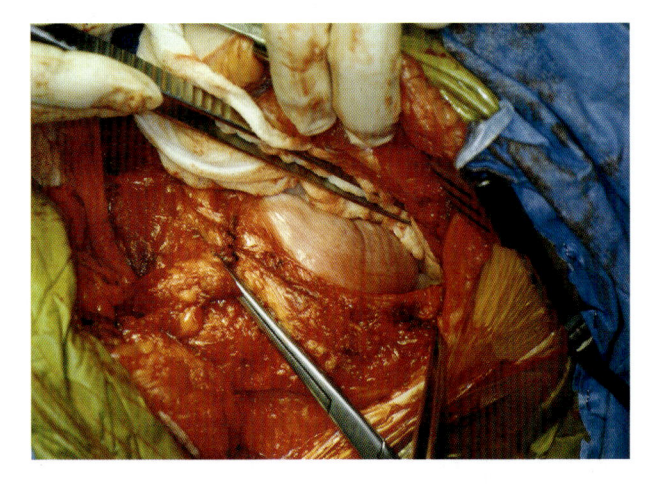

Fig. 10-12 Continuing pushing the lung with wet sponge.

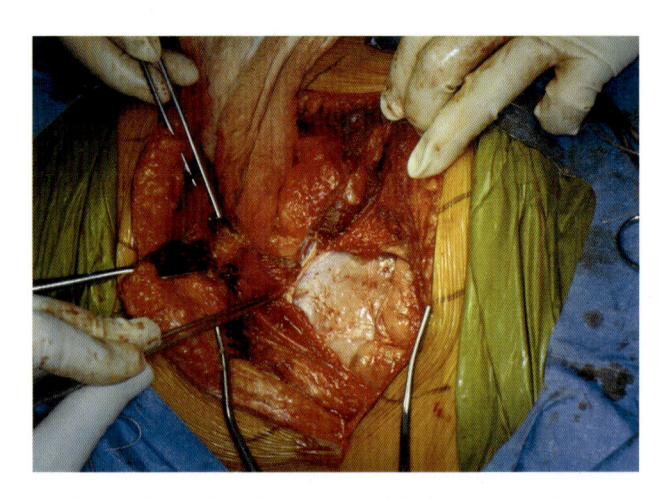

Fig. 10-13 Concentration is turned to abdominal disssection.

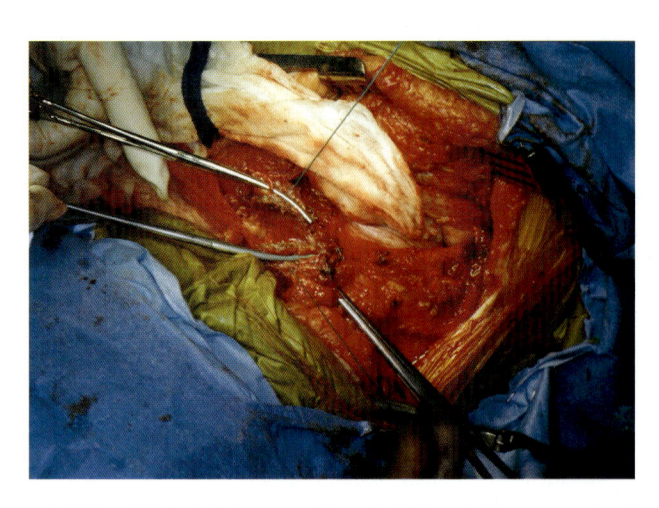

Fig. 10-14 The costal cartilage is splitted and serves as a landmark for closure. Careful dissection underneath the splitted cartilage will expose the peritoneal fat, which will lead to the retroperitoneal space.

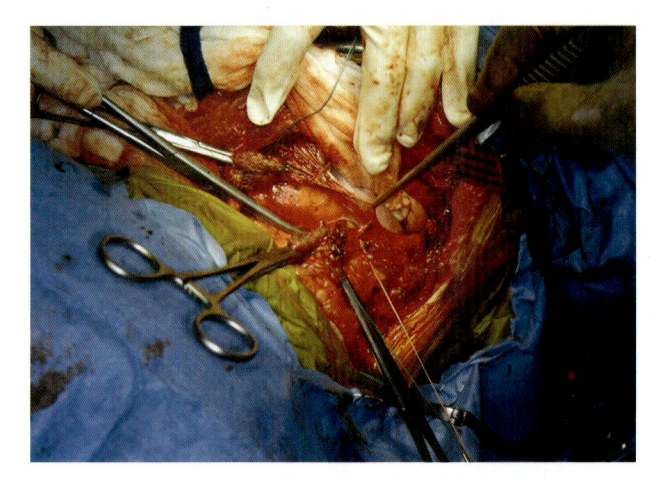

Fig. 10-15 The splitted costal cartilage is tagged temporarily. The retroperitoneal fat is identified.

CHAPTER 10 Thoracoabdominal Approach 95

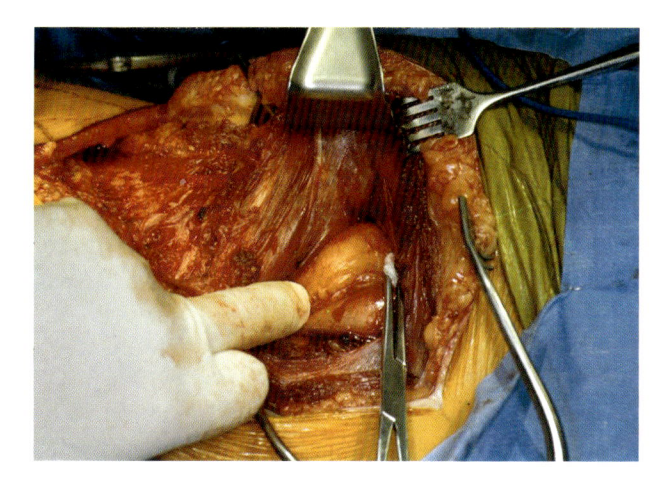

Fig. 10-16 Retroperitoneal space is entered by pushing the peritoneal fat along with the peritoneal content toward the midline.

- Simple hand pressure may be used to push on the central diaphragm to cause tension along the periphery of the diaphragm.
- Using electrocautery, first the parietal pleura is reflected at the subcostal diaphragmatic angle where the costal arch has been resected or the cartilage split is incised, followed by cutting the subjacent insertion fibers of the diaphragm, leaving about 5 to 8 mm of the diaphragmatic muscle in line of attachment.
- The critical concern at this point is to avoid entering the peritoneal cavity by staying close to the chest wall when cutting the insertion fibers, which will lead to extraperitoneal fat layer.
- Once the peritoneal fat is visualized, finger or manual dissection is carried out, separating the preperitoneal fat, peritoneum, and peritoneal contents from the abdominal muscles.
- Tagging sutures along the divided diaphragm should be placed in order to reapproximate the diaphragm later (Figs. 10-17 and 10-18).
- At this point, the self-retaining retractor system is carried in and appropriately placed to give the best view of exposure.
- In some situations, when further exposure is necessary, further dividing the lateral and medial arcuate ligaments over the quadratus lumborum and psoas muscles can be performed.
- Last, the crus can be divided or detached from the lumbar vertebrae.
- The retroperitoneal space is entered using the sweeping motion until one feels the vertebra beneath. Peritoneal contents are pushed away across the quadratus lumborum and psoas muscle.
- If the peritoneum is inadvertently opened, it is simply repaired with a 3-0 chromic catgut suture.

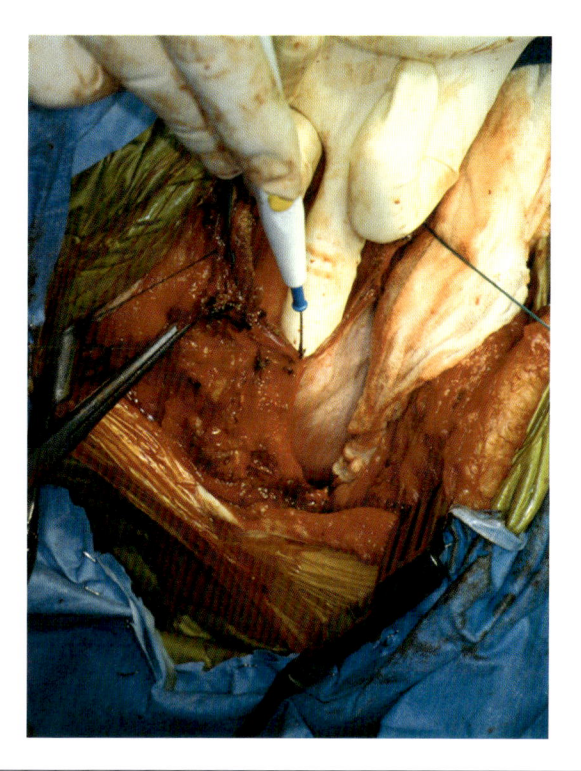

Fig. 10-17 Diaphragm is carefully cut peripherally.

- Self-retaining retractor system may be adjusted at this point to give a better view of the prevertebral and vertebra area.
- Segmental vessels are exposed and ligated or suture tied and then divided (Fig. 10-19).
- Then the affected vertebra or disk should be easily identified and confirmed using intraoperative x-rays or C-arm (Fig. 10-20).
- Next, perform the intended procedure.

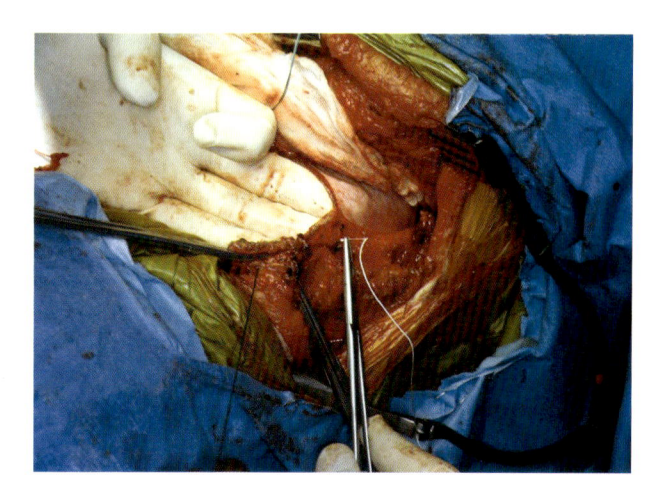

Fig. 10-18 Temporary tagged sutures are used while cutting the diaphragm and will serve as a landmark for closure.

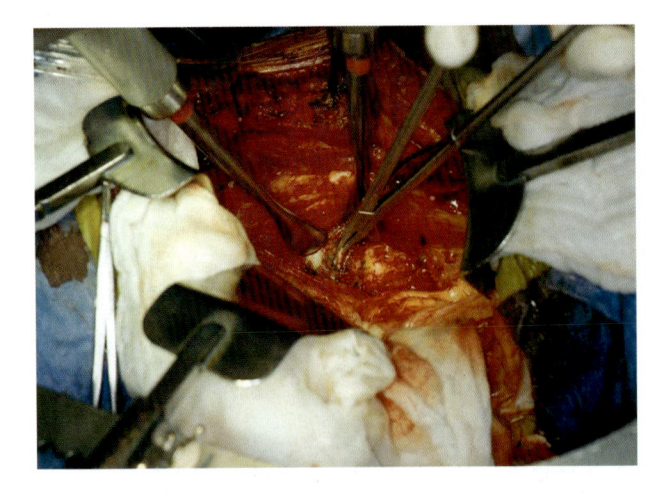

Fig. 10-19 After the diaphragm is cut, the retroperitoneal space and thoracic cavity become one space. Now attention is turned to expose and identify the vertebral body. Carefully identify and ligate the segmental vessels that lie on the center of the vertebral body.

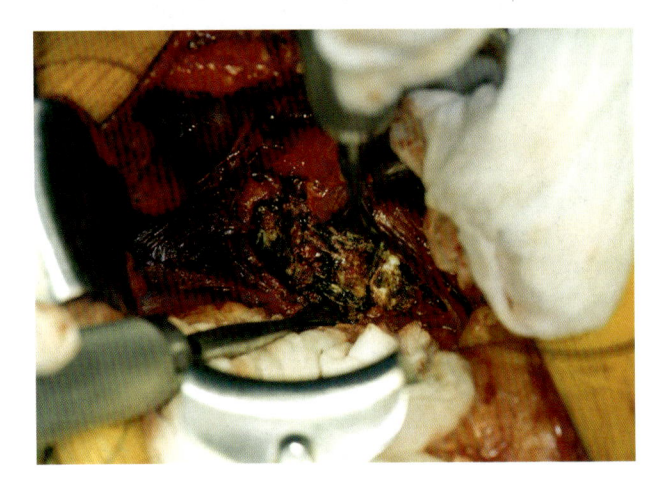

Fig. 10-20 The vertebral body is nicely exposed, and the surgeon is ready to perform intended procedure.

TRANSPLEURAL-RETROPERITONEAL APPROACH

This approach is less invasive compared to the traditional transdiaphragmatic approach. It can give nice exposure of the L1 vertebral body; however, with the retraction system it can be extended from T12 vertebral body to L2 vertebral body. It is most appropriate for treatment of localized pathology (two or one vertebral segments).[5,9] The key is to enter the pleural cavity and then identify posterior insertion and crus of diaphragm.

INCISION

The skin incision begins posteriorly near the midline of the back, follows the course of the 10th rib as far as the costal cartilage, and then continues obliquely downward on the upper and middle abdomen (see Fig. 10-4A and B).

Intrathoracic Dissection[8,18–20]

- After the skin incision is made, soft tissue and subcutaneous tissue are dissected along the course of the tenth rib.
- Posteriorly, the latissimus dorsi and anterior serratus muscles are divided with electrocautery along the course of the selected rib.
- The 10th rib is dissected subperiosteally using the Alexander periosteal elevator. Intercostal neurovascular bundle is carefully dissected and protected by using Alexander periosteal elevator and doyen.
- Then, the rib is removed using a rib cutter. The removed rib can be the best source of bone graft (Fig. 10-21).
- The pleural cavity is entering carefully through its bed.
- The lung is packed and retracted cranially.
- Identify the diaphragm (Fig. 10-22) and gradually retract caudally to expose the crus of the diaphragm.
- Palpate the vertebral body and check the level with intraoperative fluoroscope.

Diaphragm Dissection

- The target area can now be exposed with the help of a self-retaining retractor system.
- The retractor holds down the diaphragm and exposes the insertion of the diaphragm on the spine.
- Compared to extensive thoracolumbar exposures with total detachment of diaphragm required for open surgery,

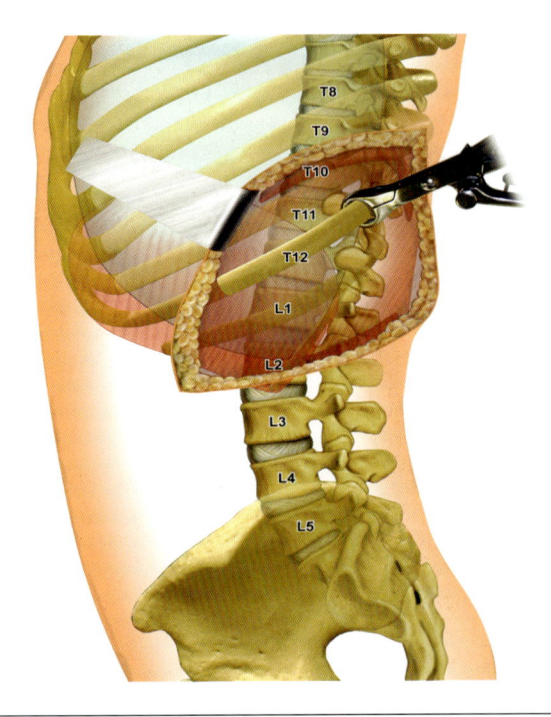

Fig. 10-21 The 10th rib was identified, isolated, and cut.

CHAPTER 10 Thoracoabdominal Approach

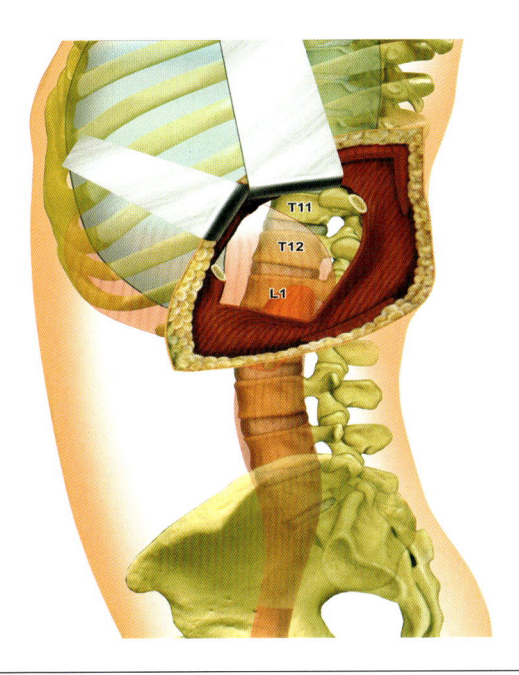

Fig. 10-22 After entering the pleural cavity and pushing the lung away from the field, the surgeon brings the diaphragm onto the field. By using the hand or retractor to push down the dome of the diaphragm, the surgeon can see and identify the diaphragmatic crus along with the psoas muscle.

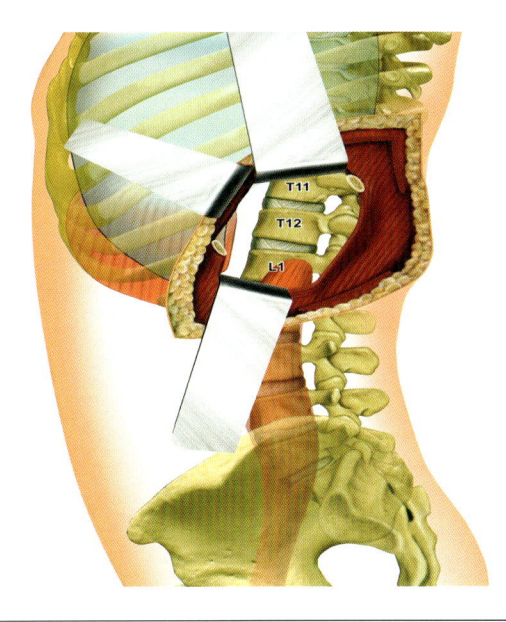

Fig. 10-23 After crus of diaphragm is dissected, further pushing down of the dissected diaphragm can expose the psoas muscle and the vertebral body underneath.

this approach requires only minimal diaphragmatic detachment, and the dissected diaphragm is held down (Fig. 10-23).
- Next, with a diaphragmatic opening of about 6 to 10 cm the L2 vertebral body can be exposed.
- A rim of 1 cm is left on the spine to facilitate closure of the diaphragm at the end of the procedure.
- The preferred incision runs along the spine and the ribs parallel to the diaphragmatic insertion and 1 to 2 cm away from it. The diaphragm is already thinner here than in the immediate area of insertion, and the remaining edge makes subsequent suturing easier.

Retroperitoneal Dissection
- Retroperitoneal fat tissue is now exposed and mobilized from the anterior surface of the psoas insertions.
- A common mistake is to reflect the retroperitoneal fat with the peritoneum; this leads to a blind space posterior to the psoas muscle.
- It is recommended that the fatty layer be separated from the peritoneum to create a plane leading down to the anterior aspect of the psoas and the vertebral bodies.
- The psoas muscle is dissected very carefully from the vertebral bodies in order not to damage the segmental blood vessels "hidden" underneath.

- The self-retaining retractor system is now readjusted and placed into the diaphragmatic gap. This usually gives a good exposure from T12 to L2 (Fig. 10-24).
- The segmental vessels are then identified over the center of the vertebral body, ligated using a hemoclip or suture tie, and divided (see Figs. 10-19 and 10-20). Then, the intended procedure can be performed.

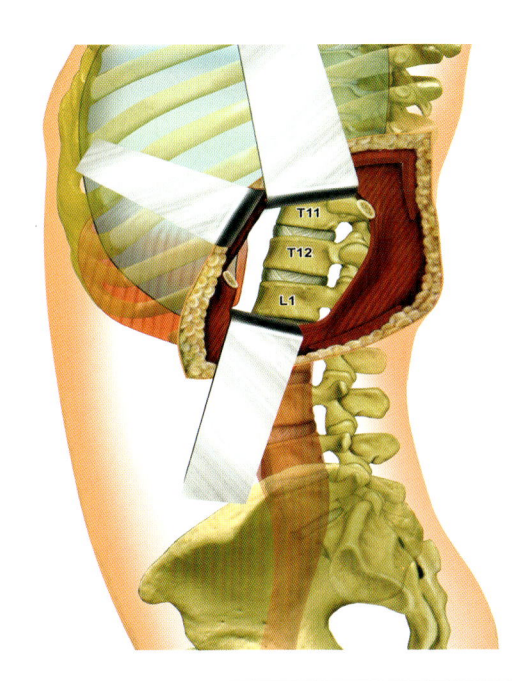

Fig. 10-24 Carefully dissect and split the psoas muscle to expose the affected vertebral body.

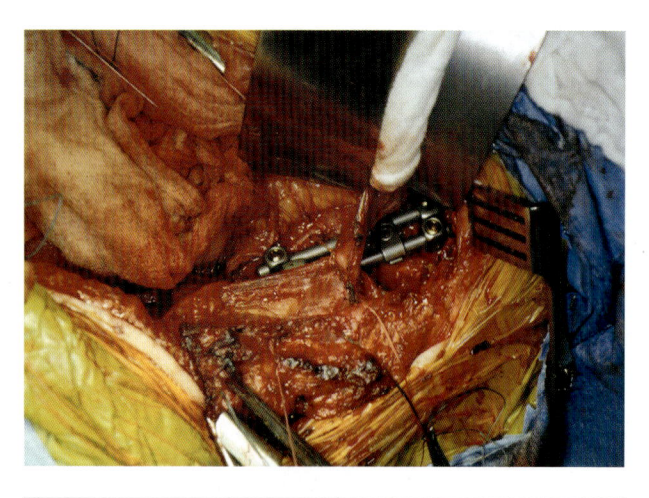

Fig. 10-25 Crus and arcuate ligament are sutured back in place.

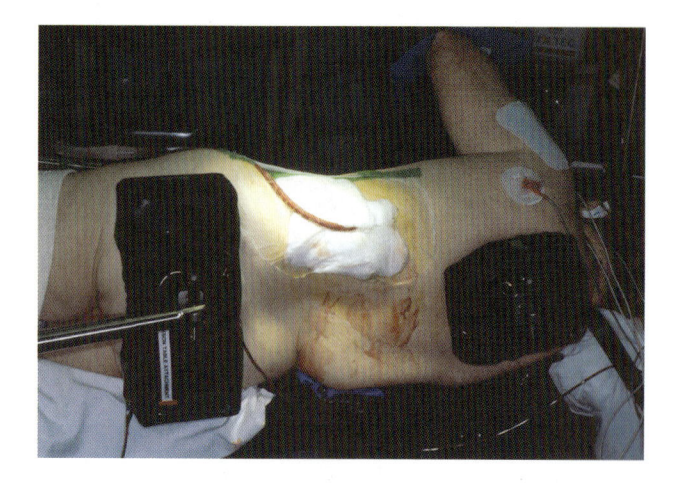

Fig. 10-27 Chest drain is placed in the thoracic cavity.

CLOSURE

Closure of the Diaphragm

- The diaphragm is reattached starting with approximation of the divided crus using a PDS 0 monofilament and proceeding as a continuous suture or interrupted suture along the periphery of divided diaphragm to the site of the division of the costal arch (Figs. 10-25 and 10-26).
- The divided costal cartilage serves as a good landmark for closure and should be reapproximated with two 0 or 1 braided polyester sutures employed as a figure eight. Then, complete closure of the diaphragm by additional stitches.
- The abdominal muscles are then approximated anatomically with a continuous suture of PDS 0. Usually, it requires two layers of closure, one for the transverse and internal oblique muscles, and a second layer for the external oblique muscles.

Retroperitoneal Closure

- After the orthopedic procedure is completed, hemostasis is secured.
- The oozing from bony surface should be stopped as the peritoneal contents are allowed to fall back in place and serve as a tamponade.
- There is no need to place a drain in the retroperitoneal space.

Intrathoracic Closure

- A chest tube is placed, a rib approximator is inserted, the parietal pleura is then closed with 3-0 running chromic catgut sutures (Fig. 10-27).
- The chest wall musculature is then closed in layers.

POSTOPERATIVE CARE

- Postoperative x-rays and chest x-ray should be obtained to determine the alignment, position of instrumentation, position of bone graft or cages, and position of chest tube, and to monitor the affected pleural cavity.
- Urine output and chest tube should be recorded in the first 48 hours.
- Underwater-seal chest suction is maintained at −15 cm H_2O.
- A chest tube should be removed when the drainage is serous and consists of 30 to 50 mL or less for two or more successive 8-hour periods.
- Advanced diet protocol should be started because the bowel may not function very well in the first 3 to 4 days.
- TLSO brace should be prescribed.

COMPLICATIONS

Many surgeons have used this approach to decompress and stabilize the spine and have obtained acceptable results.[21–27] Although this approach does provide excellent exposure, the major disadvantages are that the diaphragm must be detached

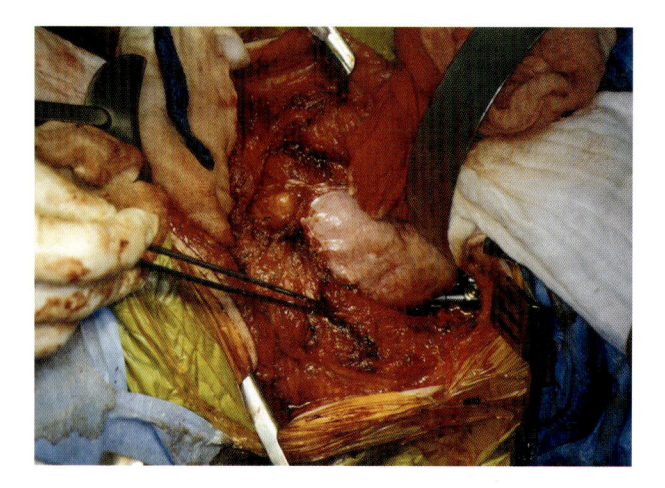

Fig. 10-26 Closure of the diaphragm using tagged suture as a landmark.

from the chest wall and that both the thoracic and retroperitoneal spaces must be entered, which adds to the morbidity of the procedure. All patients who undergo this approach require insertion of a chest tube postoperatively for varying lengths of time, often prolonging their period of immobilization and adding a risk of pulmonary empyema.

The morbidity associated with the standard thoracoabdominal approach has been well documented, and the major complications associated with this procedure are pulmonary. In a report by McDonnell and associates,[27] 34% of the patients who underwent surgery via the thoracoabdominal approach suffered complications. The most common major complication was of a pulmonary nature, including pneumonia, respiratory failure necessitating reintubation, and prolonged postoperative intubation.[27] For the elderly and many cancer patients whose life expectancy is relatively short and for whom the goal of surgery may be palliative, the violation of the diaphragm may be a considerable source of morbidity.

INTRAOPERATIVE COMPLICATIONS

- Injury to the lung, including hemopneumothorax
- Lung or respiratory complications
- Injury to the major vessels
- Injury to the ureter
- Injury to the sympathetic chain, which lies on the dorsal aspect of the vertebral body and on the most medial aspect of the psoas muscle
- Injury to the genitofemoral nerve, which lies on the anterior medial surface of the psoas muscle, attached to its fascia
- Injury to the nerve root or lumbar plexus during splitting the psoas muscle to access the lumbar vertebra
- Accidentally entering the peritoneum
- Accidental injury to intra-abdominal organs
- Bleeding from unidentified injured segmental vessels

POSTOPERATIVE COMPLICATIONS

- Diaphragmatic hernia from poorly repairing the diaphragm
- Hypoesthesia or hyperesthesia along the resected rib
- Hypoesthesia along the distribution of the genitofemoral nerve
- Postoperative infection

CONCLUSION

The thoracolumbar junction presents a unique challenge to surgeons because of the complex anatomy and the nature of a transitional zone. Understanding of the complex anatomy in this area will help spine surgeons perform this procedure without complications. Decompression, correction of the deformity, and instrumentation can be performed via these approaches.

REFERENCES

1. Mirbaha MM: Anterior approach to the thoraco-lumbar junction of the spine by a retroperitoneal-extrapleural technic. Clin Orthop 1973;91:41–47.
2. Amgwerd R: [The thoracolumbar approach to large retroperitoneal tumors]. Helv Chir Acta 1965;32:525–528.
3. Burrington JD, Brown C, Wayne ER, et al: Anterior approach to the thoracolumbar spine: Technical considerations. Arch Surg 1976;111:456–463.
4. Higai GA: [Extraperitoneal-diaphragmatic approach to the thoraco-lumbar spine in tuberculous spondylitis]. Ortop Travmatol Protez 1968;29:54–58.
5. Barone GW, Eidt JF, Webb JW, et al: The anterior extrapleural approach to the thoracolumbar junction revisited. Am Surg 1998;64:372–375.
6. Barone GW, Hudec WA: The Rumel technique. An aid for difficult diaphragmatic closures. J Cardiovasc Surg (Torino) 1999;40:463–464.
7. Juraniec J, Szostakiewics-Sawicka H: Crura of the lumbar part of the diaphragm in primates. Folia Morphol (Warsz) 1977;36:117–133.
8. Aronskii AS: [Transthoracic approach with detachment of the diaphragm in surgery of tuberculosis of the thoracolumbar portion of the spine (anatomic-surgical investigation)]. Probl Tuberk 1973;51:44–50.
9. Moskovich R, Benson D, Zhang ZH, et al: Extracoelomic approach to the spine. J Bone Joint Surg Br 1993;75:886–893.
10. de Peretti F, Hovorka I, Fabiani P, et al: New possibilities in L2-L5 lumbar arthrodesis using a lateral retroperitoneal approach assisted by laparoscopy: Preliminary results. Eur Spine J 1996;5:210–216.
11. Dulchavsky SA, Diebel LN: Retroperitoneal approach to first lumbar vertebral body. J Am Coll Surg 1995;180:495–496.
12. Kocis J, Wendsche P, Visna P, et al: [A less invasive retropleural-retroperitoneal approach to the thoraco-lumbar spine]. Acta Chir Orthop Traumatol Cech 2002;69:285–287.
13. Kim M, Nolan P, Finkelstein JA: Evaluation of 11th rib extrapleural-retroperitoneal approach to the thoracolumbar junction: Technical note. J Neurosurg 2000;93:168–174.
14. Moro T, Kikuchi S, Konno S, et al: An anatomic study of the lumbar plexus with respect to retroperitoneal endoscopic surgery. Spine 2003;28:423-428; discussion 427–428.
15. Shah AA, Memon IA: Anterolateral decompression for traumatic spinal cord compression. J Pak Med Assoc 1994;44:242–243.
16. Kossmann T, Ertel W, Platz A, et al: [Combined surgery for fractures of the thoraco-lumbar junction using the inlay-span method]. Orthopade 1999;28:432–440.
17. Boriani S, Biagini R, De Iure F, et al: Lumbar vertebrectomy for the treatment of bone tumors: Surgical technique. Chir Organi Mov 1994;79:163–173.
18. Anderson TM, Mansour KA, Miller JI Jr: Thoracic approaches to anterior spinal operations: Anterior thoracic approaches. Ann Thorac Surg 1993;55:1447–1451; discussion 1451–1442.
19. Dribinskii MB, Kashkov Iu V: [Thoracodiaphragmal approach in surgery on the lower thoracic and upper lumbar vertebrae]. Khirurgiia (Mosk) 1970;46:112–116.
20. McElvein RB, Nasca RJ, Dunham WK, et al: Transthoracic exposure for anterior spinal surgery. Ann Thorac Surg 1988;45:278–283.

21. Clohisy JC, Akbarnia BA, Bucholz RD, et al: Neurologic recovery associated with anterior decompression of spine fractures at the thoracolumbar junction (T12-L1). Spine 1992;17:S325–S330.
22. Eismont FJ, Bohlman HH, Soni PL, et al: Pyogenic and fungal vertebral osteomyelitis with paralysis. J Bone Joint Surg Am 1983;65:19–29.
23. Fidler MW: Anterior and posterior stabilization of the spine following vertebral body resection: A postmortem investigation. Spine 1986;11:362–366.
24. Kostuik JP: Anterior fixation for burst fractures of the thoracic and lumbar spine with or without neurological involvement. Spine 1988;13:286–293.
25. Kostuik JP: Anterior fixation for fractures of the thoracic and lumbar spine with or without neurologic involvement. Clin Orthop 1984;(189):103–115.
26. Kostuik JP: Anterior Kostuik-Harrington distraction systems. Orthopedics 1988;11:1379–1391.
27. McDonnell MF, Glassman SD, Dimar JR 2nd, et al: Perioperative complications of anterior procedures on the spine. J Bone Joint Surg Am 1996;78:839–847.

CHAPTER 11

ADEBUKOLA ONIBOKUN

LARRY T. KHOO

LANGSTON HOLLY

Anterior Retroperitoneal Approach to the Lumbar Spine

INTRODUCTION

Anterior surgical exposure of the lumbar spine was first reported in the literature in the 1930s by Capener and Burns who detailed their experience with transperitoneal approaches for the treatment of spondylolisthesis.[1,2] Since that time, anterior lumbar procedures have evolved with increasingly frequent use for a variety of pathologies including trauma, deformity, infection, degenerative disease, sympathetectomy, failed back syndrome, and primary or metastatic neoplasms. Direct access to ventral pathology, sparing of the lumbar paraspinal musculature and improved postoperative mobility, decreased chronic muscular pain, avoidance of previous posterior surgical scars, and the ability to place bone graft in the predominant load-bearing column of the spine are but some of the attractive features that have helped to popularize anterior techniques. The recent growth of minimally invasive and laparoscopic interbody fusion techniques have placed facility with these ventral lumbar operations at an even higher premium.

A number of complications are associated with this approach. In order to keep complications to a minimum, the surgeon must become intimately familiar with the anatomy of the retroperitoneum. A clear understanding of the anatomy of the retroperitoneum and the thoracoabdominal junction is critical for the surgeon to appropriately and safely operate in this region. In this chapter we will carefully delineate and elaborate on the anatomic landmarks that are important during this procedure

SURGICAL ANATOMY

ANTERIOR VIEW OF RETROPERITONEAL CONTENTS (Fig. 11-1)

The abdominal viscera, peritoneum, and retroperitoneal fat have been removed. The great vessels are in close proximity to the disk spaces and vertebral bodies, and visualizing their association, we can see how vascular injury can occur from both anterior and posterior approaches. The psoas muscle lies along the anterolateral aspect of the spine between the transverse processes and the lateral vertebral bodies and disk. The kidney, ureter, and perinephric fat are located anterior to the psoas and are usually mobilized medially during retroperitoneal exposures. The ureter passes along the psoas muscle and then lies anterior to the iliac vessels. The crura of the diaphragm lie along the anterolateral aspect of the upper lumbar vertebral bodies, and their tendinous fibers merge with the anterior longitudinal ligament. They must be incised and mobilized during exposure of the upper lumbar spine. The sympathetic chain enters the abdominal cavity from under the medial arcuate ligament and can be seen along the anterolateral aspect of the vertebral bodies along the entire length of the lumbar spine. The superior hypogastric plexus and inferior hypogastric plexus can be seen in this specimen along the aorta and near the L5-S1 disk space. Injury to this structures may cause retrograde ejaculation, infertility, and incontinence.

ANTEROLATERAL VIEW OF UPPER LUMBAR AREA (Fig. 11-2)

The diaphragm comprises a central tendinous portion and a muscular portion. The central tendinous portion has no bony attachment and exerts its effects through the attachments of the muscular portions. Each side of the body has three muscular portions. The costal portion attaches to the six costal cartilages and the lower four ribs. The sternal portion attaches the central tendon to the back of the xiphoid process.

The lumbar muscular portion is located near the anterolateral aspect of the upper lumbar spine and must be

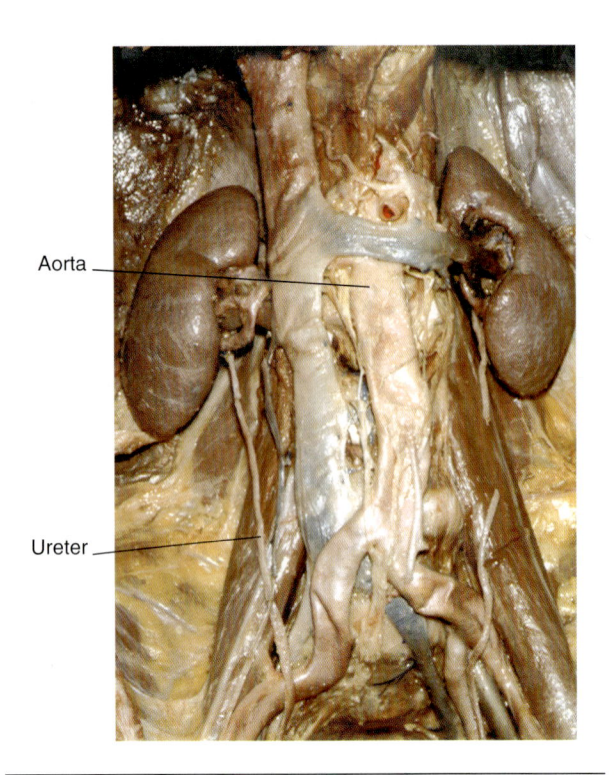

Fig. 11-1 Anterior view of retroperitoneal contents.

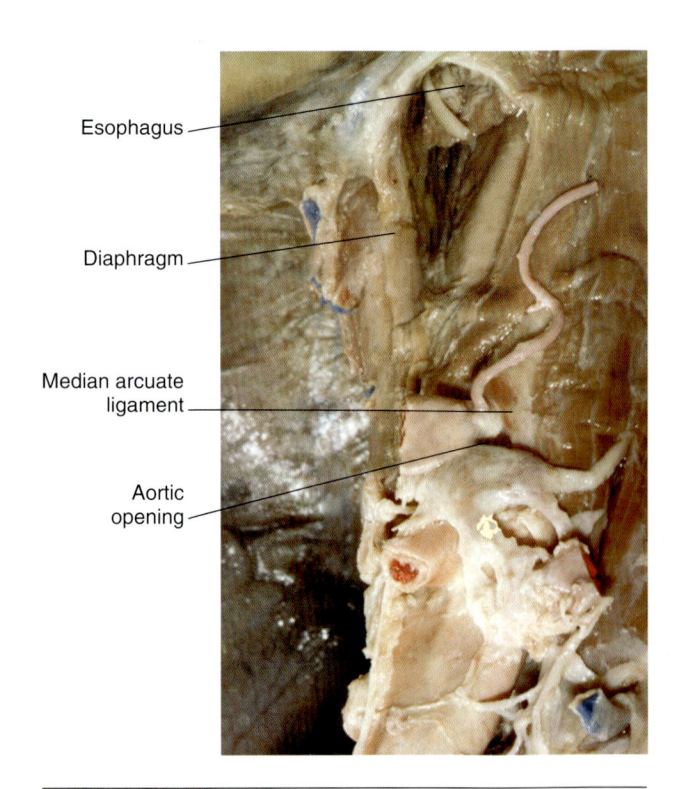

Fig. 11-2 Anterolateral view of upper lumbar area.

mobilized during operations in this area. This lumbar muscular portion has two origins. One origin is the median and lateral arcuate ligaments, which are fibrous arches over the psoas and quadratus muscles, respectively. The other origin is from the crura, which arise from the bodies of the upper lumbar vertebrae and ascend to attach to the central tendon. The right crus arises from the upper three lumbar vertebrae and the left crus arises from the upper two. As the crura join, they form the aortic opening, which also passes the thoracic duct and greater splanchnic nerves. The surgeon exposing the upper lumbar spine often must divide the crura and reflect them laterally to gain exposure. The nerve supply is via the phrenic nerve, which enters medially and innervates the diaphragm toward the periphery. Thus, the diaphragm should be incised peripherally with a small cuff left for closure.

LATERAL VIEW OF THE PSOAS MUSCLE AND ITS ORIGIN (Fig. 11-3)

The psoas muscle is a long fusiform muscle that occupies the anterolateral aspect of the lumbar spine between the lateral vertebral bodies and the transverse processes and can be of formidable size in young athletic patients. The origin of the psoas is from (1) the anterior and lower borders of the lumbar transverse processes, (2) five slips from the sides of the bodies and the corresponding intervertebral disks of the last thoracic and all the lumbar vertebrae, and (3) from a series of tendinous arches that extend across the constricted parts of the bodies of the lumbar vertebrae between the previously described slips. The lumbar radicular arteries and veins pass beneath these tendinous arches. The insertion of the psoas, by passing beneath the inguinal ligament, anterior to the capsule of the hip joint, is onto the lesser trochanter of the femur. The psoas is innervated by branches of the lumbar plexus, which contain fibers from L2, L3, and L4. The psoas functions as a powerful flexor of the thigh at the hip joint. It may assist in maintaining an erect posture by preventing

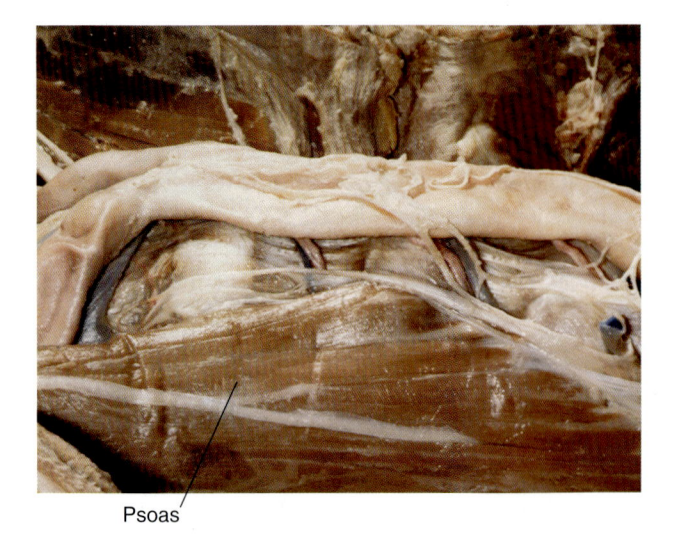

Fig. 11-3 Lateral view of the psoas muscle and its origin.

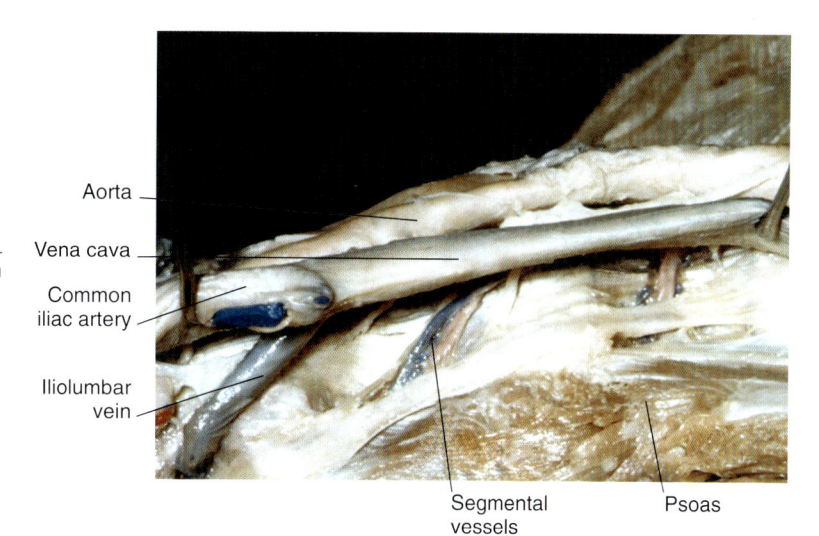

Fig. 11-4 Lateral view of the aorta and vena cava.

LATERAL VIEW OF THE AORTA AND VENA CAVA (Fig. 11-4)

The aorta has paired segmental vessels at the lumbar levels that pass laterally over the vertebral body at the midportion of the vertebral body. The disk spaces are prominent and the midvertebral levels appear as valleys when looking from this view. The segmental vessels are attached by soft tissues and can be mobilized and tied off. The segmentals actually arise from the dorsal surface, as seen in Figure 11-4. If the vessel is ligated too close to the aorta, it may retract underneath the aorta and be very difficult to locate if it continues to bleed. The blood supply to the spinal column is derived from these segmental vessels, which supply two networks. One which feeds the bony elements of the vertebrae, the paraspinal muscles, and the extradural space, and the inner network nourishes the spinal cord itself.

The segmental arteries hug the vertebral bodies, giving off a main dorsal branch as they approach the neural foramina. This main dorsal branch continues posteriorly below the transverse process and supplies the bone of the posterior elements and the paraspinal muscles. Shortly after its origin, the dorsal branch gives off an intraspinal branch, which feeds the nerve root and dura. At certain levels separate vessels arise from the dorsal segmental artery and supply the anterior two thirds of the spinal cord. These branches are known as anterior segmental medullary arteries. One large vessel occurs commonly at the upper lumbar or lower thoracic levels and is called the *artery of Adamkiewicz* and may cause paraplegia if ligated.

The bifurcation of the great vessels is variable. The bifurcation of the vena cava occurs lower than that of the aorta and is usually located above the L5-S1 disk space. The vena cava bifurcation is to the right of the aorta, and the left common iliac vein passes through the aortic bifurcation. Injury to the left common iliac vein is common during approaches to this area. The median sacral artery is the third branch or the termination of the artery and can be safely ligated for approaches to the L5-S1 disk space. It is generally small and easily mobilized.

ANTEROLATERAL VIEW OF THE SYMPATHETIC CHAIN (Fig. 11-5)

The sympathetic chain consists of a series of ganglia connected by intervening chords and extending along the lateral aspect of the vertebral column from the base of the skull to the coccyx. The trunk contains ganglia, preganglionic myelinated fibers, and postganglionic unmyelinated fibers. All fibers may run up and down the trunk for several levels before synapsing. White rami communicantes contain spinal nerve outflow to the chain and gray rami are the branches to the spinal nerves and postganglionic fibers. The gray rami are in all the nerves and the white are only on the thoracic and upper two lumbar levels. The sympathetic trunk enters the abdominal cavity from within the psoas behind the medial arcuate ligament. It descends on the vertebral bodies with close approximation to the psoas.

LATERAL VIEW OF THE SYMPATHETIC CHAIN (Fig. 11-6)

The specimen in Figure 11-6 shows the sympathetic chain with rami communicantes going to and from the spinal nerves. Identification of this chain can be difficult when there is inflammation of the prevertebral soft tissue either from disease, prior trauma, infection, or surgery. Inadvertent

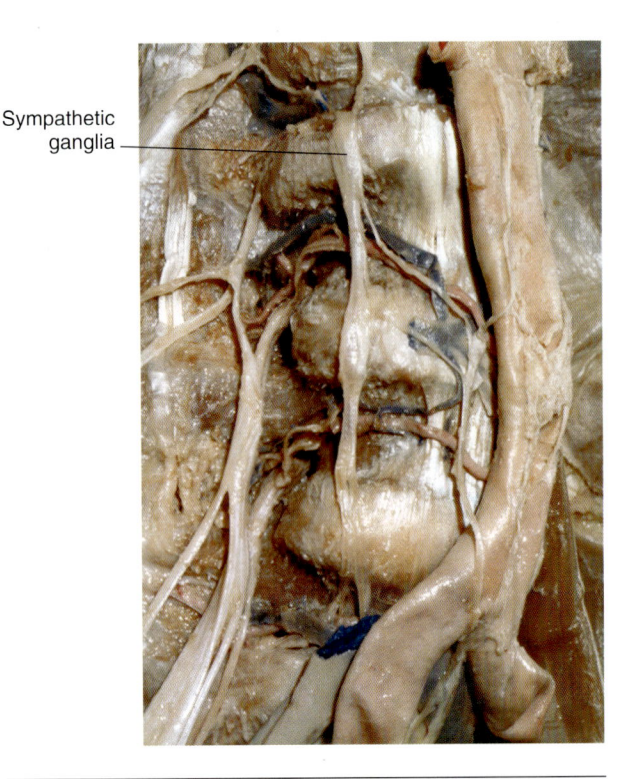

Fig. 11-5 Anterolateral view of the sympathetic chain.

transection and injury of the sympathetic chain near the disks and bodies during exposure and decompression is not uncommon.

ANTEROLATERAL VIEW OF THE PRESACRAL (SUPERIOR) HYPOGASTRIC PLEXUS (Fig. 11-7)

The urogenital system is innervated by three basic nerve complexes—the sympathetic, the parasympathetic, and the

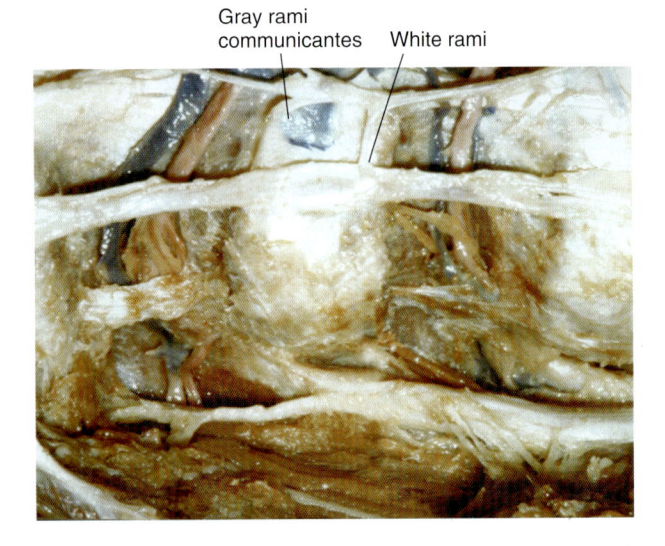

Fig. 11-6 Lateral view of the sympathetic chain.

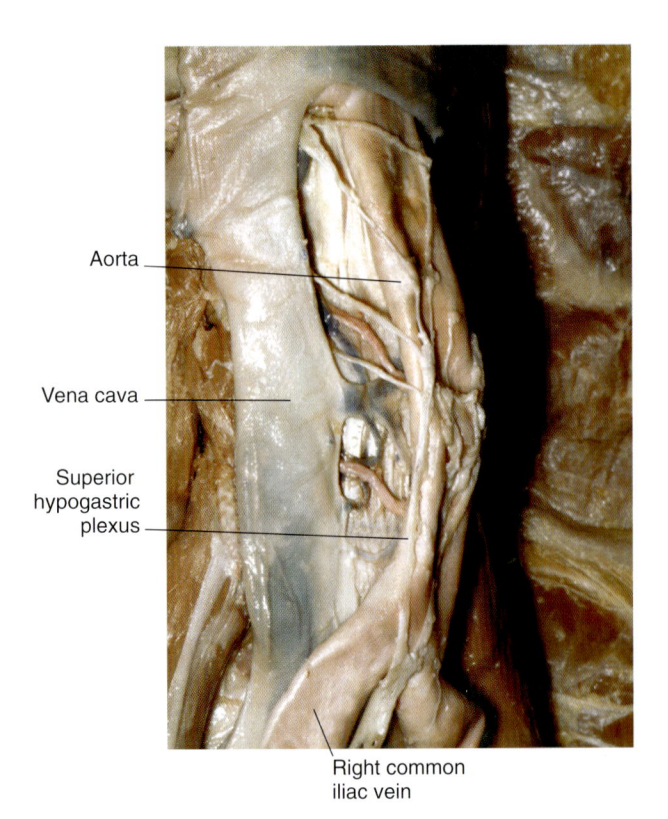

Fig. 11-7 Anterolateral view of the presacral (superior) hypogastric plexus.

somatic—through the pudendal nerve. Sexual function is directly affected by these nerves. Sympathetic nerve supply is a directed continuation of the thoracolumbar sympathetic nerves coursing along the anterolateral aspect of the lumbar vertebral bodies. At the level of the third and fourth lumbar vertebrae these ramify about the inferior mesenteric artery and the inferior mesenteric ganglion (inferior mesenteric plexus). Almost 80% of the ramifications occur on the left side of the aorta. Once ramified, these fibers are referred to as the superior hypogastric plexus as they course distally. These superior hypogastric fibers are found in the retroperitoneal space along the left side of the aorta. They cross the left common iliac artery and vein and lie anterior to the fifth lumbar vertebra within the prevertebral space. These sympathetic fibers control the normal transport of sperm and delivery of sperm ejaculation. They prevent retrograde ejaculation by closing the bladder neck during ejaculation.

Anterior View of the L5-S1 Disk Space, Aorta, Vena Cava, and Presacral Hypogastric Plexus (Fig. 11-8)

The specimen in Figure 11-8 demonstrates the precarious proximity of the presacral hypogastric plexus to the L5 and S1 bodies and the vascular anatomy. Some authors have recommended a transperitoneal approach with opening of the posterior peritoneum on the right side of the aorta and sub-

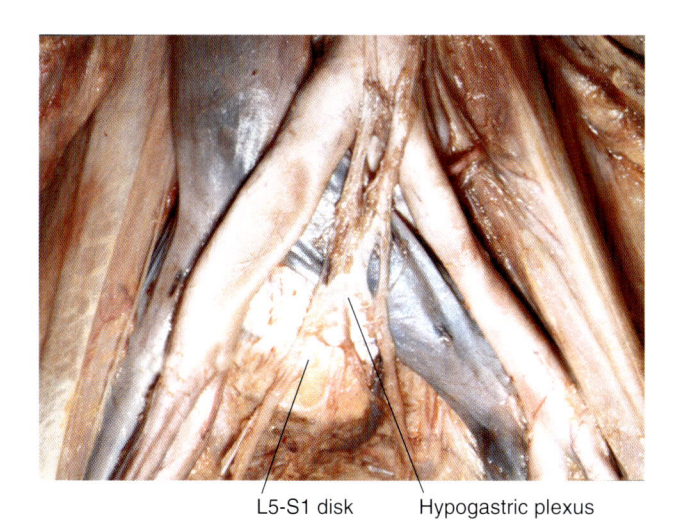

Fig. 11-8 Anterior view of L5-S1 disk space and presacral hypogastric plexus.

sequent mobilization of the plexus to the left as a means to prevent injury to the plexus. The termination of the aorta and the origin of the inferior vena cava each form a Y-shaped bifurcation. The aorta is typically anterior and left with the vena cava lying posterior and right. From our dissections, we found that the aortic bifurcation is usually immediately anterior to the body of the L4 vertebrae and the origin of the common iliac veins was observed mainly at the L5 body.

The Retroperitoneal Approach to the Lumbar Spine

The optimal side of exposure is determined predominantly by the anatomic confines dictated by vascular and other visceral structures.[3-7] Vena cava mobilization is often difficult and dangerous owing to its friability and location. Aortic mobilization provides a safer and more substantial ventral vertebral body exposure. This is similarly true for the iliac vessels. The liver, as a result of its mass and location, is more difficult to retract and mobilize than the spleen. Excessive splenic retraction, however, may result in injury to this organ. Therefore, an exposure from the left side is usually preferred.

The retroperitoneal approach to the ventral lumbar spine is dictated by the anatomic confines of the particular region of the spine to be explored. Exposures involving the resection of the eleventh or twelfth rib may be used to gain access to the thoracolumbar and upper lumbar spine.[8-10] The vertebral column is accessed via the retroperitoneal space, and subsequently, subperiosteal dissection is carried out along the vertebral body. The exposure is achieved by approaching the vertebral body immediately ventral to the quadratus lumborum muscle. The crus of the diaphragm must be detached from the anterior longitudinal ligament to provide upper lumbar exposure. Segmental arterial branches are ligated, thus providing access to the ventral spine. Following this, one can then approach the spinal canal.

The retroperitoneal approach to the midlumbar spine allows access to the ventrolateral spinal canal from L2 to below the pelvic brim. The dissection proceeds in an anatomic manner by splitting through the external oblique, internal oblique, and transverses abdominus muscles along the muscle fibers of each muscle layer, except the internal oblique muscle layer, which may be transected across its muscle fibers. If the internal oblique muscle layer is not divided in this fashion, the width of the exposure is significantly limited. The incision is then carried into the retroperitoneal space. The sympathetic chain can be visualized in the groove between the psoas muscle and the vertebral body. This exposure is limited rostrally by the crus of the diaphragm and caudally by the pelvic brim. In order to expose the neural foramina via this approach, psoas muscle retraction or incision is required.

When ventral lower lumbar exposure is planned, an incision beginning lateral to and slightly above the anterior superior iliac spine can be carried medially and caudally, parallel and rostral to the iliac crest and inguinal ligament. Access to the muscular plane below this level is thus provided. An incision along the external oblique muscle fibers and across the internal oblique and transversus abdominis muscle fibers, in turn, provides access to the extraperitoneal pelvic structures. The peritoneum and renal fascia are swept medially, taking care to prevent injury to the retroperitoneal nerves and ureter. The vertebrae beneath the aorta and iliac arteries are thus exposed.

REFERENCES

1. Capener N: Spondylolisthesis. Br J Surg 1932;19:374–386.
2. Burns BH: An operation for spondylolisthesis. Lancet 1933;1:1233–1239.
3. Found EM, Weinstein JN: Surgical approaches to the lumbar spine. In Frymoyer JW (ed): The Adult Spine: Principles and Practice. New York, Raven Press, 1991, pp 1523–1534.
4. Johnson RM, Mcguire EJ: Surgical approaches to the spine. In Rothman RH, Simeone FA (eds): The Spine, Vol 2. Philadelphia, WB Saunders, 1992, pp 1607–1738.
5. Riseborough EJ: The anterior approach to the spine for correction of deformities of the axial skeleton. Clin Orthop 1973;93:207–214.
6. Southwick WO, Robinson RA: Surgical approaches to the vertebral bodies in the cervical and lumbar regions. J Bone Joint Surg Am 1957;39:631–643.
7. Watkins RG (ed): Surgical Approaches to the Spine. New York, Springer-Verlag, 1983.
8. Digby KH: The twelfth rib incision as an approach to the kidney. Surg Gynecol Obstet 1941;73:84–85.
9. Harmon PH: Anterior excision and vertebral bone fusion operation for intervertebral disk syndromes of the lower lumbar spine: Three to five year results in 244 cases. Clin Orthop 1963;26:107–127.
10. Hodgson AR, Wong SK: A description of a technic and evaluation of results in anterior spinal fusion for deranged intervertebral disk and spondylolisthesis. Clin Orthop 1968;56:133–162.

CHAPTER 12

ADEBUKOLA ONIBOKUN

LANGSTON HOLLY

Posterior and Posterolateral Approaches to the Thoracic and Lumbar Spine

POSTERIOR APPROACHES

Posterior approaches to the spine are the most commonly employed surgical exposures and represent the most familiar technique to most spine surgeons. Early spine surgery consisted predominantly of dorsal exposures to the spine. Dorsal techniques are employed in cases of trauma and degenerative, neoplastic, vascular, and congenital disorders of the spine. The details of the dorsal midline approach are familiar to all spine surgeons and will not be covered elsewhere in the book.

SURGICAL ANATOMY

Despite spine surgeons' familiarity with the general anatomic features of the dorsal spine, certain nuances warrant emphasis. The spinal musculature encountered with the dorsal spine approaches consists predominantly of the erector spinae muscle column, which is invested by fascia, both ventrally and dorsally. The dorsal layer constitutes the thoracolumbar fascia. Laterally, the thoracodorsal fascia fuses with the aponeurosis of the transversus abdominis muscle; caudally, it attaches to the iliac crest and the lateral crest of the sacrum.

The surgical anatomy of the lamina is important for laminectomy, posterior sublaminar wire or hook instrumentation, and translaminar facet screw fixation. In the lumbar spine the laminar is very thin at its superior portion and thicker inferiorly. The ligamentum flavum inserts on top of the inferior lamina. The sagittal orientation of the lumbar facets allow for flexion/extension in each motion segment. At L5 the facets have to resist shearing forces across the lumbosacral junction and therefore will be more coronal in orientation.

The transverse processes are thin, composed of both cortical and cancellous bone, and oriented in the coronal plane (Fig. 12-1). Care must be taken during retraction or decortication to prevent fracture (Fig. 12-2). The anatomic relationships of the transverse processes are the nerve root anterior and superior and the branches of the dorsal rami found anteroinferiorly (Fig. 12-3). Complete exposure of the transverse process may lead to section of these branches with subsequent paraspinal muscle atrophy and facet denervation.

The pars interarticularis is a strong cortical region of the posterior arch joining the superior and inferior facets. In most laminectomies for spinal stenosis one should attempt to keep the pars intact to preserve the continuity between the superior and inferior facets. The pars is thin in its superomedial portion and thickest in its inferolateral portion.

The nerve roots coursing out of the lumbar spine pass immediately ventral to the transverse processes of the next lower spinal level. The intertransverse muscle and its aponeurosis form a bridge between each adjacent pair of transverse processes; therefore, dissection to expose the transverse processes carries very little risk of nerve root injury if the plane of dissection is maintained dorsal to this muscle layer. The innervation of the facet joints is provided by dorsal branches of the nerve roots as they exit the foramina.

POSTEROLATERAL APPROACHES

THE TRANSPEDICULAR APPROACH

The indications for use of the transpedicular approach include spinal neoplasm, infection, deformity, trauma, or an eccentrically herniated disk.[1-4]

Entry into the pedicle can be achieved by drilling through the dorsal aspect of the pars interarticularis at its junction with the superior articular process. Performing a laminectomy or laminotomy can also help localize the pedicle.

CHAPTER 12 Posterior and Posterolateral Approaches to the Thoracic and Lumbar Spine

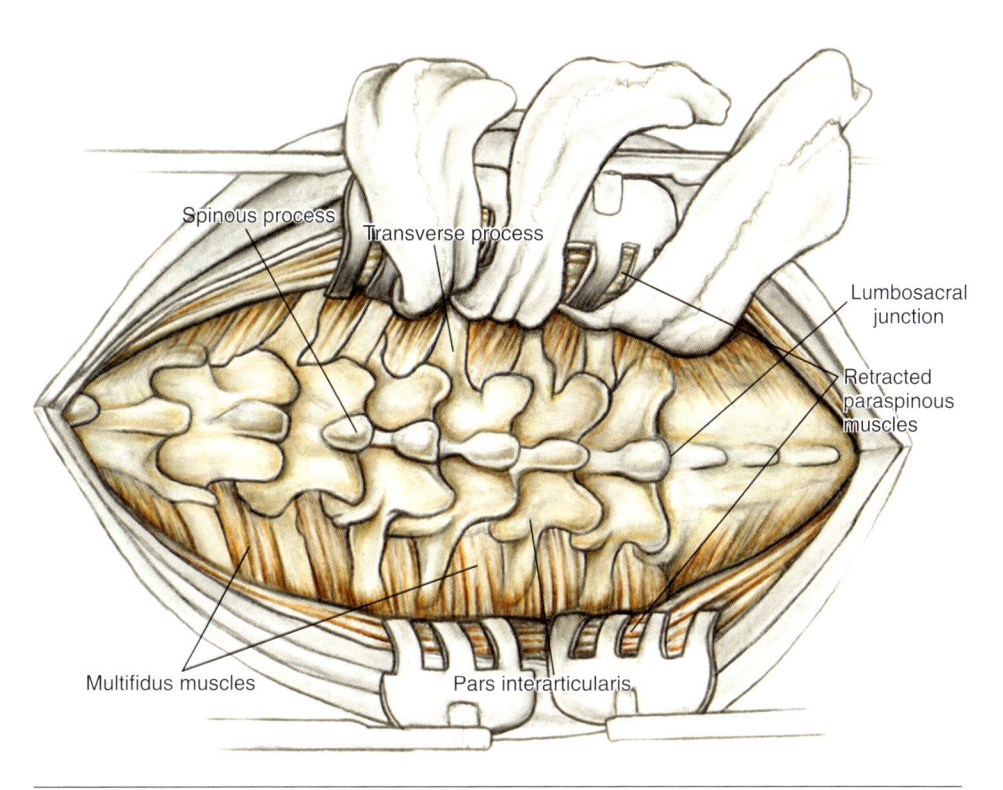

Fig. 12-1 Schematic drawing showing the posterior lumbar bony anatomy.

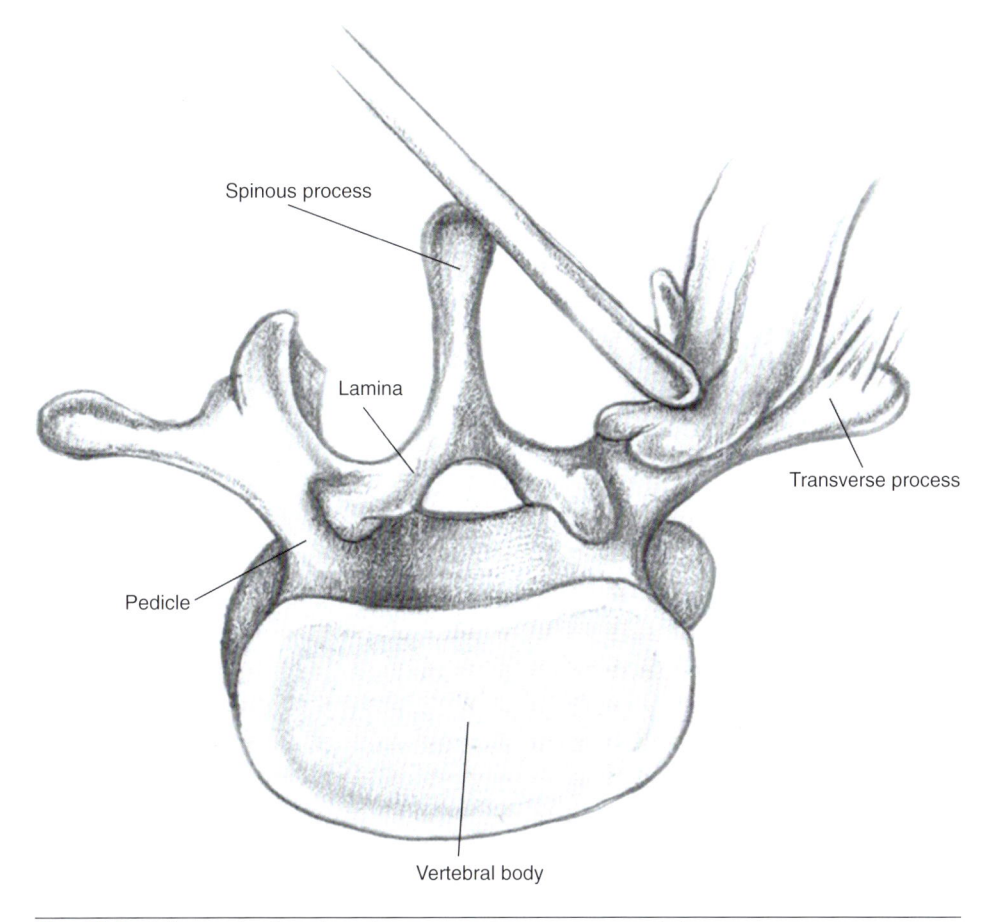

Fig. 12-2 Schematic drawing demonstrating exposure of the transverse process.

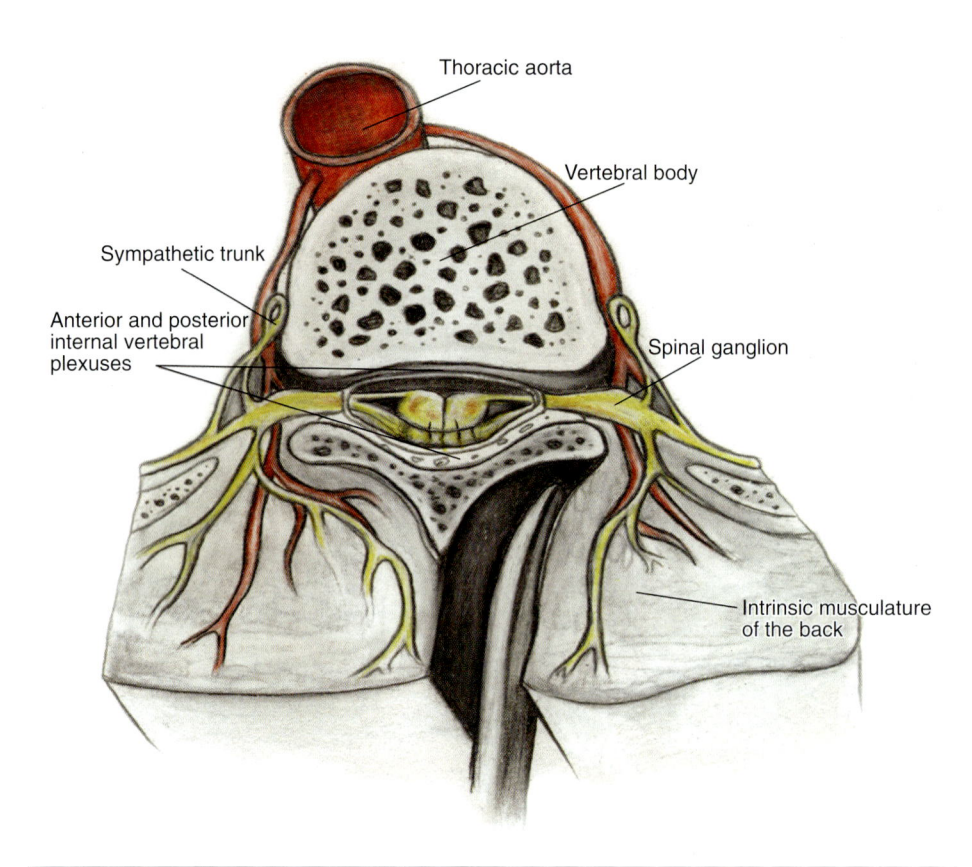

Fig. 12-3 Cross-section drawing demonstrating the vascular and nerve supply of the intrinsic muscles of the back.

Remnants of the ligamentum flavum are removed to fully expose the lateral margin of the thecal sac, the nerve roots, and the pedicle. Once the pedicle has been entered, a characteristic "pedicle blush" is encountered and corresponds to the cancellous portion of the pedicle lumen. Drilling should be initially in the internal portion of the pedicle and then should proceed to the outer cortical part. This reduces the likelihood of injury to nearby structures. Intraoperative fluoroscopy or image guidance can be used to assist in localization and surgeon orientation. Following thinning of the cortical bone from the inner cancellous surface, pituitary forceps or curettes can be used to remove the remainder of the pedicle. Upon completion of the pediculectomy, the vertebral body and the disk space are readily entered. Fractured bony fragments can easily be impacted ventrally using a reverse-angle curette. Biopsy or tumor resection can be performed with ease as well.

LATERAL EXTRACAVITARY APPROACH

In 1976, Larson and his team at the Medical College of Wisconsin defined a method in which the surgeon could safely approach lateral and anterior spine disease and perform posterior stabilization during the same procedure through the same incision.[5,6] This procedure, called the *lateral extracavitary approach* (LECA) was initially devised for the treatment of Pott's disease and vertebral osteomyelitis. During the past 30 years, this approach, along with modifications, has been used in the management of spinal disorders of the thoracic and lumbar spine due to trauma, neoplasm, degenerative disease, and infection.[7,8]

The lateral extracavitary approach is quite flexible in that it is easily combined with other procedures to allow for maximum neural decompression. The advantage of this procedure is that it provides the surgeon with access to both the posterior and lateral aspects of the spinal canal through a single incision. Because of this, the surgeon is able to decompress both the ventral and dorsal aspects of the spinal canal, while having the ability to perform posterior spinal fusion and instrumentation (Figs. 12-4 to 12-8). In addition, the exposure provided by this procedure allows the surgeon to identify the dura and the floor of the spinal canal simultaneously. This allows for the removal of the lesion with instruments that move away from the dura rather than toward it.

Surgical indications include tumor, trauma, degenerative disease, and infectious involvement of the ventral or ventrolateral aspect of the spinal column or dural sac. More laterally located pathology may be ideally addressed via this approach. Thoracic disk herniations are amenable to treatment utilizing this approach. The LECA is also well suited for thoracolumbar junction lesions.

CHAPTER 12 Posterior and Posterolateral Approaches to the Thoracic and Lumbar Spine

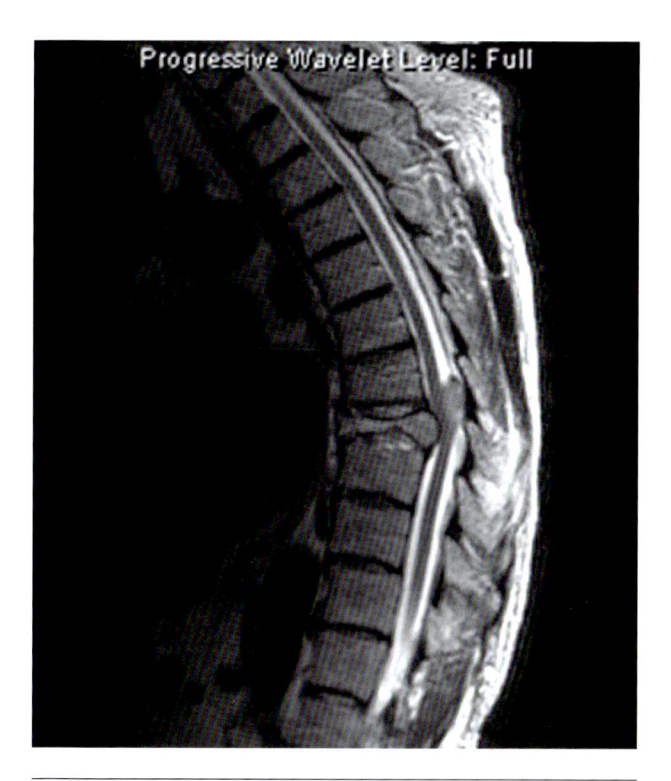

Fig. 12-4 Sagittal T$_2$-weighted magnetic resonance image demonstrating a T7 multiple myeloma lesion causing spinal cord compression in a 60-year-old male.

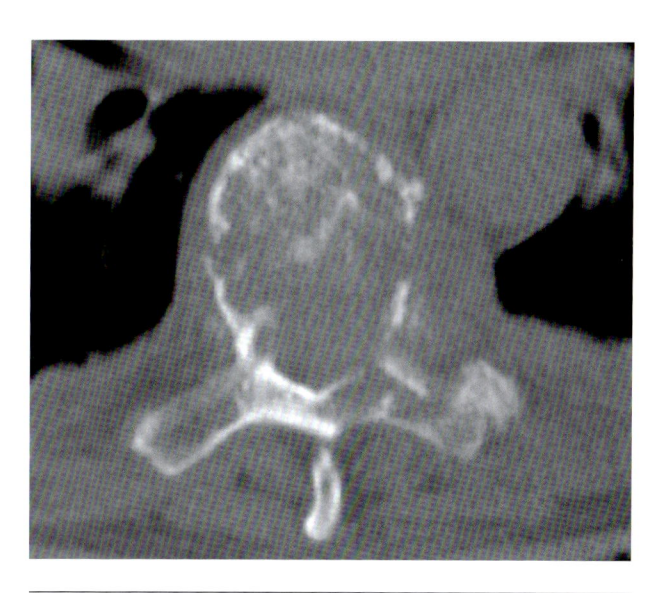

Fig. 12-6 Axial computed tomographic scan showing bony infiltration and destruction by multiple myeloma lesion.

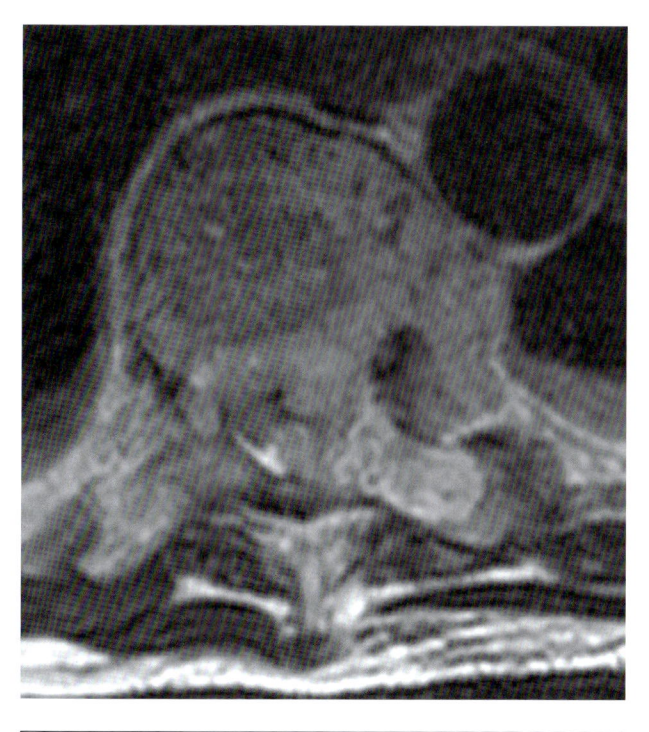

Fig. 12-5 Axial T$_2$-weighted magnetic resonance image showing circumferential spinal cord compression that is most prominent on the left side.

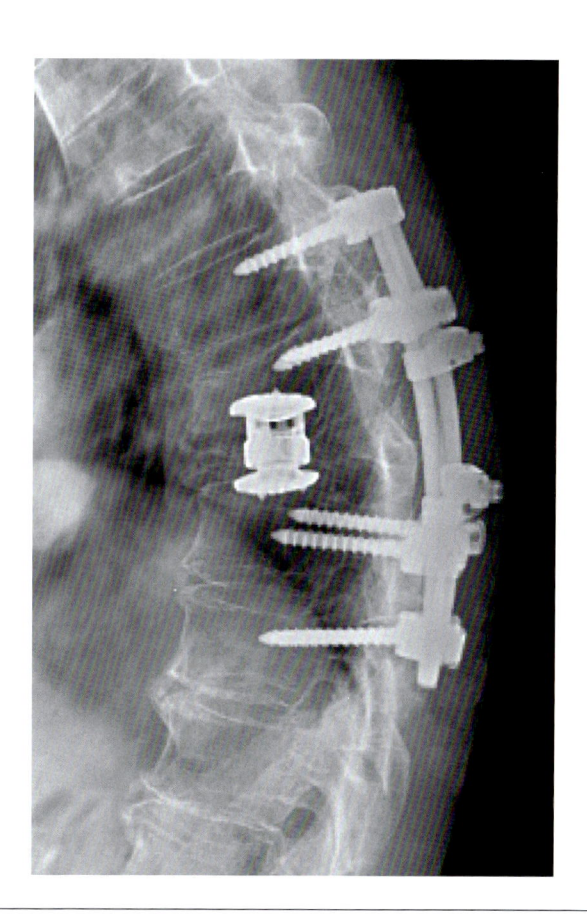

Fig. 12-7 Lateral radiograph following T7 corpectomy with intervertebral cage and posterior pedicle screw placement via a left-sided lateral extracavitary approach.

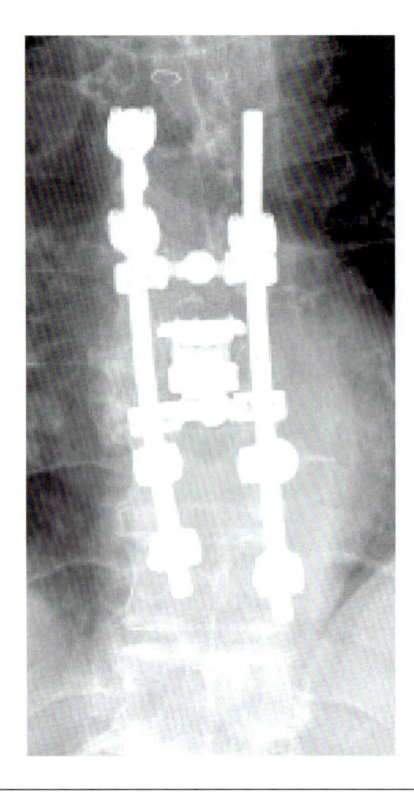

Fig. 12-8 Anteroposterior radiograph following resection of the tumor and T5-T9 spinal stabilization.

Related Anatomy

For the surgeon employing this approach, a clear understanding of the regional anatomy is imperative. Safe and effective exposure may be accomplished at all levels by the surgeon with a thorough knowledge of the paraspinal anatomy.

Dorsal to the upper thoracic spine are three nearly contiguous muscle groups: the trapezius, rhomboid, and erector spinae. These muscles constitute the dorsal plane, ventral to which the spine is approached through the LECA. The dorsolateral plane in the midthoracic spine is defined by the trapezius and longissimus muscles dorsally and the rhomboid and external intercostals muscles ventrally (Fig. 12-9). In the lower thoracic spine, dorsolaterally the erector spinae muscles remain as a discrete bundle that includes the iliocostal, transversospinal, and longissimus muscles.

In the upper lumbar spine, the dorsolateral plane in the upper lumbar spine lies between the erector spinae muscle group, dorsal to the transverse processes and the quadratus lumborum muscle. In the lower lumbar spine the plane between the erector spinae muscle group and the quadratus lumborum muscle leads to the transverse process and subsequently the neural foramen.

Each thoracic segment is accompanied by a pair of ribs. The first, eleventh, and twelfth pair typically articulate solely with their named vertebra. The second through tenth ribs articulate primarily with their named vertebral body but also with the rostral disk and to the rostral neighbor via a small demifacet on the inferolateral surface of the vertebral body. In addition, each pair of ribs articulates with the anterior surface of the transverse process of its named vertebra. The ribs are connected to the vertebral column by the costotransverse ligaments, a dense, complex, multilayered ligamentous construct.

The space between the transverse process, lateral edge of the pedicle, and the medial edge of the rib forms a roughly triangular osteoligamentous zone through which a posterolateral approach to the anterolateral and anterior aspect of the spine can be performed. Surgery within this space can be performed without entry into the pleural space.

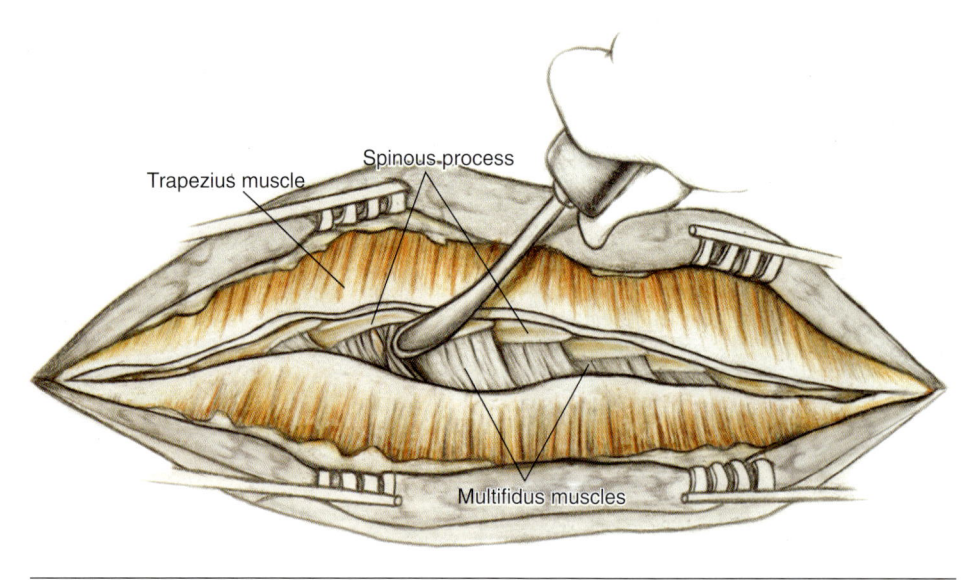

Fig. 12-9 Schematic drawing showing superficial posterior muscle dissection during exposure of the spine.

CHAPTER 12 Posterior and Posterolateral Approaches to the Thoracic and Lumbar Spine

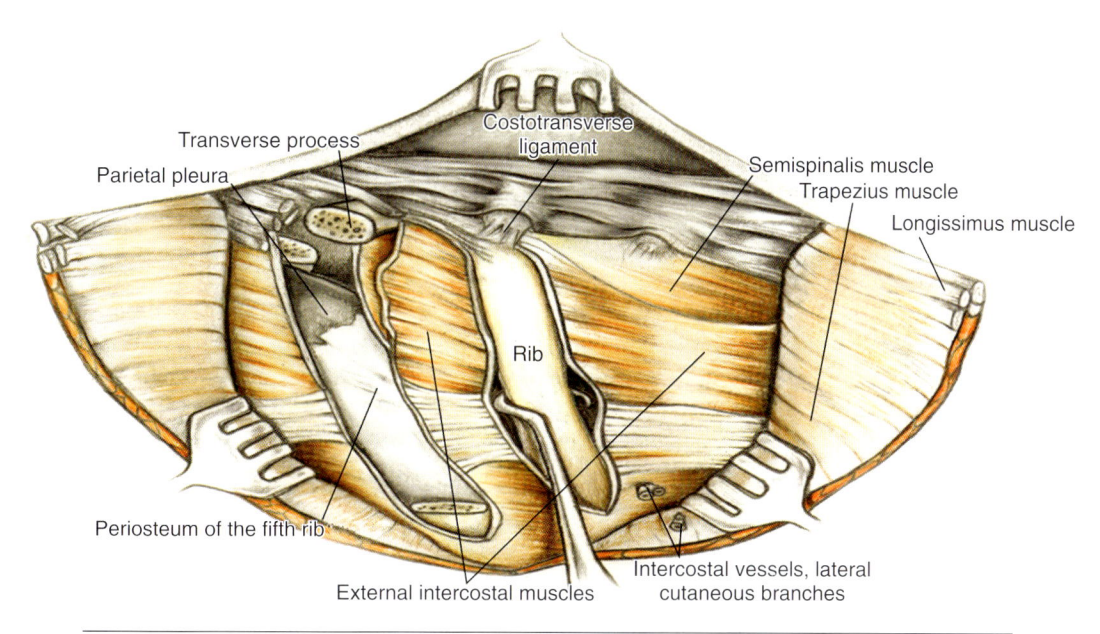

Fig. 12-10 Lateral extracavitary approach after removal of one rib and preparation of adjacent rib removal.

The neural foramen is bounded by the rostral margin of the pedicle below, the caudal margin of the pedicle above, the dorsal margin of the vertebral body and disk, and the ventral portion of the corresponding facet joint. The corresponding intercostal vein and artery arise from the aorta and the azygos vein on the right. This vascular bundle lies in the middle portion of the vertebral bundle. The intercostal vessels join the intercostal nerves exiting the neuroforamen and form the subcostal neurovascular bundle below the corresponding rib.

The Surgical Approach

This approach to the thoracic or lumbar spine can be made from either side. Regional anatomic nuances and the side of the pathology predominantly dictate the side of the surgical exposure. A variety of incisional options are available. A long midline incision mandates a significant subcutaneous dissection in order to acquire adequate lateral exposure. A hockey stick incision allows the use of a shorter incision but necessitates the performance of a significant subcutaneous flap. Next, the thoracodorsal fascia is incised. In the thoracic region, the dorsal upper back musculature (trapezius, latissimus dorsi, and rhomboid muscles) is flapped from the midline or split along its fibers in order to gain access to the underlying rib cage in the paramedian region (Fig. 12-10).

The erector spinae muscles, which lie immediately under the thoracodorsal fascia, are then retracted medially. The dissection proceeds from lateral to medial, underneath the erector spinae muscles. In the thoracic region, these muscles overlie the rib cage, whereas in the lumbar region, they overlie the quadratus lumborum. In the thoracic region, the medial 6 to 12 cm of one to three ribs are resected. The surrounding soft tissues around these ribs are first dissected off in a subperiosteal fashion. A rib cutter is used to incise the ribs laterally. Medially, the costotransverse and costovertebral joints are disarticulated by careful, sharp dissection and manipulation.

Care must be taken to aggressively dissect the parietal pleura off the undersurface of the ribs, the costovertebral joints, and the lateral aspect of the vertebral bodies in order to minimize the chance of acquiring a pleural tear during the disarticulation. During subperiosteal dissection, care must be taken to avoid injury to the subcostal neurovascular bundle. The resected ribs should be preserved for bone grafting.

In the lumbar region, the pathway to the transverse process is via the window between the erector spinae and the quadratus lumborum muscles. The appropriate transverse processes are sharply freed from the surrounding soft tissues. A subperiosteal dissection is then carried out along the underside of the transverse processes, the lateral aspect of the pedicles and vertebral bodies. The exiting nerve roots are located within the muscles juxtaposed to the vertebral bodies and take off at a minimal angle from the vertical.

In the thoracic region, the nerve roots are incised distally and tagged with a suture. Following completion of the operation, intercostal nerves are sacrificed and tied or coagulated proximal to the dorsal root ganglion in order to prevent symptomatic neuroma formation. The nerve roots in the lumbar region cannot be sacrificed because of their eloquence.

COMPLICATIONS

The posterior and posterolateral approaches to the spine are associated with a variety of well-known complications. Cerebrospinal fluid leak can occur during decompression of the neural elements. This is treated with primary closure if possible or with placement of collagen sponge and fibrin glue if primary closure is unfeasible. Neurologic injury can occur during any spinal decompression, and care must be taken to perform this maneuver safely. Infection is not uncommon in posterior spinal surgical procedures, and can be minimized with the use of perioperative antibiotics. Although the LECA is a retropleual and retroperitoneal procedure, injury to viscous or vascular structures can occur if the proper anatomic planes are not maintained during dissection.

References

1. Bilsky MH: Transpedicular approach for thoracic disc herniations. Neurosurg Focus 2000;9(4):1–4.
2. Bilsky MH, Boland P, Lis E, et al: Single-stage posterolateral transpedicle approach for spondylectomy, epidural decompression, and circumferential fusion of spinal metastasis. Spine 2000;25(17):2240–2249.
3. Chien IH, Chien JT, Yu TC: Transpedicular wedge osteotomy for correction of thoracolumbar kyphosis in ankylosing spondylitis: Experience with 78 patients. Spine 2001;16:E354–E360.
4. Murrey DB, Brigham CD, Kiebzak GM, et al: Transpedicular decompression and pedicle subtraction osteotomy (eggshell procedure): A retrospective review of 59 patients. Spine 2002;27(21):2338–2345.
5. Larson SJ: Unstable thoracic fractures: Treatment alternatives and the role of the neurosurgeon. Clin Neurosurg 1980;27:624–640.
6. Larson SJ, Holst RA, Hemmy DC, et al: Lateral extracavitary approach to traumatic lesions of the thoracic and lumbar spine. J Neurosurg 1976;45:628–637.
7. Benzel EC: The lateral extracavitary approach to the spine using the three quarter prone position. J Neurosurg 1989;71:837–841.
8. Benzel EC, Larson SJ: Operative stabilization of the posttraumatic thoracic and lumbar spine: A comparative analysis of the Harrington rod and the modified Weiss spring. Neurosurgery 1986;19:378–385.

SECTION E
Lumbar Sacral Junction

CHAPTER 13

BRIAN M. LEO
D. GREG ANDERSON

Transperitoneal Approaches to the Lumbosacral Junction

INTRODUCTION

Even before the initial description of spinal fusion by Hibbs[1] and Albee[2] in 1911, Müller had described the anterior transperitoneal approach to the spine in 1906.[3] It was, however, the work of Hodgson[4] in Hong Kong on the treatment of Pott's disease (spinal tuberculosis) that popularized the anterior approach to the thoracolumbar spine. In his 1956 article, Hodgson noted the ease with which the spinal cord could be decompressed from the anterior approach allowing evacuation of the infectious material and fusion of the spine. Sidney Sacks of South Africa was an early advocate of the anterior approach to the lumbosacral junction and used this approach to treat a variety of pathologic conditions. He was one of the first to recognize the condition of retrograde ejaculation as a complication of this approach.[5] Although the transperitoneal approach has become less popular in recent years and has been supplanted to some degree by the retroperitoneal approach, the transperitoneal approach continues to be a useful strategy for accessing the anterior aspect of the lumbosacral spine. With the advent of laparoscopic spinal procedures, this approach has seen a resurgence, especially for accessing the L5-S1 disk level.

The benefits of less invasive surgery have led to the rapid advancement of new instruments and techniques. As laparoscopic techniques have become more accepted in the fields of general and urologic surgery, these techniques have been adapted to spinal surgery. Beginning in the mid-1990s, laparoscopic surgery has been used successfully in some centers to access the lumbosacral junction. The theoretical advantages of laparoscopy over the more traditional open approaches are improved visualization of surgical anatomy, decreased postoperative pain, and early hospital discharge. Potential disadvantages of a laparoscopic approach include increased surgical time and in some series a higher rate of vascular injury. As with any new technology, these procedures are associated with a steep learning curve. Patients with multiple abdominal operations are generally considered poor candidates for laparoscopic approaches to the spine.

In this chapter we will describe the transperitoneal surgical approaches to the lumbosacral junction using both the traditional open and the newer laparoscopic approach.

ANATOMY REVIEW

The transperitoneal approach to the lumbar spine involves three stages of dissection. The *superficial stage* involves the dissection from the skin to the peritoneum. The *intraperitoneal stage* traverses the peritoneal cavity and involves packing or retracting the viscera out of the way. The *retroperitoneal stage* consists of mobilizing the retroperitoneal structures including the great vessels (aorta, vena cava, or common iliac vessels), ureters, and presacral plexus.

The anterior abdominal wall consists of the skin, subcutaneous fat, Scarpa's fascia, rectus abdominus (with the rectus sheath), the transversalis fascia, preperitoneal fat, and the peritoneum. At the midline, between the right and left rectus muscles, is a fascial condensation called the *linea alba*. The linea alba becomes less distinct caudal to the umbilicus. Lateral to the rectus abdominis muscles are the three sheet-like muscles that make up the lateral abdominal wall. These muscles include the external oblique, internal oblique, and transverse abdominis muscles (from superficial to deep). It is the fascia of these muscles that encases the rectus abdominis muscle giving rise to the rectus sheath.

The long flat rectus abdominis muscle extends the full length of the abdomen. The rectus sheath is the investing fascia of this muscle. Above the umbilicus, the internal oblique fascia splits to encase the rectus abdominis muscle. The external oblique fascia traverses anterior to the rectus, making up the anterior rectus sheath, while the transversus

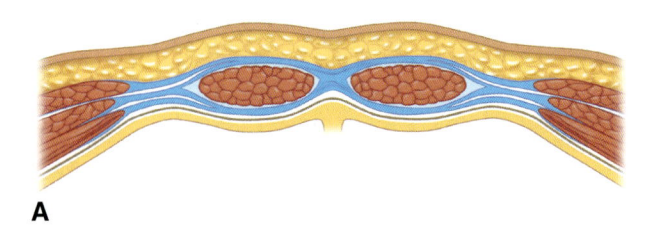

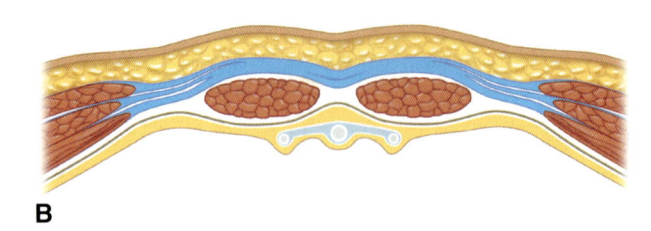

Fig. 13-1 The anatomy of the rectus sheath differs below the umbilicus. *A,* Above the umbilicus the aponeurosis of the internal oblique splits to encase the rectus abdominis muscle before joining with the aponeuroses of the external oblique and transverses abdominis to form the linea alba. *B,* Below the umbilicus all three aponeuroses pass anterior to the rectus sheath, leaving only the transversalis fascia along the posterior wall of the rectus muscle.

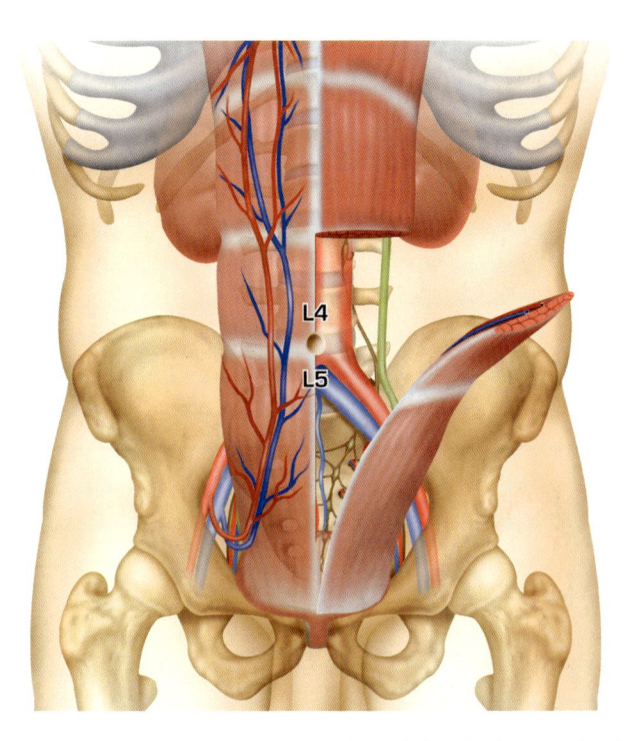

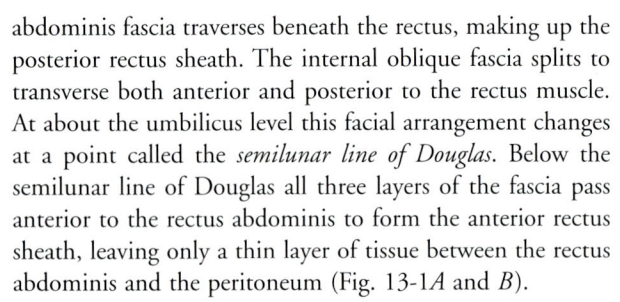

Fig. 13-2 A superior view of the intraperitoneal cavity demonstrating the location of the inferior epigastric artery and vein branching off the external iliac vessels and traveling superomedially between the transversalis fascia and the rectus abdominis muscle. These vessels may be injured if a transverse (Pfannenstiel) incision is used or during endoscopic portal placement.

abdominis fascia traverses beneath the rectus, making up the posterior rectus sheath. The internal oblique fascia splits to transverse both anterior and posterior to the rectus muscle. At about the umbilicus level this facial arrangement changes at a point called the *semilunar line of Douglas*. Below the semilunar line of Douglas all three layers of the fascia pass anterior to the rectus abdominis to form the anterior rectus sheath, leaving only a thin layer of tissue between the rectus abdominis and the peritoneum (Fig. 13-1*A* and *B*).

The inferior epigastric vessels lie between the abdominal wall muscles and the transversalis fascia. These vessels course obliquely upward from lateral to medial. Owing to their lateral position, they are rarely at risk during a midline approach but may be injured during a more lateral approach or abdominal laparoscopic portal placement (Fig. 13-2).

During the intraperitoneal stage the viscera are encountered. During exposures of the lower abdominal cavity, the small intestine and sigmoid colon are generally visualized. These may be packed or retracted out of the way to allow visualization of the posterior peritoneum. The bladder generally lies at the inferior aspect of the field. The small intestines are superficial and should be packed or retracted first upon entry into the abdominal cavity. The sigmoid colon is generally retracted toward the left, allowing access to the retroperitoneal space.

During the retroperitoneal stage of dissection, the major vessels and ureter must be identified and protected. The aortic bifurcation most commonly occurs at the L4-L5 disk level (Fig. 13-3). Thus, the approach to the L5-S1 disk is generally between the common iliac vessels. The small middle sacral vessel should be identified and ligated for access to the L5-S1 disk. The approach to the L4-L5 disk is generally more difficult than the L5-S1 level because of the vascular anatomy. To access the anterior aspect of the L4-L5 disk space, the segmental vessels that run over the lateral body of L4 generally require ligation. The ascending lumbar vein, which is the first branch of the common iliac vein, should also be sought and controlled (Fig. 13-4). This vessel lies close to the L5 vertebral body. If the vessels are retracted laterally without controlling the ascending lumbar vein, it can be avulsed from the posterior aspect of the iliac vein, leading to heavy bleeding, which is difficult to control. Variations in the bifurcation and location of the great vessels are common and should be anticipated.

The ureters are loosely attached in the retroperitoneal space. The ureters cross the common iliac vessels at the level of the sacroiliac joint and then lie on the anterior psoas as they enter the pelvis. A surgical trick to identify the ureter is

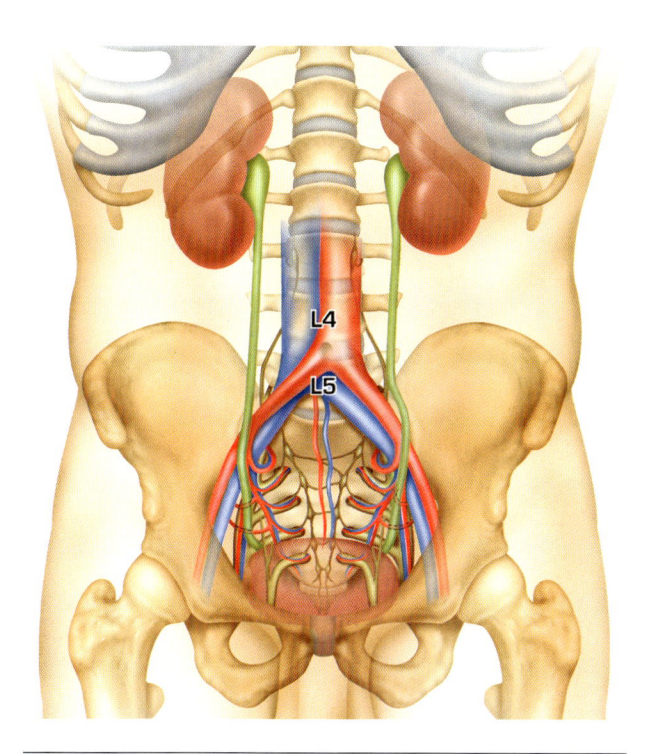

CHAPTER 13 Transperitoneal Approaches to the Lumbosacral Junction

Fig. 13-3 The aortic bifurcation most commonly occurs at the L4-L5 disk level. The inferior vena cava is located posterior and to the right of the aorta and typically bifurcates at the L5 body. The middle sacral vessels should be identified and ligated to avoid excessive bleeding.

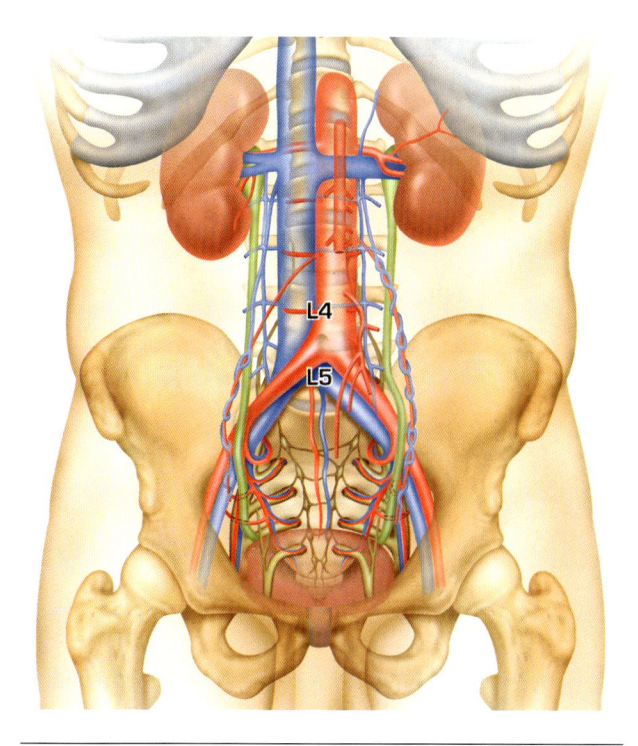

Fig. 13-4 The ascending lumbar vein is the first branch off the common iliac vein. This vessel is found near the L5 vertebral body and travels cephalad. It should be identified and ligated when accessing the L4-L5 disk space to avoid injury to this vessel resulting in heavy bleeding.

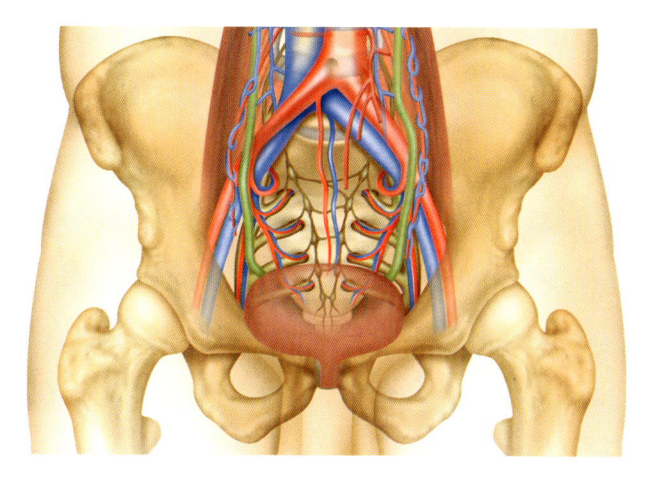

Fig. 13-5 The ureters travel in the retroperitoneal space crossing over the common iliac vessels at the bifurcation into the internal and external branches. It can be identified by gently stroking the ureter and watching for peristaltic contractions.

to gently squeeze this structure with an instrument, leading to contraction of the ureter (Fig. 13-5).

The superior hypogastric plexus lies on the anterior surface of the aorta, the sacral promontory, and the left common iliac artery. These autonomic nerves supply the internal vesicle sphincter, which contracts during ejaculation to prevent the backflow of semen into the bladder. Injury to these nerves can lead to retrograde ejaculation in males (Fig. 13-6).

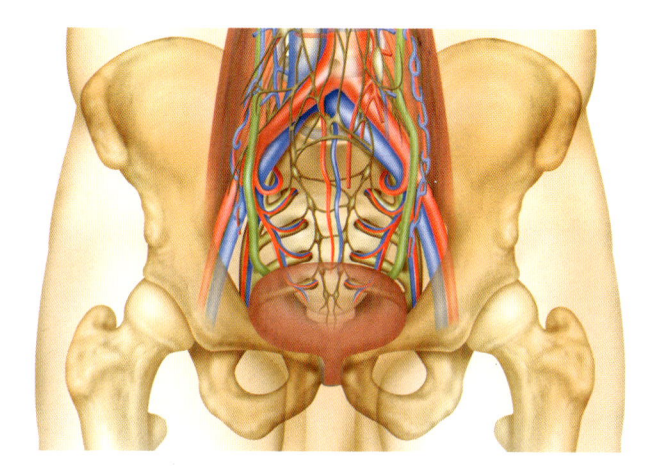

Fig. 13-6 The superior hypogastric plexus overlies the L5-S1 disk space and sacral promontory. If this autonomic nerve plexus is damaged during the dissection, impotence or retrograde ejaculation may result. Sharp dissection and electrocautery, especially monopolar, should be avoided in order to preserve this nerve supply.

INDICATIONS AND CONTRAINDICATIONS

INDICATIONS

- Intractable radiculopathy and disk pain requiring L4-L5 and L5-S1 fusion
- L5 vertebral body tumor
- Spondylolisthesis
- Spinal infections
- Failed spinal operations (posterior nonunions)
- Spinal trauma and cauda equina injury
- Correction of spinal deformities (anterior release)

RELATIVE CONTRAINDICATIONS

- No absolute contraindications
- Concurrent thoracic and abdominal trauma
- Preexisting pulmonary disease or limited pulmonary reserve
- Prior intra-abdominal infection
- Prior intraperitoneal surgery
- Morbid obesity impairing safe exposure and visualization

OPERATIVE TECHNIQUE

EQUIPMENT

- Radiolucent operating table
- Fluoroscopy or intraoperative radiograph
- Headlamps
- Optical loupes
- Abdominal self-retaining retractor (Fig. 13-7)
- Bladder blade
- Malleable retractors
- Bipolar electrocautery
- 5-mm Steinmann pins
- Red rubber catheter
- Kittner swabs
- Straight and angled curettes
- 2-to 5-mm Kerrison punches
- Bone graft (autograft, allograft, cage)
- Three-dimensional radiographic study such as magnetic resonance imaging (MRI) or computed tomography (CT) to assess the pathology and determine the level of aortic and vena cava bifurcation relative to the intervertebral disk space

PATIENT POSITIONING
Open Technique

- A bowel preparation is given to the patient on the night prior to surgery.
- The patient is placed supine with Trendelenburg positioning used to push the intra-abdominal contents superiorly away from the surgical field (Fig. 13-8).
- A Foley catheter should be used to empty bladder.
- A nasogastric (NG) tube is placed to decompress the abdomen and to diminish postoperative ileus.
- Compressive stockings are placed to diminish the risk of deep venous thrombosis.
- Some advocate placement of a pulse oximetry probe on the toes of the patient to monitor vascular flow to the lower extremities during the approach.
- The anterior iliac crests are draped into the field if autograft bone is needed for the spinal procedure (Fig. 13-9).
- To open the anterior aspects of the disk spaces, the operating table can be flexed or a surgical bump can be placed beneath the lumbar region to enhance lumbar lordosis and improve visualization of the lumbosacral junction (Fig. 13-10).

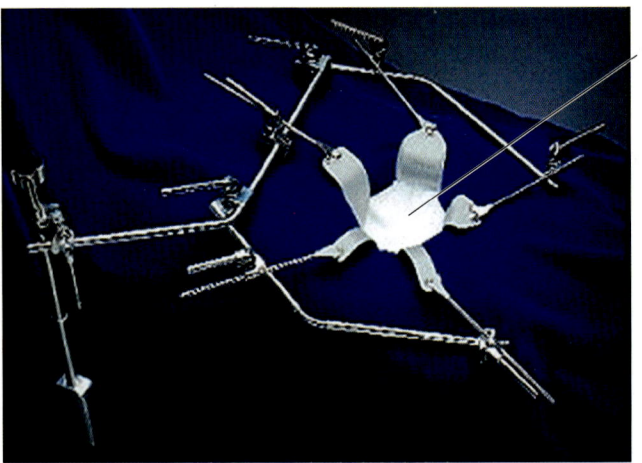

Fig. 13-7 Self-retaining abdominal retractor. A variety of blades can be used to optimize exposure to the anterior spine while protecting the intra-abdominal contents.

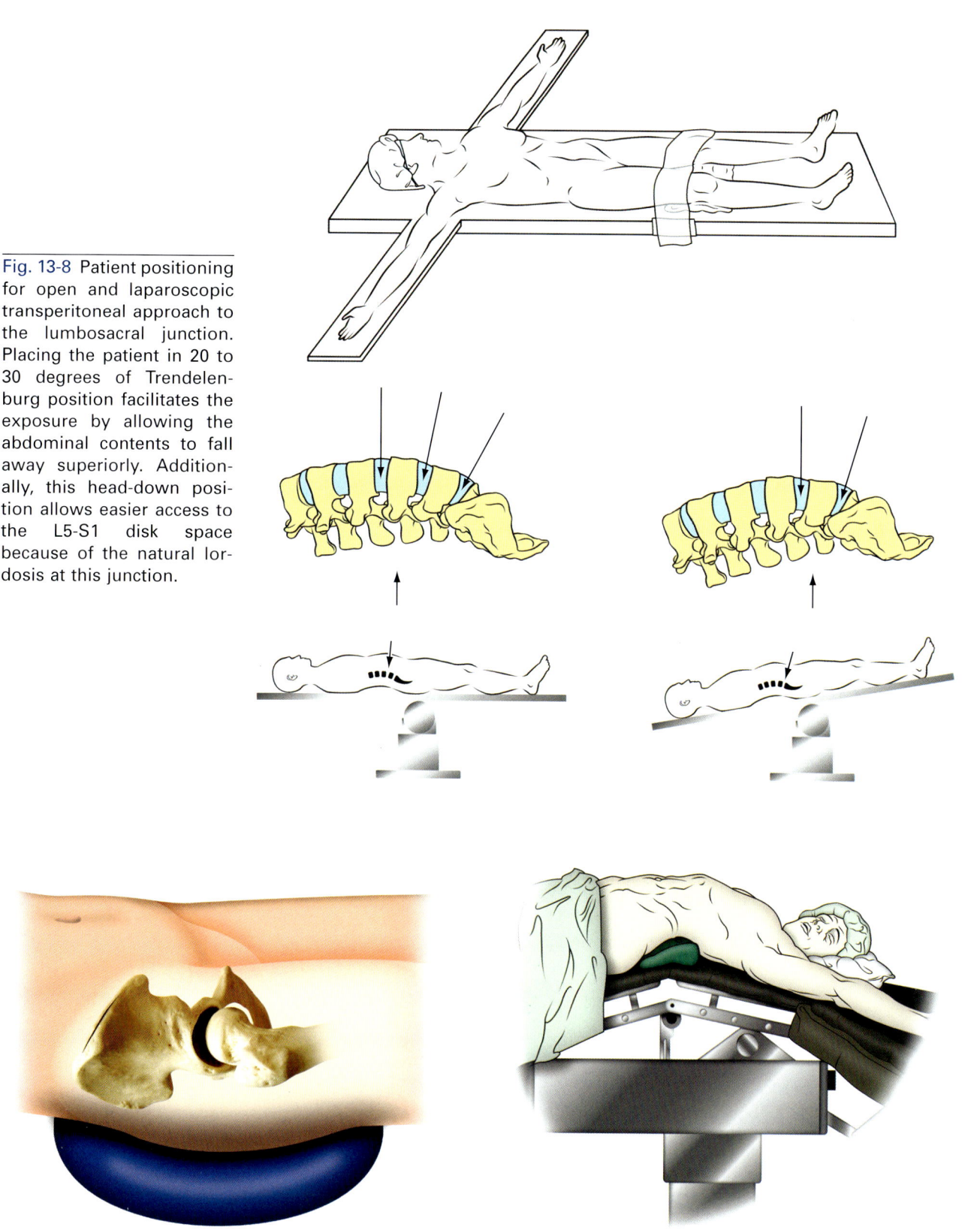

CHAPTER 13 Transperitoneal Approaches to the Lumbosacral Junction

Fig. 13-8 Patient positioning for open and laparoscopic transperitoneal approach to the lumbosacral junction. Placing the patient in 20 to 30 degrees of Trendelenburg position facilitates the exposure by allowing the abdominal contents to fall away superiorly. Additionally, this head-down position allows easier access to the L5-S1 disk space because of the natural lordosis at this junction.

Fig. 13-9 Autologous bone graft. The patient's abdomen must be prepped widely to include the anterior iliac crest for harvesting tricortical bone graft for structural support during fusion.

Fig. 13-10 Open disk space anteriorly. To help open the lower lumbar segments during the anterior approach, a small roll may be place in the small of the patient's back and the table may be flexed to create hyperlordosis.

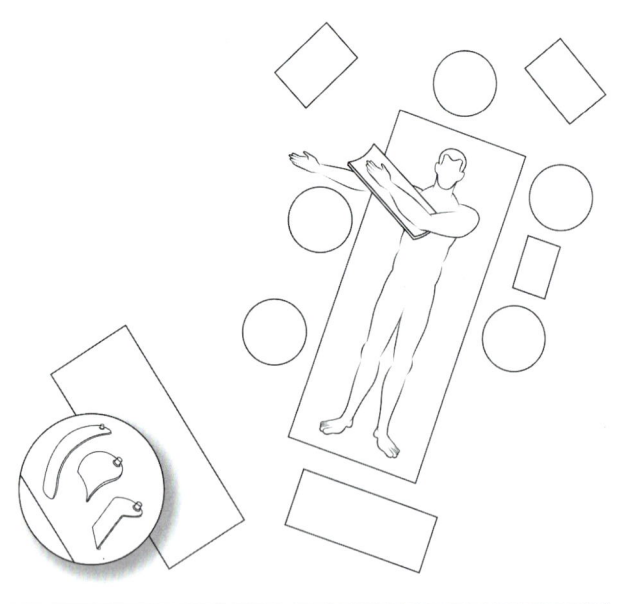

Fig. 13-11 Operating room setup for a laparoscopic approach. The right-handed surgeon generally stands to the patient's right viewing a video monitor above the patient's left shoulder. The second assistant (camera operator) stands to the patient's left above the C-arm fluoroscopy unit viewing the monitor to the patient's right, and the first assistant stands below the C-arm. Instrumentation including large retractors are available on the back table should an emergent laparotomy be necessary.

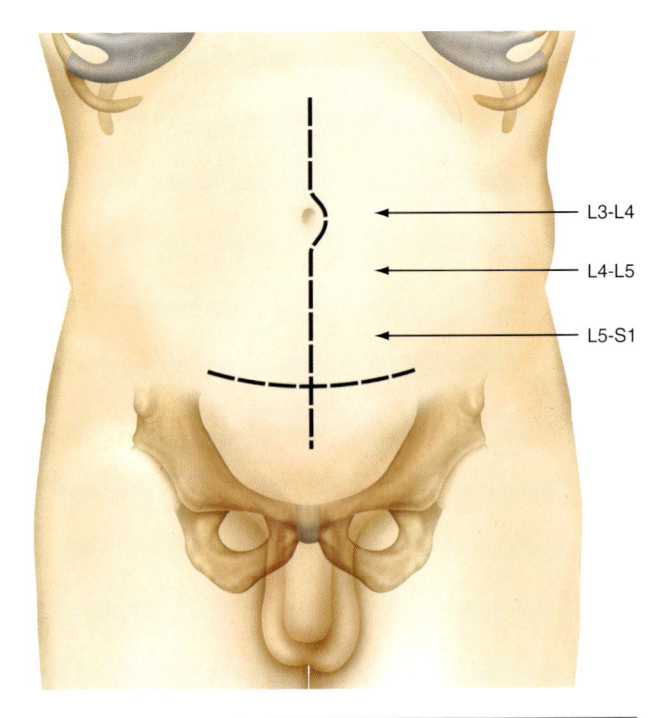

Fig. 13-12 Location of the open approach incision. A classic midline incision is made from just above the umbilicus curving to left of the umbilicus to approximately 2 to 3 cm from the pubic symphysis. A more cosmetic open approach is the transversely oriented Pfannenstiel incision.

LAPAROSCOPIC APPROACH

- A bowel preparation is given to the patient on the night prior to surgery.
- The patient is placed on a radiolucent operating table in 20 to 30 degrees of Trendelenburg position to facilitate exposure of the lumbar spine.
- A bolster is placed beneath the lumbar spine to enhance lumbar lordosis.
- A Foley catheter should be placed to empty the bladder.
- The abdomen should be prepped and draped widely.
- The surgeon generally stands to the patient's right while the assistants stand on the left above the fluoroscope to operate the camera and on the left below the fluoroscope to manipulate instruments. All necessary instruments for an open approach should be readily available in the event that rapid conversion to an open laparotomy is required (Fig. 13-11).

LOCATION OF INCISION

Open Midline Approach

- The umbilicus is generally located at the L3-L4 disk space.
- The L5-S1 disk space is located one to two fingerbreadths above the pubic symphysis, and the L4-L5 disk space located halfway between these two points.
- Owing to variability of patient anatomy, a preoperative C-arm fluoroscopy unit is useful in localizing the exact location of the incision relative to the spinal anatomy (Fig. 13-12).

Endoscopic Approach

- The classic portal strategy for L5-S1 surgery involves a 10- to 15-mm periumbilical incision for placement of the laparoscopic camera (12-mm portal).
- Two 5-mm portals are placed laterally midway between the umbilicus and the pubis to allow for retraction or suction as needed.
- A larger working portal is placed in the suprapubic region in line with the disk space. For the L5-S1 level this is approximately two fingerbreadths above the pubic symphysis.
- In obese patients a left-sided lateral portal halfway between the left lower costal margin and the umbilicus may be needed to retract the sigmoid colon (Fig. 13-13).

CHAPTER 13 Transperitoneal Approaches to the Lumbosacral Junction

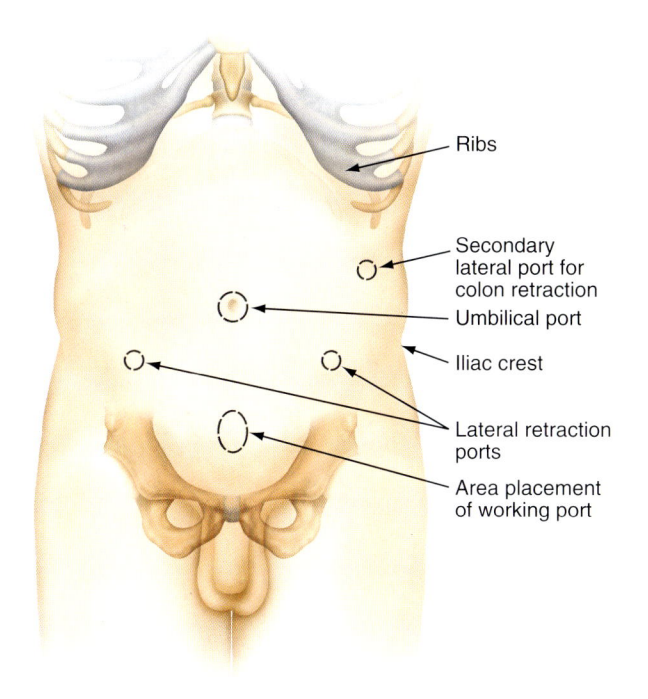

Fig. 13-13 Location of the portals for the endoscopic approach. A camera is inserted in the periumbilical portal. The lower quadrant retraction portals are placed and the low suprapubic "working" portal lies 2 to 3 fingerbreadths above the symphysis. In larger patients, an additional portal may be needed to aid with retraction.

Preparation and Draping

- The incision is marked on the skin when performing an open approach, or the portal sites are marked if performing an endoscopic approach.
- The abdomen is shaved at the incision site, and the skin is prepared sterilely.
- Draping is carefully performed to ensure bony landmarks are able to be visualized and the anterior iliac crest is available for harvesting bone graft.
- The headlamp light source is placed on the surgeon's side of the table while the fluoroscopy unit (if used) is located on the contralateral side.

INCISION AND SOFT TISSUE DISSECTION

Open Surgical Approach

- A longitudinal midline incision provides the most extensile exposure to the lower lumbar spine and lumbosacral junction (Fig. 13-14).
- If the approach is limited to the L5-S1 level, a transverse Pfannenstiel incision is useful and more cosmetic than the midline extensile incision. With the Pfannenstiel incision, care must be taken to avoid injury to the inferior epigastric vessels (Fig. 13-15).

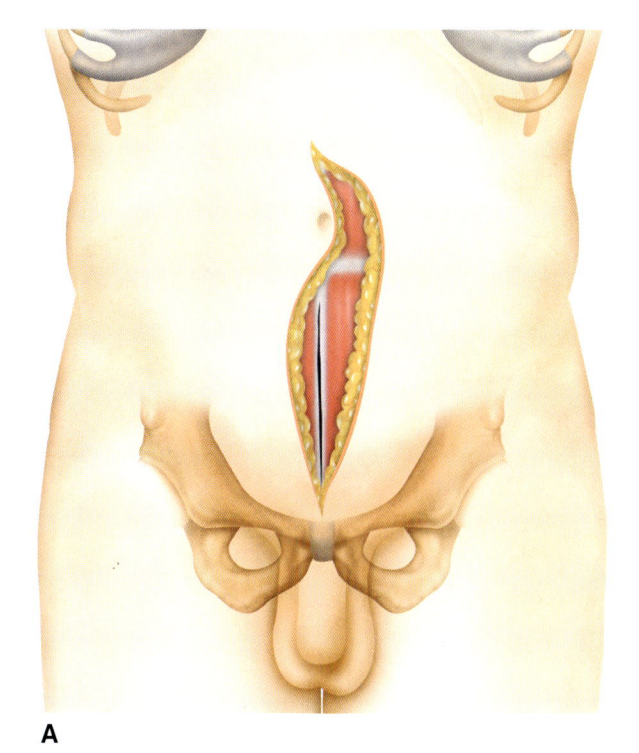

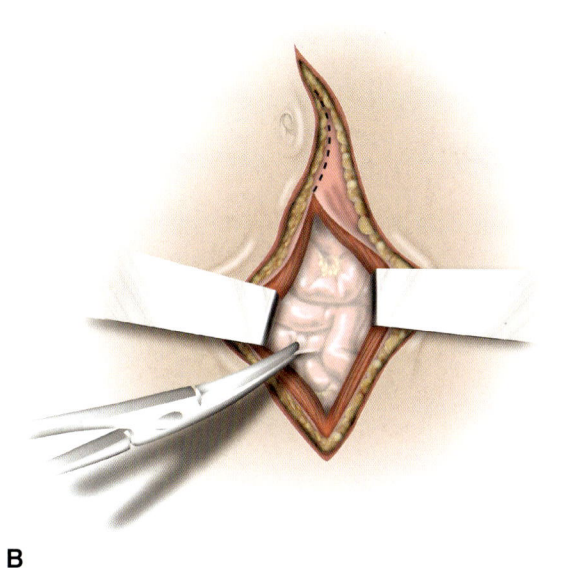

Fig. 13-14 *A* and *B*, Open midline approach. The midline longitudinal incision is most commonly used and provides the greatest anterior exposure to the lumbosacral junction.

SECTION I   SURGICAL ANATOMY AND APPROACHES

A

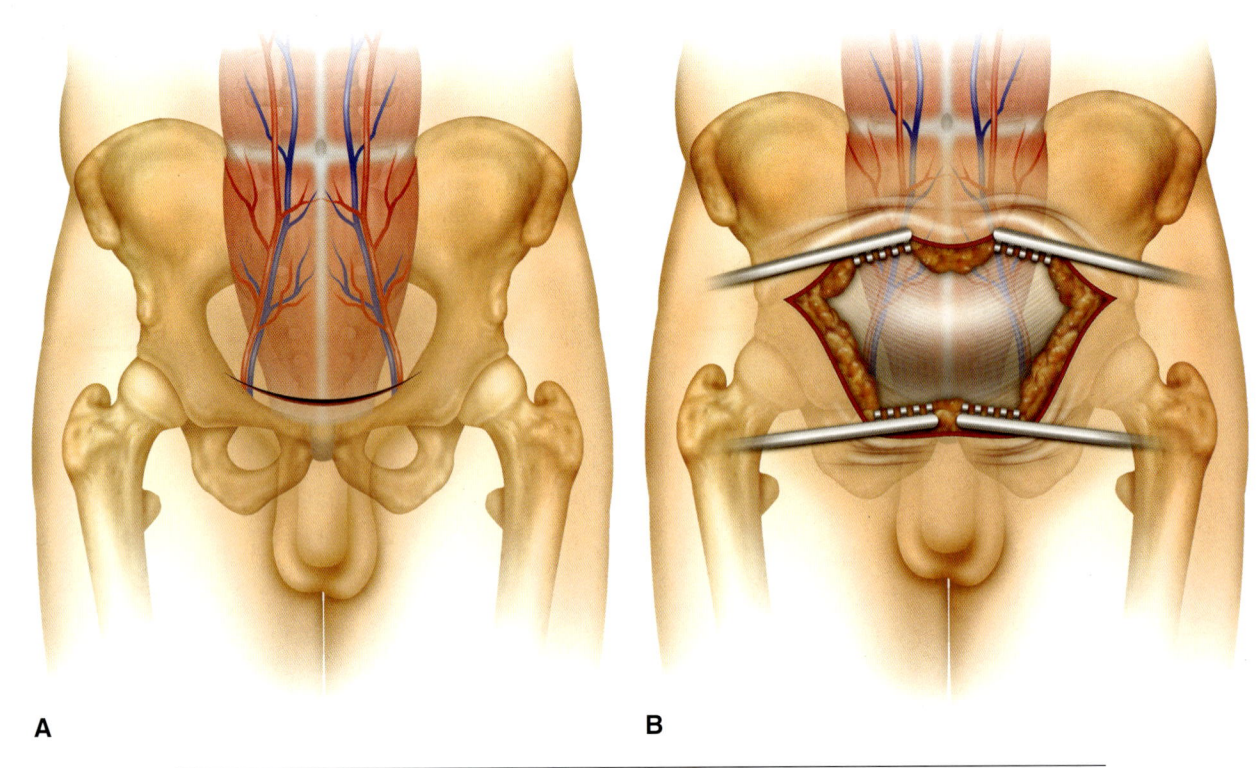

B

Fig. 13-15 *A* and *B*, Open Pfannensteil incision. The transverse Pfannensteil incision is more cosmetic than the longitudinal midline incision. It is made by palpating the pubic symphysis and making a curved incision 1 cm above in line with the skin crease. Despite the less noticeable scar, it does limit exposure to the L5-S1 disk space, and care must be taken to avoid damaging the inferior epigastric vessels, which are lateral to the midline.

- For the open transperitoneal approach the incision should be carried down in the midline between the abdominal musculature along the linea alba to avoid damage or deinnervation of the rectus muscles whose nerve supply is derived from the segmental branches of the seventh through twelfth intercostal nerves.
- Great care must be taken as the peritoneum is opened because of the risk of visceral injury. In patients with prior peritonitis or abdominal surgery, the viscera can be adherent to the anterior abdominal wall, making intraperitoneal dissection difficult.
- Once the rectus sheath is incised and the two halves are retracted laterally, the peritoneum should be elevated and a small incision is made (Fig. 13-16*A*). The hand should be placed in the abdominal cavity to protect the viscera while dividing the peritoneum (see Fig. 13-16*B*).

Intraperitoneal Dissection

- Once the peritoneal cavity has been entered, the small bowel is retracted laterally and superiorly and the sigmoid colon is identified and retracted toward the left.

- Large moist sponges are used to pack the viscera away from the operative field, and a self-retaining retractor with large malleable blades is placed (see Fig. 13-7). The small bowel and root of the mesentery are packed superiorly. The colon is retracted to the left and the bladder is protected and retracted in an inferior direction (Fig. 13-17).

LAPAROSCOPIC APPROACH

The transperitoneal technique uses carbon dioxide to insufflate the intraperitoneal space. Instruments are then introduced through special ports that prevent the insufflating gas from escaping. Because of the excellent visualization of intraperitoneal structures, this technique is ideal for addressing L5-S1 pathology.

- A Veres needle is used to insufflate the peritoneum with carbon dioxide to approximately 15 mm Hg.
- The first portal is placed at the level of the umbilicus. An incision (generally 10 to 15 mm) that allows direct visual-

CHAPTER 13 Transperitoneal Approaches to the Lumbosacral Junction

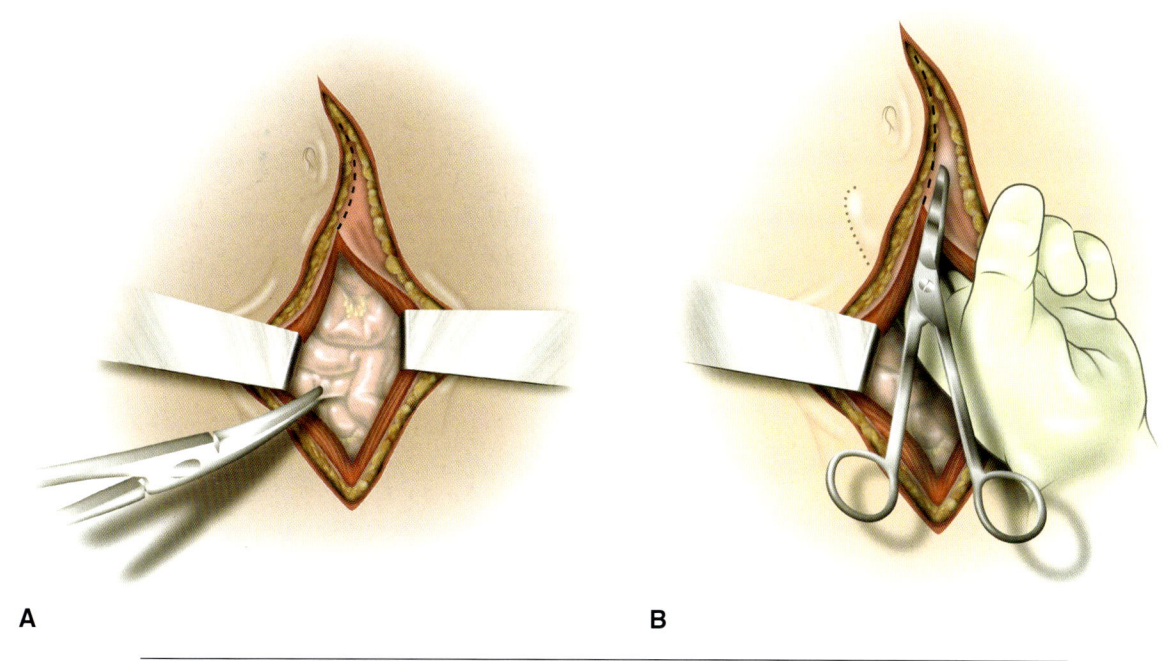

Fig. 13-16 *A* and *B*, Opening the abdominal cavity. Once the rectus sheath is incised and the musculature and transversalis fascia are retracted laterally, forceps should be used to elevate the exposed peritoneum. Prior to incising the peritoneum it is important to ensure that the bowel is not adhered or captured by the forceps (*A*). Fingers or a malleable retractor should be placed in the cavity to guide the remainder of the incision to avoid injury to the abdominal contents (*B*).

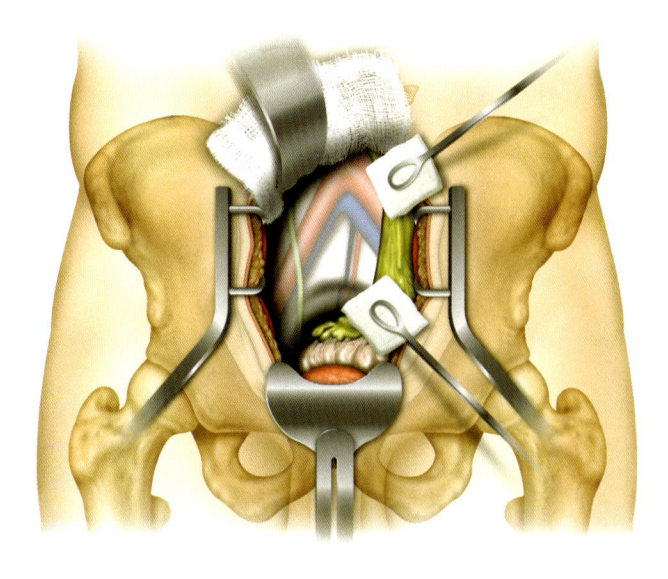

Fig. 13-17 Intraperitoneal dissection. Large moist sponges are used to pack the bowel, and self-retaining retractors with broad blades are used to maintain the operative field. The small bowel is packed superiorly while the colon is retracted to the left and caudally to expose the posterior peritoneum.

ization of the peritoneum is made. Great care is taken during placement of the sharp trochar to prevent inadvertent penetration of the abdominal viscera. A 30-degree laparoscope is then inserted into this portal.
- Additional portals are made under direct visualization with the laparoscope.
- Intraoperative fluoroscopy is helpful to position the suprapubic portal in line with the L5-S1 disk space (Fig. 13-18).
- Exposure of the disk space may require mobilization of the sigmoid colon. If necessary, the sigmoid colon can be temporarily tacked to the abdominal wall with intraabdominal sutures.
- As with open surgery, the bifurcation of the great vessels and the ureters should be identified. After division of the posterior peritoneum, the middle sacral vessels should be identified, ligated, and divided.
- The presacral autonomic plexus should be bluntly dissected over the disk space to avoid injury to these nerves.
- The diskectomy and fusion procedure then proceed with the use of instruments similar to an open approach. The 0-degree laparoscope is useful when placed through the suprapubic portal to visualize the posterior aspect of the disk space and determine the adequacy of the diskectomy.

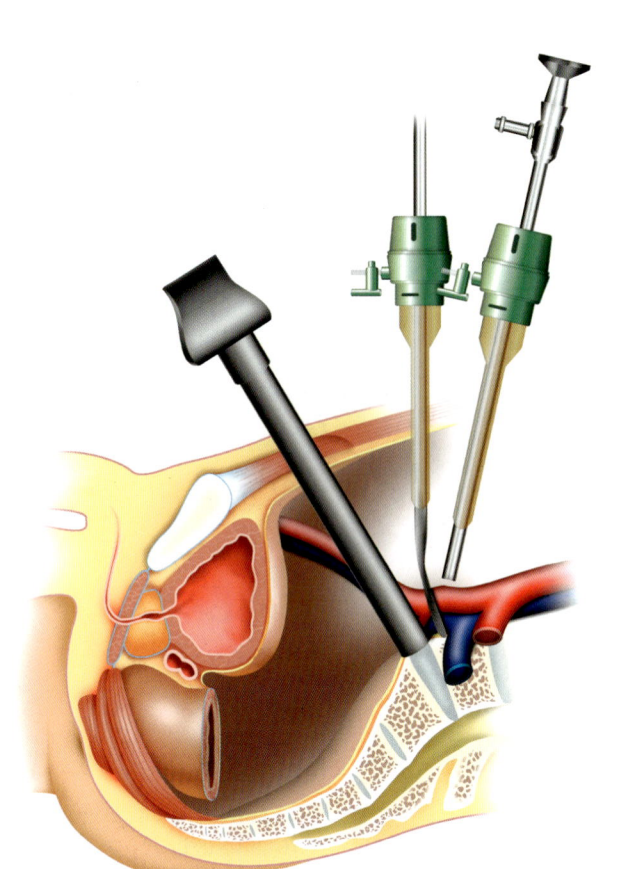

Fig. 13-18 Laparoscopic instrumentation. A 30-degree laparoscope is place in the periumbilical portal and is used to visualize placement of the remainder of the portals. A large working portal is "docked" into the L5-S1 disk space. Fluoroscopy is useful to obtain the appropriate angle and depth.

- The C-arm fluoroscopy unit is also helpful in controlling the depth and position of instruments within the disk space.

EXPOSURE OF THE VERTEBRA
Retroperitoneal Dissection

- The posterior peritoneum overlying the lumbosacral junction is identified and gently elevated using forceps and opened with Metzenbaum scissors.
- The incision is best performed lateral to the midline to avoid inadvertent injury to the middle sacral artery prior to ligation (Fig. 13-19).
- The presacral nerve plexus (hypogastric plexus) is found directly over the L5-S1 disk space. In order to minimize damage to this structure, which can result in genitourinary dysfunction, electrocautery should be avoided.
- One technique is to infiltrate the retroperitoneal space with sterile saline using a fine needle prior to entering the retroperitoneum to achieve hydrodynamic detachment of the tissue.

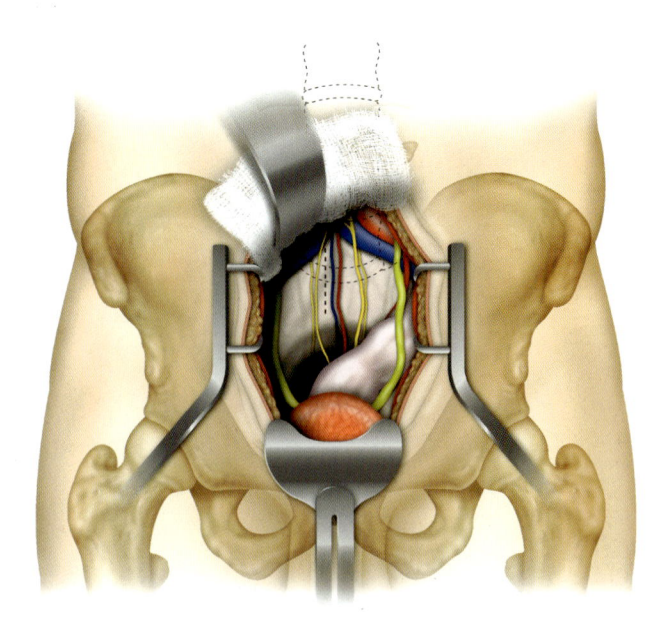

Fig. 13-19 Entering the retroperitoneum. Once the posterior peritoneum is identified, a small volume of sterile saline should be injected to hydrodynamically elevate the tissue from the underlying neurovascular structures. A longitudinal incision, avoiding the use of electrocautery, is made lateral to the midline to enter the retroperitoneal space. Blunt dissection using Kittner swabs should be used to gain exposure.

- Blunt dissection using Kittner sponges can be used to mobilize the tissue from midline toward the lateral aspect of the intervertebral disk.
- The middle sacral artery and vein, which are frequently adherent to the L5-S1 annulus, should be ligated (Fig. 13-20).
- Once the vascular structures have been mobilized and moved out of the operative field, they will need to be protected as they are retracted during the procedure. One to two stout Steinmann pins covered with a red rubber catheter can be driven into the L5 vertebral body to retract the vascular structures cephalad and laterally.

DISKECTOMY AND OSTEOPHYTECTOMY

- After exposure of the spine, a radiograph should be obtained to confirm that the correct level has been exposed.
- The disk margins are incised with a scalpel.
- A Cobb elevator is used to delaminate the cartilaginous end plate from the bony end plate. The disk is then removed with rongeurs and curettes. Vertebrectomy can be achieved following removal of the surrounding disks by resecting the bone with a rongeur or high-speed drill. If needed, the posterior annulus and posterior longitudinal ligament can be resected, allowing visualization of the dura.

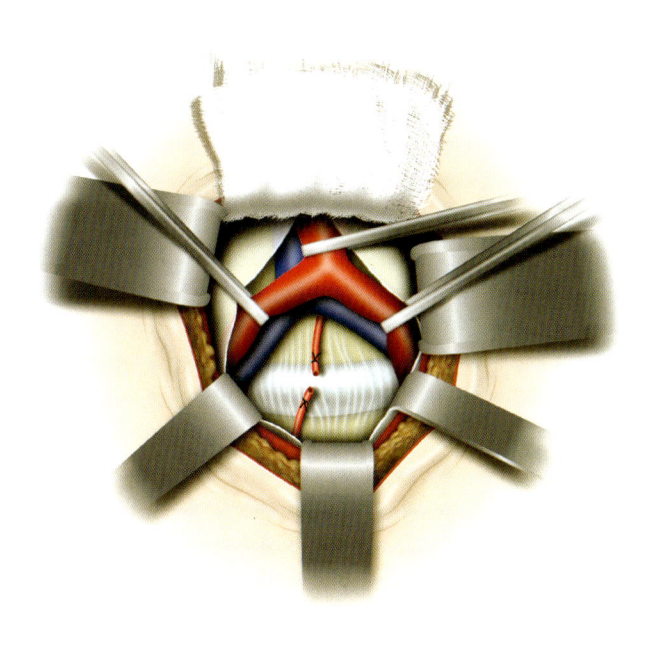

Fig. 13-20 Ligating the middle sacral artery. Once the retroperitoneum is entered, the middle sacral artery and vein should be identified and clipped.

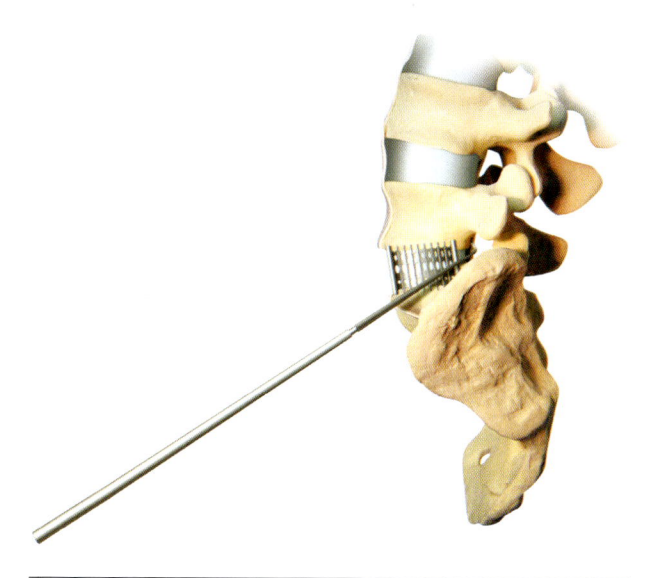

Fig. 13-21 Graft placement. Once the graft (autograft, allograft, or cage) has been placed and the distraction removed, a blunt nerve hook should be used to palpate the posterior edge of the graft to confirm that it is not compressing the dura.

- Reconstruction and fusion are then achieved using a load-bearing bone graft or structural cage packed with an appropriate osteoconductive/osteoinductive material.

BONE GRAFT

- Autologous tricortical bone harvested from the anterior iliac crest, femoral ring allograft, and a structural cage are common options used for fusion of the disk space.
- Using distraction, the L5-S1 disk space should be measured and the graft prepared.
- Under direct visualization, the graft should be tamped into place. Care must be taken not to force the graft and to protect the vascular structures during this maneuver.
- The graft should be 1 to 2 mm taller than the disk space to allow for foraminal opening and indirect decompression.
- Once the graft is in place and the distraction released, it should not move when force is applied.
- A blunt nerve hook can be used to palpate the posterior margin of the graft to ensure that it is not compressing the dural sac (Fig. 13-21).
- Once the graft is in place, anteroposterior and lateral x-rays of the lumbosacral junction should be performed to verify graft positioning.

AUTOGRAFT HARVESTING

- Iliac crest autograft is commonly used for spine fusion.
- The anterior iliac crest should be approached from a separate incision.

- The anterior superior iliac spine (ASIS) is an easily palpable bony landmark.
- A 5-cm oblique incision should be made parallel to the crest two fingerbreadths proximal to the ASIS and centered over the iliac tubercle.
- Muscle attachments are reflected subperiosteally using Bovie electrocautery on both the inner and outer tables of the ilium.
- Once the crest is exposed, Homan retractors can be used to retract the soft tissues (Fig. 13-22). Either structural tricortical or cancellous graft can be harvested.
- If a cage or femoral ring allograft is to be used with morselized autograft, a small window should be made in the cortical iliac crest over the iliac tubercle. Curved curettes can then be used to scoop out cancellous graft.
- The graft site should then be closed using heavy (such as No. 0) sutures in the fascia, followed by fine interrupted absorbable sutures superficially.
- Care should be used to avoid injury to the lateral femoral cutaneous nerve, which typically crosses the brim of the pelvis 2 cm distal to the ASIS. It is also important to avoid making a cut in the pelvis too close to the ASIS, which can result in a fracture.

CLOSURE

- At the conclusion of the procedure, the retractors are removed and the vessels and viscera are allowed to fall back to their anatomic position.
- Hemostasis should be ensured.

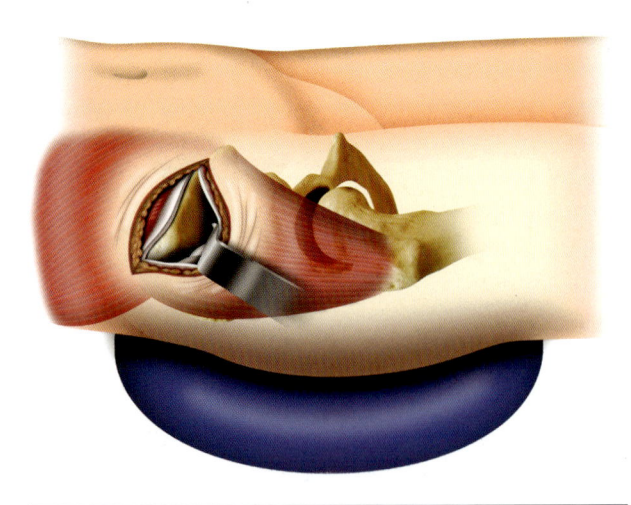

Fig. 13-22 Anterior iliac crest autograft. Autograft from the anterior iliac crest remains the gold standard for spinal fusion. The iliac crest is easily palpable, even in patients with a large body habitus. Careful surgical technique must be used to avoid complications such as nerve injury, fracture, or infection.

- The peritoneum over the retroperitoneal space can be closed with fine absorbable suture.
- The abdominal viscera are inspected to be sure that no signs of injury are present.
- The deep rectus sheath, including the peritoneum, is closed using a running No. 1 polyglycolic (Dexon) or polyglacetin (Vicryl) suture.
- The abdominal fascia is closed with heavy (No. 1) running suture.
- The subcutaneous tissue is closed with fine absorbable suture.

POSTOPERATIVE CARE

- The patient who has undergone a transperitoneal exposure for anterior spine surgery can expect to remain in the hospital for 2 to 6 days, depending on whether the approach was done laparoscopically or open.
- Intravenous antibiotic is usually given for 24 hours postoperatively and laboratory tests may be monitored as needed.
- Deep venous thrombosis prophylaxis using mechanical devices are recommended.
- When evidence of bowel function returns, the diet may be slowly advanced.
- Bracing may be used if desired.

COMPLICATIONS

In addition to the complications inherent with any surgical approach, there are a number of specific complications that occur with anterior transperitoneal surgery of the lumbosacral junction. These complications include injuries to the vessels, urogenital structures, intra-abdominal viscera, or neurologic elements and the formation of abdominal wall hernias.

VASCULAR

- Injury to the great vessels is undoubtedly one of the most feared complications. This rare complication has been reported in 0.01% to 20% of cases and is much more likely during revision surgery.
- The venous structures are more commonly injured than the arterial structures. The left common iliac vein and ascending lumbar vein are among the most commonly injured structures.
- An incidental venotomy may be unnoticed until retraction is released. The preferred treatment for these injuries is direct repair of the laceration. When this is not possible, ligation of the vessel may be required.
- Other vascular complications can include pelvic and retroperitoneal venous thrombosis and arterial thrombosis. Venous thrombosis is often unrecognized until the patient manifests with symptoms of a pulmonary embolism. However, the use of chemical prophylaxis in the postoperative spinal population remains controversial. Arterial thrombosis may result in lower extremity ischemia or arterial embolism. Complete thrombosis of the iliac or femoral arteries is a devastating complication requiring emergency vascular intervention.

UROGENITAL

- Urogenital complications include injuries to the ureter and bladder. The ureter can be divided or lacerated inadvertently during the approach resulting in kidney dysfunction.
- In revision cases, the placement of ureteral stents preoperatively is helpful to identify and prevent ureteral injury. Direct repair and stenting of ureteral injuries is recommended.
- Bladder injuries are most commonly encountered during the placement of trochars for laparoscopic surgery. Any bladder laceration should be treated with direct repair and drainage of urine using a bladder catheter.

NEUROLOGIC

- Although the cauda equina can theoretically be injured during anterior surgery of the lumbosacral junction, the sympathetic and parasympathetic plexus structures are most commonly injured.
- The sympathetic plexus runs along the lateral sides of the lumbar spine and is commonly partially disrupted during anterior approaches to the lumbar spine above the L5-S1 disk space. This may result in warmth and flushing of the

ipsilateral limb in the postoperative period but has a benign and indolent course.
- The superior hypogastric plexus is involved with male (and perhaps female) sexual function. Damage to this structure can result in retrograde ejaculation (due to loss of bladder neck innervation) and sterility. This complication is seen in 4% to 20% of male patients following anterior exposures of the lumbosacral spine.[6]
- This complication appears to be more common in transperitoneal than retroperitoneal approaches. Retrograde ejaculation can be transient but may take up to 2 years to resolve. Injury to the parasympathetic plexus and somatic innervation of the urogenital system resulting in neurologic impotence is rare during anterior exposures to the lumbosacral junction as these structures lie well below the pelvis brim.

VISCERAL

- Organ injury can occur during both open and transperitoneal approaches to the anterior lumbar spine.
- Vigilant dissection and careful instrument placement should be used to diminish the risk of this complication.
- Injuries to the bowel generally require open repair and decompression with placement of a nasogastric tube and no oral intake to allow healing.

CLOSURE

- Inadequate closure or breakdown of the abdominal wall repair may result in abdominal hernia formation.
- This complication may be detected in the postoperative period and requires hernia repair or abdominal wall reconstruction.

References

1. Hibbs RH: An operation for progressive spinal deformities: A preliminary report of three cases from the service of the orthopaedic hospital. NY Med J 1911;93:1013–1016.
2. Albee FH: Transplantation of a portion of the tibia into the spine for Pott's disease: A preliminary report. JAMA 1911;57:885–886.
3. Müller W: Transperitoneale freilegung der wirbeisaule bei tuberkuloser spondylitis. Deutsch Z Chir 1906;85:128–137.
4. Hodgson AR, Stock FE: Anterior spinal fusion: A preliminary communication on the radical treatment of Pott's disease and Pott's paraplegia. Br J Surg 1956;44:266–275.
5. Sacks S: Anterior interbody fusion of the lumbar spine. J Bone Joint Surg Br 1965;47:211–233.
6. Johnson RM, McGuire EJ: Urogenital complications of anterior approaches to the lumbar spine. Clin Orthop 1981;154:114–118.

CHAPTER 14

STEVEN C. ZEILLER

TODD J. ALBERT

Anterior Retroperitoneal Approach

INTRODUCTION

The anterior approach to the lumbar spine was initially popularized by Hodgson and associates for the treatment of tuberculosis infections of the spine.[1,2] This approach to the spine provided access for thorough débridement and bony reconstruction. The anterior approach to the lumbar spine has evolved to treat a wide variety of clinical conditions including infection, neoplasm, trauma, deformity, and degenerative disease. Access to the anterior spine is critical in these conditions to decompress the spinal canal, provide anterior column reconstruction, or perform anterior releases in cases of spinal deformity.[3]

Traditionally, two surgical approaches have been used to access the anterior lumbar spine: the transperitoneal and retroperitoneal approaches. The retroperitoneal approach has gained popularity over the transperitoneal approach for several reasons. The retroperitoneal approach can be used effectively to access any of the levels from T12 to L5, whereas the transperitoneal approach is less effective above the level of L4. The retroperitoneal approach provides a relatively avascular plane to the lumbar spine with less manipulation of the intra-abdominal contents directly.[4] This results in less intraoperative bleeding, postoperative ileus, and chance of intra-abdominal content injury. In addition, the incidence of injury to the superior hypogastric plexus has been found to be lower with the retroperitoneal approach when compared to the transperitoneal approach.[5]

The anterior retroperitoneal approach can be performed in the supine or lateral decubitus position. Patient positioning is largely dependent on the type and location of spinal pathology that is going to be treated and should be addressed on an individual basis. For example, a patient with an L1 comminuted burst fracture that requires surgery should be placed in the lateral decubitus position. This will allow for optimal visualization during decompression and placement of instrumentation. In contrast, a patient with discogenic back pain at L4-L5 undergoing anterior surgery should be placed in the supine position. This approach to the anterior lumbar spine allows for the best visualization of the major vascular structures and a complete anterior release, which allows for restoration of disk height.

INDICATIONS AND CONTRAINDICATIONS FOR ANTERIOR LUMBAR RETROPERITONEAL APPROACH

INDICATIONS

- Infection
- Trauma
- Neoplasm
- Deformity
- Degenerative disease

RELATIVE CONTRAINDICATIONS

- Significant medical comorbidities that would preclude surgery
- Previous retroperitoneal approach with excessive adhesions

OPERATIVE TECHNIQUE

EQUIPMENT

- Radiolucent operating table
- Side braces or bump for patient positioning
- Headlight system
- General surgical retractors—Buckwalter retractor or Omni retractor, Dever retractor, Wiley renal vein retractor or rubber shadded pins
- Vascular clamps

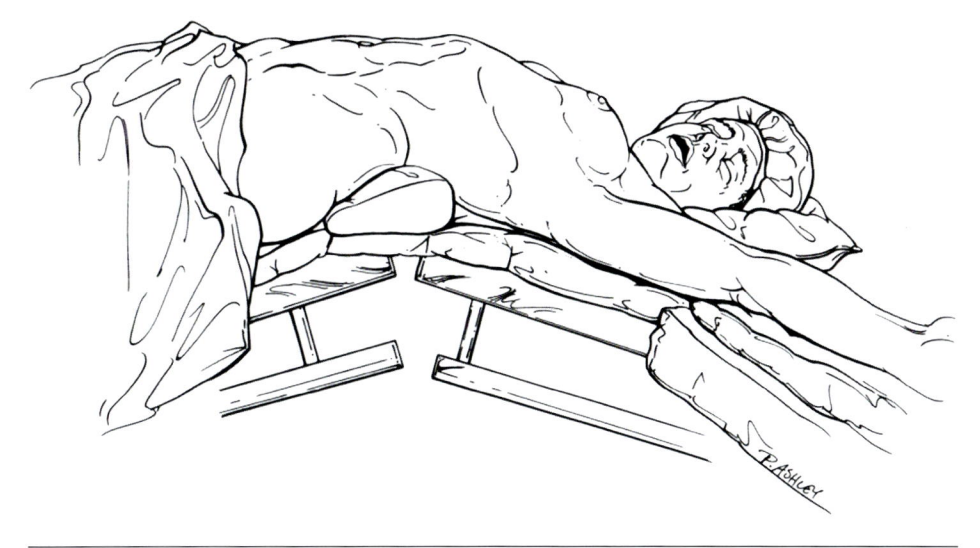

Fig. 14-1 The anterior retroperitoneal approach in the supine position. The patient is hyperextended by placing a roll under the anterior superior iliac spine, and the head and foot of the table are lowered to facilitate extension. (From Adams P, Cotler H: Alternative anterior lumbar exposures. In Albert T, Balderston B, Northrup B (eds): Surgical Approaches to the Spine. Philadelphia, WB Saunders, 1997, pp 157–171.)

- Fluoroscopy or plain films
- Cell saver
- 18-g spinal needle for localization

PATIENT POSITIONING AND DRAPING
Retroperitoneal Approach via the Supine Position

- Place patient supine on radiolucent operating table
- The patient's anterior superior iliac spine (ASIS) should be at the level of the kidney rest if possible. A bump should be placed under the patient at the level of the ASIS, and the kidney rest should be raised to facilitate extension (Fig. 14-1). It is the authors' preference to obtain maximal extension of the patient by lowering the head and foot of the table, especially in degenerative conditions. The patient can then be leveled with use of reverse Trendelenburg positioning.
- Shave the incision area and square off with plastic drapes.
- The patient is then prepped and draped in standard fashion.

RETROPERITONEAL APPROACH VIA THE LATERAL DECUBITUS POSITION

- Place the patient on the radiolucent table in the right lateral decubitus position. A left-sided approach is preferred to avoid the inferior vena cava, which is more fragile and difficult to repair than the aorta.
- The patient can be secured in the lateral decubitus position by using side braces. The patient should be placed on the table such that the operative area is over the break in the table so that it may be jackknifed (Fig. 14-2). This will facilitate the exposure by creating more room between the ribs and the superior portion of the pelvis. Care should be taken to place the patient in a true lateral position on the operative table. This will maintain the surgeons' anatomic orientation, which is critical for identifying major vessels, decompressing the spinal canal, and placing instrumentation.
- The leg on the operative side should be flexed at the hip to release any tension on the psoas muscle to facilitate with the exposure.
- Time should be taken to ensure all dependent areas are well padded, and a blanket or pillow can be placed between the legs to provide protection during the operation.
- Remainder of prepping and draping is carried out in the usual fashion.

Location of Incision

- In the lateral decubitus position to access the upper lumbar spine segments L1-L3, the incision should begin over the twelfth rib, which may need to be resected. The incision should then curve anteriorly and end at the level of the umbilicus at the lateral border of the rectus abdominis. If the lower lumbar spinal segments L4-L5 are going to be accessed, the incision can start midway between the ribs and the pelvis curve anteriorly and end below the umbilicus again at the lateral border of the rectus abdominis (Fig. 14-3).
- In the supine position a paramedian vertical incision should be used at the lateral border of the rectus

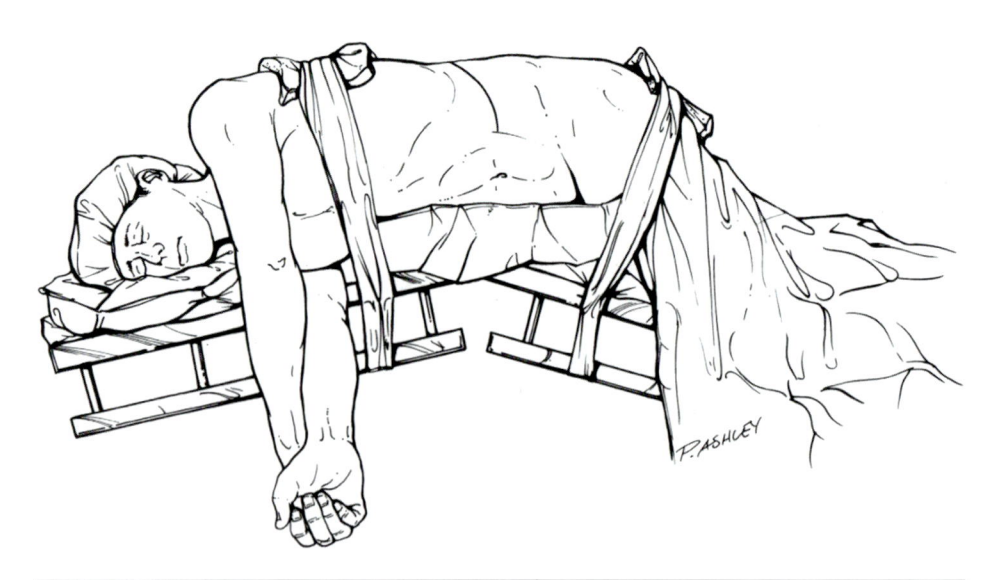

Fig. 14-2 The anterior retroperitoneal approach in the lateral decubitus position. The operative area is placed over the break in the table to jackknife the patient to facilitate with exposure. (From Emery S: Anterior retroperitoneal lumbar exposures. In Albert T, Balderston B, Northrup B (eds): Surgical Approaches to the Spine. Philadelphia, WB Saunders, 1997, pp 145–155.)

abdominis. The length of the incision will depend on the number of levels that will need exposure. The level of the incision can be determined by using anatomic landmarks as well as the anteroposterior lumbar spine to see the relationship of the superior portion of the pelvis to the lumbar spine. Typically, the superior iliac crest is at the level of L4-L5 and L5-S1 is located midway between the umbilicus and the pubic symphysis (Fig. 14-4). The use of fluoroscopy or a plain film can help prior to skin incision if there is any question.

Incision and Soft Tissue Dissection

- In the supine position a vertical paramedian or horizontal incision incision is made and hemostasis is achieved. The lateral border of the rectus abdominis should be palpated, and the rectus sheath should be opened in line with the

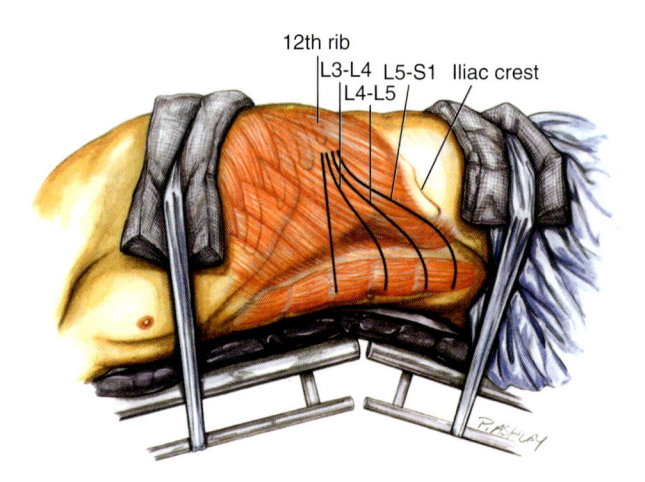

Fig. 14-3 Skin incisions, depending on operative level, for the lateral decubitus approach. (From Adams P, Cotler H: Alternative anterior lumbar exposures. In Albert T, Balderston B, Northrup B (eds): Surgical Approaches to the Spine. Philadelphia, WB Saunders, 1997, pp 157–171.)

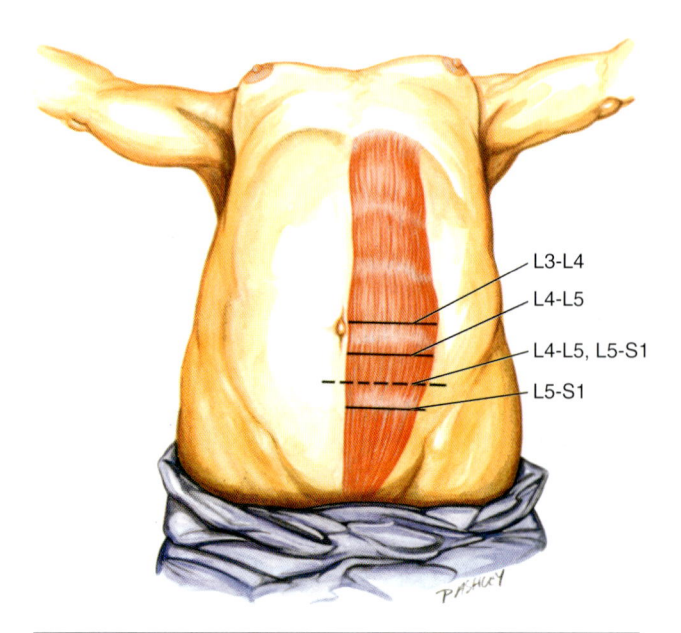

Fig. 14-4 Skin incisions, depending on operative level, for the supine approach. (From Adams P, Cotler H: Alternative anterior lumbar exposures. In Albert T, Balderston B, Northrup B (eds): Surgical Approaches to the Spine. Philadelphia, WB Saunders, 1997, pp 157–171.)

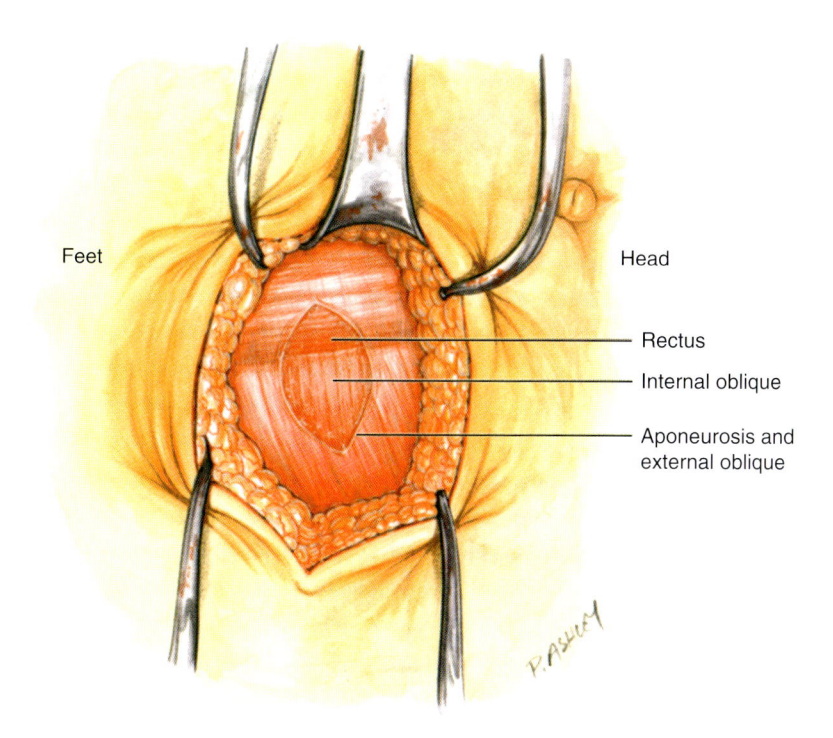

Fig. 14-5 Anterior rectus sheath is divided exposing the external oblique muscle. (From Adams P, Cotler H: Alternative anterior lumbar exposures. In Albert T, Balderston B, Northrup B (eds): Surgical Approaches to the Spine. Philadelphia, WB Saunders, 1997, pp 157–171.)

incision along the lateral border of the rectus abdominis (Fig. 14-5).
- In the lateral decubitus position an oblique incision is made and hemostasis is achieved. From here the layers of the dissection are the same, regardless of patient position.
- The external oblique muscle is then dissected in line with the incision to expose the internal oblique muscle (Fig. 14-6).
- The internal oblique muscle is divided in line with the incision to expose the transverse abdominis muscle (Fig. 14-7).
- Divide the transverse abdominis muscle to expose the transversalis fascia (see Fig. 14-7) and in the supine position (Fig. 14-8).
- Incise the transversalis fascia to expose the underlying peritoneum.
- Once the peritoneum is exposed, use blunt dissection to develop a plane between it and the fascia. Any rent that is made in the peritoneum should be repaired at that time to prevent any future possibility of an abdominal hernia.
- Retract the retroperitoneal fat and intra-abdominal contents medially exposing the psoas muscle. A Dever retractor with a wet laparotomy sponge is used for this retraction. It is important to locate the ureter during the dissection to ensure that it is included in the tissue that is retracted medially, thus minimizing the chance of injury.

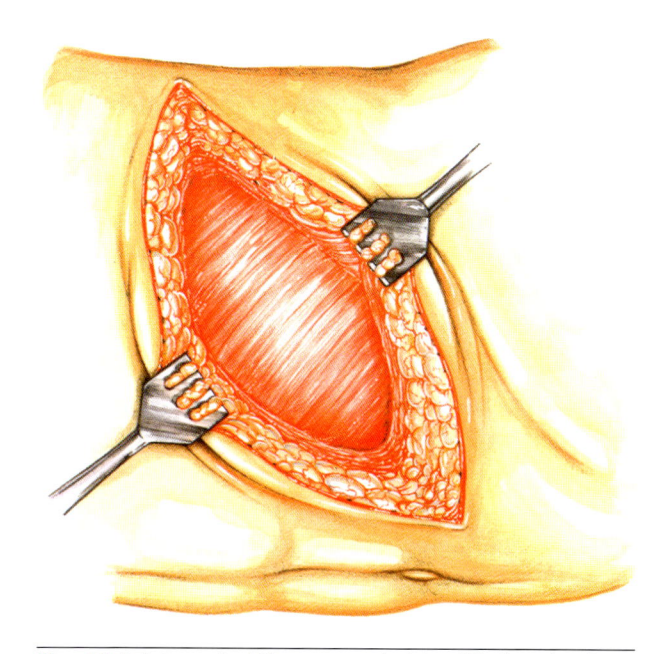

Fig. 14-6 Internal oblique muscle identified and subsequently divided to expose the transverse abdominis muscle. (From Emery S: Anterior retroperitoneal lumbar exposures. In Albert T, Balderston B, Northrup B (eds): Surgical Approaches to the Spine. Philadelphia, WB Saunders, 1997, pp 145–155.)

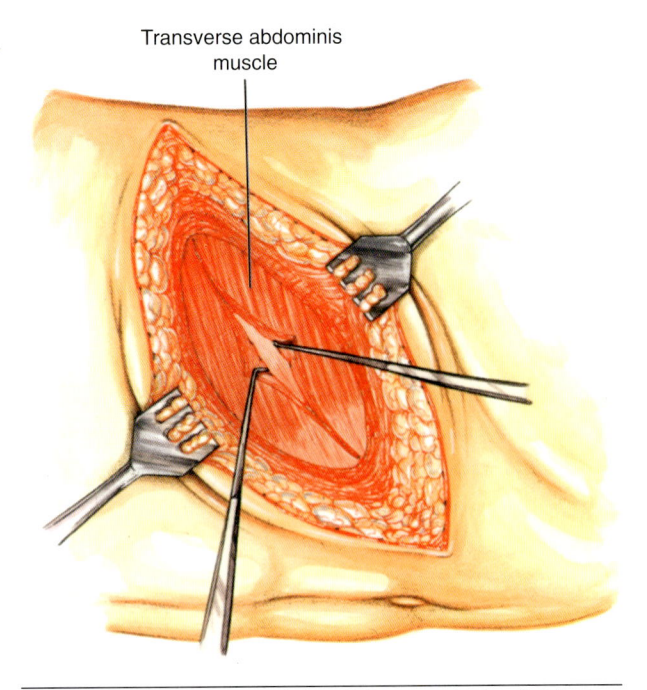

Fig. 14-7 Transversus abdominis muscle is divided to expose the transversalis fascia. (From Emery S: Anterior retroperitoneal lumbar exposures. In Albert T, Balderston B, Northrup B (eds): Surgical Approaches to the Spine. Philadelphia, WB Saunders, 1997, pp 145–155.)

- In the upper lumbar spine segments the psoas will need to be reflected off the anterior portion of the vertebral body. This can be done with a Cobb elevator and should be started at the midline and carried posteriorly. Once the psoas has been retracted, the anterior spine is visualized along with the segmental vessels and the sympathetic trunk (Fig. 14-9).
- In the lower lumbar spine less psoas dissection will be necessary. The structures that will need to be identified include the common iliac veins and arteries and all their branches. In addition, the superior hypogastric plexus will be present at these levels.
- In the upper lumbar spine it is critical to ligate all segmental vessels around the operative level or levels. This will allow the surgeon to work safely without causing unnecessary bleeding.
- In the lower lumbar spine levels care must be taken to identify all branches of the common iliac arteries and veins. The left common iliac vein, which is frequently injured, crosses at the L4-L5 disk space (Fig. 14-10). Ligating all branches will allow the vessels to be mobilized to access the spine. The middle sacral artery and vein are routinely ligated during the operation to facilitate with exposure. It

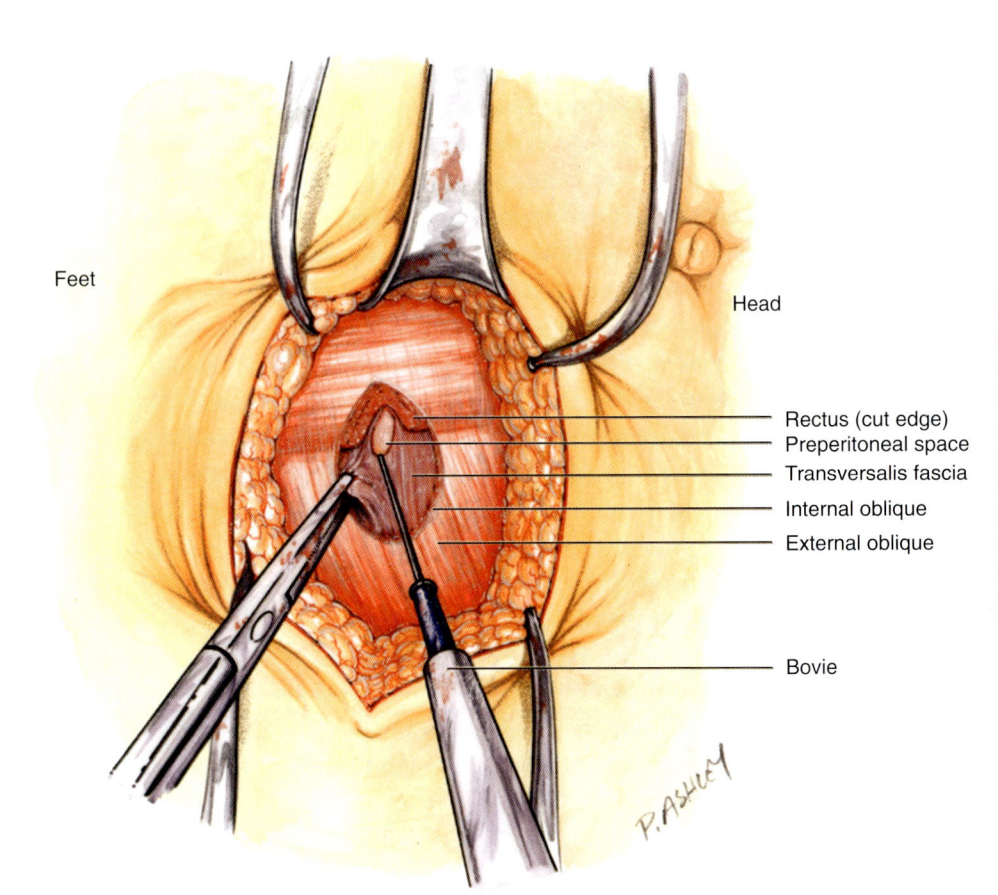

Fig. 14-8 Supine approach with division of transverse abdominis to expose the transversalis fascia. (From Adams P, Cotler H: Alternative anterior lumbar exposures. In Albert T, Balderston B, Northrup B (eds): Surgical Approaches to the Spine. Philadelphia, WB Saunders, 1997, pp 157–171.)

CHAPTER 14 Anterior Retroperitoneal Approach   131

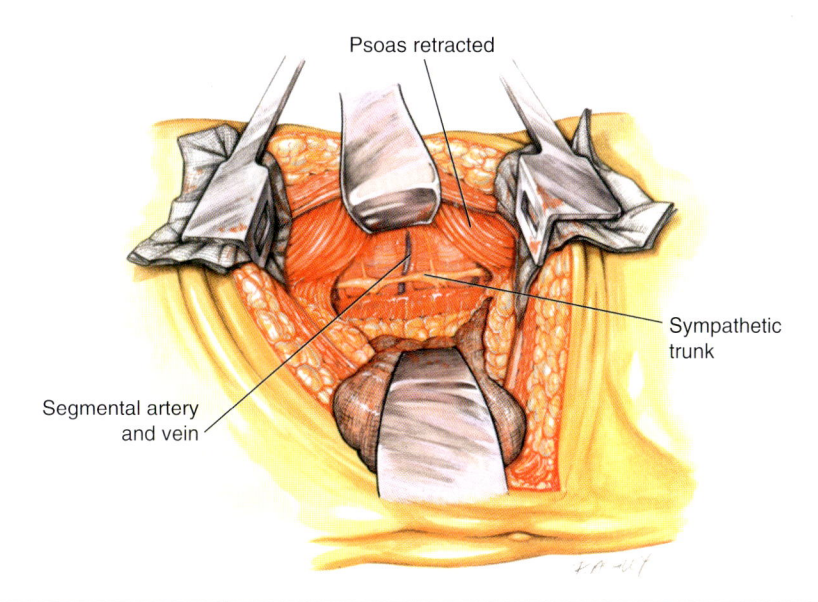

Fig. 14-9 The peritoneal contents are retracted anteriorly and the psoas is retracted posteriorly exposing the segmental vessels and the sympathetic trunk. (From Emery S: Anterior retroperitoneal lumbar exposures. In Albert T, Balderston B, Northrup B (eds): Surgical Approaches to the Spine. Philadelphia, WB Saunders, 1997, pp 145–155.)

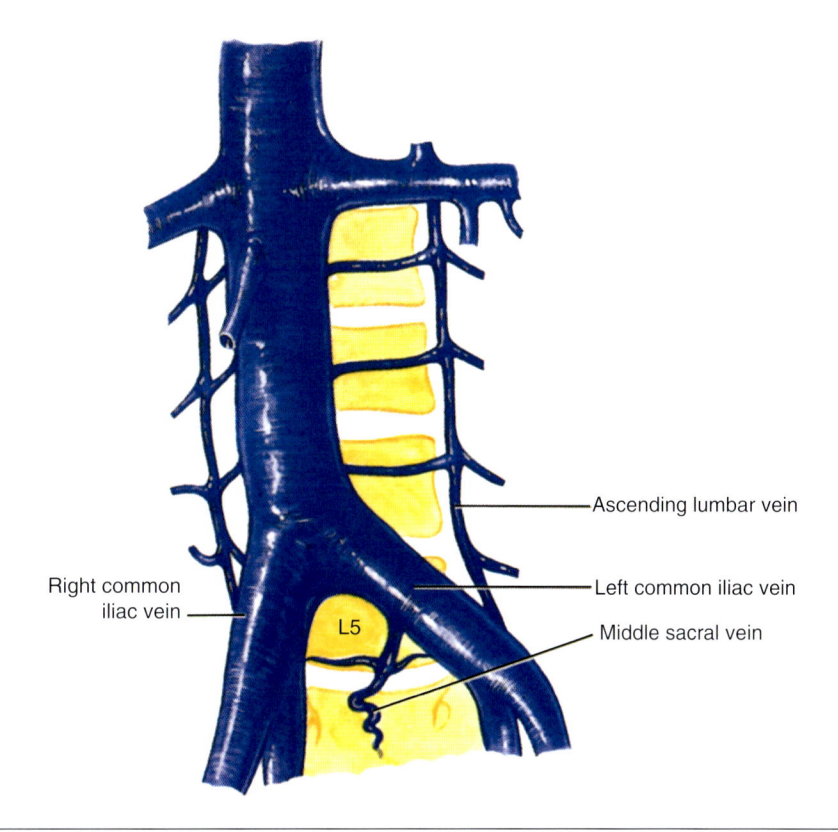

Fig. 14-10 Venous anatomy at the level of L4-L5. (From Adams P, Cotler H: Alternative anterior lumbar exposures. In Albert T, Balderston B, Northrup B (eds): Surgical Approaches to the Spine. Philadelphia, WB Saunders, 1997, pp 157–171.)

is recommended to use either vascular clamps or suture ligation to achieve this and keep the use of monopolar cautery to a minimum. The use of electrocautery can cause damage to the superior hypogastric plexus, which in males can result in retrograde ejaculation.
- Once the vessels have been identified either Wiley vein retractors can be used or rubber shadded pins can be placed into the vertebral bodies to hold the vessels clear of the operative level.

Closure

- The wound is inspected thoroughly to make sure adequate hemostasis has been achieved and then copiously irrigated.
- The transversalis fascia and muscular layers can then be individually closed with 1-0 PDS suture.
- The subcutaneous tissue can be approximated with 3-0 Vicryl suture and the skin can be closed with staples.

POSTOPERATIVE CARE

- The patient may require a monitored bed overnight, and this decision should be individualized based on the patient's comorbidities.
- The patient should be mobilized as quickly as possible. A physical therapist or occupational therapist should be consulted.
- The patient should remain NPO (nothing by mouth) until passing flatus per rectum.
- Depending on the complexity of the procedure and the patient's medical condition, the hospital stay can vary but usually ranges from 2 to 5 days.

COMPLICATIONS

- Vascular injury can be one of the most devastating complications when operating on the anterior lumbar spine. These injuries will almost exclusively be recognized intraoperatively. A general surgeon or vascular surgeon should always be available in the event of such an injury. In particular, the surgeon should be especially cautious when working on the lower lumbar spine because the left common iliac vein crosses the L4-L5 disk space and is commonly injured. Intraoperative vascular injury during anterior lumbar surgery is not infrequent and in one series was as high as 16%.[6]
- The sympathetic trunk can be injured during the operation during dissection of the psoas.[7] This injury will manifest itself as an ipsilateral warm extremity and is usually not a significant clinical injury. In the lower lumbar spine the superior hypogastric plexus can be injured. This injury is of special concern in male patients because it can lead to retrograde ejaculation. The exact incidence of retrograde ejaculation varies in the literature from 0.42%[8] to 5.9%.[9] Male patients should be counseled regarding this possible complication preoperatively.
- The ureter may be injured during the surgery if it is not identified and retracted medially with the other peritoneal contents.[7] This type of injury may not manifest itself acutely and thus a high degree of suspicion must be maintained throughout the patient's postoperative course.

References

1. Hodgson AR, Stock FE: Anterior spine fusion for the treatment of tuberculosis of the spine. J Bone Joint Surg Am 1960;42:295–310.
2. Hodgson AR, Stock FE, Fang HS, Ong GB: Anterior spine fusion: The operative approach and pathologic findings in 412 patients with Pott's disease of the spine. Br J Surg 1960;44:172–178.
3. Emery S: Anterior retroperitoneal lumbar exposures. In Albert TJ, Balderston RA, Northrup BE (eds): Surgical Approaches to the Spine. Philadelphia, WB Saunders, 1997, pp 145–155.
4. Adams PR, Cotler H: Alternative anterior lumbar exposures. In Albert TJ, Balderston RA, Northrup BE (eds): Surgical Approaches to the Spine. Philadelphia, WB Saunders, 1997, pp 157–171.
5. Sasso R, Burkus K, LeHuec JC: Retrograde ejaculation after anterior lumbar interbody fusion: Transperitoneal versus retroperitoneal experience. Spine 2003;28(10):1023–1026.
6. Baker JK, Reardon PR, Reardon MJ, Heggeness MH: Vascular injury in anterior lumbar surgery. Spine 1993;18(15):2227–2230.
7. Hoppenfield S, de Boer P: Anterolateral (retroperitoneal) approach. In Surgical Exposures in Orthopaedics: The Anatomic Approach, 2nd ed. Philadelphia, JB Lippincott, 1994, pp 235–241.
8. Flynn JC, Price CT: Sexual complications of anterior fusion of the lumbar spine. Spine 1984;9:489–492.
9. Tiusanen H, Seitsalo S, Osterman K, et al: Retrograde ejaculation after anterior interbody fusion. Eur Spine J 1995;4:339–342.

CHAPTER 15

TODD APPLEGATE

CHRISTOPHER M. BONO

Posterior Approaches to the Sacrum

INTRODUCTION

The posterior approach can be used to address a number of different pathologic conditions. The midline approach is the most utilitarian and is most frequently used. It is an extensile approach that can be continued cranially to include the lumbar, thoracic, and cervical spine. It is most commonly utilized for stabilization and fusion of the lumbosacral junction for degenerative, traumatic, infectious, or neoplastic conditions. It can also be used to perform a midline laminectomy of the posterior sacral spinal canal. More extensive lateral exposure is often used to access the posterior aspect of the iliac wing/sacroiliac joints for placement of iliac screws or rods to stabilize concomitant lumbosacral and sacroiliac fracture-dislocations. In these cases, making an additional transverse "T" incision, located at the level of the iliac crests, can facilitate exposure. Rarely, the most caudal extent of the midline approach can be used to access the coccyx for excision.

The paramedian posterior approach is useful for open reduction and internal fixation of vertical sacral fractures that pass through or lateral to the sacral foramina (zone II or I, respectively) (Fig. 15-1). One advantage over the midline approach is that it allows more direct exposure of such fractures, however, it is less easily converted to an extensile approach of the lumbar spine. Direct open plating of vertical sacral fractures can be performed through the paramedian approach. Although open reduction of displaced transforaminal sacral fractures through this approach is critical to avoid iatrogenic nerve or vascular injury, placement of iliosacral screws is typically performed percutaneously through separate lateral stab incisions through the gluteal muscles. A single transverse incision can also be used to expose the sacrum. Like the paramedian approach, this is not an extensile maneuver. It is most useful for reduction and fixation of transverse sacral fractures.

INDICATIONS AND CONTRAINDICATIONS

INDICATIONS

- Fusion of the lumbosacral junction, as may be performed for L5-S1 degenerative or isthmic spondylolisthesis, painful discogenic back pain from degenerative disk disease, lumbar scoliosis with degeneration or coronal obliquity of the L5-S1 disk space, or stabilization of impending pathologic fractures of the lower lumbar vertebrae
- Posterior decompression of the sacral spinal canal (e.g., epidural abscess, intracanal bone fragments after fracture, epidural tumors, pseudomeningocele)
- Vertical sacral fractures (paramedian approach)
- Reduction, stabilization, and fusion of lumbosacral fracture dislocations (traumatic spondylolisthesis), transverse sacral fractures, complex H-pattern sacral fractures (bilateral vertical sacral fractures through the alae with concomitant transverse upper sacral fracture)
- Incision and débridement of osteomyelitis (e.g., associated with sacral decubiti)
- Excision of posterior sacral tumors (rare)
- Coccygectomy

RELATIVE CONTRAINDICATIONS

- No absolute contraindications
- Local soft tissue infection (e.g., superficial decubiti over otherwise noninfectious pathology)
- Pulmonary, hemodynamic, intra-abdominal, or any other medical contraindication that might be worsened or complicated by prone positioning
- Resection of primarily anterior sacral tumors

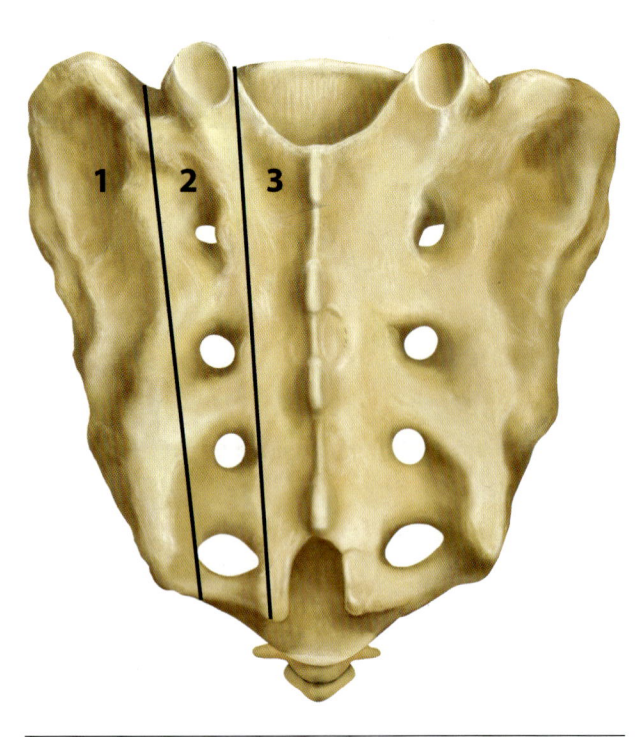

Fig. 15-1 Figure outlining the three zones of the sacrum. Zone 1 is lateral to the sacral foramina. Zone 2 is transforaminal. Zone 3 is the region medial to the foramina.

OPERATIVE TECHNIQUE

EQUIPMENT

- Radiolucent operating table enables the abdomen to be freely decompressed and facilitates control of lumbar lordosis. It is the authors' preference to use a Jackson table (OSI, Inc.) with one chest pad, two hip pads, two thigh pads, and either a sling or padded platform to support the legs (the former allows the lower pelvis to rotate forward).
- Intraoperative fluoroscopy (C-arm) is used for instrumentation cases.
- Surgical magnifying glasses (loupes).
- Headlight.
- Cobb elevators.
- Handheld retractors (Hibbs).
- Deep self-retaining soft tissue retractors: large 90-degree and 45-degree Wiltse-Gelpi retractors, Adson-Beckman retractors.
- Monopolar electrocautery (for initial exposure and periosteal dissection).
- Irrigating bipolar cautery (for dissection/hemostasis around the sacral foramina and epidural space).
- For decompression:
  - Kerrison rongeurs, 2 to 5 mm
  - Straight-ahead and angled-up pituitary rongeurs
  - Small-straight, angled-up, and down-going curettes
  - High-speed burr with 5- to 6-mm round cutting bit
- Penfield 4 elevator
- Woodson (small hockey stick) elevator
- Thrombin-soaked gelatin sponges (for hemostasis)
- ½-inch-by-½-inch cotton pledgets

PATIENT POSITIONING

- The patient is induced and intubated in the supine position on the stretcher.
- General anesthesia is initiated.
- Foley catheter is placed.
- The patient is then carefully logrolled as a unit onto the operating table.
- The chest pad should be centered on the sternum (for women, ensure that the breasts are moved to the sides so that there is no direct pressure on the nipples).
- Hip pads are just distal to the anterior superior iliac spine (to avoid undue pressure on the lateral femoral cutaneous nerve).
- Thigh pads are along the upper, anterior thigh (well-padded, to avoid femoral nerve pressue and postoperative palsy).
- The arms are placed at the patient's side flexed 90 degrees at the elbow and shoulder.
- The knees should be flexed about 30 degrees by placing two to three pillows below the leg (to avoid tension of the sciatic nerve).
- All other pressure-sensitive areas must be checked, including genitals, knees, elbows, wrists.
- The head/neck should be placed in a neutral position, and the eyes, nose, and chin must be well padded.
- Padded leg platforms (instead of the sling) are preferred if lumbosacral fixation is planned as they help approximate physiologic lordosis.
- A circulating air upper body warmer should be placed well above the proposed incision site.

LOCATION OF INCISION
Midline Incision

- The spinous processes of the lumbar spine are palpated. A surgical marker is used to mark the spinous process tips of the lower levels (L2 to L5).
- The lower sacral spinous processes (medial crest) are then marked.
- A longitudinal line is then drawn connecting the lumbar and sacral markings. If extended distally, this should be centered within the midline gluteal cleft.
- The proximal and distal extent of the incision depends on the extent of surgery. This is best marked using lateral intraoperative fluoroscopy.
- If the exposure must be taken out laterally to widely expose the sacroiliac joints or posterior ilium, the incison can be crossed ("T" incision) at the level of the iliac crests[1]

CHAPTER 15 Posterior Approaches to the Sacrum

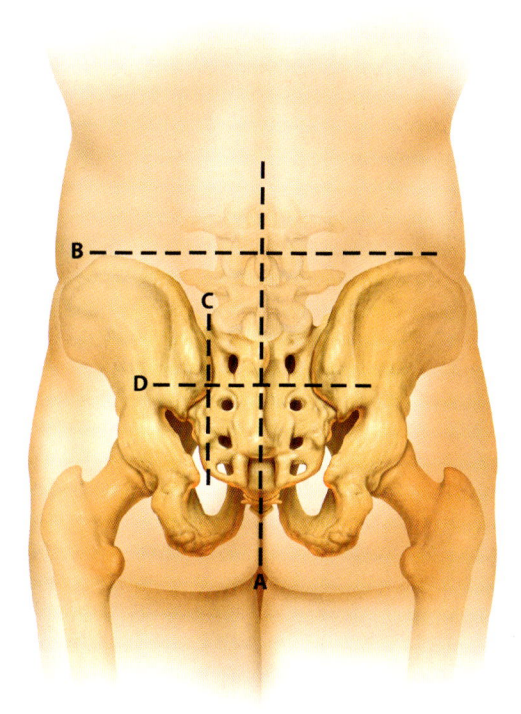

Fig. 15-2 The midline incision is created along the spinous processes of the lower lumbar spine and the midline ridge of the median sacral crest (A). This incision can be crossed with a perpendicular incision at the level of the iliac crests to allow more lateral access (B). The paramedian incision is aligned with the posterior superior iliac crest (C). The location of the incision for a transverse approach is determined by the level of pathology (D).

(Fig. 15-2). Care should be taken to maintain an adequate fasciocutaneous soft tissue flap to maintain blood supply and avoid postoperative necrosis.

Paramedian Incision
- The incision is aligned with posterior superior iliac crest (see Fig. 15-2).
- This can usually be palpated, even in obese patients.

Transverse Incision
- The transverse incision must be placed at the level of pathology/fracture. This should be exactly localized and marked by intraoperative fluoroscopy.
- The lateral extent of the incision should also be marked by fluoroscopy. Care must be taken not to extend too far lateral when working in the lower sacrum. This can endanger the neurovascular structures within the greater sciatic notch.

PREPARATION AND DRAPING
- Prior to sterile prepping, an impermeable sticky drape (1000 drape) should be placed transversely at the gluteal cleft to avoid potential fecal microbial contamination. The sides of the drape should be angled inferiorly, creating an apex just below the coccyx.
- Skin is prepared using a one-step povidone-alcohol solution. In cases of open fracture, gross contamination, or ulcerous skin lesion a surgical scrub followed by povidone paint is preferred.
- Two half-sheets are placed: one below and one above the prepared surgical site.
- The perimeter of the surgical site is draped using towels. The inferior towel is secured using staples.
- An iodine-impregnated surgical adhesive film is then placed over the surgical site. This helps seal the operative field from potential contaminants, in particular from the anal/rectal area.
- Next, a laparatomy drape is placed, centered over the surgical incision site.

INCISION AND SOFT TISSUE DISSECTION
- The skin is incised with a No. 10 scalpel blade.
- Once through the dermis, electrocautery is used to dissect through the subcutaneous fascia.
- The deep lumbosacral/paravertebral fascia is then exposed.

Midline Approach
- The deep lumbar/lumbosacral/sacral fascia is visualized (Fig. 15-3). Any spina bifida defects should be recognized preoperatively so as to avoid inadvertent entrance into the spinal canal with midline dissection.
- The fascia is incised on either side of the midline, just lateral to the spinous processes. In the lower lumbar spine, this plane is easily identified. Over the sacrum, however, the spinous processes are small and coalesce to form a median crest. The fascia should be incised just lateral to the decussation (or convergence) of the deep fascial fibers.
- The paraspinal muscles are subperiosteally elevated from the posterior sacral cortex. Cobb elevators can be used to avoid damage to the multifidus, longissiumus, and sacrospinalis muscles, which attach in this region. At this stage, cerebellar retractors can be inserted.
- Dissection is carried laterally to the level of the sacral foramina (Fig. 15-4). The dorsal sacral foramen contains numerous small epidural blood vessels and the segmental dorsal rami, which innervate the overlying skin and paraspinal musculature. Entering the sacral foramina must be avoided because of risk of injury to the cauda equina or epidural bleeding. If bleeding occurs, meticulous hemostasis should be maintained with bipolar cautery.
- The lateral sacral crest is found just lateral to the foramina.[2] The posterior superior iliac spine (PSIS) is located just

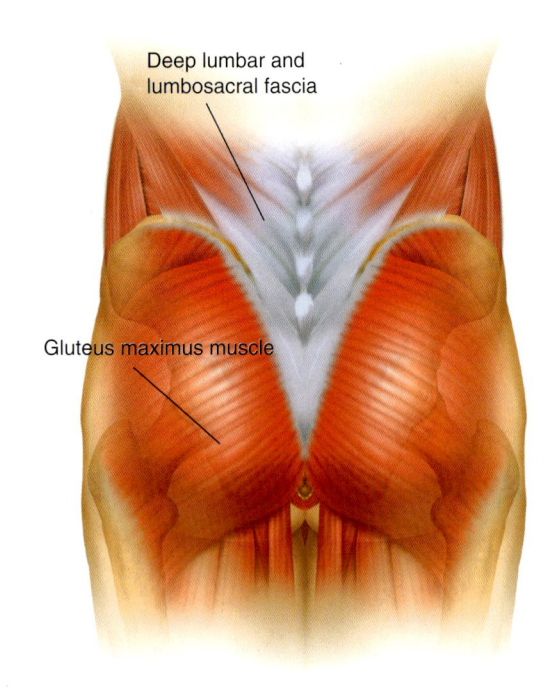

Fig. 15-3 Once through the skin and subcutaneous fascia, the deep lumbar and lumbosacral fascia is visualized.

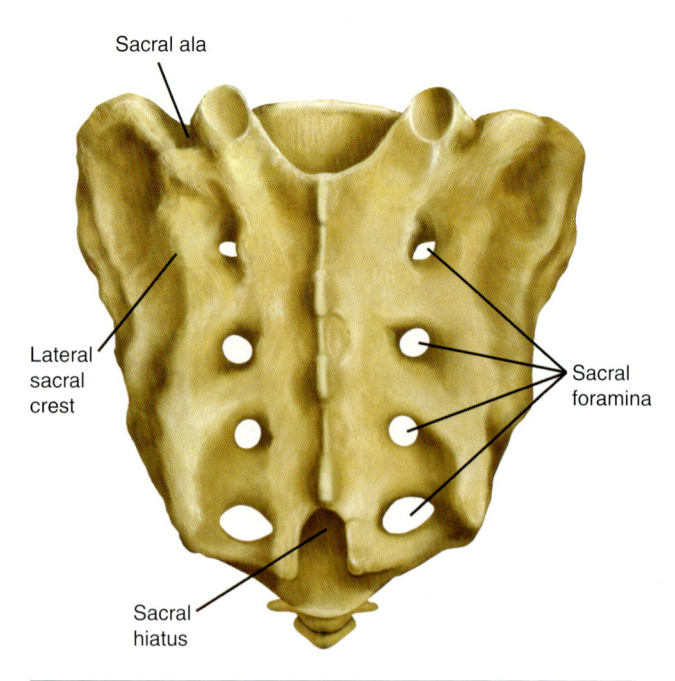

Fig. 15-5 With caudal exposure, the surgeon must be cognizant of the sacral hiatus, which is the most distal aspect of the spinal canal.

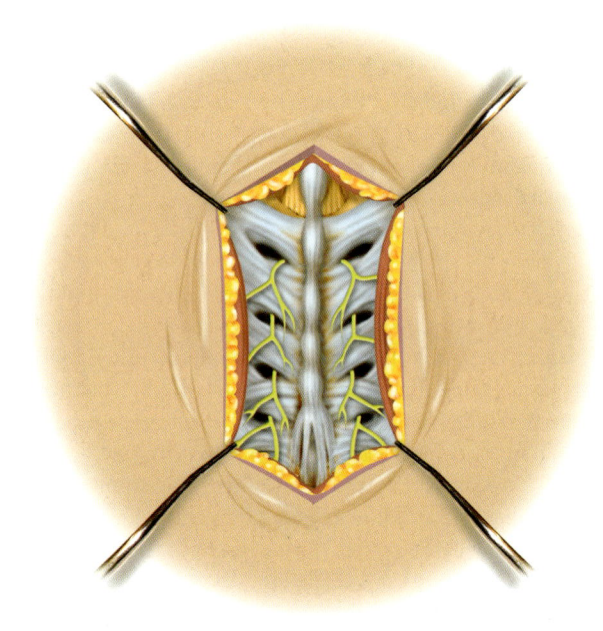

Fig. 15-4 The exiting posterior branches of the dorsal sacral rami can be visualized with dissection of and lateral to the sacral foramina. Inadvertent entrance into the foramina with electrocautery or an instrument can lead to epidural bleeding or nerve injury.

lateral to this crest. The exiting posterior neural branches usually cannot be salvaged with exposure of this region of the sacrum (zone I).
- Inferior to the PSIS is the greater sciatic foramen and its contents. The gluteus maximus muscle attaches along the lateral border of the sacrum through the posterior sacroiliac ligament.
- When exposing the most lateral aspects of the distal sacrum, care must be taken to avoid injuring the structures within the greater sciatic foramen (piriformis muscle, superior gluteal artery and vein, and sciatic nerve).
- When exposing the most distal aspect of the sacrum, the midline sacral hiatus must be identified (Fig. 15-5). It represents the point through which the final sacral nerves exit. It is important to note that there is no overlying bone in this terminal region of the spinal canal.
- Distal dissection can be extended to expose the coccyx. The anal sphincter has fascial attachments to the coccyx inferior and anteriorly.
- Exposure of the sacral ala:
  - Subperiosteal dissection is extended along the superior lamina border of S1.
  - The superior articular process of S1 is identified, along with the adjacent facet joint.
  - A Cobb elevator or Hibbs retractor is used to retract the paraspinal muscle just lateral to the joint.
  - Dissection is continued lateral to the inferior articular process, which is confluent with the posteromedial aspect of the sacral ala.

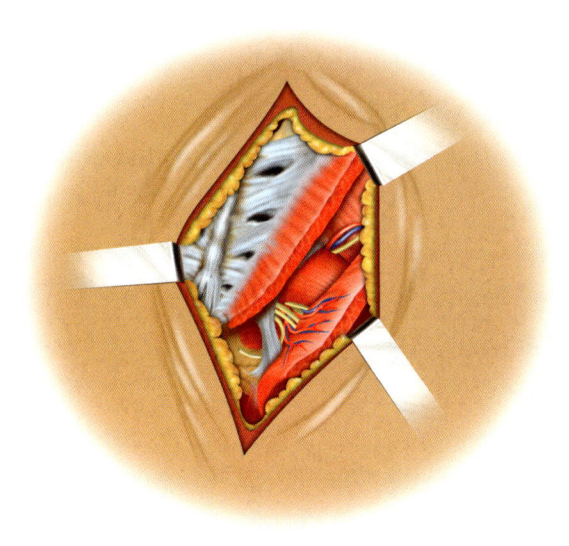

Fig. 15-6 The paramedian approach allows more direct lateral exposure. After crossing the subcutaneous layer, the posterior superior iliac spine (PSIS) will be palpable. The posterior sacroiliac ligament extends from the PSIS toward the inferolateral pole of the sacrum and is confluent with the sacrotuberous ligament. Using this approach, the sacral foramina will be first encountered at their lateral aspects.

- As the deepest region of dissection, vigorous retraction is often necessary to expose the remainder of the ala. Wiltse-Gelpi retractors can aid in maintaining exposure of the sacral alae during the remainder of the operation.

Paramedian Approach

- After crossing the subcutaneous layer, the PSIS will be palpable. The posterior sacroiliac ligament (Fig. 15-6) extends from the PSIS toward the inferolateral pole of the sacrum. It is confluent with the sacrotuberous ligament.
- The paraspinal muscles (medial) and the gluteus maximum (lateral) share a common insertion along the posterior sacroiliac ligament. The decussation of these muscles should be identified.
- The paraspinal muscle is carefully dissected from the ligament with gentle medial retraction.
- The sacral foramina will be first encountered at their lateral aspects.
- Depending on the extent of the pathology, dissection can be extended toward the midline. For reduction of vertical sacral fractures, it is usually not necessary to extend further medial than the fracture line.

Transverse Approach

- Subcutaneous dissection is taken down to the deep thoracolumbar/lumbosacral fascia.
- The deep fascia is incised longitudinally in the midline.
- Periosteal dissection is carried laterally as described previously.
- As this approach is most often used for transverse sacral fractures, a rent in the overlying muscle and fascia usually facilitates exposure of the bone.

CLOSURE

- Retractors should be released every 30 to 60 minutes during the procedure to avoid muscle necrosis.
- Retractors are removed and the wound is copiously irrigated with normal saline solution.
- Retractors are briefly replaced for final inspection.
- The wound, bony borders, and epidural regions are inspected for adequate hemostasis. If this is confirmed, the retractors are then removed.
- Watertight closure of the deep lumbosacral fascia layer is achieved with one absorbable suture applied with interrupted figure-of-eight stitches.
- Deep subcutaneous fascia is closed with 0 absorbable suture using interrupted simple stitches.
- Dermal layer is closed with 2-0 absorbable suture using inverted (buried) interrupted stitches.
- Skin is closed with staples, and sterile dressings are applied.

POSTOPERATIVE CARE

- Postoperative orders include neurologic checks every 2 hours, thromboembolic stockings, and sequential compression device applied to the calves.
- Diet can be advanced as tolerated. In cases in which multilevel lumbar laminectomy or retroperitoneal procedure has also been performed, this can be delayed by a postoperative ileus.
- Mobilization is dependent on final stability of the reconstructive construct. At minimum, the patient should be log rolled from side to side every 2 hours to avoid skin breakdown, particularly in the sacral region.
- Antibiotics are continued for 24 to 48 hours postoperatively
- Patient-controlled anesthesia (PCA) is administered until the patient has begun to ambulate. Afterward, oral pain medicine is initiated.
- The first dressing change is routinely performed on postoperative day 3 unless it has been excessively soiled.
- Prolonged recumbency may warrant chemical thromboprophylaxis. After a spinal decompression, this should be initiated no earlier than postoperative day 4.

COMPLICATIONS

INTRAOPERATIVE

- Dorsal rami injury is an expected complication with sacral exposure beyond the foramina.

- Sacral root injury can occur with associated procedures such as pedicle screw insertion, ilosacral screw placement, and decompressive laminectomy.
- Superior gluteal artery injury can occur with overly aggressive exposure of the lateral sacrum. This can lead to intraoperative hemorrhage. As the transected artery usually retracts into the pelvis, an emergent anterior pelvic exploration is usually necessary to gain control of the bleeder.
- Superior and inferior gluteal nerve injury can dennervate the gluteus muscles, leading to ambulation difficulty.

POSTOPERATIVE

- Thromboembolism (especially in patients with pelvic trauma)
- Epidural hematoma leading to neurologic compromise
- Wound infection
  - Infection is more often seen in patients who have sustained high-energy fractures associated with extensive soft tissue injuries.
- Superficial infections (persistent redness, swelling, pain with palpation) may be treated with a brief course of oral antibiotics. Surgical débridement should be considered in those who do not respond clinically.
- Deep wound infection (persistent pustulous drainage more than 7 to 10 days from surgery) should be treated with open surgical débridement and irrigation in the operating room.
- Prophylaxis for potential fecal contaminants (*Escherichia coli*) might be considered if sterility may have been breached during surgery.

REFERENCES

1. Williams RP, Heckman JD: Contemporary Extensile Exposures in Orthopaedic Surgery. Philadelphia, Williams & Wilkins, 1997, pp 230–236.
2. Netter FH: Atlas of Human Anatomy. Summit, Ciba-Geigy Corporation, 1989.

SECTION II

DEGENERATIVE DISEASE OF THE SPINE

SECTION A
Cervical Disk Herniation

CHAPTER 16

HO-YEOL ZHANG

DANIEL H. KIM

Anterior Cervical Diskectomy and Fusion

INTRODUCTION

The anterior cervical diskectomy and fusion (ACDF) technique is a ventral cervical approach designed to treat conditions that impair function of cervical nerve roots and the spinal cord at one or more levels. These conditions include acute and chronic degenerative disk disease, as well as traumatic dislocations and compression fractures. The ACDF procedure, which includes either the Cloward or Smith-Robinson technique, allows for removal of the nucleus pulposus and its annulus, posterior vertebral body osteophytes, and the adjacent calcified posterior longitudinal ligament. The Cloward technique utilizes a cylindrical bony removal and dowel placement for fusion (Fig. 16-1). The Smith-Robinson technique, however, achieves decompression and fusion via a rectangular intervertebral bony resection and intraforaminal as well as ventral midline lesions are surgically accessible via this approach (Fig. 16-2). Depending on surgeon or patient preference, either autologous or allograft bone may be used for fusion using either technique.

INDICATIONS AND CONTRAINDICATIONS

INDICATIONS

- Intractable progressive or recurrent cervical radiculopathy
- Myelopathy
- Intractable cervical-brachial or occipital pain syndromes (less common)

RELATIVE CONTRAINDICATIONS

- No absolute contraindications
- Previous anterior cervical operations resulting in extensive scarring
- Anterior cervical wound infection
- Dorsal pathology
- Patients needing more extensive decompression with corpectomy and fusion
- Severe osteoporosis associated with vertebral body collapse
- Patients with a tracheostomy and attendant increased risk of developing an infection at the surgical site
- Previous radiation therapy to the neck
- Short, thick neck and high shoulders and clavicles resulting in possibly difficult lower cervical disk space exposure

OPERATIVE TECHNIQUE

EQUIPMENT

- X-ray compatible operating table
- Fluoroscopy
- Operating microscope

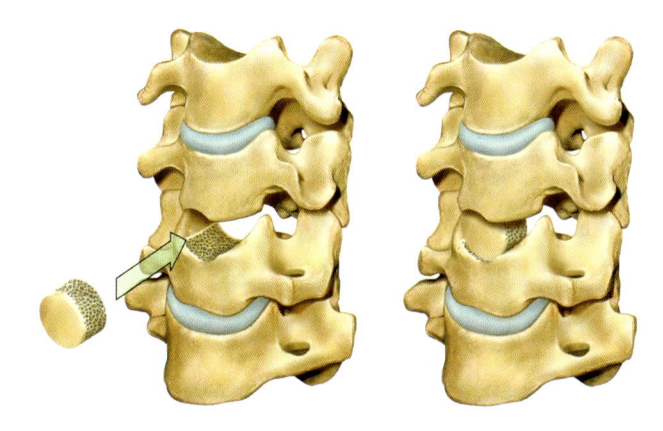

Fig. 16-1 The Cloward procedure utilizes a cylindrical bony removal and dowel placement for fusion. This technique has some limitations with regard to the approach to the intraforaminal area.

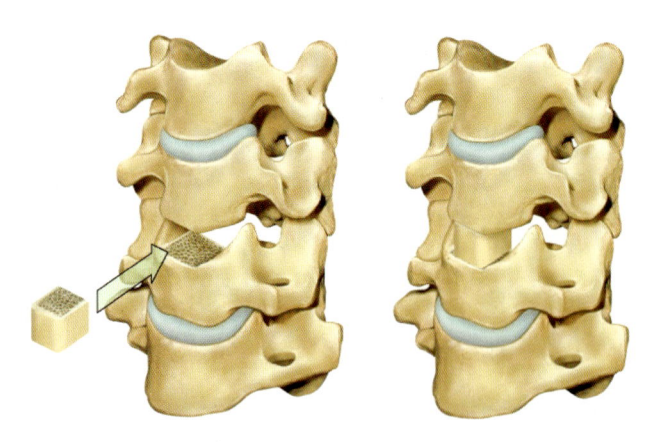

Fig. 16-2 The Smith-Robinson procedure achieves decompression and fusion via a rectangular intervertebral bony resection. Ventral midline and intraforaminal lesions are surgically accessible via this approach.

- Headlight system
- Cervical retractor system
- Caspar distraction pins, 12 to 14 mm
- Straight and angled curettes
- Kerrison punches, 1 to 3 mm
- Bone graft source
- Optional anterior plating system

PATIENT POSITIONING

- The patient is placed in a supine position (Fig. 16-3).
- General endotracheal anesthesia is used. The patient is asked to extend the neck to the point of pain or onset of radicular or myelopathic symptoms before the induction of anesthesia. If maximum neck extension necessary for oral intubation causes the onset of symptoms, then intubation or fiberoptic bronchoscopy is performed with the patient awake.

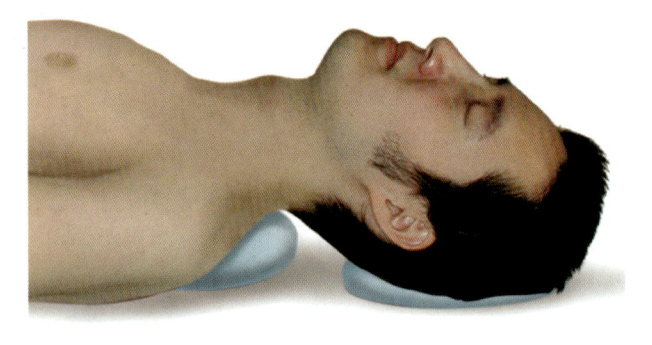

Fig. 16-3 The patient is positioned supine. After general endotracheal anesthesia, the head is placed in a foam headrest. A rolled sheet is placed behind the shoulders to extend the neck and support the lordotic cervical curve.

- A shoulder roll to facilitate neck extension is used in most cases; the head is placed in a foam cradle headrest and the arms are tucked to the sides.
- If autograft harvesting is anticipated, the iliac crest site is elevated by placing a pillow under the buttock. The planned incision should be lateral to the anterior superior iliac spine so that the lateral femoral cutaneous nerve is not injured.
- The shoulders can be taped to better visualize the lower cervical segments.

LOCATION OF INCISION

- A left-sided approach is preferred to minimize recurrent laryngeal nerve injury.
- Fluoroscopy can help with incision planning.
- For C5-C6 and C6-C7 levels, the incision is placed at the level of the cricoid cartilage. A prominent bony tubercle on the C6 transverse process can be palpated to help guide incision placement.
- At C4-C5, the incision is placed a few centimeters higher.
- At C3-C4, a separate incision is made 1 cm above the thyroid cartilage.
- At C1-C2 and C2-C3, the transverse incision is made 1 cm below the angle of the jaw from the midline to the mastoid bone.
- To expose the C7-T1 level, the transverse incision is placed as low as possible above the clavicle (Fig. 16-4).

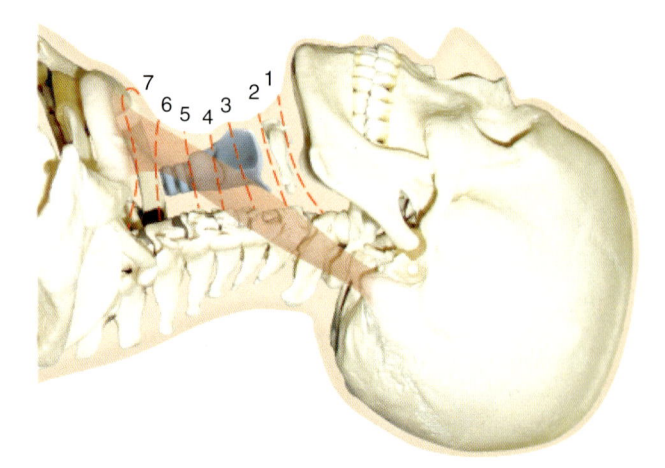

Fig. 16-4 The dotted lines are numbered according to the skin locations of the appropriate named vertebral bodies underneath. A C1-C2 and C2-C3 transverse incision is made 1 cm below the angle of the jaw from the midline to the mastoid bone. For lesions at C3-C4, an incision is made 1 cm above the thyroid cartilage (= dotted line 4, which represents the C4 level). The C5-C6 disk lies beneath the cricoid cartilage (located between dotted lines 5 and 6). If the C7-T1 level is to be exposed, the transverse incision is placed as low as possible above the clavicle.

- A transverse incision is made from the midline to the lateral border of the sternocleidomastoid muscle. If possible, the incision should be planned within a natural skin crease closest to level of pathology.

PREPARATION AND DRAPING

- The incision is marked and the cervical skin area is sterilely prepared.
- Draping is carried out in the usual manner.
- The iliac crest incision site is draped separately and covered.
- The anesthesiologist is at the head of the table, and the scrub nurse is below the iliac crest.
- The headlight and microscope are based on the side of the incision.
- Fluoroscopy is based on the contralateral side.

Illustrative case

A 52-year-old man presented with symptoms of neck pain and left shoulder pain. The neurologic examination showed left biceps muscle strength of grade 4 and a decreased biceps reflex. Sagittal and axial cervical T_2-weighted magnetic resonance imaging (MRI) scans show a C5-C6 disk, which has protruded posterocentrally to the left and has compressed the spinal cord and left C5-C6 neural foramen (Fig. 16-5). The diagnosis was a C5-C6 disk protrusion. The patient was admitted and the decision was made to perform a C5-C6 diskectomy and fusion with placement of an allograft. The patient is shown positioned supine with the neck in moderate extension (Fig. 16-6). The skin incision was made along the shown line, which is aligned with the skin crease. A left-sided approach is carried out to avoid recurrent laryngeal nerve injury.

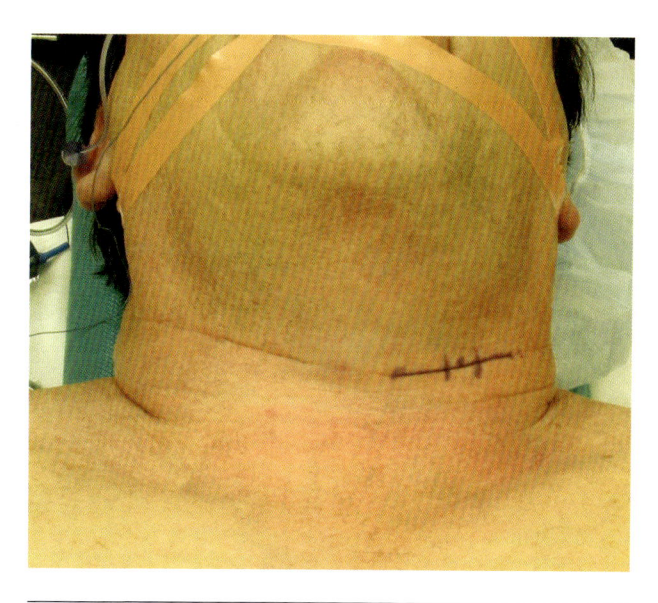

Fig. 16-6 The patient is positioned supine with the neck in moderate extension. The skin incision will be done along the drawn line, which is aligned with the skin crease. A left side approach is carried out to avoid recurrent laryngeal nerve injury.

- The operation room set-up is as follows:
  - The anesthesiologist is positioned at the head of the patient (Fig. 16-7).
  - Fluoroscopy is located transversely to the level of the operating field, so as to check the exact lesion level before surgery.
  - The patient is covered with a warm air blanket to conserve body temperature.

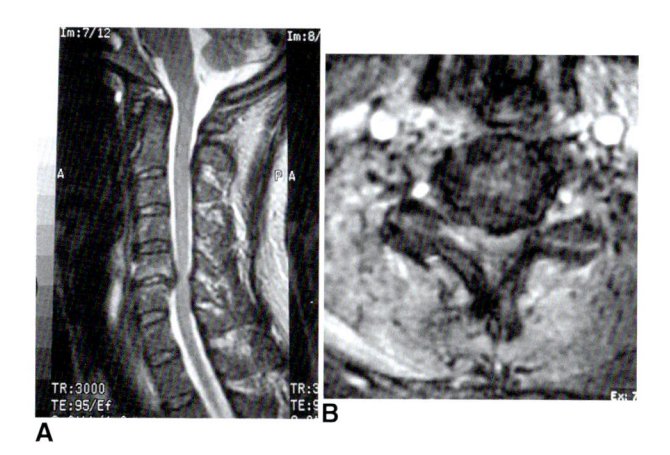

Fig. 16-5 Sagittal (A) and axial (B) cervical T_2-weighted magnetic resonance images show a C5-C6 disk, which has protruded posterocentral to the left side and has compressed the spinal cord and left C5-C6 neural foramen.

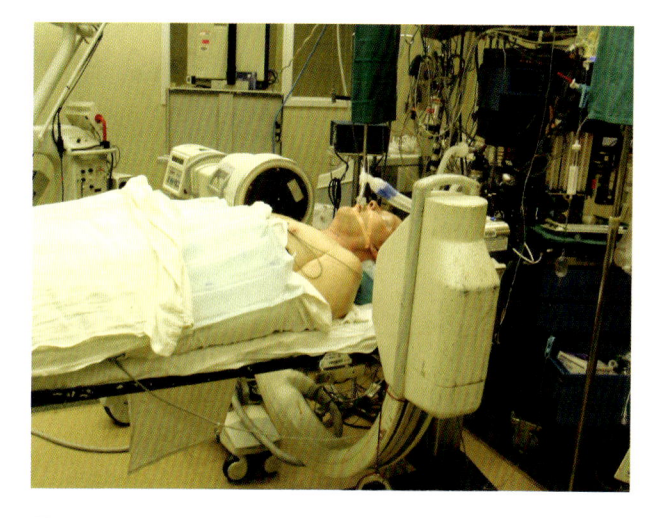

Fig. 16-7 The operation room set-up: the anesthesiologist is placed at the head of the patient. Fluoroscopy is located transversely at the level of the operating field, so as to check the exact lesion level before surgery. The patient is covered with a warm air blanket to conserve body temperature.

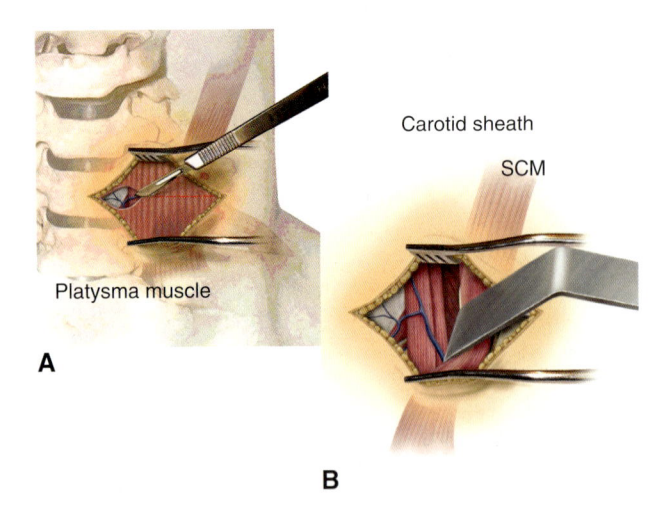

Fig. 16-8 *A*, A transverse skin incision is made from the midline to the lateral edge of the sternocleidomastoid muscle (SCM). The platysma muscle is divided transversely. *B*, The medial border of the SCM and the carotid sheath are retracted laterally, in this case to the patient's left side. The omohyoid and sternothyroid muscles are then retracted medially along with the trachea and esophagus.

INCISION AND SOFT TISSUE DISSECTION

- Local anesthetic is injected subcutaneously at the incision site.
- A transverse skin incision is made from midline to the lateral edge of the sternocleidomastoid (SCM) muscle (Fig. 16-8).
- The subcutaneous layer is divided, and hemostasis is obtained.
- The platysma muscle is identified, undermined, and divided transversely.
- The subplatysmal areolar layer is then dissected to facilitate retraction.
- The medial border of the SCM muscle is identified.
- The anterior cervical fascia on the medial border of the SCM muscle is incised, exposing the areolar plane between the SCM muscle and the omohyoid and sternothyroid muscles.
- The carotid artery pulse is palpated, freed from surrounding connective tissue medially by blunt dissection, and retracted laterally.
- The omohyoid and sternothyroid muscles are then retracted medially along with the trachea and esophagus.
- The prevertebral space can be palpated in the midline.

EXPOSURE OF THE VERTEBRA

- With blunt dissection, the prevertebral fascial layer is exposed and incised in the midline to reveal the longus colli muscles.
- An 18-gauge needle is inserted into the intervertebral disk space selected and fluoroscopy is used to localize the desired level (Fig. 16-9).
- The longus colli muscles are elevated from their medial attachments to the anterior longitudinal ligament. Electrocautery dissection should remain underneath the longus colli muscles to prevent injury to the esophagus, trachea, and neurovascular structures. Enough dissection beneath the longus colli muscles will facilitate self-retaining retractor placement.

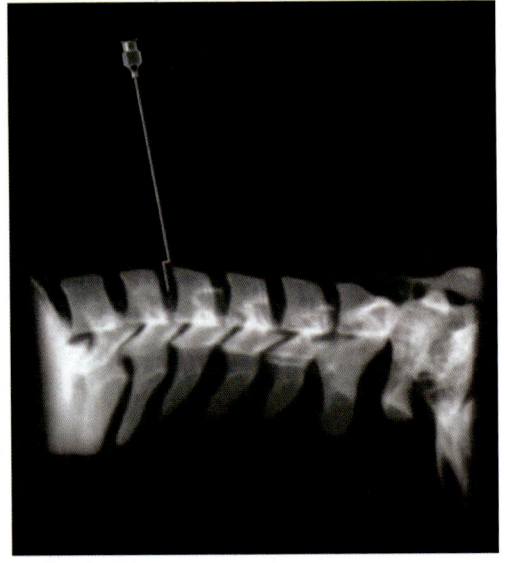

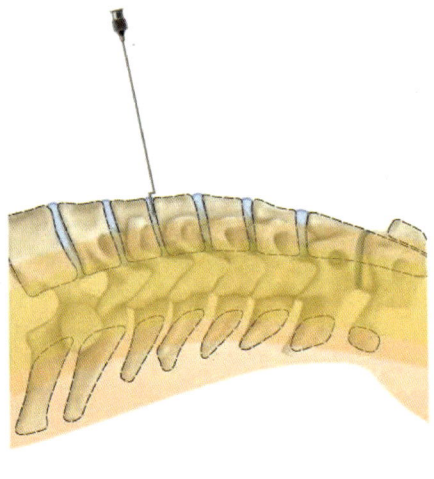

Fig. 16-9 An 18-gauge needle is inserted into the C5-C6 intervertebral disk space (*right*) and fluoroscopy is used to localize the desired level (*left*).

CHAPTER 16 Anterior Cervical Diskectomy and Fusion

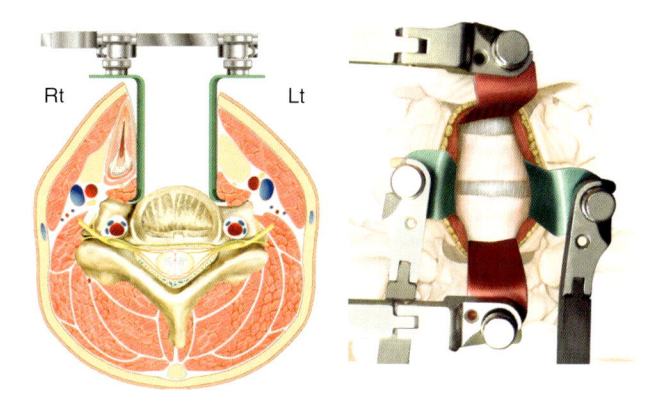

Fig. 16-10 A self-retaining retractor system is positioned as shown. Blade teeth are inserted underneath the longus colli muscles. Midline must be firmly established to avoid an asymmetrical approach to the posterior portion of the disk and the vertebrae and vertebral artery injury. A second retractor with longer smooth-tipped blades is positioned perpendicular to the placed retractors to complete the exposure.

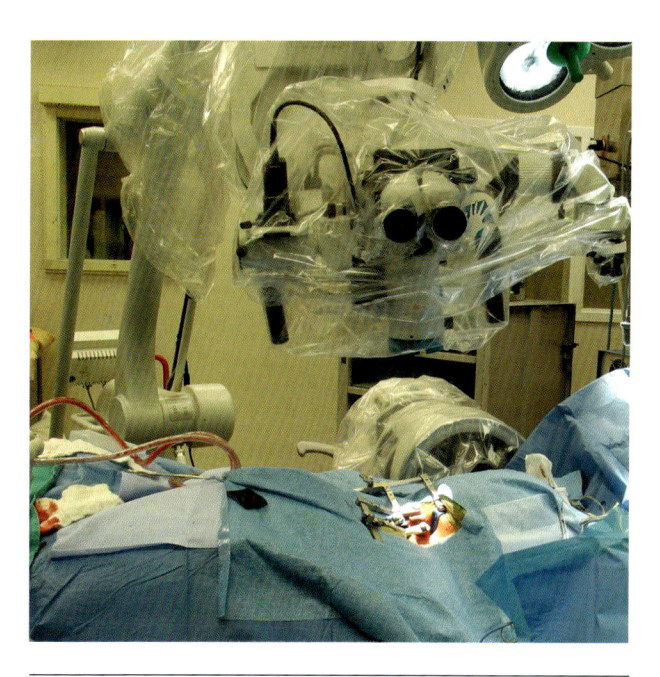

Fig. 16-11 A surgical microscope is used after Caspar retractor placement.

RETRACTOR PLACEMENT

- Attention to midline is important during longus colli muscle dissection and is guided by the contour of the vertebral bodies and the original sites of attachment of the longus colli muscles.
- The inferior thyroid vein and artery may also be encountered, especially if the dissection is extended toward C4-C5. If necessary, they may be ligated.
- The superior laryngeal nerve near the C3-C4 and C4-C5 spaces can be identified coursing inferomedially from the region of the carotid sheath toward the thyroid cartilage and should be preserved.
- A self-retaining retractor system is then positioned and secured. Blade teeth are inserted underneath the longus colli muscles (Fig. 16-10).
- A vertical line of sight to the vertebral column and midline must be firmly established to avoid an asymmetrical approach to the posterior portion of the disk and the vertebral osteophytes and a potential for vertebral artery injury.
- A second retractor with longer smooth-tipped blades is positioned longitudinally to complete the exposure.
- A surgical microscope may be used after Caspar retractor placement (Fig. 16-11).
- Intervertebral bridging osteophytes should be removed.
- Caspar distraction pins (12 to 14 mm) are placed into the midportions of the vertebral bodies above and below the operative disk space with a cephalad angle.
- The disk space is distracted via use of distractor pins (Fig. 16-12).

DISKECTOMY AND OSTEOPHYTECTOMY

- A rectangular opening 10 to 12 mm wide is created by incising the anterior longitudinal ligament and annulus at the desired level (Fig. 16-13).
- The remaining procedure is done under the operating microscope.
- To maintain midline positioning during microscopic surgery, the microscope should be aligned perpendicular to the anterior surface of the spinal column.

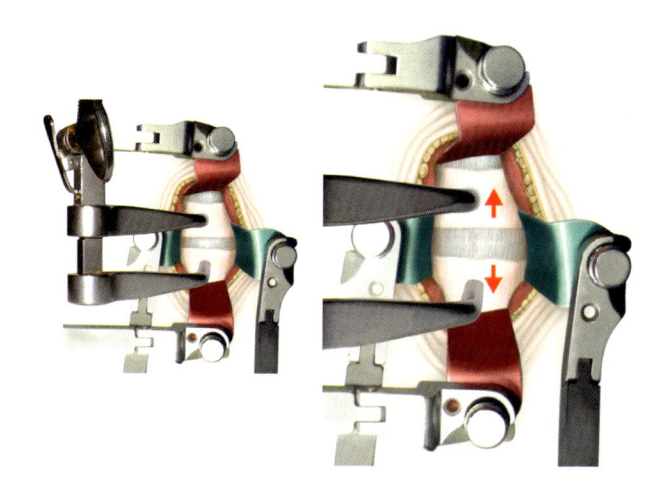

Fig. 16-12 Caspar 12- to 14-mm distraction pins are placed into the midportions of the vertebral bodies above and below the operative disk space in a cephalad angle (i.e., parallel to the alignment of the vertebral bodies as seen on lateral fluoroscopy). The disk space is distracted via the use of distractor pins.

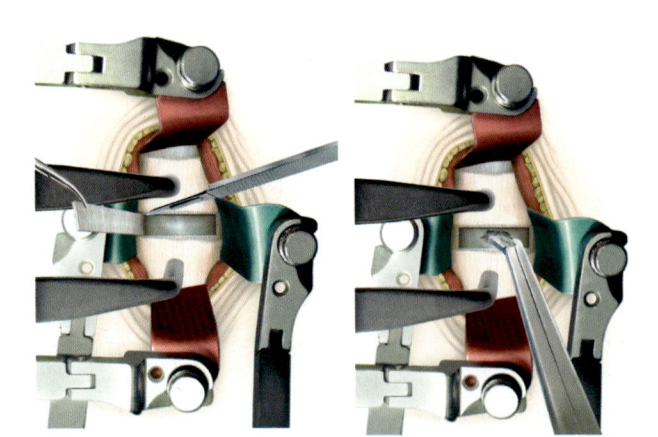

Fig. 16-13 A rectangular opening 10 to 12 mm in length and width, the disk height, is created by incising the anterior longitudinal ligament and annulus at the desired level. The remaining procedure is done under the operating microscope, which should be aligned perpendicular to the anterior surface of the spinal column. This provides magnification and enhances illumination posteriorly in the depths of the disk space.

- Curettes and rongeurs are used to remove the fibrocartilage of the annulus and disk.
- The anterior vertebral body lips and marginal osteophytes that usually overhand the disk space should be drilled away.
- The curved surfaces of the cartilaginous plates of the upper and lower vertebral bodies are drilled maintaining the rectangular shape of the bony opening (Fig. 16-14).

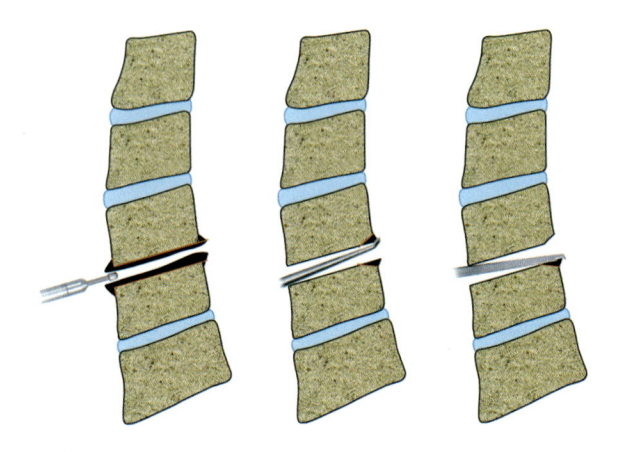

Fig. 16-14 The anterior and marginal osteophytes should be drilled away. The curved cartilaginous plate surfaces of the upper and lower vertebral bodies are drilled. The rectangular shape of the bony opening is maintained. A power drill is used to remove the posterior osteophyte(s). Complete osteophyte removal should be performed by undercutting the osteocytes with the drill and Kerrison rongeur.

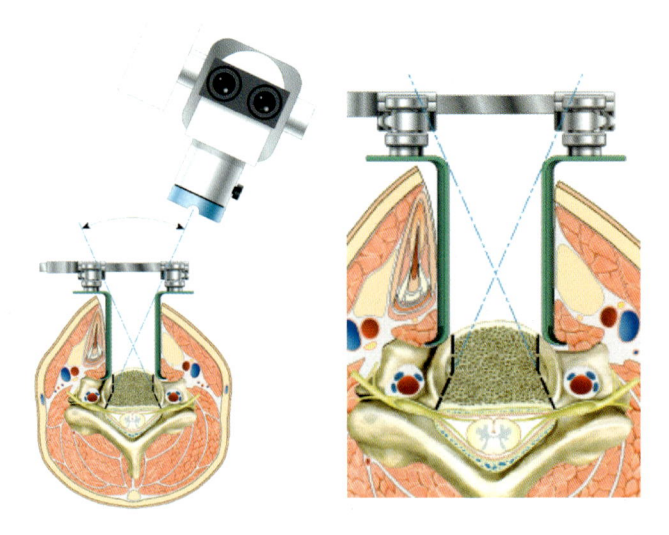

Fig. 16-15 We orient the microscope obliquely to see the uncinate process. We can remove the posterior third of the uncinate process to decompress the neural foramen and to remove the laterally herniated disk and spurs.

- Straight 2-0 curettes are used to remove the residual annulus from the posterior aspect of the disk space.
- A power drill is used to remove the posterior vertebral body lip and attached osteophyte.
- Posteriorly and inferiorly, complete osteophyte removal should be performed by undercutting with a drill and Kerrison rongeurs.
- The amount of osteophyte removal can be estimated from preoperative imaging studies and noting decompression at the time of surgery.
- We orient the microscope obliquely to see the uncinate process. We can remove the posterior third of the uncinate process to decompress the neural foramen and to remove the laterally herniated disk and spurs (Fig. 16-15).
- If complete decompression is uncertain, the posterior longitudinal ligament should be opened and the epidural space inspected.
- Residual osteophyte(s) may still be present if the ventral dura is not pulsatile and has not expanded into the space created by diskectomy.
- Palpating the floor of the neural canal and foramina with a blunt hook can help confirm the completeness of decompression (Fig. 16-16).
- In the illustrative case, lateral fluoroscopy showed the position of the blunt hook in the C5-C6 disk space. This hook is introduced to confirm the osteophytectomies, removal of disk particles, and complete decompression of both neural foramen. The Caspar pins must parallel the anteroposterior diameter of the cervical vertebrae and be located in the center of the vertebral bodies (Fig. 16-17).
- Epidural venous bleeding can be coagulated with a bipolar forceps or controlled by gentle packing with thrombin-soaked Gelfoam.

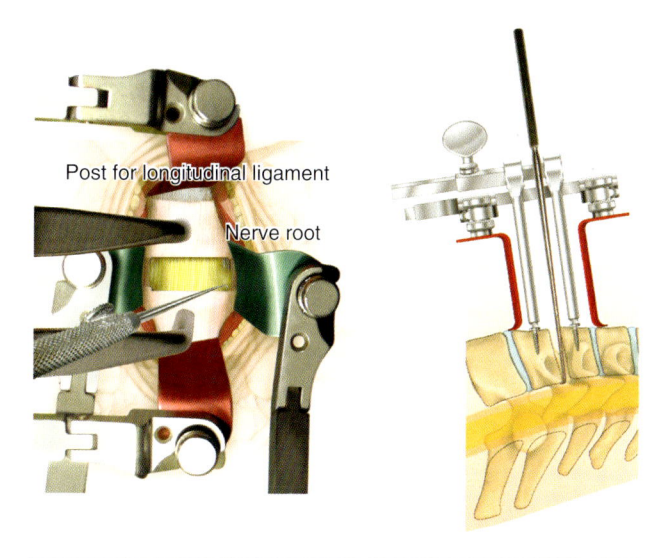

CHAPTER **16** Anterior Cervical Diskectomy and Fusion   147

Fig. 16-16 If complete decompression is uncertain after palpating the floor of the neural canal and foramen with a blunt hook, the posterior longitudinal ligament should be opened and the epidural space inspected. Palpating again as described can help confirm completeness of decompression. Epidural venous bleeding can be coagulated with a bipolar forceps or controlled by gentle packing with thrombin-soaked Gelfoam.

BONE GRAFT

- Bone wax should be avoided because it may interfere with the fusion process.
- Under distraction, the rectangular bed prepared for the bone graft is measured.

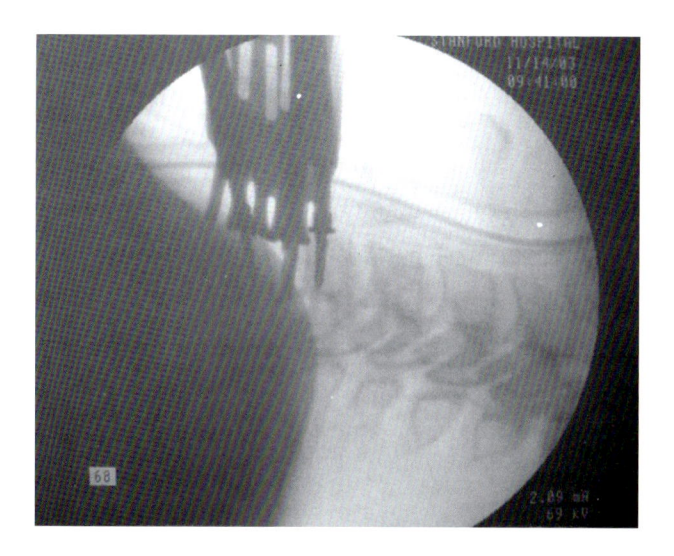

Fig. 16-17 After a C5-C6 diskectomy, a blunt hook dissector is introduced to confirm the osteophytectomies, removal of disk particles, and complete decompression of both neural foramina. The Caspar pins must parallel the anteroposterior diameter of the cervical vertebrae and be located in the center of the vertebral bodies.

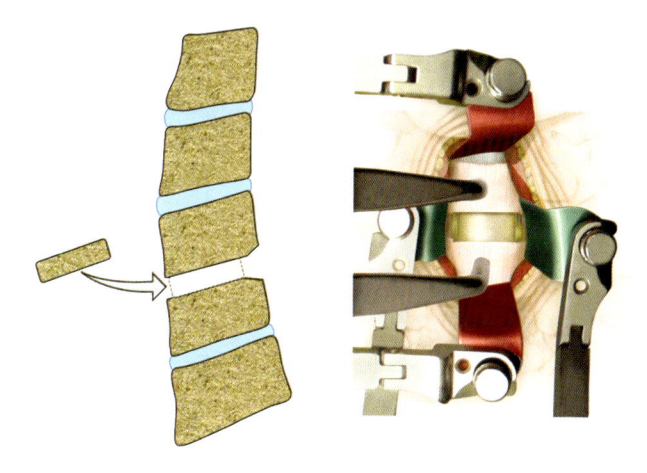

Fig. 16-18 The appropriate-sized bone graft is tamped into the diskectomy site, which is under distraction. Once the distraction is released, it should not be possible to move the graft using reasonable force.

- The appropriate size bone graft is tamped into the diskectomy site under distraction (Fig. 16-18).
- In the illustrative case, after diskectomy, allograft bone material is inserted into the C5-C6 disk space. Allograft bone should be somewhat wider than the disk space. This allows for foraminal widening, firm placement of the bone graft, and reasonable disk space maintenance, even if subsidence occurs.
- If the graft does not start to enter the intervertebral space, it should be removed and inspected for oversized surfaces or protruding points that need to be trimmed.
- Once distraction is released, it should not be possible to move the graft with reasonable force.
- Palpation of the posterior margin of the bone graft with a blunt nerve hook should verify lack of dural compression.
- Final lateral cervical films are taken to verify graft placement and correct level.

AUTOGRAFT HARVESTING

- For harvesting of a tricortical iliac crest autograft, an oblique incision is made extending on the lateral side of the crest posterior to the anterior superior iliac spine.
- Muscle attachments are reflected subperiosteally, and all soft tissue is cleared from the exposed portion of the iliac crest.
- Straight osteotomes are used to make two parallel perpendicular cuts to the surface of the iliac crest and are separated by a distance that is several millimeters larger than the measured height of the graft space during distraction.
- A cross cut along the base connecting the two perpendicular cuts using angled osteotomes will be required to free the bone graft.

SECTION II DEGENERATIVE DISEASE OF THE SPINE

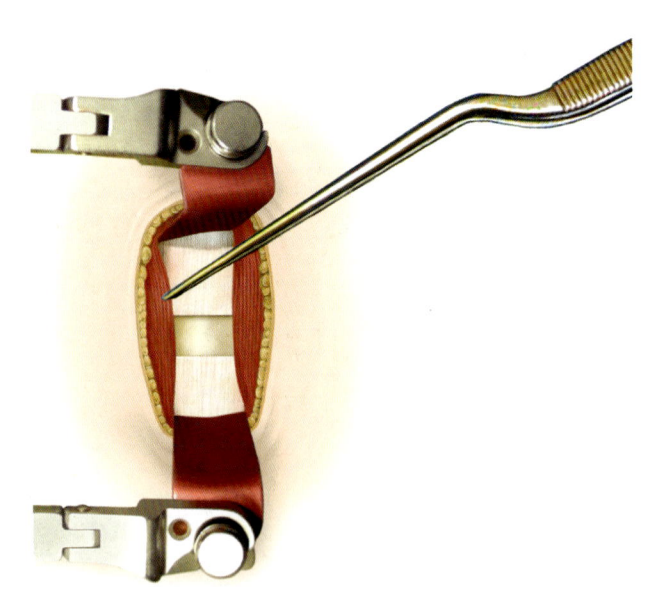

Fig. 16-19 Distraction pins and retractors are removed, and hemostasis is carefully carried out. The esophagus should be checked for possible injury due to retraction. A subplatysmal drain should be placed if the amount of epidural and bony oozing was significant.

- The graft size required for the average patient is 12 mm in the transverse plane and 8 to 12 mm in the anteroposterior plane.
- The vertical height of the graft is usually 6 to 10 mm, depending on initial disk space collapse.

CLOSURE

- Distraction pins and retractors are removed.
- Hemostasis is carefully performed (Fig. 16-19).
- The esophagus should be checked for injury due to retraction.
- A subplatysmal drain should be placed if the amount of epidural and bony oozing is significant.
- The platysma layer is closed separately with fine absorbable sutures.
- Fine interrupted subcuticular stitches are used to cosmetically reapproximate the skin (Fig. 16-20).
- In the illustrative case, postoperative anteroposterior and lateral cervical spine x-rays show good position of the allograft in the C5-C6 disk space with some widening of the intervertebral gap (Fig. 16-21).
- If cervical plating is not contemplated, a rigid collar should be applied at the end of the case.

POSTOPERATIVE CARE

- Postoperative orders are written for monitoring of airway and neurologic deterioration.

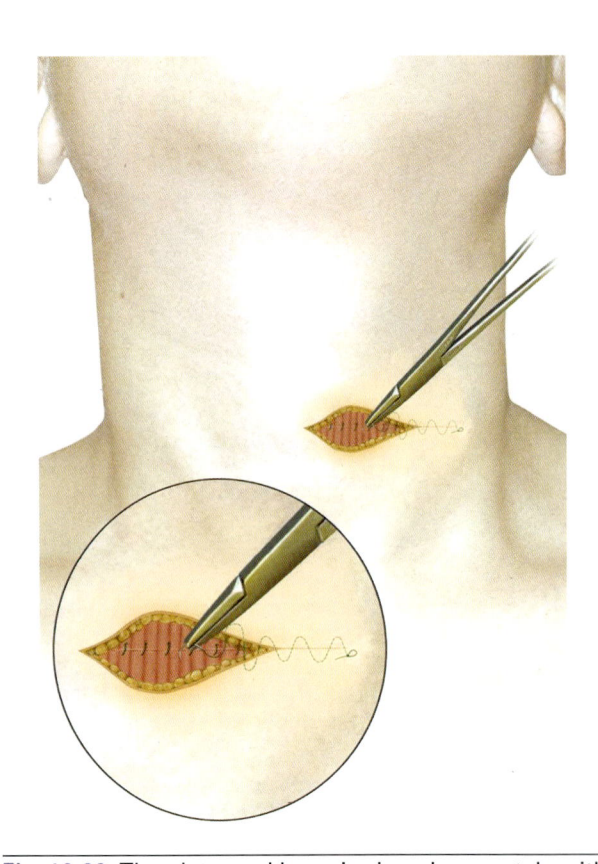

Fig. 16-20 The platysmal layer is closed separately with fine, absorbable sutures. Fine interrupted subcuticular stitches are used next, to cosmetically reapproximate the skin.

- Early ambulation is encouraged.
- The diet can be advanced as tolerated, depending on esophageal edema and swallowing difficulties.
- Paratracheal edema can give a sensation of upper airway tightness.

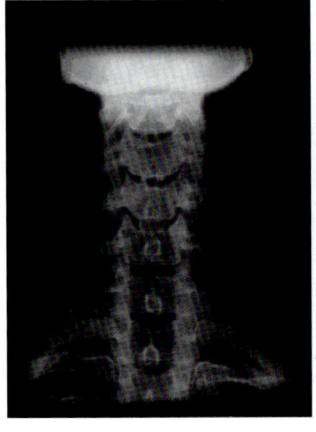

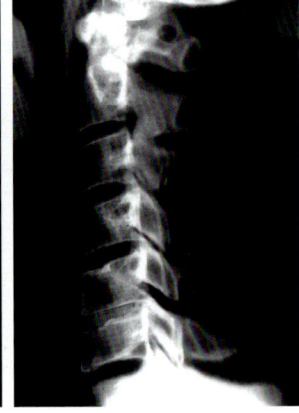

Fig. 16-21 Postoperative anteroposterior (A) and lateral (B) cervical spine x-rays showing good position of the allograft in the C5-C6 disk space with some widening of the intervertebral gap.

- Head elevation can reduce cervical edema.
- Oral pain control is usually sufficient but can be patient dependent.
- Posterior cervical and shoulder pain can be an initial response to ligamentous and facet capsule stretching during the surgery.
- Patients are usually discharged from the hospital the following day if there are no complications.
- A postoperative cervical film can be obtained before discharge to verify maintenance of spinal alignment and bone graft position and to provide a baseline for follow-up visits.

COMPLICATIONS

- A new neurologic deficit may develop after recovery from anesthesia secondary to nerve root injury or edema, spinal cord concussion, or rapid release of chronic compression.
- Acute deficits may develop as a result of mechanical problems such as intervertebral subluxation, migrated bone graft, residual compressive disk fragment, residual osteophyte, or an acute epidural hematoma, all of which should be surgically treated.
- For nonprogressive mild neurologic deficits not associated with swelling, or mechanical causes, including hematoma, further imaging studies will help with surgical treatment options.
- Early delayed deficits are usually due to postoperative edema, in which case prognosis for recovery is good.
- Progressive deficit after the first week of surgery may indicate spinal instability or an epidural abscess.
- Severe cervical pain occurring weeks or months after surgery may be secondary to vertebral osteomyelitis.
- Carotid thrombosis from lateral retraction can be a risk factor with patients who have a history of transient ischemic attacks. These patients should be treated for significant carotid stenosis before undergoing anterior cervical fusion.
- Persistent postoperative hoarseness due to injury of the recurrent laryngeal nerve may occur. Care must be taken initially to prevent aspiration postoperatively.

CHAPTER 17

HO-YEOL ZHANG

DANIEL H. KIM

Anterior Cervical Microforaminotomy

INTRODUCTION

In 1934, Mixter and Barr[1] published a report on 19 cases of ruptured intervertebral disks treated successfully with a posterior laminectomy. Four of these patients had cervical disk herniation. Since then, the approach for discogenic cervical radiculopathy has evolved into a small keyhole foraminotomy via posterior approach with or without diskectomy. Although the posterior procedure preserves a functioning motion segment, decompression of the nerve root is indirect, leaving the compressive lesion untouched.

Compressive pathologic lesions causing cervical radiculopathy (soft disk fragment herniation or spondylotic bone spurs) are most often located anterior to the nerve root. These anterior pathoanatomic features logistically justify anterior approaches, despite the feasibility of the posterior approaches. Anterior diskectomy procedures described by Robinson and Smith[2] in 1955 and Cloward[3] in 1958 represented significant new technical advances that provided direct access to the ventral aspect of the cervical root where the pathology is most frequently located.

However, surgical access to compressive pathologic lesions via conventional anterior approaches requires complete removal of the remaining disk in the intervertebral disk space. The ideal surgical treatment for impaired organs would restore their original anatomic features and function. Such surgical treatment for diskcogenic cervical radiculopathy is called "functional cervical disk surgery" or "functional spine surgery."[4] Anterior microforaminotomy was developed by Jho to preserve the remaining disk in the intervertebral space as much as possible while directly eliminating the compressive pathologic lesion.[5]

The operative procedure has the advantages of direct anterior decompression of a lesion impinging on the nerve without a fusion procedure and results in minimal operative morbidity. The success of outpatient anterior cervical diskectomy and fusion procedures has been established recently and is a relatively painless procedure with few complications. Anterior cervical microforaminotomy represents a technical evolution in treating cervical radiculopathy and is a procedure that can be used successfully in an outpatient setting because it involves even less tissue exposure, retraction, and procedural time. The disadvantages include unfamiliarity with the procedure, and the long-term issues related to disk degeneration and unilateral removal of an uncovertebral joint.[6]

INDICATIONS AND CONTRAINDICATIONS

INDICATIONS[4,7]

- Unilateral cervical radiculopathy with predominant radicular symptoms
- Imaging studies corresponding to the clinical symptoms
- No previous cervical spine surgery
- Minimal neck pain
- No significant spondylotic stenosis causing spinal cord compression
- No contralateral foraminal stenosis
- No spinal instability

CONTRAINDICATIONS[4]

- Asymptomatic spondylotic spinal cord compression, necessitating spinal cord decompression at the time of anterior foraminotomy
- Previous cervical spine surgery

OPERATIVE TECHNIQUE

EQUIPMENT

- X-ray-compatible operating table
- Fluoroscopy
- Operating microscope
- Standard anterior cervical disk surgery instruments

CHAPTER 17 Anterior Cervical Microforaminotomy

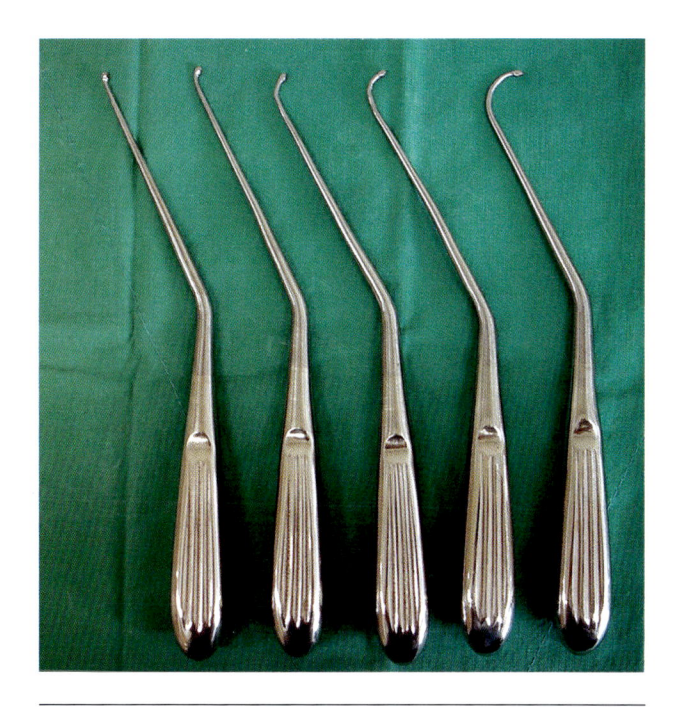

Fig. 17-1 Microcurette sets show various sizes and angles.

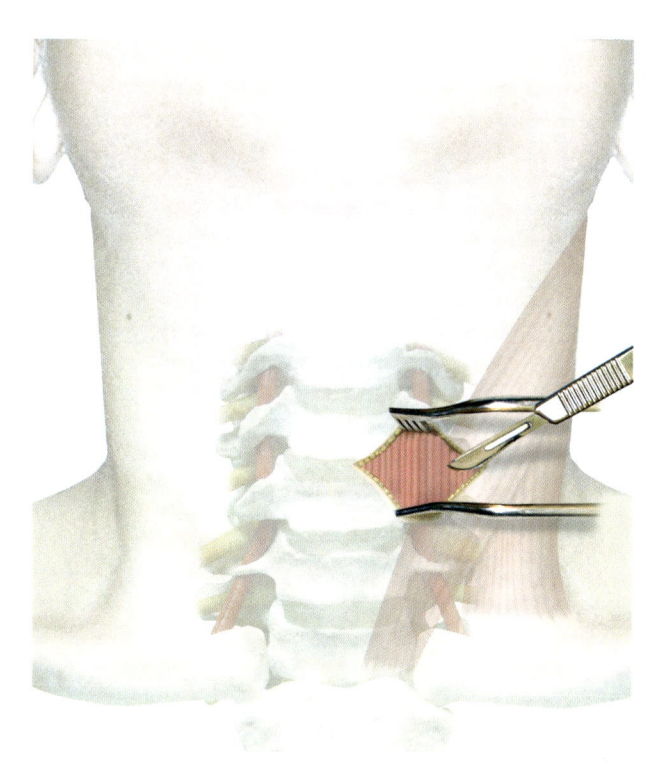

Fig. 17-2 Incision—A transverse skin incision is made around the medial border of the sternocleidomastoid muscle within 2 cm under the fluoroscopy guidance.

- High-speed drill for telescope surgery or microsurgery
- Microsurgical tools
- Microcurettes (Fig. 17-1)

PATIENT POSITIONING
- The patient is placed in a supine position as a standard anterior cervical exposure.
- General endotracheal anesthesia is used.
- In most cases, a shoulder roll to facilitate neck extension is used.
- The incision area is prepared and sterilized.
- Draping is carried out in the usual manner.

LOCATION OF INCISION
- The surgical entry site on the anterior aspect on the spine is located at the uncovertebral junction.
- Fluoroscopy is located transversely to the level of the operating field, so as to check the exact lesional level before surgery.
- Under fluoroscopic guidance, the incision area is marked at the medial border of the sternocleidomastoid (SCM) muscle perpendicular to the disk space angle.

INCISION AND SOFT TISSUE DISSECTION
- Local anesthetic is injected subcutaneously at the incision site.
- A transverse skin incision is made around the medial border of the SCM muscle within 2 cm (Fig. 17-2).
- The platysma muscle is identified, undermined, and divided transversely.
- The medial border of the SCM muscle is identified.
- The anterior cervical fascia on the medial border of the SCM muscle is incised, exposing the areolar plane between the SCM and the omohyoid and sternothyroid muscle.
- The carotid artery pulse is palpated, freed from surrounding connective tissue medially by blunt dissection, and retracted laterally.
- The omohyoid and sternothyroid muscles are then retracted medially along with the trachea and esophagus.
- The prevertebral space can be palpated in the operating side.
- The operation level is again confirmed by fluoroscopy.

EXPOSURE OF THE UNCOVERTEBRAL JUNCTION
- After identifying the longus colli muscles, the surgeon palpates the lateral border of the vertebral body and the lateral border of the transverse process.
- The longus colli muscles are covered and attached around the uncovertebral joint (Fig. 17-3).

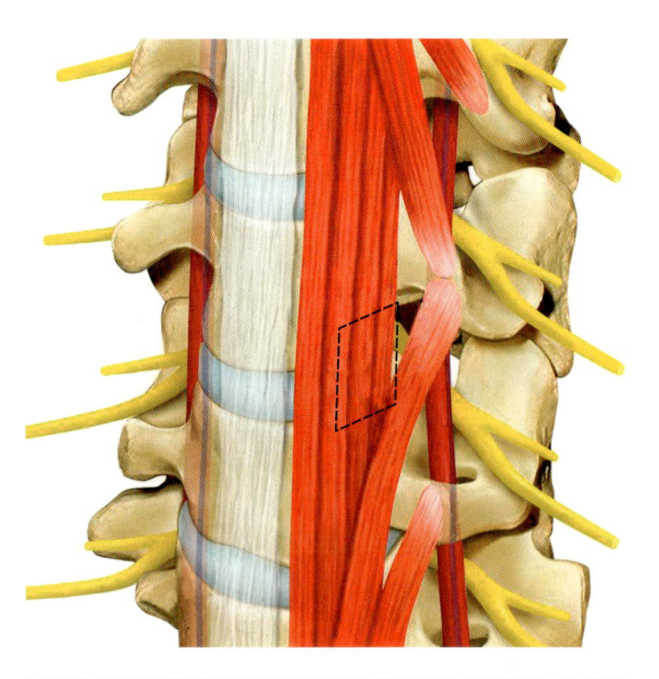

Fig. 17-3 After identification of the longus colli muscles, locate the lateral border of the vertebral body and the lateral border of the transverse process by palpation. Longus colli muscles are covered and attached around the uncovertebral joint.

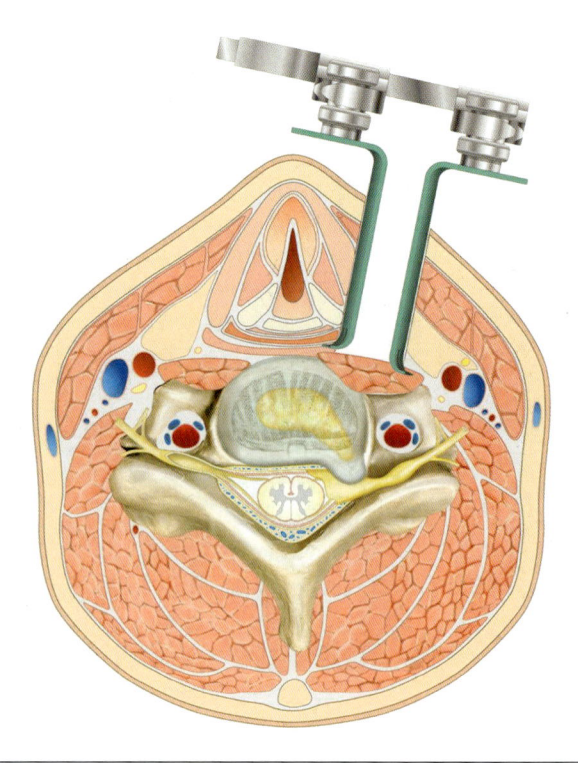

Fig. 17-4 A Caspar retractor with thin blades or tubular retractor or METRx system is introduced on the uncovertebral joint area.

RETRACTOR PLACEMENT

- A Caspar retractor with thin blades or tubular retractor is introduced on the uncovertebral joint area (Fig. 17-4).
- A tubular retractor is commonly used with a METRx system or the syringe, in which the funneled end was cut.

PARTIAL REMOVAL OF LONGUS COLLI MUSCLE

- Use the knife to cut the longus colli muscle in a rectangular shape, then remove it. Bleeding is controlled by bipolar Malis coagulator (Fig. 17-5).
- The sympathetic trunk of the cervical vertebrae runs on the longus colli muscle above the transverse foramen. Therefore, the muscle cutting medial of the uncovertebral joint is safe to the sympathetic damage of the sympathetic chain (Fig. 17-6).[8]
- Bear in mind that peeling off the longus colli muscles around the uncinate process can be a difficult task owing to the small working area.

DRILLING OF UNCINATE PROCESS

- A long and thin malleable retractor is placed between the uncinate process and vertebral artery to protect the vascular injury (Fig. 17-7). This retractor is attached to a table-mounted retractor system (e.g., Thompson, Greenberg, or Leyla type).

- The vertebral artery is located just lateral to the uncovertebral joint and is not seen during the procedure.
- The surgical microscope is now introduced, and partial removal of uncinate process is started.
- As indicated in Jho's original technique, the uncinate process is removed and a hole approximately 5 mm in diameter is created in the medial wall of the neural foramen.
- The foraminotomy hole is performed in a medial-to-lateral direction, bone removal is started at the most lateral margin of the uncovertebral junction, next to the vertebral artery, and then advanced medially.
- Because of the cephalad inclination of the intervertebral disk in the sagittal plane, the upper margin of the foraminotomy hole must be higher than the uncovertebral junction on the anterior aspect of the spine (Fig. 17-8).
- When the formation of a foraminotomy hole is advanced more posteriorly with this superior entry on the anterior spine, the appropriate portion of the neural foramen, where the nerve root is located, is revealed.

DECOMPRESSION OF THE NERVE ROOT

- For this task, a 2-mm cutting drill is used.
- The drilling is continued with the decompression centered over the uncovertebral joint until the posterior rim of the uncovertebral joint remains (Fig. 17-9).

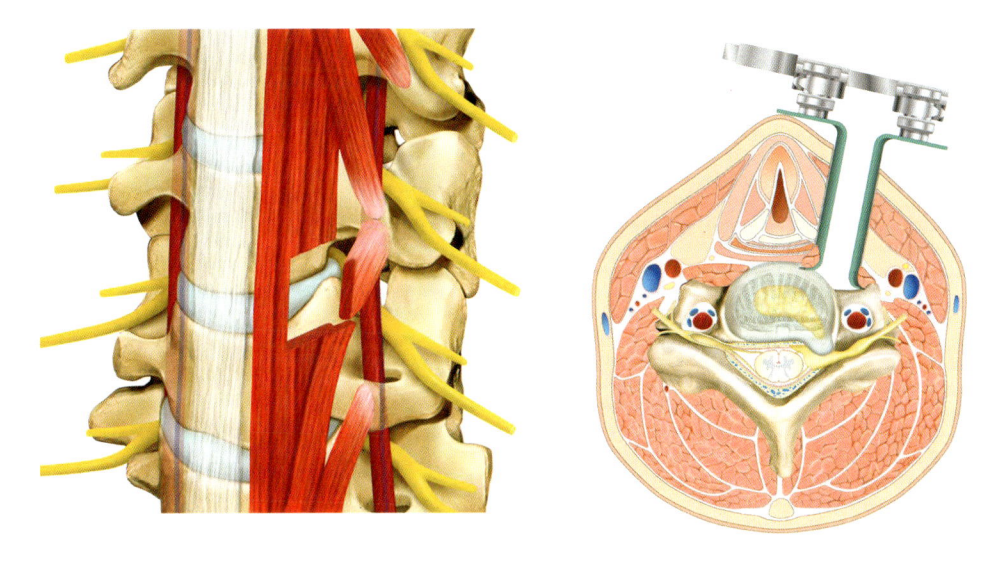

CHAPTER **17** Anterior Cervical Microforaminotomy   153

Fig. 17-5 Use the knife to cut the longus colli muscle in a rectangular shape, and then remove it. Bleeding is controlled by a bipolar Malis coagulator.

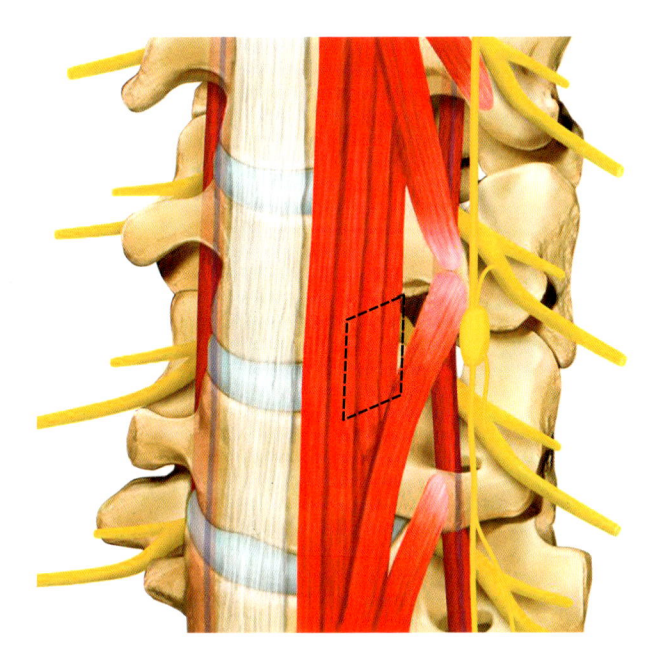

Fig. 17-6 The sympathetic trunk of the cervical vertebrae runs on the longus colli muscle above the transverse foramen. Therefore, the muscle cutting medial of the uncovertebral joint is safe to the sympathetic damage of the sympathetic chain.

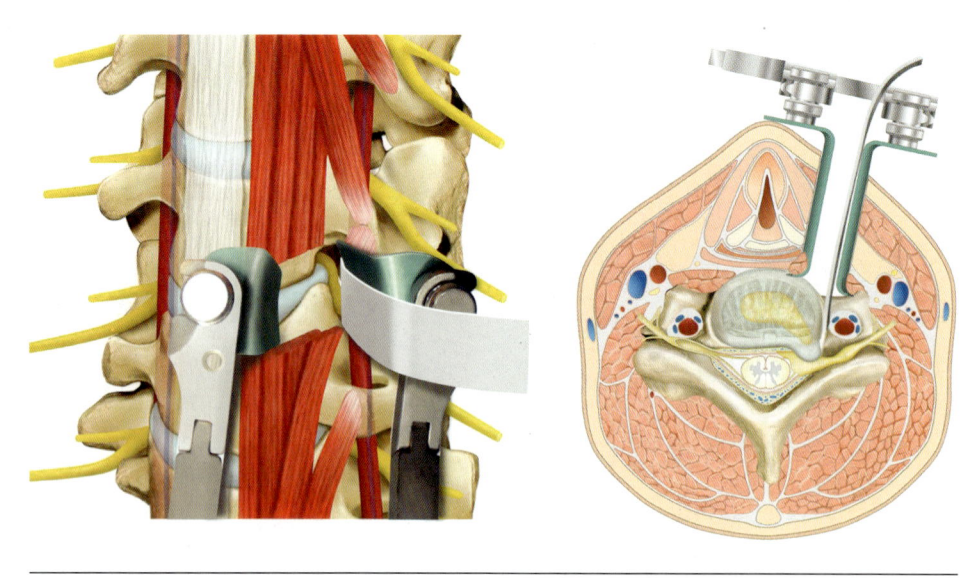

Fig. 17-7 A long and thin malleable retractor is placed between the uncinate process and vertebral artery to protect the vascular injury.

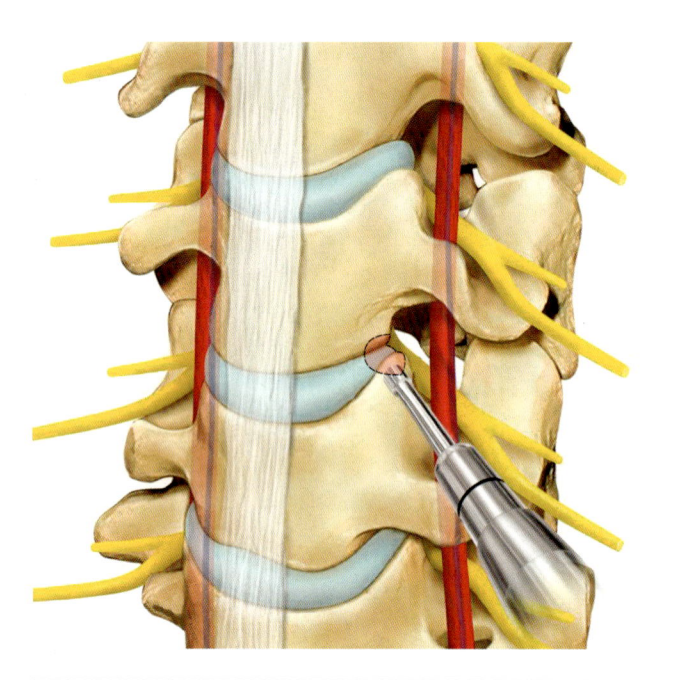

Fig. 17-8 The uncinate process is removed and a hole approximately 5 mm in diameter is created in the medial wall of the neural foramen. Bone removal is started at the most lateral margin of the uncovertebral junction, next to the vertebral artery, and then advanced medially. Because of the cephalad inclination of the intervertebral disk in the sagittal plane, the upper margin of the foraminotomy hole must be made higher than the uncovertebral junction.

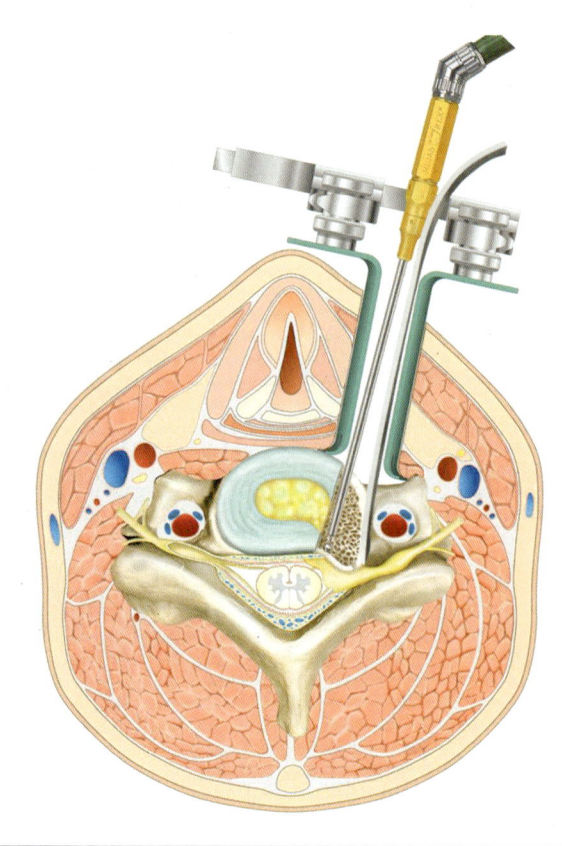

Fig. 17-9 A 2-mm cutting drill is used and drilling is continued with the decompression centered over the uncovertebral joint until the posterior rim of the uncovertebral joint remains.

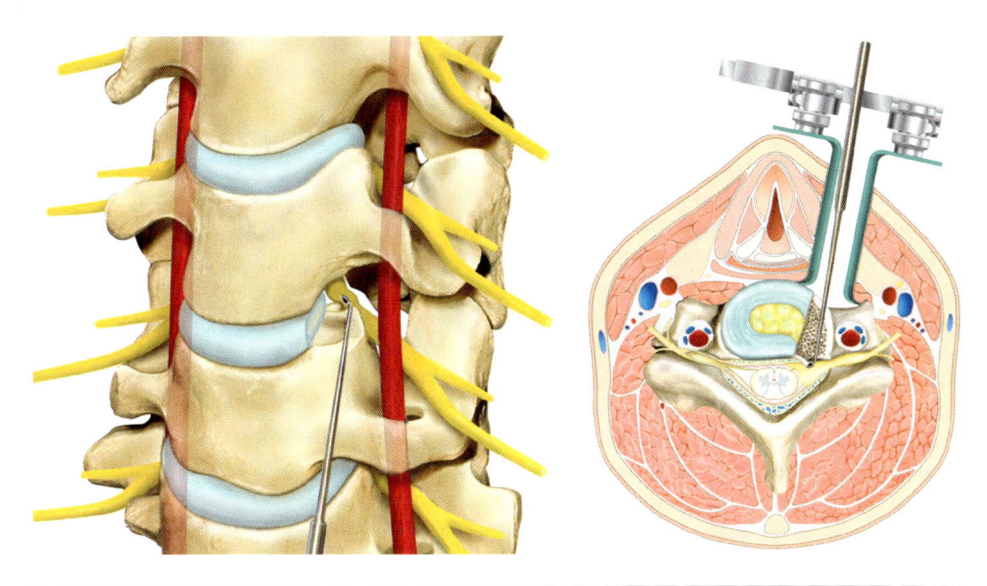

Fig. 17-10 Spondylotic spurs compressing the nerve root are drilled until they are thin and can be removed with sharp curettes and Kerrison rongeurs.

- Spondylotic spurs compressing the nerve root are drilled until they are thin and can be removed with sharp curettes and Kerrison rongeurs (Fig. 17-10).
- In cases with soft disk fragment herniation, the disk fragments are excised via a microforaminotomy hole (Fig. 17-11).

- Treatment of a ruptured and migrated disk herniation requires further exploration to remove the particles, which can occur in several locations. The preoperative magnetic resonance imaging (MRI) scan is often useful to guide the search. A subligamentous disk at the level of the disk should be readily apparent.
- Often, a migrated fragment is found in the axillary region of the nerve root and requires opening the posterior longitudinal ligament to locate the fragment in the same manner as a cervical diskectomy and fusion procedure.
- After the decompression procedure, the entire foramen can be palpated with a blunt nerve hook or 4-0 curved curette to ensure complete removal of osteophytes or disk material and complete decompression of nerve root (Fig. 17-12).

WOUND CLOSURE

- The retractors are removed with great care to prevent carotid artery and esophagus damage.
- Hemostasis is carefully performed.
- The platysma layer is closed separately with fine absorbable sutures.
- Fine interrupted subcuticular stitches are used to cosmetically reapproximate the skin.

POSTOPERATIVE CARE

- Postoperatively, the patient is assessed for airway and neurologic deterioration.
- A cervical orthosis is not used postoperatively.
- Oral pain control is sufficient.

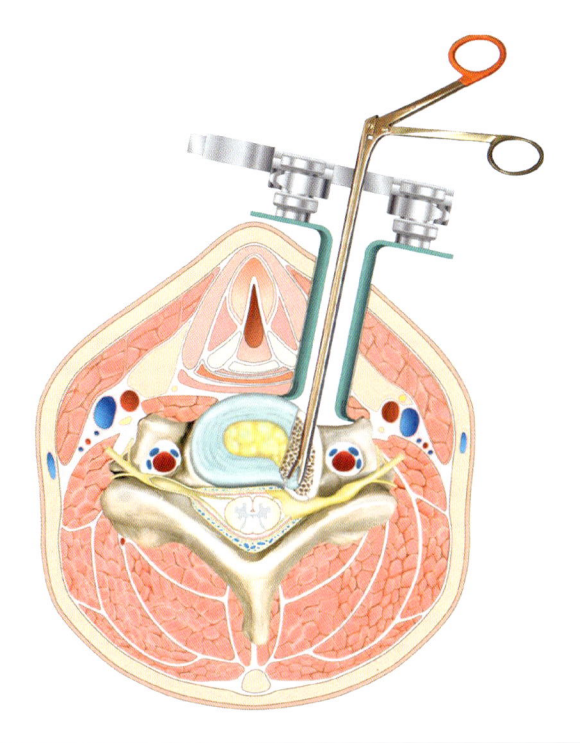

Fig. 17-11 In cases with soft disk fragment herniation, the disk fragments are excised via a microforaminotomy hole.

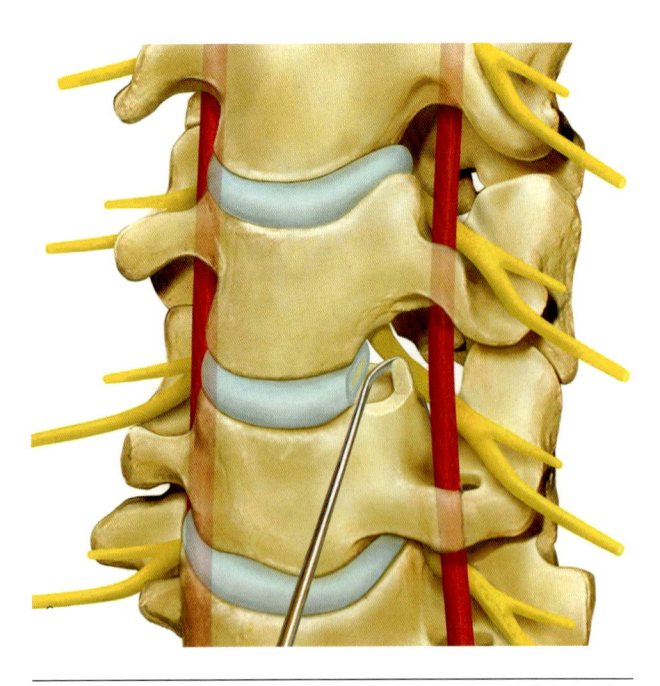

Fig. 17-12 After the decompression procedure, the entire foramen can be palpated with a blunt nerve hook to ensure the complete removal of osteophytes or disk material and complete decompression of the nerve root.

- Patients are usually discharged from the hospital within a few hours after being fully awake and ambulating independently.

COMPLICATIONS[7]

- Potential complications include bleeding or injury to the adjacent vertebral artery, bleeding from the perivertebral venous plexus, Horner's syndrome due to injury to the sympathetic chain, and inadequate decompression of the nerve root.
- Other complications are usually related to poor patient selection.
  - A patient with severe mechanical neck pain due to degenerative joint disease may not respond well to simple nerve root compression.
  - A patient with severe mechanical neck pain associated with functional levels (i.e., cervicothoracic junction and adjacent to previous fusions) may develop increased mechanical neck pain after partial unilateral removal of the uncovertebral junction.
  - A patient with new radicular symptoms at the contralateral side due to asymptomatic contralateral foraminal narrowing at the same level may develop new contralateral radicular symptoms, most likely as a result of some hypermobility after the procedure.

REFERENCES

1. Mixter WJ, Barr JS: Rupture of the intervertebral disc with involvement of the spinal canal. N Engl J Med 1934;211:210–215.
2. Robinson RA, Smith GW: Anterolateral cervical disc removal and interbody fusion for cervical disc syndrome. Bull Johns Hopkins Hosp 1955;96:223–224.
3. Cloward RB: The anterior approach for removal of ruptured cervical discs. J Neurosurg 1958;15:602–614.
4. Jho HD, Kim WK, Kim MH: Anterior microforaminotomy for treatment of cervical radiculopathy: Part 1—Disc-preserving "functional cervical disc surgery." Neurosurgery 2002;51(5)S2:46–53.
5. Jho HD: Microsurgical anterior cervical foraminotomy for radiculopathy: A new approach to cervical disc herniation. J Neurosurg 1996;84:155–160.
6. Johnson JP, Filler AG, McBride DQ, Batzdorf U: Anterior cervical foraminotomy for unilateral radicular disease. Spine 2000;25:905–909.
7. Johnson JP: Anterior cervical foraminotomy. In Perez-Cruet MJ, Fessler RG (eds): Outpatient Spinal Surgery. St. Louis, Quality Medical Publishing, 2002, pp 95–105.
8. Clemente CD: Axilla and shoulder. In Clemente CD (ed): Clemente's Anatomy—A Regional Atlas of the Human Body, 4th ed. Baltimore, Williams & Wilkins, 1997, plate 16.

CHAPTER 18

HO-YEOL ZHANG

DANIEL H. KIM

Anterior Cervical Fusion and Instrumentation Techniques

INTRODUCTION

Anterior cervical diskectomy and fusion is a commonly employed procedure for the treatment of radiculopathy, myelopathy, and myeloradiculopathy. It may include excision of a soft disk herniation or, more radically, the removal of osteophytes. To alleviate symptoms, one or more levels may require decompression and fusion. After adequate neural decompression is achieved, a fusion can be accomplished. The goals of fusion should include the stabilization and maintenance of normal cervical lordosis to diminish the chance of axial pain and instability.

Autogenous iliac crest bone graft or allograft bone have historically been used to achieve fusion.[1,2] Significant donor site complications have been described with autogenous graft techniques.[3] Decreased fusion rates, graft collapse, and resorption can be associated with the use of allografts.[4–6]

In the late 1960s, Simmons and associates described a graft in the shape of a keystone that was intended to enhance the stability of the graft by providing a larger area for potential fusion.[7] The anterior cervical plating system was first used by Hermann, who subsequently published his experience in 1975.[8] After this time, supplemental cervical plates were able to provide more rigid stabilization, prevent graft dislodgement, and even improve fusion rates.[9]

However, plates may cause stress shielding of the graft/donor bed interface.[10,11] This may prevent normal subsidence, which is necessary for graft incorporation. If a fusion does not occur, plates can loosen, break, and dislodge, thereby causing injury to the esophagus or surrounding soft tissues. The placement of a plate too close to an adjacent normal disk space may cause periplate ossification.[12] This idea prompted the development of intervertebral cages.

Intervertebral cages can function like bone graft for structural stability and provide an advantageous environment for osteosynthesis. Cages do not require additional plate fixation and eliminate other potential fixation and graft complications. Various intervertebral cages can provide immediate stabilization; they carry osteoconductive and osteoinductive graft material, maintain lordosis, and are considered low profile.

The objective of this chapter is to present the anterior cervical plating system and the use of cervical intervertebral cages.

INTERBODY FUSION WITH ANTERIOR CERVICAL PLATING SYSTEM

INDICATIONS

- Diskectomy (degenerative disk disease)
- Corpectomy (cervical spondylosis, neoplasm of the cervical spine or spinal cord)
- Instability of the cervical spine (trauma, fracture, rheumatoid instability)
- Deformity of the cervical spine
- Pseudoarthrosis or other previous failed cervical spine surgery

RELATIVE CONTRAINDICATIONS

- Disorders of hemostasis
- Acute local infection
- Severe osteoporosis

OPERATIVE TECHNIQUE
Equipment

- X-ray-compatible operating table
- Fluoroscopy

- Operating microscope
- Cervical retractor system
- Caspar distraction pins, 12 to 14 mm
- Straight and angled curettes
- Kerrison punches, 1 to 3 mm
- Bone graft source
- Optional anterior plating system

Plate Fixation Technique

After proper diskectomy or corpectomy and bone grafting, plate system is introduced to create a more tight fusion. If the surgeon elects internal fixation, four basic constructs are available: (1) single-level diskectomy and plating, (2) multiple-level diskectomy and plating, (3) partial corpectomy and plating, and (4) corpectomy and plating.

- *Single-level diskectomy and plating.* This construct consists of a diskectomy and interbody graft with a plate extending over two vertebral bodies, fusing a single motion segment (Fig. 18-1).
- *Multiple-level diskectomy and plating.* This procedure is essentially an extension of a single-level diskectomy and plating and involves fusion across multiple motion segments (Fig. 18-2).
- *Partial corpectomy and plating.* Multiple diskectomies are performed. However, if the posterior third of the vertebral body is intact, a trough corpectomy is not necessary. The anterior half to two thirds of the affected vertebral body can be removed following the diskectomy at the levels above and below. A graft can then be placed across multiple motion segments and secured with screws placed through the plate into the posterior cortex of the remaining vertebral body. This results in the most stable construct possible (Fig. 18-3).
- *Corpectomy and plating.* Diskectomies are performed on at least two levels, with removal of the midportion of the vertebral body. Similarly, multiple trough corpectomies can be performed. However, it is essential that diskectomies be performed at all levels of the intended fusion. In this construct, the plate is affixed to intact vertebral bodies above and below the extent of corpectomy (Fig. 18-4).

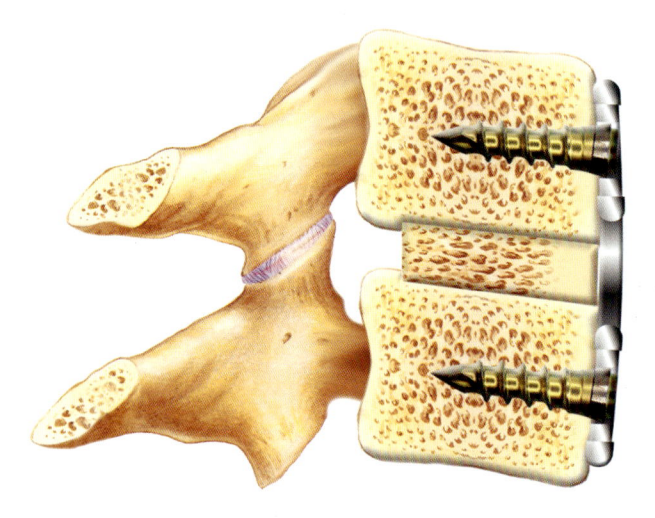

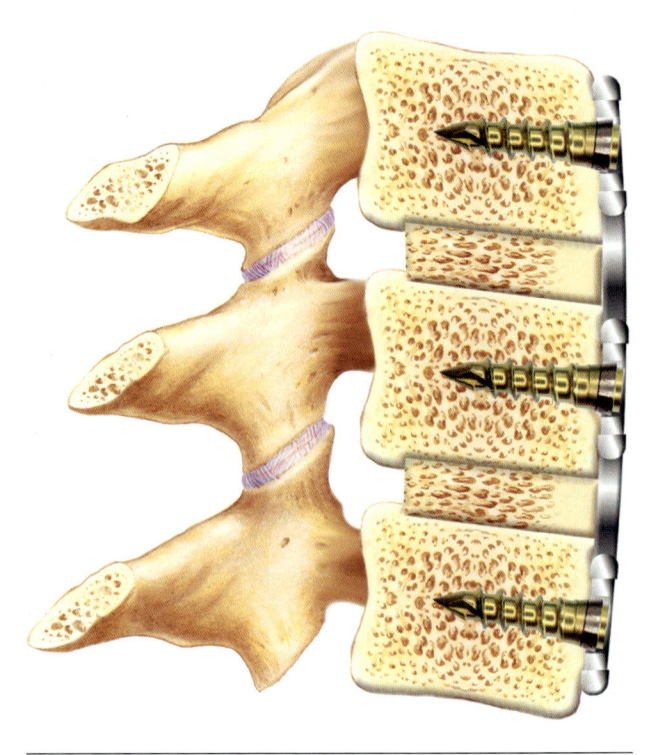

Fig. 18-2 Multiple-level diskectomies and plating.

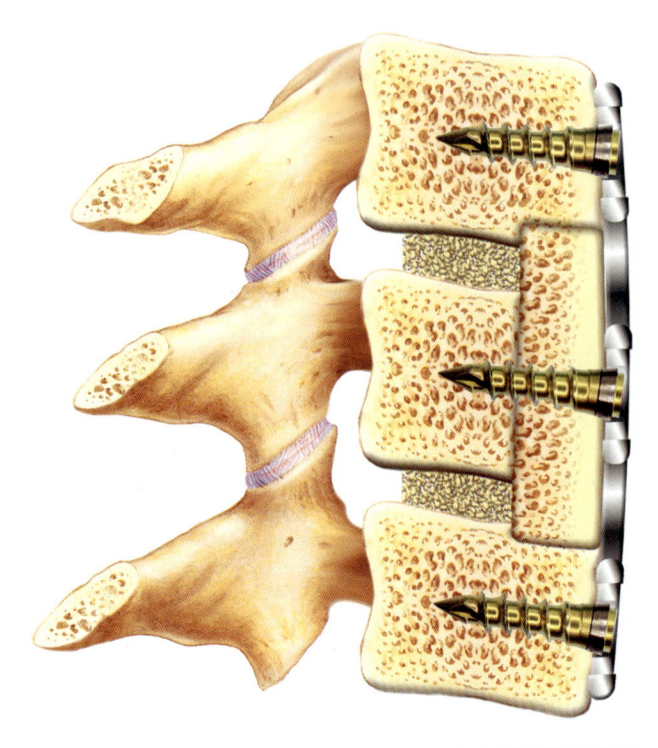

Fig. 18-1 Single-level diskectomy and plating.

Fig. 18-3 Partial corpectomy and plating.

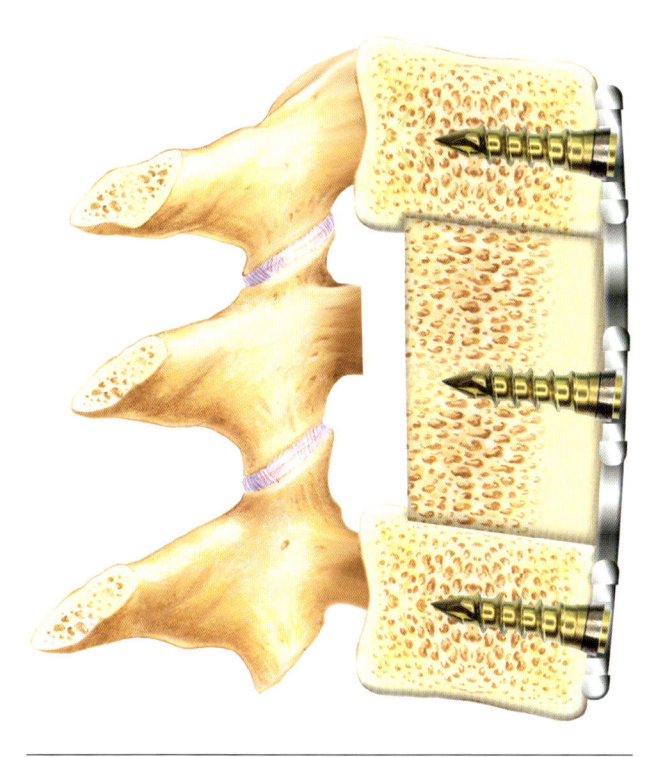

Fig. 18-4 Corpectomy and plating.

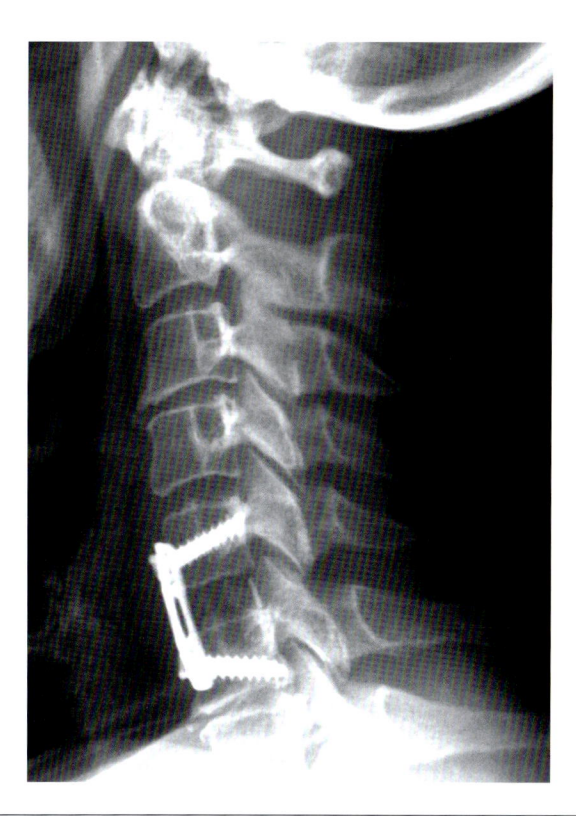

Fig. 18-5 Caspar plate is a bicortical screw type and allows settling of the graft by the shape of the holes.

Selection of Proper Plating System

Selection of the plate system is dependent on the surgeon's preference, characteristic of the disease, level of operation, and patient's general condition.

For plate osteosynthesis of the cervical vertebrae, various implant types are available in assorted sizes. Each implant is fastened with two screws per vertebra. These can be classified as bicortical screw or unicortical screw with locking system, constrained or semiconstrained (dynamic), and metal or bioabsorbable plate. Brief introductions of each system are described here. These descriptions will help facilitate the choice of the proper plate for each patient.

- *Bicortical screw type* [Example: Caspar plate system (nonconstrained type, Fig. 18-5)]. In this system, the screws are not locked to the spine. Classically, it has been fixed onto the anterior aspect of the cervical spine by titanium. Non-self-tapping screws are also placed into the posterior cortex of the vertebral body. Be aware that there is a potential risk of damaging the thecal sac or the spinal cord and of causing intraspinal hematoma. This plate allows settling of the graft by the shape of the holes.
- *Unicortical screw with locking system* [Examples: CSLP (cervical spine locking plate, constrained type), Orion plate (constrained type)]. In this system, locked cephalad and caudal screws (1) provide a secure constrained construct with the bone, (2) minimize the risk of screw back-out, and (3) minimize the need for intraoperative fluoroscopy, and (4) the locking mechanism prevents the screw migration even if there is screw breakage.
- *Semi-constrained (or dynamic) plate system* (Examples: PEAK polyaxial anterior cervical plate, Ant-Cer Dynamic Plate, SLIM-LOC, DOC, ABC, Premier, Atlantis). Dynamic plating systems are defined as semiconstrained and are characterized by the inherent motion that exists between some of its components. It functions as a load-sharing (nonconstrained) rather than load-bearing (constrained) device. This system is designed to provide some resistance to subsidence in the early phase of graft incorporation while maintaining the most effective biomechanical function of an anterior plate as a tension band. It allows for loading to be present across the remodeling bone graft later in the course of bone healing and enables stress to fortify the fusion as predicted by the Wolff law.
- *Bioabsorbable system* [Example: anterior cervical graft containment system from OS reconstructive mesh and screws (MacroPore Biosurgery, Inc., San Diego, CA)]. Resorbable polylactide polymer compounds are known as alpha-polyesters or poly (alpha-hydroxy) acids. Alpha-polyesters are a family of chemical compounds, including PLA and PGA, based on the lactic acid and glycolic acid monomer, respectively. PGA has a propensity to produce more of an inflammatory tissue reaction than PLA.[13] Polylevolactic acid, a stereoisomer of PLA, has exhibited the slowest rate of degradation with a half-life of 6 months.[14] This system is not intended to be load-bearing device. There is a lack of postoperative imaging artifact, although it allows for more physiologic osseous healing. There is a possibility

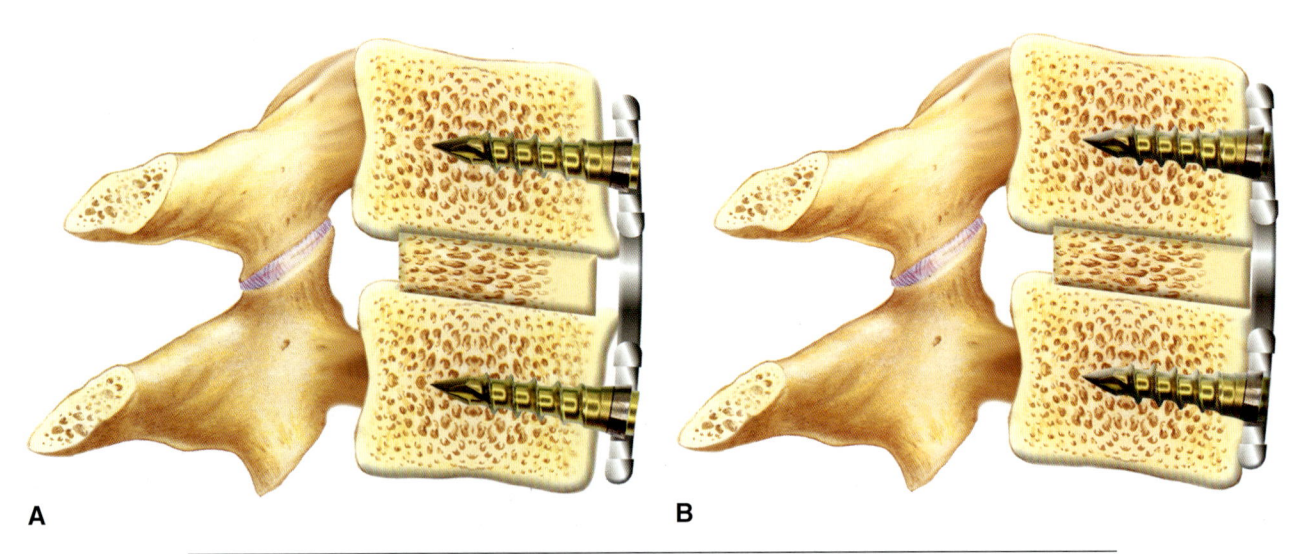

Fig. 18-6 Removal of anterior osteophytes. *A,* Osteophytes can lead to hardware failure. *B,* Proper removal of the anterior osteophytes and flattening of the spinal surface are important to fix the plate securely.

of sterile local inflammatory reaction.[13] Complications include sterile sinus tract formation, osteolysis, synovitis, and hypertrophic fibrous encapsulation.

Anterior Surface of Spine Preparation

The underlying bone surface should be inspected for elevated bony ridges. If the plate is applied on the irregular surface, it can lead to screw pullout or screw breakage and fusion failure. These ridges should be removed with a drill or rongeur, and the anterior surface of the spine (plating bed) must be flattened or bent in the same way as the bent plate curvature to contact the whole surface of the plate (Fig. 18-6*A* and *B*).

Selection of Proper Size Plate and Position on the Anterior Surface of the Spine

After proper placement of the graft on the diskectomy or corpectomy site, the appropriate length plate is then selected and positioned. If the plate length is correct, then (1) two pairs of holes on either end of the plate should lie just beyond the ends of the bone graft and over the adjacent vertebrae, and (2) this length will permit the anchor screws to be positioned optimally in the center of the vertebrae.

The plate should not overlap with an intact disk space. An overlap increases the risk of screw loosening and fixation failure. If the plate must be bent to conform better to the curvature of the anterior cervical spine, a slightly longer plate should be selected because any bending will reduce the plate length.

Excessive bending of the plate should be avoided because bending can fatigue the metal and compromise its structural integrity. Furthermore, excessive bending may cause the plate center to ride too high over the underlying bone graft, compromising fixation of the plate to the graft.

The plate should be centered medially and laterally on the spine. The uncinate process is an excellent reference point.

Drill Holes for Taps and Screws

Most current plate systems have drill guides. In the case of using the Orion plate, seat the drill guide into the plate at the 15-degree cephalad/caudal angle and 6-degree convergent angle.[15] Other current plate systems adopt the polyaxial screw, in which the angulation is not fixed strictly, but the principal inserting angle is somewhat cephalad/caudad.

When inserting the appropriate drill bit into the drill guide, the screw length is determined by the depth of bone purchase required. For standard unicortical purchases, 13 mm in length, the adjustable drill bit and adjustable drill stop are used.

Remove the drill guide and insert the appropriate tap into the predrilled hole at the same angulation. The appropriate length of screw is over two thirds of the vertebral length. The 12-mm or 14-mm screw usually fits in this size.

The preferred method of screw insertion is as follows:
- Drill, tap, and place one screw securely through the plate (if concerns requiring mediolateral tilt or positioning arise, obtain an anteroposterior [AP] radiograph prior to drilling the screw hole).
- Drill, tap, and place one screw securely at the opposite end of the plate diagonally from the first screw position.
- Drill the remaining two screw implant sites and tap until the screws are securely inserted[15] (Fig. 18-7).
- Apply a final tightening of the screws to ensure screw seating below the surface of the plate for the appropriate locking screw application. Confirm the plate and screw position using x-rays.

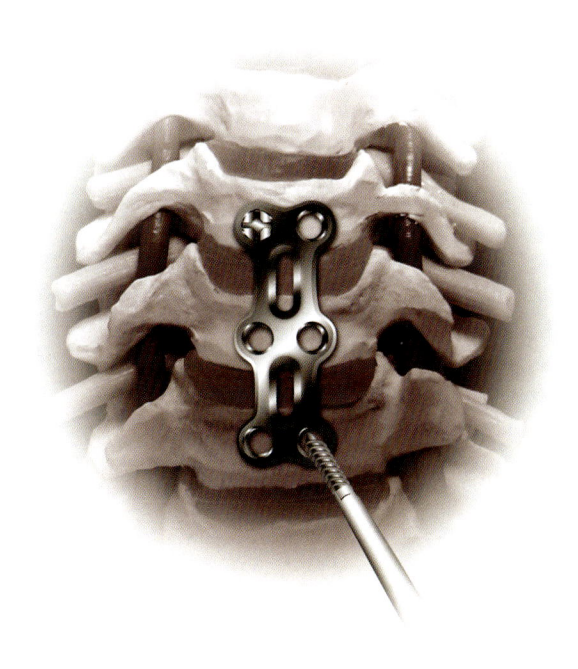

CHAPTER 18 Anterior Cervical Fusion and Instrumentation Techniques

Fig. 18-7 A second screw is placed at the opposite end of the plate diagonally from the first screw.

Locking Screw Application

Insert the locking screw or carry the locking mechanism of each screw. If the blocking mechanism of the plate is not properly engaged at the conclusion of this procedure, there is a potential for the fixation screw to back out. Apply a final tightening of the locking screw.

Closure

Finally, irrigate the wound and close the wound with a drain.

COMPLICATIONS

Complications may include the following:
- Infection, instrument migration, or nonunion of the graft
- Violation of adjacent disk space
- Risk of retropharyngeal structure damage (esophageal perforation)
- Dysphagia (note that low-profile plates can reduce the dysphagia)
- Damage to the thecal sac or spinal cord
- Intraspinal hematoma in bicortical screw procedures
- Nerve root injury (if plate is placed out of midline, a malpositioned screw can damage the nerve root)
- Hardware failure (e.g., screw back-out, screw or plate fracture)
- Kyphosis because of adjacent level instability or collapse at the pseudoarthrosis

INTERBODY FUSION WITH VARIOUS CERVICAL CAGES

Two types of cages may be used: (1) the cylindrical and threaded type (e.g., BAK/C, Affinity cage) and (2) a cubic cage such as a tricortical bone block (e.g., Bengal system, PEEK spacer, Conerstone HSR).

BAK/C CAGE

Indications

This cage is typically used with the ACDF (anterior cervical diskectomy and fusion) procedure.

Relative Contraindications

Contraindications can include systemic infections, metabolic bone disease such as osteoporosis or osteomalacia, circulatory or cardiopulmonary disorders, active malignancies, and rheumatoid disease.

Operative Techniques

CHARACTERISTICS OF BAK/C INSTRUMENT SET
- Hollow, cylindrical cage with circumferential holes between the inside and the outside wall of the device (Fig. 18-8).
- Titanium alloy (Ti_6Al_4V).
- Five diameters of implants (6 mm, 7 mm, 8 mm, 10 mm, and 12 mm) and all 12 mm in length.

PREPARATION AND POSITIONING
- Position the patient in the desired cervical lordosis.
- After confirming the pathologic operative level, an incision is made to expose the disk space.
- The diskectomy is performed using standard surgical techniques. (See Chapters 16 and 17 for more details on this procedure.)

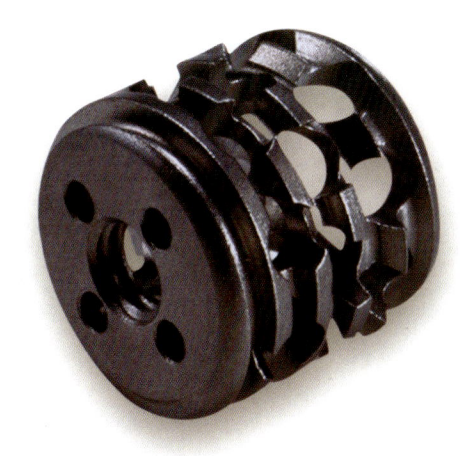

Fig. 18-8 BAK/C cage is a hollow, cylindrical cage with circumferential holes between the inside and the outside wall of the device with titanium alloy.

Establishing a Working Channel in the Disk Space

Based on the presurgical templating, an appropriately sized distraction guide is inserted into the disk. In the case of single-cage insertion, the guide should be located in the disk space midline of the spine.

With the distraction guide in place, the selected guide tube is advanced over the guide and the paddles of the guide tube are inserted into the disk space. Once the guide tube has been centered midline on the spine, the distraction guide is removed, and a guide starter is inserted into the tube.

The impaction of the proximal end of the starter will position the paddles of the guide tube properly in the disk space and set the teeth of the tube into the vertebral bodies. A working channel has then been established after removal of the guide tube starter.

Using a depth gauge and ruler, measure the margins of the vertebral bodies from anterior to posterior. This measurement is referenced during the subsequent reaming step to safely ream to within 2 to 3 mm of the posterior edge of the vertebral body.

Preparing the Disk Space for the Implant

- An adjustable-depth reaming tool is advanced into the working channel through the guide tube.
- Ream with a clockwise advancement until the reamer meets the top of the guide tube. Initial reaming depth should not exceed 12 mm to ensure that the end of the reamer is adequately retained with the guide tube.
- Clean bone fragments from the channels of the reamer, which will be placed inside the BAK/C. If additional reaming is desired to obtain deeper cage implantation, the reamer can be adjusted and reinserted.
- To prevent excessive reaming and to maintain the appropriate 2 to 3 mm distance to the posterior margin, make adjustments in increments and inspect the area intraoperatively using a lateral fluoroscopy or x-ray.
- Any additional decompression needed can be performed with the guide tube removed. If reinsertion of the guide tube is needed, it is best to use the distraction guide.
- After the reaming is completed, the disk space is prepared to accept the threaded implant by tapping. The size-specific taps are designed to form an initial thread pattern in the bone prior to inserting the device.
- The clockwise rotation of the tap is advanced only until the positive stop is in contact with the guide tube. The tap is then removed in a counterclockwise rotation.

Insertion of the Implant

- The cage is attached to the implant driver assembly and can be packed with bone graft obtained during the decompression as well as the bone reamings.
- When the desired driver depth is reached, the attached BAK/C implant is inserted and advanced in a clockwise rotation. At this point, the implant is then released from the driver.
- If the implant is positioned above the superior margin of the vertebral bodies, the driver can be reattached, and the implant rotated clockwise until the desired depth of implantation is obtained.
- If a double implantation is being performed, the bilateral placement of side-by-side BAK/C implants is accomplished by modifying the technique described with use of dual barrel guide tubes. The smaller diameter cages are most typically used in this bilateral procedure.

Complications

Complications may include the following:
- Dural tear
- Neural or vascular injury
- Dysphagia
- Implant migration or subsidence
- Vocal cord paresis

BENGAL CAGE

The Bengal cervical cages are carbon fiber reinforced polymer cages designed to separate the mechanical aspect from the biologic aspect of fusion in the traditional graft (Fig. 18-9). These carbon fiber cages have a modulus of elasticity similar to that of cortical bone, which results in better load sharing through the graft and a more physiologic distribution of load onto the graft as compared with other cages. The cages are filled with cancellous autograft from a less extensive harvest procedure than that for a tricortical graft. Furthermore, the cage morphology prevents disk space collapse, provides foraminal decompression, and assists in the preservation of lordosis.

This operation is likely very familiar to many surgeons. The procedure of selecting a cage is not unlike the procedure

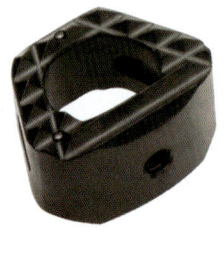

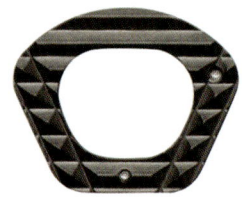

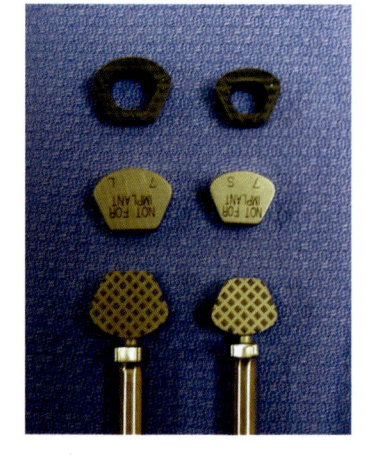

Fig. 18-9 The Bengal cervical cages are carbon fiber reinforced polymer cages designed to separate the mechanical from the biologic aspect of fusion of the traditional graft.

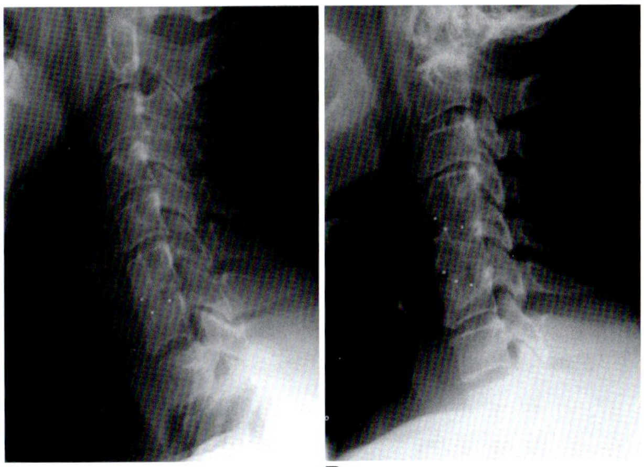

CHAPTER 18 Anterior Cervical Fusion and Instrumentation Techniques

Fig. 18-10 Postoperative x-rays of Bengal cages without instrumentation. Radiographic evidence of fusion was readily obtained owing to the radiolucent nature of the graft.

for an allograft spacer. The harvest procedure is much simpler than for a tricortical graft, and no additional instruments are generally needed. The dissection is also less extensive. The preshaped grafts have the advantage of being in predictable and familiar shapes, thereby simplifying the preparation of the end plates.

In our experience, we have implanted over 20 Bengal cages without instrumentation. The only slightly increased operative time was due to the graft harvest. The patient outcomes with respect to clinical improvement and fusion status are at least as good as for patients treated with allograft and plating. After 6 months after surgery, donor site pain was of no significant morbidity. Radiographic evidence of fusion was readily obtained owing to the radiolucent nature of the graft (Fig. 18-10).

Biomechanical evaluation of existing cages suggests that the hollow carbon fiber cages have the highest stabilizing effect and resistance to subsidence due to the geometry of the wedge, as opposed to titanium mesh cylinders and threaded cages.[16]

It is also possible to use bone extenders or allograft with the cage. Anterior instrumentation could be applied to stabilize the cage and decrease the potential for pseudoarthrosis.

The PEEK cage has several advantages:
- Carbon fiber reinforcement results in a material 200% stronger than PEEK polymer alone.
- Radiolucence facilitates evaluation of fusion.
- Teeth prevent migration.
- Large center opening offers more bone graft to end plate contact.
- Lateral openings facilitate fusion and vascularization.
- Tantalum beads allow rapid localization.
- Trapezoidal shape achieves proper sagittal alignment.
- Simple instrumentation offers preparation and insertion.

References

1. Robinson RA, Smith GW: Anterolateral cervical disc removal and interbody fusion for cervical disc syndrome. Bull Johns Hopkins Hosp 1957;96:223–224.
2. Cloward RB: The anterior approach for removal of ruptured disc. J Neurosurg 1959;8:93–132.
3. Selber JS, Anderson DJ, Daffner SD, et al: Donor site morbidity after iliac crest bone harvest for single-level anterior cervical discectomy and fusion. Spine 2003;28:134–139.
4. Brown MD, Malinin TI, Davis PB: A rank demographic evaluation of frozen allografts versus autografts in anterior cervical fusion. Clin Orthop Relat Res 1976;119:231–236.
5. Hanley E, Harvell J, Shapiro D, Kranz D: Use of allograft in cervical spine surgery. Semin Spine Surg 1989;1:262–270.
6. An HS, Simpson JN, Blever JN, Stephany J: Comparison between allograft plus demineralized bone matrix versus autograft in anterior cervical fusion: A prospective multicenter study. Spine 1995;20:2211–2216.
7. Simmon EH, Bhalla SK: Anterior cervical discectomy and fusion: A clinical and biomechanical study with eight years follow-up. J Bone Joint Surg Br 1969;51:225–237.
8. Hermann MD: Metal plate fixation after anterior fusion of unstable fracture dislocation of the cervical spine. Acta Neurochir 1975;32:101–111.
9. Ibraheim MA, DeTroye RJ, Rupp RE, et al: Osteosynthesis of the cervical spine with an anterior plate. Orthopedics 1995;18:141–147.
10. Epstein NE: Re-operation rates for acute graft extrusion and pseudoarthrosis after one-level anterior corpectomy and fusion with and without plate instrumentation: Etiology in corrective management. Surg Neurol 2001;56:73–81.
11. DiAngelo DJ, Foley KT, Vassell KA, et al: Anterior cervical plating reverses load transfer through multilevel strut grafts. Spine 2000;25:783–795.
12. Riew DK, Park JB, Cho YS: Adjacent-level ossification disease, ALOD (secondary to anterior cervical plates). Proc North Am Spine Soc 18th Ann Meeting 2003;3,5S:92S.
13. Bostman O, Pihlajamaki H: Adverse tissue reactions to bioabsorbable fixation devices. Clin Orthop 2000;371:216–227.
14. Stroman P, Dorvil J, Marois Y, et al: In vivo time course studies of the tissue responses to resorbable polylactic acid implants by means of MRI. Magn Reson Med 1999;42:210–214.
15. Lowery GL: Stabilization of the cervical spine utilizing the orion anterior cervical plate system. In Fessler RG, Haid RW (eds): Current Techniques in Spinal Stabilization. New York, McGraw-Hill, 1996, pp 35–42.
16. Kandziora F, Pflugmacher R, Schafer J, et al: Biomechanical comparison of cervical spine interbody fusion cages. Spine 2001;26:1850–1857.

CHAPTER 19

AZADEH FARIN

MICHAEL Y. WANG

Posterior Keyhole Cervical Foraminotomy

INTRODUCTION

This chapter describes posterior keyhole foraminotomy for cervical spondylosis. In this procedure, a posterior paramedian approach is used to perform a foraminotomy in order to relieve cervical nerve root compression caused by a laterally herniated soft cervical disk or spondylotic spur.

Although most cases of radiculopathy will resolve with conservative treatment, severe or persistent symptoms warrant surgical decompression. In these cases nerve root entrapment can be addressed from either an anterior or posterior approach. Anterior cervical diskectomy is a highly effective treatment for both central and lateral disk herniations. However, because virtually the entire disk must be removed in order to reach the neural elements, the decompression itself is destabilizing and requires a subsequent fusion. A posterior approach for nerve root decompression preserves the majority of the disk. This avoids the need for a fusion, simplifying the operation. Several advantages result: (1) operative time and blood loss are reduced, (2) there is no risk of a pseudarthrosis, (3) there is no need for bone allograft or autograft, (4) adjacent segment disease is prevented, and (5) the complications and costs of metallic implants are avoided. In addition, in patients with multiple levels of compression tandem foraminotomies avoid the need for long segment spinal fusions.

DIAGNOSIS

Patients with cervical radiculopathy present with neck, shoulder, scapular, or arm pain associated with weakness or numbness. The diagnosis is typically confirmed by magnetic resonance imaging demonstrating either bony foraminal narrowing or a lateral disk herniation. Computed tomographic scanning can be useful to differentiate between compression from bony osteophytes and soft disk material. In cases in which multiple nerve roots appear trapped and the clinical correlation is difficult, electromyography or selective anesthetic nerve root injections can be useful for determining the most severely compromised levels. When metallic instrumentation causes substantial imaging artifact or a cardiac pacemaker precludes magnetic resonance imaging a myelogram is the study of choice.

INDICATIONS AND CONTRAINDICATIONS

INDICATIONS

Intractable, progressive, or recurrent cervical radiculopathy with correlative imaging findings showing neuroforaminal compression indicate the need for this procedure.

RELATIVE CONTRAINDICATIONS

- Large central herniated cervical disks
- Cervical instability at the pathologic level
- Axial neck pain
- Cervical myelopathy
- Severe preoperative cervical kyphosis

OPERATIVE TECHNIQUE

EQUIPMENT

- Mayfield skull clamp
- Lateral fluoroscopy
- Illumination and visualization system (loupes and headlight, microscope, or endoscope)
- Retractor system (Williams retractor, modular retractor system, or tubular dilator retractor)
- Bovie and bipolar cautery
- Microcurettes

- Kerrison rongeurs
- Microdissectors
- Micro pituitary rongeurs
- High-speed drill with a diamond burr

PATIENT POSITIONING

- General endotracheal anesthesia and a Mayfield skull clamp are utilized to prevent any intraoperative motion during the procedure. Patients may be placed in either the prone or sitting position. The sitting position reduces venous pressure and intraoperative bleeding but requires greater preoperative preparation (Fig. 19-1).
- For patients in the sitting position, a Doppler probe is placed over the precordium by the anesthesiologist to detect air emboli. A central venous line may also be inserted for monitoring of central venous pressure and for air aspiration, if necessary.
- For prone positioning the head should be kept elevated at 30 degrees to reduce the pressure in the cervical venous plexus.
- The neck is kept in a slightly flexed position.

PREPARATION AND DRAPING

- Lateral fluoroscopy is used to plan a small incision targeted over the laminar interspace of interest. The machine is placed with the C-arm under the table for prone positioning and over or in front of the head for sitting position.
- For cases in which the pathologic level is too low to be visualized on fluoroscopy the incision will have to be extended cranially to a level that can be definitively visualized by x-ray.
- The midline is marked.
- The posterior neck is prepped and sterilely draped.

INCISION AND SOFT TISSUE DISSECTION

- Lidocaine with epinephrine is injected subcutaneously into the dermal layer. Expansion of the skin prior to incision will result in smaller scars and also reduces skin bleeding.
- A small 2-cm incision is made 2 cm lateral to the midline over the affected level.
- The fascial layer is then incised vertically with Mayo scissors.
- A retractor is then placed down to the level of the laminae and proper positioning is confirmed with fluoroscopy.
- Muscle is dissected off the bone using a periosteal elevator and bovie cautery to expose the junction between the lamina above, the lamina below, and the facet joint (Fig. 19-2).
- The lateral aspect of the superior lamina and medial portion of the facet are clearly identified to ascertain the location of the neuroforamen.
- Alternatively, if multiple foraminotomies are performed, then a larger open exposure is necessary. For multiple levels on the same side a unilateral soft tissue exposure will leave the contralateral neck undisturbed.

LAMINECTOMY, FACETECTOMY, AND FORAMINOTOMY

- The operating microscope, loupe magnification, or endoscope is then employed to improve magnification and illumination.
- The medial one third of the facet joint and lateral one third of the superior and inferior laminae are then thinned with

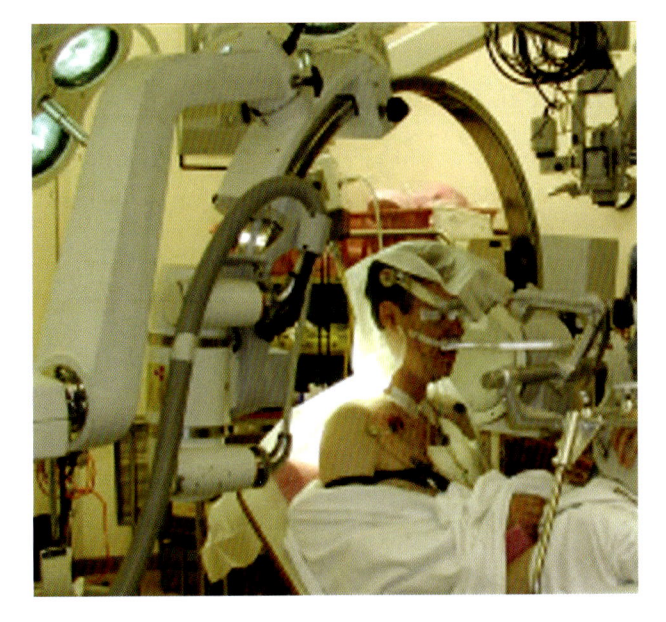

Fig. 19-1 Sitting position with lateral fluroscopy over and in front of the patient's head.

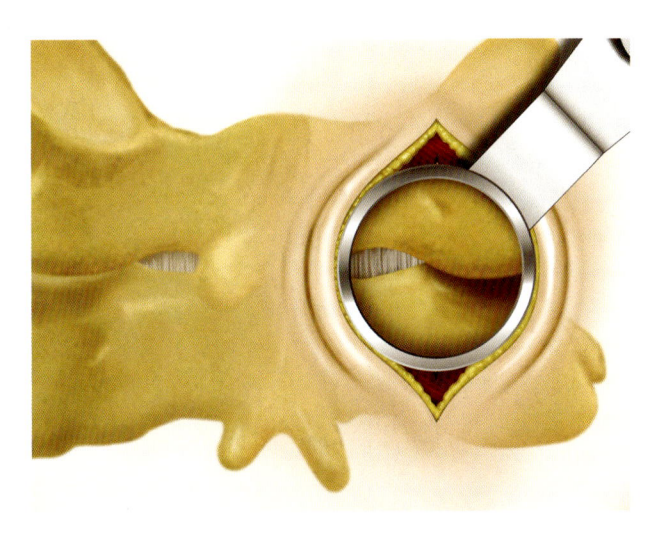

Fig. 19-2 Surgical exposure of the lamina facet junction.

Fig. 19-3 Drilling of the lamina facet junction to expose the underlying ligamentum flavum and exiting nerve root.

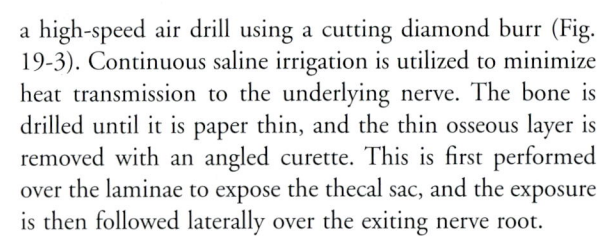

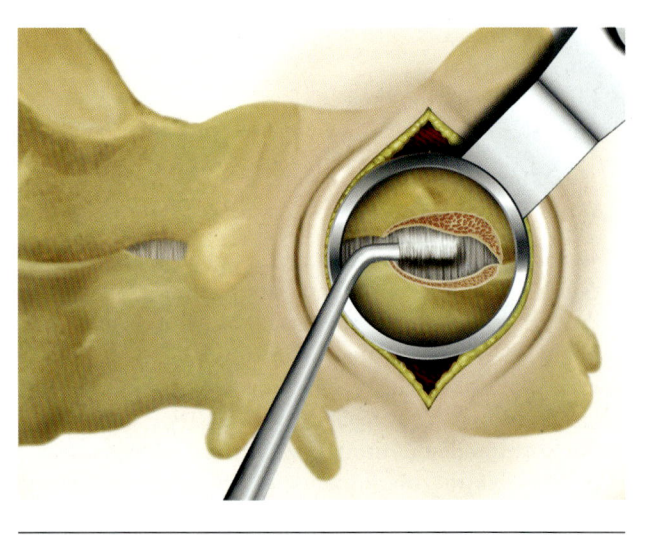

Fig. 19-5 Isolation of the ligamentum flavum medially over the spinal dura.

a high-speed air drill using a cutting diamond burr (Fig. 19-3). Continuous saline irrigation is utilized to minimize heat transmission to the underlying nerve. The bone is drilled until it is paper thin, and the thin osseous layer is removed with an angled curette. This is first performed over the laminae to expose the thecal sac, and the exposure is then followed laterally over the exiting nerve root.
- A Kerrison rongeur with a thin footplate is then used to open and complete the small laminotomy medially, which is then extended laterally over the exiting nerve root (Fig. 19-4).
- The ligamentum flavum is identified medially and incised with a No. 15 scalpel. A 0.5-cm vertical incision allows placement of a small Woodson or dental dissector to lift the ligamentum away from the dura (Fig. 19-5). Removal of this layer of ligamentum can be accomplished with a No. 15 blade or Kerrison rongeur.
- The lateral thecal sac, as well as the exiting nerve root, are thus exposed.
- A plexus of epidural veins will commonly cover the nerve root. These can be coagulated with bipolar forceps. Persistent bleeding can be controlled with Gelfoam powder soaked in thrombin until the source of hemorrhage is identified and cauterized.
- Lateral decompression of the nerve root is completed when the lateral aspect of the cervical pedicle can be palpated using a small nerve hook.

DISKECTOMY AND OSTEOPHYTECTOMY

- The pedicle below the exiting nerve should be identified and palpated with a small dissector.
- The nerve root is very gently mobilized and retracted upward (if the herniated disk is below the root) or downward (if the disk is above the root) to expose the herniated disk (Fig. 19-6). The sensory and motor roots may not have fused in some cases, and the root may still therefore be a double root; otherwise, there is a large sensory component superiorly and posteriorly and a smaller motor portion inferiorly and anteriorly. In some cases, the nerve root sleeve is displaced posteriorly and draped around the herniated disk. It is imperative to manipulate the root carefully and to avoid injuring the anterior motor division, which may be stretched. Any free disk fragments may be carefully removed with a small pituitary rongeur.
- For contained soft disks, a small cruciate incision is made in the posterior longitudinal ligament and disk capsule using a No. 11 scalpel blade. Small disk fragments may then be removed with a small pituitary rongeur.

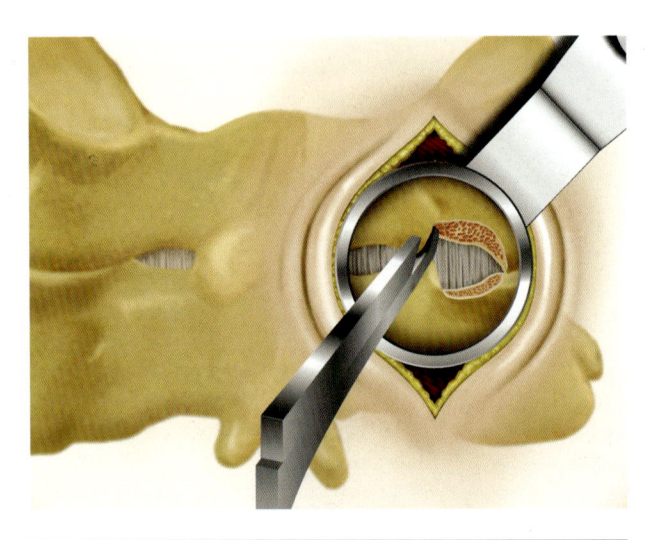

Fig. 19-4 Completion of bone removal using a Kerrison rongeur.

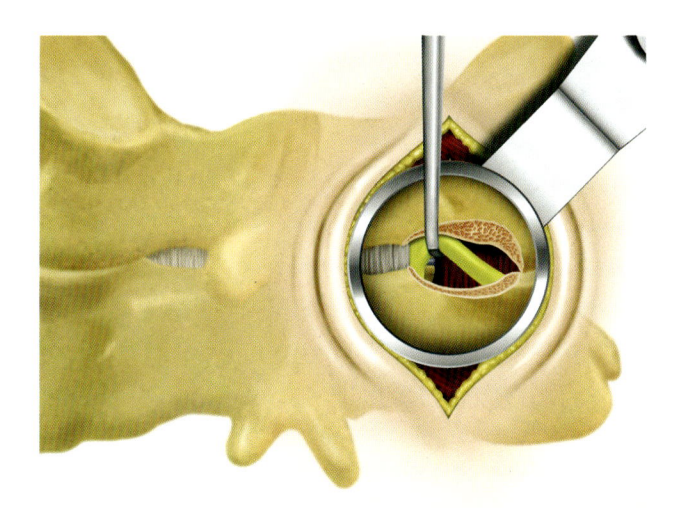

Fig. 19-6 Upward retraction of the exiting nerve root to expose the disk space for possible disk fragment removal.

- Anterior osteophytes may be drilled away from below the root axilla and above the root shoulder with a 2-mm diamond-tipped burr. This maneuver should be undertaken only when there is marked root deformation or compression after unroofing the foramen.
- A small hook is used to explore the nerve root axilla ventral to the dural sac superiorly, medially, and inferiorly. A circular motion with the tip of the hook can retrieve any remote fragments. Typically, extensive extrusion of disk material does not take place in cervical disk disease. More medial disk fragments may be accessed by drilling away the pedicle to increase the working space in the axilla. It is important to avoid retraction of the spinal dura during these maneuvers.
- Epidural venous bleeding can be coagulated with bipolar forceps or controlled by gentle packing with thrombin-soaked powdered Gelfoam.
- Additional levels or sides may be decompressed in cases with multiple nerve root compression.

CLOSURE

- The wound is irrigated and all cottonoids are removed.
- Hemostasis is carefully ensured.
- The fascia is closed in layers (ligamentum nuchae and subcutaneous fascia) with absorbable interrupted sutures.
- Fine interrupted stitches are used to cosmetically reapproximate the skin.

POSTOPERATIVE CARE

- Oral opiates are sufficient for pain control.
- A soft cervical collar may be applied for 1 day but is not required, and patients typically have full range of neck motion.
- Ambulation is begun the evening of surgery.
- Some patients are sent home the same day, but most spend 1 night in the hospital.
- Sutures or staples are removed 5 to 7 days postoperatively.

COMPLICATIONS

- Intraoperative hemorrhage may occur as a result of inadvertent vertebral artery injury from extending the dissection too far laterally.
- Air emboli may occur with the sitting position.
- Cerebrospinal fluid leakage may occur from a tear in the dura.
- New neurologic deficits immediately following surgery may be due to nerve root injury, spinal cord manipulation, or local hematoma formation. Transient increased root deficits are more common when more than one root is exposed.
- Progressive deficits after the first week of surgery may indicate an epidural abscess.
- Persistent symptoms of radiculopathy can be due to residual nerve compression, perineural scarring, recurrent disk herniations, or neuropathic pain from long-standing compression.
- Postoperative wound infection or dehiscence.

CONCLUSION

The posterior keyhole foraminotomy is indicated for the safe and effective treatment of lateral cervical disk herniation with radiculopathy. This procedure is associated with a success rate of over 90% and a complication rate of less than 3%. Because this approach can be performed in a minimally invasive manner, recovery periods are short, and the surgical procedure is well tolerated.

SECTION B
Cervical Stenosis

CHAPTER 20

UNGKYU CHANG

MAX C. LEE

DANIEL H. KIM

Anterior Corpectomy and Fusion

INTRODUCTION

Anterior cervical corpectomy is an extensive surgical procedure in which intervertebral disks and the intervening vertebral bodies are removed. This procedure is used for anterior decompression of the spinal cord. The indicated diseases are degenerative spondylotic myelopathy, ossified posterior longitudinal ligament (OPLL), spondylitis due to infection, vertebral body tumor, and vertebral body bursting fractures. Also, in some patients with spondylotic radiculopathy on multiple levels, a corpectomy may be applied, but not as a general principle.[1-4]

OPERATIVE TECHNIQUE

POSITION, PREPARATION, AND DRAPING

The position for the anterior corpectomy is similar to that for the anterior diskectomy. The wider operative field should be provided. The procedures of preparation and draping are the same as in a diskectomy operation (see Chapters 16 to 18).

SKIN INCISION

There are two choices for the skin incision—horizontal and longitudinal. A horizontal incision can be used for one level corpectomy. However, for individuals who are short and stocky with chronic obstructive pulmonary disease and a kyphotic deformity of the neck, a longitudinal incision gives a more comfortable exposure of the cervical spine. For a multilevel corpectomy, a longitudinal incision along the anterior margin of the sternocleidomastoid muscle is usually used. If the lower part of C2 needs to be exposed, a horizontal incision in the submandibular area may be added at the top of the longitudinal incision.

EXPOSURE OF VERTEBRAE

The cervical spine is exposed using the routine anterior approach (as described in Chapters 5 and 16 to 18). Retractors are placed under the medial border of the longus colli muscle bilaterally, as well as in a cranial and caudal direction (Fig. 20-1). After Caspar screws are inserted onto the midportion of the vertebral bodies above and below the spondylectomy level, Caspar distractors are slipped over the screw shafts, and gradual distraction is performed (Fig. 20-2).

VERTEBRECTOMY

When a corpectomy is performed, diskectomies are performed above and below the corpectomy sites (Figs. 20-3 and 20-4). This provides enough room to use a high-speed drill to remove the cortical end plates of the vertebral bodies and a visual gauge of where the spinal canal lies. After disk material is cleared from each of the disk spaces, the cortical end plates are drilled away using a high-speed drill cutting burr. The diskectomy and removal of the cortical end plates minimizes blood loss.

After the end plates are drilled out, the vertebrectomy begins. A longitudinal groove of 10 to 15 mm width is first made in, or a little lateral to, the midline, according to the size of the lesion. Through the emptied interspaces above and below, the vertebral body is resected by use of a Leksell rongeur.

The width of the corpectomy should not exceed 15 mm in the anterior half of the vertebral body because the remaining lateral body will help with bony fusion. If a wide epidural decompression is needed, the corpectomy in the posterior half of vertebral body can be widened (see Fig. 20-6).

Bleeding from the cancellous bone, especially from the nutrient artery, may be controlled by applying bone wax on the tip of a peanut gauze held in a hemostat. Bone wax can be applied on the floor of the trough, which is created during the corpectomy, but should not be applied on the side walls of the trough, where it could interfere with bone fusion. The successive corpectomy can be achieved by use of an air drill with a cutting burr (Fig. 20-5). As the posterior longitudinal

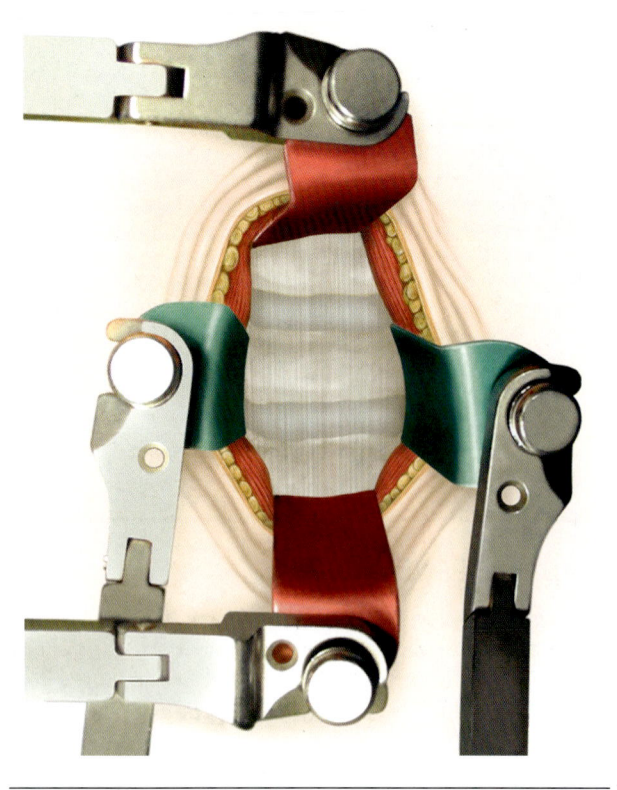

Fig. 20-1 The exposure of vertebral bodies. Retractors are placed under the medial border of the longus colli muscle bilaterally, as well as in a cranial and caudal direction.

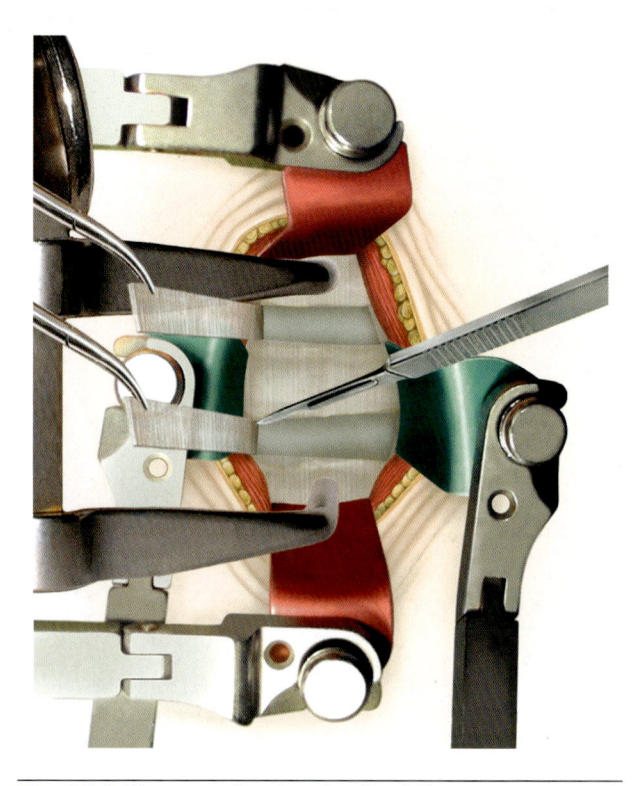

Fig. 20-3 The anterior longitudinal ligament removal. With the aid of the surgical microscope, the anterior longitudinal ligament is incised according to the shape of disk.

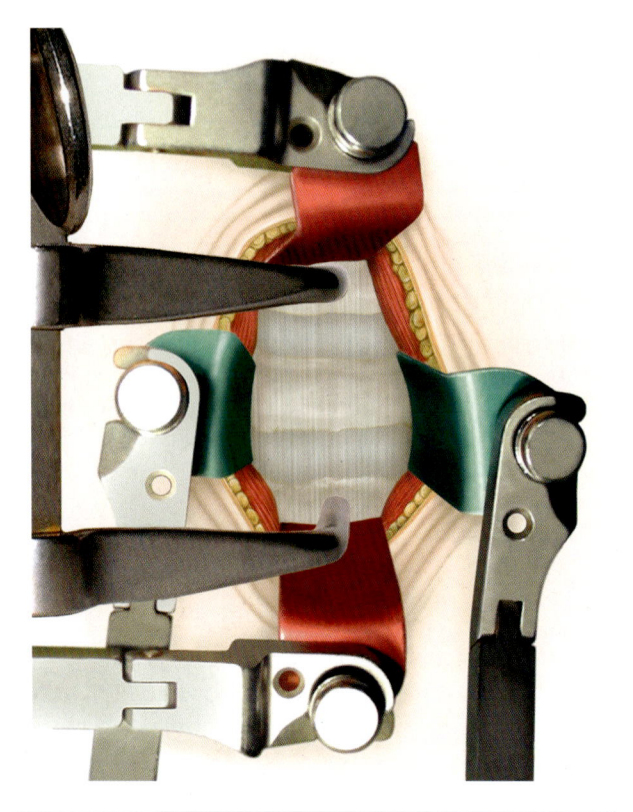

Fig. 20-2 The application of the Caspar retractor. Caspar screws are inserted onto the midportion of vertebral body; distractors are slipped over the screw shafts, and gradual distraction is performed.

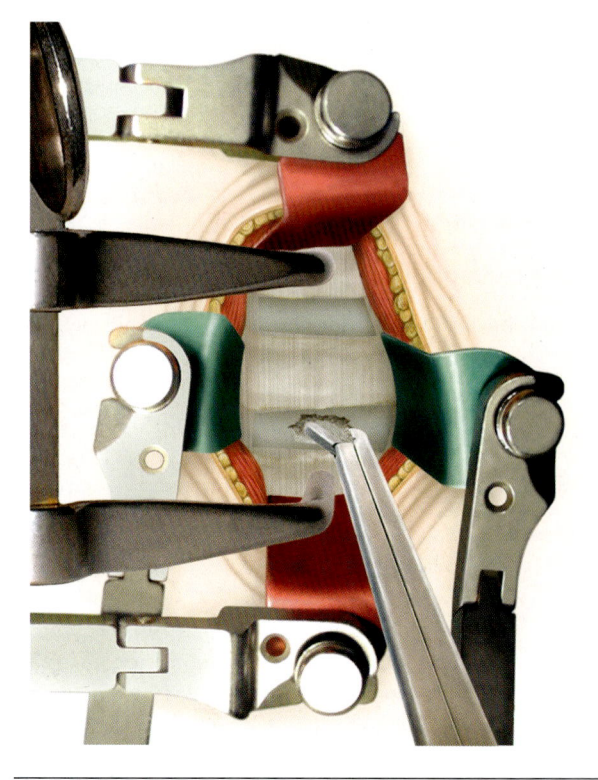

Fig. 20-4 Removal of nucleus and annulus. The disk material is cleared with pituitary forceps and curette until the posterior longitudinal ligament is seen.

CHAPTER 20 Anterior Corpectomy and Fusion   171

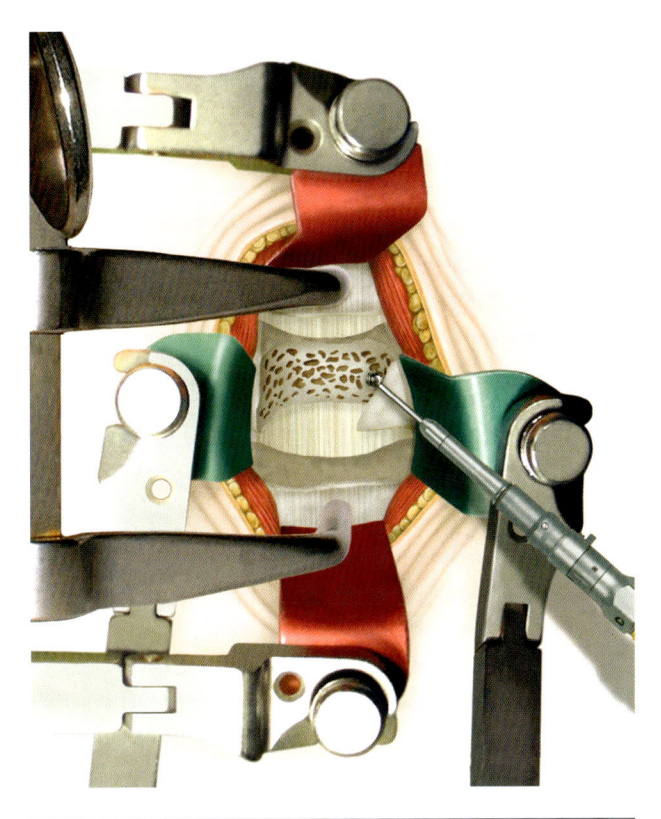

Fig. 20-5 Drilling in anterior portion of the vertebral body. At first, vertebral body is resected by use of a Leksell rongeur and then with a high-speed drill.

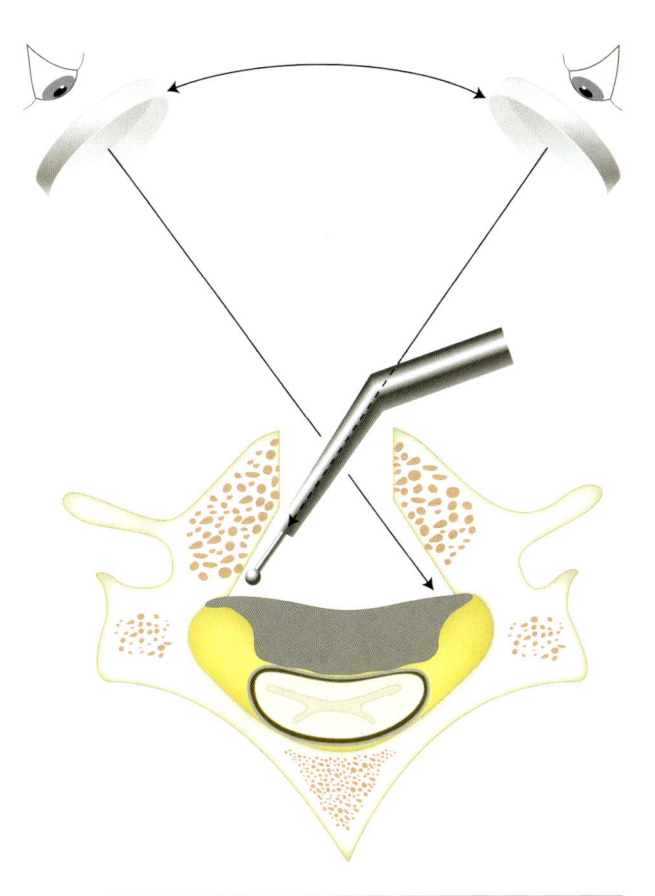

Fig. 20-6 Vertebrectomy in posterior half of the vertebral body. The drilling is directed toward the epidural space lateral to the ossified posterior longitudinal ligament, minimizing the risk of the cord damage. To obtain an adequate visual field, the angle of microscope as well as the position of the operating table must be adjusted frequently.

ligament (PLL) is reached, it may be safer to use a diamond burr. At this point, the cortical bone in the posterior aspect of the vertebral bodies is elevated by using up-biting curettes, and the PLL is identified posteriorly (Fig. 20-6).

FUSION BED PREPARATION

Initially, end plates were prepared by perforating them with curettes to enhance fusion. New modifications use a drill to create bleeding surfaces without complete resection of the end plates. These are for the placement of bone graft. A 1- to 2-mm posterior shelf of bone is created in the superior aspect of the inferior vertebral body to prevent migration of the graft. Careful preparation of the end plate ensures successful incorporation of the graft and prevents it from being dislodged.

POSTERIOR LONGITUDINAL LIGAMENT REMOVAL

The PLL is incised with a No. 15 blade or Beaver blade perpendicular to the direction of the ligament fiber. After the repeated shallow incisions are performed, bipolar coagulation is applied to the incised defect. The ligament fibers are cut away to the longitudinal direction, and the underlying dura is exposed. The biplolar coagulator is used with a power of 5 or 10.

Remember that the PLL has two layers—a very tough anterior layer containing longitudinal fibers and a thin, transparent posterior layer closely resembling the dura. Sometimes the posterior layer may be mistaken for the dura. To make sure that the exposed membrane is in fact the dura, a Penfield No. 4 dissector is inserted between the dura and the overlying membrane. If the dissector moves smoothly between the two layers, the space is epidural space. When the epidural space is confirmed, the PLL is excised piecemeal using a small Kerrison rongeur. When the dura is tightly adherent to the thickened PLL or the OPLL, it may be torn during the PLL removal, and the underlying arachnoid space and the cord may be seen.

When the PLL is removed, the dura is exposed and cerebrospinal fluid pulsation may be seen (Fig. 20-7). As the PLL is removed from the midline to root exit zone, the epidural bleeding becomes severe. Any epidural bleeding can be controlled by one of two methods: (1) elevate the head of the

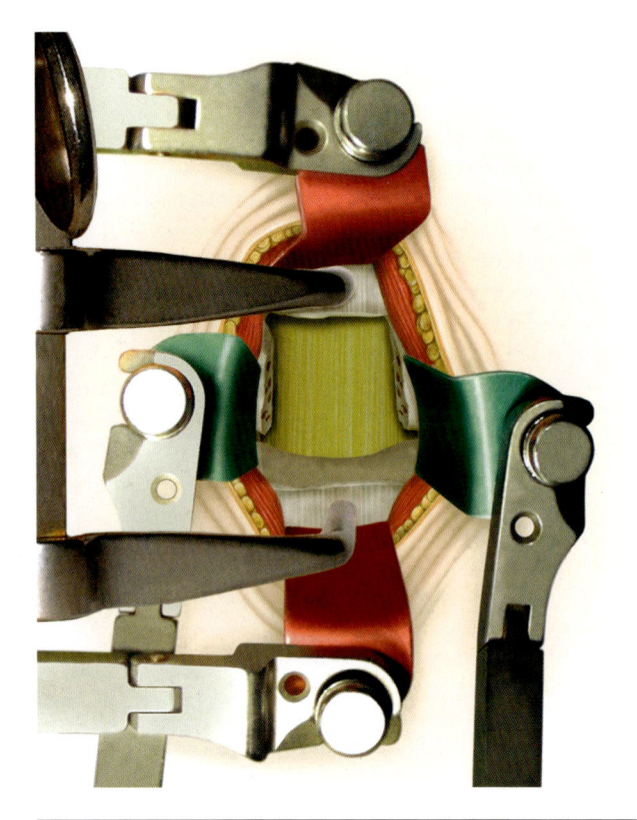

Fig. 20-7 Exposed posterior longitudinal ligament (PLL) after vertebrectomy. The posterior cortical shell adherent to PLL is removed with up-biting curettes. There can be an undulating surface and several spotty bleeding focus on the PLL.

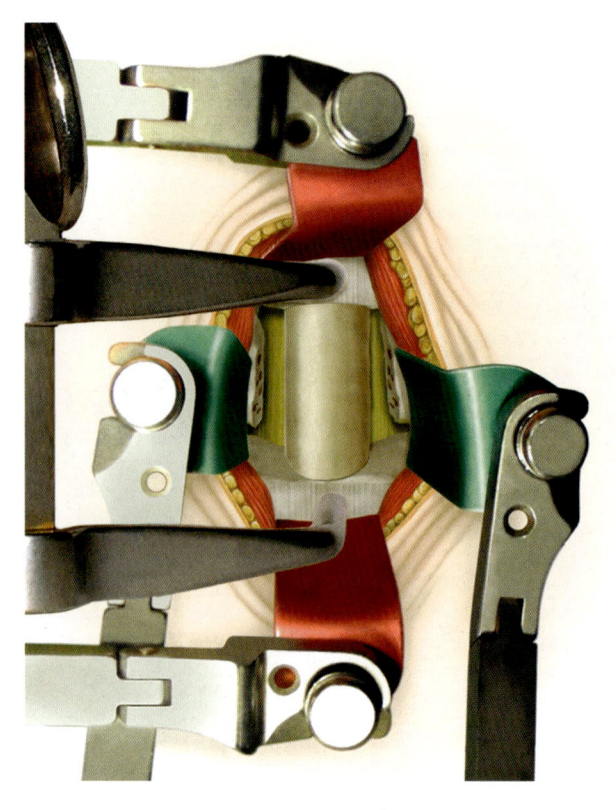

Fig. 20-8 Exposed dura after posterior longitudinal ligament (PLL) removal. The PLL is removed from the midline to root exit zone. The exposed dura is seen to be glistening and shows pulsatile flow of cerebrospinal fluid.

operating table such that the venous bleeding will be minimal with low venous pressure, and (2) place a strip of Gelfoam soaked in topical thrombin over the dura temporarily to stop the venous bleeding.

CORPECTOMY IN THE OSSIFIED POSTERIOR LONGITUDINAL LIGAMENT: ISOLATION-ELEVATION TECHNIQUE

The cortical bone in the posterior aspect of the vertebral bodies is contiguous with the OPLL. This part of the OPLL is flattened, and the drilling is advanced toward the epidural space abutting the lateral border of the OPLL. In this procedure, the optical axis must be kept in the right direction. Both the microscope and the operating table should be manipulated frequently to obtain an adequate visual field (Fig. 20-8). If the drilling within the vertebral body has proceeded in the right direction, the epidural space is opened. After the OPLL is bilaterally isolated from the vertebral bodies, the rostral end is drilled thin so that it can bend like a hinge. Then, the caudal end of the OPLL is elevated gradually by use of a small, curved bone curette as a lever, while the dura is separated from the OPLL.[5,6]

Alternatively, the OPLL may be resected by the use of an air drill, leaving a paper-thin layer of bone attached on the dura. The drilling must be carried out all over the posterior surface of the OPLL in close proximity to the underlying dura and the spinal cord.

BONE GRAFT INSERTION

Autologous bone graft can be harvested from the iliac crest, tibia, and fibula. Fibula allografts are also frequently used. The bone graft is shaped to fit the bone defect and is placed while the end plates are distracted. After the graft is placed, the distraction is removed slowly to provide compression along the graft site to enhance fusion according to Wolfe's law. The interspaces and the slit between the graft and the vertebral bodies are amply filled with the previously harvested bone chips.

PLATING

Anterior vertebral body surfaces are undulating, with concave surfaces at the midvertebral bodies and convex ridges near the anterior osteophytes. In addition, the sharp corners of the graft may be projecting as well. Using a high-speed drill, the osteophytes and anterior beaks are drilled down, as is any part of the graft that is projecting outward.

In choosing the appropriate plate length, the plate should extend onto the vertebral body above and the vertebral body below but without encroaching on the normal motion segments. Once a plate of suitable length has been chosen, it is then bent gently in the sagittal plane with a plate bender to fit the contour of the cervical spine. The plate is bent in small increments with repeated checking rather than in a single move.

The plate is then seated over the proposed site and preferably in direct contact with the bone without intervening soft tissues. After the plate is anchored, two drill holes are made into the vertebrae above and below the spondylectomy level. After the length of the drill canal has been measured, which should almost reach the posterior vertebral cortex, four screws are inserted after the tapping procedure. The screw tip should lie in the posterior vertebral cortex or as close to it as possible. The locking screws are then tightened.

References

1. Bartolomei J, Sonntag VKH: Anterior approach including cervical corpectomy. In Winn RH, Youmans JR (eds): Youmans Neurological Surgery, 5th ed, Vol. 4. Philadelphia, WB Saunders, 2004, pp 4431–4443.
2. Rengachary SS: Partial median corpectomy with fibular grafting for cervical spondylotic myelopathy. In Rengachary SS, Wilkins RH (eds): Neurosurgical Operative Atlas, Vol. 2. Baltimore, Williams & Wilkins, 1991, pp 421–434.
3. Rengachary SS: Anterior stabilization of the cervical spine. In Rengachary SS, Wilkins RH (eds): Neurosurgical Operative Atlas, Vol. 3. Baltimore, Williams & Wilkins, 1991, pp 425–434.
4. Seifert V: Anterior approaches in multisegmental cervical spondylosis. In Schmidek HH, Sweet HW (eds): Operative Neurosurgical Technique. Indications, Methods and Results, 4th ed, Vol. 2. Philadelphia, WB Saunders, 2000, pp 1987–2002.
5. Asano T, Tsuzuki N: Surgical management of ossification of the posterior longitudinal ligament. In Schmidek HH, Sweet HW (eds): Operative Neurosurgical Technique. Indications, Methods and Results, 4th ed, Vol. 2. Philadelphia, WB Saunders, 2000, pp 2003–2015.
6. Cloward RB: Removal of cervical ossified posterior longitudinal ligament at single and multiple levels. In Rengachar SS, Wilkins RH (eds): Neurosurgical Operative Atlas, Vol. 1. Baltimore, Williams & Wilkins, 1991, pp 175–181.

CHAPTER 21

CARL SPIVAK

DANIEL H. KIM

Laminotomy and Laminectomy for Cervical Stenosis

INTRODUCTION

Cervical spondylotic myelopathy is the most common cause of spinal cord dysfunction among people over age 55 in North America.[1] The aging process results in degenerative changes in the cervical spine that, in advanced stages, can cause compression of the spinal cord. Symptoms are characterized by neck and arm pain associated with weakness and numbness of the hands and unsteadiness of gait. Signs may include Lhermitte's sign, atrophy of the hands, and spastic weakness of the lower extremities. Treatment options may include conservative management as well as anterior, posterior, or combined surgery.

PATHOPHYSIOLOGY

Cervical spondylotic myelopathy is spinal cord dysfunction resulting from spinal stenosis. The exact mechanism is unknown, although both mechanical and vascular mechanisms have been hypothesized.[2-4] Spinal stenosis is the narrowing of the spinal canal and is usually acquired, but may have a congenital predisposition. This degenerative process begins with the drying out and collapse of the intervertebral disk. The collapsed disk changes the force and motion across the disk and facet complexes resulting in osteophytosis, facet hypertrophy, and thickening of the ligamentum flavum.[3,5]

This process may progress to symptomatic compression resulting in myelopathy or radiculopathy.

CLINICAL EVALUATION

Patients typically have a long history of neck and shoulder pain and stiffness, either with or without arm pain. Flexion of the neck may produce "electrical shocks" shooting down the back (Lhermitte's sign). The arm pain is typically a result of nerve root compression, usually at the foramen. It may be characterized as sharp, shooting, burning, or a dull ache. It can be worsened by certain neck positions or activities. It is usually associated with numbness and tingling in the hand and the location of this sensation suggests the nerve root is involved—for example, the thumb (C6), middle finger (C7), and little finger (C8). There may be associated weakness in the arm affecting the deltoid (C5), biceps (C6), triceps (C7), and grip (C8) and hand intrinsics (T1). The hallmark symptom of cervical spondylotic myelopathy is an unsteady gait associated with weakness and stiffness in the legs.[6]

Upon examination, the patient typically has reduced range of motion in the neck and pain with motion. Certain positions may elicit arm (radicular) or back pain (Lhermitte's sign). Strength in the upper extremity may reveal weakness in the deltoid, biceps, triceps, grip (flexor digitorium profundus), or intrinsics (first dorsal interossi), with the corresponding root involvement. Reflexes may be decreased or increased, depending on the location of the cervical stenosis. Nerve roots affected at the level of the stenosis by compression will demonstrate decreased or absent reflexes. Nerve roots below the level of the compression have increased reflexes.

For example, the patient may present absent brachioradialis and biceps reflexes (C5 and C6), but increased (hyperactive) triceps reflex (C7). Sensory loss may localize to the shoulder (C5), thumb (C6), middle finger (C7), little finger (C8), or medial arm (T1). Examination of lower extremities will demonstrate upper motor neuron (myelopathic) weakness secondary to spinal cord compression. The flexor muscles, iliopsoas (hip flexion), and tibialis anterior (foot dorsiflexion) are weaker than the gluteus maximus (hip extension) and gastrocnemius (dorsiflexion). Reflexes in the legs are exaggerated and may show increased reflexes, clonus, extensor plantar reflexes, and clasp-knife rigidity. Patients may reveal a spastic gait; the types of gaits at presentation have been previously graded by Nurick[2] (Table 21-1).

CHAPTER 21 Laminotomy and Laminectomy for Cervical Stenosis

TABLE 21-1 Disability Classification of Cervical Spondylotic Myelopathy Related to Gait

GRADE	DESCRIPTION OF MOVEMENT AND GAIT
0	Signs/symptoms of root involvement; no evidence of cord disease
1	Signs of spinal cord disease; normal gait
2	Slight difficulty walking; full-time employment
3	Difficulty in walking preventing full-time employment
4	Ambulation only with assistance
5	Chairbound or bedridden

Source: Modified from Nurick S: The pathogenesis of the spinal cord disorder associated with cervical spondylosis. Brain 1972;95: 87–100.

NATURAL HISTORY

The natural history of cervical spondylotic myelopathy is not completely understood, but there is a preference to surgical management with the development of myelopathy or hyperintense T2 cord signal change on magnetic resonance imaging (MRI). Recent prospective randomized study has found no benefit to surgery in mild to moderate cervical myelopathy.[7]

SURGICAL DECISION MAKING

Cervical spondylotic myelopathy may be treated by either anterior or posterior approaches. There are advantages and disadvantages to both approaches as well as controversy over the surgical indications. In general, the anterior approach is preferred for involvement of a few levels (one or two, and possibly three) and in the setting of straightening or kyphotic deformity of the spine (Fig. 21-1), and the posterior approach is preferred for multiple spinal levels (three or more).

ANTERIOR APPROACH

The anterior approach to the cervical spine can be complex and difficult. It requires dissection between the internal carotid artery, esophagus, and trachea, and mobilization of the longus colli. There is greater potential for complications because of the close proximity of major vasculature (internal carotid artery and vertebral artery), spinal cord and nerves (hypoglossal, superior laryngeal nerve, recurrent laryngeal nerve, and sympathetics), and esophagus. Furthermore, fusion of this level promotes accelerated degenerative changes immediately above and below (adjacent level disease) and may be associated with significant donor site morbidity (osteomyelitis, chronic pain, and pelvic instability).

POSTERIOR APPROACH

The posterior approach to the cervical spine is through laminotomy or laminectomy, which may be done through

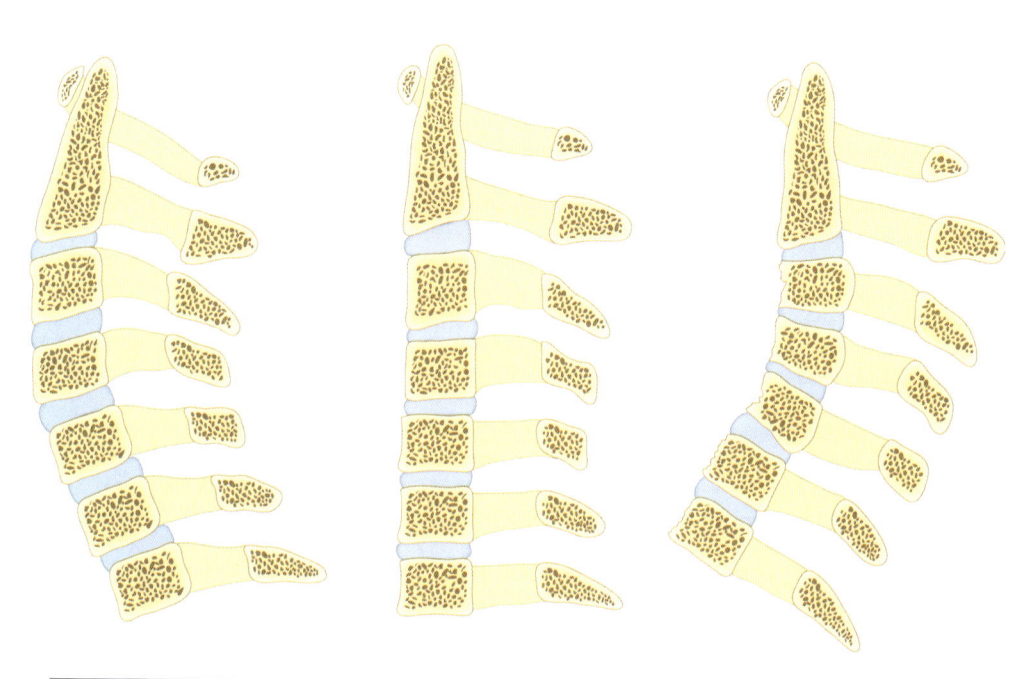

Fig. 21-1 Lordotic (*left*), straight (*center*), and kyphotic (*right*) cervical spines. Stand-alone posterior approach would not be recommended for straight or kyphotic cervical spines.

minimal invasive access. The advantages of the posterior approach include safer access to the spine, shorter surgery, and easy decompression of multiple levels. Furthermore, it eliminates the risks of instrumentation and fusion, including donor site morbidity. The major disadvantages include neck pain, postoperative seroma or infection, nerve root injury, and delayed kyphosis. The risk of delayed kyphosis can be minimized by proper patient selection, eliminating patients with loss of lordosis or kyphosis.

OPERATIVE PROCEDURE

The patient is placed under general endotracheal anesthesia and the head is secured in the Mayfield head clamp. The patient is positioned prone on the operating table and prophylactic antibiotics are given prior to incision (Fig. 21-2). The cervical area of interest is shaved, prepped, and draped in the standard fashion. The spinous process of C2 can be palpated in the upper spine and C7 in the lower spine at the cervical thoracic junction. The level may be confirmed by cross table lateral roentgenogram or fluoroscopy prior to incision.

A midline skin incision is made over the appropriate levels with a scalpel. The incision is then taken down through the midline avascular raphe to the spinous process, and a subperiosteal exposure of the spinous process, lamina, and medial facet joints is completed (Figs. 21-3, 21-4, and 21-5). The subperiosteal dissection may be unilateral or bilateral, depending on the access needed. The monopolar cautery should be held vertically and should strip the muscular attachments off the spine with a rostral caudal brush stroke, parallel to the spinal processes.

To prevent muscular bleeding and injuries to the vertebral artery, spinal nerves, and spinal cord, the monopolar cautery should hug the bone and should not plunge into poorly visualized areas. Lateral roentgenogram should be obtained with a towel clip attached to the spinous process to verify the correct level.

Afterward, self-retaining retractor is positioned to provide maximum exposure of the operation site. After exposure of the bony spine, efforts are made to decompress the spinal cord and nerve roots. This may be done by bilateral laminotomies or laminectemies.

CERVICAL LAMINOTOMY

A cervical laminotomy is better suited for unilateral, single-level disease but can be used for multilevel or bilateral spinal

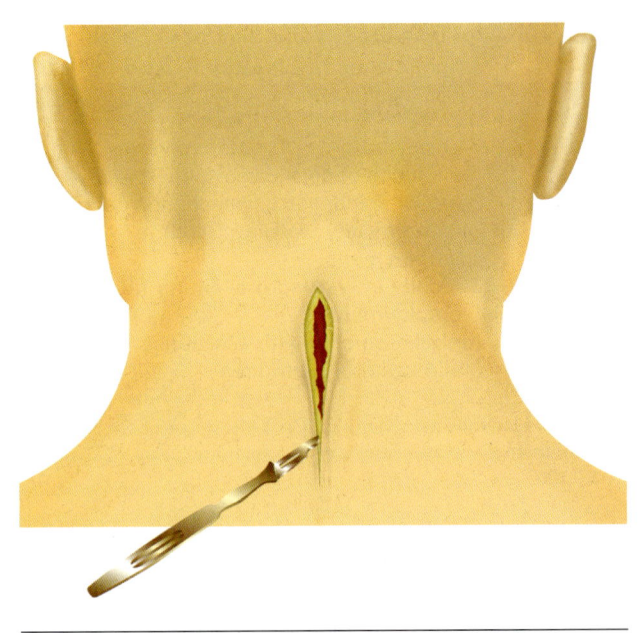

Fig. 21-3 Midline incision with a scalpel.

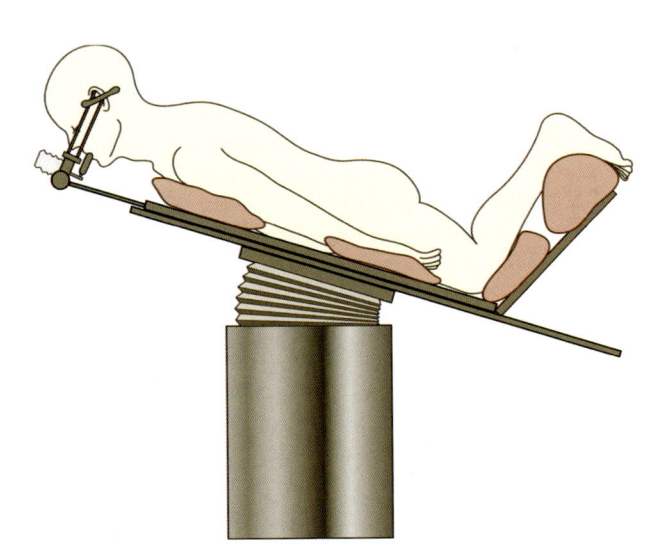

Fig. 21-2 Patient is positioned in the prone position with the head secured with Mayfield head pins.

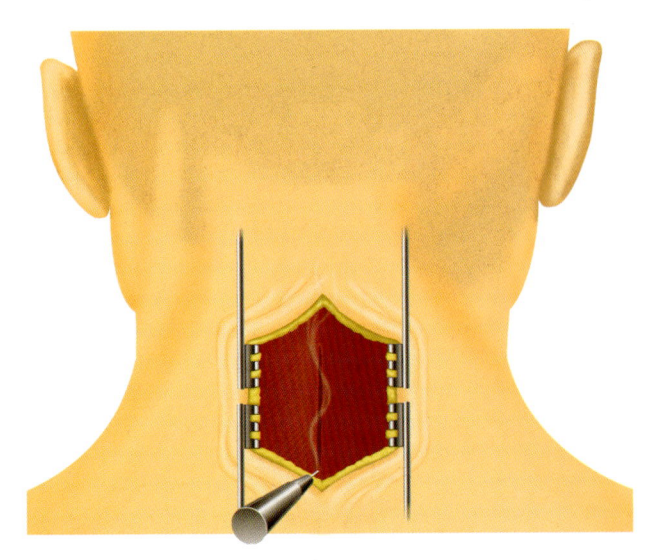

Fig. 21-4 Division of the midline raphe with monopolar cautery.

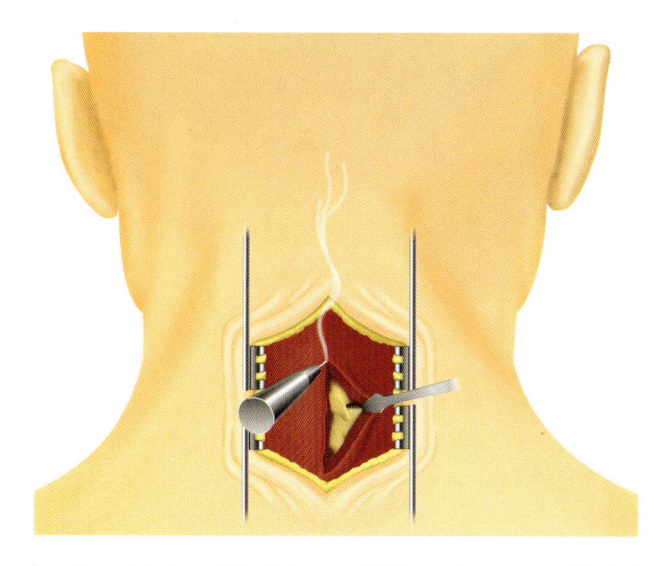

Fig. 21-5 Subperiosteal dissection of the spinous process, lamina, and facet joints.

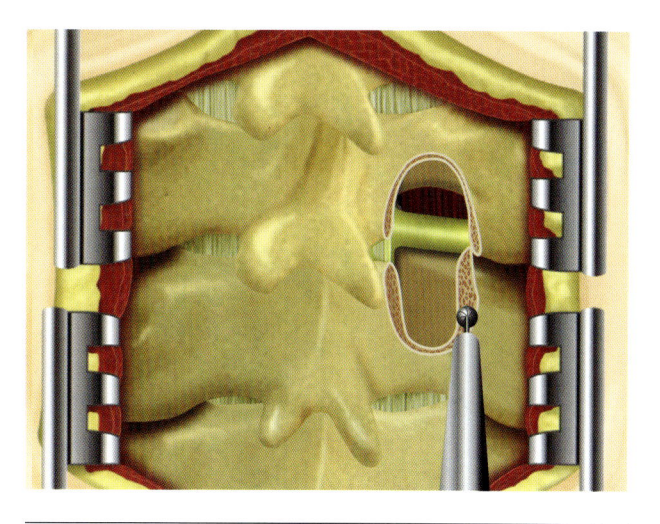

Fig. 21-7 Cervical laminotomy done with a Midas Rex drill.

stenosis. It is a less destructive and potentially less destabilizing operation to the spine than laminectomy. The purpose of a cervical laminotomy operation is to decompress the spinal cord by partial removal of the superior and inferior laminae (Figs. 21-6 and 21-7). This can be accomplished with a curette and Kerrison punches or power drill.

Using the curette, the ligamentum flavum is carefully separated from the lamina. The thickened lamina and ligamentum flavum are then removed with Kerrison rongeurs in order to form a "window" into the cervical spine. After formation of a "window," the remaining lamina and ligamentum flavum are undercut. Initially, small (1 to 2 mm) Kerrison rongeurs are used in the decompression to prevent trauma to the nervous structures; these are later exchanged for larger Kerrison punches as space is made available.

The medial facet may be removed to decompress a symptomatic foraminal stenosis, keeping in mind that removal of greater than one third to one fourth of the medial facet may cause instability (Fig. 21-8). Bilateral stenosis may be treated by repeating the foraminotomy on the opposite side.

CERVICAL LAMINECTOMY

A cervical laminectomy is the complete removal of the lamina and spinous process and may include the medial facet for foraminal decompression. The patient is set up as described earlier.

After completion of the bilateral subperiosteal muscle dissection, the lamina and spinous processes are removed. They can be removed en bloc or in piecemeal fashion. Generally,

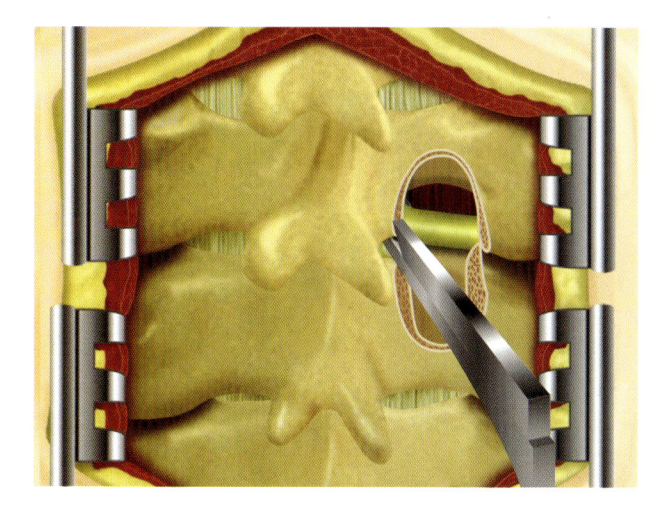

Fig. 21-6 Cervical laminotomy done with a curette and Kerrison punches.

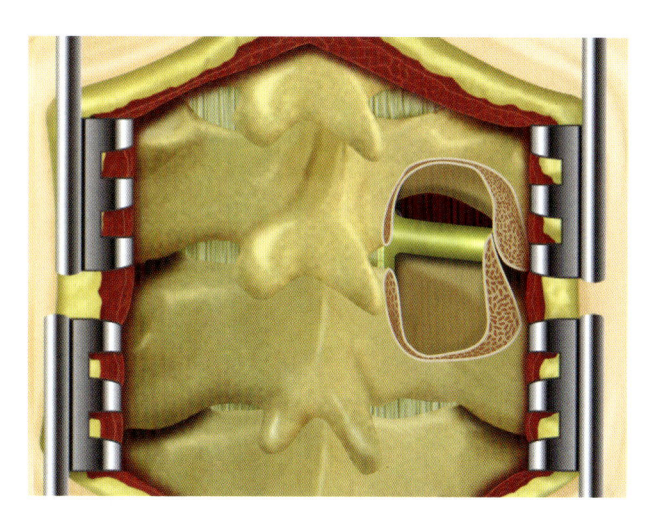

Fig. 21-8 Removal of medial facet to decompress the exiting nerve root (foraminotomy).

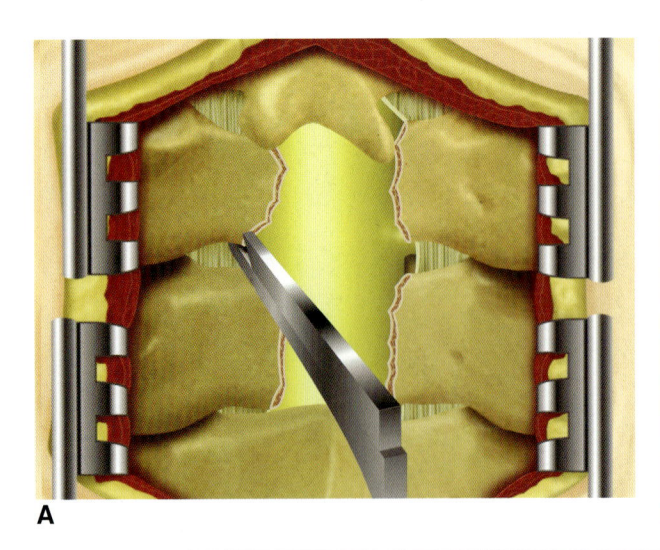

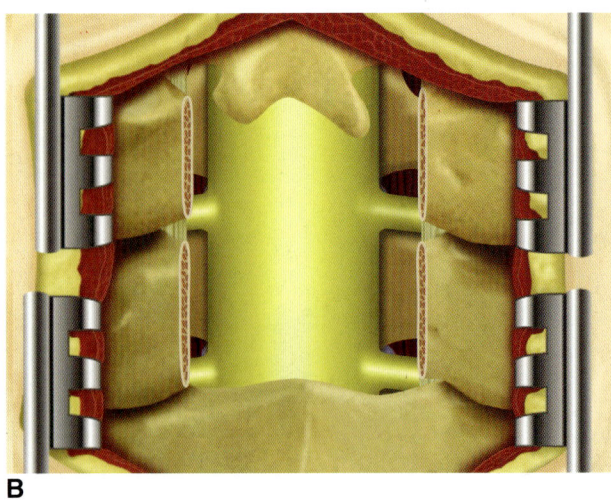

Fig. 21-9 *A* and *B*, Piecemeal removal of the spinous process and lamina. The lamina should be removed laterally to the lamina-facet junction in order to completely uncover the thecal sac.

piecemeal removal is favored unless laminoplasty is being contemplated.

This procedure begins with removal of the spinous process and lamina with Lexal rongeur, followed by use of curettes and Kerrison punches (Fig. 20-9*A* and *B*). The lamina should be removed up to the facet joint (the junction of the lamina and facet) in order to completely uncover the thecal sac. The facet joint is normally not removed. Removal of the facet joint may compromise spinal stability. En bloc removal of the lamina and spinous process can be done with the use of a high-power drill, such as the Midas Rex drill (Fig. 20-10*A* and *B*). The laminae are cut at the lamina facet junction at each side with the high-power drill. The ligamentum flavum is disrupted with the Kerrison punch or scalpel to allow the removal of the lamina and spinous process as one unit.

Once satisfied with the spinal decompression, a Jackson Pratt (JP) drain is placed through a stab wound and sutured into position. The wound is closed in layers beginning with the paraspinal muscles, dorsal lumbar fascia, subcutaneous tissue, and skin. The JP drain is usually removed the following day. Prophylactic antibiotics are continued for three postoperative doses.

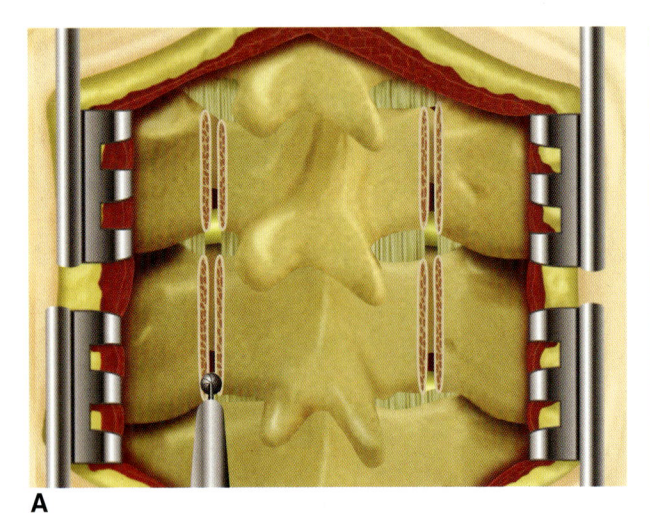

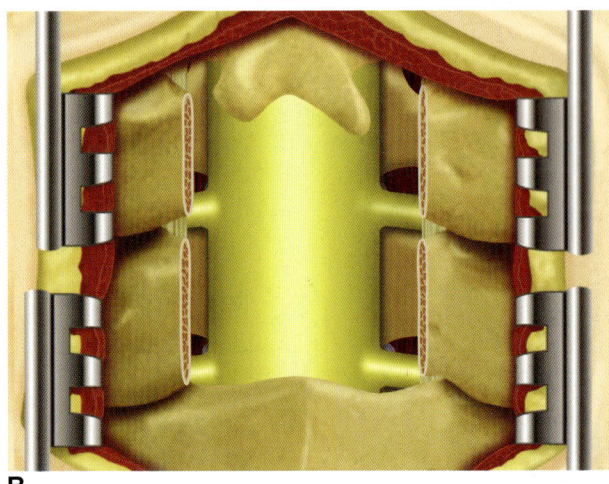

Fig. 21-10 *A* and *B*, En bloc removal of the lamina and spinous process.

References

1. Cooper PR: Cervical spondylotic myelopathy. Contemp Neurosurg 1997;19(25):1–7.
2. Nurick S: The pathogenesis of the spinal cord disorder associated with cervical spondylosis. Brain 1972;95:87–100.
3. Parke WW: Correlative anatomy of cervical spondylotic myelopathy. Spine 1988;13:831–837.
4. Panjabi MM, White AA: Biomechanics of nonacute cervical spinal cord trauma. Spine 1988;13:838–842.
5. MacNab I: The traction spur. J Bone Joint Surg 1971;53A:663–670.
6. Montgomery DM, Brower RS: Cervical spondylotic myelopathy. Orthop Clin North Am 1992;23:487–493.
7. Kadanka Z, Mares M, Bednarik J, et al: Approaches to spondylotic cervical myelopathy conservative versus surgical results in a 3-year follow-up study. Spine 2002;20:2205–2211.

CHAPTER 22

HOWARD S. AN
AMIR H. FAYYAZI
ASHOK BIYANI

Laminoplasty Techniques

INTRODUCTION

Laminoplasty was originally developed in Japan in the early 1970s for treatment of ossification of posterior longitudinal ligament (OPLL). It was developed to prevent the complications associated with laminectomy (instability, kyphosis, neural scarring, and delayed progressive neurologic compromise). However, despite its popularity in Japan, its use in North America was limited to the low prevalence of OPLL. With increased expertise and the application of this procedure to other causes of cervical spinal stenosis, its acceptance has increased in North America.

Laminoplasty is a canal enlargement procedure that decompresses the spinal cord indirectly by allowing the dural sac to drift away from anterior spondylotic bars. It appears to avoid some of the complications and morbidity associated with laminectomy (i.e., instability, kyphosis, and delayed neurologic compromise). The technique of laminoplasty is relatively simple, and avoids the prolonged anesthesia time necessary for anterior decompression and fusion. Because laminoplasty does not destabilize the spine, concomitant fusion is therefore not necessary. Preservation of range of motion improves functional outcome and may also theoretically decrease the incidence of adjacent segment degeneration at C2-C3. The protective function of the lamina is retained and there is less perineural scarring. Because fusion is not necessary and the spine remains stable, earlier and more aggressive rehabilitation is possible. Finally, cost of the implant for anterior or posterior fusion procedures is saved.

TYPES OF LAMINOPLASTY

Hittori *Z-plasty* was initially described in 1973 in Japanese for treatment of OPLL.[1] This procedure is performed by thinning the lamina and performing a Z-shaped cut between adjacent thinned laminae, which are then opened and secured with a suture (Fig. 22-1A). Despite its elegance, this procedure is quite time consuming and labor intensive. Hirabayashi in 1977 simplified the procedure by describing the *open door expansive laminoplasty*.[2] In this procedure, the

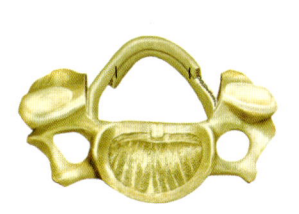

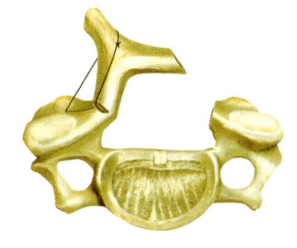

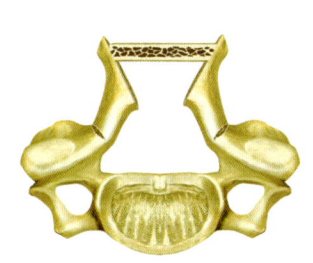

Fig. 22-1 *A*, Hittori Z-plasty: The spinous processes are removed, the lamina is thinned, troughs are drilled laterally, a Z-cut is then made between adjacent lamina, and the laminae are secured by sutures. *B*, Hirabayashi expansive laminoplasty: The spinous processes are removed; bilateral troughs are made in the facet lamina junction; on one side the lamina is separated while the other side is hinged open and secured to the facets using sutures. *C*, Kurokawa French door laminoplasty: The spinous processes are split and troughs are made on both sides of the laminofacet junction; the spinous processes are split in midline and stabilized.

decompression is performed by lifting up a side of the lamina without complete resection of the lamina and stabilizing it in place with the help of sutures through the facet capsule (see Fig. 22-1*B*). A third technique, described by Kurokawa in 1984, in which the lamina is split in the midsagittal plane and is opened bilaterally (see Fig. 22-1*C*), is commonly named the *French door technique*.[3]

Since their initial descriptions, each of these procedures has been modified by a number of different authors. The majority of these modifications are with regard to stabilization of the laminae. Some of these options include the use of heavy sutures through the facet capsule, use of wires, bone anchors, bone blocks, hydroxyapatite blocks, miniplating systems, or a combination of any of these options.

This chapter describes a modification of Hirabayashi type open door laminoplasty in which the lamina is held in place with the help of a wedge structural allograft without the addition of other anchoring devices.

INDICATIONS AND CONTRAINDICATIONS

INDICATIONS

- Cervical myelopathy due to cord compression that extends more than three intervertebral spaces (e.g., developmental canal stenosis, multiple disk lesions, or ossification of the posterior longitudinal ligament)[4,5]
- Myelopathy due to posterior compression such as thickening, calcification, or ossification of ligamentum flavum

CONTRAINDICATIONS

- *Kyphotic deformity*: In the presence of kyphotic deformity, laminoplasty will not remove the anterior pressure on the cord and may decrease stability of the spine resulting in progression of kyphosis.[6]
- *Spinal instability*: In the presence of spinal instability, laminoplasty must be supplemented with spinal arthrodesis to prevent further progression.
- *Relative contraindication*: Patients with severe forms of rheumatoid arthritis may be at risk for postoperative instability.[7]

ADVANTAGES AND DISADVANTAGES OF LAMINOPLASTY

Advantages

- The spinal cord may be decompressed without removal of anterior protrusions.[8]
- Spinal canal is expanded without compromising the stability of the cervical spine.[9]
- The risk of postlaminectomy kyphosis or listhesis is decreased.[5,10,11]
- Hemostasis is easily accomplished within the spinal canal.
- Laminoplasty prevents invasion of the scar tissue around the dura.
- It can be combined with posterior lateral mass fusion for increased stability of the cervical spine.[12]
- It can be combined with posterior foraminotomy.[9,13]
- Laminoplasty preserves some range of motion in the cervical spine, although this range of motion is diminished postoperatively.[4–6,8,9,14–17]
- Preservation of subaxial motion may prevent degenerative changes at adjacent segments.[18]

Disadvantages

- Range of motion is reduced following laminoplasty, particularly in extension, lateral bending, and rotation.
- Neck discomfort may be persistent after laminoplasty. If the patient presents with significant neck pain prior to surgery, then posterior fusion combined with laminoplasty is advantageous.

OPERATIVE TECHNIQUE

EQUIPMENT

- Operating table with Mayfield tong attachment arm
- Fluoroscopy/x-ray for localization
- Headlights and surgical loops
- Retractors (e.g., cerebellar, Adson-Beckman)
- 3-mm cutting and diamond burrs
- Saw blade
- Kerrison punches (1 to 3 mm)
- Fresh-frozen or freeze-dried allograft (ilium)
- Floseal Matrix Hemostatic Sealant (Baxter Healthcare Co., Fremont, CA) or thrombin-soaked Surgifoam (Johnson and Johnson, Somerville, NJ) for hemostasis

PREOPERATIVE EVALUATION

- Extensive history and a complete neurologic evaluation are necessary prior to surgery.
- Clinical symptoms must be correlated with advanced radiographic studies (e.g., postmyelography computed tomographic scan, magnetic resonance imaging scan)
- In presence of significant radiculopathy, foraminotomy should be considered.
- Flexion and extension radiographs should be obtained to evaluate instability.
- In presence of instability, additional instrumented fusion is necessary.

PATIENT POSITIONING

- The patient is placed in the supine position.
- Because of underlying myelopathy, fiberoptic intubation is preferred.

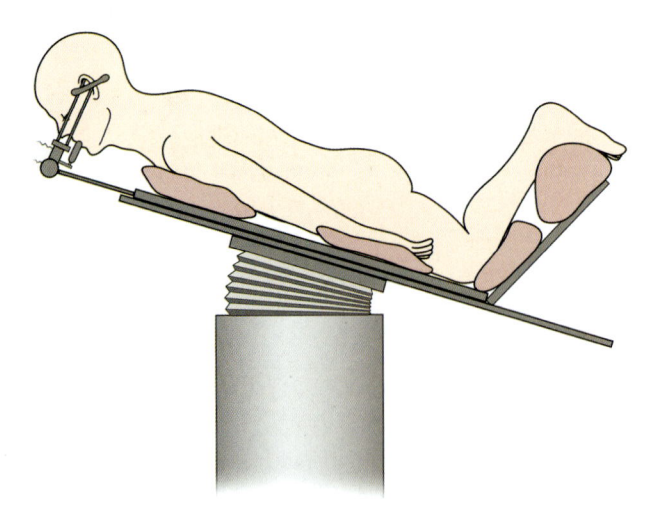

Fig. 22-2 The patient is positioned prone with the head and neck extending over the edge of table. The head is stabilized with Mayfield tongs in a neutral position. All bony prominences are padded. The knee is bent in order to prevent sliding while the table is placed in reverse Trendelenburg position to decrease venous bleeding.

- Following intubation, neuromonitoring electrodes are placed and baseline somatosensory and motor evoked potentials are measured.
- Mayfield tong retractor is placed.
- The patient is log rolled onto the operating table in the prone position with the head and neck extending over the edge of the table. The neck is kept in neutral position during the transfer to prevent iatrogenic spinal cord injury.
- The Mayfield tong is stabilized to the table via the attachment arm (Fig. 22-2). The arms are then padded and placed at the patient's sides and held in place with a draw sheet. The knees are padded using gelfoam and are bent to prevent distal migration of the patient. The table is finally placed in reverse Trendelenburg position in order to facilitate venous drainage. The shoulders may be taped down.
- It is optimal to place the neck in slight flexion to increase the interlaminar space. However, if posterior fusion is required, the neck needs to be brought into slight extension either after laminoplasty is completed or during initial positioning.
- Once the patient is positioned, the somatosensory and motor evoked potentials are again measured. If there is any change in the evoked potentials, the neck may need to be repositioned to decrease compression of the spinal cord.
- Alternative positioning/table:
  - Jackson frame with Mayfield tong attachment
  - Stryker frame with Gardner tong traction

PREPARATION AND DRAPING

- If posterior arthrodesis is planned in addition to laminoplasty, then once the patient is positioned, a lateral fluoroscopic view or x-ray is taken to evaluate the position of the neck. The posterior iliac crest is also prepped and draped for autogenous bone graft harvest.
- The bony landmarks are then palpated. In majority of patients, the spinous process of C2 and C7 are quite prominent and can be palpated easily beneath the skin. Additionally, the occipital protuberance can be palpated.
- A razor is used to shave the inferior aspect of the scalp covering the occipital protuberance.
- Posterior cervical spine is then prepped and draped in a sterile fashion so that the occipital protuberance and the spinous process of T3 are within the operative field.

INCISION AND SOFT TISSUE DISSECTION

- A midline longitudinal incision is then made from the occipital protuberance to the spinous process of T1. Generally, a longer incision is needed in posterior cervical spine due to ligamentum nuchae and its tight elastic fibers. (Fig. 22-3)
- Dissection is advanced through the ligamentum nuchae that is dividing and is achieved using electrocautery, and the dissection is kept in the midline.

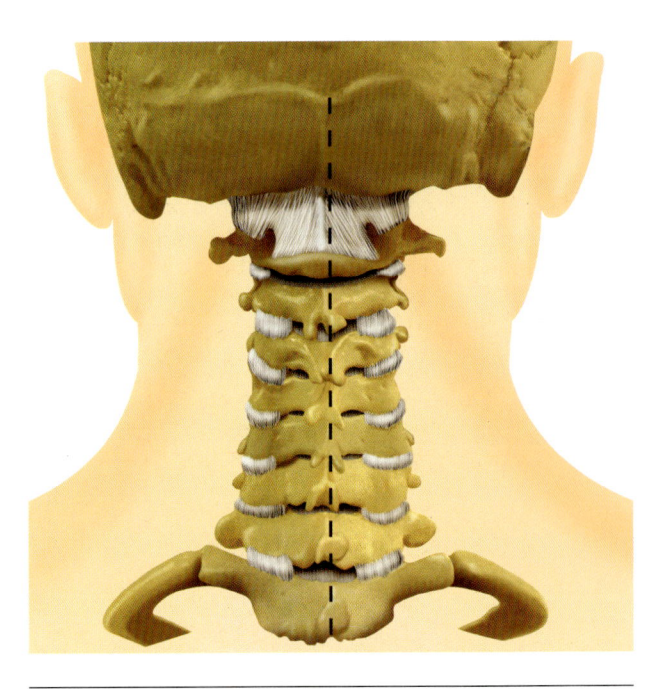

Fig. 22-3 Bony prominences are palpated beneath the skin. The occipital protuberance and C2, C7, and T1 spinous processes are easily palpated. An incision is made from the inferior occipital protuberance to the T1 spinous process.

CHAPTER 22   Laminoplasty Techniques   183

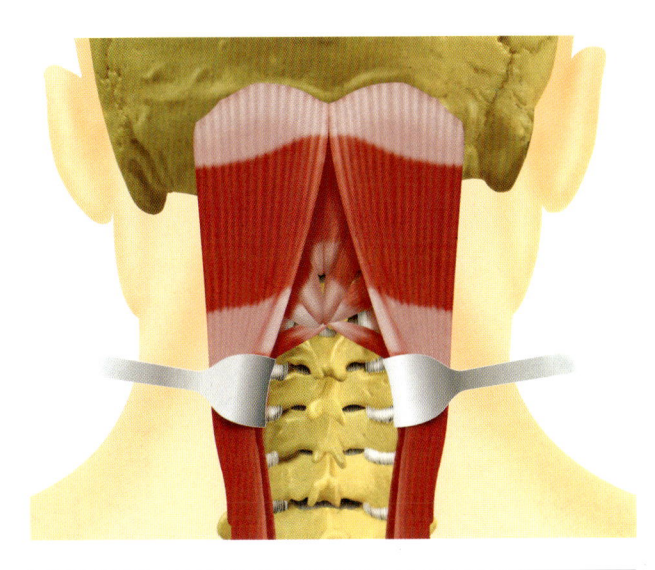

Fig. 22-4 The ligamentum nuchum is incised in the midline followed by the subperiosteal dissection of the paravertebral muscles exposing the facet joints. The muscle attachments of C2 are not released.

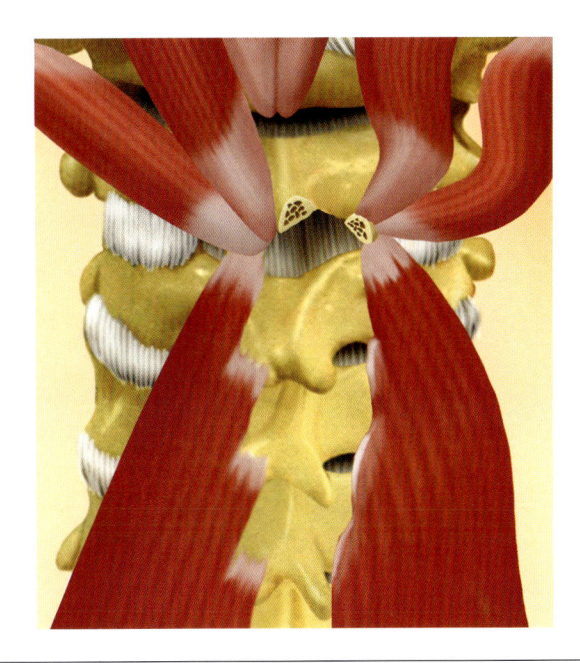

Fig. 22-5 Alternatively, the C2 muscle attachments can be released as a sleeve that can later be sutured back down to the C2 spinous process.

- The spinous processes of C2 to T1 are exposed. The supraspinous and the interspinous ligaments should be preserved during the dissection.
- Paravertebral muscles are then dissected subperiostally of the spinous processes of C3 to C7 and are retracted laterally (Fig. 22-4). The dissection is extended to the lateral masses of C3 to C7. Care is required during the subperiosteal elevation of the paravertebral muscles to avoid plunging through the interlaminar space, which, unlike the thoracic and the lumbar spine can be wide, with less overlap between laminae.
- The facet capsule is kept intact; the lateral margin of the facet joints does not need to be exposed unless arthrodesis is planned.
- It is not necessary to release the muscular attachments off C2. If these attachments are released, then they should be sutured back down to the C2 spinous process. Alternatively, they can be taken off with a thin osseous sleeve that can be reattached during closure (Fig. 22-5).

RETRACTOR PLACEMENT

- We prefer to use two cerebellar retractors for exposure. The retractors should be placed at either end of the wound.
- An additional retractor may be placed vertically to widen the visual field in the cephalad-caudad direction.

OPEN HINGED LAMINOPLASTY

- Prior to performing the laminoplasty, adequate visualization is essential. This can be accomplished by appropriate use of retractors and meticulous hemostasis.

- In order to limit blood loss, the opening side of the lamina should be cut first, followed by the hinged side. We prefer to place the opening on the side of the laminoplasty with more significant radiculopathy. This allows additional foraminotomy to remove foraminal stenosis, discussed in the next section.
- With a help of a 3-mm cutting burr, a trough is made at the lamina-lateral mass junction from C3 to C7 (Fig. 22-6A). The burr should be used in a side-to-side sweeping manner, avoiding downward force toward the canal. The burr can be used more aggressively on the inferior aspect of the lamina because the dura is protected by ligamentum flavum.
- Once the lamina is sufficiently thinned, a 1-mm Kerrison punch is used to complete the cut (see Fig. 22-6B). It is safer to start at the inferior aspect of C7 lamina and to move in a cephalad direction. To enter a canal, a small curette can be used to lift the ligamentum flavum off the inferior edge of the C7 lamina. At times, brisk bleeding can occur but can be controlled easily by thrombin-soaked Surgifoam or Floseal.
- Attention is then directed to the hinged side of the laminoplasty (Fig. 22-7). We prefer to perform the cut at the lamina-lateral mass junction with minimal resection of the facets to prevent postoperative instability and neck pain. A 3-mm cutting burr is used to first thin the lamina. It is essential not to overheat the bony edges, which can be accomplished with frequent irrigation.

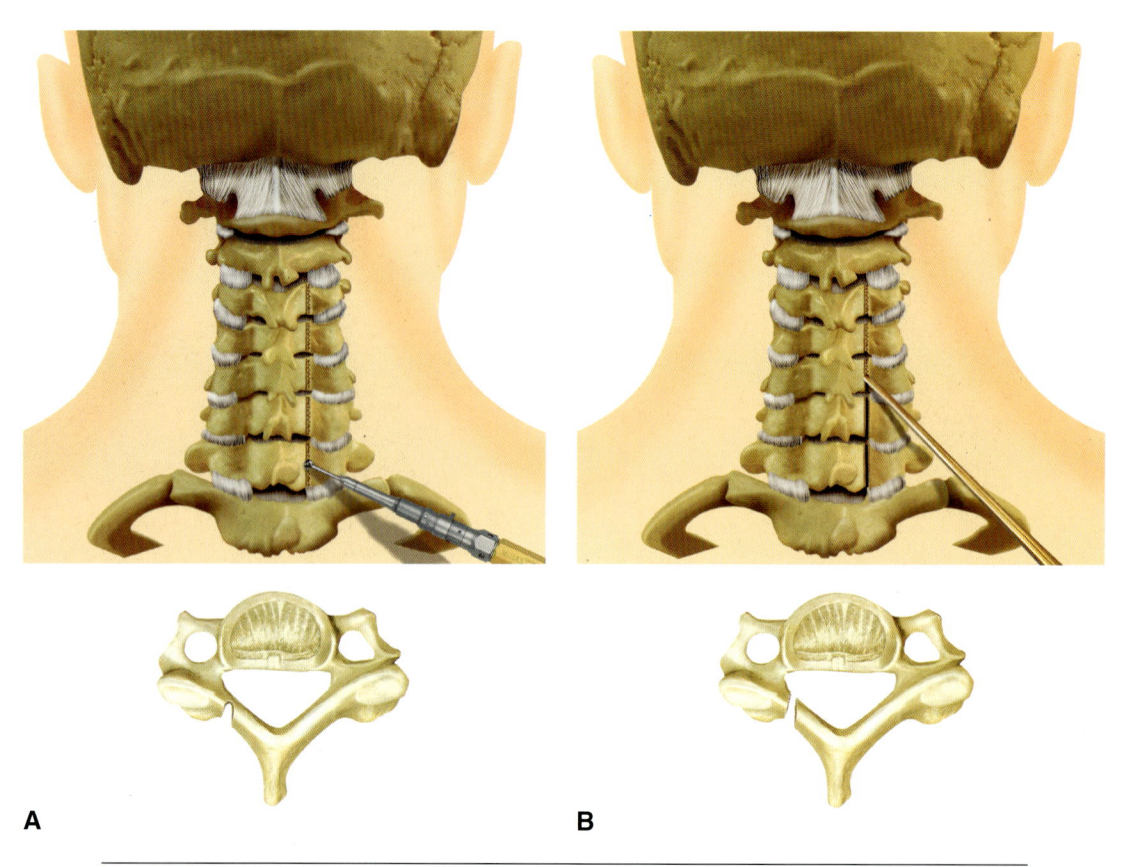

Fig. 22-6 *A,* With the help of a 3-mm burr, a trough is made on the opening side of the laminofacet junction. *B,* A 1-mm Kerrison punch is then used to detach the lamina from the facet.

- As the lamina is thinned, the posterior element becomes more flexible and can be opened with pressure on the spinous processes of the corresponding lamina. This maneuver of lamina opening must be done cautiously and gradually by thinning the hinged bone incrementally and by allowing creep deformation of the hinged bone. If too much force results in fracture at the hinged side, laminectomy and fusion should be carried out. To further loosen the posterior elements, the interspinous ligaments at C2-C3 and at C7-T1 are divided. Additionally, to allow the lamina to hinge open, the ligamentum flavum needs to be released at the open side of the lamina (Fig. 22-8).
- To release possible adhesions, a Woodsen probe is gently swept under the lamina as it is deflected away from the canal. Hemostasis can be achieved by Gelfoam or Floseal. In cases in which the epidural bleeding site is visualized, bipolar electrocautery may be used for hemostasis.

GRAFT PREPARATION

- The source of graft may be autograft, allograft, ceramic blocks, and the like. Typically, a freeze-dried or fresh-frozen allograft such as rib grafts or tricortical iliac crest is obtained and prepared. Fresh-frozen grafts should be thawed slowly and meticulously washed with antibiotic irrigation prior to use. Freeze-dried grafts need to be rehydrated prior to use. This can be accomplished by placing then in saline for 10 minutes prior to use.
- Three parallel segments, each 4 × 15 mm, are cut out of the ileal wing. The cuts should be perpendicular to the surface of the ileum (Fig. 22-9).
- With the help of a cutting burr, troughs are made on either side of the graft. One side of the trough is kept more prominent. This prominence prevents accidental dislodgement into the canal either during graft placement or postoperatively.

GRAFT FIXATION

- The fabricated allografts are carefully wedged into place (Fig. 22-10*A*). If sized appropriately, the graft can easily be wedged with minimal force and at the same time be quite resistant to pullout or dislodgement. The laminar opening can be exaggerated by traction on the spinal process.

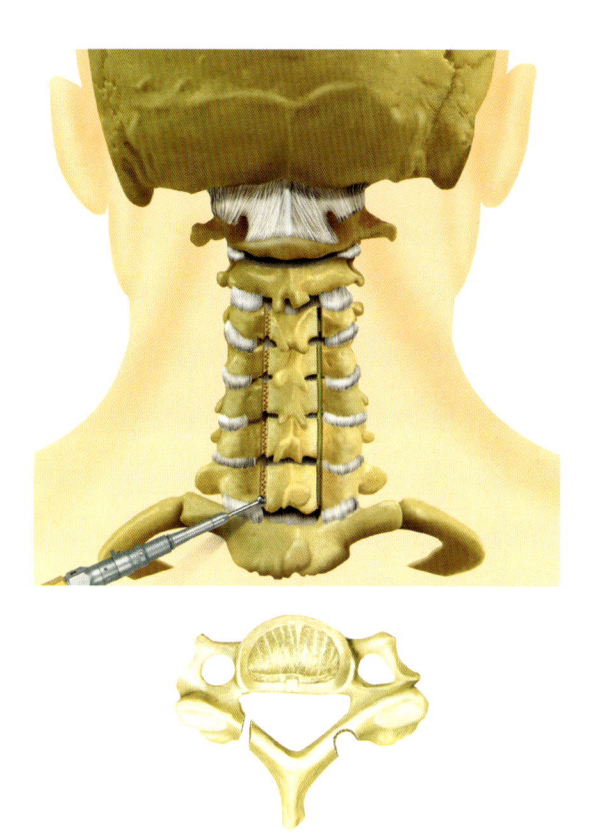

Fig. 22-7 A trough is then made in the hinged side of the lamina at the laminofacet junction. This trough needs to be wider than the opposite side to allow the lamina to hinge.

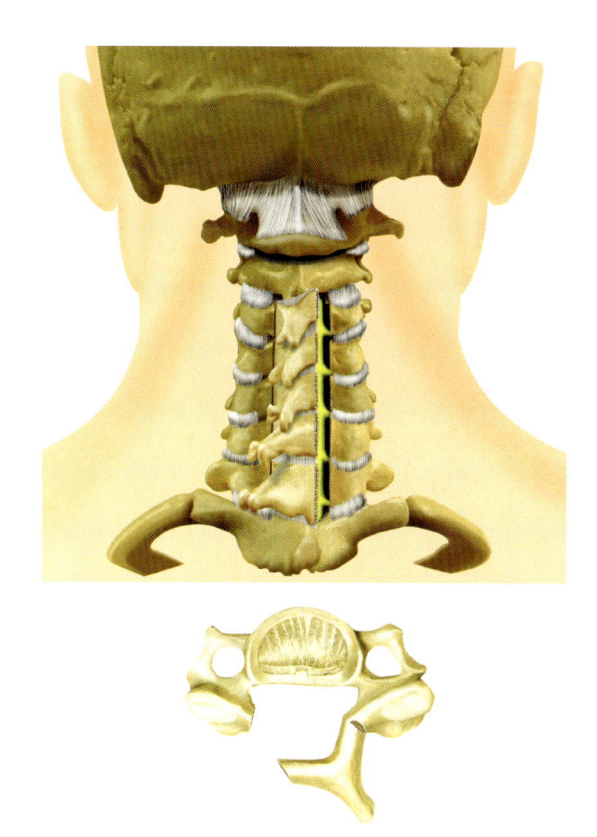

Fig. 22-8 Once the interspinous ligaments at C2-C3 and at C7-T1 are released, the lamina is hinged open.

- We prefer to place the wedge grafts at the C3, C5, and the C7 laminar openings. The graft at C5 is slightly larger than the ones at C3 and C7.
- Other methods of lamina stabilization: The lamina may be stabilized with a suture that is passed through the facet capsule and tied to the spinous process (see Fig. 22-10*B*) or by a bone anchor that is placed through the lateral mass (see Fig. 22-10*C*).

FORAMINOTOMY TECHNIQUE

- The indication for foraminotomy in addition to laminoplasty is the presence of significant radiculopathy on the opening side of the laminoplasty.
- This approach can be accomplished by excising the medial third of the facet using first a cutting burr, followed by a diamond burr, while protecting the exposed dura (Fig. 22-11)
- Once the facet is sufficiently thinned, then a 1-mm Kerrison punch can be used to excise the foraminal roof, exposing the exiting nerve root.
- The foraminal opening should be checked with the help of a nerve hook to assess the decompression. If the nerve

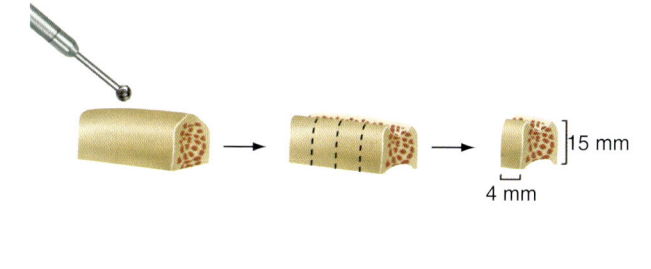

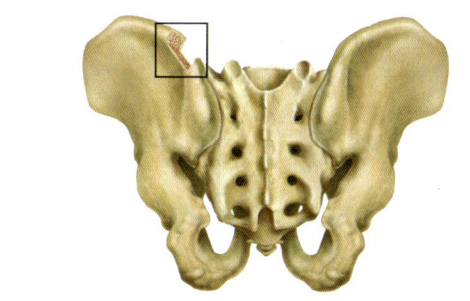

Fig. 22-9 Three 4 × 15-mm segments are cut out of the anterior ileal crest using a sagittal saw.

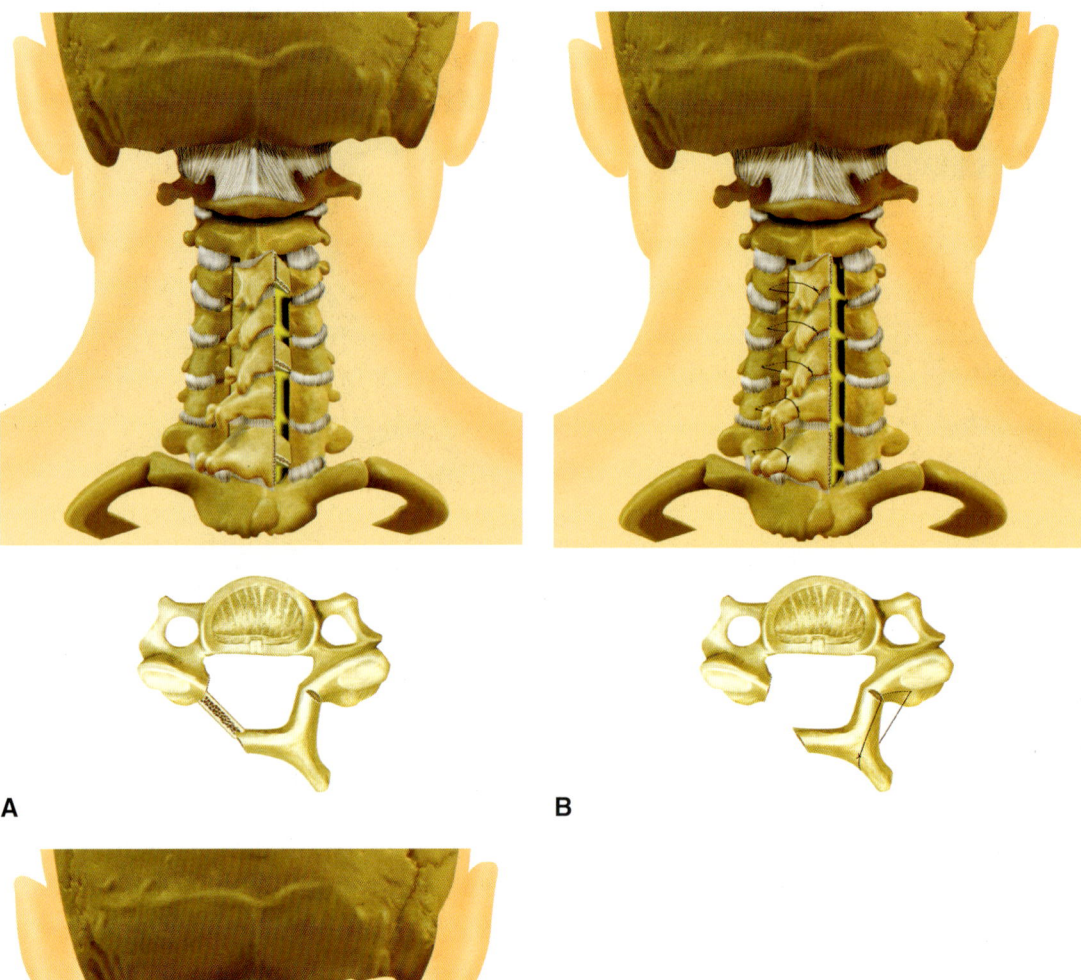

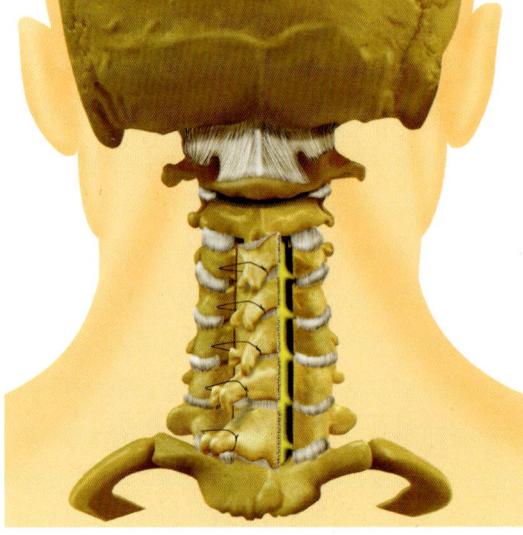

Fig. 22-10 *A*, The prepared grafts are wedged into place at C3, C5, and C7 laminar openings. Some degree of work is needed to fashion the grafts into appropriate sizes that allow the tension of the lamina to hold it in place. The beveled edge prevents the graft from dislodging into the canal. The lamina may be stabilized with a suture through the facet capsule (*B*) or with a bone anchor placed in the lateral mass (*C*).

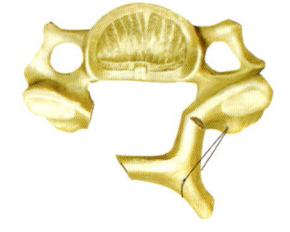

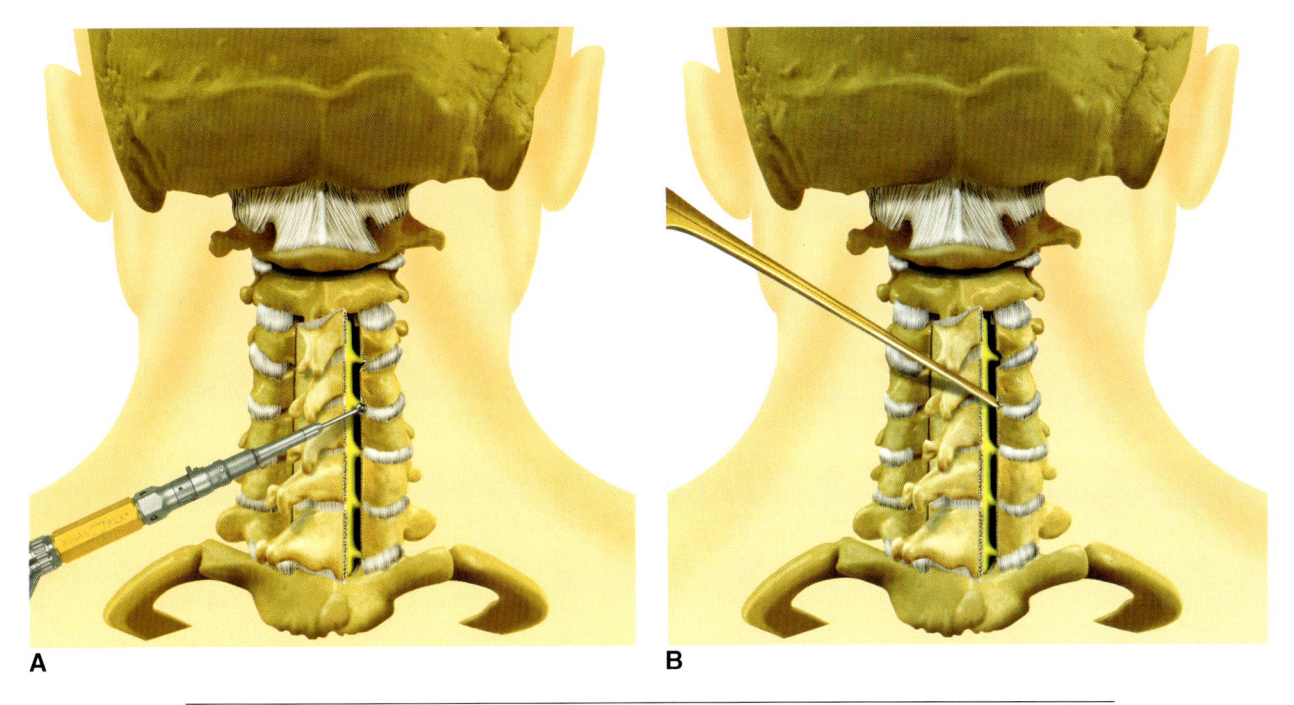

Fig. 22-11 *A* and *B*, The foraminotomy can be performed on the opening side of the laminoplasty. This is accomplished by thinning out the medial third of the facet with a burr followed by a 1-mm Kerrison punch.

hook can be inserted easily into the foramen, then the decompression is adequate (Fig. 22-12).

ARTHRODESIS TECHNIQUE

- The indication for arthrodesis in addition to laminoplasty includes severe axial neck pain, evidence of spondylotic instability, or bilateral radiculopathy in addition to myelopathy
- In cases with planned arthrodesis, the lateral side of the facet joint must be exposed using electrocautery. Additionally, the facet capsule at the C3-C4, C4-C5, C5-C6, and C6-C7 are excised during the initial exposure. The facet capsules at the C2-C3 and the C7-T1 junctions must be preserved to prevent postoperative degeneration and instability.
- Following the completion of the laminoplasty, lateral mass screws are place at C3 to C7 lateral masses. We prefer to start the screw at a point 1 mm medial to the center of the lateral mass. The screws are then directed at a 15-degree cephalad and 30-degree lateral vector.[19] Alternatively, a pedicle screw can be placed at C7 for better bony purchase.[20]
- Following screw placement, the lateral masses are decorticated and packed with cancellous autograft harvested from the posterior iliac crest.

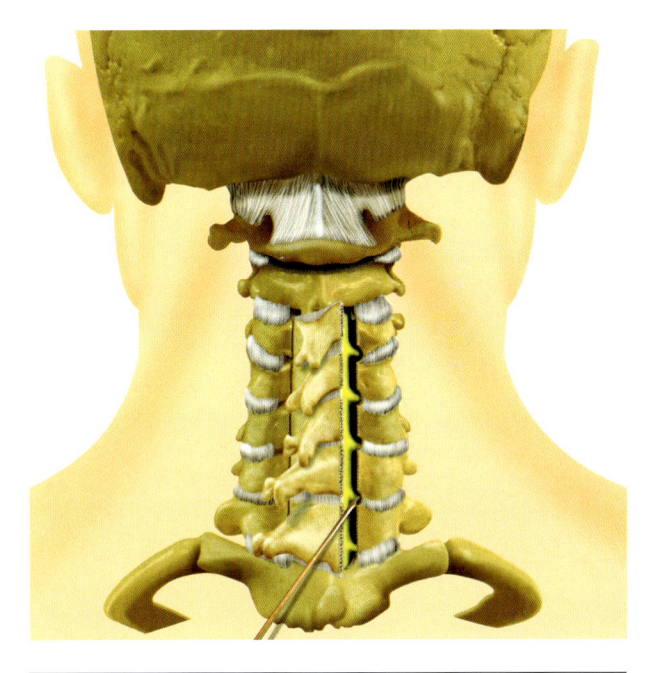

Fig. 22-12 The adequacy of the foraminotomy can be measured by passing a nerve hook through the foramen.

WOUND CLOSURE

- Prior to wound closure, the spinous processes of the lower cervical vertebra are excised in order to decrease the pressure on the wound edges. This may decrease the rate of postoperative wound dehiscence.
- The retractors are then removed and hemostasis is achieved via electrocautery.
- A deep drain is then placed to decrease postoperative hematoma formation.
- The paravertebral muscle layer is reapproximated with a thick absorbable suture in a running fashion. This suture serves two purposes: It obliterates the dead space and decreases the tension at the facial closure.
- The ligamentum nuchum is then reapproximated with interrupted absorbable figure-eight sutures in a watertight fashion followed by the closure of the subcutaneous tissue.
- We prefer a subcuticular closure of the skin.
- The patient is placed in a hard cervical collar (Aspen, Miami-J, or Philadelphia) prior to extubation.

POSTOPERATIVE CARE

- We prefer to keep the head of the bed at 30 to 45 degrees during the first 24 hours after surgery in order to decrease venous bleeding.
- The patient is initially treated using patient-controlled analgesia and later changed to oral narcotics.
- The patient stands and ambulates on postoperative day 1 with the help of the nurse or the physical therapist.
- The patient is discharged home on postoperative day 3 or 4. In cases of severe myelopathy, transfer to a dedicated rehabilitation center is advantageous.
- Hard cervical collar will be worn for 6 weeks. Following this initial immobilization, the patient is started on range of motion and strengthening exercises. A brief period of transition to a soft collar is necessary for patient comfort.

COMPLICATIONS

The complications associated with laminoplasty can be divided into soft tissue complications and neurologic complications.

SOFT TISSUE COMPLICATIONS

Soft tissue complications include postoperative wound infection and wound dehiscence. Wound infections can be minimized by delicate soft tissue technique, meticulous hemostasis, intraoperative irrigation, excision of necrotic muscle prior to closure, pre- and postoperative antibiotics, and appropriate wound care. It is essential to perform a watertight closure of the ligamentum nuchum. In our experience, the rate of posterior cervical wound infection with or without hardware is very low. Although, we have not had a wound dehiscence in our patients, the increased risk of wound dehiscence has been described in the literature. It is hypothesized that this is due to the elevated posterior lamina. We prefer to excise the spinous processes prior to wound closure in order to decrease the tension on the facial closure. Hematoma formation is relatively common, and meticulous hemostasis is important. Prior to closure, the operating table should be shifted back to neutral from the reverse Trendelenburg position to detect any additional bleeding. Subfascial drain is routinely recommended to avoid epidural and soft tissue hematoma.

NEUROLOGIC COMPLICATIONS

Neural injury can be divided into intraoperative causes and postoperative causes. Intraoperatively, the nerve roots can be injured by direct pressure during mechanical decompression or by thermal injury from the burr. It is essential to use a 1-mm Kerrison punch and to keep the lamina cool by constant irrigation while using the high-speed burr.

Postoperative nerve root palsy is a well-described entity associated with both laminectomy and laminoplasty. It has been reported in 5% to 12% of cases,[21-24] and is hypothesized to be due to the tethered nerve root and dorsal shift of the cord. The palsy usually presents in the first 24 to 48 hours and most commonly affects the C5 nerve root followed by the C6 nerve root. The associated weakness usually recovers within 24 months.[5]

The most common cause of a bad result following laminoplasty is due to postoperative axial back pain and is reported in 6% to 60% of the patients.[16,22,25-29] This complication can be limited by appropriate patient selection. If there is significant preoperative axial symptoms or in the presence of instability, laminoplasty alone is contraindicated and should be accompanied by arthrodesis.

ILLUSTRATIVE CASE

The patient is a 53-year-old female who presented with early signs and symptoms of myelopathy. Preoperative cervical spine x-rays were suggestive of diffuse spondylosis involving multiple segments (Fig. 22-13A). No evidence of instability was noted on flexion and extension views. Preoperative MRI scan confirmed the presence of multilevel spinal stenosis with cord compression (see Fig. 22-13B). The patient underwent C3-C7 laminoplasty without complications. Postoperative radiographs demonstrated the increase in the size of the canal (see Fig. 22-13C). Postoperative computed tomography demonstrates the position of the allograft spacer (see Fig. 22-13D).

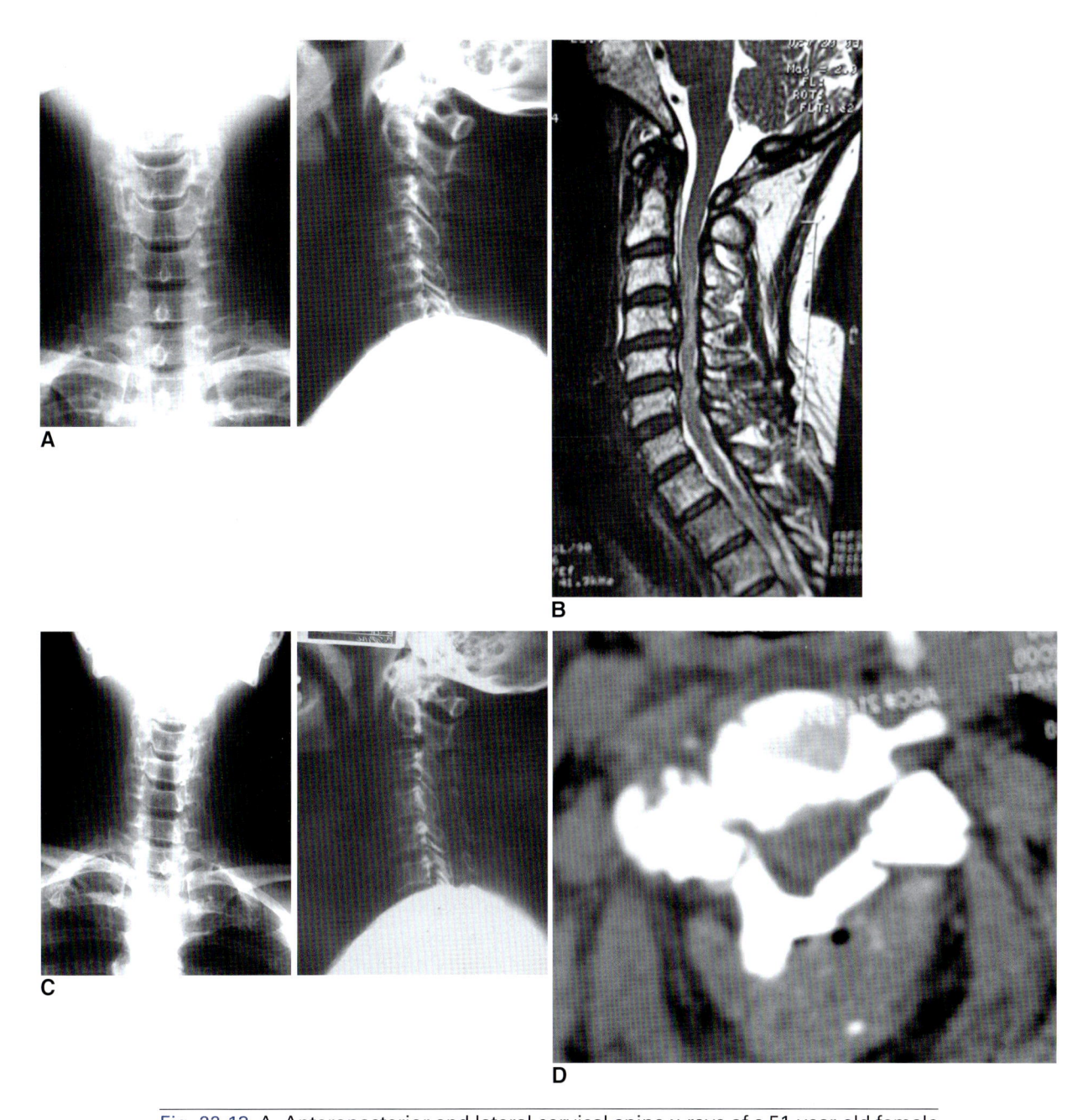

Fig. 22-13 **A**, Anteroposterior and lateral cervical spine x-rays of a 51-year-old female with diffuse spondylosis. **B**, Sagittal T_2-weighted magnetic resonance image of the cervical spine demonstrates severe multilevel stenosis with cord compression. **C**, Anteroposterior and lateral views following C3-C7 laminoplasty demonstrating the increased size of the canal. **D**, Transverse computed tomography reconstruction demonstrating the enlarged canal and the allograft block keeping the door open.

References

1. Kawai S, Sunago K, Doi K, et al: Cervical laminoplasty (Hattori's method). Procedure and follow-up results. Spine 1988;13(11): 1245–1250.
2. Hirabayashi K, Watanabe K, Wakano K, et al: Expansive open-door laminoplasty for cervical spinal stenotic myelopathy. Spine 1983; 8(7):693–699.
3. Kurokawa T, Tsuyama N, Tanaka H, et al: Enlargement of spinal canal by the sagittal splitting of spinal processes for cervical spondylotic myelopathy. Rinsho Seikeigeka 1984;19:483–490.
4. Hirabayashi K, Satomi K: Operative procedure and results of expansive open-door laminoplasty. Spine 1988;13(7):870–876.
5. Hirabayashi K, Toyama Y, Chiba K: Expansive laminoplasty for myelopathy in ossification of the longitudinal ligament. Clin Orthop 1999;(359):35–48.

6. Fujimura Y, Nishi Y, Nakamura M: Dorsal shift and expansion of the spinal cord after expansive open-door laminoplasty. J Spinal Disord 1997;10(4):282–287.
7. Mukai Y, Hosono N, Sakaura H, et al: Laminoplasty for cervical myelopathy caused by subaxial lesions in rheumatoid arthritis. J Neurosurg 2004;100(1 Suppl):7–12.
8. Chiba K, Toyama Y, Watanabe M, et al: Impact of longitudinal distance of the cervical spine on the results of expansive open-door laminoplasty. Spine 2000;25(22):2893-2898.
9. Herkowitz HN: Cervical laminoplasty: Its role in the treatment of cervical radiculopathy. J Spinal Disord 1988;1(3):179–188.
10. Baba H, Imura S, Kawahara N, et al: Osteoplastic laminoplasty for cervical myeloradiculopathy secondary to ossification of the posterior longitudinal ligament. Int Orthop 1995;19(1):40–45.
11. Inoue A, Ikata T, Katoh S: Spinal deformity following surgery for spinal cord tumors and tumorous lesions: Analysis based on an assessment of the spinal functional curve. Spinal Cord 1996;34(9):536–542.
12. Miyazaki K, Tada K, Matsuda Y, et al: Posterior extensive simultaneous multisegment decompression with posterolateral fusion for cervical myelopathy with cervical instability and kyphotic and/or S-shaped deformities. Spine 1989;14(11):1160–1170.
13. Snow RB, Weiner H: Cervical laminectomy and foraminotomy as surgical treatment of cervical spondylosis: A follow-up study with analysis of failures. J Spinal Disord 1993;6(3):245-50; discussion 50–51.
14. Herkowitz HN: A comparison of anterior cervical fusion, cervical laminectomy, and cervical laminoplasty for the surgical management of multiple level spondylotic radiculopathy. Spine 1988;13(7):774–780.
15. Hirabayashi K, Miyakawa J, Satomi K, et al: Operative results and postoperative progression of ossification among patients with ossification of cervical posterior longitudinal ligament. Spine 1981;6(4):354–364.
16. Satomi K, Nishu Y, Kohno T, et al: Long-term follow-up studies of open-door expansive laminoplasty for cervical stenotic myelopathy. Spine 1994;19(5):507–510.
17. Hirabayashi K, Bohlman HH: Multilevel cervical spondylosis. Laminoplasty versus anterior decompression. Spine 1995;20(15):1732–1734.
18. Morimoto T, Matsuyama T, Hirabayashi H, et al: Expansive laminoplasty for multilevel cervical OPLL. J Spinal Disord 1997;10(4):296–298.
19. An HS, Gordin R, Renner K: Anatomic considerations for plate-screw fixation of the cervical spine. Spine 1991;16(10 Suppl):S548–S51.
20. Xu R, Ebraheim NA, Yeasting R, et al: Anatomy of C7 lateral mass and projection of pedicle axis on its posterior aspect. J Spinal Disord 1995;8(2):116–120.
21. Koshu K, Tominaga T, Yoshimoto T: Spinous process-splitting laminoplasty with an extended foraminotomy for cervical myelopathy. Neurosurgery 1995;37(3):430–434; discussion 34–35.
22. Edwards CC 2nd, Heller JG, Silcox DH 3rd: T-saw laminoplasty for the management of cervical spondylotic myelopathy: Clinical and radiographic outcome. Spine 2000;25(14):1788–1794.
23. Roselli R, Pompucci A, Formica F, et al: Open-door laminoplasty for cervical stenotic myelopathy: Surgical technique and neurophysiological monitoring. J Neurosurg 2000;92(1 Suppl):38–43.
24. Yue WM, Tan CT, Tan SB, et al: Results of cervical laminoplasty and a comparison between single and double trap-door techniques. J Spinal Disord 2000;13(4):329–335.
25. Hosono N, Yonenobu K, Ono K: Neck and shoulder pain after laminoplasty: A noticeable complication. Spine 1996;21(17):1969–1973.
26. Iwasaki M, Ebara S, Miyamoto S, et al: Expansive laminoplasty for cervical radiculomyelopathy due to soft disc herniation. Spine 1996;21(1):32–38.
27. Hidai Y, Ebara S, Kamimura M, et al: Treatment of cervical compressive myelopathy with a new dorsolateral decompressive procedure. J Neurosurg 1999;90(4 Suppl):178–185.
28. Kawaguchi Y, Matsui H, Ishihara H, et al: Surgical outcome of cervical expansive laminoplasty in patients with diabetes mellitus. Spine 2000;25(5):551–555.
29. Wada E, Suzuki S, Kanazawa A, et al: Subtotal corpectomy versus laminoplasty for multilevel cervical spondylotic myelopathy: A long-term follow-up study over 10 years. Spine 2001;26(13):1443–1447; discussion 48.

CHAPTER 23

FARROKH R. FARROKHI

ANDREW DAILEY

Ossification of the Posterior Longitudinal Ligament

INTRODUCTION

Ossification of the posterior longitudinal ligament (OPLL) can present with myelopathy, radiculopathy, or myeloradiculopathy. Calcification and thickening of the posterior longitudinal ligament (PLL) in this disease leads to reduction in cross-sectional area of the spinal canal and subsequent compression of the neural elements.

Reported first in 1838, OPLL was not recognized as a pathologic condition until the 1960s.[1] Recent advances in radiographic techniques, particularly computed tomography (CT) and magnetic resonance imaging (MRI), have made it easier to diagnose. A number of surgical options for the treatment of OPLL have been developed over the past 2 decades. This chapter will review the disease process, details of available surgical techniques, and their current predicted outcomes.

EPIDEMIOLOGY

Asian populations are most affected by OPLL. A study by Tsuyama found that 2% to 3% of asymptomatic Japanese individuals have radiographic evidence of the disease. Other ethnic groups reveal much lower rates, with asymptomatic white North Americans having an incidence of 0.12% to 0.2%.[1] Despite the low incidence, OPLL accounts for 20% to 25% of cervical myelopathy seen in the United States and 27% of that observed in Japan.[2] The primary focus of OPLL is in the cervical spine in 70% to 95% of patients, with the remainder divided between the midthoracic and upper lumbar spine.[2,3] The spinal levels most often affected are C4-C6, T4-T7, and L1-L2.[1]

PATHOPHYSIOLOGY

Although the exact etiology of OPLL remains to be determined, evidence is mounting that genetic susceptibility plays the most significant role in disease development.[4,5] Familial studies show the disease in as many as 25% of first-degree relatives of affected individuals.[6] Multiple chromosomal abnormalities have been shown in vitro and in vivo to contribute to more rapid ossification under conditions of repetitive strain in ligaments.[7] Clinical associations have also been reported between OPLL and other disorders, including diffuse idiopathic skeletal hyperostosis, ankylosing spondylitis, obesity, diabetes, acromegaly, and hyperparathyroidism.[1,3,8]

In an early and commonly used classification system developed by Hirabayashi, four types of OPLL were identified: (1) continuous, with the ossified mass extending over several levels, (2) segmental, with ossification only behind each vertebral body, (3) mixed, which is a combination of types 1 and 2, and (4) localized, which may present as anterior or circumferential ossification and stenosis (Fig. 23-1). In a study of Japanese patients, these types of OPLL were found in 39%, 27%, 29%, and 7.5% of patients, respectively.[1]

CLINICAL PRESENTATION AND NATURAL COURSE

Myelopathy, radiculopathy, and neck pain are the most common presenting symptoms of OPLL. In a meta-analysis of six series, compiling data from 120 patients (including 51 of her own patients), Epstein reported that 84% presented with myelopathy causing severe neurologic dysfunction in Ranawat classes IIIA and IIIB.[2] Radiculopathy with dysesthesias was seen in 47% and neck pain was found in 42%. These symptoms were present an average of 13.3 months (range, 7.5 to 22 months) at the time of presentation.

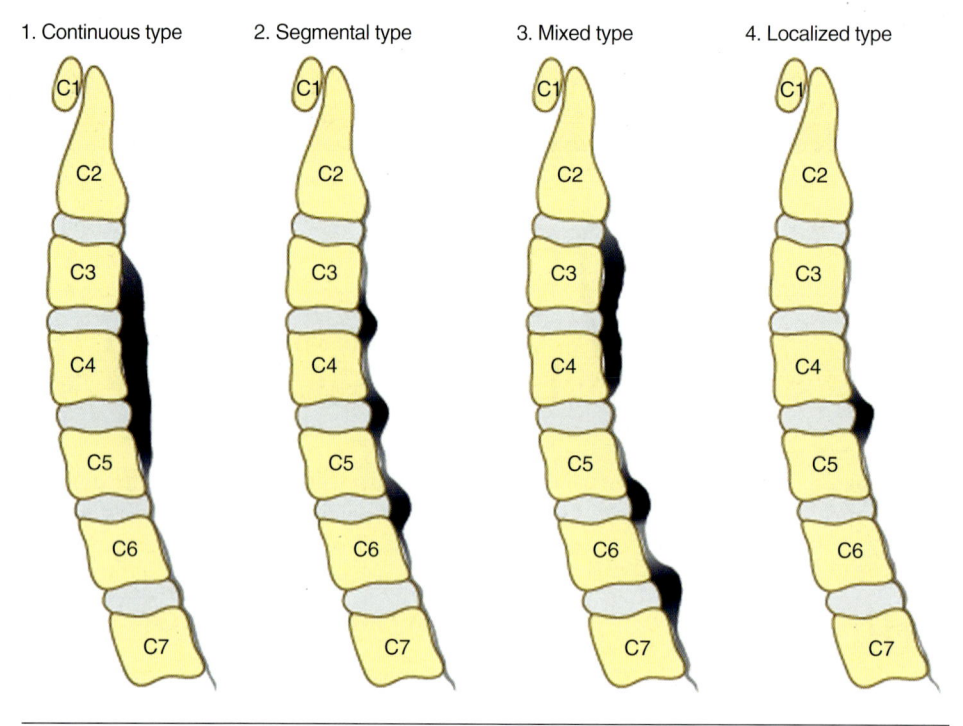

Fig. 23-1 Classification of the four types of ossification of the posterior longitudinal ligament (OPLL).

The majority of patients with OPLL (70% to 85%) report a very gradual onset of symptoms.[1] Another subset (15% to 30%) present with sudden deterioration of neurologic function, often after only minor cervical trauma.[2,9] While following 207 patients, Matsunaga found that of those who presented with myelopathy, 37% experienced worsening of symptoms during a 10-year observation period.[9] In 170 patients who were initially free of myelopathy, only 16% developed myelopathy over the same time course. In multiple reports, duration of symptoms correlated inversely with recovery.[10,11]

DIAGNOSTICS AND RADIOGRAPHIC FINDINGS

Prior to the advent of CT, diagnosis of OPLL was based on true lateral spinal x-rays. Dynamic lateral cervical spine x-rays remain a critical part of the evaluation of stability in the workup of OPLL, with instability defined by greater than 3.5 mm of subluxation, more than 20 degrees of angulation, or over 2 mm of motion between adjacent spinous processes.[12]

High-resolution CT with sagittal reconstructions represents the definitive diagnostic tool for OPLL (Fig. 23-2). CT also permits calculation of canal diameter and transverse area of the spinal cord, factors which may predict recovery after surgery.[11] CT myelography allows more detailed evaluation of the level and location of compression on neural elements.

MRI contributes significantly to the evaluation of patients with OPLL by delineating the amount of cord compression

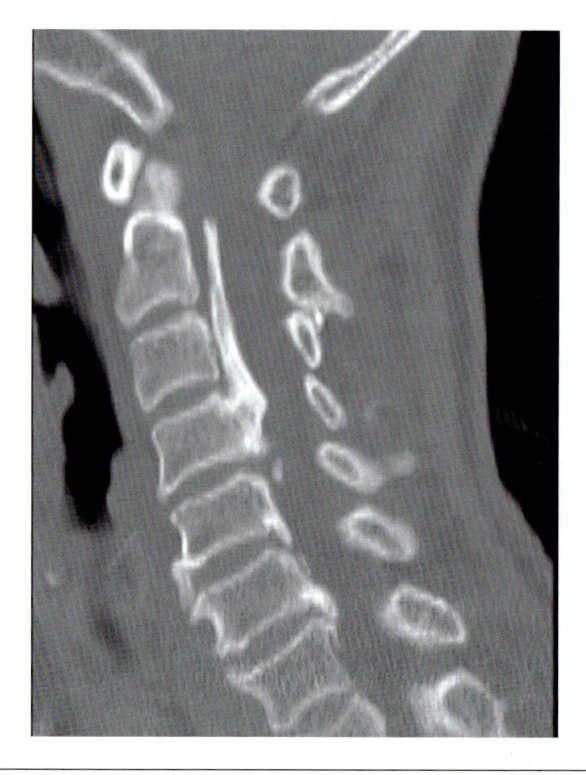

Fig. 23-2 Sagittal reconstruction of cervical ossification of the posterior longitudinal ligament (OPLL).

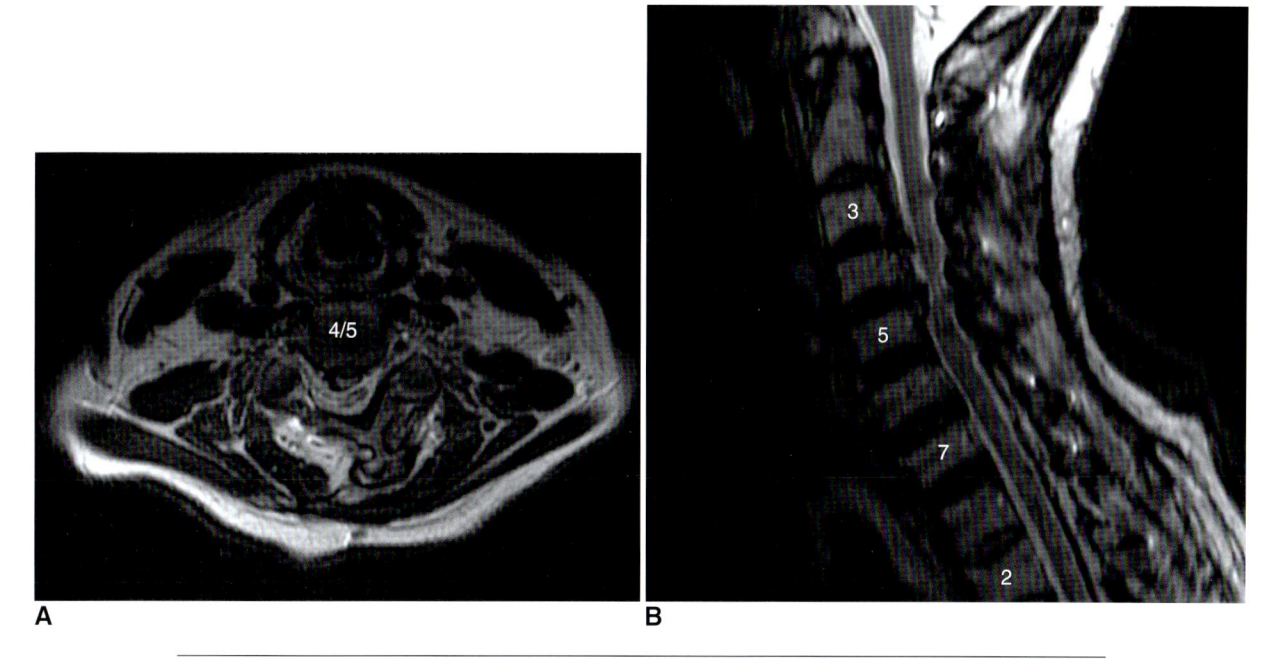

Fig. 23-3 Axial (*A*) and sagittal (*B*) T$_2$-weighted magnetic resonance imaging sequences of cervical ossification of the posterior longitudinal ligament.

and spinal cord edema, which when present on T$_2$-weighted sequences has been shown to correlate with worse outcomes[2,13] (Fig. 23-3*A* and *B*). The ossified ligament usually appears as an area of low-signal intensity in the anterior aspect of the canal on both T$_1$- and T$_2$-weighted images. Flexion and extension MRI can also be obtained to evaluate the dynamic changes on canal diameter and cord compression.

SURGICAL OPTIONS AND OUTCOMES

In those patients whose symptoms progress despite conservative therapy, surgical options include laminectomy, laminectomy plus fusion, laminoplasty, and anterior decompression and fusion. The decision on the most appropriate surgical approach is complex, with no data currently available to define a standard. Multiple factors must be considered in each case, including the patient's age, anatomy of the lesion, degree of stenosis, extent of lordosis or kyphosis, and symptomatology.

LAMINECTOMY

Laminectomy provides a relatively safe and simple approach to decompression of the neural elements in cases in which the normal cervical lordosis is preserved.[12,14] Posterior decompression in a lordotic spine allows the spinal cord to settle always from the compressive mass of the calcified PLL. However, the same procedure in a kyphotic spine will provide little relief, as the cord remains draped over the anterior elements. In addition, 30% to 40% of patients risk progression of the kyphotic deformity after the elimination of the posterior tension band.[10,15] This result is of particular concern in some younger patients, who have a higher tendency for development of postlaminectomy kyphosis. Laminectomy is best reserved for older patients with multisegmental disease, preserved lordosis, and limited cervical range of motion. The details of laminectomy are described in Chapter 21.

LAMINECTOMY PLUS FUSION

The addition of posterior instrumentation and fusion after decompressive laminectomy should be considered in cases of segmental instability, cervical kyphosis, or decompression extending across the cervicothoracic junction.[12] Fusion can best be achieved by employing a screw-plate or screw-rod fixation system. Although facet wiring techniques had been used extensively in the past, the recent developed instrumentation systems provide more stable constructs with higher fusion rates and lower complication rates.[12] The techniques for placement of lateral mass screws and posterior cervical fusion techniques are described in Chapter 18.

ANTERIOR APPROACHES

Anterior decompression of the spinal canal by partial or complete vertebrectomy and subsequent grafting and fusion represented an alternative to posterior approaches.[15-17] Anterior corpectomy and fusion may help prevent progressive kyphotic deformity and allow direct decompression of the calcified ligament. However, it does have drawbacks, such as increased intraoperative blood loss, significant risk of dural damage, cerebrospinal fistula formation, and high pseudoarthrosis rates in greater than three-level fusions.[18] In light of the risks, anterior approaches should be reserved for segmental OPLL involving three spinal segments or less, greater than 7 mm PLL thickness, and greater than 50% canal compromise.[18,19]

Several modifications to the standard anterior approach should be considered. Preoperative placement of a lumbar drain and preparation for dural repair or grafting are recommended. The use of a small diamond burr with the high-speed drill and an operative microscope aid in minimizing dural and spinal cord injury. Although some surgeons advocate removal of all calcified elements, this increases the risk of dural violation. Therefore, an alternative technique which may provide adequate decompression, is the generation of a floating segment of bone.[17] This can be achieved by thinning the posterior vertebral body and ossified PLL, followed by the drilling of small troughs at the lateral aspects of the canal (Fig. 23-4).

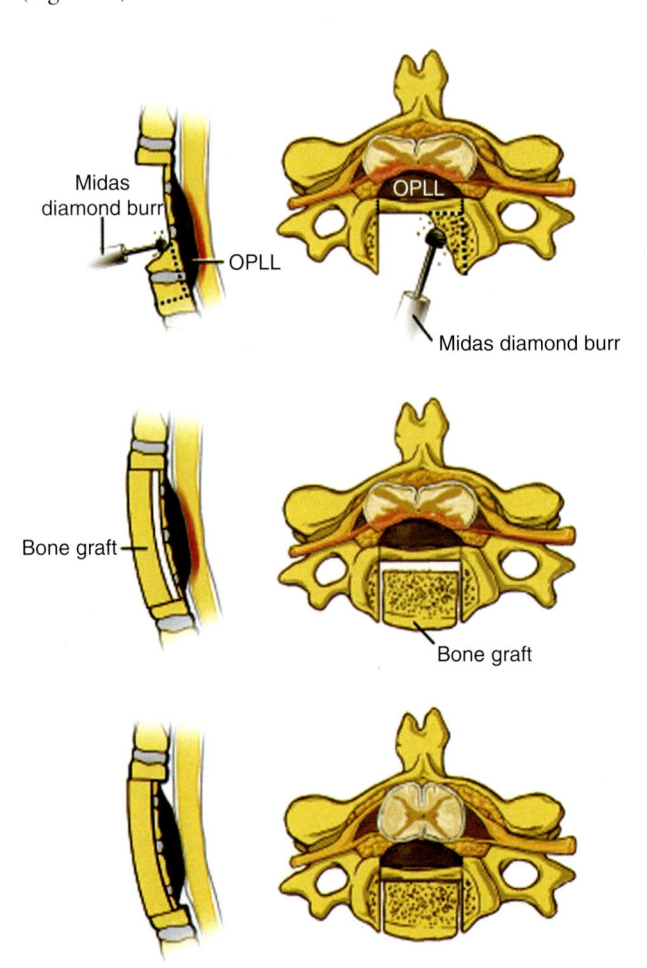

Fig. 23-4 Anterior "floating segment" approach.

COMBINED ANTERIOR AND POSTERIOR APPROACHES

In cases of multisegmental OPLL in younger patients, Epstein advocates circumferential surgery.[12] She reports 25 successful fusions in 26 patients with multilevel anterior corpectomy with fusion followed by decompressive laminectomies and posterior fusion. Improvements of +3 Nurick grades were noted with most patients rated at Nurick grades 0 to I at follow-up. These promising reports must be weighed against the cumulative risks of combined procedures, and as always, the choice must be tailored to individual cases.

LAMINOPLASTY

In an effort to prevent postlaminectomy kyphosis and repeat compression from postlaminectomy membranes, laminoplasty was developed as an alternative. In a recent review of the laminoplasty data, Ratliff and Cooper attempted to evaluate the benefits of laminoplasty the using Japanese Orthopedic Association (JOA) scale for assessing myelopathy.[20] They found wide-ranging results, with recovery rates of 20% to 80%, and an average recovery rate of 55% in a meta-analysis of 41 series. These data were compared with laminectomy outcomes, which had similar recovery rates of 54% (immediate) and 48% (at 5 years).

Other findings in Ratliff and Cooper's review included a 10% rate of postlaminoplasty kyphosis and a 35% rate of worsening cervical alignment, although these data were not defined as loss of lordosis or progression of present kyphotic deformity. A 50% reduction in cervical range of motion and 40% restenosis rate was also seen. Rates of postoperative axial neck pain were noted to range from 6% to 60%. The common finding of C5 root injury, seen in 8% of patients, was similar in most series reviewed.[21] No evidence was found to indicate a slowing of the patient's posterior cervical muscle atrophy with laminoplasty versus laminectomy. As much as 70% reduction in the cross-sectional area of cervical musculature has been noted after laminoplasty, with no correlation between the degree of atrophy and spinal curvature. Similarly, it is unclear to what degree preservation of the posterior tension band preserves range of motion. From their review, the authors concluded that the literature has yet to support the benefits of laminoplasty as a standard in all patients with OPLL. As with other procedures, laminoplasty must be applied and tailored to the individual patient and pathology.

LAMINOPLASTY TECHNIQUES

Laminoplasty techniques were first popularized by Hirabayashi in the late 1970s.[22,23] Since that time many variations have been offered in order to lower the rates of postlaminectomy kyphosis.[22,24–26] Many modifications of the original laminoplasty technique have subsequently been

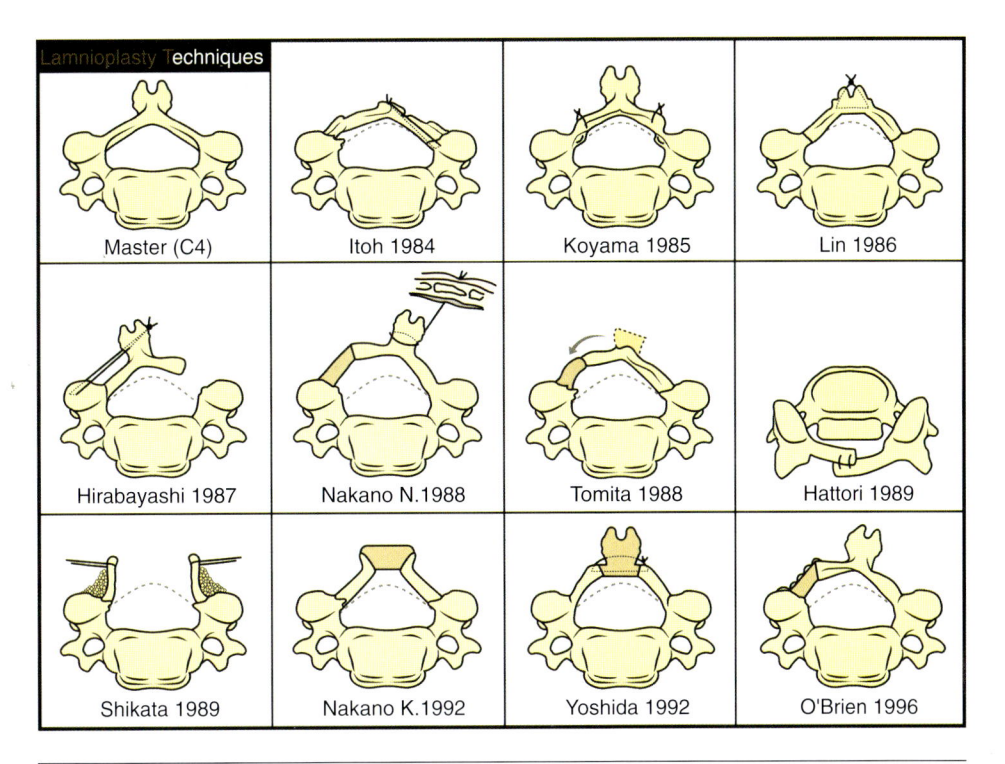

Fig. 23-5 Laminoplasty techniques.

described in the literature and are schematically represented here (Fig. 23-5).

Development of these earlier methods, in many cases, was driven by the lack of appropriate implantable stabilization hardware. Recent availability of allograft bone spacers and small titanium plating systems allows for a simple and effective fixation. Open door laminoplasty using titanium miniplates avoids the use of stainless steel implants and allows for improved visualization on postoperative MRI. Precut allograft eliminates the morbidity of autograft. The detailed procedure for open door laminoplasty using grafts and a plating system is outlined next. However, outcomes of a particular type of laminoplasty may be more a function of an individual surgeon's experience with a given technique.

INDICATIONS AND CONTRAINDICATIONS FOR LAMINOPLASTY

Indications
- Myelopathy
- Progressive or recurrent cervical radiculopathy
- Minimum of 10 degrees of cervical lordosis from C2 to C7[12,14]
- Less than 7 mm of ventral OPLL[19]
- Less than 50% canal stenosis[19]
- Multilevel disease
- Younger patients (age <60 years)[14]
- Preserved cervical mobility

Relative Contraindications
- Cervical kyphosis[12,19]
- Single or short segment disease
- Segmental instability
- Older patients with other comorbidities

OPERATIVE TECHNIQUE: OPEN DOOR LAMINOPLASTY

Equipment
- X-ray-compatible operating table
- C-arm fluoroscopy
- Somatosensory evoked potential (SSEP) and motor evoked potential (MEP) monitoring
- Headlight system
- Self-retaining retractors
- High-speed drill with fine cutting and diamond burrs
- Straight and angled curettes: 3-0, 4-0, and 5-0 sizes
- Kerrison punches (1 to 3 mm)
- Bone graft source
- Autograft (spinous process, rib, iliac crest)
- Allograft (precut and sized fibula)
- Titanium laminar plating system

Patient Positioning and Intubation
- General endotracheal anesthesia is used. The use of awake, nasotracheal, or fiberoptic-aided intubation is preferred to

minimize cervical extension and potential spinal cord injury.
- Baseline spinal cord monitoring is performed prior to turning into the prone position.
- Mayfield three-pin head holder is placed.
- Patient is placed in the prone position and the Mayfield head holder is attached to the bed, taking particular care to maintain neutral positioning of the neck.
- The shoulders are gently taped down to maximize visualization under fluoroscopy.
- Spinal cord monitoring is repeated to confirm maintenance of signals.
- If autograft harvesting is anticipated, the site is appropriately selected and prepped.

Location of Incision
- C-arm is moved into position for verification of appropriate cervical positioning and marking of appropriate level.
- A midline incision is marked from one spinous process above to the one spinous process below the planned levels of laminoplasty.

Preparation and Draping
- The incision is marked and the cervical skin area is sterilely prepared.
- Draping is carried out in the usual manner.
- If autograft is to be used, a harvest site is draped separately and covered.
- The anesthesiologist is at the head of the table and the scrub nurse is at the lower half of the table.
- The headlight and microscope are based on the side of the primary surgeon.
- Fluoroscopy is based on the contralateral side to the primary surgeon.

Incision and Soft Tissue Dissection
- Local anesthetic is injected subcutaneously at the incision site.
- A midline skin incision is made along the appropriate levels.
- Monopolar electrocautery is used to carry the dissection through the midline raphe to the spinous processes (Fig. 23-6A).
- Paraspinous musculature is dissected off the spinous processes and lamina in a subperiosteal fashion. Care is taken to preserve the intraspinous ligaments.
- Particular care should be taken to avoid damage to the facets, which can lead to instability and kyphosis.[12]
- Fluoroscopy-guided confirmation of the level of exposure is made by applying towel clips to the upper and lower most exposed spinous processes.
- Two self-retaining retractors are placed in the cranial and caudal aspects of the wound to spread laterally the paraspinous musculature.

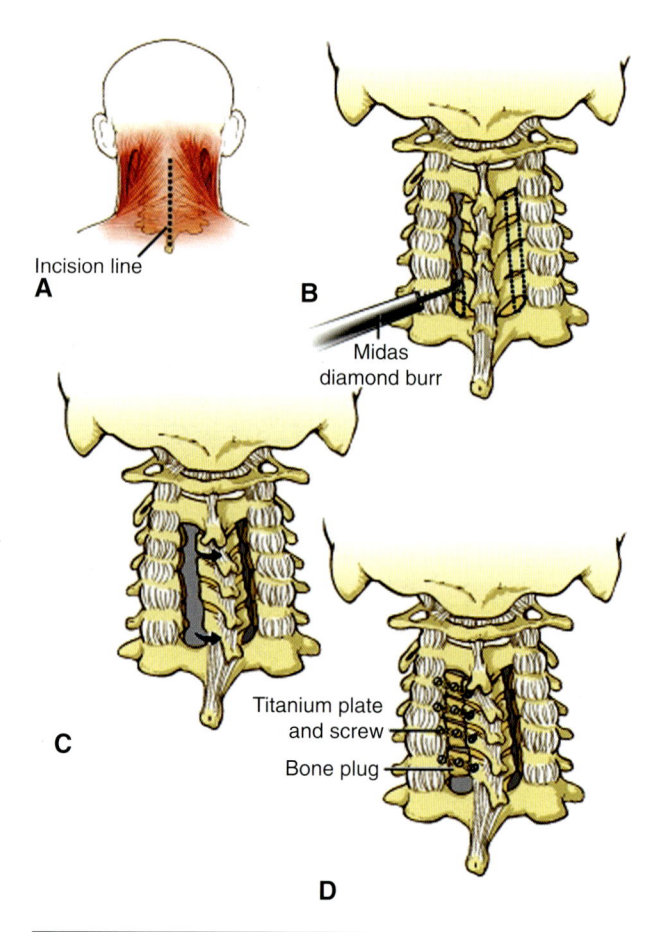

Fig. 23-6 Incision and approach (*A*), drilling troughs (*B*), spreading of lamina (*C*), and placement of bone plugs, plates, and screws (*D*).

Laminoplasty
- A high-speed drill with a fine-cutting burr is used to generate troughs bilaterally at the junctions of the lamina and lateral masses. The ventral cortex should not be penetrated. Unintentional entry in to the canal can be prevented by creating a small shelf on the medial aspect of the lateral mass to a depth that exposes the ventral cortex of the lamina (see Fig. 23-6B).
- Right- or left-sided opening of the laminoplasty should be dictated by eccentricity of the bony pathology and radiculopathy (see Fig. 23-6C).
- The remaining bone is preferentially removed with careful drilling or with the use of a 1-mm Kerrison rongeur and up-angled curettes.
- The unicortical trough on the "hinge" side of the lamina is then thinned to a point that allows posterior rotation of the released bony mass.
- Partial release of the intraspinous ligaments and ligamenta flava are performed at the cranial and caudal extents of the laminoplasty.
- The posterior elements are rotated posteriorly using the lamina spreader in an en bloc fashion, keeping the inter-

CHAPTER 23 Ossification of the Posterior Longitudinal Ligament

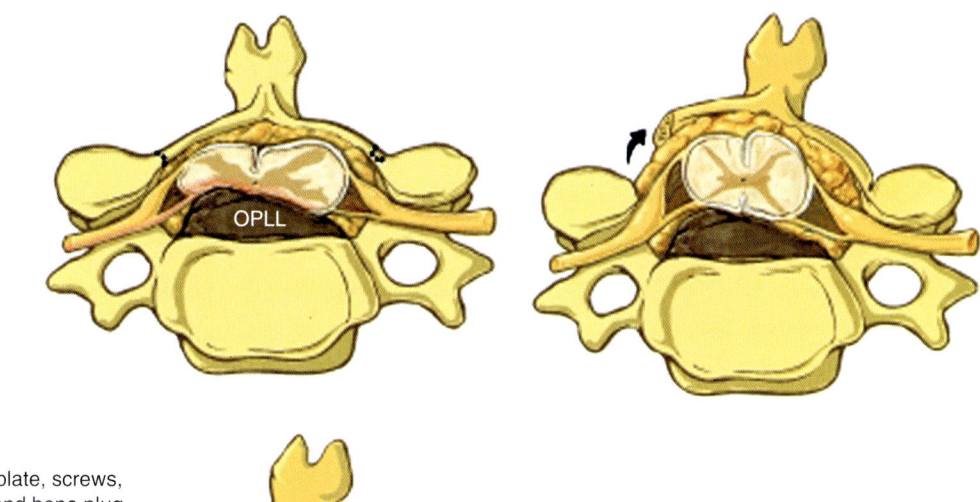

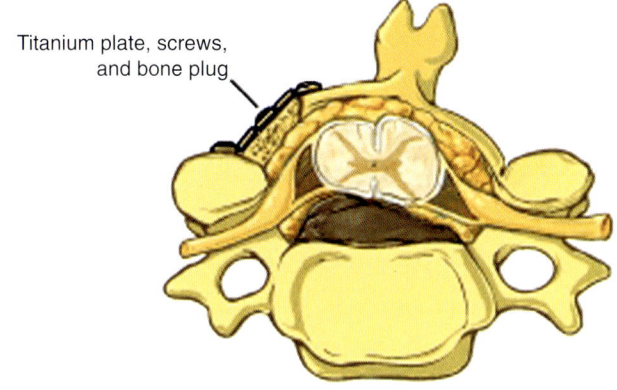

Fig. 23-7 Axial views of laminoplasty technique.

spinous ligaments and ligamentum flava intact. Care should be taken not to fracture the ventral cortex on the "hinge" side of the lamina.
- Epidural adhesions and the venous plexus should be freed at this time. This may result in significant bleeding, which is best treated with powdered Gelfoam and bipolar electrocautery.

Bone Graft and Instrumentation
- Bone wax should be avoided, as it may interfere with the fusion process.
- Allograft spacers or appropriately cut autografts are then placed at each exposed level to maintain the open position of the lamina.
- Miniplates are secured to the lamina, graft, and lateral mass using screws. Screws should be directed into the lateral mass at an angle to avoid penetration of the facets (Figs. 23-6D, 23-7, and 23-8).

Closure
- Careful hemostasis is achieved.
- A drain should be placed and tunneled out a few centimeters caudal to the inferior aspect of the incision.
- The muscle layer is gently apposed using 0 vicryl suture.
- A secure fascial closure is achieved with interrupted 0 vicryl suture.
- The deep dermal layer is approximated using interrupted 2-0 vicryl suture.

- The skin is closed with a 4-0 monocryl absorbable suture in a running subcuticular fashion.
- A rigid collar should be applied at the end of the case.

POSTOPERATIVE CARE
- Cervical x-rays are obtained in the recovery room to confirm cervical alignment, verify graft and hardware

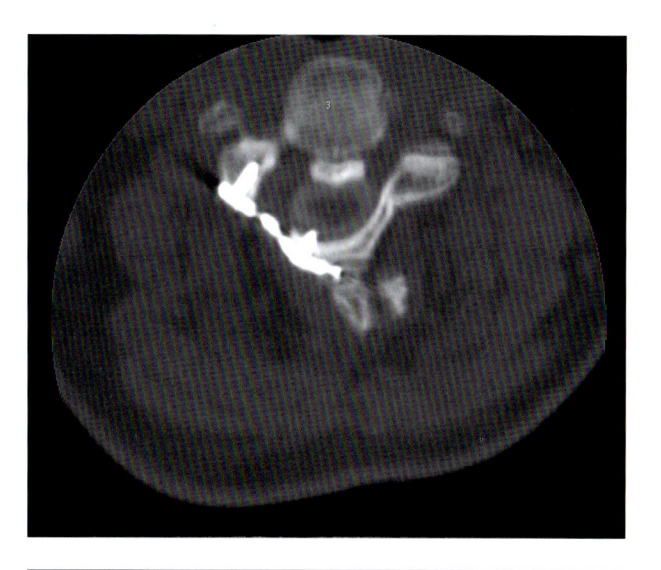

Fig. 23-8 Axial computed tomograph of postlaminoplasty cervical spine myelogram.

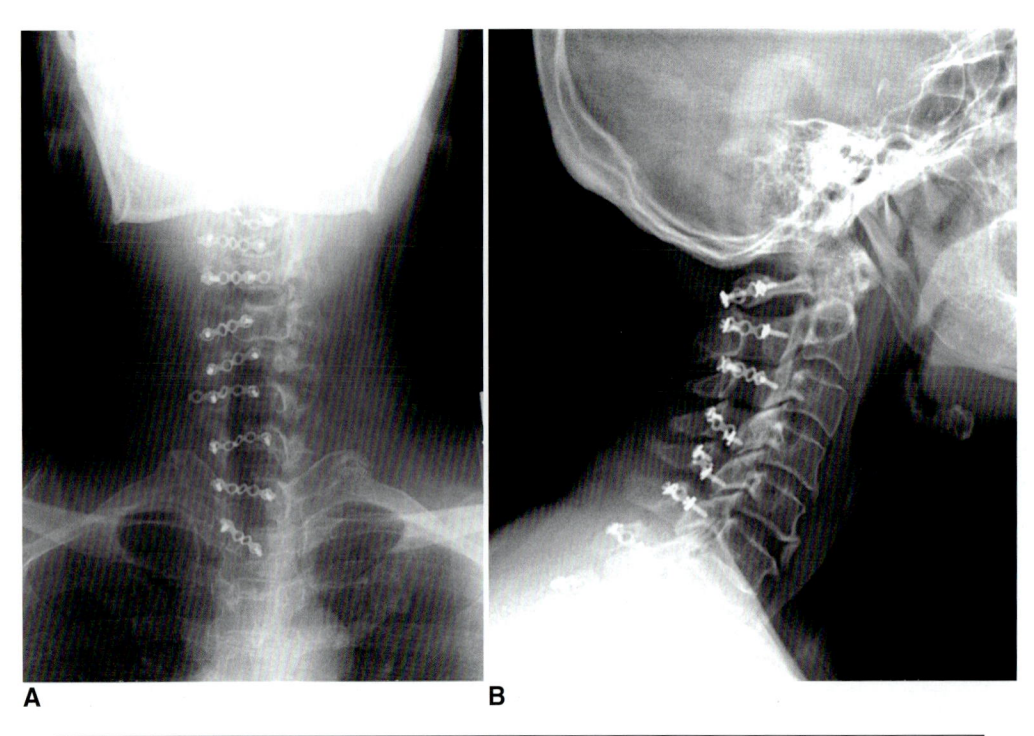

Fig. 23-9 Anteroposterior (A) and lateral (B) cervical spine x-rays after laminoplasty.

position, and as a baseline for follow-up (Fig. 23-9A and B).
- Early ambulation and pulmonary toilet is encouraged.
- Oral pain control is usually supplemented with a short course of intravenous narcotics and muscle relaxants.
- Upright cervical spine x-rays are obtained after patient has been ambulating to confirm stability.
- Patients are usually discharged from the hospital in 2 or 3 days if there are no complications.

COMPLICATIONS

- New neurologic deficit may occur after recovery from anesthesia secondary to nerve root injury or edema, spinal cord concussion, or rapid release of chronic compression.
- Acute deficits may result from mechanical etiologies such as intervertebral subluxation, migrated bone graft, or an acute epidural hematoma, all of which should be surgically treated.
- Early delayed deficits, including C5 root symptoms, are usually due to postoperative edema or stretch with a good prognosis for recovery.[21]
- Postoperative axial symptoms of neck pain and shoulder may be seen in as many as 60% of laminoplasty patients.[17,27]
- Progressive deficit after the first week of surgery may indicate spinal instability or an infection.

CONCLUSIONS

As a general guideline, older patients with multisegment OPLL, preserved cervical lordosis, and no obvious instability will do well with simple laminectomy. Fusion or laminoplasty may be employed in younger patients and in cases in which preservation of a posterior tension band would prove beneficial. Anterior decompression should be reserved for short segment disease or accompanied by a posterior decompression and fusion.

The variety of options available for the surgical treatment of OPLL is a testament to challenges presented by this difficult disease. As with most pathology, the therapy must be directed at the individual patient. Careful consideration of the patient's symptoms, anatomy, pathology, and comorbidities should direct the approach rather than strict criteria and routines.

REFERENCES

1. Tsuyama N: Ossification of the posterior longitudinal ligament of the spine. Clin Orthop 1984;184:71–84.
2. Epstein N: The surgical management of ossification of the posterior longitudinal ligament in 51 patients. J Spinal Disord 1993; 6:432–454; discussion 454–435.
3. Trojan DA, Pouchot J, Pokrupa R, et al: Diagnosis and treatment of ossification of the posterior longitudinal ligament of the spine: Report of eight cases and literature review. Am J Med 1992; 92:296–306.
4. Koga H, Sakou T, Taketomi E, et al: Genetic mapping of ossification of the posterior longitudinal ligament of the spine. Am J Hum Genet 1998;62:1460–1467.
5. Matsunaga S, Yamaguchi M, Hayashi K, et al: Genetic analysis of ossification of the posterior longitudinal ligament. Spine 1999; 24:937–938; discussion 939.
6. Terayama K: Genetic studies on ossification of the posterior longitudinal ligament of the spine. Spine 1989;14:1184–1191.

7. Iwasaki K, Furukawa KI, Tanno M, et al: Uni-axial cyclic stretch induces cbfa1 expression in spinal ligament cells derived from patients with ossification of the posterior longitudinal ligament. Calcif Tissue Int 2004;74:448–457.
8. Ramos-Remus C, Russell AS, Gomez-Vargas A, et al: Ossification of the posterior longitudinal ligament in three geographically and genetically different populations of ankylosing spondylitis and other spondyloarthropathies. Ann Rheum Dis 1998;57:429–433.
9. Matsunaga S, Sakou T, Taketomi E, et al: The natural course of myelopathy caused by ossification of the posterior longitudinal ligament in the cervical spine. Clin Orthop 1994;305:168–177.
10. Hamanishi C, Tanaka S: Bilateral multilevel laminectomy with or without posterolateral fusion for cervical spondylotic myelopathy: Relationship to type of onset and time until operation. J Neurosurg 1996;85:447–451.
11. Koyanagi T, Hirabayashi K, Satomi K, et al: Predictability of operative results of cervical compression myelopathy based on preoperative computed tomographic myelography. Spine 1993;18:1958–1963.
12. Epstein NE: Laminectomy for cervical myelopathy. Spinal Cord 2003;41:317–327.
13. Ramon S, Dominguez R, Ramirez L, et al: Clinical and magnetic resonance imaging correlation in acute spinal cord injury. Spinal Cord 1997;35:664–673.
14. Kawai S, Sunago K, Doi K, et al: Cervical laminoplasty (Hattori's method): Procedure and follow-up results. Spine 1988;13:1245–1250.
15. Herkowitz HN: A comparison of anterior cervical fusion, cervical laminectomy, and cervical laminoplasty for the surgical management of multiple level spondylotic radiculopathy. Spine 1988;13:774–780.
16. Kojima T, Waga S, Kubo Y, et al: Anterior cervical vertebrectomy and interbody fusion for multi-level spondylosis and ossification of the posterior longitudinal ligament. Neurosurgery 1989;24:864–872.
17. Tateiwa Y, Kamimura M, Itoh H, et al: Multilevel subtotal corpectomy and interbody fusion using a fibular bone graft for cervical myelopathy due to ossification of the posterior longitudinal ligament. J Clin Neurosci 2003;10:199–207.
18. Cheng WC, Chang CN, Lui TN, et al: Surgical treatment for ossification of the posterior longitudinal ligament of the cervical spine. Surg Neurol 1994;41:90–97.
19. Yamazaki A, Homma T, Uchiyama S, et al: Morphologic limitations of posterior decompression by midsagittal splitting method for myelopathy caused by ossification of the posterior longitudinal ligament in the cervical spine. Spine 1999;24:32–34.
20. Ratliff JK, Cooper PR: Cervical laminoplasty: A critical review. J Neurosurg 2003;98:230–238.
21. Sakaura H, Hosono N, Mukai Y, et al: C5 palsy after decompression surgery for cervical myelopathy: Review of the literature. Spine 2003;28:2447–2451.
22. Hirabayashi K, Miyakawa J, Satomi K, et al: Operative results and postoperative progression of ossification among patients with ossification of cervical posterior longitudinal ligament. Spine 1981;6:354–364.
23. Hirabayashi K, Satomi K: Operative procedure and results of expansive open-door laminoplasty. Spine 1988;13:870–876.
24. Nakano N, Nakano T, Nakano K: Comparison of the results of laminectomy and open-door laminoplasty for cervical spondylotic myeloradiculopathy and ossification of the posterior longitudinal ligament. Spine 1988;13:792–794.
25. O'Brien MF, Peterson D, Casey AT, et al: A novel technique for laminoplasty augmentation of spinal canal area using titanium miniplate stabilization: A computerized morphometric analysis. Spine 1996;21:474–483; discussion 484.
26. Seichi A, Takeshita K, Ohishi I, et al: Long-term results of double-door laminoplasty for cervical stenotic myelopathy. Spine 2001;26:479–487.
27. Hosono N, Yonenobu K, Ono K: Neck and shoulder pain after laminoplasty: A noticeable complication. Spine 1996;21:1969–1973.

SECTION C
Thoracic Disk Herniation

CHAPTER 24

DEAN G. KARAHALIOS
ERIC A. POTTS

Thoracic Diskectomy

INTRODUCTION

Patients with thoracic disk disease may present with pain, radiculopathy, or myelopathy. When indicated, diskectomy may be performed via a posterior or anterior approach, depending on the location and consistency of the disk herniation. Posterior approaches include the transpedicular, costotransversectomy, and lateral extracavitary techniques (Fig. 24-1). Diskectomy by a midline posterior laminectomy approach alone is associated with a relatively high risk of neurologic morbidity and is generally contraindicated. An anterolateral approach can be facilitated by open thoracotomy, or by a minimally invasive thoracoscopic technique.

The level, position, and consistency of the disk herniation will dictate the optimal approach. Additional factors such as patient age and medical comorbidities may favor a posterior approach to avoid pulmonary complications.

In general, lateral or soft disk herniations may be safely approached posteriorly. Midline or broad-based disk herniations or densely calcified disk herniations may favor an anterior or anterolateral approach.

Disk herniations in the upper thoracic spine may be more easily approached by a posterolateral approach, or by a straight anterior approach via manubrial window or sternotomy. An anterolateral open thoracotomy or thoracoscopic approach can be performed; however, visualization into the disk space may be cumbersome or limited, given the tangential angle of approach toward the apex of the chest cavity from a more inferior entry. Midthoracic disk herniations lend themselves well to either posterolateral or anterolateral approaches. Lower thoracic disk herniations can be approached posteriorly in a straightforward manner. Anterolateral approaches can also be performed but can increase the complexity in that a retroperitoneal extension may be necessary.

This chapter describes the most commonly performed anterior and posterior approaches:
- Posterior transpedicular approach
- Posterior costotransversectomy approach
- Posterior lateral extracavitary approach
- Anterolateral transthoracic approach
- Anterolateral video-assisted thoracoscopic approach

COSTOTRANSVERSECTOMY AND LATERAL EXTRACAVITARY APPROACH

RATIONALE

The three posterior approaches can be thought of as a continuum of the same procedure. Each builds on the other, with further exposure and bone removal, to gain better access to the ventral thecal sac. A posterior transpedicular approach will gain the least access to the ventral epidural space, and a

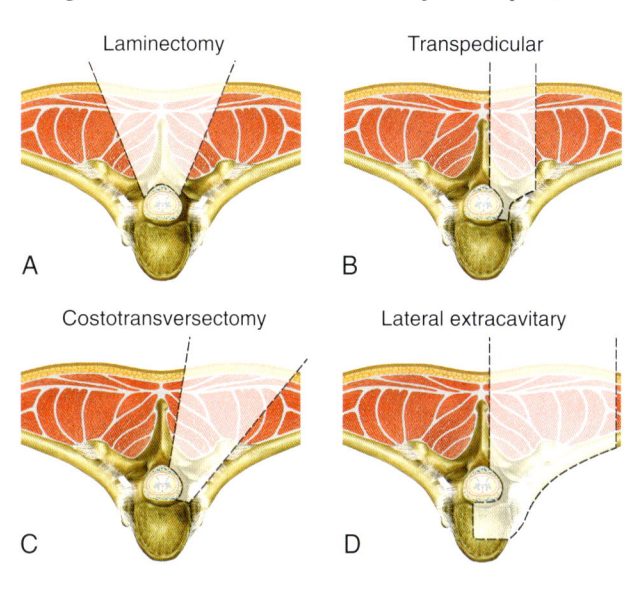

Fig. 24-1 A laminectomy (A) is inadequate for approaching a thoracic disk herniation. Safe posterior approaches include the transpedicular (B), costotransversectomy (C), and lateral extracavitary (D) techniques.

lateral extracavitary will gain the most. The straight posterior laminectomy for thoracic disk herniation has an unacceptably high morbidity rate and poor clinical results. As such, it is not recommended. A transpedicular approach can be accomplished through a midline exposure, laminectomy, and subsequent resection of the desired pedicle and proximal transverse process. This procedure will not be discussed in detail here. Both costotransversectomy and lateral extracavitary approaches involve the same preoperative considerations and preparations. They will be considered together here.

INDICATIONS AND CONTRAINDICATIONS
Indications
- Paracentral, soft thoracic disk herniations
- Myelopathy
- Refractory radiculopathy

Contraindications
- Calcified, midline thoracic disk herniations
- Medical comorbidities
- Spinal instability requiring anterior column reconstruction

OPERATIVE TECHNIQUE
Special Requirements
- Preoperative imaging
- Magnetic resonance imaging (MRI) to characterize the involvement of the neural elements
- Computed tomography (CT) to estimate the density or degree of calcification of the herniated disk
- Scout views such as a T_2-weighted sagittal survey (includes the level of the lesion and landmarks, such as the lumbosacral junction, and may be helpful for comparison during intraoperative localization)
- Intraoperative electrophysiologic monitoring
  - Somatosensory evoked potentials
  - Motor evoked potentials

Equipment
- Radiolucent operating table
- Fluoroscopy
- Headlight system
- Operating microscope
- High-speed drill
- Thoracotomy instruments
- Kerrison punches
- Curettes, including down-pushing curettes
- Instrumentation for fixation, optional
- Image guidance, optional

Patient Positioning
- General anesthesia is used.
- Intraoperative electrophysiologic monitoring baseline is obtained.
- The patient is prone on chest rolls or radiolucent spinal operating table.
- Abdomen should hang freely to decrease epidural venous congestion.
- The patient is taped to the table to facilitate table rotation.

Location of Incision
- Multiple skin incisions have been described:
  - Paramedian incision is made 3 to 6 cm off the midline.
  - Curvilinear incision is made with the apex centered over the area of interest, 3 to 6 cm off midline. This type of incision will allow access to the dorsal midline structures.
  - Lateral extracavitary incision may be made several centimeters further laterally.
- A lateral fluoroscopic image may be obtained with a radiopaque marker over the chest to confirm the level and appropriateness of the trajectory. Typically, the incision is centered over the target level.

Preparation and Draping
- Duraprep is used.
- Draping is routine.
- The table is not turned. The anesthesiologist is at the head of the table. The scrub nurse is at the foot.
- Surgeon works from the side of the approach.
- Microscope, if needed, is brought in from the side opposite the surgeon.

Incision and Soft Tissue Dissection
- Local anesthetic is infiltrated prior to incision.
- Incision is made. Subcutaneous tissue, latissimus dorsi, and thoracodorsal fascia are divided with electrocautery.
- Erector spinae muscles are dissected in a subperiosteal fashion and reflected medially to expose the transverse process and ipsilateral hemilamina (Fig. 24-2).
- Large fishhooks on rubber bands can be very effective in retracting this muscle mass (Fig. 24-3).

Spinal Dissection
- Rib is identified and stripped using electrocautery on the dorsal surface. Subperiosteal dissection circumferentially around the rib is accomplished using various elevators and Doyene rib dissector.
- Transverse process is identified, costotransverse ligament is divided, and transverse process is removed (Figs. 24-4 and 24-5).
- Rib is cut 3 to 6 cm from its origin and dissected from underlying pleura.
- Rib should be mobile, and can be disarticulated after dividing the costovertebral ligament (see Fig. 24-4).
- Pedicle should now be visible.
- Neurovascular bundle can be followed to the foramen (Fig. 24-6).
- Pedicle can be removed with a high-speed drill and Kerrison punches.

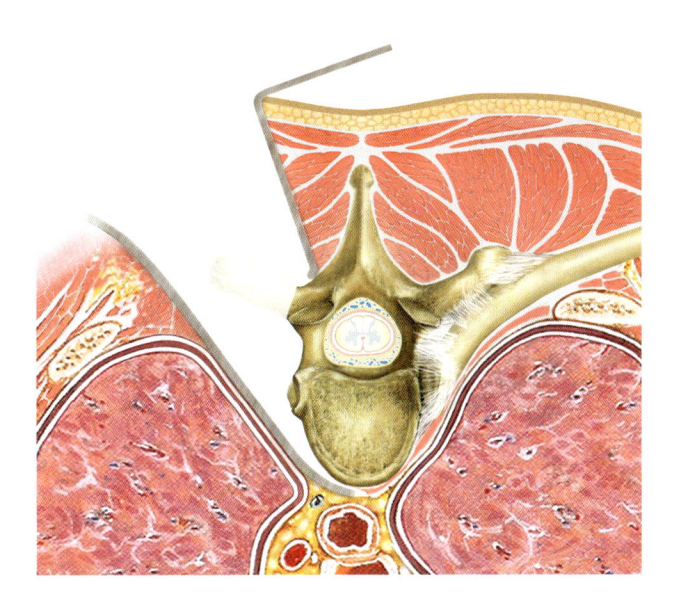

Fig. 24-2 Erector spinae are dissected in a subperiosteal fashion and reflected medially. The dissection is taken laterally to expose the ipsilateral hemilamina, transverse process, and rib.

- This approach will gain access to the spinal canal, and lateral thecal sac should be visible.

Decompression

- Posterior vertebral body immediately adjacent to the disk space can be drilled and removed. This creates a trough into which the disk herniation can be pushed with various curettes (Fig. 24-7).
- This trough can be developed further toward the midline with further lateral exposure. Herein lies the distinction between costotransversectomy and lateral extracavitary approaches. The amount of rib resected in the former is approximately 6 cm, whereas in the latter it is up to 12 cm.
- The table can be rotated away from the surgeon to give better visualization toward midline structures (Fig. 24-8).

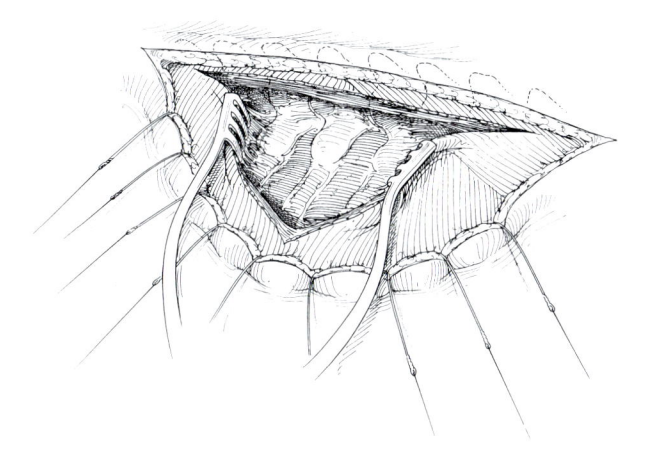

Fig. 24-3 Fish-hook retraction is very effective in retracting tissues laterally while keeping the profile flat. This will facilitate a tangential view of anterior spine structures, especially once the operating table is turned to the contralateral side. (Used with permission from Barrow Neurological Institute.)

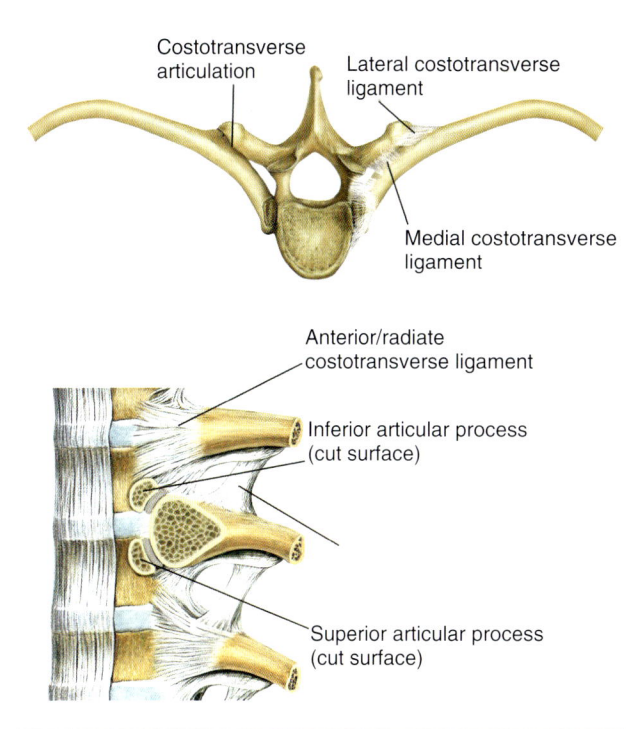

Fig. 24-4 The rib is attached to the vertebral body at two points: the costotransverse and costovertebral articulations. Understanding the triangular anatomic relationship between the transverse process, pedicle, and rib head is critical to the safe exposure of the disk space and spinal canal.

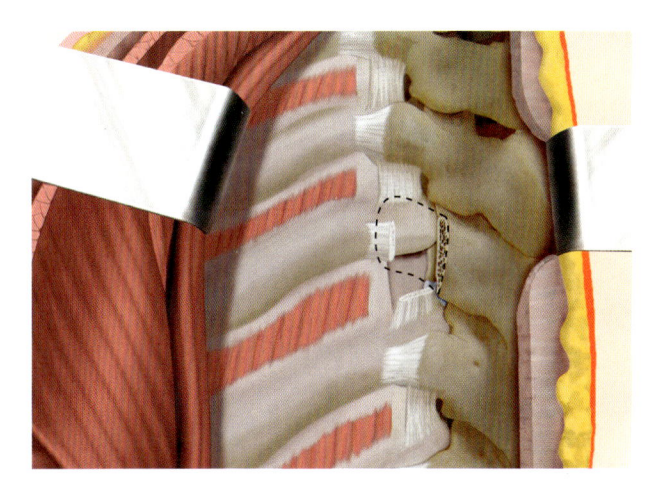

Fig. 24-5 The costotransverse ligament is divided, and the transverse process is removed, exposing the pedicle and underlying rib head.

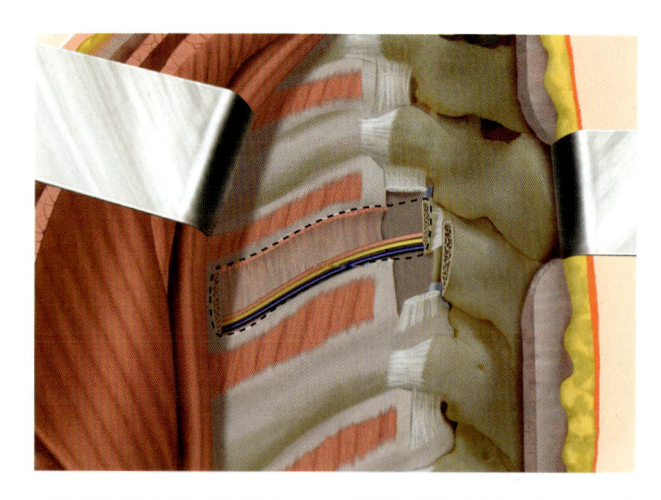

Fig. 24-6 Once the rib head is removed, the neurovascular bundle can be followed to the foramen. Care should be taken in manipulating this structure to avoid bleeding and postoperative intercostal neuralgia.

- Epidural bleeding is controlled with bipolar cautery and Gelfoam powder mixed with thrombin to create a "paste."
- For midline calcified disks image guidance, utilizing 3-D fluoroscopic image guidance can be quite helpful.
- As decompression proceeds, real-time navigation can show if the exposure encompasses the disk herniation.
- After decompression of a calcified disk, postoperative images with 3-D fluoroscopic image guidance can confirm disk removal.

Stabilization

- Arthrodesis and fixation are optional, but should be considered with more aggressive bone removal.
- If significant amounts of vertebral bodies are removed, pieces of harvested rib can be cut to size and impacted into the newly created defect. Troughs can be drilled to allow the rib graft to be seated more securely to reduce the chances of migration.
- If bone graft is placed, its location should be verified with anteroposterior and lateral fluoroscopy.
- A separate midline fascial incision can give access to place pedicle instrumentation.
- Once decompression—and, if undertaken, arthrodesis and instrumentation—is complete, then the field is irrigated with antibiotic solution. The pleura is inspected for any breaches. Small defects can be closed primarily. Large defects require tube thoracostomy.
- Wound is then closed in multiple layers. Subcutaneous drains are not routinely employed.

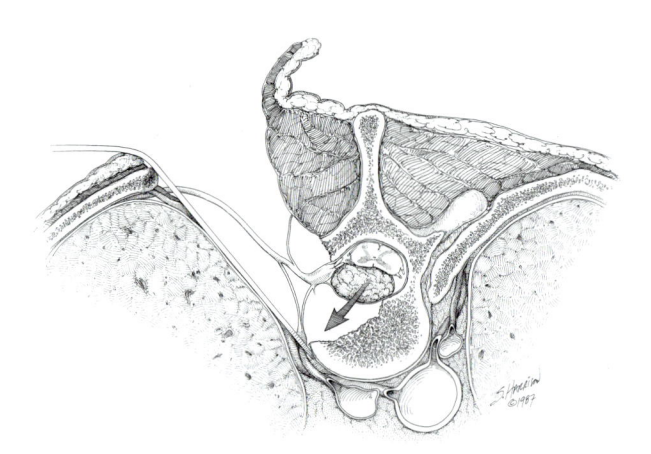

Fig. 24-7 Once a trough has been created in the vertebral body, disk material can be safely dissected away from the cord and into the defect. (Used with permission from Barrow Neurological Institute.)

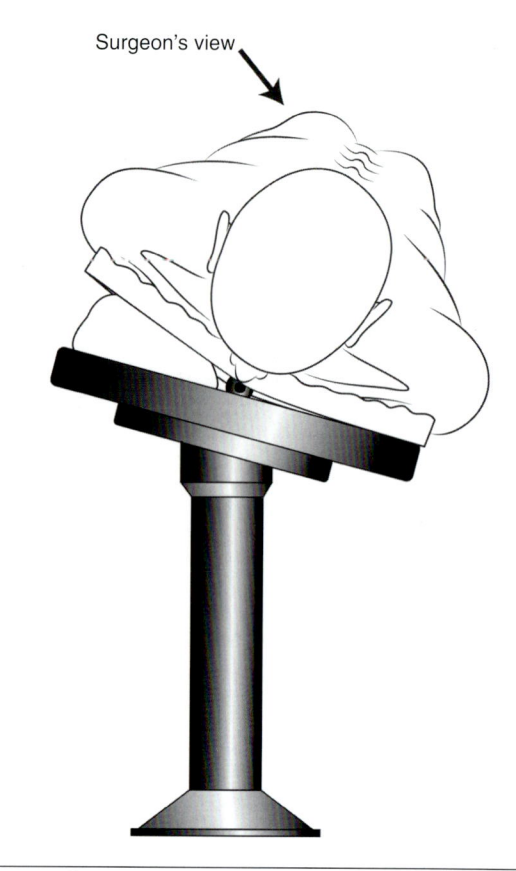

Fig. 24-8 Rotating the operating table to the contralateral side of the exposure facilitates the surgeon's view ventral to the thecal sac and across the midline.

COMPLICATIONS

- Neurologic deficit may be due to hematoma, graft dislodgement, or direct cord trauma. Any deficit should be evaluated with STAT radiographs and MRI.
- Pleural effusion may require thoracentesis or tube thoracostomy.
- Pneumothorax may develop.

- Cerebrospinal fluid leak may be repaired primarily with 5-0 prolene suture. If suture is not possible, fibrin glue can be used to seal leaks.

POSTOPERATIVE CARE

- Patient is monitored overnight in the intensive care unit (ICU).
- PCA (patient-controlled analgesia) pump is utilized for analgesia.
- Postoperative cross-sectional imaging is performed to ensure adequate decompression and appropriate positioning of instrumentation.
- Early ambulation is encouraged.

ANTEROLATERAL OPEN THORACOTOMY APPROACH

RATIONALE

Advantages over posterior approaches include (1) direct and full visualization of the disk herniation, (2) possibly less neurologic morbidity, and (3) facilitation of reconstruction and internal fixation over a shorter segment. The disadvantages include (1) increased risk of medical morbidity, (2) the need for a chest tube, (3) longer hospitalization and recovery, and (4) difficulty in repairing durotomy/cerebrospinal fluid leak.

INDICATIONS AND CONTRAINDICATIONS

Indications

- Debilitating radiculopathy refractory to conservative management
- Myelopathy
- Incapacitating discogenic back pain refractory to conservative management
- Midline or calcified disk herniations

Relative Contraindications

- Lateral or paramedian soft disk herniation (best approached posteriorly)
- Advanced age or medical comorbid conditions
- Inability to tolerate one-lung ventilation
- Previous thoracotomy or pleural infection
  - An extrapleural dissection can be used in this scenario
- Lower thoracic level herniations (may require a combined transthoracic/retroperitoneal approach)

OPERATIVE TECHNIQUE

Special Requirements

- Preoperative imaging
- MRI to characterize the involvement of the neural elements
- CT to estimate the density or degree of calcification of the herniated disk
- Scout views such as a T_2-weighted sagittal survey (includes the level of the lesion and landmarks, such as the lumbosacral junction, which may be helpful for comparison during intraoperative localization)
- Intraoperative electrophysiologic monitoring
  - Somatosensory evoked potentials
  - Motor evoked potentials
- Thoracic surgeon to perform approach

Equipment

- Double-lumen endotracheal tube
- Radiolucent operating table
- Fluoroscopy
- Headlight system
- Operating microscope
- Thoracotomy retractor system
- Thoracotomy instruments
- Long spinal dissection instruments
- Curettes
- Cobb periosteal elevators
- Kerrison punches
- High-speed drill with long attachments
- Optional interbody fusion device (allograft, cage, etc.)
- Optional anterolateral fixation device
- Chest tube

Patient Positioning

- The patient is first positioned supine over a beanbag on the operating table
- Intubation is performed with a double-lumen endotracheal tube to facilitate one-lung ventilation.
- The patient is placed in the lateral decubitus position.
- Side of approach is typically dictated by the eccentricity of the disk herniation. For a midline disk herniation:
  - A left-sided approach is chosen for herniations in the lower third of the thoracic spine, as the aorta at this level is easier to manipulate and protect than the azygous vein.
  - A right-sided approach is chosen for herniations in the upper and middle thirds of the thoracic spine to avoid the aortic arch.
- An axillary roll is placed under the dependent arm.
- The beanbag is deflated with suction. In addition, tape and straps are used to further secure the patient to maintain position.

Location of Incision

- Ribs are identified by palpation and counting.
- A lateral fluoroscopic image may be obtained with a radiopaque marker over the chest to confirm the level and appropriateness of the trajectory. Typically, the incision is centered over the target level.
- Rib resection may be performed to facilitate exposure, or to obtain autologous bone graft material. Given the caudal

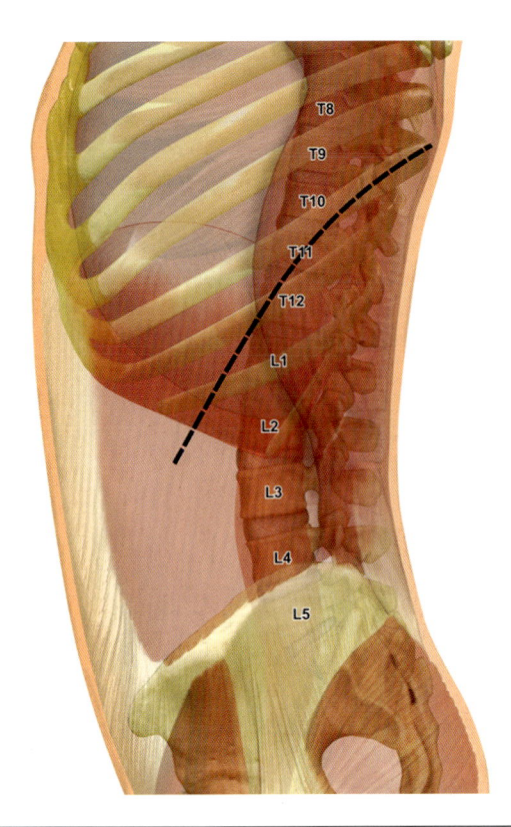

Fig. 24-9 A curvilinear incision is planned. It is centered over the level of the pathology.

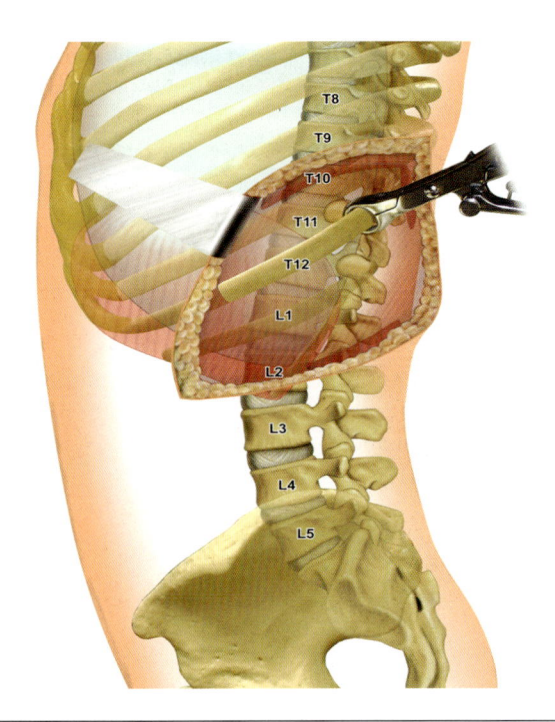

Fig. 24-10 A rib may be removed to facilitate the exposure and to obtain graft material. One to two additional ribs may be "hinged" to expand the aperture as needed.

orientation of the ribs in the lower half of the thorax, an incision may be required one to two levels above the target level, with resection of the rib below.
- A curvilinear incision is planned (Fig. 24-9).

Soft Tissue and Chest Wall Dissection
- The skin is incised in a curvilinear fashion.
- The muscle layers of the chest wall are incised with an electrocautery over the superior aspect of the rib to avoid injury to the neurovascular bundle.
- The parietal pleura is divided.
- A rib may be removed to facilitate the exposure and to obtain graft material. One to two more ribs may be hinged to expand the aperture as needed (Fig. 24-10).
- A self-retaining retractor is placed to spread the ribs and maintain the exposure.

Deep Soft Tissue Dissection and Localization
- The ipsilateral lung is collapsed by the cessation of ventilation. Suction may be applied to collapse the lung further. Direct retraction on the lung is rarely required, but may be accomplished using lap sponge packs or a coiled malleable retractor.
- The parietal pleura overlying the spinal column is divided in a U-shaped fashion, revealing the underlying sympathetic chain and segmental vessels.
- A spinal needle is inserted into the exposed disk space, and a lateral fluoroscopic image is obtained. The level should be confirmed by counting from the lumbosacral junction up to the level of the marker. Anatomic variations or defects in the vertebral bodies may be used as cues as well. The images are compared to the preoperative imaging to confirm the level of the pathology, which is otherwise still obscured. One can also count ribs internally, from the apex of the chest (the second rib is the first visualized in the thoracic cavity) down to the marker (Fig. 24-11).
- The disk is marked to confirm the appropriate level. The overlying sympathetic chain is divided. The segmental vesicles are typically left intact for simple diskectomy, but may be sacrificed if internal fixation is applied to the anterolateral spine.

Spinal Dissection
- A high-speed drill or sharp osteotome is used to transect the rib overlying the disk space approximately 3 cm from the spine. The rib head is mobilized with a Cobb periosteal and curettes, which divides the costovertebral and costotransverse ligamentous attachments. Upon removal of the rib head, the pedicle of the inferior vertebra is exposed.
- The remaining bony dissection and diskectomy should be performed with the aid of the microscope or loupe magnification to adequately visualize the neural elements.

CHAPTER 24 Thoracic Diskectomy

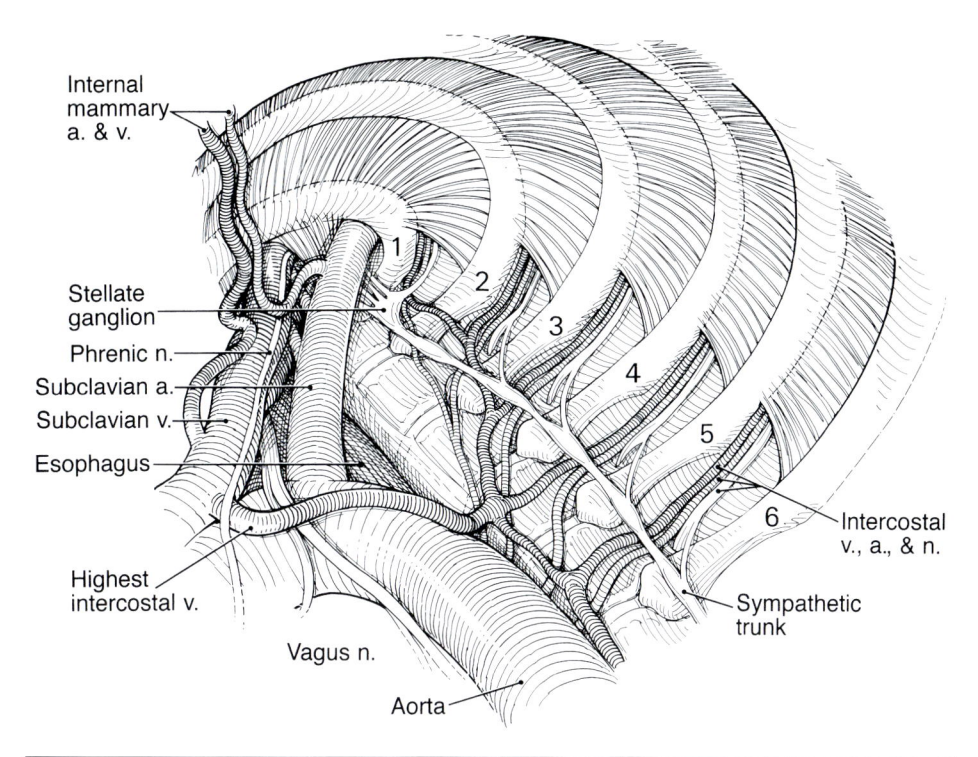

Fig. 24-11 A view into the apex of the left hemithorax. Typically, the second rib is the first seen. The first rib is usually covered by the fat pad. Understanding the anatomic relationship between the sympathetic chain, rib head, and neurovascular bundle with the disk space is of critical importance. (Used with permission from Barrow Neurological Institute.)

- The pedicle is drilled down to a thin shell, and Kerrison rongeurs are used to remove the remaining bone, thus exposing the spinal canal and dura of the thecal sac. Once the neural elements are revealed, the procedure moves along expeditiously.
- The end plates of the vertebral bodies above and below the disk are drilled down, creating a cone-shaped trough based at the level of the spinal canal.
- A series of microcurrettes and pituitary rongeurs are then used to mobilized the disk material off the thecal sac and into the trough (Fig. 24-12). Once the disk is removed, the decompression can be assessed using a nerve hook or Penfield dissector to ensure there is no significant compressive material remaining.

Interbody Arthrodesis and Fixation

- For diskectomies requiring extensive partial vertebrectomies or those near the lumbosacral junction, one may elect to perform an interbody arthrodesis and internal fixation procedure.
- Autologous bone grafting material harvested during the exposure (ribs) and decompression (vertebral body bone dust) may be used alone or in conjunction with an interbody appliance or cage.
- Internal fixation may be achieved by using a screw-plate or screw-rod fixation device.

Closure

- A chest tube is placed with its tip at the apex of the chest cavity, and exited through a separate intercostal stab incision. The chest tube will be placed to 40 cm H_2O suction.

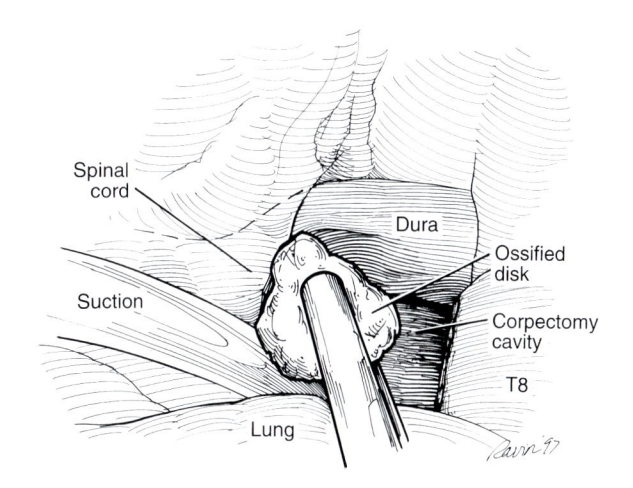

Fig. 24-12 As in the posterior approach, disk material is safely dissected away from the spinal cord by manipulating it into a partial corpectomy defect created in the adjacent vertebral bodies. (Used with permission from Barrow Neurological Institute.)

- A multilayered closure is performed, and sterile dressings are applied.
- Subcutaneous narcotic infusion catheters may be placed to help manage postoperative pain.
- If an interbody arthrodesis was performed without instrumentation, the patient may be braced with external orthoses.

COMPLICATIONS

- A durotomy with cerebrospinal fluid leakage can be closed primarily with sutures or dural clips. Fibrin glue may be used to reinforce the closure, or to manage smaller pinhole leaks. If a cerebrospinal fluid leak is encountered, the chest tube should be placed to water seal, and a lumbar drain should be used until the chest tube is removed.
- Postoperative atelectasis can be minimized by periodically reinflating the lung every 15 to 30 minutes during surgery.

POSTOPERATIVE CARE

- Postoperative imaging should be performed to ensure that the neural elements have been adequately decompressed, that there is no significant residual disk material, and that interbody grafts/devices and instrumentation are in adequate position.
- The chest tube is removed once it is determined that the lung has completely reinflated, and fluid drainage has resolved.
- An external orthoses may be used to manage patients with uninstrumented fusions and to help with pain management.

ANTERIOR VIDEO-ASSISTED THORACOSCOPIC APPROACH

RATIONALE

The advantages over open thoracotomy include less normal tissue disruption, less postoperative pain, less postoperative pulmonary dysfunction, less blood loss, faster recovery, and better cosmetic result. The disadvantages over open thoracotomy include the steep learning curve, longer initial procedure times, and the need for specialized equipment.

INDICATIONS AND CONTRAINDICATIONS

Indications

Indications are the same as for the open thoracotomy technique.

Contraindications

Contraindications are the same as for the open thoracotomy technique, including the following:
- Adhesions from a previous thoracotomy
- Empyema
- Pleurodeisis

OPERATIVE TECHNIQUE

Special Requirements

- Special requirements are the same as for the open thoracotomy technique.
- A thoracic surgeon should be on stand-by in the event of a vascular complication or the need to convert to open thoracotomy.

Equipment

- Double-lumen endotracheal tube
- Radiolucent operating table
- Fluoroscopy
- Thoracotomy instruments (must be prepared to convert to open thoracotomy in an emergency!)
- Access and dissection tools
  - Portals, rigid and flexible (Flexible portals may have a lower incidence of postoperative intercostal neuralgia.)
  - Soft tissue dissection tools (lung retractors, suction, irrigators, forceps, scissors, cotton-tipped dissectors)
- Endoscopic imaging tools
  - 10-mm rigid lenscope (0 and 30 degree)
  - High-resolution digital camera (Three-dimensional endoscopic imaging systems may be used to enhance spatial resolution and depth perception.)
  - Light source (halogen or xenon)
- Endoscope holder
  - Mechanical articulated arm
  - Robotic voice-controlled endoscope holder
- Long spinal dissection instruments (long versions of common instruments used in open procedures with graduated depth markings)
- High-speed drill with long attachments
- Hemostatic tools
  - Unipolar and bipolar cautery
  - Hemoclips
  - Cotton-tipped applier with bone wax
  - EndoAvitene (Davol, Cranston, RI)
  - Sponge stick for large vessel bleeding
- Optional interbody fusion device (allograft, cage, etc.)
- Optional anterolateral fixation device
- Chest tube

Patient Positioning

- Positioning is the same as for the open thoracotomy technique.
- Portal sites are marked.
- An incision for possible emergent thoracotomy is marked.

Portal Placement

- A portal for the endoscope is placed between the posterior and midaxillary lines (Fig. 24-13).

CHAPTER 24 Thoracic Diskectomy

- Difficult on the right side where diaphragm rides higher.
- Use reverse Trendelenburg position to allow abdominal viscera to retract with gravity.
- The diaphragm may be retracted.
- For T10-T12, may need to take down pulmonary ligament and crus of the diaphragm. Retroperitoneal portals may be placed.

Incisions

- 15-mm skin incisions are made for the portals.
- The fascia is incised with electrocautery.
- A blunt clamp is used to dissect through the muscle layers and through the parietal pleura. This is done over the superior aspect of the rib to avoid injury to the neurovascular bundle, which courses along the inferior margin of the rib.
- The endoscope portal is placed first. Subsequent portal placements are performed under direct visualization from within the thoracic cavity to avoid injury to the underlying vascular and visceral structures (Fig. 24-14).

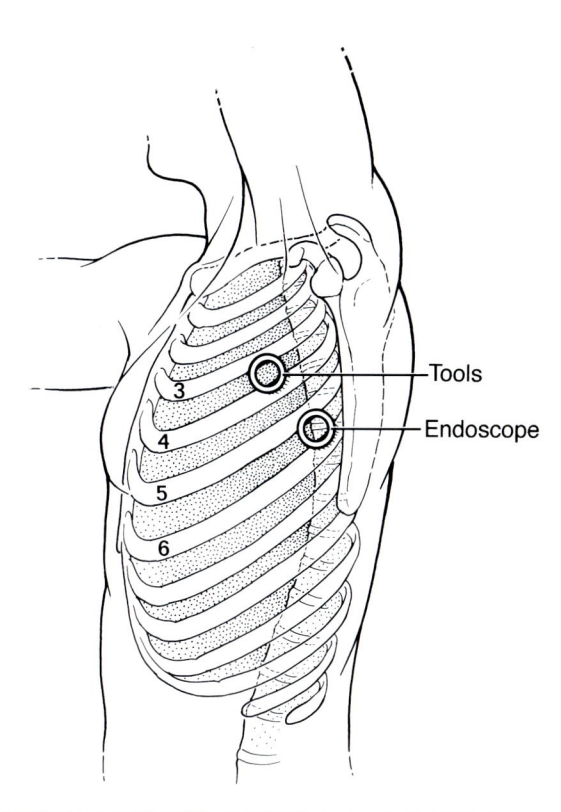

Fig. 24-13 The endoscope portal is typically placed between the mid- and posterior axillary line, immediately overlying the spine at the level of the pathologic lesion. (Used with permission from Barrow Neurological Institute.)

- Instrument portals are placed between the middle and anterior axillary lines. Two to three working portals are typically used. One portal is used for a lung retractor, and two are used for other instruments.
- The portals should be triangulated directly over the level of the pathology.
- The portals should be adequately spaced to avoid interference or "fencing" of instruments and the endoscope within the thoracic cavity.
- Various portal configurations may be employed.
  - In a T-shaped configuration, a 0-degree endoscope is positioned directly over the pathology.
  - In an L-shaped configuration, a 30-degree endoscope is positioned above or below the surgical level. This can be used to avoid "fencing" of instruments, or to avoid portal placement near critical structures.
- T1-T4 levels
  - Position portals near inferior edge of axilla.
  - Do not enter axillary space to avoid injury to brachial plexus and axillary vessels.
  - Avoid entering first or second intercostal space to protect subclavian vessels.
- T5-T9 levels: straightforward T- or L-shaped configuration is employed.
- T10-L1 levels

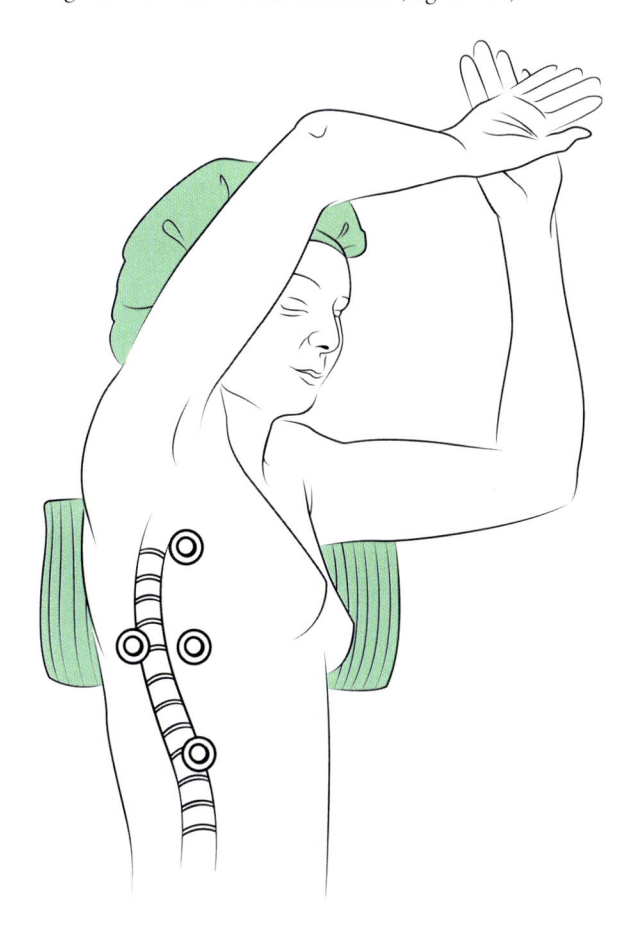

Fig. 24-14 The endoscope portal is placed first. Subsequent portal placements are performed under endoscopic visualization from within the thoracic cavity to avoid injury to the underlying vascular and visceral structures. Instrument portals are placed more anteriorly, and spaced appropriately to avoid crowding or "fencing" of instruments within the thoracic cavity.

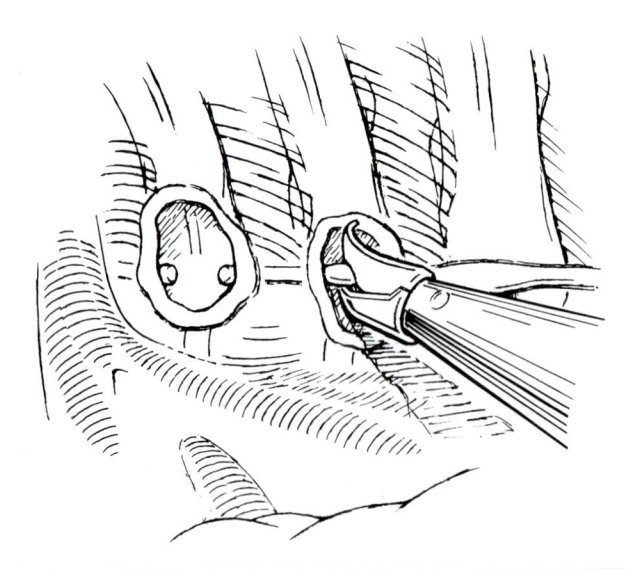

Fig. 24-15 As in the open approach, the exposure of the spine begins by mobilizing the parietal pleura and exposing the underlying structures. The safest approach is to begin over the rib head. The subpleural dissection should be undertaken with caution to avoid injury to the neurovascular bundle and great vessels. (Used with permission from Barrow Neurological Institute.)

Exposure
- Lung retraction can be accomplished in a number of ways.
- The lung may be deflated by the anesthesiologist with cessation of ventilation through a double-lumen endotracheal tube or by the use of a blocker.
- A fan retractor can be used to further retract the lung.
- The bed may be turned to allow the lung to fall away from the spine.
- If encountered, pleural adhesions can be taken down with monopolar cautery scissors.

Localization
- Ribs may be counted from within the thoracic cavity. The second rib is consistently seen at the apex, just below the fat pad.
- Once exposed, a disk space can be marked with a long K-wire, and fluoroscopic imaging is used to count to the appropriate level, as in the open technique.

Deep Soft Tissue Dissection
- The parietal pleura is incised over the rib head with the monopolar cautery scissors (Fig. 24-15).
- The edge of the pleura is grasped with forceps and the incision is extended with a pleural hook dissector. As the disk space and adjacent vertebral bodies are exposed, care is taken to avoid injury to the underlying segmental vessels.
- Soft tissue hemostasis can be achieved with monopolar or bipolar cautery.

Spinal Dissection
- The rib head is mobilized using a rib dissector to transect the costoverterbral and costotransverse ligaments and articulations.
- An osteotome or high-speed drill is used to transect the rib head approximately 3 cm from the spine.
- The rib head is removed, revealing the underlying dorsal aspect of the disk space and the pedicle of the inferior vertebral body.
- A curette is used to incise the foraminal ligaments along the inferior edge of the pedicle.
- A Kerrison rongeur is used to remove the inferior portion of the pedicle to expose the dura of the thecal sac in the spinal canal (Fig. 24-16).
- A high-speed drill is used to drill a trough into the adjacent dorsal vertebral bodies along the edge of the disk.
- An irrigation/suction instrument is used to clear debris and blood.
- Herniated disk material is pulled back into the trough using microcurettes.
- Bone bleeding is controlled with bone wax applied on a cotton-tipped applicator. Epidural venous bleeding can be readily controlled with EndoAvitene or a thrombin/Gelfoam mixture.

Spinal Reconstruction and Internal Fixation
- A graft or cage may be introduced through one of the portals and mortised within the defect using an impactor and mallet.

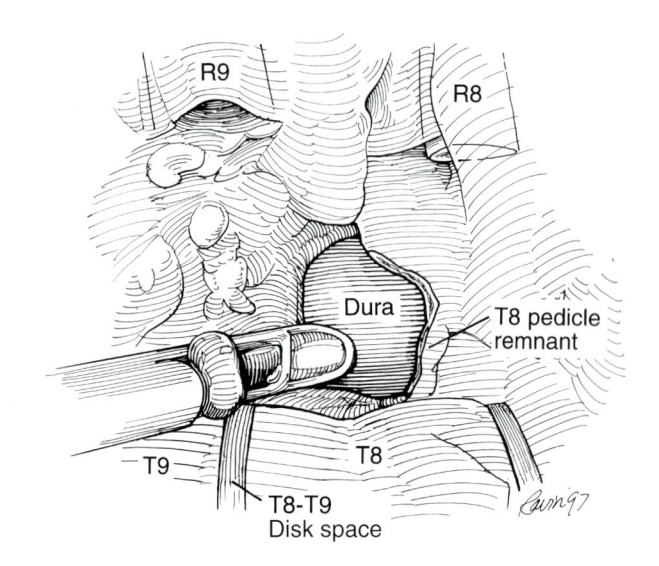

Fig. 24-16 As in the open approach, the rib heads are removed first. The underlying pedicles are then exposed. By removing some bone from the inferior aspect of the cephalad pedicle, the spinal canal and dura can be identified. Only after these structures are identified can the dissection and decompression proceed safely. (Used with permission from Barrow Neurological Institute.)

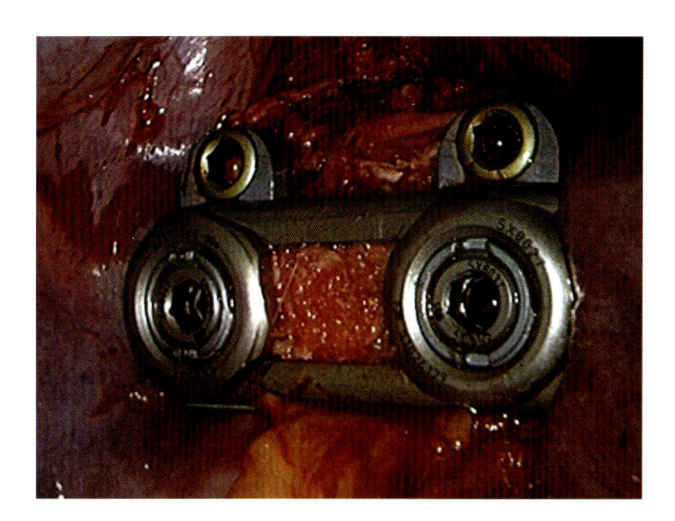

Fig. 24-17 Conventional screw-plate or screw-rod instrumentation may be used for internal fixation. Additional portals may be needed to facilitate a perpendicular trajectory over the vertebral levels to be fixated for the placement of the screws.

- Screw-plate or screw-rod instrumentation may be used for internal fixation. Additional portals may be needed to facilitate a perpendicular trajectory over the vertebral levels to be fixated for the placement of screws. Rods or plates may be introduced through one of the portals as well (Fig. 24-17).

Closure

- A chest tube is inserted through one of the portal sites and secured.
- The other portal sites are closed. The fascia and skin are closed separately.

COMPLICATIONS

- Durotomy with cerebrospinal fluid leak may be managed as in open thoracotomy.
- A large durotomy can be closed with suture using endoscopic needle holders and knot-tying device. Endoscopic clip appliers for dural closure are also available.
- Fibrin glue may also be applied.
- As previously mentioned, a lumbar drain should be placed and chest tube kept on water seal only.

SECTION D
Lumbar Disk Herniation

CHAPTER 25

ARTHUR J. ULM, III
ERICH O. RICHTER
DAVID A. PEACE
JEFFREY S. HENN

Lumbar Microdiskectomy: Midline Open and Far-Lateral Techniques

INTRODUCTION

Several large clinical series have been published detailing the clinical features, indications,[1-3] operative results,[4-19] and potential complications[2,20-24] of lumbar disk surgery. The goal of this chapter is to describe the surgical technique and pertinent anatomy of lumbar disk surgery.

ANATOMY

In the normal spine there are five lumbar vertebrae. However, in some instances L5 may be "sacralized," or conversely, the S1 vertebral body may be "lumbarized," making precise localization dependent on the nomenclature of the radiologist reading the imaging study. In these instances, disagreement by one level may occur when one observer counts down from T12 and another counts up from S1.

The bony spinal canal is made up of three parts: the vertebral body anteriorly, the pedicles laterally, and finally the posterior bony elements. These bony constituents are connected to each other by ligaments, muscles, and the intervertebral disk (Figs. 25-1 and 25-2). As a major source of both flexibility and weight bearing in the spine, the lumbar vertebrae are relatively large structures compared to their counterparts in the thoracic and cervical regions.

The intervertebral disk consists of three parts: a cartilaginous base covering the end plates of adjacent vertebral bodies, a semigelatinous nucleus pulposis, and the anulus fibrosis, which surrounds the nucleus and resists lateral forces produced by axial compression. The posterior longitudinal ligament attaches to the disk space posteriorly and to the margins of the vertebral bodies above and below the disk space. The posterior longitudinal ligament tends to thin out laterally and is thickest at the midline.

The posterior elements of the lumbar vertebral unit consist of the pedicles, transverse and spinous processes, facet surfaces, lamina, and the pars interarticularis (see Fig. 25-2). There are two superior and two inferior facet surfaces. The superior facet surface lies dorsal to the disk space above the vertebral segment and articulates with the inferior facet surface of the next superiorly placed vertebral body. The inferior facet lies dorsal to the disk space below the vertebral segment and articulates with the superior facet of the next inferiorly placed vertebra (see Fig. 25-2). The pedicles extend from the dorsolateral surface of the vertebral body just below the superior end plate. The pedicles lie ventral and slightly inferior to the superior articular facet surface. The pars interarticularis or isthmus is a bony bridge connecting the superior and inferior facet surfaces and is continuous medially with the hemilamina of the vertebral segment (see Fig. 25-2). The two hemilaminae converge in the midline to form the dorsally projecting spinous process. The transverse process projects from the dorsolateral surface of the pedicle. The mammillary process is a raised bony prominence on the proximal dorsal aspect of the transverse process that serves as an external landmark for the long axis of the underlying pedicle. The intertransverse ligaments connect adjacent transverse processes.

The ligamentum flavum, or yellow ligament, attaches to the undersurface of adjacent lamina and overlies the spinal epidural space. The ligamentum flavum ends laterally at the level of the facet joint. The yellow ligament is often hypertrophied in degenerative diseases of the lumbar spine.

Nerve roots exit the spinal canal at the level of the corresponding pedicle. For example, the L4 nerve root crosses the L3-L4 disk space and exits the spinal canal beneath the L4 pedicle prior to crossing the L4-L5 disk space. After exiting the foramen, the L4 nerve root crosses the L4-L5 disk space

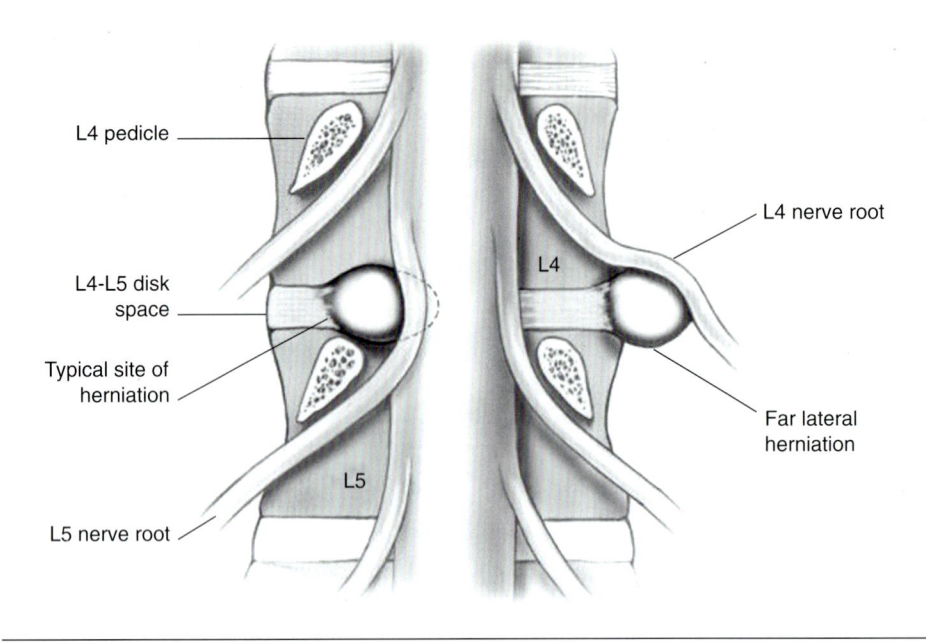

Fig. 25-1 The bony spinal canal.

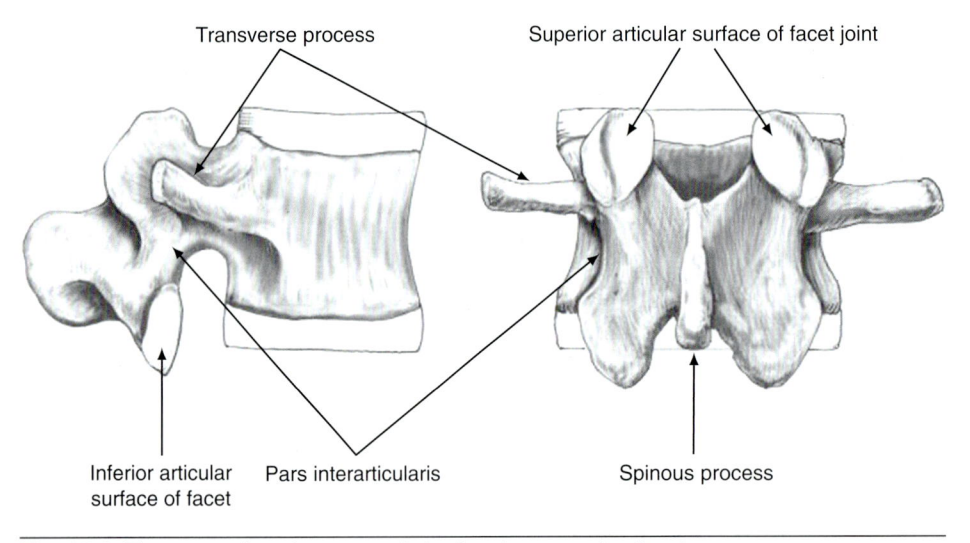

Fig. 25-2 The posterior elements of the lumbar vertebral unit.

at its lateral margin (see Fig. 25-1). Therefore, typical paramedian disk herniations affect the lower spinal nerve root so that an L4-L5 disk herniation would result in compression of the L5 nerve root. However, the L4 nerve root can be compressed by a foraminal disk herniation or by an extraforaminal or far lateral disk herniation at L4-L5.

TECHNIQUE

Lumbar disk surgery can be performed under local, spinal, or general anesthesia. The most common position for patients undergoing a lumbar diskectomy is prone; however, a variation of the lateral decubitus postion can also be used. When the patient is prone, an attempt to reduce intrathoracic and intra-abdominal pressure should be undertaken to reduce epidural venous congestion and bleeding during the procedure. We prefer the use of the Wilson frame, although simple bolstering with large gel rolls can accomplish the task.

OPEN STANDARD MICRODISKECTOMY

The first step in any lumbar diskectomy is localization of the appropriate level. In an attempt to perform surgery through as small an opening as possible, an intraoperative x-ray or fluoroscopic localization is standard practice. Once localized, a 1- to 2-inch midline incision incorporating the appropriate spinous process is performed. The initial incision is carried through the skin and subcutaneous tissues down to the level of the lumbar spinal fascia. A self-retaining retractor is inserted and unipolar electrocautery or a scalpel is used to make a linear midline incision through the lumbar fasica. The next step in the dissection is the removal of the paravertebral muscle from the spinous process, laminae, and medial portion of the facet joint overlying the affected intervertebral disk space. There are several methods for performing the muscle dissection. We employ unipolar electrocautery to minimize bleeding, but many surgeons prefer periosteal dissectors. The key is to stay in the subperiosteal plane in order to limit muscular trauma and bleeding. Once the muscle has been dissected free, a deep retractor is placed. The choice of retractor is determined by surgeon preference and familiarity. The goal of the dissection so far has been to expose half of the lamina above and below the interspace, as well as the entire intralaminar and intraspinous space out to the medial facet joint (Fig. 25-3A).

The next step in the procedure is to perform a hemilaminotomy by removing the inferior edge of the superior lamina overlying the disk space. In some cases, when the interlaminar space is wide, it is possible to perform a diskectomy without performing the hemilaminotomy. However, it has been our experience that the additional exposure added from the bony removal outweighs any advantage in operative time gained by skipping the step. The added exposure allows for better visualization and usually results in less retraction of the nerve root. The traditional technique for performing the hemilaminotomy involves stripping the ligamentum flavum from the undersurface of the lamina using a curette, followed by removal with a punch such as a Kerrison rongeur (see Fig. 25-3B to D). Another approach is to use a high-speed drill, usually under the microscope, to complete the exposure of the underlying ligament. The ligament is opened sharply with a scalpel and is excised or removed piecemeal with a rongeur (see Fig. 25-3E). Removal of the ligament exposes the epidural space with a variable amount of fat covering the dura of the thecal sac medially and the nerve root inferior and lateral to the thecal sac. Bipolar cautery is used to coagulate epidural veins and shrink epidural fat, allowing the identification of the exiting nerve root. Palpation of the dorsal vertebral body with a blunt dissecting instrument provides a means for identifying the disk space. At this point an intraoperative x-ray is taken to confirm that the dissector is at the appropriate interspace. Inspection of the nerve takes place prior to diskectomy. Free fragments of disk may be located beneath the exiting nerve root and may be displaced caudally or rostrally in relation to the interspace. If a disk fragment is found, it should be removed prior to retraction of the nerve root to prevent a retraction injury caused by retracting a root that is already mechanically deformed by a herniated disk fragment. Some surgeons do not enter the disk space if a large free fragment is found. We typically enter the space and remove what disk "comes easily" to minimize the likelihood of recurrent herniations (see Fig. 25-3F).

After radiographic confirmation, the disk space is entered sharply using a scalpel. A small window is made through the anulus to allow access to the disk space. Up and down facing right-angle curettes and various sizes of pituitary punches are used to perform the diskectomy (see Fig. 25-3G). Care must be taken not to violate the anterior disk margin, as catastrophic vascular injuries could occur. After the diskectomy is performed the visible course of the nerve is inspected and palpated with blunt right-angled instruments to ensure adequate decompression. The disk space is copiously irrigated with an angiocath to flush out any free intradisk fragments. Likewise, the foramen is palpated to assess for foraminal narrowing due to bony overgrowth or disk protrusion. If needed, a foraminotomy can be performed at this point to further decompress the nerve.

The wound is copiously irrigated and bleeding is stopped with hemostatics and bipolar cautery. The fascia of the lumbar musculature, the dermis, and the skin are closed as separate layers.

TRANSMUSCULAR FAR LATERAL DISKECTOMY

Foraminal and extraforaminal disk herniations present unique challenges to the spine surgeon. Approaching these lesions from a midline exposure requires extensive muscular retraction and often extensive removal of the facet joint and pars interarticularis in order to access the disk fragment. We prefer to approach these lesions through a paramedian muscle-splitting route.[25] In the transmuscular approach, the patient is positioned prone on a Wilson frame. The incision is placed 5 to 8 cm from the midline to allow for an oblique approach to the foramen and disk space. The exposure is centered over the pars or isthmus of the affected level. For example, in the case of an L4-L5 lateral disk herniation causing L4 radiculopathy, the trajectory would be from lateral to medial and the L4 isthmus would be the center of the operative field. In addition, the L4 transverse process would be the upper limit of the exposure.

The initial steps of the technique include intraoperative confirmation of the level with fluoroscopy, a 3- to 4-cm skin incision 5 to 8 cm off the midline centered over the pars interarticularis (Fig. 25-4A). The superficial lumbar musculature is divided longitudinally between the muscle fibers, and a self-retaining retractor is placed. At this point surgical landmarks, including the isthmus and transverse process as well as the intertransverse ligament, are clearly defined (see Fig. 25-4B). The intertransverse ligament is detached from the trailing edge of the rostral transverse process and retracted laterally. A crescent-shaped area of bone, which includes the angle between the superior aspect of the isthmus and the inferior portion of the rostral transverse process, is removed using a high-speed drill (see Fig. 25-4C). The removal of bone should expose the lateral ligamentum flavum and the inferior aspect of the pedicle underlying the transverse process. At this

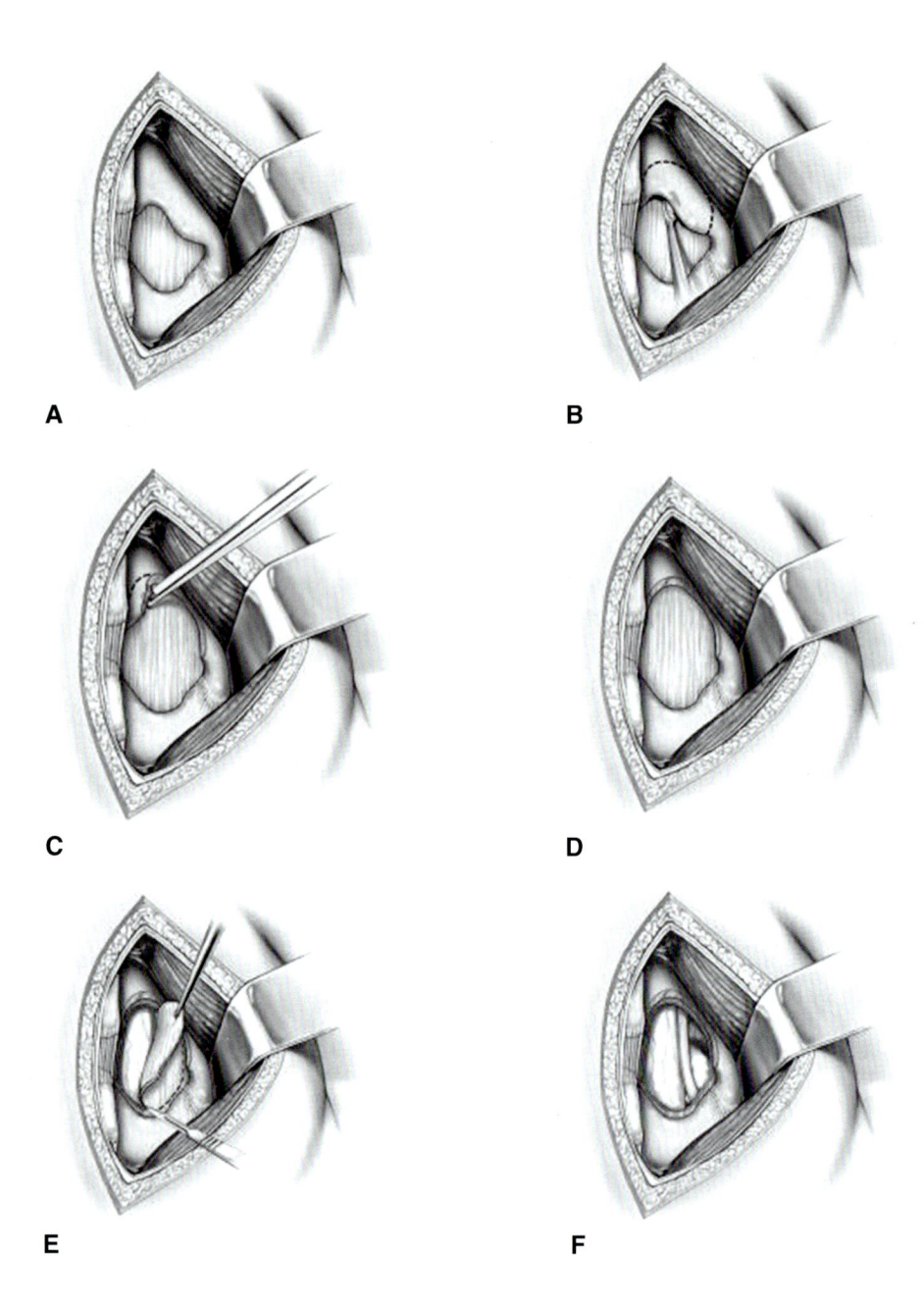

Fig. 25-3 *A*, The dissection exposes half of the lamina above and below the interspace, as well as the entire intralaminar and intraspinous space out to the medial facet joint. *B* to *D*, The traditional technique for performing the hemilaminotomy involves stripping the ligamentum flavum from the undersurface of the lamina using a curette followed by removal with a punch such as a Kerrison rongeur. *E*, The ligament is opened sharply using a scalpel and excised or removed piecemeal with a rongeur. *F*, Enter the space and remove what disk "comes easily" to minimize the likelihood of recurrent herniations. *G*, Up- and down-facing right-angle curettes and various sizes of pituitary punches are used to perform the diskectomy.

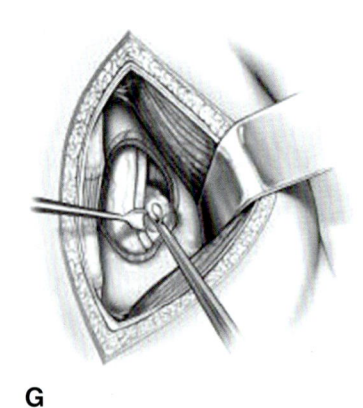

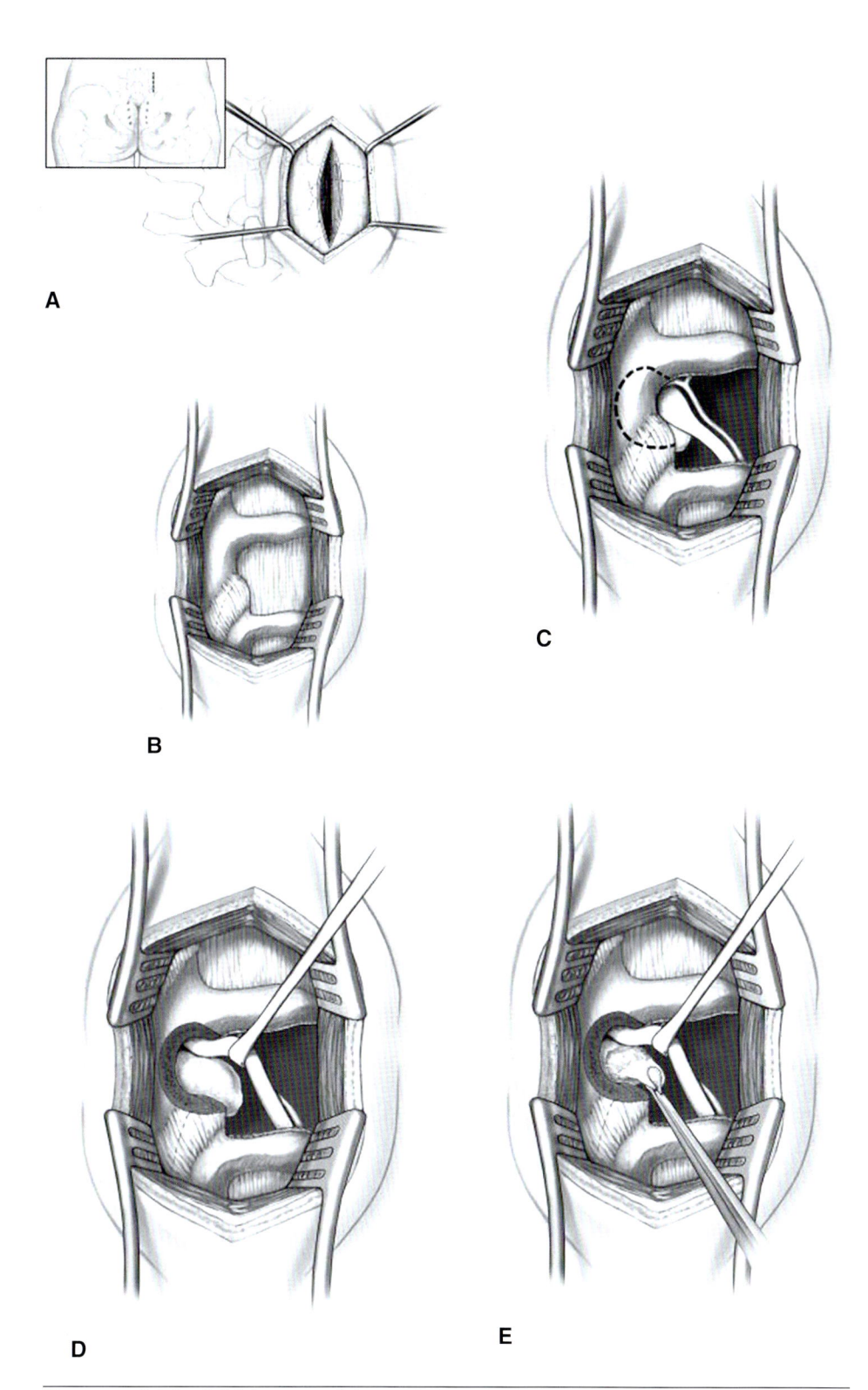

Fig. 25-4 *A,* The initial steps of the technique include intraoperative confirmation of the level with fluoroscopy, a 3- to 4-cm skin incision 5 to 8 cm off the midline centered over the pars interarticularis. *B,* Surgical landmarks, including the isthmus and transverse process, as well as the intertransverse ligament, are clearly defined. *C,* A crescent-shaped area of bone, which includes the angle between the superior aspect of the isthmus and the inferior portion of the rostral transverse process, is removed using a high-speed drill. *D,* Begin the inspection of the nerve medially using a blunt microinstrument to gently retract the nerve in a lateral direction. *E,* The disk space is opened sharply medial to the nerve, and a limited diskectomy is performed.

point the lateral ligamentum is resected using a Kerrison rongeur, which exposes the dorsal root ganglion of the affected nerve (see Fig. 25-4C).

The ganglion and nerve are often displaced superiorly and laterally by the underlying disk herniation. Therefore, we begin our inspection of the nerve medially using a blunt microinstrument to gently retract the nerve in a lateral direction (see Fig. 25-4D). The free fragment or disk bulge is usually found medial and inferior to the exiting root. The nerve can be followed distally if a fragment has migrated from the usual position. Extensive distal dissection should be undertaken with care because of the presence of lumbar arteries and veins entering the lower foramen as well as the presence of the dorsal primary ramus exiting from the more distal nerve root. The disk space is opened sharply medial to the nerve, and a limited diskectomy is performed (see Fig. 25-4E). The final step in the procedure is to explore the foramen where the nerve exits just below the pedicle. The maneuver is carried out using a blunt nerve hook and assures that no sequestered fragments are left in the foramen.

The wound is copiously irrigated, and bleeding is stopped with hemostatics and bipolar cautery. The fascia of the lumbar musculature, the dermis, and the skin are closed as separate layers.

References

1. Nygaard OP, Kloster R, Solberg T: Duration of leg pain as a predictor of outcome after surgery for lumbar disc herniation: A prospective cohort study with 1-year follow up. J Neurosurg Spine 2000;92:131–134.
2. Schaller B: Failed back surgery syndrome: The role of symptomatic segmental single-level instability after lumbar microdiscectomy. Eur Spine J 2004;13:193–198.
3. Tureyen K: One-level one-sided lumbar disc surgery with and without microscopic assistance: 1-year outcome in 114 consecutive patients. J Neurosurg Spine 2003;99:247–250.
4. Findlay GF, Hall BI, Musa BS, et al: A 10-year follow-up of the outcome of lumbar microdiscectomy. Spine 1998;23:1168–1171.
5. Gaetani P, Aimar E, Panella L, et al: Surgery for herniated lumbar disc disease: Factors influencing outcome measures: An analysis of 403 cases. Funct Neurol 2004;19:43–49.
6. Asch HL, Lewis PJ, Moreland DB, et al: Prospective multiple outcomes study of outpatient lumbar microdiscectomy: Should 75 to 80% success rates be the norm? J Neurosurg Spine 2002;96:34–44.
7. Barlocher CB, Krauss JK, Seiler RW: Central lumbar disc herniation. Acta Neurochir (Wien) 2000;142:1369–1374; discussion 1374–1365.
8. Ferrer E, Garcia-Bach M, Lopez L, et al: Lumbar microdiscectomy: Analysis of 100 consecutive cases: Its pitfalls and final results. Acta Neurochir Suppl (Wien) 1988;43:39–43.
9. Goffin J: Microdiscectomy for lumbar disc herniation. Clin Neurol Neurosurg 1994;96:130–134.
10. Haglund MM, Moore AJ, Marsh H, et al: Outcome after repeat lumbar microdiscectomy. Br J Neurosurg 1995;9:487–495.
11. Hirabayashi S, Kumano K, Ogawa Y, et al: Microdiscectomy and second operation for lumbar disc herniation. Spine 1993;18:2206–2211.
12. Ng LC, Sell P: Predictive value of the duration of sciatica for lumbar discectomy: A prospective cohort study. J Bone Joint Surg Br 2004;86:546–549.
13. Pappas CT, Harrington T, Sonntag VK: Outcome analysis in 654 surgically treated lumbar disc herniations. Neurosurgery 1992;30:862–866.
14. Patel N, Pople IK, Cummins BH: Revisional lumbar microdiscectomy: An analysis of operative findings and clinical outcome. Br J Neurosurg 1995;9:733–737.
15. Postacchini F, Cinotti G, Perugia D: Microdiscectomy in treatment of herniated lumbar disc. Ital J Orthop Traumatol 1992;18:5–16.
16. Quigley MR, Bost J, Maroon JC, et al: Outcome after microdiscectomy: Results of a prospective single institutional study. Surg Neurol 1998;49:263–267; discussion 267–268.
17. Schoeggl A, Maier H, Saringer W, et al: Outcome after chronic sciatica as the only reason for lumbar microdiscectomy. J Spinal Disord Tech 2002;15:415–419.
18. Schoeggl A, Reddy M, Matula C: Functional and economic outcome following microdiscectomy for lumbar disc herniation in 672 patients. J Spinal Disord Tech 2003;16:150–155.
19. Wang JC, Shapiro MS, Hatch JD, et al: The outcome of lumbar discectomy in elite athletes. Spine 1999;24:570–573.
20. Gaston P, Marshall RW: Survival analysis is a better estimate of recurrent disc herniation. J Bone Joint Surg Br 2003;85:535–537.
21. Kotilainen E: Long-term outcome of patients suffering from clinical instability after microsurgical treatment of lumbar disc herniation. Acta Neurochir (Wien) 1998;140:120–125.
22. Kotilainen E, Valtonen S: Clinical instability of the lumbar spine after microdiscectomy. Acta Neurochir (Wien) 1993;125:120–126.
23. Leung PC: Complications in the first 40 cases of microdiscectomy. J Spinal Disord 1988;1:306–310.
24. Solberg TK, Nygaard PO, Sjaavik K, et al: The risk of "getting worse" after lumbar microdiscectomy. Eur Spine J 2005;14:49–54.
25. Tessitore E, de Tribolet N: Far-lateral lumbar disc herniation: The microsurgical transmuscular approach. Neurosurgery 2004;54:939–942; discussion 942.

CHAPTER 26

ERICH O. RICHTER
ARTHUR J. ULM, III
DAVID A. PEACE
JEFFREY S. HENN

Percutaneous and Endoscopic Diskectomy

INTRODUCTION AND HISTORICAL PERSPECTIVE

The anatomy and techniques of lumbar microdiskectomy have been extensively discussed in a previous chapter. In this chapter, we will explore the reasons to employ a minimally invasive approach, and the technical differences from the open approach.

The first to use an endoscope to approach the lumbar disk was Poole in 1938.[1,2] Over the ensuing decades, several authors experimented with minimally invasive procedures such as chymopapain injections,[3] percutaneous lumbar nucleotomy,[4] intradiskal electrothermy,[5] and laser diskectomy.[6-8] Beginning in 1983, Kambin worked extensively with arthroscopic techniques to perform lumbar microdiskectomy from a posterolateral approach.[9-11] The use of endoscopic techniques continued to develop throughout the next decade with Schreiber and Suizawa's biportal endoscopic approach,[12] Smith's far lateral approach,[13] and Matthews and Ditsworth's transforaminal uniportal approach.[14,15] Advances in instrumentation also provided better visualization and ease of manipulating tissue through these small working channels.[16] Despite the advantages of each of these approaches, none could surpass the excellent results and low morbidity of standard microdiskectomy.[16,17]

In 1997, Smith and Foley introduced the MED (microendoscopic diskectomy) system, a muscle-dilating, minimally invasive posterior approach to perform the same decompression and exploration that was offered by standard microdiskectomy.[18] The system was rapidly followed by the second generation version, called the METRx (microscopic endoscopic tubular retractor) system, which incorporated several improvements, including a choice of retractor diameter, improved optics, and versatility in allowing the surgeon to use the operating microscope to visualize along the retractor instead of the endoscope.[19]

One advantage of the endoscope is the availability of angled scopes that with developed exposure may yield visualization beyond the edge of the retractor. However, the instrumentation currently in widespread use may not truly allow the surgeon to operate in this increased visual range without employing techniques such as wanding (discussed later), which would also bring these areas within the view of the operating microscope. The operating microscope has the advantage of being stereoscopic, but technologic advances are producing smaller and more functional stereoscopic endoscopes, and these instruments may make stereoscopic endoscopic diskectomy a reality in the near future. The need to visualize from a vantage point proximal to the working channel for the instruments may cause difficulty with either the visualization or lighting when using the operating microscope. These difficulties are usually overcome easily with the use of bayoneted instrument sets, or occasionally with the use of readily available retractor-mounted fiberoptic illumination sources. The use of an endoscope makes bayoneted instrumentation unnecessary, and eliminates the ergonomic issues related to head position, because the display is positioned to the preference of the surgeon regardless of the position of the retractor, whereas the operating microscope must be positioned coaxially with the retractor. These relatively minor benefits of the endoscope are often outweighed by the learning curve required to master these techniques,[20] whereas the operating microscope is very familiar to neurosurgeons. No clear advantage has been demonstrated for one technique over the other, and the use of one or the other remains essentially a matter of surgeon preference. The authors routinely use the minimally invasive approach with the operating microscope, and this chapter has been written primarily from this perspective.

The advantages of a minimally invasive approach to lumbar diskectomy include (1) the smallest skin incision possible for the exposure obtained and (2) the use of muscle dilators for the soft tissue approach.

TABLE 26-1 Complication Rates, Length of Hospitalization, and Average Time to Return to Work with Minimally Invasive Microdiskectomy

AUTHOR/YEAR	NO. OF PATIENTS	COMPLICATION RATES	LENGTH OF HOSPITALIZATION	AVERAGE LENGTH OF TIME TO RETURN TO WORK
Perez-Cruet et al, 2002[23] (MED)	150	Total 9%: 5% dural tears 0.7% delayed pseudomeningocele 0.7% superficial wound infection 2.6% recurrent disk herniation	Average 7.7 hours	17 days
Palmer, 2002[24] (METRx)	135	0.7% superficial wound infection 2.9% recurrent disk herniation 0.7% spinal stenosis	Average 24 hours	32.1 days
Brayda-Bruno & Cinnella, 2004[21] (METRx)	68	4% intraoperative cerebrospinal fluid leak	18–24 hours	No data
Muramatsu et al, 2002[22] (MED)	110	No data	8.1 days	2–3 months (physical), less time for return to "desk jobs"

The use of a muscle-dilating exposure, as opposed to a muscle incision, minimizes disruption of fascia, ligament, and muscle, which may lead to a shorter hospital stay.[20-22] This decreased recovery time has been demonstrated in endoscopic posterior cervical laminoforaminotomy,[23] and it is hoped that reduced recovery time will be demonstrated for lumbar diskectomy as well. Outcomes have been shown to be equivalent to open diskectomy,[21,22,24] though there was a learning curve to the technique[19,20] with a higher incidence of dural tears earlier in the process.[20] One series demonstrated earlier postoperatrive ambulation, a reduction in intraoperative blood loss, and decreased need for postoperative pain medications.[22] Average lengths of hospital stays have been reported to be short, and patient recovery quick[20,22] (Table 26-1). Series have shown very short hospital stays with minimally invasive lumbar diskectomy[20–22] (as little as 7.7 hours[17]) that compare favorably with traditional microdiskectomy, but it cannot be denied that there is an increasing trend toward outpatient traditional microdiskectomy, although no randomized trial has yet been published.

SURGICAL TECHNIQUE

The primary difference between a standard microdiskectomy and a minimally invasive diskectomy lies in the exposure prior to the hemilaminotomy. Thereafter, the operation is essentially the same.

For a minimally invasive lumbar diskectomy, the patient is typically positioned prone on a radiolucent operating table, and the correct level is identified with intraoperative lateral C-arm fluoroscopy. The midline is marked, and the appropriate trajectory is determined using a spinal needle and lateral fluoroscopy, with attention that the tip of the needle is never inserted below the depth of the lamina. The needle should be in line with the disk space to be explored.

Once the appropriate entry site has been determined, a Steinmann pin is inserted approximately 2.5 cm from midline on the side of the disk herniation. The pin is advanced to the junction of the lamina and facet under continuous lateral fluoroscopic guidance (Fig. 26-1). Although

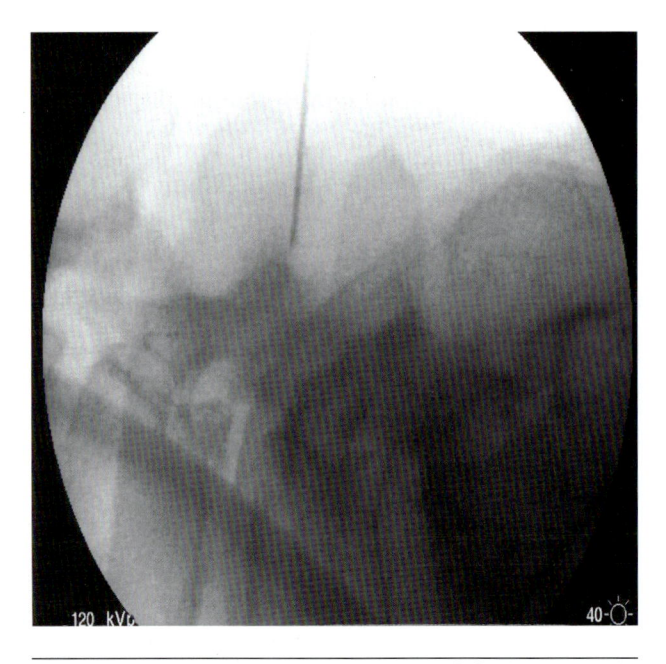

Fig. 26-1 Lateral fluoroscopic view of Steinmann pin placement. The Steinmann pin is placed under continuous fluoroscopic guidance until it is docked firmly against bone.

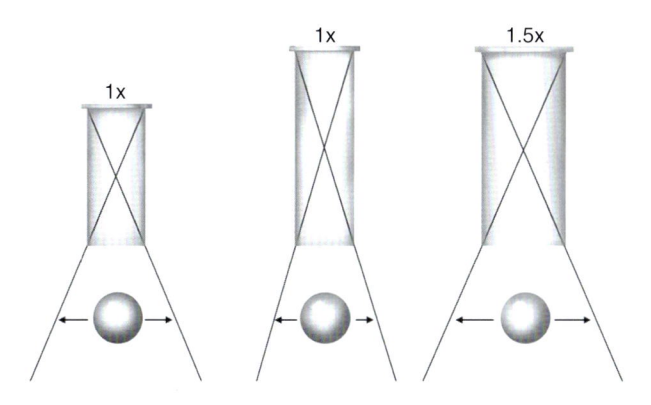

CHAPTER 26 Percutaneous and Endoscopic Diskectomy

Fig. 26-2 Relationship of working angle and field of view to retractor length and width. As the length of the retractor increases at a given width, the working angle and field of view decrease. In order to maintain the working angle and the field of view, the width of the tubular retractor must be increased as well.

This process is repeated sequentially with a series of larger dilators (Fig. 26-3). It is important to keep each dilator firmly docked on the bone. There is a tendency for a slight loss of depth with each progressive dilator, usually because the muscle is compressed under the advancing edge of the dilator rather than passing around it. This can be avoided by rotating each dilator into place rather than simply pushing it in, and by sweeping slightly back and forth as each dilator is fully inserted. This sweeping motion as the dilators are inserted dissects the muscle from the bony surface of the lamina as well, and minimizes the need for excessive monopolar dissection of muscle once the final tubular retractor is in place.

When the final dilator is placed, the depth is read off the scale on the side of the dilator, and the appropriate tubular retractor is placed with the same rotating motion. This allows the final trajectory of the dialators and retractor will have a slightly medial orientation, it is best at this stage to maintain a more vertical orientation and contact the medial facet surface with the Steinmann pin. The pin should not be advanced beyond the junction of the facet and lamina, as the sharp tip of the pin can damage structures such as the exiting nerve root laterally, or the dura and nerve roots medially.

Once the Steinmann pin is in firm contact with bone, a skin incision centered on the pin is made of a length sufficient for the intended tubular retractor. Usually, an 18- to 22-mm incision suffices for a lumbar diskectomy. This length will be partially dictated by the depth of the exposure, as tubular retractors become progressively more difficult to work through as they get longer. This is partially due to the decreased working angle available with increasing retractor length (Fig. 26-2).

For example, in a thinner patient, an 18-mm tubular retractor provides sufficient exposure at an operating depth of 5 cm—this provides a working angle of 19.7 degrees. In a slightly more obese patient, requiring a 6-cm retractor, this angle is reduced to 16.7 degrees. In order to obtain the equivalent exposure in the larger patient, the width of the retractor would need to be increased to 21.6 mm.

The lumbodorsal fascia is strong, and may be very resistant to the initial placement of the dilators. A No. 15 blade may be passed along the Steinmann pin to make a generous opening in the fascia, which greatly increases the ease of the insertion of the sequential dilators.

The first dilator is then placed over the Steinmann pin, and when it is firmly docked on bone, the pin is removed. Once the sharp pin is removed, the risk of injury is greatly diminished. Under fluoroscopic guidance, the dilator is swept medially off the facet and back and forth along the trailing edge of the lamina to dissect the muscle from the lamina. If necessary, this may be monitored with fluoroscopy.

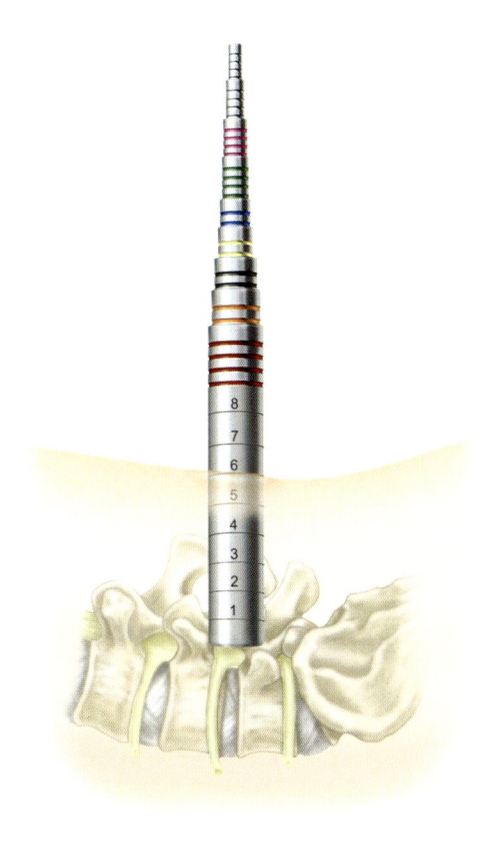

Fig. 26-3 Muscle dilators. Once the Steinmann pin has been verified to be in correct position, a series of muscle dilators are sequentially passed over each other until the working channel is the desired width. The Steinmann pin is removed after the first dilator is placed to reduce the risk of injury, particularly dural puncture. As the dilators are placed, it is important to check intermittently with fluoroscopy to verify that they remain in correct position. The dilators are marked with a depth scale on the outer surface that indicates the appropriate length of the tubular retractor. (Courtesy of Medtronic Sofamor Danek, Memphis, TN.)

the shortest possible tubular retractor to be used, maximizing the working angle. The tubular retractor is connected to the table with an adjustable attachment device.

It is usually recommended that the mounting device be attached to the table on the contralateral side from the surgeon, but the important point is that it is positioned in such a way as to not be in the surgeon's way during the operation. Some have felt that it holds its position better in the arc made when they position it ipsilaterally. It is very important to place it out of the line of fluoroscopy for the operative levels, as it is not radiolucent. Of note, it is a rail-mounted device, and an adapter is necessary when using it with a Jackson table.

It is important to note that patients with lumbar pathology have a high incidence of significant facet hypertrophy, which may hamper placement of the tubular retractor of the desired width at the desired depth (Fig. 26-4A and B). This problem is addressed by simply replacing the tubular retractor with a longer retractor later in the dissection after a medial facetectomy allows deeper placement (see Fig. 26-4C). When a change of retractors is necessary, it is easily accomplished by replacing the largest dilator within the retractor. The retractor can then be removed, and the new retractor is replaced into the same position over the dilator.

The exposure at this point (Fig. 26-5A to C) consists of a tubular retractor centered over the interlaminar space with the base of the spinous process medially, the medial facet laterally, the trailing edge of the upper lamina rostrally, and the leading edge of the lower lamina caudally. There will generally be some remaining muscle tissue on the lamina and there may be some muscle bleeding.

The exposure is probed with a nerve hook to clearly identify these landmarks, the bone is cleaned, and hemostasis is obtained with unipolar electrocautery with a long insulated bayoneted Teflon tip. Because the instruments are bayoneted, there are separate left, right, and forward angled nerve hooks available. Any cauterized muscle tissue may be removed with pituitary rongeurs. When the bony anatomy is clearly delineated, the operating microscope is brought onto the field, or the endoscope is inserted, and the remainder of the operation proceeds as discussed in Chapter 25.

The exposure is centered on the trailing edge of the superior lamina (see Fig. 26-5A). Some portion of the medial aspect of the facet is typically visible in the lateral aspect of the field and may have been partially resected to achieve proper placement of the retractor. Depending on the patient and the size of the retractor being used, the superior edge of the lamina of the level below may be clearly visible, or may be only palpable below the area visualized using a nerve hook. The base of the spinous process should be readily palpable just medial to the retractor edge.

Once the bony surface has been cleared with monopolar electrocautery, the hemilaminotomy (see Fig. 26-5B) and removal of the ligamentum flavum expose the thecal sac. A long drill extension is helpful for the bone work, and when using the operating microscope, an angled drill is nearly essential. The lateral aspect of the thecal sac and the disk space is then explored, with bipolar electrocautery of the

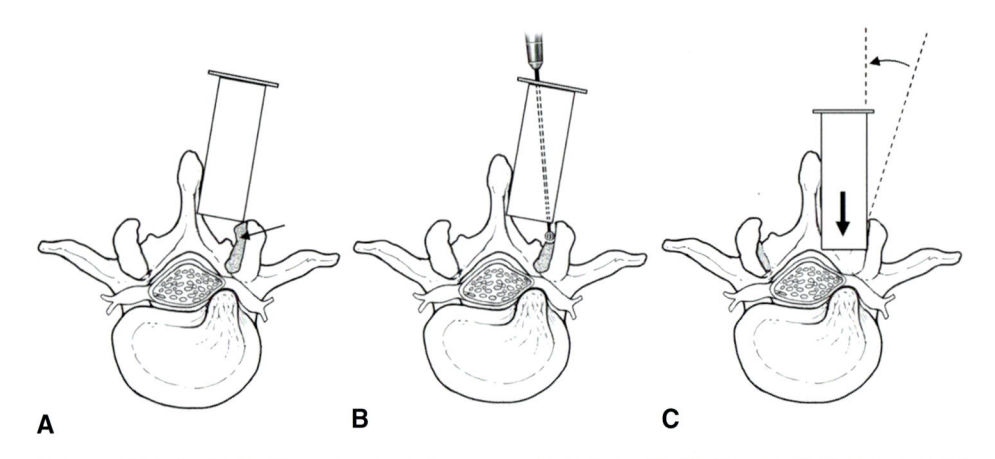

Fig. 26-4 Effect of facet hypertrophy on retractor placement. *A,* Facet hypertrophy is common in the population that requires surgical decompression for disk herniation. This facet hypertrophy can make appropriate placement of the tubular retractor virtually impossible. *B,* Through the exposure gained by the initial placement of a shorter tubular retractor, a judicious medial facetectomy can be performed, usually without destabilizing the level. *C,* With removal of the hypertrophied medial facet, the path is clear for exchange over dilators of the shorter retractor for the appropriate length retractor that reaches to the trailing edge of the lamina. This retractor can now be positioned appropriately without obstruction.

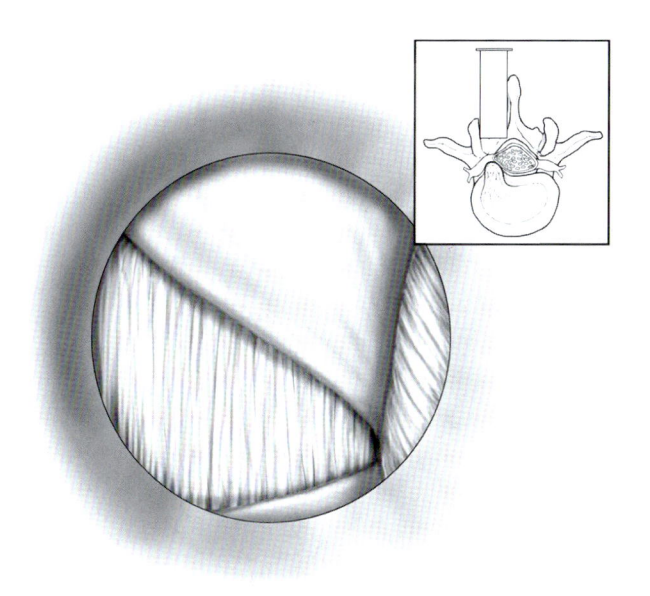

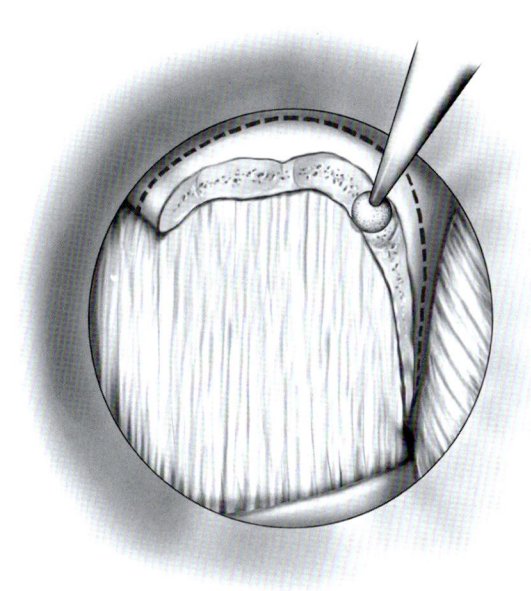

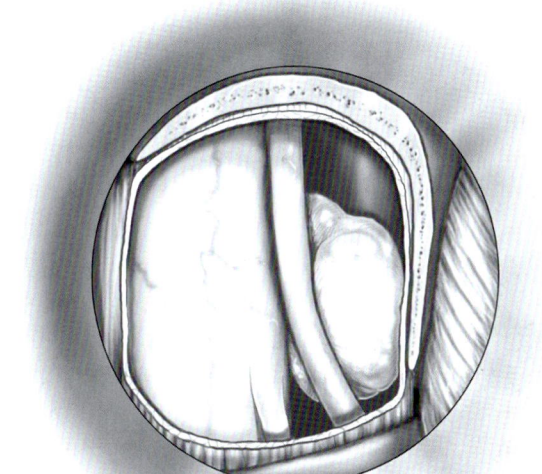

CHAPTER 26 Percutaneous and Endoscopic Diskectomy

Fig. 26-5 Operative exposure through tubular retractors. *A*, The trailing edge of the superior lamina and upper edge of the inferior lamina are exposed. Laterally, the medial aspect of the facet is visible, although it may have been previously removed to gain appropriate placement of the retractor. The spinous process is medial, and cannot typically be seen, though the lamina can be seen making its characteristic upward sweep into it. The spinous process should be palpable with a nerve hook. *B*, The laminotomy is performed as in a standard open microdiskectomy. *C*, After removal of the ligamentum flavum and standard dissection of the nerve root and coagulation of epidural veins, the disk herniation is identified and removed as in a standard open microdiskectomy.

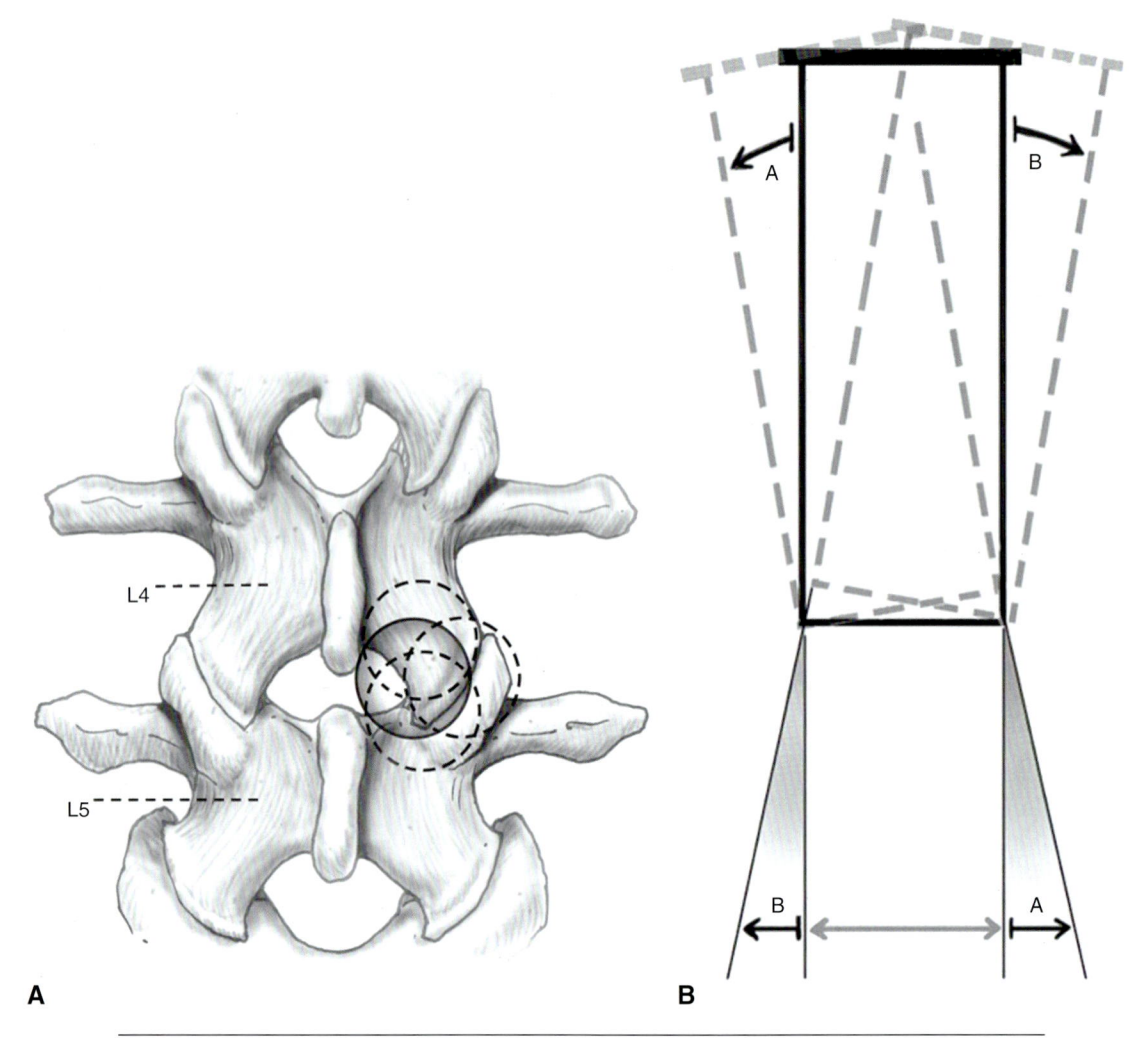

Fig. 26-6 The operative exposure can be significantly increased in a sequential fashion by the technique known as "wanding." Although only the portion at the end of the retractor is visible at any one moment, at different times during the operation the surgeon may angle the retractor differently (*B*) to provide a view of different parts of the operative field (*A*).

epidural veins. The disk herniation is identified and annulotomy and disk removal are as in a standard open diskectomy (see Fig. 26-5*C*).

The exposure at the depth of the wound may be maximized by "wanding" (Fig. 26-6*A* and *B*). When used with the operating microscope, it is impossible to visualize more of the operative field than the area just around the end of the tubular retractor. However, the retractor can be reangled to provide a different view. This is accomplished by reinserting the largest dilator to act as a handle, loosening the snake-type retractor holder, redirecting the tubular retractor, and retightening the holder. This allows a progressive adjustment in view angle throughout the procedure and effectively allows the operative field to be significantly larger than the area of the tip of the retractor, though only a portion of that field can be visualized at any given time.

Retractors also exist that are expandable distally, increasing the exposure.

After obtaining adequate local hemostasis, the retractor is withdrawn slowly, and the walls of the dilated muscle are examined carefully for any bleeding. If any bleeding is identified, it is stopped with brief monopolar or bipolar electrocautery. One or two absorbable sutures in the lumbodorsal fascia are sufficient, and the skin may be closed according to the surgeon's preference. Patients are observed in the recovery room and discharged according to routine same-day surgery criteria.

CONCLUSION

Although this is a new technique, it is clear that the clinical results are at least comparable to open microdiskectomy in terms of reduction of pain and length of hospital stay. In addition, the cost effectiveness of minimally invasive diskectomy should be taken into account. Palmer has reported an 18% mean savings per case over the traditional microdiskectomy.[24] Indications for minimally invasive dissection are virtually the same as for the open approach, and patients may benefit from the decreased tissue disturbance of the muscle-dilating approach. Minimally invasive diskectomy provides an excellent alternative to standard microdiskectomy for some patients. The trend toward minimally invasive techniques has been largely patient-driven, and we await studies that will clarify the perceived benefits in terms of hospital stay, cost, and return to activity.

References

1. Pool J: Myeloscopy: Intraspinal endoscopy. Surgery 1942;11:169–82.
2. Pool JL: Direct visualization of dorsal nerve roots of the caude equina by means of a myeloscope. Arch Neurol Psychiatr 1938;39:1308–1312.
3. Smith L: Enzyme dissolution of the nucleus pulposus in humans. JAMA 1964;265:137–140.
4. Hijikata S, Yamagishi M, Nakayama T, Oomori K: Percutaneous discectomy: A new treatment method for lumbar disc herniation. J Toden Hosp 1975;5:5.
5. Saal JS, Saal JA: Management of chronic discogenic low back pain with a thermal intradiscal catheter: A preliminary report. Spine 2000;25:382–388.
6. Hellinger J: Technical aspects of the percutaneous cervical and lumbar laser-disc-decompression and -nucleotomy. Neurol Res 1999;21:99–102.
7. Choy DS, Case RB, Fielding W, et al: Percutaneous laser nucleolysis of lumbar disks. N Engl J Med 1987;317:771–772.
8. Liebler WA: Percutaneous laser disc nucleotomy. Clin Orthop 1995;311:58–66.
9. Kambin P, O'Brien E, Zhou L, et al: Arthroscopic microdiscectomy and selective fragmentectomy. Clin Orthop 1998;347:150–167.
10. Kambin P, Savitz MH: Arthroscopic microdiscectomy: An alternative to open disc surgery. Mt Sinai J Med 2000;67:283–287.
11. Kambin P: Arthroscopic microdiscectomy. Arthroscopy 1992;8:287–295.
12. Schreiber A, Suezawa Y: Transdiscoscopic percutaneous nucleotomy in disk herniation. Orthop Rev 1986;15:35–38.
13. Smith MM, Foley KT, Ondra SL: Endoscopic working channel diskectomy for far lateral disk herniation. Annual Meeting of the Congress of Neurological Surgeons. San Francisco, CA, 1995.
14. Ditsworth DA: Endoscopic transforaminal lumbar discectomy and reconfiguration: A postero-lateral approach into the spinal canal. Surg Neurol 1998;49:588–597; discussion 97–98.
15. Mathews HH: Transforaminal endoscopic microdiscectomy. Neurosurg Clin North Am 1996;7:59–63.
16. Mayer HM, Brock M: Percutaneous endoscopic discectomy: Surgical technique and preliminary results compared to microsurgical discectomy. J Neurosurg 1993;78:216–225.
17. Gibson JNA, Grant IC, Waddell G: Surgery for lumbar disc prolapse. Cochrane Database of Systematic Reviews Database, 05-26-04. Accessed Oct. 27, 2004.
18. Foley KT, Smith MM: Microendoscopic discectomy. Tech Neurosurg 1997;3:301–307.
19. Thongtrangan I, Le H, Park J, et al: Minimally invasive spinal surgery: A historical perspective. Neurosurg Focus 2004;16:E13.
20. Perez-Cruet MJ, Foley KT, Isaacs RE, et al: Microendoscopic lumbar discectomy: Technical note. Neurosurgery 2002;51:S129–S136.
21. Brayda-Bruno M, Cinnella P: Posterior endoscopic discectomy (and other procedures). Eur Spine J 2000;9(Suppl 1):S24–S29.
22. Muramatsu K, Hachiya Y, Morita C: Postoperative magnetic resonance imaging of lumbar disc herniation: Comparison of microendoscopic discectomy and Love's method. Spine 2001;26:1599–1605.
23. Perez-Cruet MJ, Fessler RG, Perin NI: Review: Complications of minimally invasive spinal surgery. Neurosurgery 2002;51:S26–S36.
24. Palmer S: Use of a tubular retractor system in microscopic lumbar discectomy: 1 year prospective results in 135 patients. Neurosurg Focus 2002;13:1–4.

SECTION E
Lumbar Stenosis

CHAPTER 27

JIN-WOO HUR

DANIEL H. KIM

Surgical Anatomy and Operative Techniques of Lumbar Stenosis

GENERAL CONSIDERATIONS

The spectrum of lumbar stenosis is broad, ranging from single nerve root compression to constriction of the cauda equina over several levels. In lumbar stenosis, the sagittal or transverse diameters of the spinal canal, or both, are reduced at one or more levels by osteophytic hypertrophy on the facet joints and by thickening of the ligamentum flavum. A sagittal diameter of the spinal canal of between 10 and 15 mm is considered a relative stenosis, and a diameter of less than 10 mm an absolute stenosis.

The nerve root coursing in the lateral recess can be compressed gradually by degenerative changes of the superior articular process, which is considered a lateral stenosis. The L4-L5 and L5-S1 joints are affected most frequently.

SYMPTOMS

The symptoms of lumbar stenosis are so typical that the diagnosis is rarely difficult to make. Typical symptoms of central stenosis include low back pain and bilateral sciatic-type pain that are experienced after the patient has walked a certain distance, forcing him or her to sit down (intermittent claudication). These symptoms are occasionally accompanied by paresthesia and weakness of the thighs. Walking uphill or while leaning forward is usually less painful than walking downhill or with an erect gait.

Unilateral radicular leg pain, which is increased under stress (walking or extension of back), is associated with a narrow lateral recess that compresses the nerve root.

Surgical relief of radicular pain and claudication can be just as dramatic for most patients, but for some patients, pain and disability remain in spite of apparently adequate surgical decompression.

SURGICAL APPROACH

The surgical approach for a patient must be planned in accordance with the level and degree of pathologic condition present. The traditional approach to spinal central stenosis is a wide total laminectomy, which preserved the pars interarticularis. Subsequently, given a possibility of postoperative instability and spondylolisthesis, the interlaminar decompression was developed (also called *laminotomy*). The interlaminar decompression allows for decompression of the central canal, lateral recess, and neural foramina above and below the disk space while keeping the part of laminar arch, spinous process, and midline ligamentous structures, and thus maintaining the spinal stability.

Compression of a single nerve root in the lateral recess may be dealt with adequately by a hemilaminectomy above and below the involved nerve root with removal of bone along the course of the nerve root laterally through its foramen.

OPERATIVE TECHNIQUES

TOTAL LAMINECTOMY

Positioning of the patient on the operating table is the same as lumbar disk surgery—providing flexion for the lumbar spine and keeping the abdomen free. A precise midline incision is made directly over the spinous processes. If a total laminectomy is planned, the fascia is opened in the midline.

Using an elevator, the paravertebral musculature is bilaterally retracted laterally over the facet joints and so that both laminae are exposed (Figs. 27-1). Because of the usually massive enlargement of facets at the L3-L4 and L4-L5 levels, the overlying paravertebral musculature is wrapped inward may adhere to the ligamentum flavum, and there is no epidural fat at the level of the compression.

The laminectomy is started at the lower margin of lamina with the Leksell rongeur and Kerrison punch, taking away bone in the midline to the upper part of the lamina and exposing the superior margin of ligamentum and the dura, which is vulnerable to tear in this region because it can be folded easily by the rongeur or punch.

A high-speed drill is then used to create bilateral troughs at the medial margin of the facets (Fig. 27-3). Using first a cutting and then a diamond-tip bit, the surgeon can safely drill through the lower two thirds of the lamina. At the superior third of the lamina, however, it is best to use the drill only to thin down the ventral cortex to avoid dural tears, where there is no protective ligamentum flavum. The remainder of the laminectomy is then performed with a fine 2- or 3-mm Kerrison punch. The surgeon should work with prudence using a fine dissector and cottonoid pads beneath the lamina.

The lateral part of the ligamentum flavum is now removed with a small 2- or 3-mm Kerrison punch. At this point, the medial third of the facet joint may be removed with the Kerrison punch or, preferably, a microdrill (Fig. 27-4). It is important not to resect the joint and the inferior articular process too extensively, and not to make the isthmus too thin. Removal of more than the medial one third of the facet is rarely required. If the facet joint removal is confined to

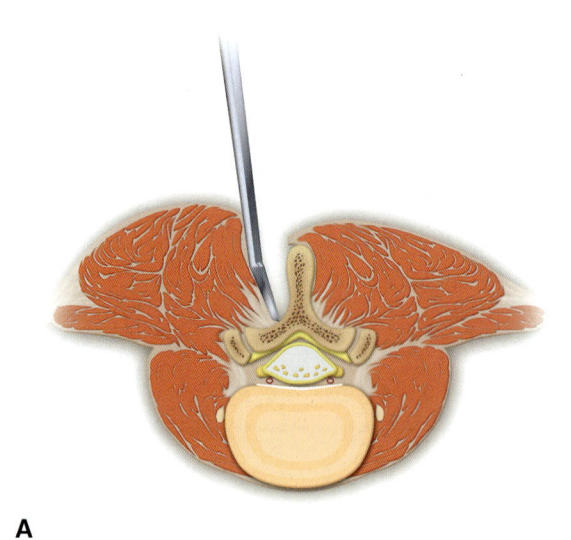

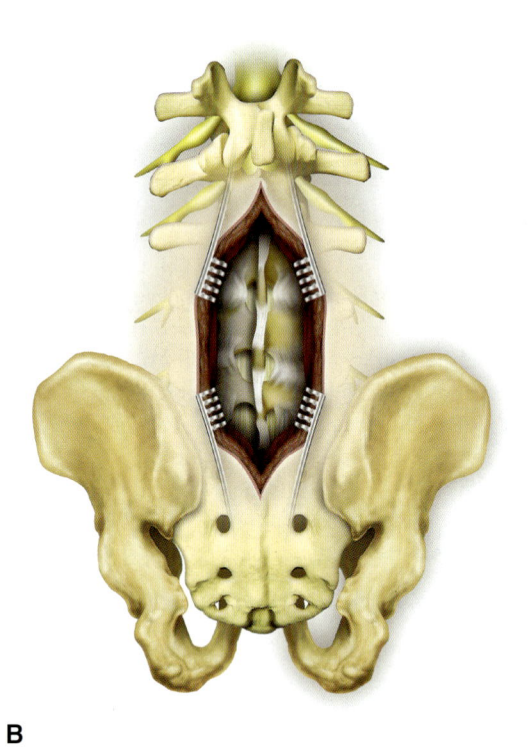

Fig. 27-1 Using an elevator, the paravertebral musculature is bilaterally retracted laterally over the facet joints to expose both laminae. *A*, Axial view of the muscular dissection. *B*, Operative view of the muscular dissection.

with hypertrophy of the facets. The fine electrocautery needle is used to minimize muscle injury with careful outward retraction.

The spinous process is removed with the part of laminae (Fig. 27-2). Using a curved dissector, the ligamentum flavum is dissected and retracted from the lower border of the arch (see Fig. 27-2). This is an important step, because the dura

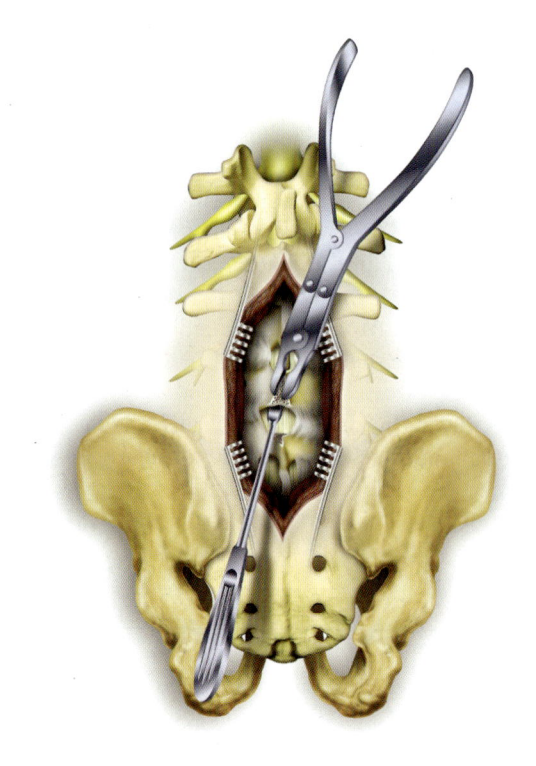

Fig. 27-2 The spinous process is removed with the part of laminae. Using a curved dissector, the ligamentum flavum is dissected and retracted from the lower border of the arch.

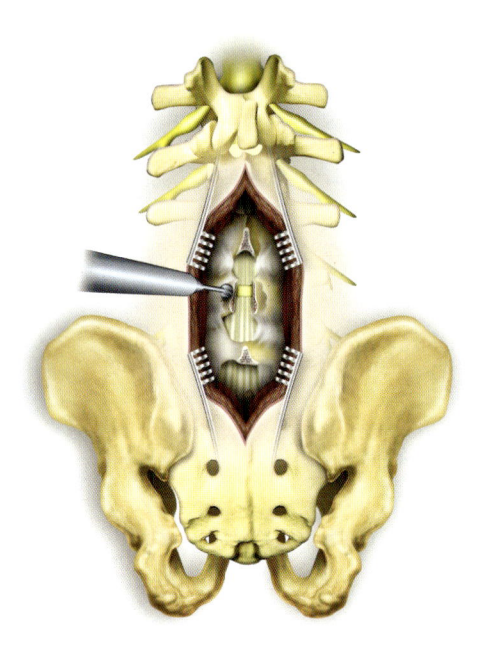

CHAPTER 27 Surgical Anatomy and Operative Techniques of Lumbar Stenosis

Fig. 27-3 A high-speed drill is used to create bilateral troughs at the medial margin of the facets.

medial one third, postoperative instability may be expected in 2% to 5% of these patients.

A foraminotomy is then performed by removing the rostral tip of the superior facet to allow each nerve root to exit freely (Fig. 27-5). Sometimes it may be difficult to dissect

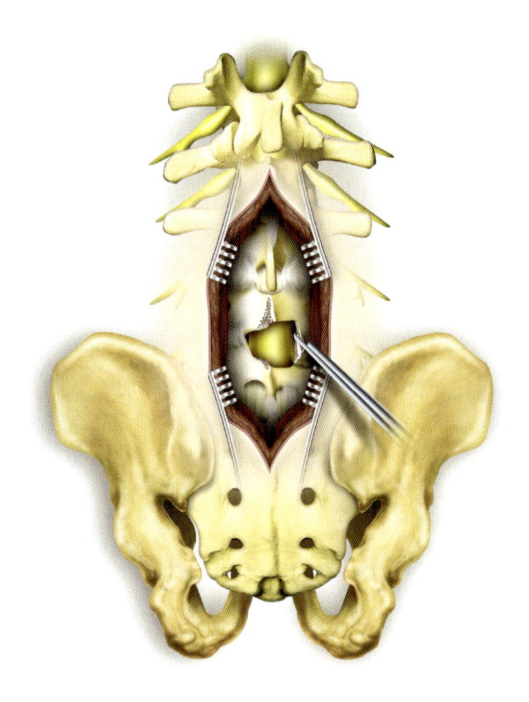

Fig. 27-4 The medial third of the facet joint may be removed with the Kerrison punch or, preferably, with a microdrill.

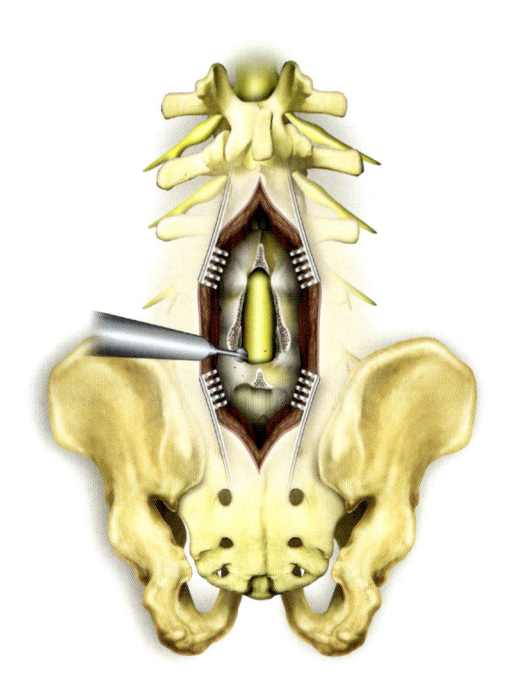

Fig. 27-5 A foraminotomy is performed by removing the rostral tip of the superior facet to allow each nerve root to exit freely.

the dura free from the lateral part of ligamentum and overlying bone, particularly in the area of the lateral recess, where it may be adherent because of chronic compression. A good plane of epidural dissection can be achieved by working well above and below the nerve root, and liberating the dura and the nerve root sleeve completely (Fig. 27-6).

During the laminectomy, frequent waxing of bone edges to limit blood loss may be required. Epidural bleeding is usually easily controlled by use of bipolar coagulation, cottonoid pads, and Gelfoam. Sometimes, however, some minor residual bleeding occurs after muscle retractors have been removed; in this case a Hemovac catheter should be left over the exposed dura beneath the muscles and brought percutaneously lateral to the wound. The muscles are approximated with three or four sutures drawn snugly but not too tightly together. The fascial layer is closed tightly and the superficial fascia and subcuticular layers are closed with Dexon.

LAMINOTOMY

If a selective interlaminar decompression (laminotomy) is planned, bilateral laminotomies, medial facetectomies, and foraminotomies at each symptomatic level should be performed using a high-speed drill, curettes, and Kerrison punches, but this procedure does not include a resection of the spinous process and interspinous, supraspinous ligamentum (Fig. 27-7). The entire ligamentum flavum is removed from beneath the laminar arch, and the arch is undercut as needed to decompress the central canal adequately.

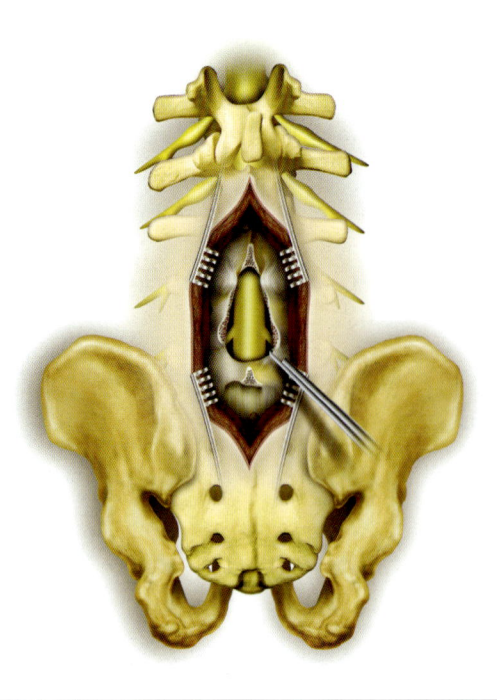

Fig. 27-6 A good plane of epidural dissection is achieved by working well above and below the nerve root to liberate the dura and the nerve root sleeve completely.

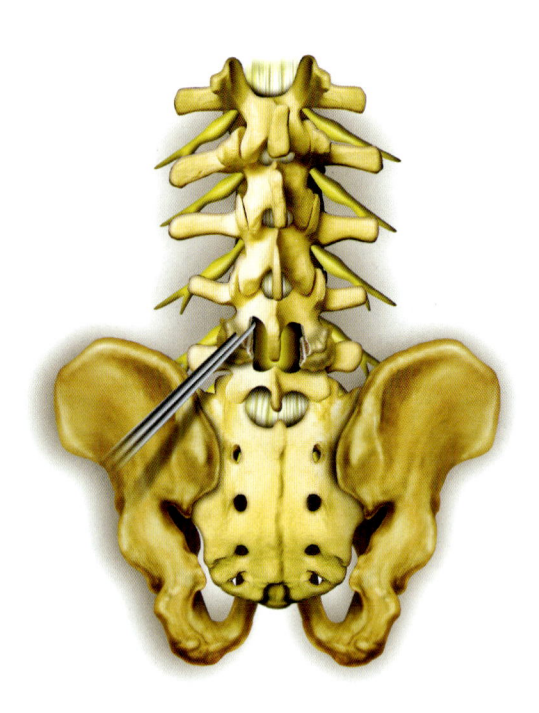

Fig. 27-8 If angulated rongeurs are employed, the resection should be carried out with fine punches (2 or 3 mm).

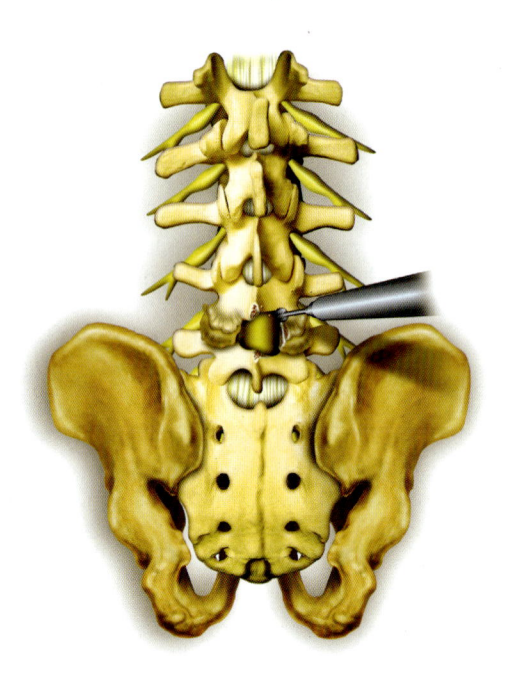

Fig. 27-7 If a selective interlaminar decompression (laminotomy) is planned, bilateral laminotomies, medial facetectomies, and foraminotomies at each symptomatic level should be performed using a high-speed drill, curettes, and Kerrison punches, but do not resect the spinous process and interspinous and supraspinous ligamentum.

HEMILAMINECTOMY AND FORAMINOTOMY

In case of a single nerve root compression in lateral recess, for decompression of the affected nerve root, the hypertrophic medial portion of the superior articular process has to be removed. At first, about 5 mm to 6 mm of the superior hemiarch is removed, followed by the medial third of the inferior articular process, down to the articular surface. Finally, the hypertrophic superior articular process is carefully removed until the subjacent nerve root is completely decompressed. The stenosis of the recess may severely compromise the nerve root; it is best protected by using a microdrill for the resection. If angulated rongeurs are employed, resection should be carried out with fine punches (2 or 3 mm) (Fig. 27-8).

The main goal is that the nerve root should be fully decompressed, and that its course should be freely visible.

CHAPTER 28

RONNIE I. MIMRAN

JEFFREY S. HENN

Minimally Invasive Lumbar Decompression

INTRODUCTION

Lumbar spinal stenosis is the most commonly diagnosed spinal disorder in the elderly population of the United States today. It is a major cause of lower back pain, leg pain, activity limitation, and disability in this population; these symptoms lead patients to consider surgery at rapidly increasing rates. In fact, rates of surgery for lumbar stenosis have increased up to eightfold in recent years.[1]

PRESENTATION

Patients presenting with lumbar stenosis characteristically complain of bilateral or unilateral leg pain, weakness, or paresthesias. Many (approximately 50%) also suffer from neurogenic claudication, a type of leg pain that is typically aggravated by standing and walking and relieved by sitting or lying down. Symptomatic relief with lumbar flexion is often a reliable characteristic that helps to distinguish so-called neurogenic "spinal" claudication from vascular claudication (caused by arterial insufficiency). The neurologic examination at rest may be fairly benign until very late stages of the disease when fixed motor or sensory deficits become evident. Sphincter disturbance is a late symptom of the condition and is usually associated with severe compression of the cauda equina, sometimes due to an acute disk herniation superimposed on preexisting spinal stenosis.

RADIOGRAPHIC EVALUATION

Radiographic imaging usually begins with plain films, which often reveal degeneration of the motion segments, loss of disk space height, narrowed neural foramina, and hypertrophy of the facet joints. Magnetic resonance imaging (MRI) scanning is the study of choice and will, with rare exception, provide diagnostic images. Typical findings include degenerative disk disease, ligamentous and facet hypertrophy, and a triangular "trefoil" spinal canal (Fig. 28-1). For the occasional patient who is not a candidate or who is uncomfortable with an MRI, myelography combined with a computed tomography (CT) scan can be obtained. Myelography will show constrictions or blocks in the dye column, and the CT scan can be used for accurate measurements of canal diameter.

TREATMENT

The most commonly performed surgical procedure for treating lumbar stenosis is a lumbar laminectomy. A

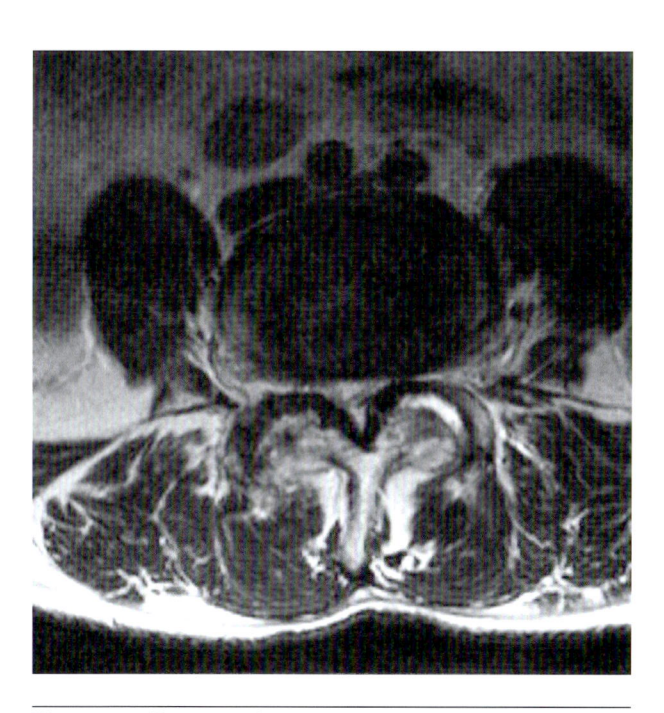

Fig. 28-1 Preoperative magnetic resonance image showing "trefoil"-shaped canal, formed by ligamentous overgrowth, intervertebral disk bulging, and facet hypertrophy. Note the narrowing of both neural foramina.

standard open laminectomy requires resection of the spinous process, the interspinous and supraspinous ligaments, the bilateral laminae, the ligamentum flavum, and often, in varying amounts, the facet complex. This method allows complete decompression of the spinal canal, including the lateral recess and intervertebral foramen. This wide resection may be considered excessive for forms of lumbar stenosis occurring solely at the level of the disk space. These forms of the disease, mainly due to intervertebral disk pathology and a combination of thickened ligaments and hypertrophic facets, are accessible through a widened interlaminar space. The recognition of this, combined with an effort to preserve midline posterior element structures, led to the introduction of the hemilaminotomy, initially performed bilaterally, to treat degenerative lumbar stenosis.[2-4]

Young and associates introduced the concept of the unilateral approach for performing a bilateral decompressive laminotomy, in which the ipsilateral side of the canal is decompressed first and the contralateral canal, lateral recess, and intervertebral foramen are decompressed *under* the midline structures.[5] This approach offered the advantage of preserving the spinous processes and midline ligamentous structures while simultaneously allowing the surgeon access to both sides of the spinal canal in order to address the main points of compression.

With the recent advent of endoscopic and minimally invasive approaches for removal of herniated lumbar disks, it became a natural progression to apply the technique to decompressive laminectomy and laminotomy. In addition to the benefits of preservation of the midline structures, this new method allowed the added advantages of a smaller skin incision, less tissue trauma, and improved visualization. After Fessler reported the feasibility of the technique in cadavers, it was later shown to be a safe, effective surgical procedure for the decompression of the stenotic lumbar spine.[6]

PATIENT SELECTION

Appropriate selection for the minimally invasive approach is an essential step toward a good outcome. Reoperative cases are relatively more difficult and should not be attempted until the surgeon has gained significant experience with minimally invasive approaches. Morbid obesity increases the working distance from the skin to the spine and increases the technical difficulty for the surgeon. These cases are best deferred until a high level of comfort and experience with tubular retractor systems is achieved.

OPERATIVE TECHNIQUE

EQUIPMENT

- Minimally invasive lumbar laminectomy is performed in a standard operating room with routinely available equipment.
- Fluoroscopy is used for the initial approach and confirmation of the correct surgical level.
- Several manufacturers market tubular retractor systems. Our group has substantial experience with the METRx system, which begins with a set of serial dilators that are used to sequentially dilate the muscle and soft tissue to the point that an adequate working channel is established through which to perform the procedure. The advantage is minimizing muscle damage and dissection. The tubular retractors are available in several working diameters, and in various lengths to accommodate variability in the depth of soft tissues (Fig. 28-2).
- Standard spinal surgery instruments are not ideal for use with tubular retractor systems due to the confined space of the retractors. If the surgeon is using a microscope for magnification and illumination, either the surgeon's hands or the back of standard instruments would tend to obscure the visual pathway. For these reasons a full set of bayoneted instruments, including Kerrison rongeurs, curettes, probes, and dissectors, are essential for enjoyable surgery (Fig. 28-3).
- A high-speed air drill is used, preferably one with a curved shaft and flexible bit to allow the surgeon's hand to remain out of the visual pathway.
- The operative microscope is employed for excellent illumination and stereoscopic visualization through the dilated working channel.
- As an alternative, a METRx set adapted for use with endoscopy is available. The specially designed instruments in this alternative set are not bayoneted (the surgeon's line of sight is not obscured by the surgeon's hands). Using an angled endoscope coupled to the tubular retractor, sur-

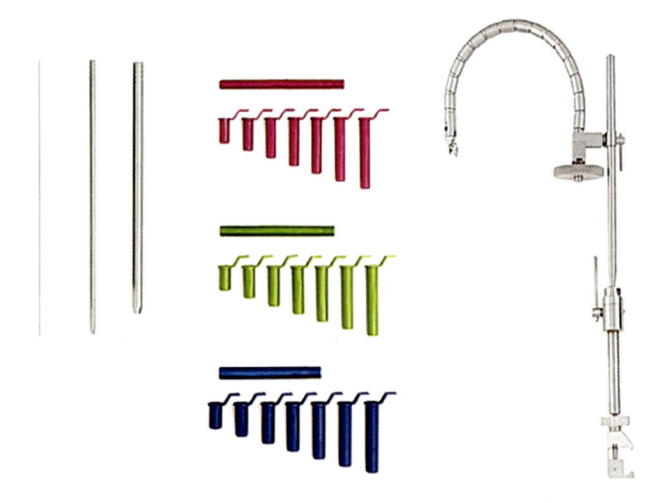

Fig. 28-2 The METRx system of sequential dilators. From left to right, the guidewire and two initial soft tissue dilators (5.3 mm and 9.4 mm), tubular retractor sets with respective dilators (14, 16, and 18 mm), and flexible arm assembly with table attachment clamp.

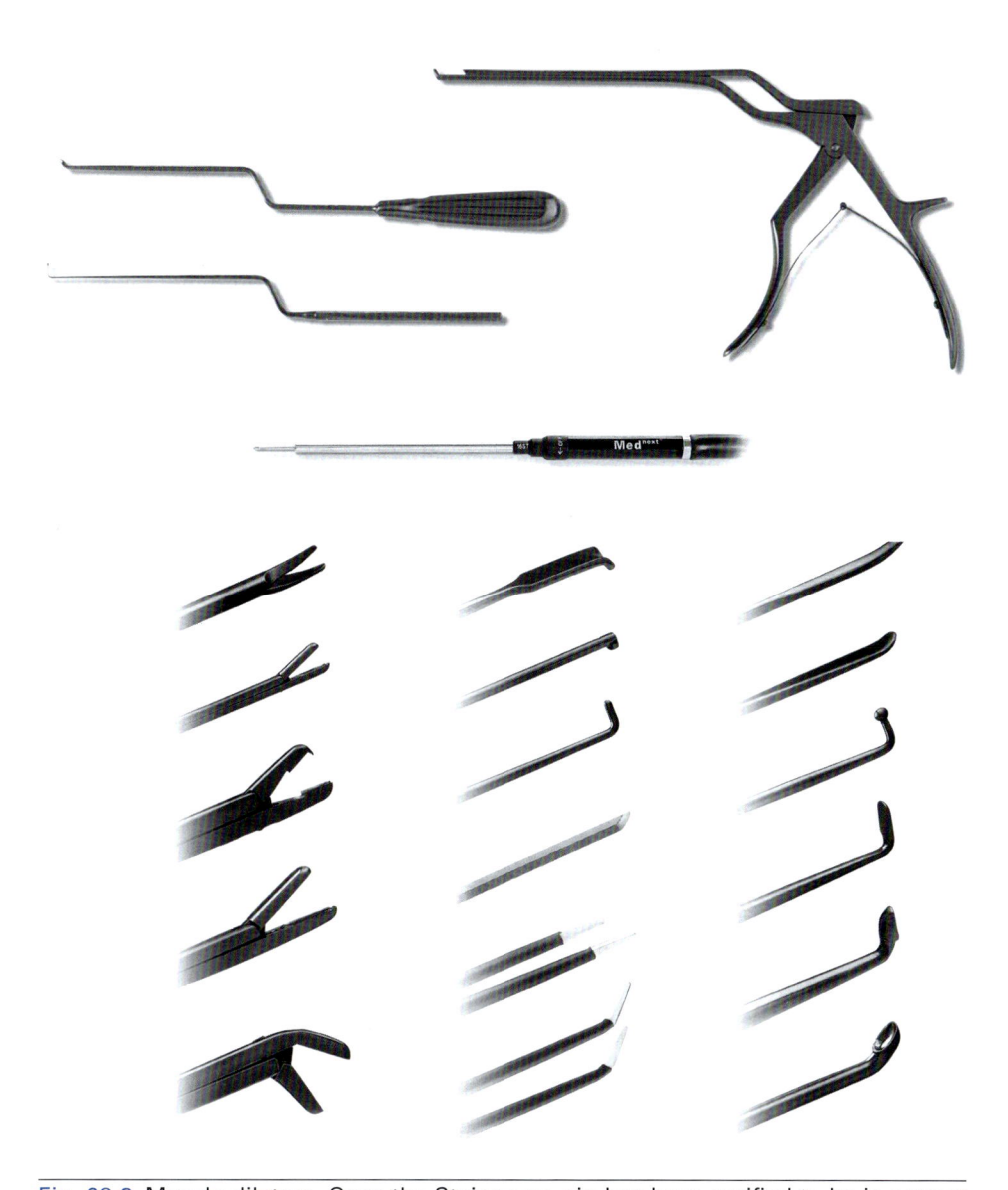

Fig. 28-3 Muscle dilators. Once the Steinmann pin has been verified to be in correct position, a series of muscle dilators are sequentially passed over each other until the working channel is the desired width. The Steinmann pin is removed after the first dilator is placed to reduce the risk of injury, particularly dural puncture. As the dilators are placed, it is important to check intermittently with fluoroscopy to verify that they remain in correct position. The dilators are marked with a depth scale on the outer surface that indicates the appropriate length of the tubular retractor. (Courtesy of Medtronic, Inc., Minneapolis, MN.)

geons have the advantage of being able to visualize anatomy outside the confines of the retractor. Surgeons using the operative microscope accomplish this by altering the angle of the working retractor.
- The shortcoming of the endoscopic technique is the somewhat steep learning curve required to learn endoscopic techniques and nuances (two-dimensional visualization, hand-eye coordination, etc.).

PATIENT POSITIONING

- After routine preoperative preparations and induction of general anesthesia, the patient is transferred to a fluoroscopy-compatible operating table in the prone position.
- Patients are positioned on a frame to allow for flexion of the hips and lumbar spine. This maneuver reverses the lumbar lordosis, widens the interspinous and interlaminar

distances, and places the vertebral canal in its widest arrangement. In addition, the abdomen is kept dependent and decompressed, which decreases venous backpressure and reduces epidural venous bleeding.
- Positioning for minimally invasive procedures is accomplished similar to standard open cases with the same precautions.
- Intraoperative C-arm fluoroscopy is positioned to provide lateral images during the procedure. When not in use, it is moved out of the way and is maintained in a position just caudal to the patient's elbows.

PREPARATION AND DRAPING

- Using the fluoroscope for guidance, an 18-gauge spinal needle is inserted approximately 4 cm lateral to midline at the appropriate level. The target is the superior aspect of the facet complex. Staying relatively lateral at this stage of the operation avoids inadvertent dural puncture.
- Once proper position has been attained, a 4- to 5-cm area around the insertion site is subcutaneously infiltrated with a solution of 0.25% bupivicaine and 1:200,000 epinephrine. This acts to reduce bleeding around the track of the dissection and to provide postoperative pain control.

INCISION AND RETRACTOR PLACEMENT

- A stab incision is made above and below the spinal needle, the total size of which should match the size of the intended final tubular retractor.
- The knife blade is inserted along the needle to make a nick in the lumbodorsal fascia, making subsequent dilator insertion easier.
- Once the stab incision is completed, a guidewire is placed alongside the spinal needle to ensure that an identical target is reached. With the guidewire in place, the spinal needle is removed.
- The first dilator is placed over the guidewire; subsequently, the guidewire is then removed to reduce the risk of inadvertent dural puncture.
- The initial dilators are "wanded" once docked on bone. Wanding is a sweeping maneuver used to subperiosteally clear the musculature from the dorsal surface of the lamina (Fig. 28-4). In this manner, the exposure is carried more medially to target the trailing edge of the superior lamina.
- Serial dilators are sequentially placed and docked firmly against the lamina (Fig. 28-5).
- Once an adequate dilation has been achieved, usually 20 mm or 22 mm, a tubular retractor is placed over the largest dilator (Fig. 28-6). The tubular retractor chosen should be as short as possible to reach the lamina, such that the outer rim of the retractor sits flush on the patient's skin. This acts to create the shortest possible channel, improving visualization and illumination.

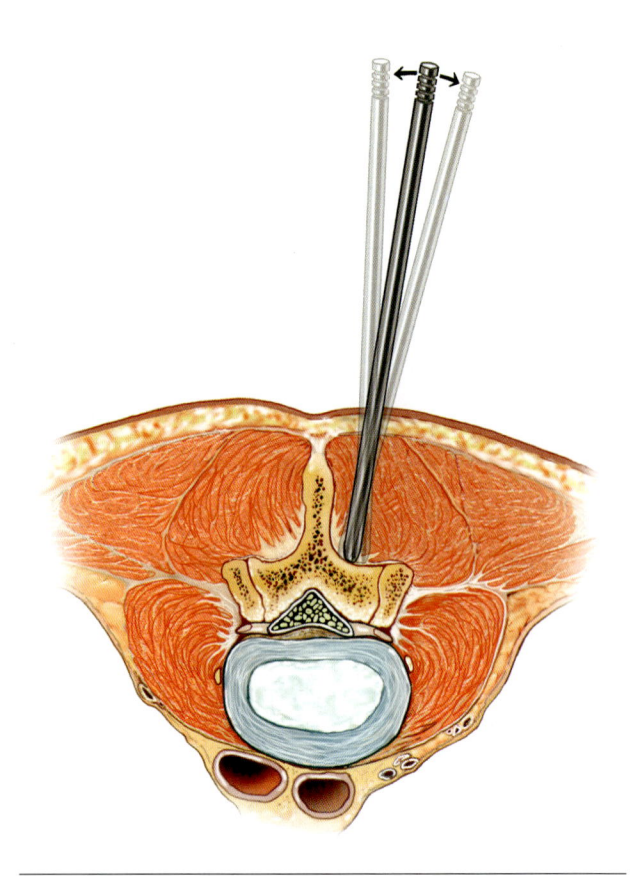

Fig. 28-4 The initial dilator is placed and "wanded" to remove excess soft tissue from the surface of the lamina and facet.

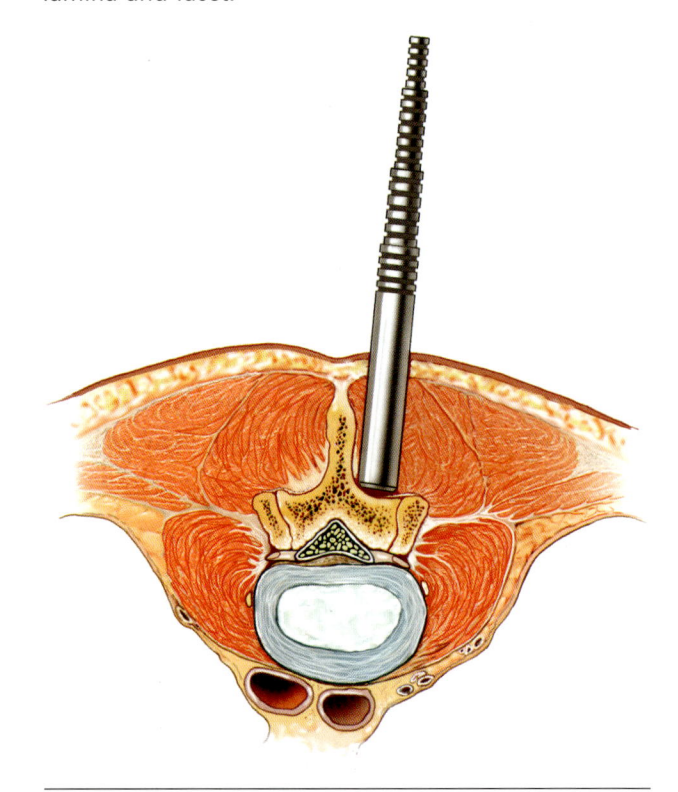

Fig. 28-5 With all dilators in place, an adequate-sized channel is created in the soft tissues.

CHAPTER 28 Minimally Invasive Lumbar Decompression   235

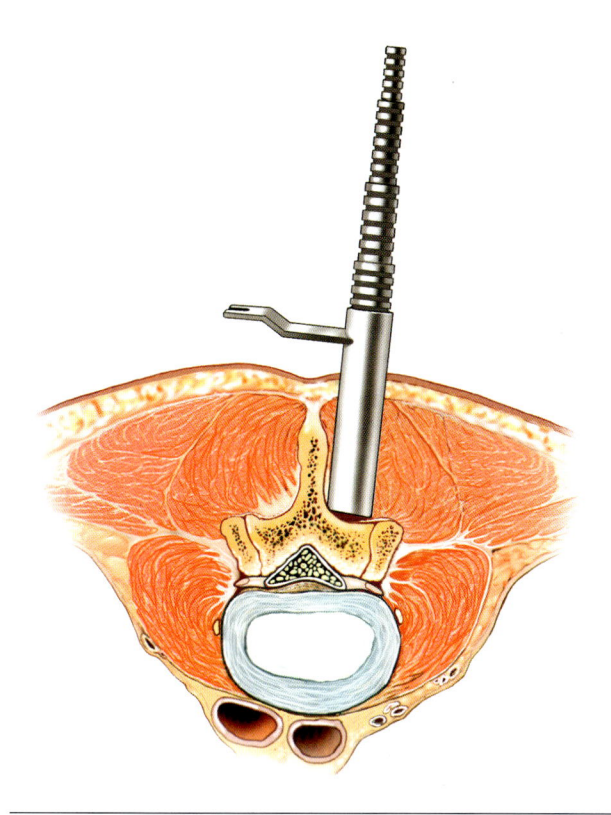

Fig. 28-6 The final tubular retractor is placed.

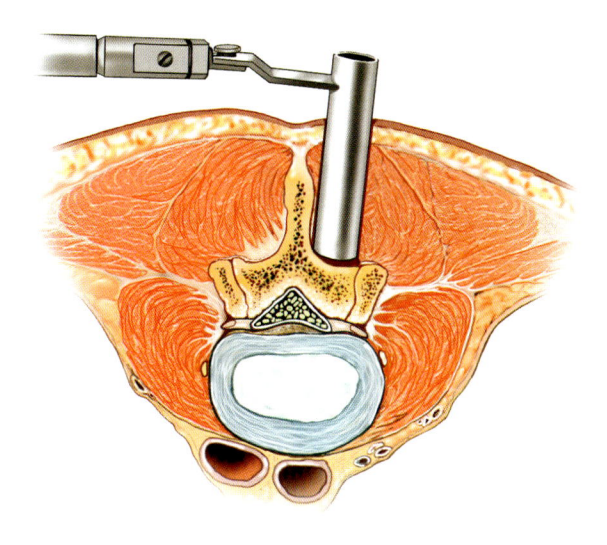

Fig. 28-7 The final retractor assembly, fixed to the flexible arm.

- The appropriate tubular retractor is secured using the flexible arm assembly, which is fastened to the side rail of the operating table, out of the path of the fluoroscopic unit (Fig. 28-7).
- The operating microscope or surgical loupes and a headlight are utilized for enhanced illumination and visualization.
- At this point, fluoroscopy should be used to definitively confirm the level of operation (Fig. 28-8).

DECOMPRESSION

- The remaining soft tissue on the laminar/facet surface is then removed with monopolar cautery. The edges of the inferior lamina and medial facet should now be seen.
- Using the high-speed air drill, a laminotomy is performed, burring through the lamina to the thickened ligamentum flavum. The tubular retractor can be repositioned, or wanded, to alter the surgeon's view and complete the hemilaminectomy.
- Any bleeding occurring from the bone edges is easily controlled with bone wax.
- Once the ipsilateral hemilaminectomy is completed, the ligamentum flavum is excised using a combination of curettes and Kerrison rongeurs.
- The lateral recess is then decompressed with as much removal of the medial facet as necessary, focusing on the superior articular process.
- The tubular retractor can be angled in a medial to lateral orientation to view the medial facet more effectively. This allows the surgeon to undercut the facet and widen the lateral recess through a combination of bony and ligamentous removal. The exiting nerve root should be identified, and the intervertebral foramen is visualized and decompressed (Fig. 28-9).
- The retractor is then angled toward the midline; the lamina beneath the spinous process is removed with the drill,

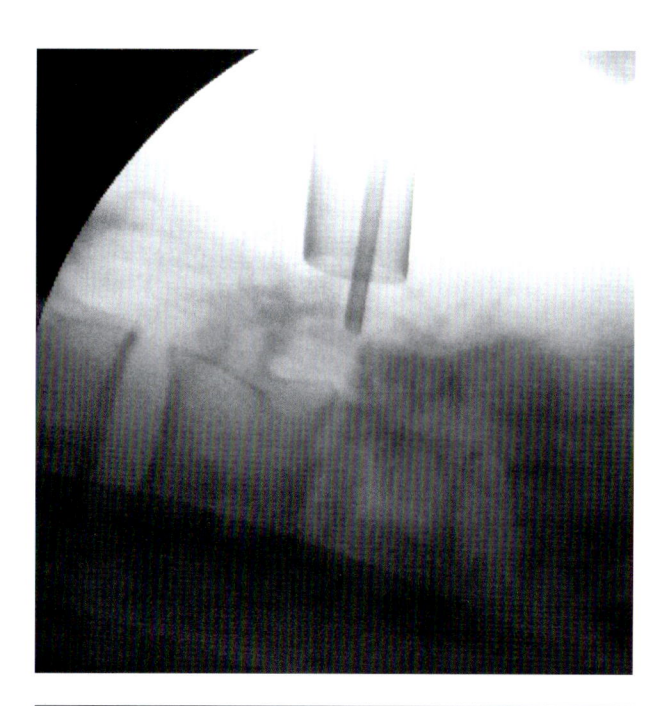

Fig. 28-8 Intraoperative fluoroscopic image showing tubular retractor docked on inferior edge of lamina.

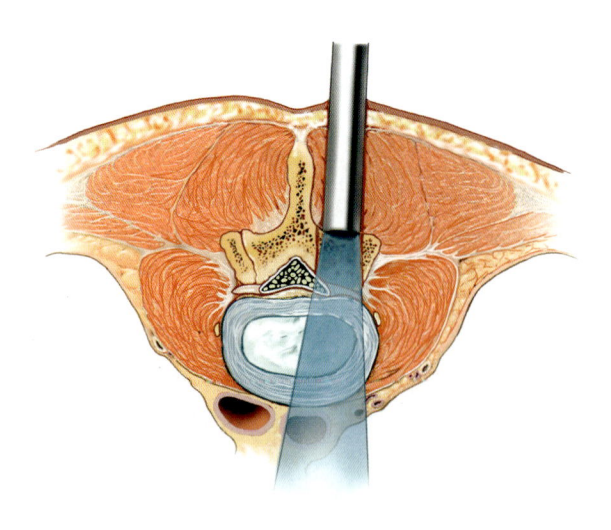

Fig. 28-9 View after the ipsilateral laminectomy is performed. Note the retractor is positioned to decompress the canal centrally and laterally, including the neural foramen.

exposing the central portion of the spinal canal. *The key maneuver in this operation is the angling of the tubular retractor medially to visualize the contralateral side* (Fig. 28-10). The angle of the tubular retractor is approximated by the medial to lateral slope of the contralateral lamina. The operating microscope is similarly positioned to view down the tubular retractor.

- Leaving the medial cut edge of the ligamentum flavum as a protective layer over the dura, the high-speed drill is used to extend the bone resection toward the contralateral side. This process is not a complete laminectomy in the same manner as the ipsilateral side, because the dorsal surface of the lamina will be left. The bony removal is an undercutting of the lamina, intended not only to decompress the neural elements, but also to facilitate visualization of the contralateral lateral recess and neural foramen. Endoscopy does confer some advantage here, as the 30-degree angled endoscope can be very useful in visualizing the opposite side of the canal, including the lateral recess and intervertebral foramen.
- The ligamentum flavum is now removed with an up-biting Kerrison punch. The dorsal surface of the dural is gently depressed with a spatula dissector and followed until the opposite exiting nerve root is identified. As the dissection is carried laterally, the thickened ligamentum flavum is removed.
- A medial facetectomy is carried out to decompress the lateral recess, with care being taken to first identify and then protect the contralateral nerve root as it exits the foramen.
- The superior articular process is typically the area of greatest compression and should be addressed if present. The full bilateral decompression is now complete (Fig. 28-11).
- The addition of a second, contiguous level for decompression can be accomplished by simply wanding the tubular retractor from the same skin incision up or down to the adjacent segment. If additional reach is needed, the tubular retractor system can be reinserted though a new fascial/muscle tract using the same skin incision. Once the tubular retractor is appropriately positioned, the procedure is identical to the first level.

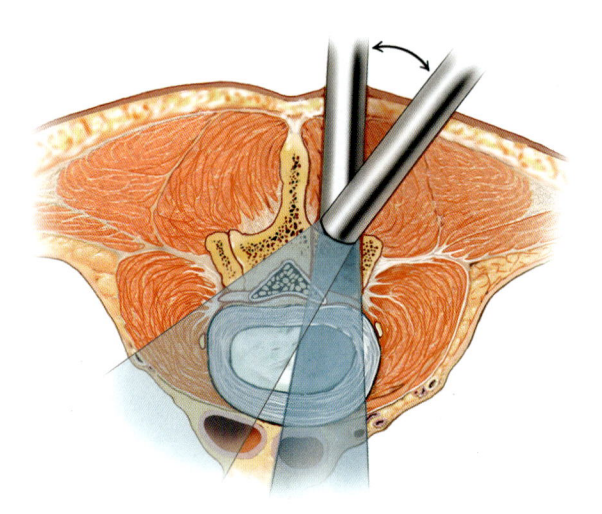

Fig. 28-10 The angling of the tubular retractor allows contralateral decompression and good visualization of the contralateral neural foramen.

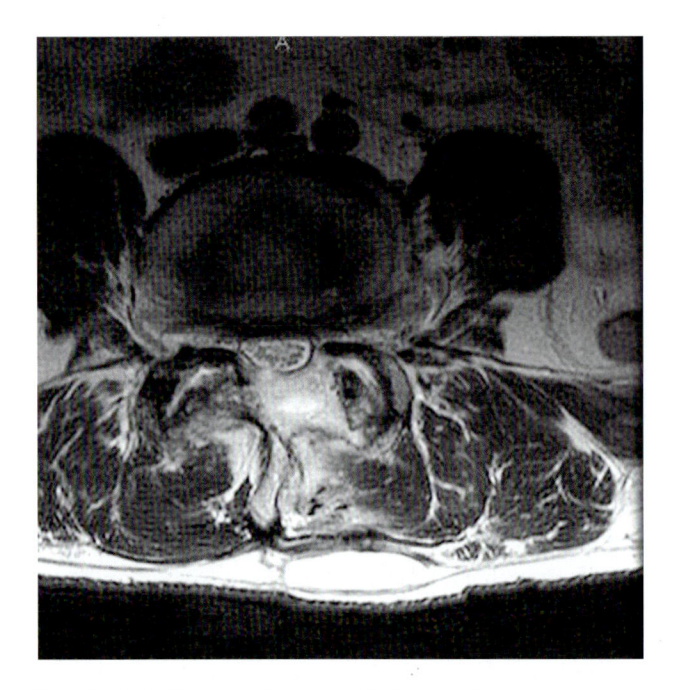

Fig. 28-11 Postoperative magnetic resonance image showing extent of resection after minimally invasive laminectomy.

CLOSURE

- Once a full decompression of the vertebral canal, lateral recesses, and nerve root foramina is complete, a broad inspection is performed and meticulous hemostasis is obtained using bipolar cautery, bone wax, and thrombin-soaked Gelfoam.
- The wound is irrigated with antibiotic solution.
- Pledgets of Gelfoam soaked with Depo-Medrol 40 mg may be placed in the epidural region to reduce inflammation and postoperative pain.
- Muscular hemostasis is ensured as the tubular retractor is withdrawn.
- Closure is accomplished with absorbable sutures in the fascia and subcutaneous layers and a small adhesive bandage.

POSTOPERATIVE CARE

- Depending on the patient's comorbidities, they are typically discharged the same day as surgery, or the following day.
- With proper local anesthetic infiltration of the surrounding tissues, there is usually no need for intravenous analgesic medications. Oral medications will suffice both in the operative recovery period and after discharge.
- Early ambulation is encouraged, with a return to light duties within a week. Full activity return is expected by 3 weeks postoperatively.

COMPLICATION AVOIDANCE

- Correct identification of the surgical level is dependent on fluoroscopy because, unlike open procedures in which familiar landmarks can be identified, exposure is limited.
- Initial opening of the ligamentum flavum is often the most difficult portion of the procedure. This is a likely time for the occurrence of a dural tear. Careful use of curettes can limit the risk.
- Suture repair of a dural tear through the tube is possible, although very tedious. Instead, a plug of Gelfoam and fibrin glue may be sufficient. The risk of cerebrospinal fluid leak is somewhat reduced (as compared to open procedures) by the muscle-dilating techniques; once the tubular retractor is withdrawn, the paraspinal tissues reapproximate nicely and "seal" the operative tract.
- Careful identification of the midline and the ipsilateral facet will help to maintain correct orientation. It is easy to enter the spinal canal on the opposite side if the tubular retractor is angled too medially during the initial bone drilling.
- When working toward the opposite side, keep the smooth heel of the Kerrison rongeurs against the dura to reduce the risk of dural laceration.
- Prior to closure, use fluoroscopy to identify the most rostral and caudal extent of the decompression to ensure that the entire segment is adequately treated.

CONCLUSION

With the ubiquity of the disease and the frequency of operations performed to correct it, lumbar stenosis represents an exciting opportunity to improve existing tenets of surgery. One such improvement is the advent of minimally invasive laminectomies. When performed properly, the procedure is a safe, effective method for decompressing the stenotic lumbar spinal canal and offers patients a smaller incision, less postoperative pain, and a more rapid recovery.

References

1. Ciol MA, Deyo RA, Howell E, et al: An assessment of surgery for spinal stenosis: Time trends, geographic variations, complications, and reoperations. J Am Geriatr Soc 1996;44:285–290.
2. Aryanpur J, Ducker T: Multilevel lumbar laminotomies: An alternative to laminectomy in the treatment of lumbar stenosis. Neurosurgery 1990;26:429–432.
3. Lin PM: Internal decompression for multiple levels of lumbar spinal stenosis: A technical note. Neurosurgery 1982;11:546–549.
4. Postacchini F, Cinotti G, Perugia D, et al: The surgical treatment of central lumbar stenosis: Multiple laminotomy compared with total laminectomy. J Bone Joint Surg Br 1993;75:386–392.
5. Young S, Veerapen R, O'Laoire SA: Relief of lumbar canal stenosis using multilevel subarticular fenestrations as an alternative to wide laminectomy: Preliminary report. Neurosurgery 1988;23:628–633.
6. Guiot BH, Khoo LT, Fessler RG: A minimally invasive technique for decompression of the lumbar spine. Spine 2002;27:432–438.

SECTION F
Lumbar Fusion and Instrumentation Techniques

CHAPTER 29

HO-YEOL ZHANG

DANIEL H. KIM

Transpedicular Screw Fixations

INTRODUCTION

The use of a pedicle screw-plating system for spinal fixation began in 1963 with Roy-Camille and associates. They described using pedicle screw fixation for treatment of lumbar fracture, malunion, lumbar metastases, primary spine tumor, lumbosacral fusion, and high-grade spondylolisthesis.[1] This technique has the advantage of requiring the least amount of normal anatomy to be involved in the fusion. However, care must be taken in the placement of the pedicle screw to prevent injury to the nerve root. The pedicle screw device can be used to provide distraction, compression, and translation. The pedicle screw-rod system was first introduced by Magerl[2] and was modified to improved fusion rate and easier handling by others. The screw-rod system allows axial, angular, and rotational adjustability, permitting instrumented segments of the spine to be held in distraction, compression, or derotation.

Pedicle screw fixation is indicated for the management of lumbar stenosis, as well as fractures, failed fusions, spondylolisthesis, and failed back syndrome. It offers the advantage of immediate stabilization, along with higher rates of fusion, easy contouring, and more available space for bone graft.[3,4] Fusion rate is reported from 88% to 95% in success cases,[5,6] and the procedure carries a 6% pseudoarthrosis rate.[5]

Pedicle screw fusion of the lumbar spine has neurologic and orthopedic goals. Neurologic goals include minimization of ongoing injury, spinal cord decompression, and functional recovery. Orthopedic goals include mechanical spinal stability, correction of malalignment and deformity, and remedy or prevention of pseudoarthrosis.[7]

INDICATIONS

- Trauma (Trauma that results in two- or three-column injury or injury to the posterior ligamentous complex is sufficiently unstable to require surgical stabilization.)
- Degenerative disease
  - Isthmic spondylolisthesis
    - Progression of slippage
    - Persistent symptom of back pain
    - Persistent neurologic symptoms
  - Degenerative spondylolisthesis
  - Disk degeneration—recurrent disk herniation and diskographic disk disruption with reproduction of symptoms
  - Degenerative scoliosis—progression of the scoliotic curve, progression of stenotic symptoms, progression to instability
  - Lumbar stenosis-wide decompressive laminectomy—destabilization of the spine.
- Osteomyelitis
  - When osteomyelitis erodes more than 50% of the vertebral body
  - When aggressive débridement would result in an unstable spine
- Tumor (Decision to use pedicle screw fixation is based on the location of the disease and the patient's medical condition.)
- Deformity corrections
- Malunion

SURGICAL TECHNIQUES

EQUIPMENT

- X-ray-compatible operating table
- Jackson table, Wilson frame, or chest rolls
- Fluoroscopy
- Headlight system
- Pneumatic compression stocking or antiembolic stocking to both legs

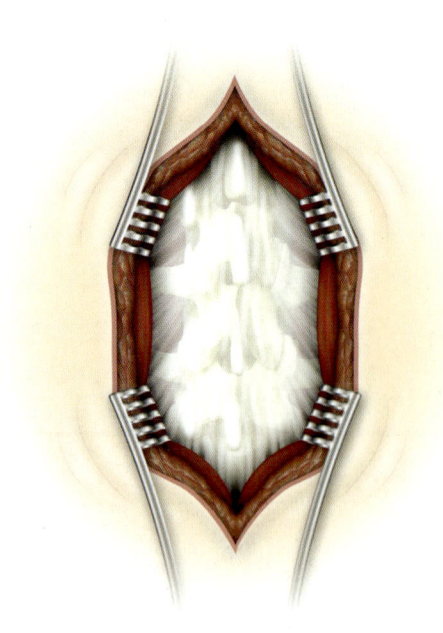

Fig. 29-1 Incise the midline of the lumbar spine under general anesthesia. Perform subperiosteal dissection of the musculature from the spinous processes. On both sides, dissection is carried out to the level of the transverse processes in the region of the intended fusion. Meticulously remove the musculature and the periosteum in the region of the segment to be fused.

- Lumbar laminectomy set
- Steinmann pins
- Bone graft source
- Lumbar pedicle screw system

PATIENT POSITIONING AND INCISION

- After endotracheal anesthesia, place the patient in a prone position to avoid epidural venous distention from abdominal compression.
- Incise the midline of the lumbar spine (Fig. 29-1).
- Perform subperiosteal dissection of the musculature from the spinous processes. On both sides, dissection is carried out to the level of the transverse processes in the region of the intended fusion. Remove the musculature and the periosteum meticulously in the region of the segment to be fused.

PEDICLE PREPARATION AND SCREW INSERTION

- Perform laminectomy and proper managements of lumbar lesion.
- Localize the external landmarks for the pedicles.
- Obtain fluoroscopic confirmation for pedicle identification, hole preparation, and screw placement.
- Two well-known methods are the Roy-Camille method and the Magerl method:

- Roy-Camille's screw entrance point is situated at the crossing of two lines on a typical bony crest. The horizontal line passes through the middle of the transverse process; the vertical line is given by the articular process 1 mm under the facet joint[1] (Fig. 29-2).
- In Magerl's method direction of the screw is 10 to 20 degrees convergent toward the sagittal plane. The point of entry is in the central axis of the pedicular tube, indicated by the intersection of the two lines. The vertical line touches the lateral border of the superior articular process. The horizontal line bisects the base of the transverse process[8] (Fig. 29-3).
- Localize the height of the pedicle and determine the pedicle entry level with the image intensifier, according to the method described by Roy-Camille or Magerl.
- Identification of the facet complex is facilitated by moving the spinous process with a Kocher clamp and removing the soft tissue from the surface of the superior facet.
- Open the pedicle and insert marking wires (Steinmann pin). Then, perform an x-ray check to determine the exact position of the drill channels in the lateral and anteroposterior projections. In slightly oblique fluoroscopic images, the pedicle and Steinmann pin appears as an oval structure with a central dot (Fig. 29-4).
- The external landmark for the first sacral pedicle is located at the inferolateral portion of the superior S1 facet. Fluoroscopy is used to confirm correct entry sites.
- Two commonly used sacral screw placements are (1) anterolaterally into the ala and (2) anteromedially into the promontory (Fig. 29-5A and B).

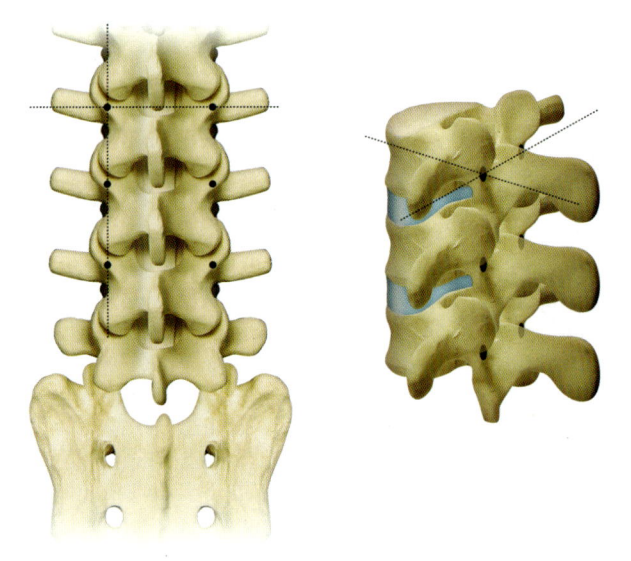

Fig. 29-2 Roy-Camille's screw entrance point is situated at the crossing of two lines on a typical bony crest. The horizontal line passes through the middle of the transverse process; the vertical line is given by the articular process 1 mm under the facet joint.

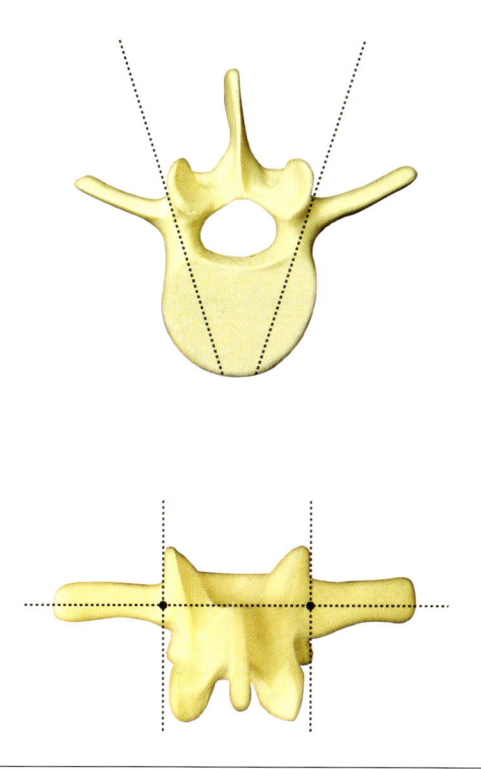

CHAPTER 29 Transpedicular Screw Fixations 241

Fig. 29-3 Magerl's method; direction of the screw is 10 to 20 degrees convergent toward the sagittal plane. The point of entry is in the central axis of the pedicular tube, indicated by the intersection of the two lines. The vertical line touches the lateral border of the superior articular process. The horizontal line bisects the base of the transverse process.

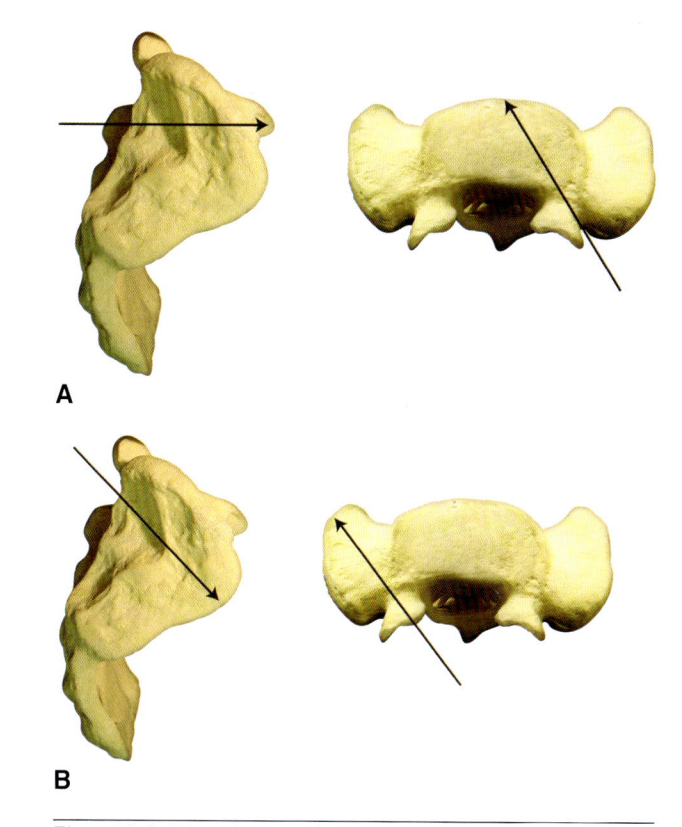

Fig. 29-5 Directions of sacral screw. Anteromedial (promontory) direction (A) and anterolateral (alar) direction (B).

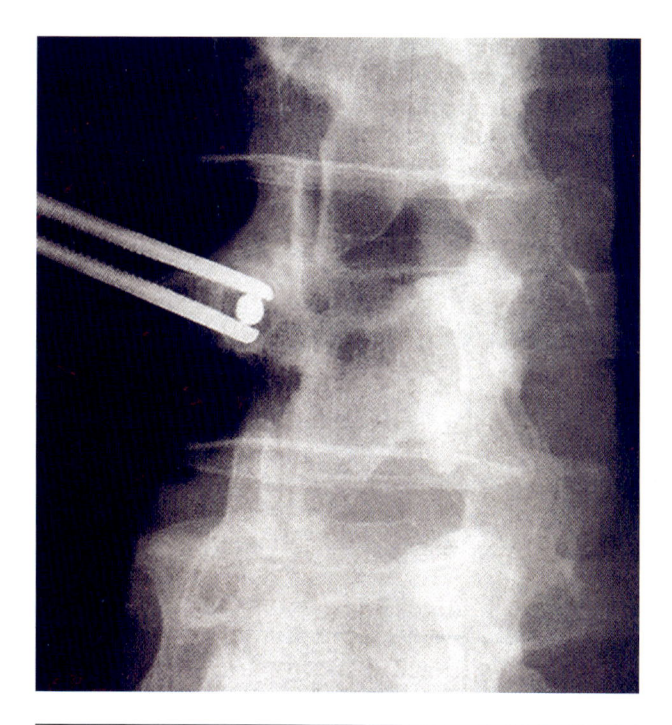

Fig. 29-4 Fluoroscopic image shows the alignment of the pedicle and Steinmann pin.

- The anteromedial (promontory) direction screw provides as strong, or stronger, fixation than the anterolateral (alar) direction screw. Because of this greater strength, and because of intraoperative radiography, the promontory can be seen more easily than the anterior-most portion of the ala.
- This procedure is repeated at each pedicle.
- The progress of pin and screw penetration into the vertebral body is monitored using lateral imaging. Each pin is driven until positioned into the end plate of the vertebrae, avoiding penetration into the disk space.
- After all pins are placed into the vertebral bodies to create paths for the pedicle screws, the Steinmann pins are removed, and the superficial 5- to 10-mm area of each track is enlarged with a drill.
- Tap a thread in the pedicles for subsequent insertion of the screws. The depth of the drilled channel can be established with the depth gauge (Fig. 29-6).
- Pedicle screw sizes are preselected on the basis of the computed tomographic images of the particular vertebra.

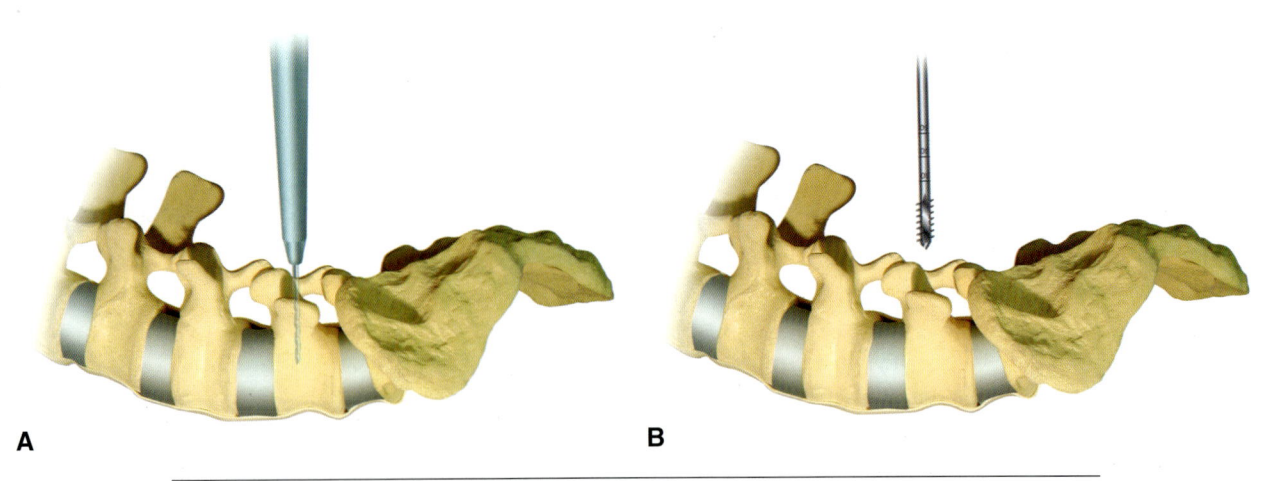

Fig. 29-6 Open the pedicles with the awl, then drill them (A). Tap a thread in the pedicles for subsequent insertion of the polyaxial screws (B).

- The screws are placed into the prepared holes with the same trajectory as that of the Steinmann pins (Fig. 29-7).
- Screw purchase is obtained by advancing the screw with a screwdriver to a depth of 70% to 80% of the vertebral body. The anterior portion of the vertebral body is not penetrated to avoid injury to vascular and visceral structures in the retroperitoneum (Fig. 29-8).
- This procedure is repeated at each pedicle (Fig. 29-9), after inserting the screws and checking their exact position with fluoroscopy.

FUSION SITE PREPARATION

- The fusion sites are prepared before rod replacement.
- After all soft tissue is removed from the surface of the fusion bed, a high-speed drill is used to decorticate the transverse processes, facet joints, and other bone fusion surfaces. The articular surfaces of the facet joints are curetted or drilled to remove cartilage (Fig. 29-10).
- Cancellous bone grafts are packed into the facets.

ROD SYSTEM ASSEMBLY

- Cut rod to the appropriate length and bend to match the lumbar curvature.
- For contour, an S-shaped curve is used for thoracolumbar rods, and a lordotic curve is used for lumbar or lumbosacral rods (Fig. 29-11).
- The rods are connected bilaterally to the pedicle screws by threading the rods through the screws (i.e., Moss-Miami system, Cotrel-Dubousset system) or attaching the eyebolts to the rods (i.e., TSRH system).

REDUCTION OR REALIGNMENT OF SPINE

- Starting caudally, apply the nut assembles on the screws at S1 and L4 to fixate the rod in the screw heads and tighten partially (Fig. 29-12).
- Perform partial reduction of the listhesis by dorsally directing tension at the cranial part of the rod overlapping the screw at L4 (Fig. 29-13).

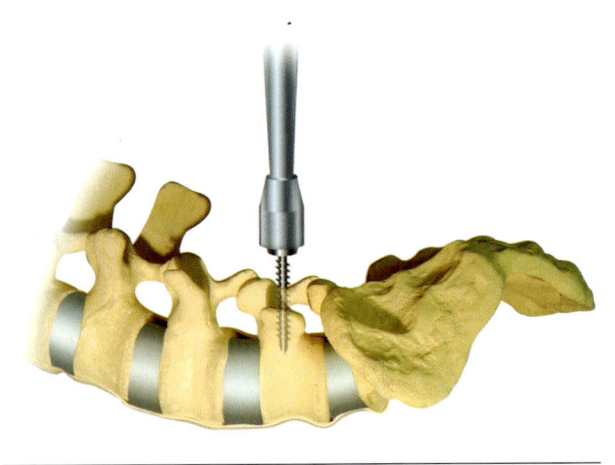

Fig. 29-7 Screw insertion.

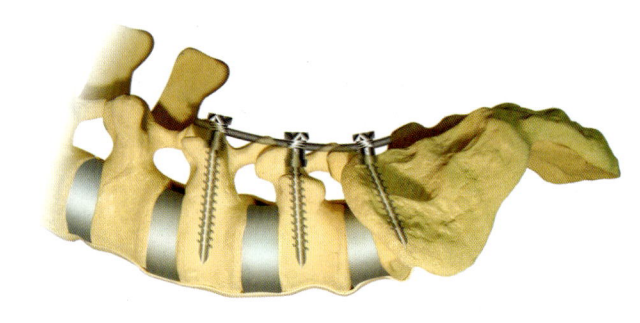

Fig. 29-8 Screw purchase is obtained by advancing the screw with a screwdriver to a depth of 70% to 80% of the vertebral body.

CHAPTER 29 Transpedicular Screw Fixations 243

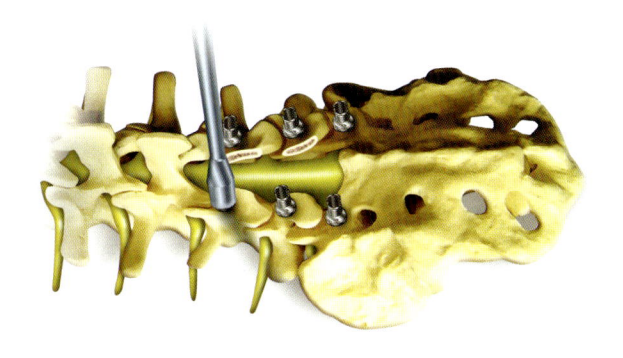

Fig. 29-9 The screws have been inserted and their exact position has been checked with fluoroscopy.

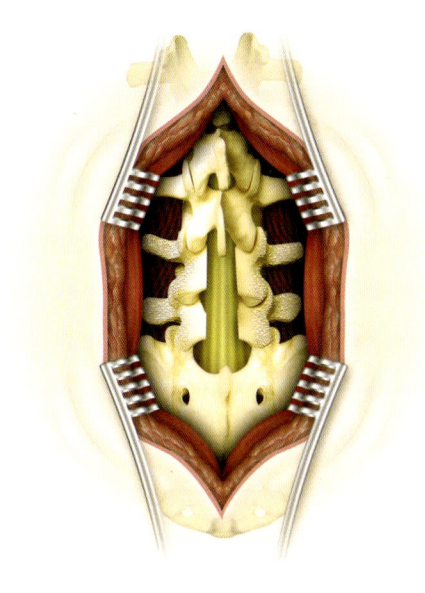

Fig. 29-10 Surfaces of decortication include the transverse process, the lateral aspect of the facet joints, the facet articular surfaces, and the remaining lamina of the levels to be fused.

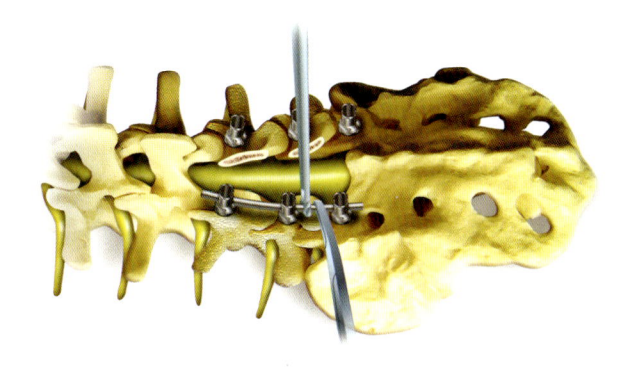

Fig. 29-11 Cut rod to the appropriate length and bend to match the lumbar curvature. Contour a lordotic curve for lumbar or lumbosacral rods.

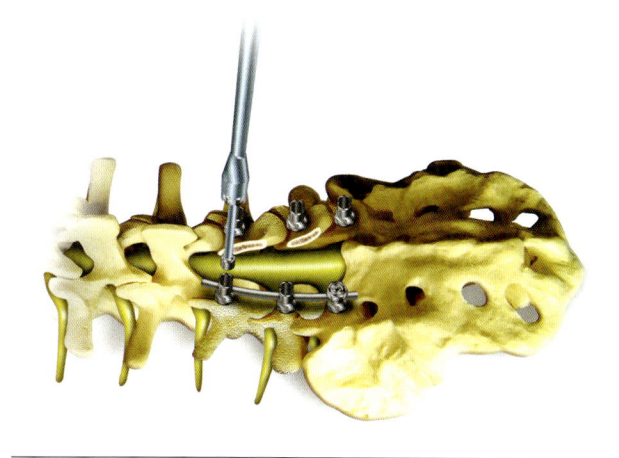

Fig. 29-12 Starting caudally, apply the nut on the screws at S1 and L4 to fixate the rod in the screw heads.

- Insert the nut for fixation of the screw at L5 and tighten partially (Fig. 29-14).
- Apply segmental distraction initially between S1 and L4 while under simultaneous posteriorly directed extension at the cranial end of the rod. Tighten partially the nut at L4 to fixate this partial reduction (Fig. 29-15).
- Apply segmental distraction or compression between S1 and L5 while still under posteriorly directed extension at the cranial end of the rod (Fig. 29-16A and B).
- A fixation of this new position is established by completely tightening the nut at the level of L5. Use an image intensifier to make an assessment of the reduction maneuver. The same procedure is now carried out on the contralateral side.

BONE GRAFT AND CLOSURE

- After rod placement and wound irrigation with antibiotic-containing solution, cancellous bone and cortical matchstick grafts are placed for a posterolateral fusion. Autogenous iliac crest bone is the preferred bone graft (Fig. 29-17).

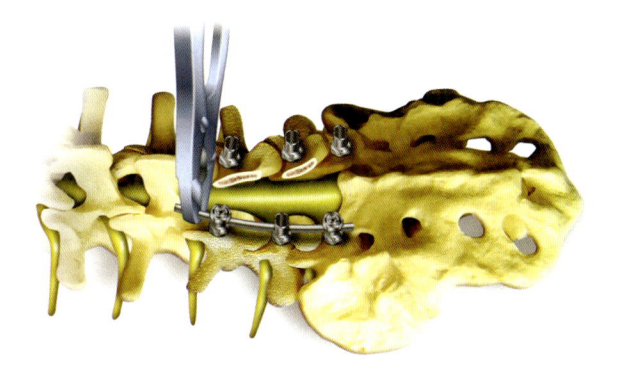

Fig. 29-13 Perform partial reduction of the listhesis by dorsally directing tension at the cranial part of the rod overlapping the screw at L4.

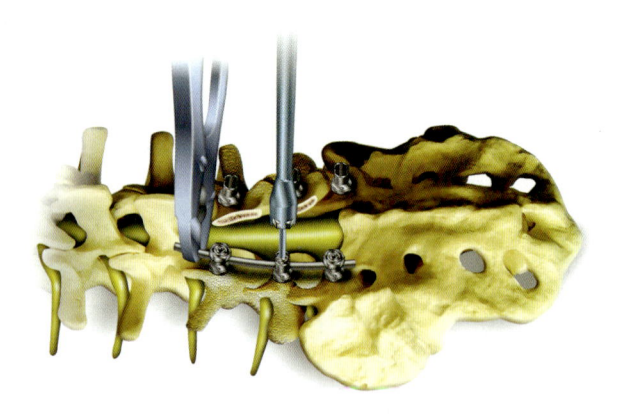

Fig. 29-14 Now insert the nut for fixation of the screw at L5.

- Closed suction drainage systems are placed into the wound, and multilayer wound closure is completed.

POSTOPERATIVE CARE

- All wound drains are removed 24 to 48 hours after surgery.
- Patients with lumbar fusions wear a thoracolumbosacral orthosis for 3 to 6 months.
- Patients are ambulatory within the first few postoperative days.
- Physical therapy for rehabilitation is then provided.
- Patients are usually discharged from the hospital at 2 to 3 days after operation if there are no complications.

COMPLICATIONS

- Hardware failure (screw breakage, pull out, rod fracture, inaccurate screw placement)
- Excessive hemorrhage
- Dural tear

A

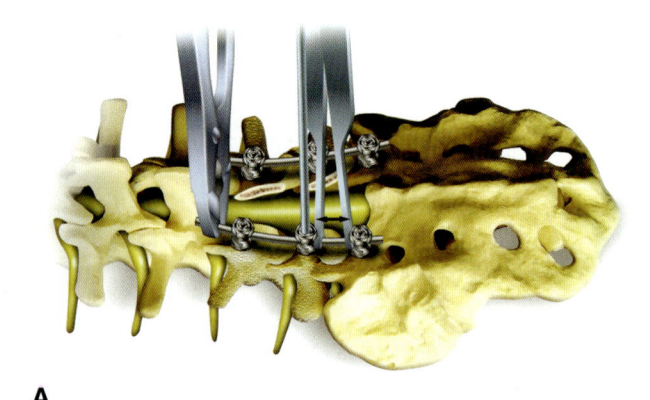

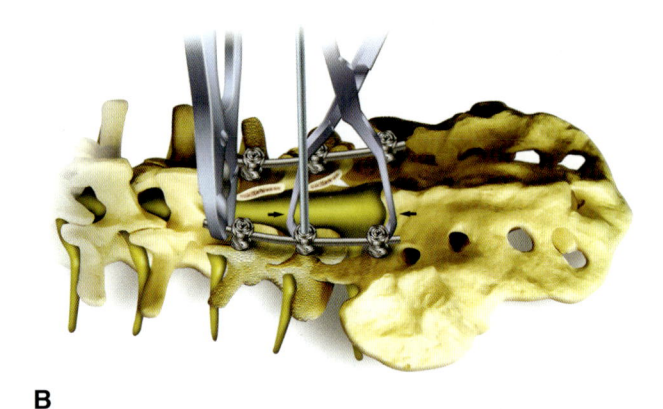

B

Fig. 29-16 Apply segmental distraction or compression between S1 and L5 while still under posteriorly directed extension at the cranial end of the rod.

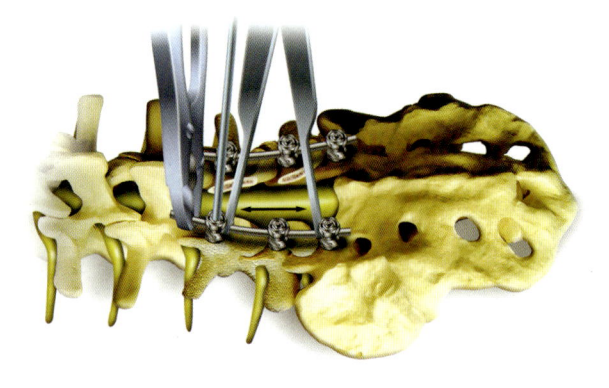

Fig. 29-15 Apply segmental distraction initially between S1 and L4 while under simultaneous posteriorly directed extension at the cranial end of the rod. Tighten the inner screw and outer nut at L4 to fixate this partial reduction.

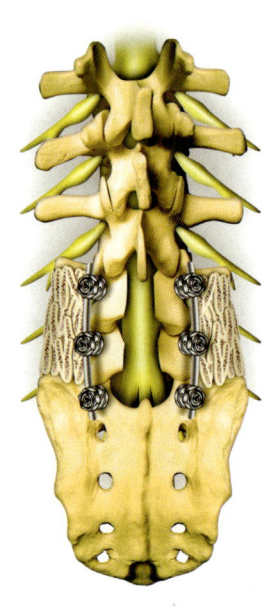

Fig. 29-17 After rod placement, cancellous bone and cortical matchstick grafts are placed for a posterolateral fusion.

- Increased incidence of disease at adjacent level (spondylolisthesis, spinal stenosis, disk herniation, stress fracture, scoliosis)[9]

REFERENCES

1. Roy-Camille R, Saillant G, Mazel C: Internal fixation of the lumbar spine with pedicle screw plating. Clin Orthop 1986;203:7–17.
2. Magerl F, Dick W, Kluger P, et al: A new device for internal fixation of thoracolumbar and lumbar spine fractures: The "fixateur interne." Paraplegia 1981;23:225–232.
3. McAfee PC, Weiland DJ, Carlow JJ: Survivorship analysis of pedicle spinal instrumentation. Spine 1991;16(Suppl):S422–S427.
4. Puno RM, Bechtold JE, Byrd JA 3rd, et al: Biomechanical analysis of transpedicular rod systems: A preliminary report. Spine 1991;16:973–980.
5. Marchesi DG, Thalgott JA, Aebi M: Application and results of the AO internal fixation system in nontraumatic indications. Spine 1991;16:S162–S169.
6. Yahiro MA: Comprehensive literature review: Pedicle screw fixation devices. Spine 1994;20(Suppl):2274S–2278S.
7. Fessler RG: Decision making in spinal instrumentation. Clin Neurosurg 1993;40:227–242.
8. Magerl FP: Stabilization of the lower thoracic and lumbar spine with external skeletal fixation. Clin Orthop 1984;1989:125–141.
9. Guigui P, Benoist M, Delecourt C, et al: Motor deficit in lumbar spinal stenosis: A retrospective study of a series of 50 patients. J Spinal Disord 1998;11:283–288.

CHAPTER 30

HO-YEOL ZHANG

DANIEL H. KIM

Posterior Lumbar Interbody Fusion

INTRODUCTION

Posterior lumbar interbody fusion (PLIF) was developed by Cloward in 1943,[1] who used iliac crest graft following radical diskectomy. Early clinical reports suggested a fusion rate of approximately 90% with very good or excellent results in the same number. The complication rate, however, was reported to be in the range of 5% to 8%, with a high incidence of nerve root injury. PLIF had largely fallen out of favor, because of the neurologic deficit occurring during decompression, as well as bone graft failures (nonunion, extrusion, disk space collapse) when performed without instrumentation.

PLIF has been resurrected in recent years because of the observation that transverse process fusion, although biomechanically effective in stabilizing the spine, often does not eliminate micromotion at the disk.[2] This observation led to the popularity of the "360-degree approach." PLIF has become particularly popular in recent years with the advent of preformed bone grafts and PLIF application sets, as well as titanium and carbon cages. Recent biomechanical data suggest advantages of the cages over bone.

Presently, PLIF is a surgical technique that allows fusion across two adjacent vertebrae by inserting grafts, titanium threaded cages, bone dowels, or carbon fiber spacers filled with bone graft into the disk space. All PLIF techniques require removal of the disk material from within the disk space. The bone grafts and spacing devices are used to heal a bony bridge and fuse the two adjacent vertebral bodies.

PLIF is a valuable way of achieving a spinal fusion. If spinal instability is present (i.e., spondylolisthesis or slippage of the vertebrae), then the PLIF should be performed with spinal stabilizing instruments such as pedicle screws or hooks and rods to immobilize the loose vertebrae.

The many advantages in instrumented PLIFs or 360-degree fusions include a decrease in pain and an increase in functional activities.[3] Compared with anterior-posterior fusions,[4] instrumented PLIFs also have equal patient satisfaction, much lower costs, and faster return to work and other activities. Furthermore, a recent biomechanical study by Bennett and associates found that PLIFs double the spinal stiffness produced by transpedicular fixation following laminectomy and facetectomy.[4]

Other theoretical advantages of PLIF are technical. They include the fact that a much larger area of bone surface exists for the fusion, with the fusion at the center of motion and at the site of maximum compression loading. The disk space is maintained in a distracted position without the collapse that is often seen in transverse process fusion using transpedicular fixation. In addition, the blood supply is better at the decorticated end plate than at the transverse process.

Although Cloward's original PLIF technique (noninstrumented PLIF) is no longer used today, this basic concept had been used to invent numerous cages and dowels for instrumented PLIF.

INDICATIONS

- Broad-based herniations
- Totally degenerated disks with marked instability (spondylolisthesis, some cases of scoliosis)
- Recurrent disk herniation
- Pseudoarthrosis of transverse process fusion (as an alternative to anterior lumbar fusion) in the absence of epidural scarring
- Back pain due to symptomatic spondylosis and/or symptomatic degenerative disk disease

PLIF is not recommended as a fusion technique if decompression of neural elements is not to be performed; there is little justification for exposing nerve roots to scarring or injury to achieve the spinal stability obtainable by transverse process or anterior lumbar fusion.[5]

CHAPTER 30 Posterior Lumbar Interbody Fusion

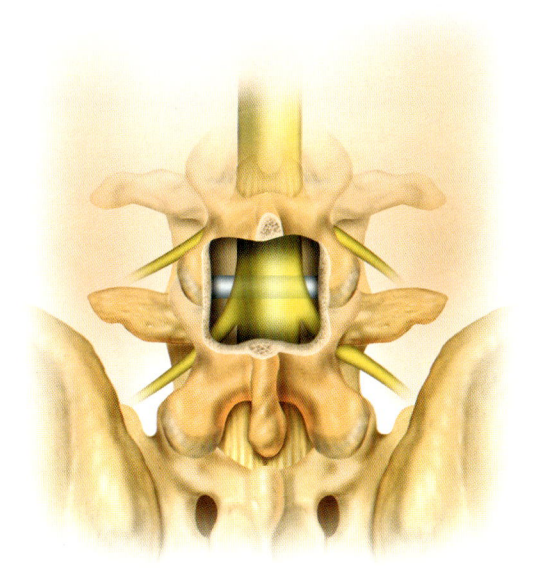

Fig. 30-1 L4 subtotal laminectomy.

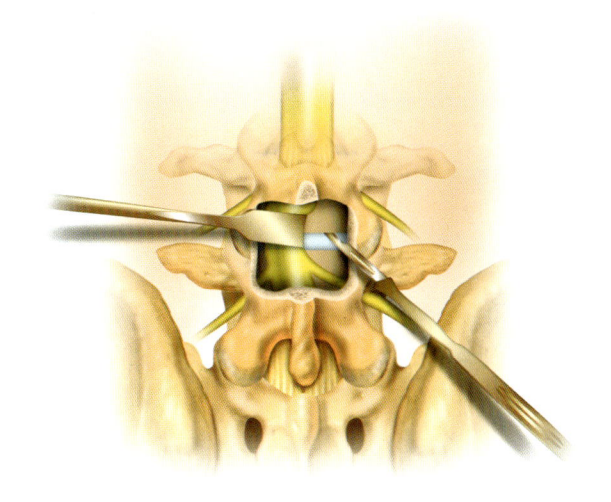

Fig. 30-2 Careful retraction of the nerve root and removal of the annulus.

OPERATIVE TECHNIQUE (CLOWARD'S METHOD)

LAMINECTOMY

- Patient is placed in prone position with chest rolls, on a Wilson frame, or using the Jackson table.
- Midline longitudinal skin incision is made.
- Subperiosteal dissection extends laterally beyond the border of the articular facet joints.
- Laminectomy and complete decompression of nerve roots are performed in the desired level. Total or subtotal laminectomy is easier than the partial laminectomy to handle the thecal sac and nerve roots (Fig. 30-1).
- Medial facetectomy is recommended for the preservation of the posterior column function.

TRADITIONAL DISKECTOMY

- After gently retracting the nerve roots and thecal sac, the epidural space is identified and epidural vessels are coagulated.
- Carefully retracting the nerve root at risk, a No. 15 blade is used to incise the annulus widely. A large rectangle of annulus and available disk is removed (Fig. 30-2).
- Traditional bilateral diskectomy requires removal of as much disk as possible to ensure that none bunches up to the midline, compressing the dural sac, when bone grafts or cages are placed laterally (Fig. 30-3).
- An up-biting pituitary forceps is used to remove disk underneath the thecal sac without manipulating it.
- Ring curettes are often used to further empty the disk space.
- Backward-angled curettes are carefully placed between the dural sac and the annulus to push down any bulging disk or osteophyte near the midline.

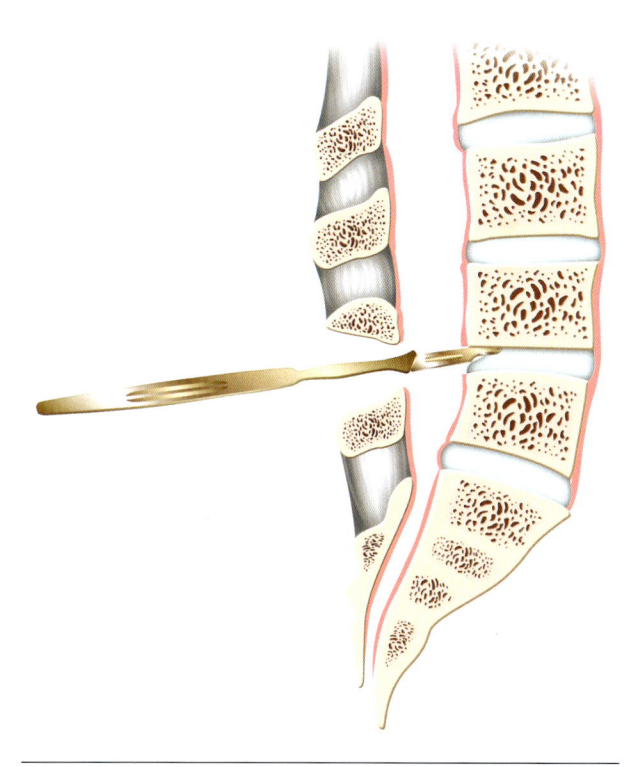

Fig. 30-3 Traditional diskectomy before end plate removal.

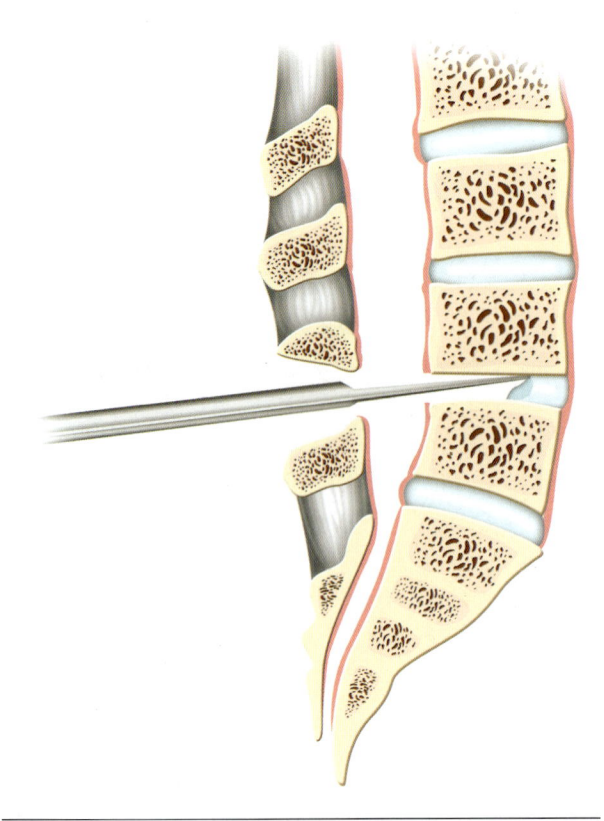

Fig. 30-4 Osteotomes are placed parallel to the end plates both at the superior and inferior aspect of the disk space, and then medial/lateral.

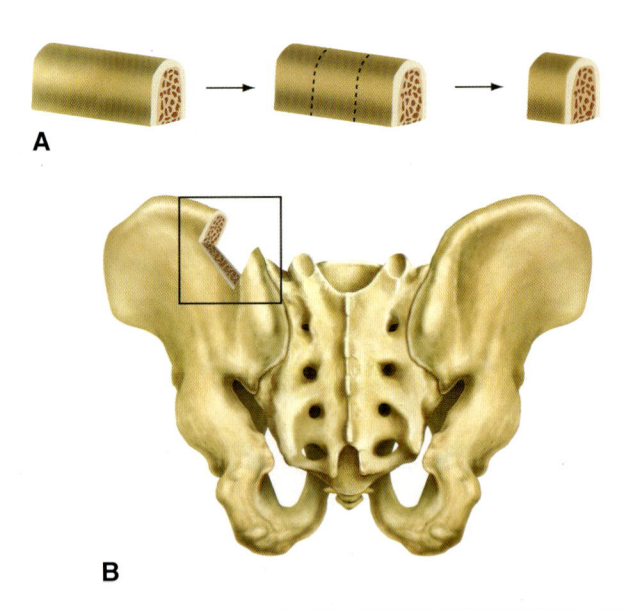

Fig. 30-5 Iliac bone harvesting. *A,* Graft harvest. *B,* Location of graft harvesting from the iliac crest.

DISK SPACE WIDENING AND END PLATE PREPARATION OR REMOVAL

- Vertebral spreader is used to widen the disk space.
- Radiographs are taken to determine how deep the osteotome cut can safely be made.
- A Penfield or ruler is placed into the disk space, and images are obtained.
- The osteotome should not be placed more than 50% to 60% through the anteroposterior diameter of the vertebral body.
- Osteotomes are placed parallel to the end plates at both the superior and inferior aspects of the disk space, and then medial/lateral (Fig. 30-4).

BONE GRAFT PREPARATION

- Separate the skin incision on the posterior superior iliac crest.
- Remove the long tricortical iliac bone.
- Shape it as three pieces of bone graft materials with the height of the distracted disk space by the vertebral spreader (Fig. 30-5).
- Donor-site bleeding control is achieved with bone wax and closure.

BONE GRAFT PLACEMENT

- The nerve root and dural sac should be very carefully protected with handheld retractors that are regularly released.
- The prepared tricortical grafts are then tapped into the widened disk space.
- A bleeding cancellous bone surface should then be available on the cephalad and caudal edges of the space, and possibly laterally as well.
- We generally prefer to place the more medial bone grafts first, to minimize total mobilization of the dural sac (Fig. 30-6).
- Others place the grafts laterally, and then push them toward the midline.
- The superior edge of the graft should be at least 5 mm ventral to the floor of the spinal canal.
- Two to three pieces can safely be placed on each side of the thecal sac (Fig. 30-7).
- After placing the grafts, be certain that the dural sac and nerve roots are not being compressed.

CLOSURE AND POSTOPERATIVE CARE

- Control bleeding of the disk space, epidural space, and paraspinal muscles.
- Place a drain for 24 hours and close the wound in layers.
- Patients are mobilized on the day of surgery and usually go home in an orthosis 1 or 2 days later.

INTERVERTEBRAL CAGES IN PLIF

The first commercial cage for PLIF in the United States is the Ray threaded fusion cage (TFC) system. Since the early 1990s, many spine surgeons have used intervertebral cages

CHAPTER 30   Posterior Lumbar Interbody Fusion   249

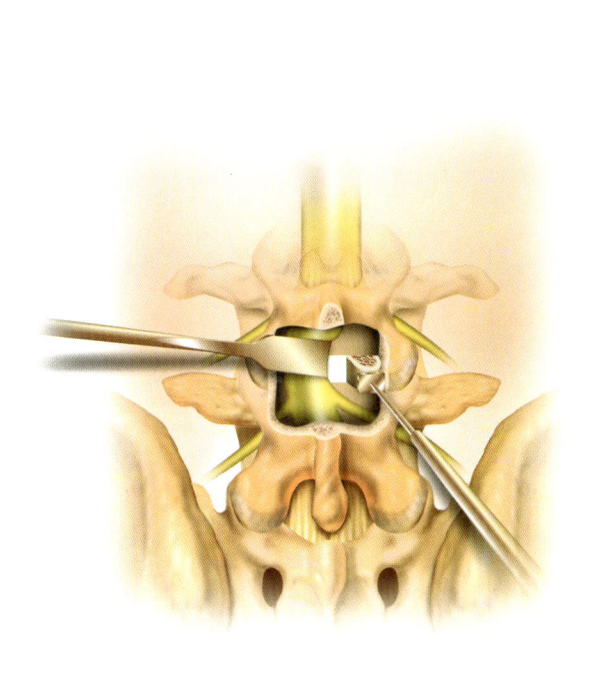

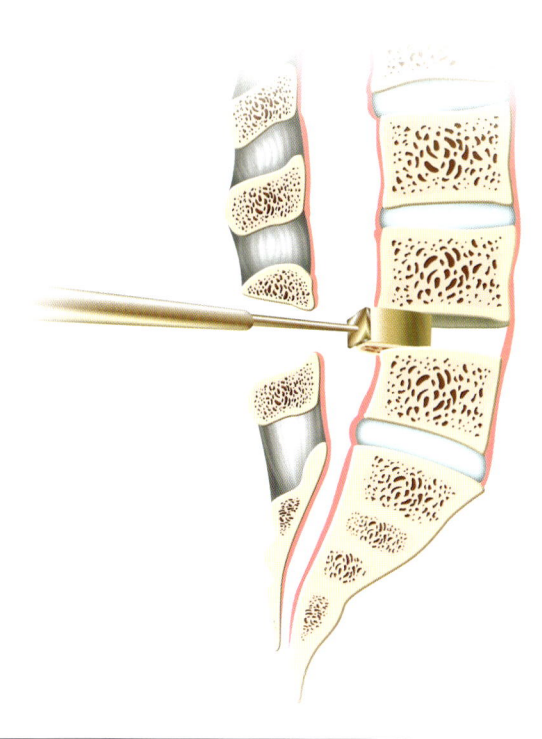

Fig. 30-6 Bone graft placement.

for most PLIFs. These cages allowed distraction of the disk space[6]; grafting using cancellous bone, which is optimal for fusion; optimal preparation of the host bone with excision of the end plates; and fixation that some feel approximates transpedicular fixation in a relatively safe and straightforward approach.[7]

Described in the following section is the Ray threaded fusion cage, marketed by Surgical Dynamics. (Note that in the case of pedicle fixations, there are surgeons who adamantly insist that one company's device is vastly superior to another. However, differences are minimal and largely technical. The choice of systems is thus dependent on the doctor's preference.)

The Ray cage was designed by Charles Ray as a hollow titanium alloy threaded cylinder that is fenestrated to promote bone growth into the vertebra adjacent to the cage.[8] Threads promote insertion, and improve pull-out strength and segmental stiffness (Fig. 30-8).

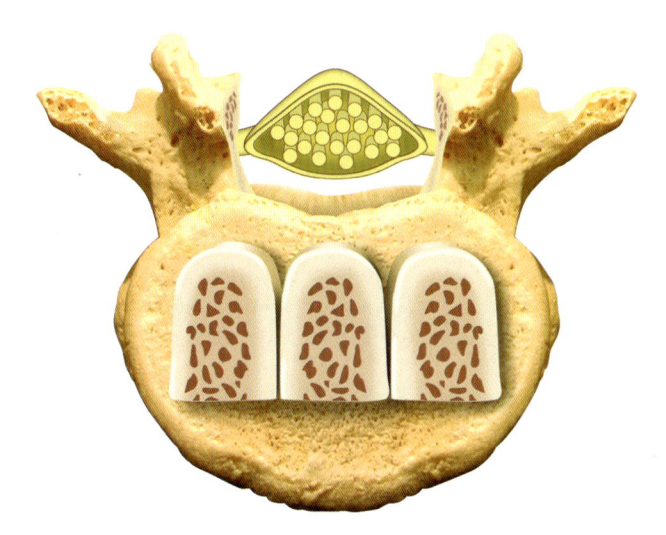

Fig. 30-7 Three bone grafts are placed.

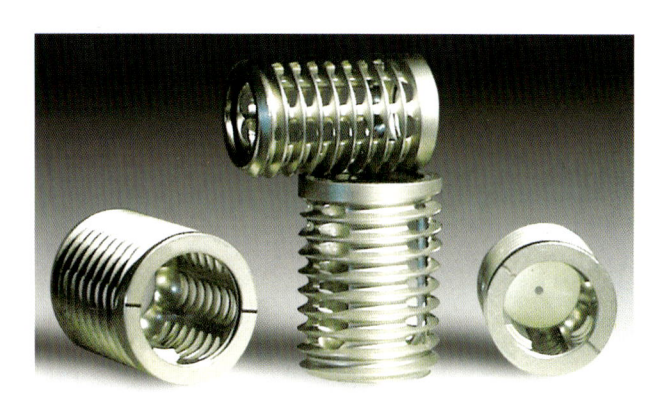

Fig. 30-8 The Ray threaded fusion cage (TFC) was designed by Charles Ray as a hollow titanium alloy threaded cylinder that is fenestrated to promote bone growth and to improve pull-out strength and segmental stiffness.

OPERATIVE TECHNIQUE: RAY THREADED FUSION CAGE

LAMINECTOMY AND DISKECTOMY

- The procedure for PLIF with intervertebral cages is the same as for original PLIF until the point of removal of the intervertebral disk.
- After the correct vertebral level has been confirmed, semicircular laminectomies are performed on both lateral sides of the disk space using standard rongeur or other tools. Medial facetectomy should be minimized to preserve the posterior column stability (Fig. 30-9). Preservation of spinous process is recommended also, but some surgeons prefer to remove it and use its pieces as bone graft materials.
- Bilateral annulotomies are then performed sufficiently wide to accommodate a tang retractor and other instrument placement (Fig. 30-10).
- The semicircular laminectomy performed on the side of the distractor tip or spacer placement should be just large enough to allow retraction of the dura and insertion of the distractor tip or spacer.
- Care must be taken to protect all neural and vascular structures throughout the procedure using the dura retractor and ganglion retractor.
- The cage size should be determined after partial diskectomy. The cages should allow at least 3 mm subcortical placement of the cage both anterior and posterior to be certain that there is no nerve root or dural sac compres-

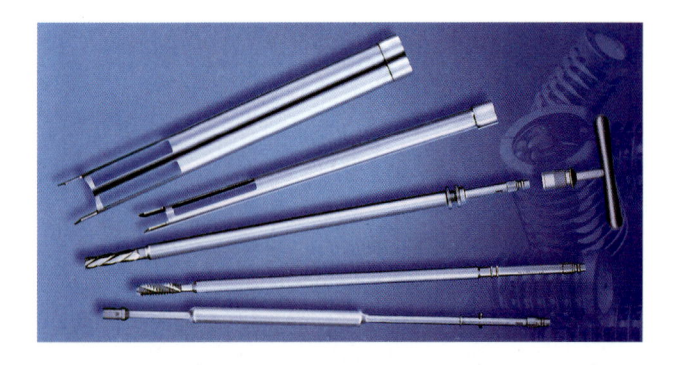

Fig. 30-10 Instruments for threaded fusion cage. From top, tang retractor for anterior lumbar interbody fusion, tang retractor for posterior lumbar interbody fusion, vertebral drill and T handle, vertebra tap and cage insertion instrument (cage holder).

sion. In addition, cage placement should be lateral enough so that the cages do not touch.
- The Ray threaded fusion cage is available in four diameters (12, 14, 16, and 18 mm) and two lengths (21 and 26 mm). It is ideal to place the largest diameter cage that safely fits.

PLACEMENT OF DISTRACTOR TIP

- All distractor, tang, and cage placements are recommended to be performed under radiographic control. On the first side approached, the distractor is placed into the disk space following disk removal.
- Before placing the blades of the distractor into the disk space, all neural structures need to be carefully retracted. The dura retractor is leveraged under the interspinous ligament from the contralateral side, and the dura is retracted medially. The ganglion retractor gently retracts the ganglion cephalad nerve root, if needed, while exposing the disk space (Fig. 30-11).
- Remove osteophytes or hypertrophied annulus to allow the distractor and tang to fit flush with the posterior vertebral margin.
- Select the largest distractor tip that safely fits, and drive it into the hole in the disk space using a mallet. Impact the distracter tip appropriately under the fluoroscopy, directing the distractor slightly medially. Then remove the handle, leaving the distractor tip in place (Fig. 30-12). The dural sac is allowed to fall back over the distractor.

PLACEMENT OF TANG RETRACTOR

- On the contralateral side, the nerve roots and thecal sac are again carefully retracted. A tang retractor of the same diameter as the distractor is impacted into place with x-ray guidance.

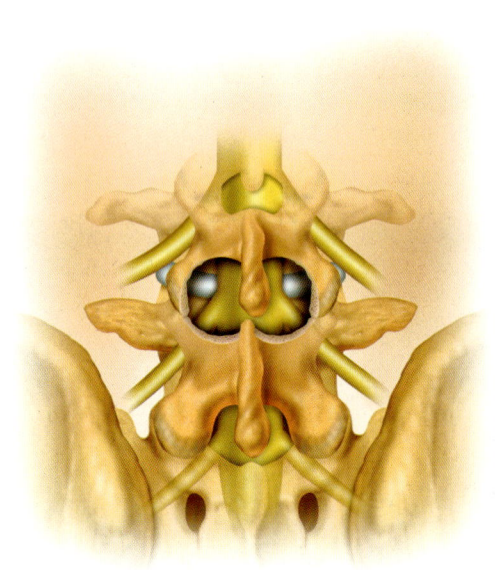

Fig. 30-9 Semicircular laminetomies are performed on both lateral sides of the disk space using standard rongeur, power drill, or chisel. Facet joint removal should be minimized to preserve the posterior column stability.

CHAPTER 30 Posterior Lumbar Interbody Fusion

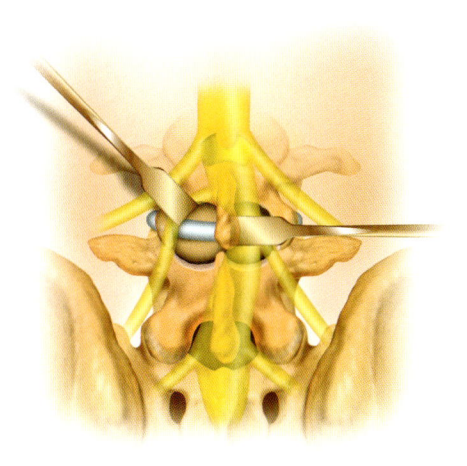

Fig. 30-11 Careful retraction of the dura and upper nerve root. Dura retractor leveraged under the interspinous ligament from the contralateral side, the dura is retracted medially. The ganglion retractor gently retracts the nerve root ganglion cephalad, if needed, while exposing the disk space.

- The tang and distractor are the right size and appropriately placed if the blades are firmly against both end plates and are well placed within the disk space itself (Fig. 30-13). The length of the blade (24 mm) of the tang allows determination of cage length as well.

DRILLING

- Before drilling, the surgeon should again be absolutely certain that the tang is seated flush on the vertebral body and annulus and that all neural elements are safely away from the barrel. This must be confirmed prior to drilling.
- The disk space is then drilled. Overdrilling greater than the cage depth is important to prevent disk bulging back against the cage from the anterior surface (Fig. 30-14). Loose disk material is removed with pituitary forceps. The tang should be controlled to prevent the blades from loosening and the tang from wobbling.

TAPPING

- The hole is then tapped. Carefully advance the tap clockwise to the desired depth. We prefer to overtap 2 mm to 3 mm beyond the marks to take further advantage of the overdrilling performed in the previous step.
- The tap is removed with equally careful counterclockwise unscrewing to prevent cross-threading.

CAGE INSERTION

- The cage is threaded clockwise to the appropriate length laser-etched on the handle. We then generally thread the cage another 3 mm (one complete turn) beyond what the tool indicates (Fig. 30-15).

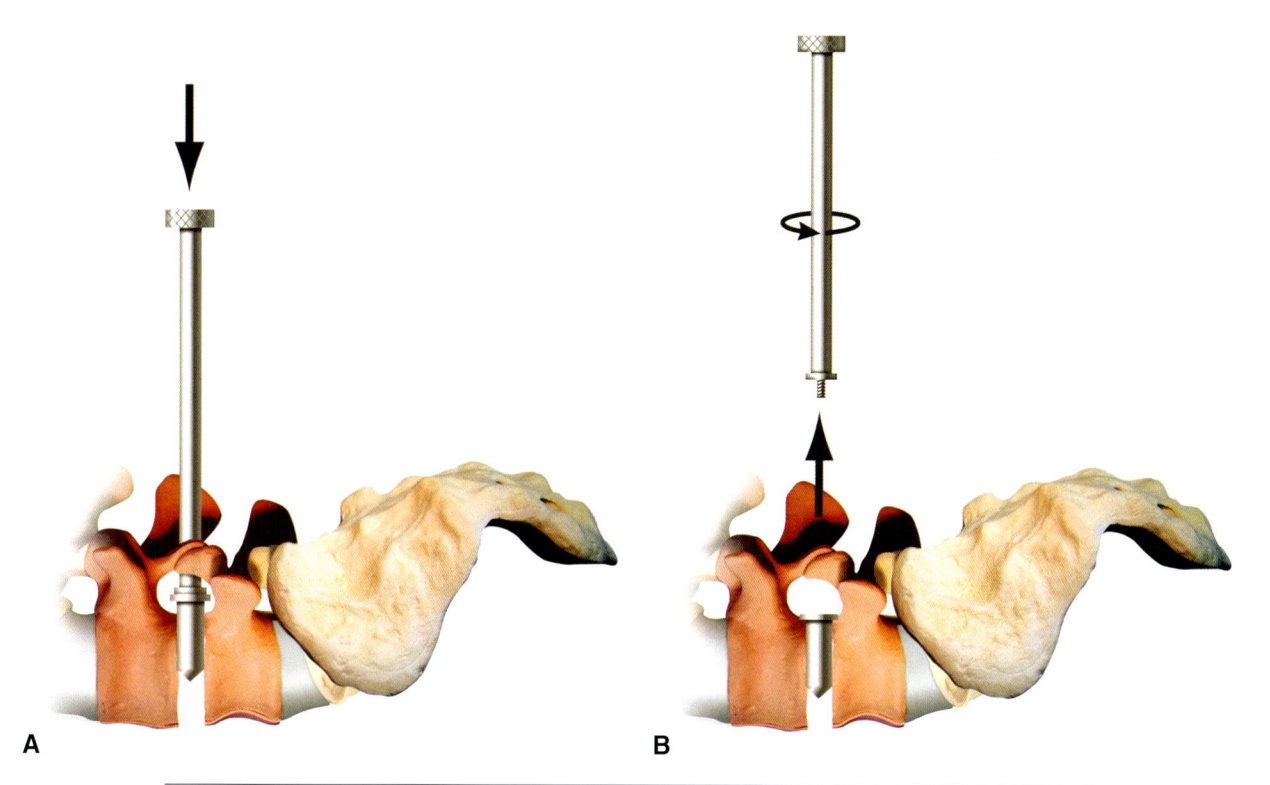

Fig. 30-12 Distractor tip placement. A, Distractor with applier. B, Removal of the distractor handle.

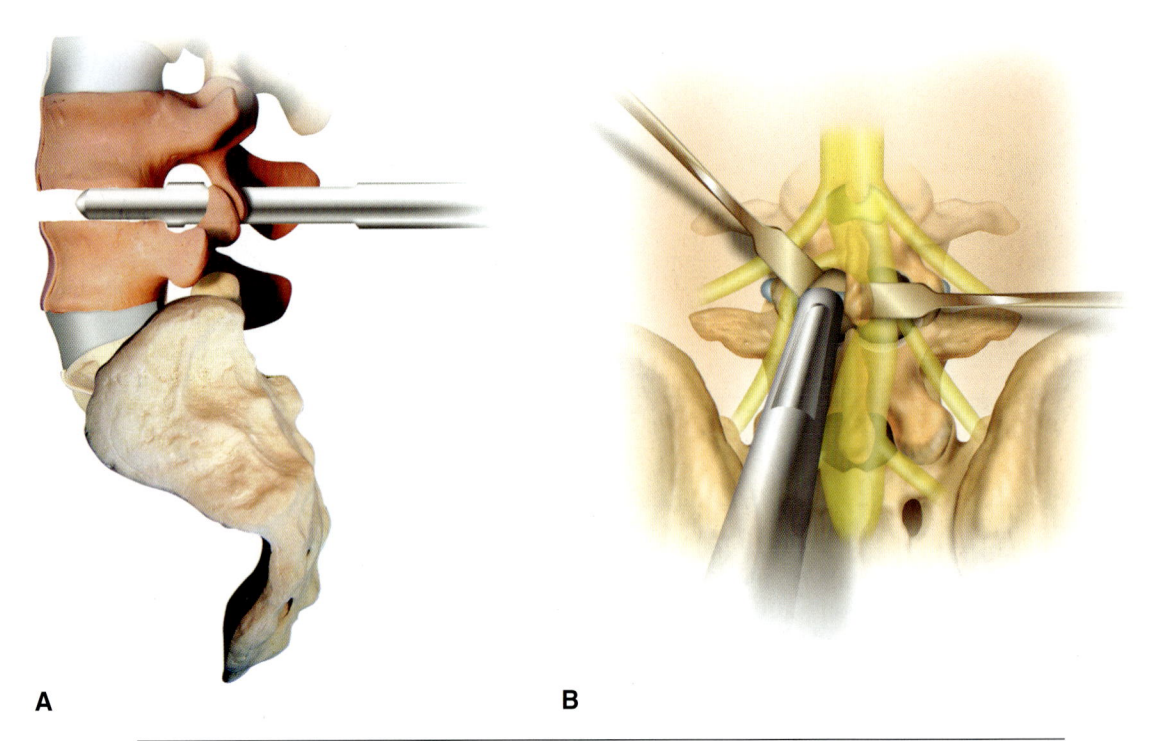

Fig. 30-13 The tang and distractor are the right size and appropriately placed if the blades are firmly against both end plates and are well placed within the disk space itself. *A*, Lateral image of the distractor. *B*, Nerve root retraction and placement of the distractor.

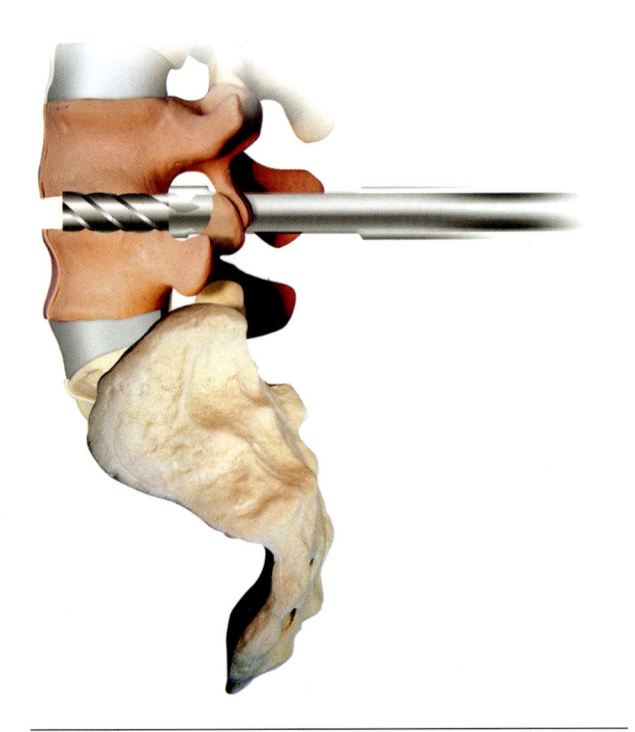

Fig. 30-14 Drilling. A shorter drill will create a 25-mm hole for the 21-mm cage, and the longer drill will make a 30-mm depth for the 26-mm cage. The tang should be controlled to prevent the blades from loosening and the tang from wobbling.

- Two small indicator pins on the insertion handle must be pointing directly cranial-caudal when insertion is complete.

BONE FRAGMENT GRAFT AND END CAP SNAPPING

- The cage is then packed with bone fragments. When local bone is being used, complete removal of soft tissue is needed. As the bone is placed, it should be packed using the instrument available in the set. Bone graft placement should stop one or two screw threads below the edge of the cage. The plastic end cap is then placed (Fig. 30-16).
- Following successful placement of this cage, the next step is the other side. Aggressive disk removal should be carried out. Remove the distractor and remove more disks than had been taken out previously. The dural retractors are again placed, and a tang is placed in the same position and alignment. The cage insertion procedure is then repeated.

CLOSURE AND POSTOPERATIVE CARE

- Bleeding is controlled in the disk space, epidural space, and paraspinal muscles.
- Place a drain for 24 hours and close the wound in layers.
- Patients are mobilized on the day of surgery and usually go home in an orthosis 1 or 2 days later.

CHAPTER 30 Posterior Lumbar Interbody Fusion 253

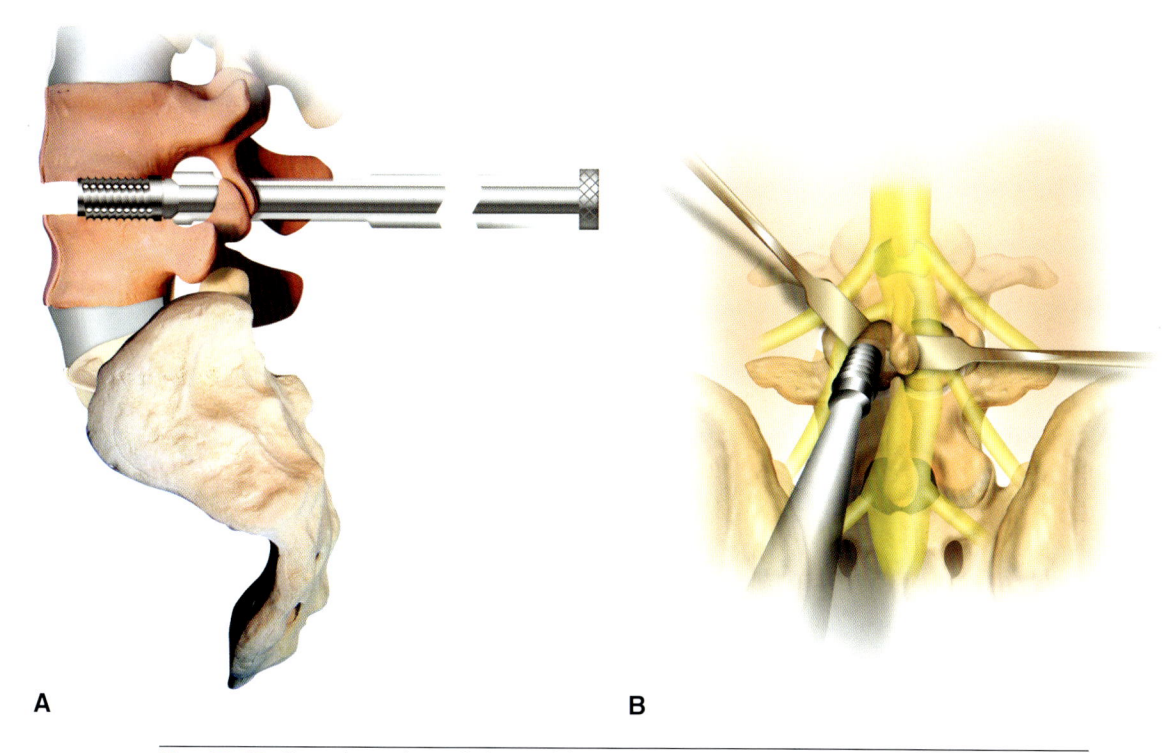

Fig. 30-15 Cage insertion. *A,* Lateral image. *B,* Anteroposterior image.

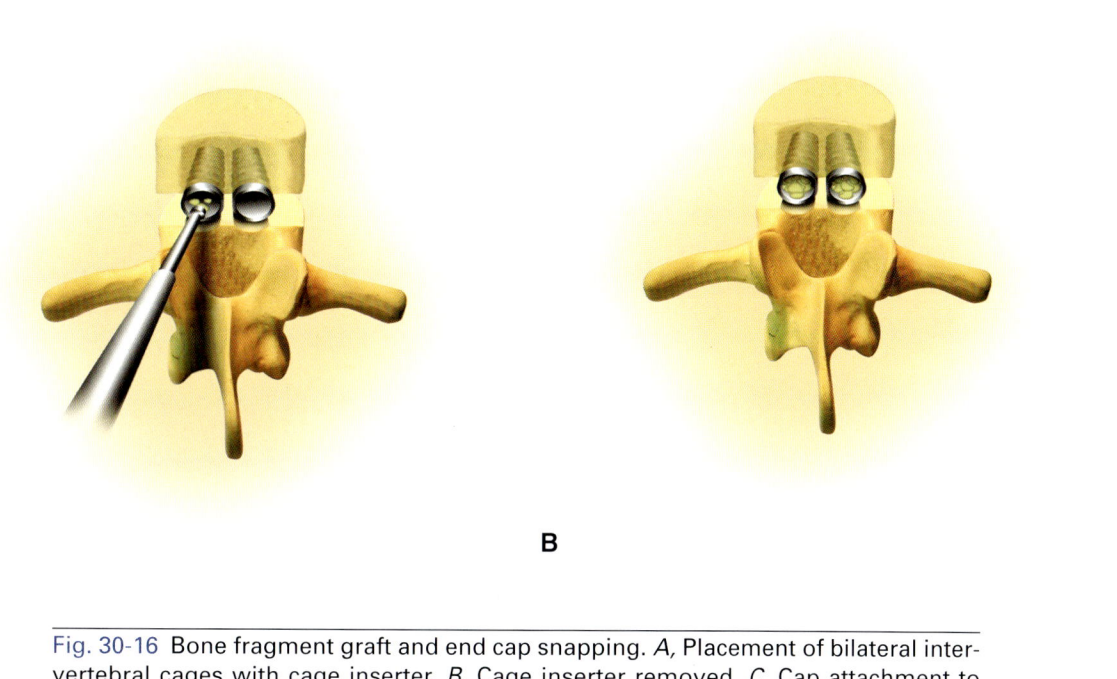

Fig. 30-16 Bone fragment graft and end cap snapping. *A,* Placement of bilateral intervertebral cages with cage inserter. *B,* Cage inserter removed. *C,* Cap attachment to intervertabral cage.

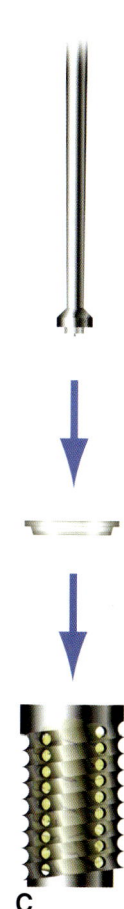

COMPLICATIONS

- Significant hemorrhage with inadequate coagulation of the epidural space
- Nerve root and cauda equina injury
- Remained central disk protrusion
- Cage retropulsion
- Nonunion
- Wound infection

References

1. Cloward RB: The treatment of ruptured lumbar intervertebral discs by vertebral body fusion: Indications, operative technique and aftercare. J Neurosurg 1953;10:154–168.
2. Christoferson LA, Selland B: Intervertebral bone implants following excision of protruded lumbar discs. J Neurosurg 1975;42:401–405.
3. Hinkley BS, Jaremko ME: Effects of 360 degree lumbar fusion in a workers' compensation population. Spine 1997;22:312–322.
4. Hacker RJ: Comparison of interbody fusion approaches for disabling low back pain. Spine 1997;22:660–666.
5. Larson JL, Maiman DJ: Surgical Approaches. In Larson JL, Maiman DJ (eds): Surgery of the Lumbar Spine. New York, Thieme, 1999, pp 267–324.
6. Sandhu HS, Turner S, Kabo JM, et al: Distractive properties of a threaded interbody fusion device: An in vivo model. Spine 1996;21:1201–1210.
7. Bagby G: Arthrodesis by the distraction-compression method using a stainless-steel implant. Orthopedics 1988;11:931–934.
8. Ray C: Threaded titanium cages for lumbar interbody fusions. Spine 1997;22:667–679.

CHAPTER 31

HO-YEOL ZHANG

DANIEL H. KIM

Unilateral Transforaminal Lumbar Interbody Fusion

INTRODUCTION

Posterior lumbar interbody fusion (PLIF) after lumbar disk removal was first reported by Jaslow[1] in 1946. Cloward[2] presented his first 100 cases at the Harvey Cushing Society meeting in 1947. More recently, Steffe,[3] Brantigan,[4] and Ray[5] have reported on the use of posterior segmental instrumentation or the use of cage implants for PLIF.

Perhaps the greatest concern with a standard PLIF is the amount of neural retraction needed. An improper amount could potentially lead to nerve root injury, cauda equina injury, dural laceration, and epidural fibrosis.[5,6]

Consequently, the unilateral transforaminal posterior lumbar interbody fusion (TLIF) was developed to address some of these problems. The concept of a unilateral approach to the anterior column was refined and popularized by Dr. Professor Jurgen Harms.[7] The purpose of this approach was to obtain the same goals as a PLIF without the potential risks and complications.

The TLIF technique allows clearance of the entire intervertebral disk compartment by opening the neural foramen on one side. After appropriate clearance, it is possible to achieve further enlargement of the cleared intervertebral compartment by posterior transpedicular distraction. This enables definitive anterior column support and certain fusion by transforaminally introduced bone material and support structures. After the introduction of these anterior fusional elements, segment stability is restored by converting the distraction force into compression force. The TLIF approach helps to avoid damage to important anatomic structures such as the nerve roots, dura, ligamentum flavum, and interspinous ligament. Preservation of the ligamentous structures is of great importance to restoring biomechanical stability of the segment and its adjacent counterparts.

The advantages over the standard PLIF include the ability to provide bilateral anterior column support through a single posterolateral approach of the disk space. The transforaminal approach preserves the anterior and most of the posterior longitudinal ligamentous complex, which provides a tension band for compression of the graft and prevents retropulsion of the graft. It avoids excessive soft tissue dissection, which may help prevent scarring and instability of adjacent segments, as well as injury to the exiting nerve root. Epidural bleeding is less of a problem than with the standard bilateral PLIF because of the unilateral transforaminal approach, and, with experience, proper cage placement within the disk space is consistently achieved.[6]

INDICATIONS AND CONTRAINDICATIONS

INDICATIONS

- Best indication is a grade I or grade II spondylolisthesis without neurologic deficit or with a deficit on one side only.[8]
- Degenerative disease with positive diskography without any intracanal pathologic condition.
- Anterior column deficiency with chronic mechanical pain related to degenerative disk disease, recurrent disk herniation, and/or spondylolisthesis.[6]
- Segmental kyphosis related to disk narrowing.
- Grade II or III spondylolisthesis can also be reduced with this technique without the need for anterior surgery.
- Patients with multiple comorbidities potentially affecting successful arthrodesis (obesity, smoking, diabetes, previous failed fusion) are also candidates for the TLIF because it provides a circumferential fusion through a posterior-only approach.
- The TLIF procedure can also be used to decrease pseudoarthrosis at the lumbosacral junction.

CONTRAINDICATION

- Tight anterior disk space with osteophyte formation in which there is no potential for disk space distraction.[8]

RELATIVE CONTRAINDICATIONS

- If there is extensive epidural scarring or history of prior infection, a TLIF may be performed; however, in this case, it is often more prudent to perform a direct anterior lumbar interbody fusion.[8]
- Severe osteopenia (bone mineral density <60% predicted).[6]
- Bilateral epidural fibrosis with pseudoarthrosis.
- Fusion of more than two levels.

OPERATIVE TECHNIQUE

EQUIPMENT

- X-ray-compatible operating table
- Jackson table, Wilson frame, or chest rolls
- Fluoroscopy
- Headlight system
- Pneumatic compression stocking or antiembolic stocking to both legs
- Lumbar laminectomy set
- Steinmann pins
- Bone graft source
- Lumbar pedicle screw system

PATIENT POSITIONING AND PEDICLE SCREW PLACEMENT

- After endotracheal anesthesia, the patient is placed in a prone position with avoidance of epidural venous distention from abdominal compression.
- Posterior spinal elements are exposed through a midline longitudinal incision.
- A subperiosteal dissection of the paraspinous muscles is completed to the transverse processes.
- Pedicle screws are sized and inserted under C-arm x-ray guidance before decompression to minimize blood loss and achieve distraction (Fig. 31-1).

UNILATERAL FACETECTOMY AND CONTRALATERAL DISTRACTION

- If radiculopathy is present, the spinal canal is entered through a unilateral laminectomy and inferior facetectomy on the side of the radicular pain. If no radiculopathy is present, the side is chosen arbitrarily.
- Apply the rod system at the contralateral side and distract the disk space (Fig. 31-2). The interspinous ligament as well as the ligamentum flavum on the opposite side is left intact. The degree of bone resection necessary for this unilateral TLIF technique is indicated in Figure 31-2.

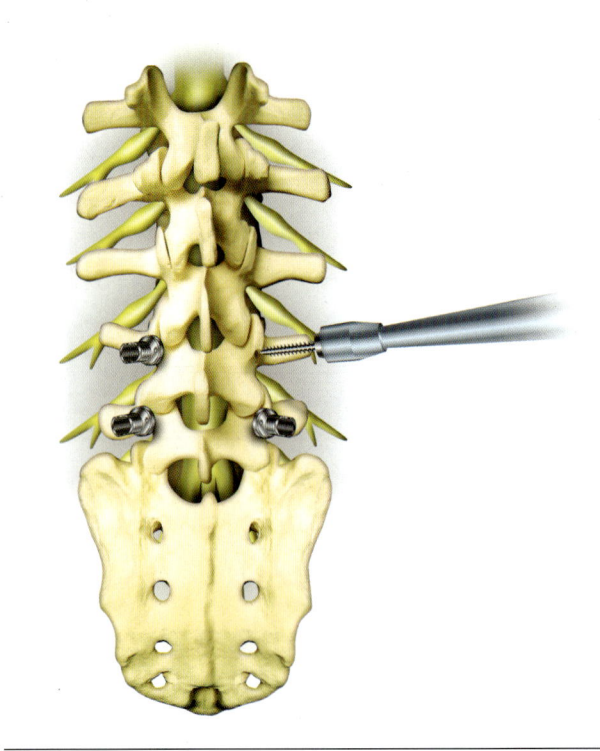

Fig. 31-1 After the subperiosteal dissection, pedicle screws are sized and inserted before decompression.

- The next step is to gain access to the disk at L4-L5 via the transforaminal approach. The inferior articular process of the cranial vertebra is now thinned out with the use of a burr, while distraction forces are applied to the contralateral side (Fig. 31-3).

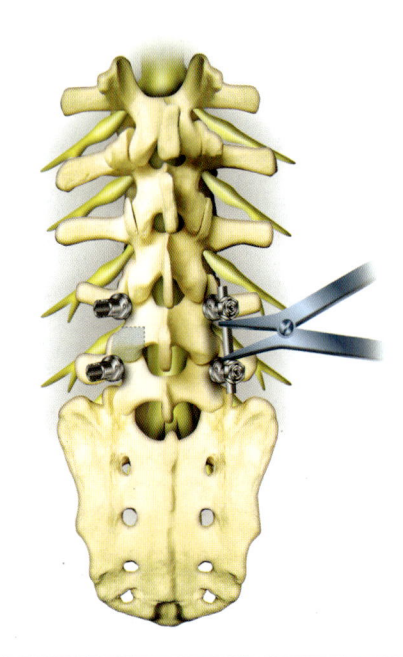

Fig. 31-2 Apply the rod system at the nonradiculopathy side and distract the disk space. A facetectomy will be done at the radiculopathy side.

CHAPTER 31 Unilateral Transforaminal Lumbar Interbody Fusion

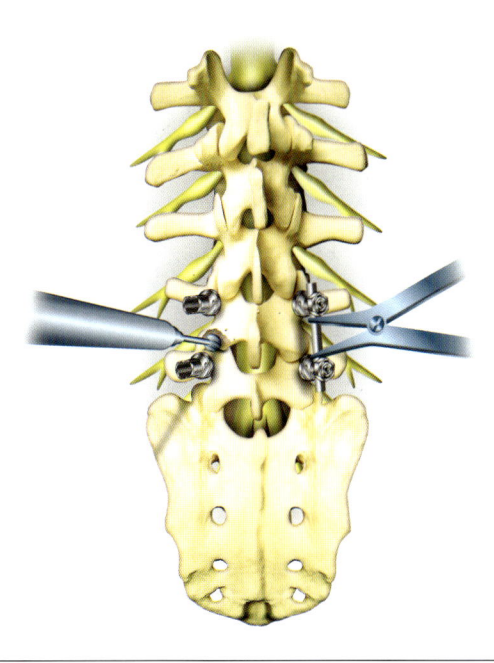

Fig. 31-3 The inferior articular process of the cranial vertebra is thinned out with the use of a burr, while distraction forces are applied to the contralateral side.

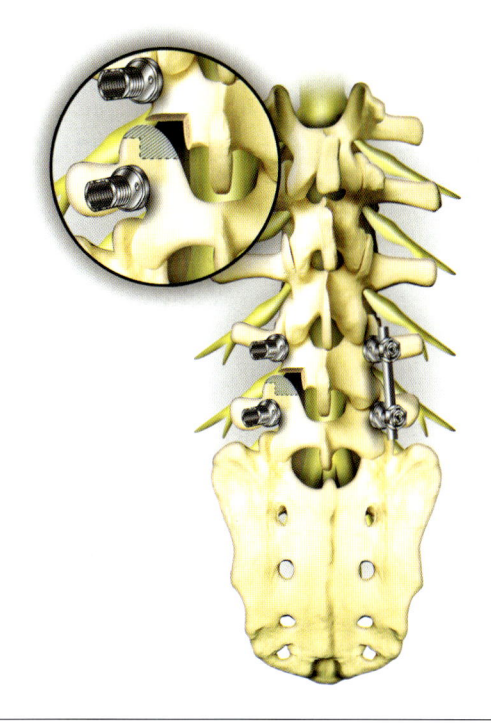

Fig. 31-4 After thinning by using a drill, resect the inferior articular process of the cranial vertebral body with a chisel or bone cutter, thereby uncovering the neural foramen. The degree of bone to be resected from the superior facet of the inferior vertebra is indicated.

- Once thinned, resect the inferior articular process of the cranial vertebral body with a chisel or bone cutter, uncovering the next stage in the approach to the neural foramen. The degree of bone to be resected from the superior facet of the inferior vertebra is indicated in Figure 31-4.
- The capsular part of the ligamentum flavum is now visible and can be resected. To avoid damage to the nervous structures, it is necessary to cut around the superior articular facet of the caudal vertebral body. Care must be taken to ensure the lateral delimitation of the ligamentum flavum is largely preserved.
- Only in exceptional cases is resection of the lateral part of the ligamentum flavum necessary. Tactile exploration of the neural foramen is recommended with palpatory identification of the cranial nerve root and the position and breadth of the pedicle of the caudal vertebral body (Fig. 31-5).
- Resect the superior facet of the inferior vertebra as the final step in gaining access to the disk at L4-L5, the posterolateral parts of the annulus fibrosus, and the longitudinal ligament (Fig. 31-6).
- The entire neural foramen is identified after resection of the upper medial parts of the superior articular facet of the lower vertebral body. The upper nerve root that passes around the pedicle of the upper vertebral body and the lateral part of the intervertebral disk can be identified. The nerve root can be identified merely by palpation in its course within the foramen, especially where it crosses over the lateral parts of the intervertebral space. The origin of the next nerve root in the caudal direction and the dural sac in the medial border can also be identified. After identification of these nervous structures, meticulous coagulation of the epidural veins in the neural foramen is carried out (Fig. 31-7).

TOTAL DISKECTOMY THROUGH UNILATERAL APPROACH

- The thecal sac is gently retracted medially, if necessary.
- A diskectomy is performed through this unilateral approach (Fig. 31-8).
- Partially clear the intervertebral disk compartment by using various rongeurs. Curettes can be used to remove the intervertebral disk remnants adhering to the upper plates. With the curettes, the cartilaginous coats of the end plates can be removed at the same time without destroying the osseous structure of the end plates.

END PLATE PREPARATION

- After the initial diskectomy, gradual distraction is applied to the pedicle screws on the opposite side.
- An osteotome is used to remove the posterior lateral lip of concave bone to achieve a flat end plate surface. This is important, because the upper plates of the lumbar vertebral bodies always have a pronounced concave shape.

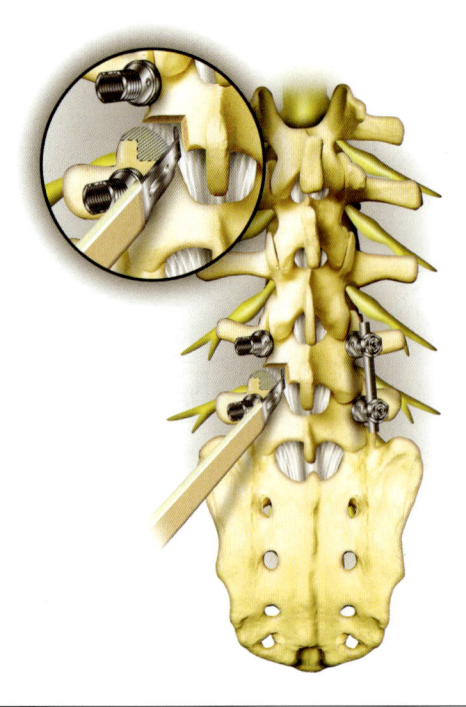

Fig. 31-5 The ligamentum flavum removal. Care must be taken to ensure that the lateral delimitation of the ligamentum flavum is largely preserved. The exiting nerve root is identified and protected from surgical trauma. Tactile exploration of the neural foramen is recommended with palpatory identification of the upper nerve root and the position and breadth of the pedicle of the caudal vertebral body.

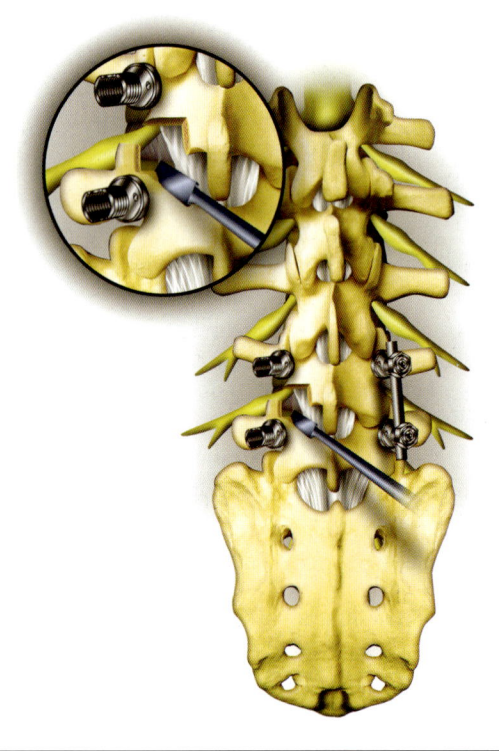

Fig. 31-6 Resect the superior facet of the inferior vertebra as the final step in gaining access to the disk at L4-L5, the posterolateral parts of the annulus fibrosus, and the longitudinal ligament.

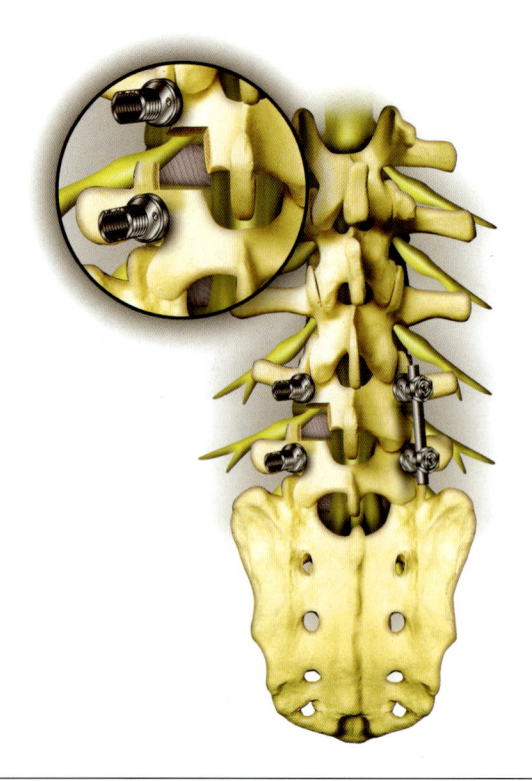

Fig. 31-7 After resection of the upper medial parts of the superior articular facet, the neural foramen is opened. The upper nerve root and the lateral part of the intervertebral disk can now be identified.

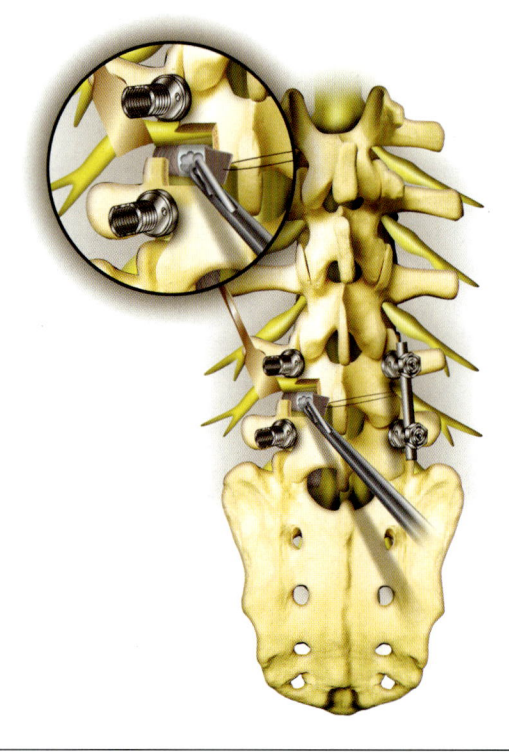

Fig. 31-8 The thecal sac is gently retracted medially, if necessary. The diskectomy is performed through this unilateral approach.

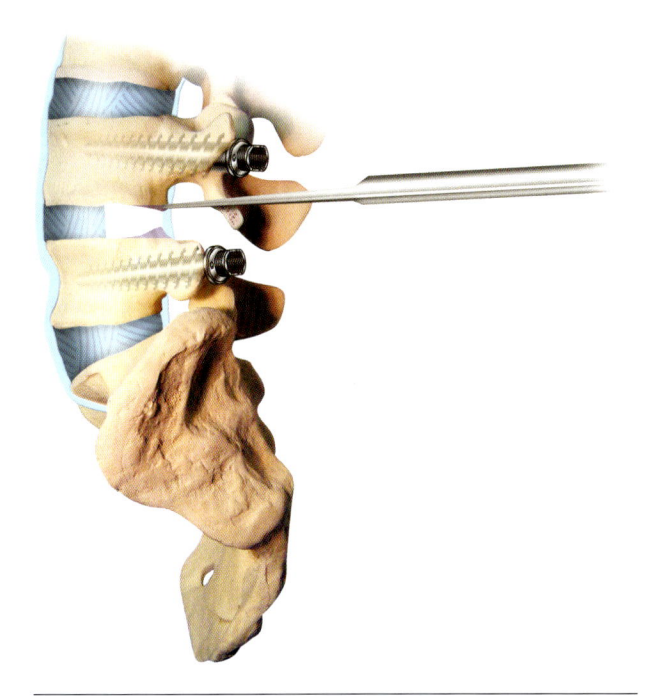

CHAPTER **31**   Unilateral Transforaminal Lumbar Interbody Fusion

Fig. 31-9 Clear the intervertebral disk compartment by using various rongeurs and curettes. An osteotome is used to remove the posterior lateral lip of concave bone to achieve a flat end plate surface. The dorsal lips of the vertebral body should be resected to form a uniform aperture.

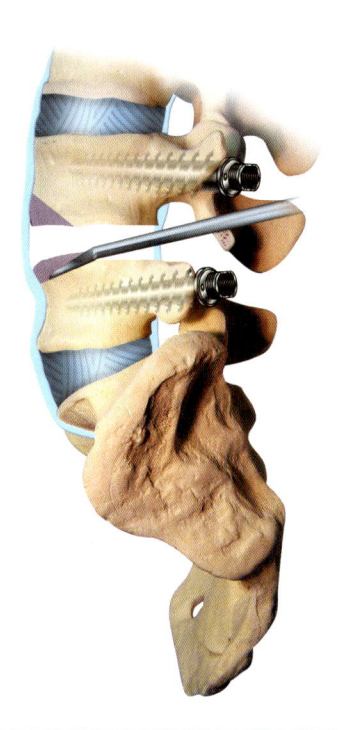

Fig. 31-10 Remove the anterior one third or one quarter of the end plates to enable osseous fusion. The remaining part of the osseous end plate must be carefully preserved to accommodate the supporting structural graft. The anterior longitudinal ligament must be preserved to prevent the vascular injury.

- By a marginal resection of the dorsal edges of the end plates, a parallel plane between the adjacent vertebral bodies can be established. This is for the introduction of the structural graft. The dorsal lips of the vertebral body should be resected to form a uniform aperture (Fig. 31-9).
- Carefully curette the remaining cartilaginous parts of the end plates. A chisel is not indicated, because it will destroy the cortical structure of the end plates.
- It is necessary to remove the anterior one third or one quarter of the opposing end plates to enable definitive osseous fusion.[9] By this resection with angular chisels, the cancellous bone structure of the vertebral body is exposed, guaranteeing rapid osteointegration. Only the anterior one third or one quarter is resected. The remaining part of the osseous end plate must be carefully preserved to accommodate the supporting structural graft, which will be inserted later. In the process of chiseling, the anterior longitudinal ligament must not be damaged, as this can result in vascular injury. A surgeon who is inexperienced in this procedure should initially use an image intensifier or fluoroscopy when completing this step (Fig. 31-10).

CANCELLOUS BONE AND STRUT BONE (OR CAGE) GRAFT

- The previously harvested cancellous bone is introduced into the retracted intervertebral disk compartment and brought to the anterior longitudinal ligament. Impact the introduced cancellous bone with straight and angled impactors. This procedure can attain a definite bone layer in the anterior one third of the intervertebral space. Also, this impacted cancellous bone prevents the structural graft from being positioned too far anteriorly (Fig. 31-11).
- Cut the structural graft to the appropriate height and insert it. A cage of the proper height and packed with cancellous bone is inserted into the disk space. For biomechanical reasons, the graft should be situated in the middle or posterior half of the intervertebral space. Insert the first graft transforaminally into the disk space and place it primarily close to the posterior wall and slide it anteriorly to the contralateral side.
- Bring the first graft over the midline to the opposite side in a rolling movement. The graft is supported on the ventrally introduced autologous bone chips, which prevents it from becoming positioned too far ventrally (Fig. 31-12).
- A second graft is seated next to the first one to line them up to the left and to the right of the midline, respectively. In this way, a good broad area of support from the adjacent vertebral bodies is attained (Fig. 31-13).
- After insertion of the bilateral strut graft or cages from a unilateral approach, the final position is checked visually

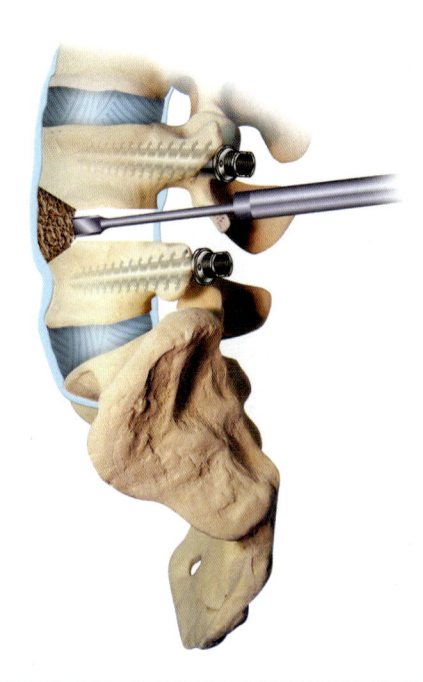

Fig. 31-11 Cancellous bone is introduced into the intervertebral disk space and brought to the anterior longitudinal ligament. This is necessary to attain a definite bone layer in the anterior one third of the intervertebral space. At the same time, this impacted cancellous bone prevents the structural graft from being positioned too far anteriorly.

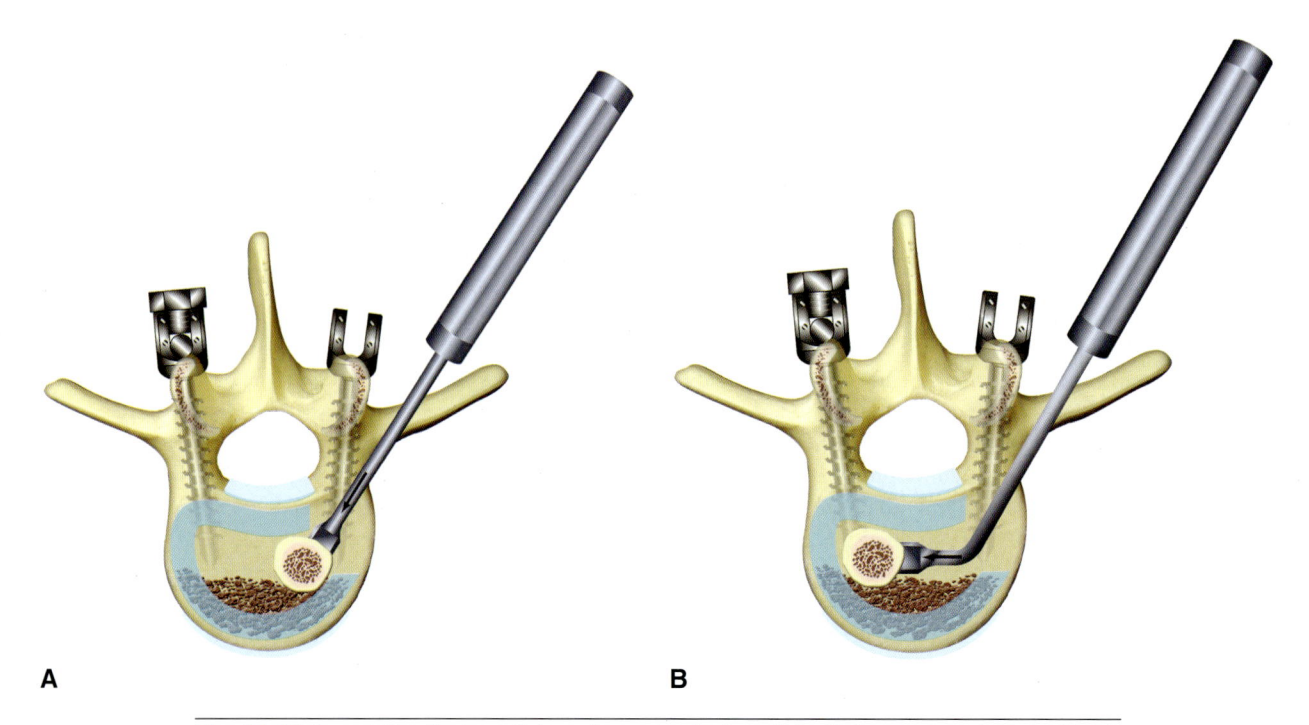

Fig. 31-12 Insert the first graft transforaminally into the disk space and place it primarily close to the posterior wall. Then slide it anteriorly to the contralateral side.

CHAPTER 31 Unilateral Transforaminal Lumbar Interbody Fusion

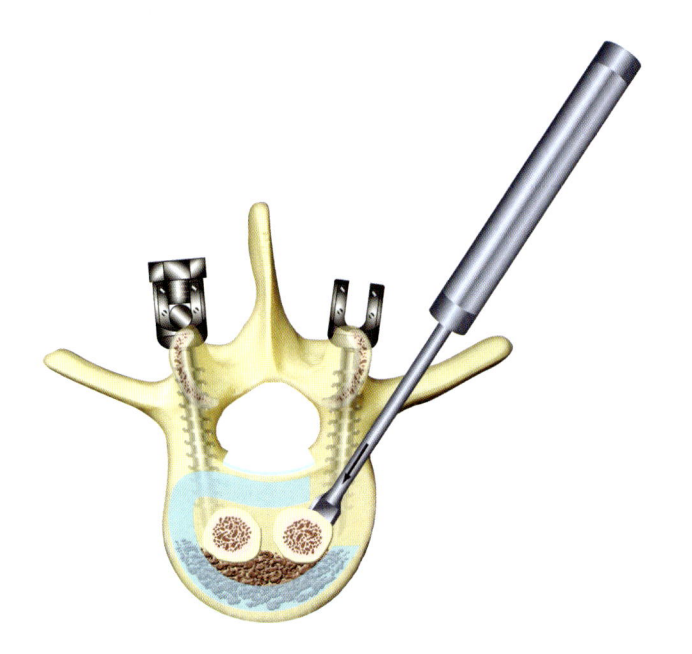

Fig. 31-13 A second graft is seated next to the first one to line these up to the left and to the right of the midline, respectively. In this way, a good broad area of support from the adjacent vertebral bodies is attained.

and radiologically. Then the disk space distraction is released.

FINAL ASSEMBLY OF ROD-SCREW SYSTEM AND CLOSURE

- The construct is compressed to establish an optimal graft-bone interface and to reestablish lumbar lordosis at the operated segments (Fig. 31-14).
- The rod-screw system is tightened and cross-linked.
- Perform a posterolateral fusion with cancellous iliac bone graft over the transverse processes after adequate decortication on both sides (Fig. 31-15).
- Insert drains and carry out the muscle closure, followed by fascia suture, subcutaneous suture, and finally skin closure.

POSTOPERATIVE CARE

- All wound drains are removed 24 to 48 hours after surgery.
- Patients with a one-level lumbar fusion do not need external orthosis.

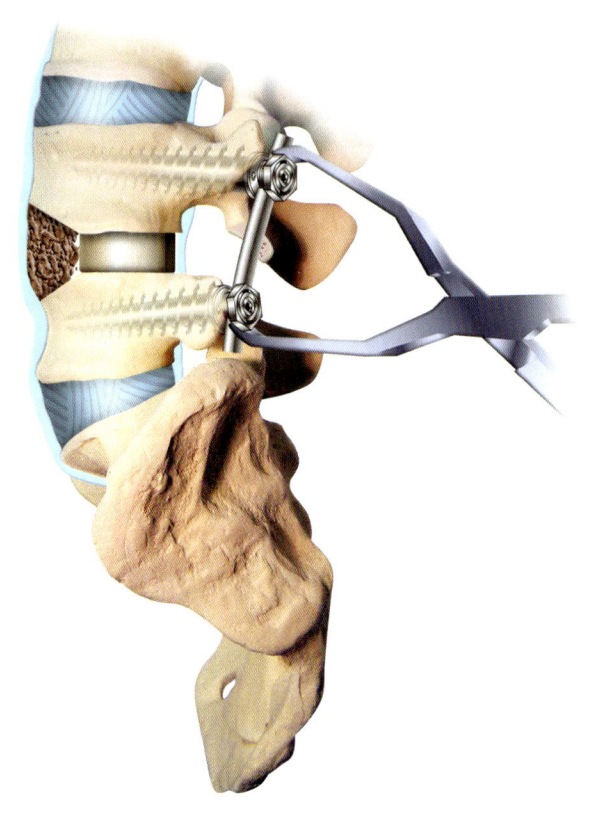

Fig. 31-14 After insertion of the bilateral cages from a unilateral approach, the final position of the structural graft is checked visually and radiologically. Then the disk space distraction is released. The construct is compressed to establish an optimum graft-bone interface and to reestablish lumbar lordosis at the operated segments.

- Patients are mobilized postoperatively on day 1.
- Physical therapy for rehabilitation is then provided.
- Patients are usually discharged from the hospital at 2 to 3 days after operation if there are no complications.

COMPLICATIONS

- Pseudoarthrosis
- Excessive hemorrhage
- Dural tear
- Infection

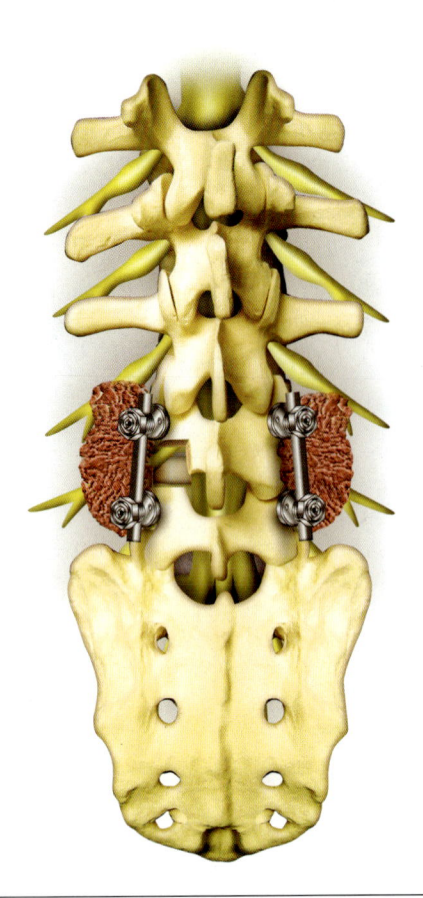

Fig. 31-15 After tightening and cross-linking of the rod-screw system, perform a posterolateral fusion with bone graft over the transverse processes.

REFERENCES

1. Jaslow LA: Intercorporal bone graft in spinal fusion after disc removal. Surg Gynecol Obstet 1946;82:215–222.
2. Cloward RB: The treatment of ruptured intervertebral disc by vertebral body fusion. Indications, operative technique, after care. J Neurosurg 1953;10:154–168.
3. Steffee AD, Sitkowski DJ: Posterior lumbar interbody fusion and plates. St. Vincent Charity Hospital, Cleveland (OH). Clin Orthop 1988;227:99–102.
4. Brantigan JW, Steffee AD: A carbon fiber implant to aid interbody lumbar fusion: Two year clinical results of the first 26 patients. Spine 1993;18:1213–1221.
5. Ray CD: Threaded titanium cages for lumbar interbody fusions. Spine 1997;22:667–680.
6. Lowe TG, Tahernia AD, O'Brien MF, Smith DAB: Unilateral transforaminal posterior lumbar interbody fusion (TLIF): Indications, technique, and 2-year results. J Spinal Disord Tech 2002;15:31–38.
7. Harms J, Roliger H: A one-stage procedure in operative treatment of spondylolisthesises: Dorsal traction-reposition and anterior fusion. Z Orthop Grenzgeb 1982;120:343–347.
8. Moskowitz A: Transforaminal lumbar interbody fusion. Orthop Clin North Am 2002;33:359–366.
9. Harms J, Jeszenszky D, Stolze D, et al: True spondylolisthesis reduction and more segmental fusion in spondylolisthesis. In Bridwell KH, Dewald RL, Hammerberg KW (eds): The Textbook of Spinal Surgery, 2nd ed. Philadelphia, Lippincott-Raven, 1997, pp 1337–1347.

CHAPTER 32

MICHAEL Y. WANG
CARL LAURYSSEN

Anterior Lumbar Interbody Fusion

INTRODUCTION

Anterior lumbar interbody fusion (ALIF) has evolved as one of the predominant surgical techniques for the treatment of diskogenic back pain. Through an anterior, retroperitoneal approach the entire ventral surface of the disk is exposed, making complete diskectomy and subsequent placement of a large intradiskcal implant straightforward.

Although various surgical techniques have been developed to access the anterior lumbar spine (open retroperitoneal, transperitoneal, endoscopic, and balloon-assisted endoscopic), the mini-open retroperitoneal approach has become the most widely accepted. Mini-open access allows wide exposure of up to three disk spaces from L3-L4 to L5-S1. Furthermore, standard open techniques and instrumentation can be utilized, allowing for direct manipulation of vascular structures. Surgeon disorientation is also kept to a minimum.

ADVANTAGES OF AN ANTERIOR APPROACH

Interbody fusion can be approached from a number of different access corridors (anterior, anterolateral, extreme lateral, transforaminal, and posterior). The anterior retroperitoneal corridor provides the most direct and complete exposure of the disk space. Through this approach the view is centered in the midline with lateral exposure to either side of the vertebral bodies. This extensive lateral exposure allows for the most extensive disk removal and placement of a single unit implant that nearly matches the vertebral end plate in surface area. Large bone surface areas allow for low nonunion rates and minimize the risk of interbody subsidence. Direct neurologic compression is not routinely performed with ALIF techniques, but posterior disk herniations and posterior longitudinal ligament removal are possible.

Another major advantage of ALIF is that the technique spares the posterior spinal musculature. This results in a reduction of the postoperative pain and disability that frequently accompanies posterior spinal fusions. In addition, because ALIF avoids the extensive stripping of the dorsal soft tissues, muscle denervation and atrophy, implicated in abnormal biomechanics and failed back surgery syndrome, are avoided.

PATIENT SELECTION

The surgical treatment of diskogenic back pain remains controversial. Although the intervertebral disk undoubtedly contains nociceptive receptors, the relationship between symptoms of back pain, diagnostic studies, and surgical outcomes remains unclear. Because of the ubiquity of back discomfort and the high incidence of disk abnormalities on magnetic resonance imaging, strict criteria in selecting patients for surgery remains critical.

Several factors do appear to be predictive of pain relief following lumbar interbody fusion: (1) the history should be consistent with mechanical symptoms of axial pain aggravated by spinal loading and motion; (2) radiographic studies should demonstrate severe disk degeneration localized to discrete levels; (3) provocative diskography should produce concordant pain only at the affected levels and demonstrate an abnormal nuclear distribution; and (4) abnormal excessive motion on dynamic studies or sagittal deformity are highly predictive of postoperative improvement.

INDICATIONS AND CONTRAINDICATIONS

INDICATIONS

- Discogenic disease at the L3-L4, L4-L5, and L5-S1 level(s)
- Revision of a failed posterior fusion at the L3-L4, L4-L5, or L5-S1 level(s)

RELATIVE CONTRAINDICATIONS

- Severe medical comorbidities
- Morbid obesity
- Retroperitoneal scarring from previous surgery
- Aortic aneurysm
- Severe peripheral vascular disease
- Solitary kidney on the side of the exposure (risk of ureteral injury, without stenting)
- Severe osteoporosis with a high risk of interbody graft settling
- Spinal infection
- High-grade spondylolisthesis in the absence of a posterior fusion

OPERATIVE TECHNIQUE (MINI-OPEN APPROACH)

EQUIPMENT

- Table-mounted abdominal retractor system
- Lateral fluoroscopy or flat film x-rays
- Vascular clips and ligature suture
- Long curettes
- Long Kerrison punches
- Laminar spreader or interbody distractor
- Tamp
- Long-handled osteotomes (for vertebrectomy)
- High-speed drill (for vertebrectomy)
- Interbody spacers
  - Bicortical iliac crest autograft
  - Femoral ring allograft
  - Cylindrical threaded allograft bone dowels
  - Cylindrical threaded titanium cages
  - Titanium mesh cage
  - Alternate material cages (carbon fiber, resorbable polylactic acid, polyetheretherketone polymer)
- Osteoconductive/osteoinductive substances to fill interbody spacers
  - Vertebral autograft
  - Cancellous iliac crest autograft
  - Cortical or cancellous allograft chips
  - Demineralized bone matrix
  - Bone morphogenetic protein
- Anterior thoracolumbar plating system (optional)

PATIENT POSITIONING

- The patient is positioned supine on a standard operating table with the arms abducted at 90 degrees.
- Careful attention should be paid to the degree of lumbar lordosis following positioning, and an inflatable bladder should be placed under the patient's back to elevate the midlumbar spine. This not only opens the anterior disk space to assist in the diskectomy, but also allows easier placement of lordotic implants.
- Abduction of the arms permits placement of the table-mounted abdominal retractor closer to the patient's torso without the risk of an upper extremity compressive neuropathy.
- The anterior abdomen and iliac crest (if autograft is to be harvested) are prepped.

EXPOSURE

- A 12-cm skin incision is made to the left of the midline over the appropriate disk space (Fig. 32-1).
- Blunt finger dissection is used to mobolize the skin and soft tissues off the left anterior rectus sheath (Fig. 32-2).
- The anterior rectus sheath is divided longitudinally near the midline.
- The medial border of the intrafascial muscle belly is mobilized over a cranial to caudal distance of 12 cm.
- The muscle is then mobilized laterally to expose the underlying arcuate line. Alternatively, a lateral incision can be made in the anterior sheath and the muscle mobilized medially (Fig. 32-3).
- Blunt dissection under the arcuate ligament (which marks the most caudal aspect of the incomplete posterior rectus sheath) and superficial to the exposed peritoneum allows access to the retroperitoneal space (Fig. 32-4).

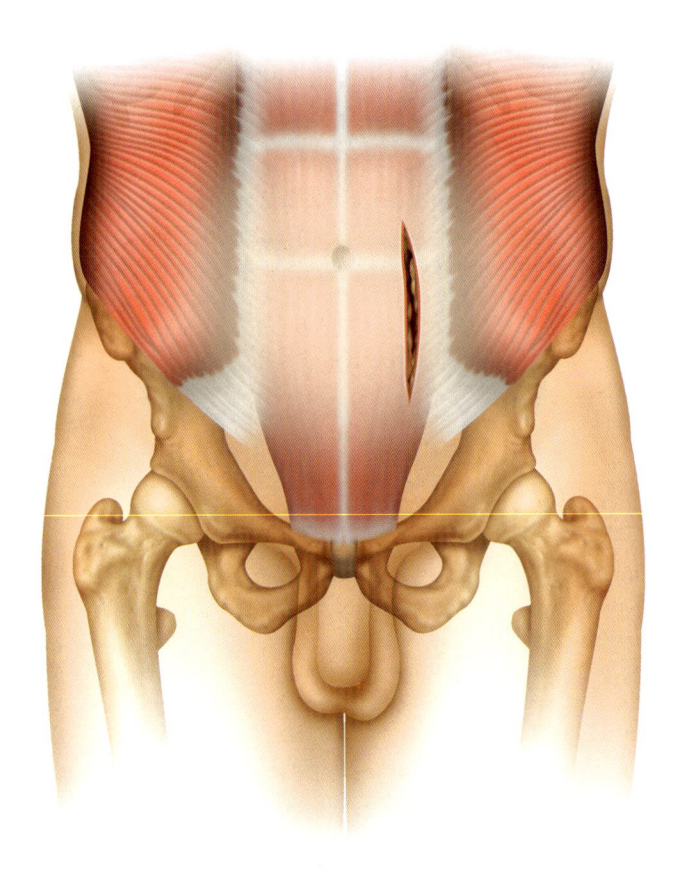

Fig. 32-1 Incision along the left lateral aspect of the rectus abdominis.

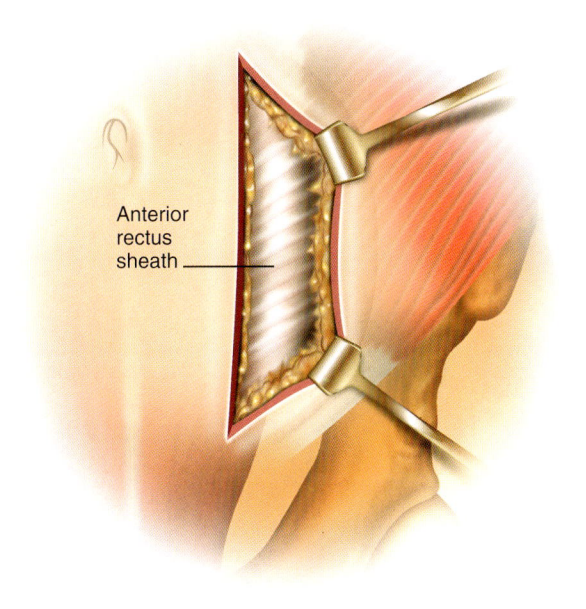

Fig. 32-2 Blunt dissection and retraction of the superficial soft tissues to expose the anterior rectus sheath.

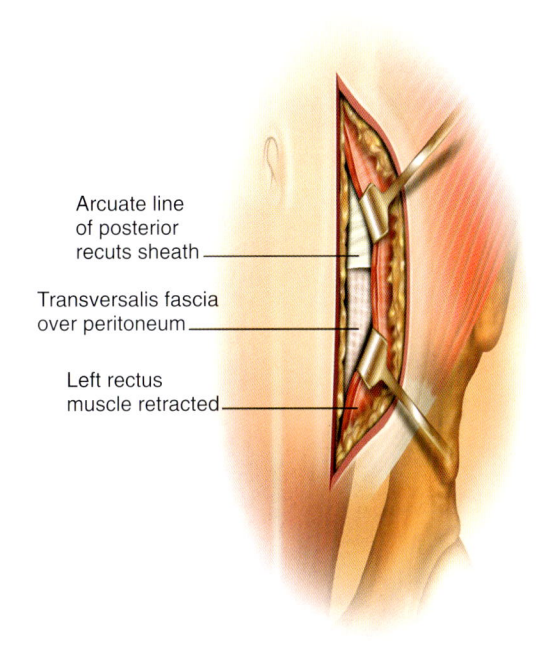

Fig. 32-3 Blunt dissection along the fibers of the rectus abdominis muscle medially to expose the posterior sheath. The arcuate line marks the transition at the lower end of the incomplete posterior rectus sheath to the peritoneum.

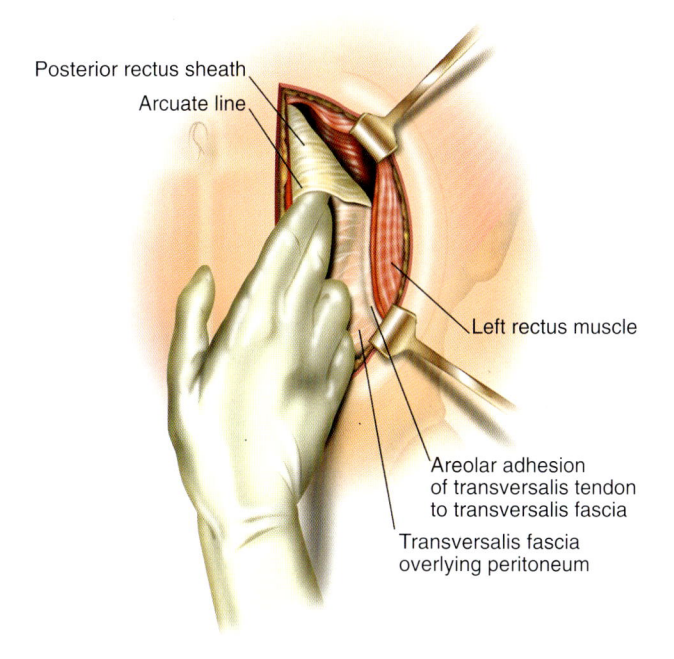

Fig. 32-4 Identification of the retroperitoneal layer is accomplished with blunt finger dissection under the arcuate line between the posterior rectus sheath and the peritoneum.

- Inserting the fingers and then the entire hand into the retroperitoneal space allows the surgeon to sweep the intraperitoneal contents superiorly, inferiorly, and medially to reveal the spinal column in the midline (Fig. 32-5). Because this technique relies on palpation and not visualization, the surgeon must be familiar with the relevant anatomy. Palpation of the great vessels helps to avoid vascular injury, and care should be exercised to avoid tears in the peritoneal lining. These tears can be either repaired primarily or opened to prevent bowel strangulation.
- The ureter must be identified to prevent inadvertent injury and is typically found on the peritoneal side of the exposure.
- Deep, self-retaining abdominal retractors can then be placed and attached to the table-mounted frame to maintain a midline corridor to the spine (Fig. 32-6).
- Proper localization is confirmed with lateral radiography.

VASCULAR DISSECTION

- The aorta and vena cava are then identified. For exposure of the L5-S1 interspace, the disk typically can be accessed below the bifurcation of the great vessels (the interiliac corridor). At the L3-L4 and L4-L5 levels the aorta and vena cava will have to be retracted left from their midline position (the left lateroaortic route).
- In the absence of scarring, blunt dissection with a sponge stick is very effective for mobilizing the vessels. Segmental

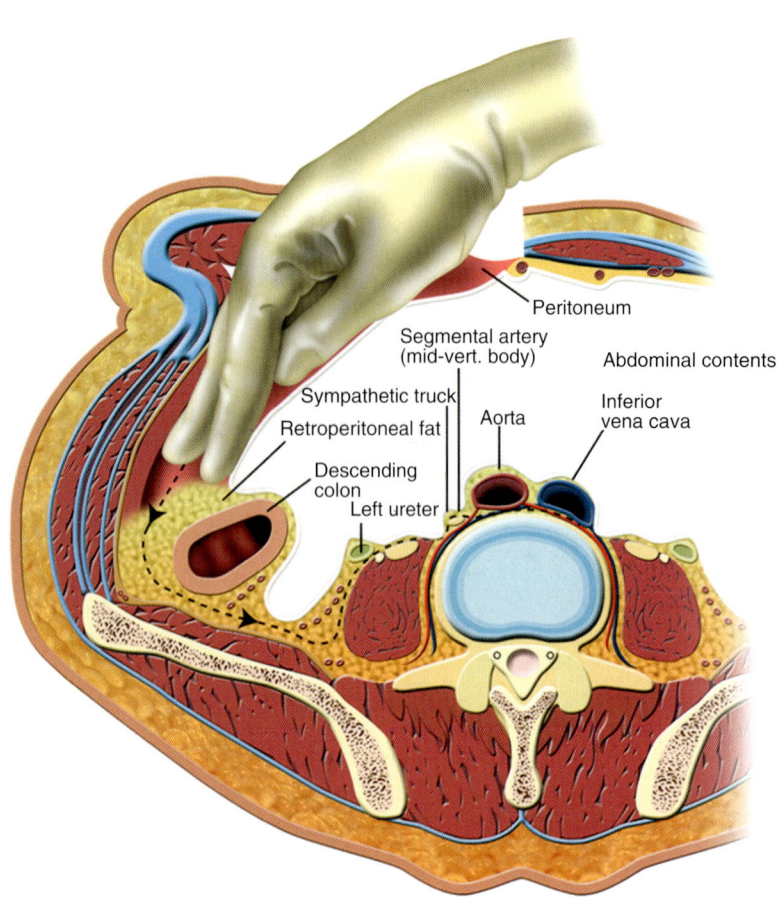

Fig. 32-5 Axial section showing the approach of the blunt finger dissection used to reach the anterior aspect of the lumbar spine.

arteries traversing the disk space or tethering the aorta need to be ligated securely. Iliolumbar veins can also be a troublesome source of bleeding. Any nearby iliolumbar veins should be prophylactically ligated, as inadvertent tearing of these vessels can be difficult to control and may lead to substantial blood loss (Fig. 32-7).

- The middle sacral artery and vein may need to be ligated for access below the bifurcations.
- The vascular anatomy of this region can be quite variable (Fig. 32-8).
- If the iliac vessels are medially located, an assistant should retract them laterally with handheld retractors to expose the disk space widely.

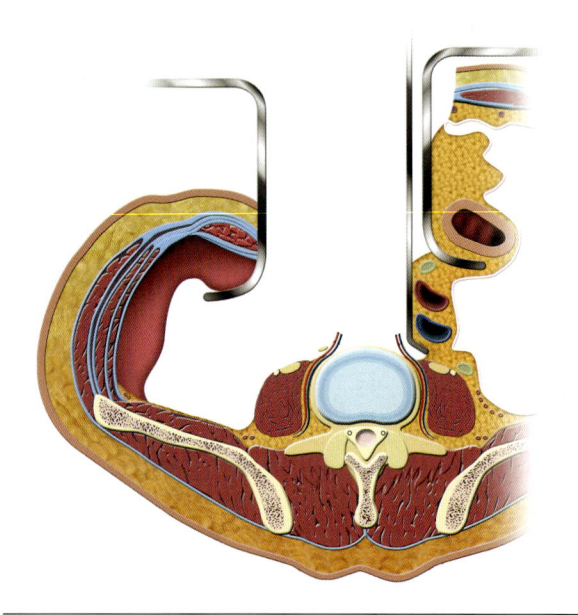

Fig. 32-6 Deep retractor placement allows for a centered, midline anterior approach to the spinal column.

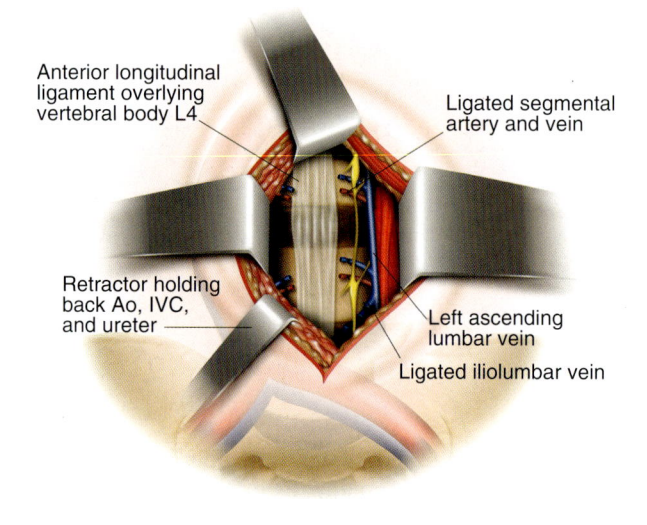

Fig. 32-7 Intraoperative view of the anterior longitudinal ligament with neighboring segmental arteries and the iliolumbar vein.

CHAPTER 32 Anterior Lumbar Interbody Fusion 267

A

B

C

D

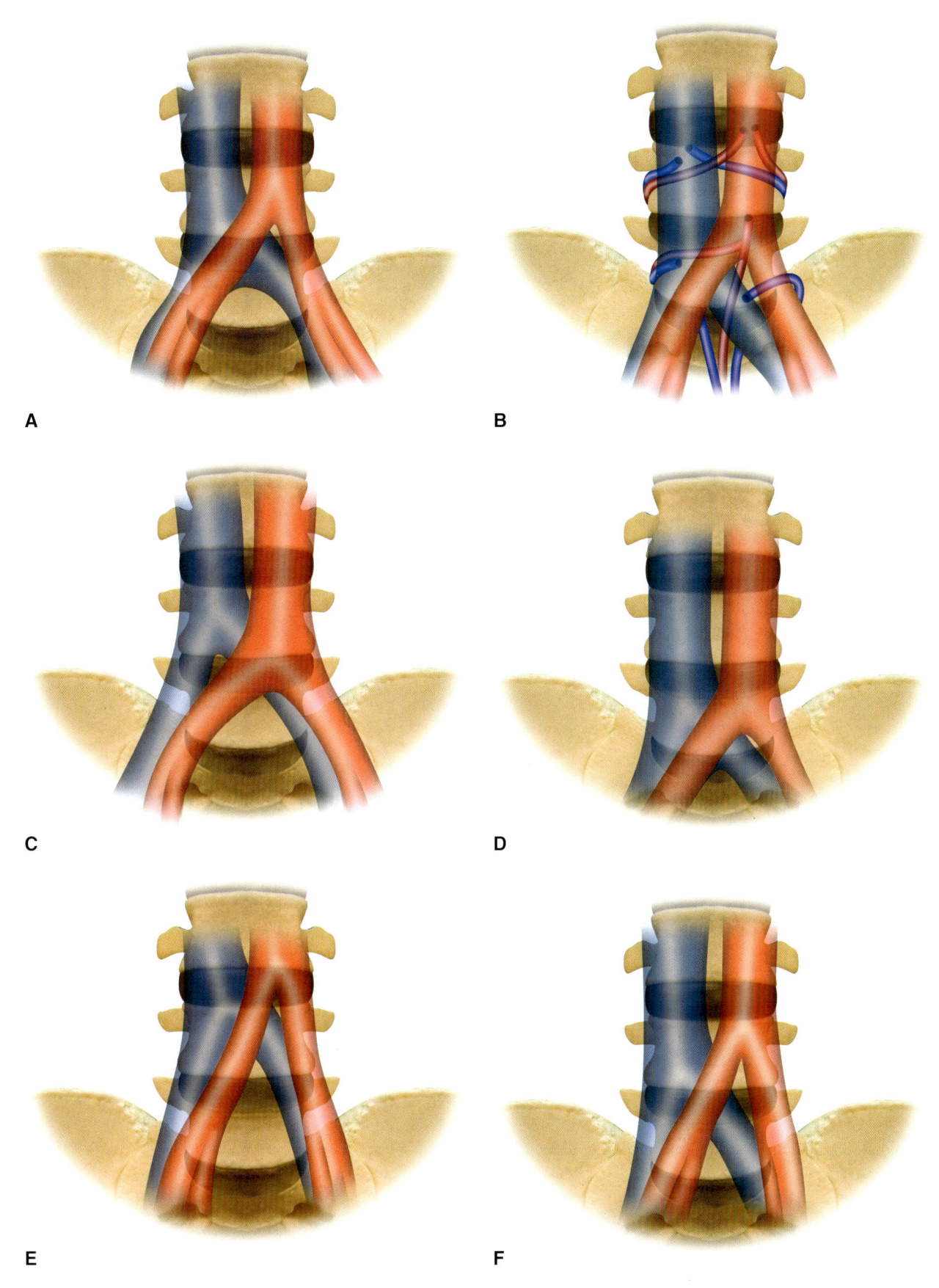

E

F

Fig. 32-8 Various relationships between the aortic and vena cava bifurcations to the L5-S1 disk space.

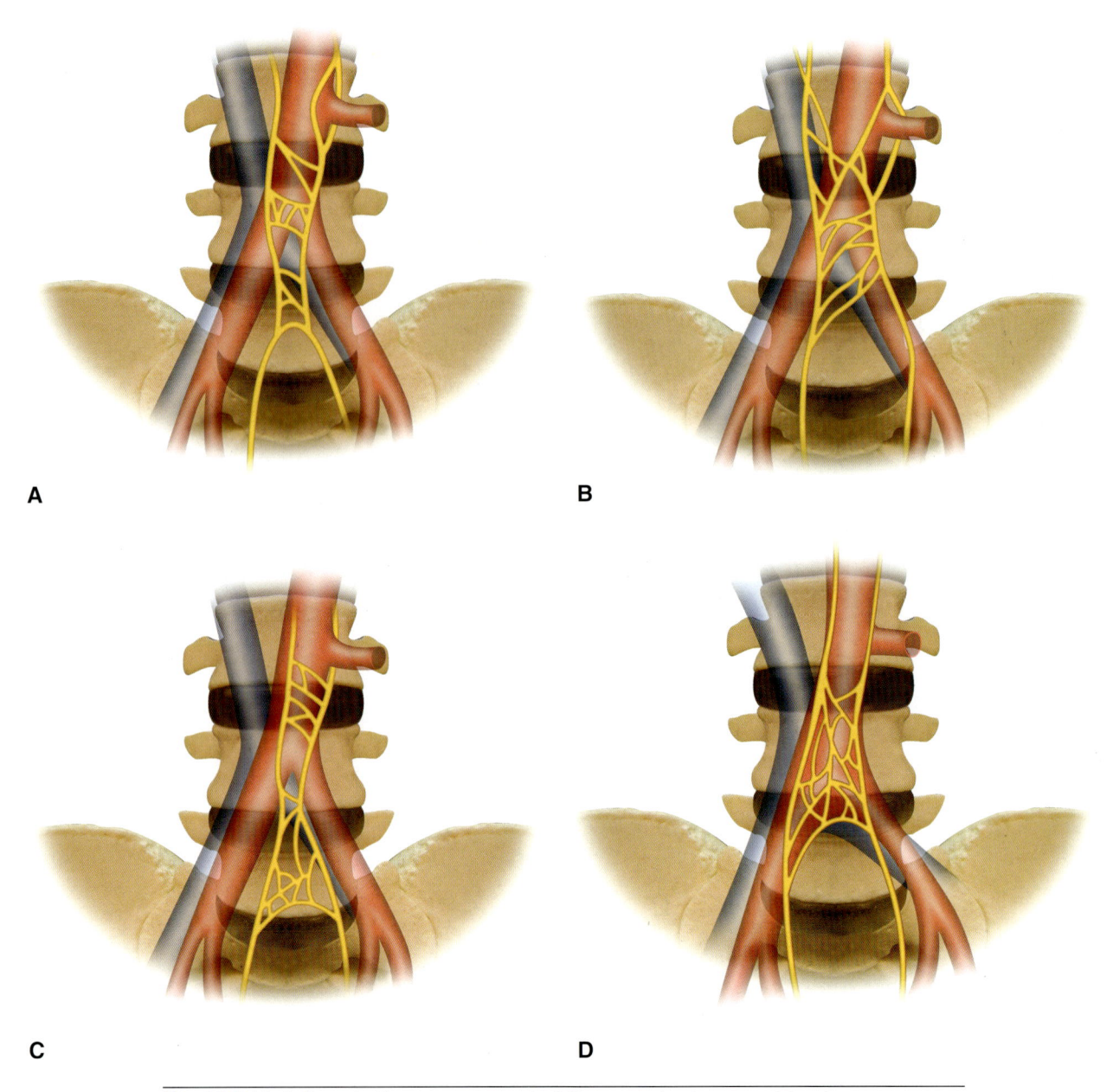

Fig. 32-9 Variations in the arrangement of the superior hypogastric plexus.

DISKECTOMY

- Excessive electrocautery along anterior longitudinal ligament should be avoided to prevent injury to the hypogastric plexus. Injury to this sympathetic plexus may result in retrograde ejaculation (Fig. 32-9). Instead, blunt dissection should be used to sweep the plexus from left to right.
- After determining the midline, the anterior longitudinal ligament is incised with a No. 10 scalpel blade on a long handle.
- Complete disk removal is then accomplished with curettes and rongeurs.
- The cartilaginous end plates should be completely removed, and the vertebral body surfaces decorticated to prepare the graft recipient site.
- In select cases the intervertebral space will then need to be increased through serial dilation of the disk space prior to implant insertion.
- Distraction between vertebral bodies can increase the foraminal height and effect an indirect neural decompression.

INTERBODY IMPLANTS

A variety of interbody spacers can then be placed to maintain disk height and promote interbody fusion:

E

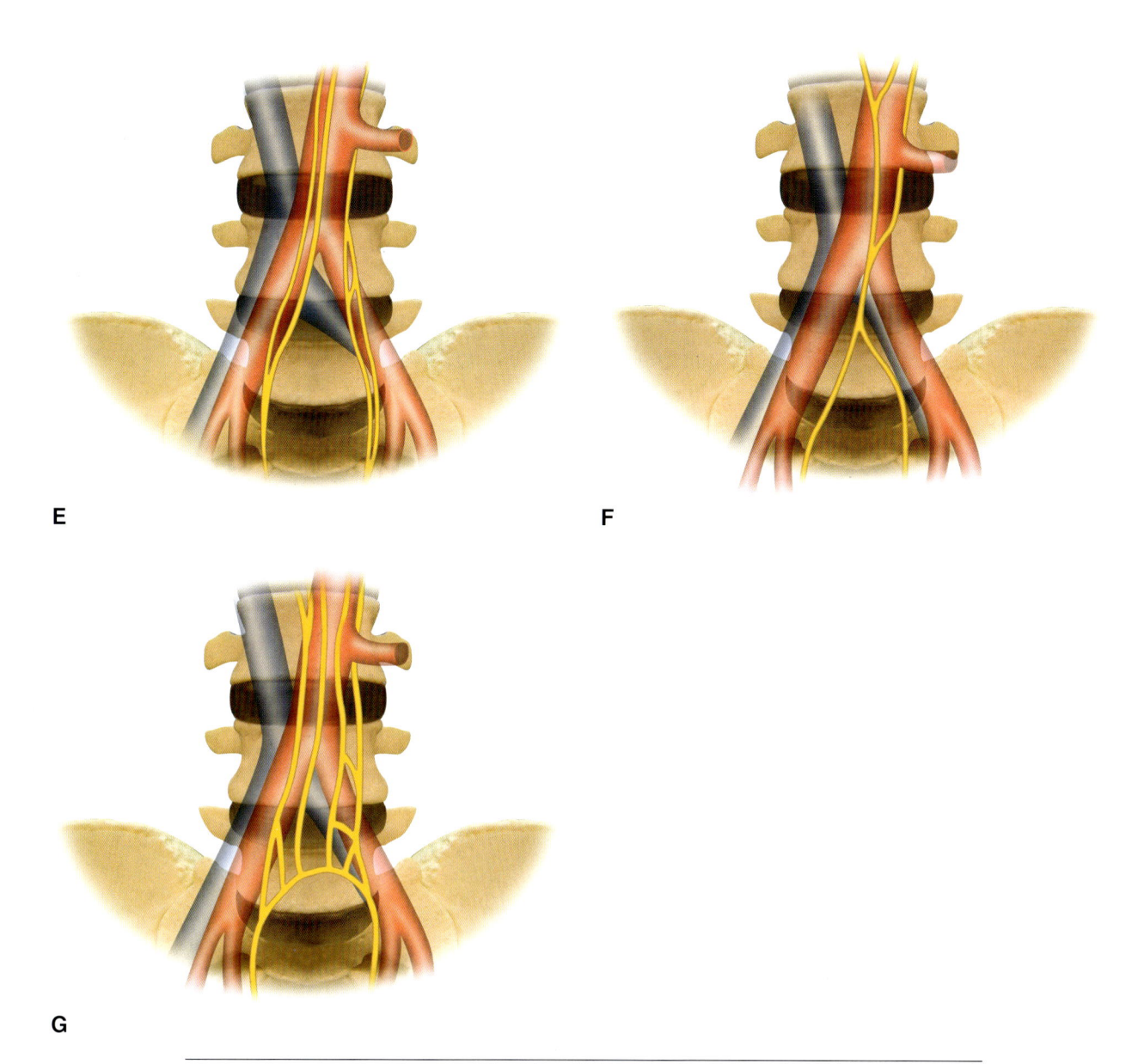

F

G

Fig. 32-9, cont'd. For legend see opposite page.

- Bicortical iliac crest autograft can be inserted with the ridge of the crest placed anteriorly. In this position cortical bone supports the interspace, maximizing contact between cancellous autograft and vertebral end plates.
- Rings of femur or humerus allograft bone can be cut to size to fit into the disk space. The cylindrical geometry of these long bones matches the vertebral end plates nicely as the strongest vertebral end plate is at the periphery. The allograft should be cut for an appropriate lordosis. The central canal should be packed with osteoconductive/osteoinductive materials as is the case with all implants except autograft bone. Commercially precision machined allograft rings are also readily available.
- Precision machined cylindrical threaded allograft bone dowels have the advantages of allograft but a reduced risk of backout because of their treaded contact with host bone.
- Titanium threaded fusion cages have been purported to provide superior stabilization when compared to impacted spacers (Fig. 32-10). This presumably decreases the need for supplemental posterior fixation.
- Titanium mesh cages have a long track record of safety and efficacy and remain a versatile option.
- Impacted cages composed of alternate materials (carbon fiber, resorbable polylactic acid, polyetheretherketone polymer) are becoming widely available.

PLATING (OPTIONAL)

- Plating of the anterior lumbar spine enhances the rigidity of the construct and decreases the risk of interbody spacer migration (Fig. 32-11).

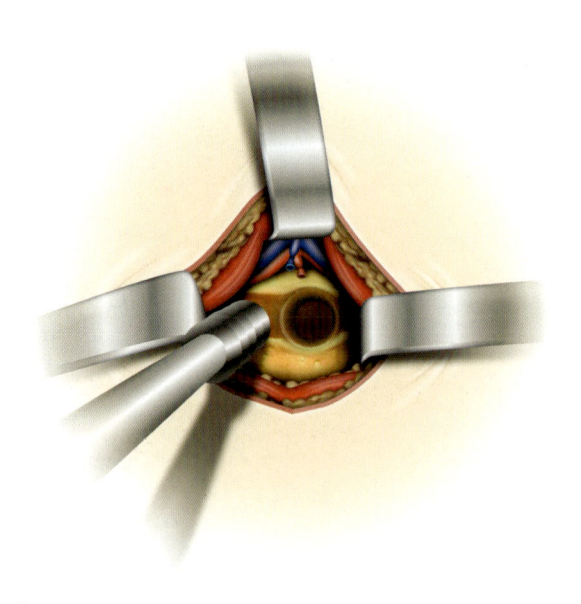

Fig. 32-10 Placement of titanium threaded fusion cages into the disk space: intraoperative (A) and sagittal (B) views.

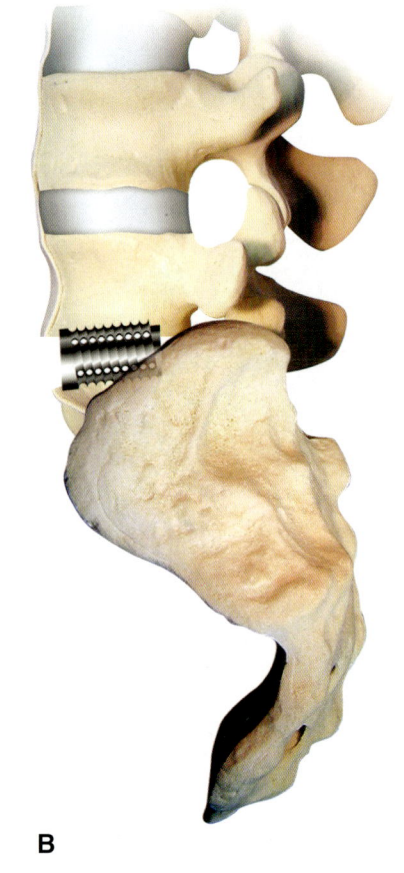

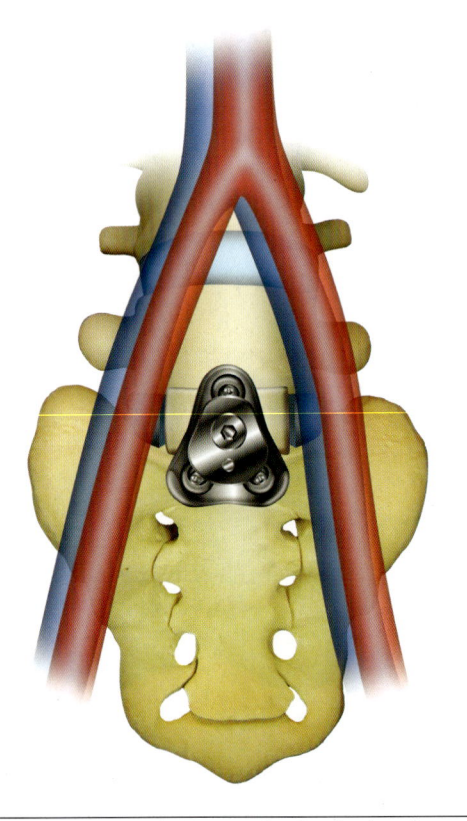

Fig. 32-11 Anterior plating at the L5-S1 level.

- Additional options include the use of buttress plates attached to only the superior or inferior vertebral body.

CLOSURE

- The wound is irrigated and all cottonoids and retractors are removed.
- A final x-ray is taken to confirm implant location and to check for retained sponges.
- The wound is inspected for any bleeding, and all vasculature ligatures are checked.
- The peritoneal lining and ureter are inspected. Small tears in the peritoneum should either be repaired primarily or be opened widely to prevent bowel strangulation.
- The rectus sheath is reapproximated with resorbable suture.
- The skin is closed with a running subcuticular stitch.

POSTOPERATIVE CARE

- Patient-controlled analgesia (PCA) is appropriate for pain control.
- The patient is mobilized the day after surgery.
- A liquid diet is begun as soon as the patient has bowel sounds.

- Depending on the number of levels treated, a 1- to 3-day hospital stay is typical.
- Weight-bearing standing x-rays are obtained prior to hospital discharge to ensure that the implants have not shifted.
- For multilevel fusions the patient should wear a rigid orthosis such as a TLSO (with thigh extension for L5-S1) for 3 months postoperatively.
- For multilevel fusions posterior supplemental instrumentation may be necessary. This can be performed under the same anesthetic or in a delayed fashion.

COMPLICATIONS

- Injury to the alimentary tract can be avoided by packing the peritoneum away from the operative corridor. Postoperative ileus is uncommon and should be treated with intravenous hydration, minimization of narcotic doses, and restricted oral intake.
- Damage to the ureter is uncommon and can be avoided by its proper identification.
- Careful manipulation of the numerous vessels encountered during ALIF will minimize the risk of vascular complications, and nearby arteries and veins should be prophylactically ligated.
- Retraction or electrocautery of the hypogastric plexus should be avoided to avoid possibility of retrograde ejaculation. Male patients are offered the opportunity to bank their sperm prior to surgery.
- Proper graft sizing and shaping are critical. Undersized grafts can lead to fusion in a kyphotic attitude. Grafts with a small surface area are prone to settling. Ideally, the interbody spacer should maintain vertebral height and physiologic lordosis with distraction across the neuroforamina.
- Telescoping of the graft into to adjacent end plates can be minimized by preserving the vertebral end plates and using a graft with the maximal cross-sectional contact area.
- Pseudarthrosis rates can be minimized by proper recipient site preparation, incorporation of osteoinductive substances, supplemental posterior stabilization, proper nutrition, and postoperative immobilization. Patients addicted to tobacco are strongly encouraged to refrain from or minimize smoking in the perioperative period.
- Abdominal wall weakness from partial denervation of the rectus abdominis muscle may result from injury of the superficial segemental nerves during exposure.

CONCLUSION

ALIF is a highly effective method for fusing the lower lumbar spine in carefully selected patients with back pain from degenerative disk disease.

CHAPTER 33

Lateral Lumbar Interbody Fusion

MICHAEL Y. WANG
BRYAN C. OH
CHRISTOPHER J. AHO

INTRODUCTION

A lateral approach to the lumbar spine offers distinct advantages over both anterior and posterior techniques. By accessing the spine through a large retroperitoneal opening, multiple levels of the lumbar spine can be exposed. This technique can thus be used to provide for neural decompression, ventral deformity correction, and anterior fusion from L2 to L5. This technique is particularly useful in the following settings.

INFECTION

Débridement of a spinal column infection allows isolation of the offending microorganisms, removal of devitalized tissues, reduction of microbial burden, revitalization of blood flow to the affected area, neural decompression, and deformity prevention. Frequently, both pyogenic and indolent infectious processes will span multiple spinal levels, and a lateral approach is appropriate if multilevel anterior column pathology is to be addressed. In addition, paravertebral abscesses can be drained and treated directly during the surgical exposure.

NEOPLASIA

Both primary and metastatic neoplasms of the spine can result in destruction of its bony integrity. Although neoplastic processes will often involve only a single vertebral level, a corpectomy for tumor often necessitates a spinal column reconstruction. Subsequent anterolateral instrumentation requires exposure of the adjacent levels for rigid fixation. This exposure is best provided through a lateral approach.

DEFORMITY

Degenerative, post-traumatic, and iatrogenic deformities can result in pain, disability, and loss of function. In advanced cases a combined approach to multiple levels of both the anterior and posterior spine is necessary. A lateral approach can thus be useful for both coronal and sagittal plane imbalance. Lateral exposure of the disk spaces allows for ventral releasing maneuvers in fixed deformities followed by fusion using interbody spacers.

INDICATIONS AND CONTRAINDICATIONS

INDICATIONS

- Fusion or instrumentation of multiple disks or vertebrae in the lumbar spine from L2 to S1

RELATIVE CONTRAINDICATIONS

- Anterior instrumentation down to the S1 vertebral body
- Severe medical comorbidities
- Retroperitoneal scarring from previous surgery
- Aortic aneurysm
- Severe lower extremity peripheral vascular disease
- Solitary kidney on the side of the exposure due to the risk of ureteral injury (without stenting)
- Severe osteoporosis with a high risk of interbody graft settling
- Morbid obesity

OPERATIVE TECHNIQUE

EQUIPMENT

- Table-mounted abdominal retractor system
- Lateral fluoroscopy or flat film x-rays
- Vascular clips and ligature suture
- Long curettes
- Pituitary rongeurs
- Long Kerrison punches
- Laminar spreader or interbody distractor
- Tamp

- Long-handled osteotomes (for vertebrectomy)
- High-speed drill (for vertebrectomy)
- Interbody spacers
  - Tricortical iliac crest autograft
  - Allograft bone dowels or rings
  - Titanium mesh or threaded cage
  - Alternate material cages (carbon fiber, resorbable polylactic acid, polyetheretherketone polymer)
- Osteoconductive/osteoinductive substances to fill interbody spacers
  - Vertebral autograft
  - Cancellous iliac crest autograft
  - Cortical or cancellous allograft chips
  - Demineralized bone matrix
  - Bone morphogenetic protein
- Anterior thoracolumbar plating system (optional)

PATIENT POSITIONING

- The patient is positioned in a true lateral position (Fig. 33-1). Careful attention to placing the body in a plane perpendicular to the floor will make obtaining lateral radiographs straightforward.
- The operative levels should be positioned over the break of the table so that flexing and re-flexing the table will mobilize the spine in the coronal plane. This will allow for efficient access and manipulation of the disk spaces. However, the spine should be restored to a physiologic position prior to any anterior plating.
- The left side is routinely positioned up so that the approach will preferentially involve retraction of the descending aorta as opposed to the vena cava, which can be quite fragile and difficult to repair in the event of a vascular tear. In addition, for surgery in the high lumbar spine the liver may prevent a right-sided exposure. For those cases in which the release of a coronal deformity will have to be performed on the right side, care must be taken to minimize trauma to the vena cava.
- The leg on the side of the incision should be flexed at the hip to reduce tension on the psoas muscle, which will have to be mobilized off of the spinal column for optimal exposure.
- The arms and neck should be positioned to avoid compressive or traction injuries. An axillary roll should be placed under the downward shoulder and the head should be supported to leave the neck in neutral position. The upward arm should be placed on pillows or an airplane.

EXPOSURE

- A standard left flank incision is used, tailored to the desired levels of exposure (Fig. 33-2A to D).
- A retroperitoneal approach will reliably provide access as high as L2. Exposure above this level is hindered by the crura of the diaphragm. Inferiorly, access to the L5-S1 disk space is limited by the ilium. In particular, instrumentation of the sacrum, which requires a direct lateral view of the S1 body, is hindered by the pelvis.
- The external oblique muscle and fascia are exposed and divided in the plane of its fibers up to the attachment of the rectus abdominis (Fig. 33-3). The underlying internal oblique and transversus abdominis muscles are transected in line with the incision.

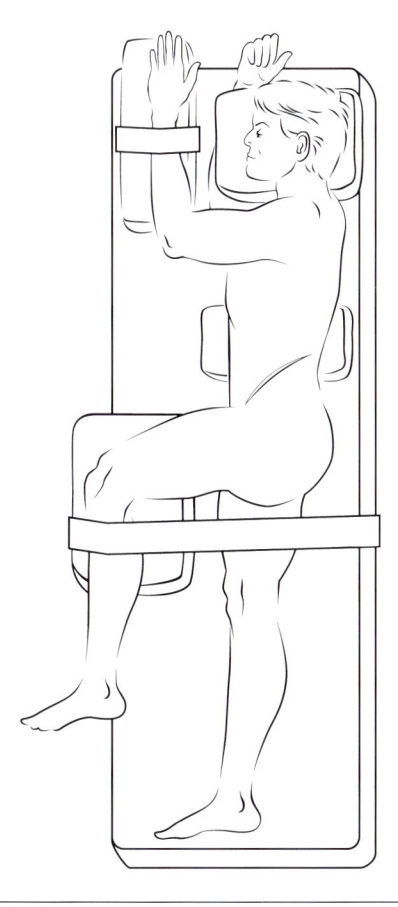

Fig. 33-1 Patient positioning in true lateral orientation.

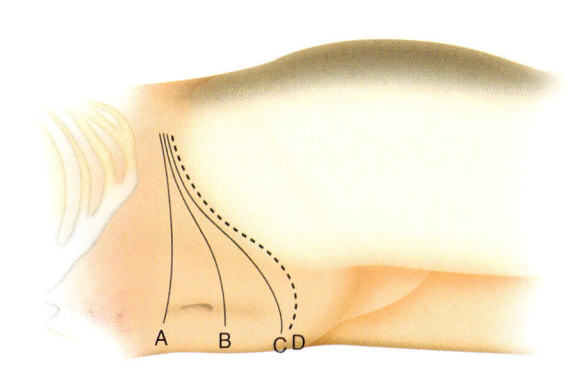

Fig. 33-2 Left flank incision for exposure of L2-L4 (A), L4-L5 (B), or L5-S1 (C). A more cosmetically sensitive incision for L5-S1 access falls below the bikini line (D).

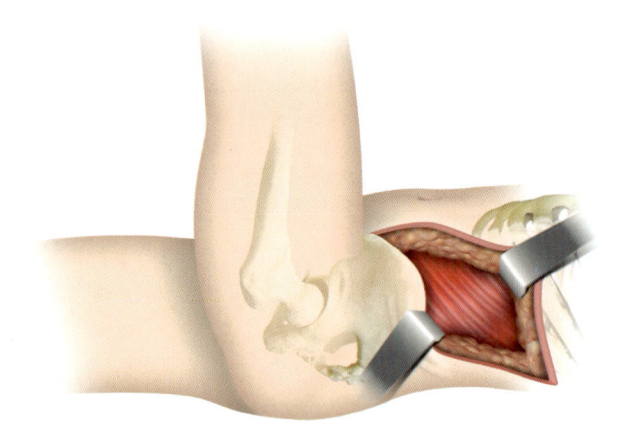

Fig. 33-3 Exposure of the external oblique muscle.

- When the deeper fascia of the transversus abdominis is encountered blunt scissors are used to make an incision in its posterolateral aspect, revealing the retroperitoneal space.
- Blunt finger dissection then proceeds anteromedially, and once the peritoneum has been stripped off the transversalis fascia, the fascia is then divided with blunt scissors.
- Blunt hand dissection then proceeds posteriorly, reflecting the kidneys anteriorly off the quadratus lumborum and psoas muscles (Fig. 33-4).
- The anterior spinal column is identified adjacent to the psoas and quadratus lumborum muscles, which should be retracted dorsally away from the vertebrae (Figs. 33-5 and 33-6).
- The ureter must be identified to prevent inadvertent injury, and a deep self-retaining table-mounted retractor is inserted. It will typically lie on the peritoneal side of the opening, but the position can vary.
- The genitofemoral nerve should be identified on the surface of the psoas muscle and be protected from injury.
- The sympathetic chain, running along the anterior aspect

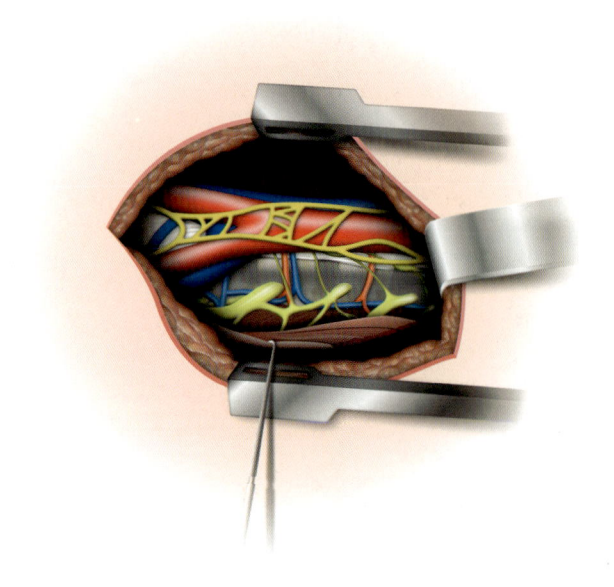

Fig. 33-5 Exposure of the great vessels and the anterolateral spinal column.

of the exposed foramina, should be preserved, if possible, by gently sweeping it dorsally.
- Following radiographic confirmation of the appropriate spinal level, care is taken to ensure adequate cranial and caudal exposure for the fusion.
- The segmental arteries and veins at each level should be ligated prophylactically midway between their origin off the great vessels and the neuroforamen. Too proximal a division can lead to great vessel side wall injury. Too distal a division can risk damage to the vascular supply of the neural elements, as some degree of collateralization occurs near the foramen.

DISKECTOMY

- Diskectomy is straightforward as the entire anterolateral aspect of the spinal column is exposed.

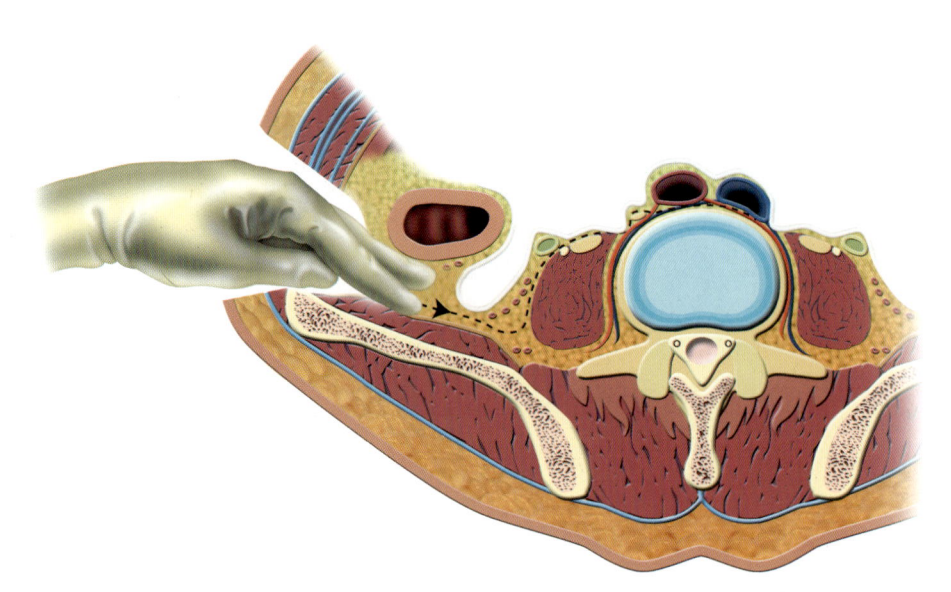

Fig. 33-4 Cross-sectional view of the abdomen showing the retroperitoneal plane of dissection to reach the anterolateral spinal column.

CHAPTER 33 Lateral Lumbar Interbody Fusion

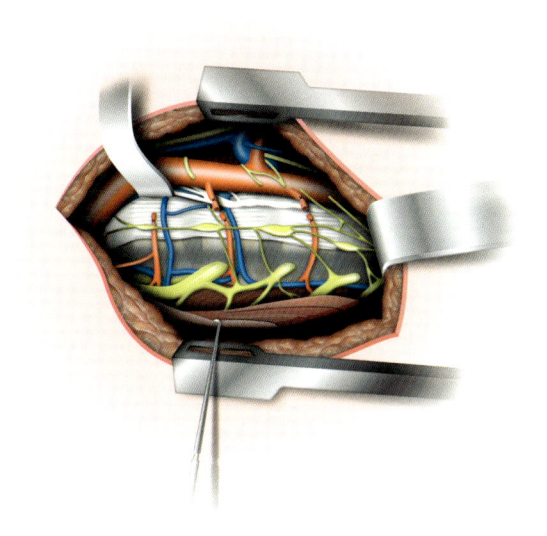

Fig. 33-6 Retraction of the psoas muscle to give access to the spinal column.

- The lateral annulus is incised and the disk is removed with pituitary rongeurs and curettes.
- It may be necessary for an assistant to retract the psoas muscle during the diskectomy or vertebrectomy.
- If decompression of the central spinal canal is necessary, magnification with loupes or the operating microscope is helpful. The posterior border of the disk is separated from the epidural space by the posterior longitudinal ligament. This should be carefully opened with Kerrison rongeurs. At the level of the conus medullaris care should be exercised, but the cauda equina is usually present below the L2 level, making central decompression relatively safe.
- With the exception of structural autograft, the intervertebral spacers should be prepared by packing the center of a weight-bearing spacer intended to maintain disk height with osteoconductive/osteoinductive material to promote fusion (cancellous iliac crest autograft, cortical or cancellous allograft chips, demineralized bone matrix, or bone morphogenetic protein).
- A wide selection of intervertebral spacers are available:
  - Iliac crest autograft
  - Rib autograft (for more rostral exposures involving rib resection)
  - Femoral/humeral allograft rings fashioned in the operating room
  - Precision machined allograft rings/ramps
  - Threaded titanium cages
  - Titanium wire mesh cages
  - Carbon fiber impacted spacers
  - Polyetheretherketone (PEEK) impacted spacers
  - Polylactic acid resorbable impacted spacers
- The vertebral end plates are decorticated with curettes or a burr to promote bony fusion followed by interspace implant insertion (Fig. 33-7A to C).

VERTEBRECTOMY

- If a vertebrectomy is to be performed, then diskectomies from rostral to caudal should be accomplished first (Fig. 33-8).
- Osteotomy and drilling should proceed to the posterior margin of the vertebral bodies, which is identified by the anterior margin of the intervertebral foramina (Fig. 33-9). This line marks the anterior margin of the spinal canal.
- Decompression of the central spinal canal necessitates identification and opening of the posterior longitudinal ligament, revealing the epidural space.
- For cases that require complete removal of the vertebral bodies to the contralateral side, a malleable retractor can be placed to create a plane between the aorta/vena cava complex and the anterior longitudinal ligament lateral

Fig. 33-7 Removal of multiple intervertebral disks (A), followed by decortication of the end plates (B), and interbody graft placement (C).

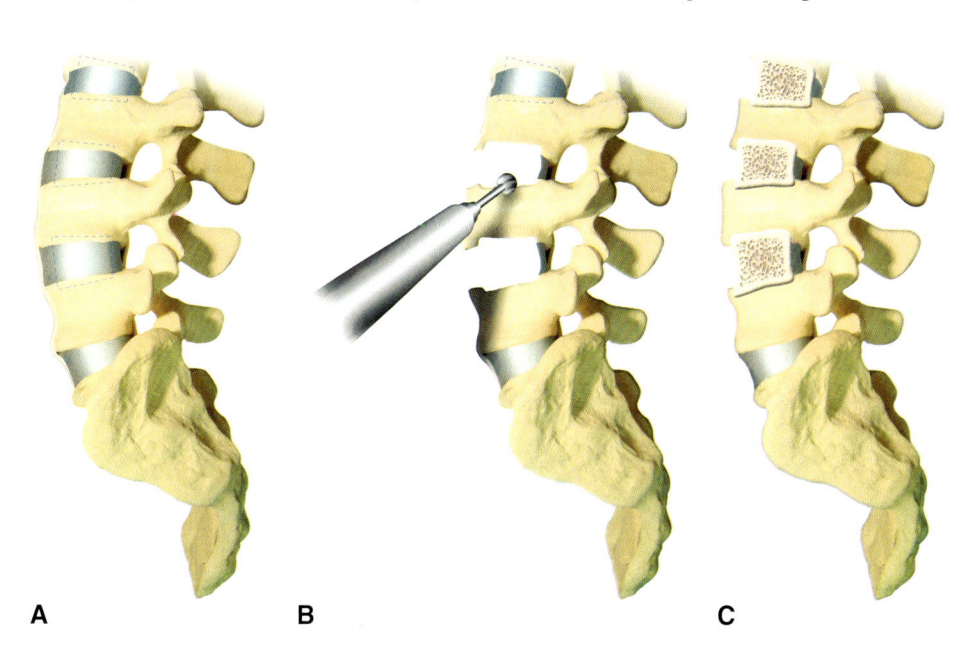

A B C

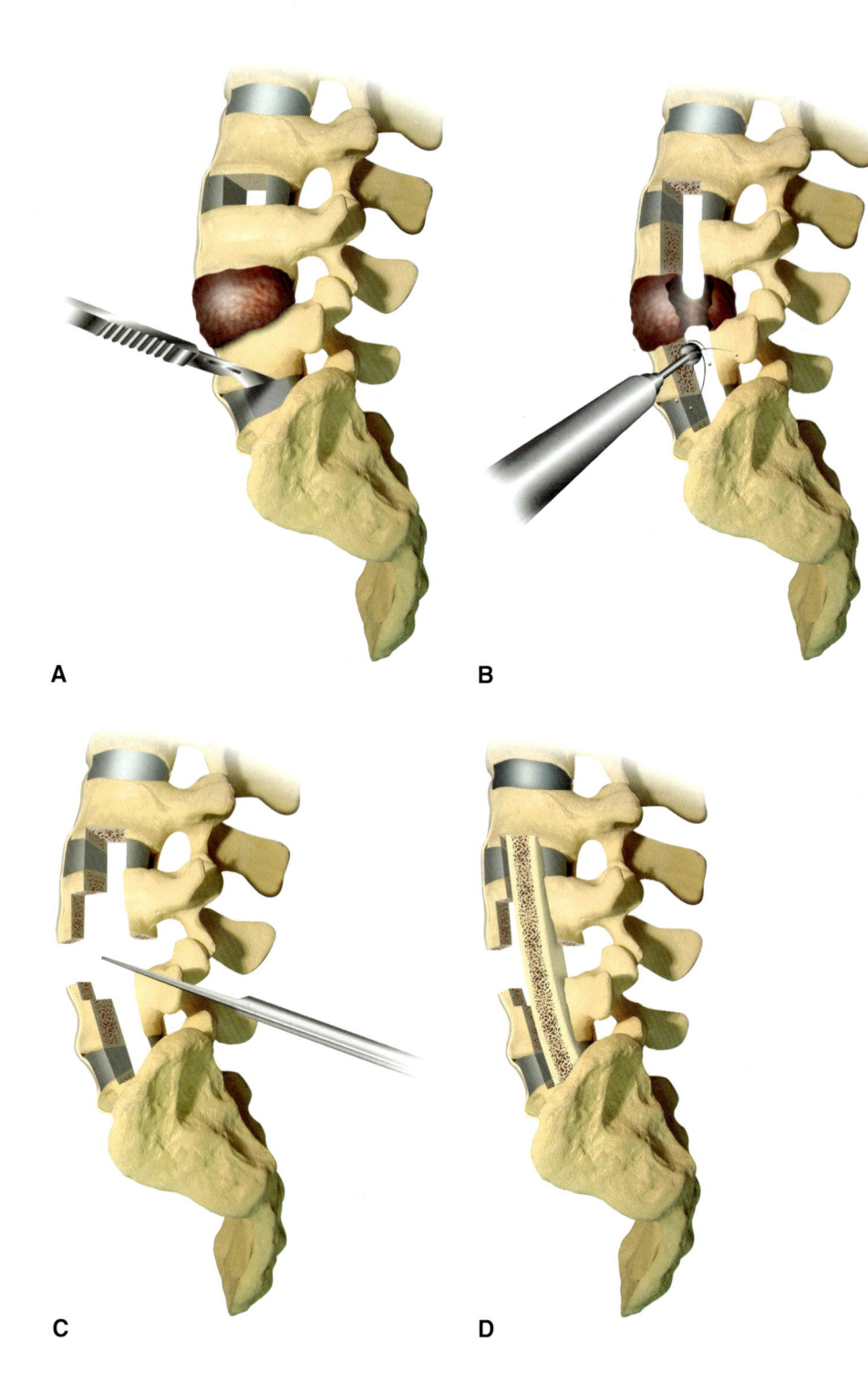

276 SECTION II DEGENERATIVE DISEASE OF THE SPINE

Fig. 33-8 *A,* For a vertebrectomy the adjacent diskectomies are first performed; *B,* removal of the vertebra is then performed with osteotomes and a drill; *C,* the graft recipient site is carefully prepared to prevent graft displacement; and *D,* the interbody graft is placed.

vertebral body. This retractor can be held by an assistant during the vertebrectomy.
- Preservation of the anterior longitudinal ligament or, alternatively, keystoning of the rostral and caudal vertebral bodies, if possible, will help to prevent implant kickout.
- The completion of the vertebrectomy should involve decortication of the rostral and caudal vertebral end plates to promote fusion. Preservation of the cortical end plates will help minimize the risk of graft settling or telescoping into the adjacent vertebral bodies.
- Decompression is followed by reconstruction of the anterior spinal column. This can be accomplished with a number of intervertebral struts, which (excepting structural autograft) should be packed with osteoconductive/osteoinductive materials (Fig. 33-10):

CHAPTER 33   Lateral Lumbar Interbody Fusion   277

- Iliac crest autograft
- Rib autograft (for more rostral exposures involving rib resection)
- Vascularized or nonvascularized fibula autograft
- Femoral humeral allograft shafts
- Titanium wire mesh cages
- Carbon fiber impacted spacers
- Polyetheretherketone (PEEK) impacted spacers
- Polylactic acid resorbable impacted spacers

INSTRUMENTATION

- Prior to instrumentation the surgeon should confirm that the patient is in true lateral position to make screw placement straightforward. In addition, the spine must be aligned in the coronal plane, particularly if the table has been reflexed at its break.
- Anterior stabilization with internal fixation can be accomplished with screw-plate or screw-rod implants (Fig. 33-11).
- When rostral/caudal exposure is inadequate, the bone is severely demineralized, or purulent infection is present, a large internal fixator may not be appropriate. To prevent anterior graft kickout, the vertebral end plates should be keystoned and the anterior longitudinal ligament left intact. To prevent leftward lateral kickout a retaining screw

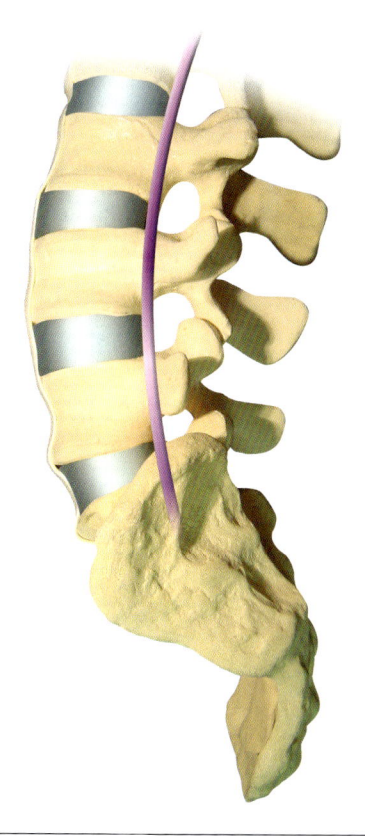

Fig. 33-9 Line at the anterior aspect of the neuroforamina demarcating the anterior margin of the spinal canal.

Fig. 33-10 Commercially available vertebrectomy spacers: titanium mesh (*A*), expandable titanium cage (*B*), and stackable modular polyetheretherketone (PEEK) (*C*).

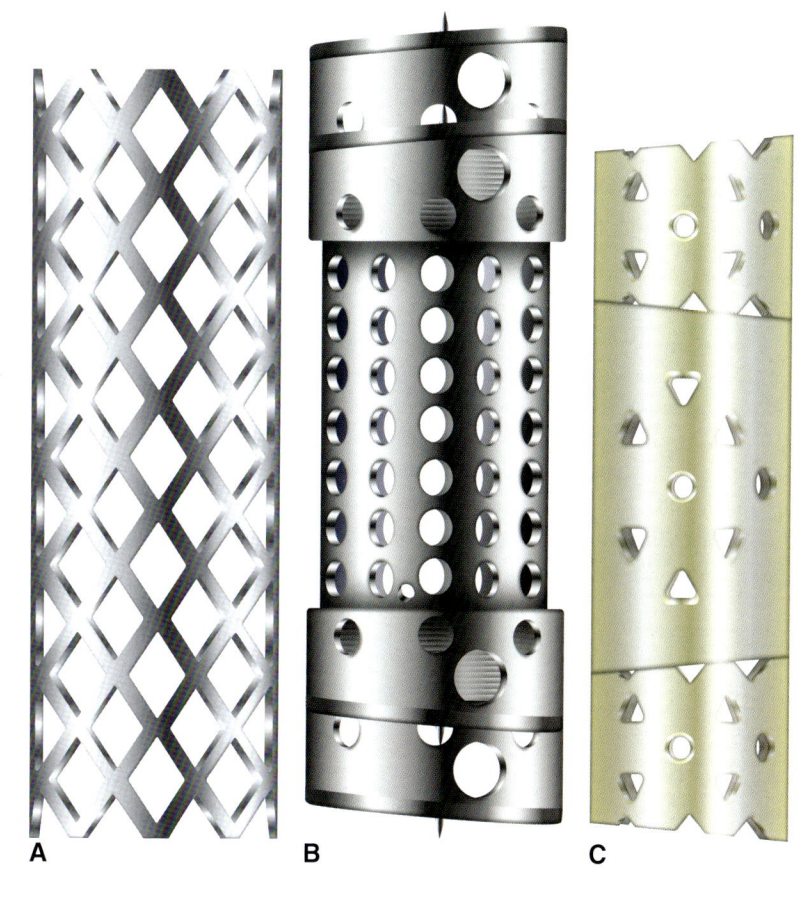

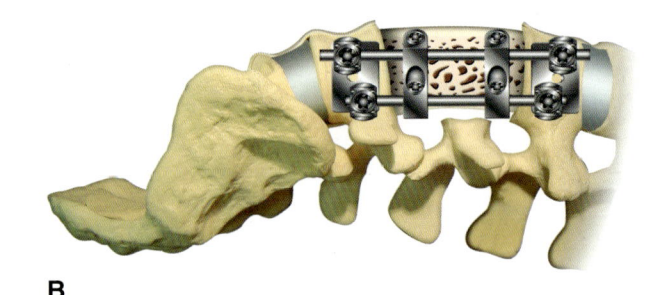

Fig. 33-11 Anterior plating with screw-plate (A) and screw-rod (B) instrumentation.

can be inserted into the rostral and caudal vertebral bodies as a buttress.

CLOSURE

- The self-retaining table-mounted retractor blades are removed and final x-rays are taken.
- The ureter, vena cava, and aorta are examined for injury, and all the ligated vessels are checked to ensure that there is no bleeding. The peritoneum is also inspected. Large openings are well tolerated. However, small tears may result in bowel herniations and strangulation and should either be closed primarily or opened widely.
- The wound is irrigated copiously.
- The transversalis fascia is closed with a running, resorbable suture.
- The external oblique fascia is closed with a running, resorbable suture.
- Continuous, running subcutaneous suture is used to reapproximate the skin.

POSTOPERATIVE CARE

- The patient is extubated. Barring significant comorbidities, care on a regular hospital ward is appropriate if the diaphragm has not been detached.
- Patient-controlled analgesia (PCA) is appropriate for pain control.
- The patient is mobilized the day after surgery.
- A liquid diet is begun as soon as the patient has bowel sounds.
- Depending on the number of levels treated, a 3- to 6-day hospital stay is typical.
- The patient should wear a rigid orthosis such as a TLSO for 3 months postoperatively.
- Weight-bearing standing x-rays are obtained prior to hospital discharge to ensure that the implants have not shifted.
- For multilevel fusions posterior supplemental instrumentation may be necessary. This can be performed under the same anesthetic or in a delayed fashion.

COMPLICATIONS

EXPOSURE

- Injury to the intra-abdominal contents is possible if the peritoneum is not securely packed out of the way with lap sponges.

- Damage to the ureter intraoperatively can be avoided by its proper identification.
- The numerous vessels encountered in the anterolateral approach mandate meticulous attention to securing and prophylactically ligating any obstructing arteries or veins. Inadvertent breach of a large iliolumbar vein can lead to several liters of blood loss in a matter of minutes. For this reason, a cell saver device is useful in cases without infection or neoplasia.
- Retraction or electrocautery of the genitofemoral nerve and hypogastric plexus should be avoided.
- Even with meticulous technique, partial denervation of the rectus abdominis muscle through injury to the superficial segmental nerves may lead to abdominal asymmetry.

DECOMPRESSION

- Injury to the conus medullaris or cauda equina can be avoided with proper identification of the posterior longitudinal ligament and careful opening of this protective layer under higher magnification and illumination.
- Similarly, dural breaches can be avoided by careful technique. In the advent of inadvertent or unavoidable dural injury a patch graft (fat, muscle, fascia, or commercially available dural substitutes) can be placed to cover the defect. Small midline tears can be repaired primarily, but lateral or large tears should be patched with a few anchoring stitches strategically placed. Fibrin glue can then be used to seal the defect. A lumbar drain should be placed to keep tension off the graft for several days.
- Incomplete decompression of the spinal canal can be avoided by palpating the pedicles on both sides of the patient. This will reveal whether the decompression has spanned the width of the spinal canal.

RECONSTRUCTION

- Proper graft sizing is critical. Undersized grafts are more easily placed but will lead to fusion in a kyphotic attitude.
- Telescoping of the graft into to adjacent end plates can be minimized by preserving the vertebral end plates and using a graft with the maximal cross-sectional contact area.
- Pseudarthrosis rates can be minimized by proper recipient site preparation, incorporation of osteoinductive substances, supplemental posterior stabilization, proper nutrition, and postoperative immobilization.

CHAPTER 33 Lateral Lumbar Interbody Fusion

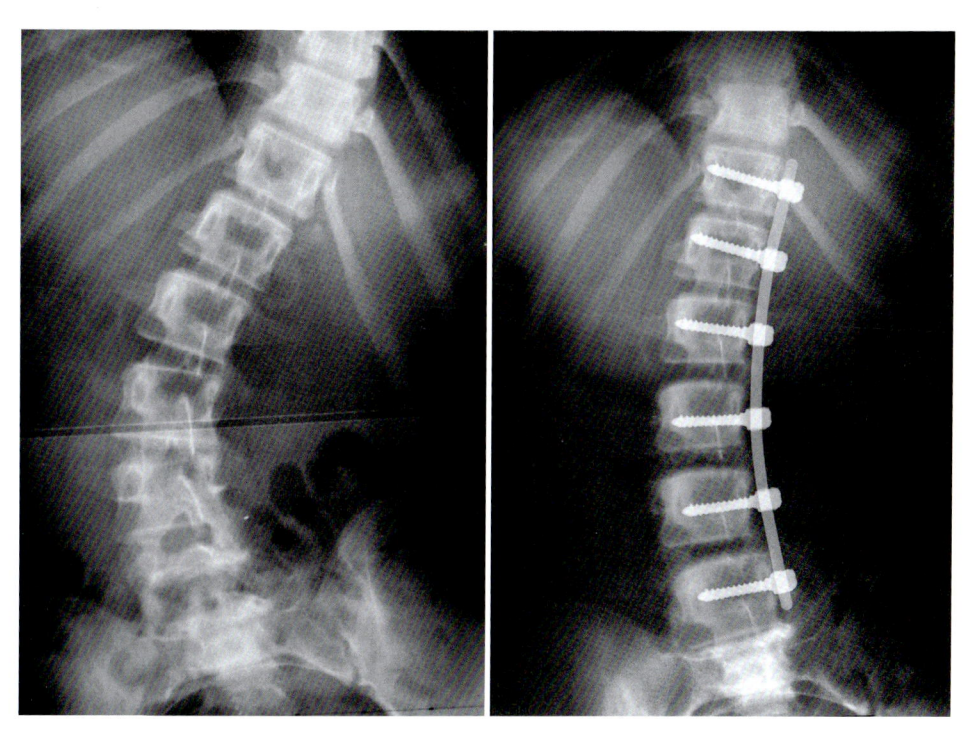

Fig. 33-12 Degenerative lumbar scoliosis correction from T12 to L5 from a standalone lateral approach.

- The critical adjacent vasculature mandates that any spinal instrumentation be of low profile. Protruding screw heads or screws tips violating the contralateral vertebral cortex should be avoided as continuous movement between metallic implants and a vessel wall can lead to a lethal vascular rupture.

ALTERNATIVE LATERAL APPROACHES

- The lateral approach to the lumbar spine is highly versatile. For treating pathology rostral to L2 the incision can be extended. Mobilization of the diaphragmatic attachments will be necessary to expose the lateral aspect of the spine.
- With modern anterior screw-rod constructs scoliotic deformity correction is now possible through a lateral-only approach (Fig. 33-12).
- Innovative lateral approaches through the psoas muscle have been developed for interbody graft placement through a minimal access tubular dilator retractor port. The extreme lateral lumbar interbody fusion (XLIF) is a minimally invasive transpsoas technique that relies on continuous electromyography to avoid damage to the nerve tissues within the psoas muscle (Fig. 33-13).

CONCLUSIONS

A lateral retroperitoneal approach is the optimal technique for multiple level interbody fusions of the lumbar spine. This technique facilitates the treatment of spinal infections, neoplasia, and deformity. Furthermore, it allows for rigid anterolateral plate or plate/rod fixation.

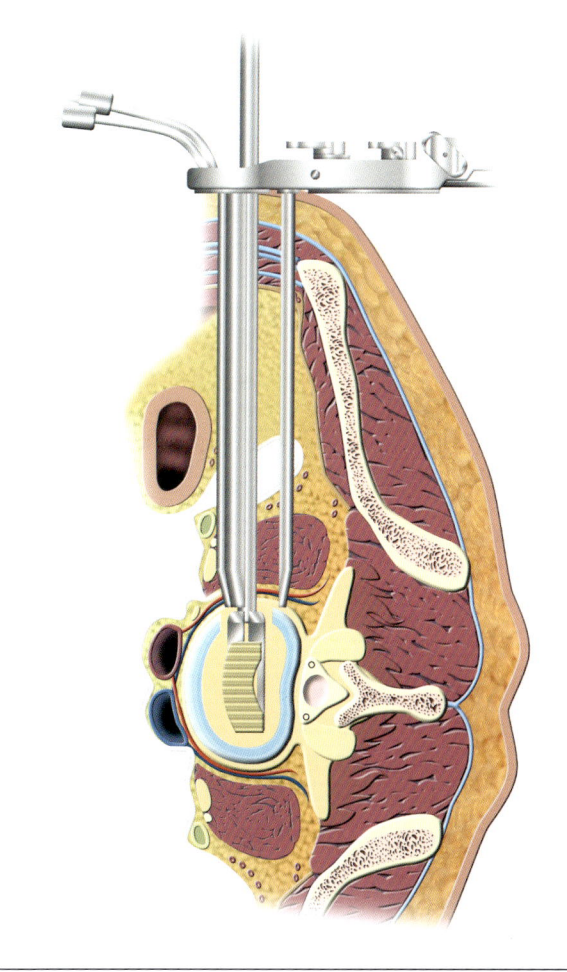

Fig. 33-13 The transpsoas or extreme lateral lumbar interbody fusion (XLIF) technique

CHAPTER 34

ENSOR E. TRANSFELDT
AMIR A. MEHBOD

Spondylolisthesis Reduction

INTRODUCTION

Spondylolisthesis was first described by Herbiniaux[1] in 1782 when he wrote about the obstetric problems associated with high-grade spondylolisthesis causing narrowing of the birth canal. In 1854, Killian[2] coined the term *spondylolisthesis* from the Greek roots of *spondylo* and *listhesis*, meaning spine and slippage, respectively. Since then, many have written about spondylolisthesis with multiple proposals for its classification. The most widely used classification is by Wiltse and associates,[3] who describe five types of spondylolisthesis, including dysplastic, isthmic, degenerative, traumatic, and pathologic. In addition to this classification, a radiographic grading system has been proposed by Meyerding.[4] In this classification, no slippage is grade 0, 1% to 25% is grade 1, 26% to 50% slippage is grade 2, 51% to 75% slippage is grade 3, and 76% to 100% slippage is grade 4. Complete slippage is called *spondyloptosis*. Another important radiographic finding is the slip angle, which represents the amount of lumbosacral kyphosis.

The initial treatment of patients with spondylolisthesis should be conservative. Surgical intervention is warranted when there is (1) significant progression of the slippage, (2) slippage of 50% with a slip angle of 55 degrees or more, or (3) neurologic deficit.[5,6] Fusion in situ is the most commonly performed surgical procedure[6-23] with pseudarthrosis rates ranging from 0% to 19%. However, there have also been many reports of noninstrumented or instrumented reductions followed by fusion, especially in patients with grade III and IV spondylolisthesis[10,24-39] with pseudarthrosis rates of 0% to 8% being reported. Recent comparative studies have shown even higher fusion rates with reduction of high-grade spondylolisthesis with addition of anterior fusion and structural grafting.[40,41]

INDICATION FOR SPONDYLOLISTHESIS REDUCTION

At our center, every case of spondylolisthesis is treated individually. The most important factor is the sagittal balance and clinical appearance of the patient (Fig. 34-1). The slip angle, or lumbosacral kyphosis, can significantly affect the patient's sagittal balance and the ability to compensate at the proximal levels. These patients can present with short trunks and transverse abdominal crease because of the reversal of lumbar lordosis. These patients usually stand with flexed hips and knees. If the sagittal balance is acceptable, then fusion in situ

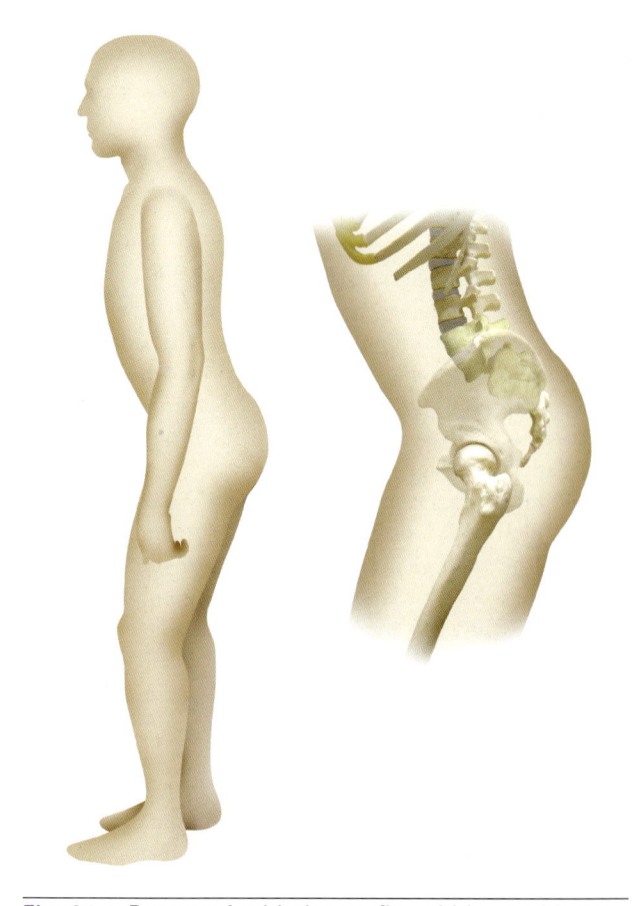

Fig. 34-1 Poor sagittal balance; flexed hips and knees.

with a 360-degree fusion technique is preferred. Indications to reduce a high-grade spondylolisthesis include (1) progression of a high-grade slip, (2) inability to stand upright with significant lumbosacral kyphosis, (3) unacceptable clinical appearance, and (4) high slip angle which if not reduced is more likely to develop a progression after fusion.[42,43]

SURGICAL TECHNIQUE

Our steps for the surgical treatment of high-grade spondylolisthesis which is to be reduced involve (1) positioning the patient on the table, (2) decompression to visualize nerve roots and bony anatomy, (3) placement of instrumentation and reduction maneuver, (4) posterior fusion, (5) anterior fusion.

POSITION

Patient position on the table is important and can aid in the reduction. As a matter of fact, on many occasions after positioning the patient on the table and obtaining a radiograph, there has already been a partial correction of both the slip angle as well as the slip itself. The patient is positioned prone on the table with hyperextension of the hips with pillows, which in turn improves the lumbar lordosis. The knees can be flexed to decrease the tension of the nerve roots. All areas of prominences, especially the fibular head, should be well padded. At this point, the neuromonitoring signal should be checked for baseline comparison.

DECOMPRESSION

We prefer to decompress the area of the spondylolisthesis in order to visualize the nerve roots and avoid unnecessary tension on them. Additionally, a lot of these patients do complain of radicular-type pain, which can be attributed to the stenosis of these nerve roots. The three main causes of compression of nerve roots are (1) fibrocartilaginous tissue due to pars defect, (2) foraminal stenosis due to hypertrophic facet capsule and ligamentum flavum, and (3) entrapment of the nerve root between the pedicle and anterolateral aspect of the superior end plate. We first begin with a laminectomy of L5. Curettes and Kerrison rongeurs are used to remove the spinous process and the lamina, thickened ligamentum flavum, and the fibrocartilaginous buildup from the area of the lysis itself. Part of this fibrocartilaginous buildup is actually at the area of the pars and into the foramen, and this should be completely removed. Typically, with the L5-S1 isthmic spondylolisthesis, there is symptomatic L5 nerve root stenosis, and the L5 nerve roots will be in a very deep position and difficult to identify. One can often find the L5 pedicles, which in turn will help find the origin of the L5 nerve roots and follow it into the foramen. Kerrison rongeurs are used over the nerve roots to decompress the fibrocartilaginous area.

Foraminal stenosis due to hypertrophy of the facet capsule and ligamentum flavum is common. Kerrison rongeurs can be used to perform foraminotomies and to remove the hypertrophied ligaments in the capsule. Occasionally, it may be necessary to remove part of the L5-S1 disk, which can compress the nerve roots from below (Fig. 34-2A).

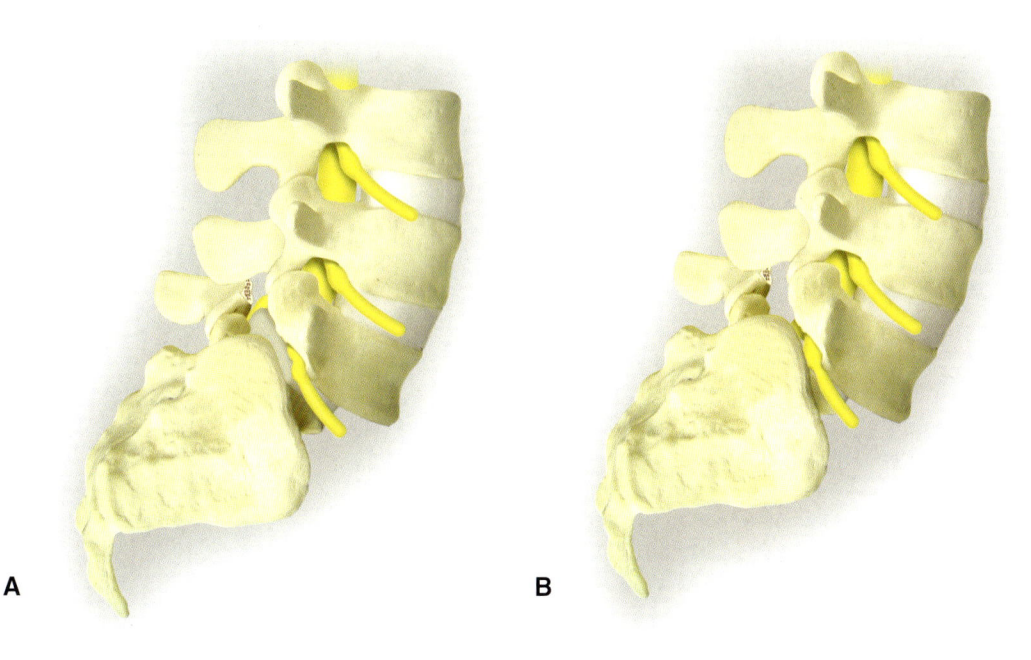

Fig. 34-2 *A*, The L5-S1 disk can cause foraminal impingement on the L5 nerve root. *B*, The nerve root can be compressed between the pedicle of L5 and the anterolateral body of S1.

Frequently, this is not enough, as there may be compression of the nerve root between the pedicles of L5 and the anterolateral aspect of the superior end plate of S1 (see Fig. 34-2B). One may need to remove that pedicle or perform a partial vertebrectomy of S1 or do both to fully decompress the nerve. To remove a pedicle, the overlying bone on the pedicle can be removed to expose the cancellous bone of the pedicle. A burr can be used into the pedicle decancellating it and leaving its walls intact to protect the nerve itself. The burring of the pedicle should be performed down to the level of the posterior vertebral body of L5. The walls of the hollowed out pedicle can then be removed with rongeurs and flattened out. The nerve can then be lying over the flat area where the pedicle used to be. If further decompression is needed, one can use a nerve root retractor and superiorly retract the L5 nerve root, exposing the anterolateral aspect of the superior end plate of S1. This potential area of compression can then be removed with small osteotomes and rongeurs. The nerve root should then be decompressed and visualized and palpated to determine the amount of tension on it.

INSTRUMENTATION AND REDUCTION

The reduction phase of the operation includes placement of the instrumentation, temporary distraction to unlock the slipped vertebral bodies, angular reduction of the kyphosis, and translational reduction.

The placement of the instrumentation is performed under fluoroscopic guidance, with the most important step being achievement of a stable base into the sacrum or pelvis. Achievement of a very stable sacral fixation is mandatory because it serves as the base on which the rest of the vertebrae are reduced. This can be performed by placement of sacral screws, preferably bicortical, engaging the anterior cortex of the sacrum. Placement of S2 screws or iliac screws adds to the stability. The authors prefer to use a sacral plate, which allows for placement of two screws into the sacrum (Fig. 34-3). The proximal screw through the sacral plate is directed into the sacral promontory, capturing the anterior cortex as well as superior cortex of S1. The distal screw through the sacral plate is directed laterally toward the sacral ala, preferably engaging the anterior cortex of the ala as well. With the establishment of a stable base, the reduction can be performed. The pedicle screws can be placed into L4 pedicles in usual fashion (Fig. 34-4). Screws can also be placed into L5 if the L5 pedicle has not been removed for the decompression. Alternatively, if the L5 pedicles are still present and are deep within the wound in a difficult angle, one can opt to place them subsequent to partial reduction, making the pedicles more visible and accessible to screw placement. The L4 screws can then be connected to the sacral fixation with rods (see Fig. 34-4). The rod is fixed to the sacral plate in a stable fashion and tightened. However, the L4 pedicle screw is attached to the rod but not tightened completely, allowing room for reduction. Distraction is applied between the L4 screws and the sacral fixation to disengage the L5 vertebra (Fig. 34-5A). This maneuver partially reduces

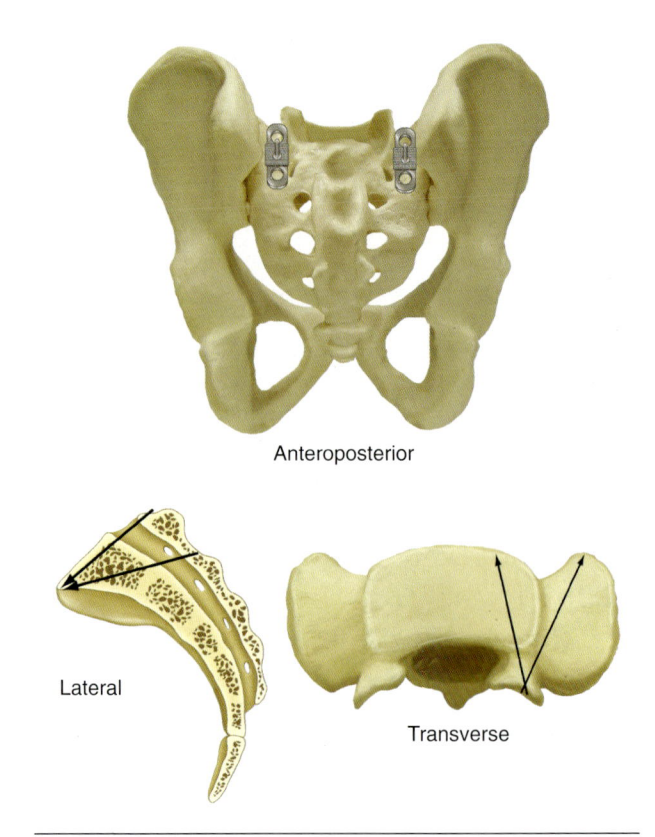

Fig. 34-3 Anteroposterior, lateral, and transverse directions of S1 screw and sacral ala screw through the sacral plots.

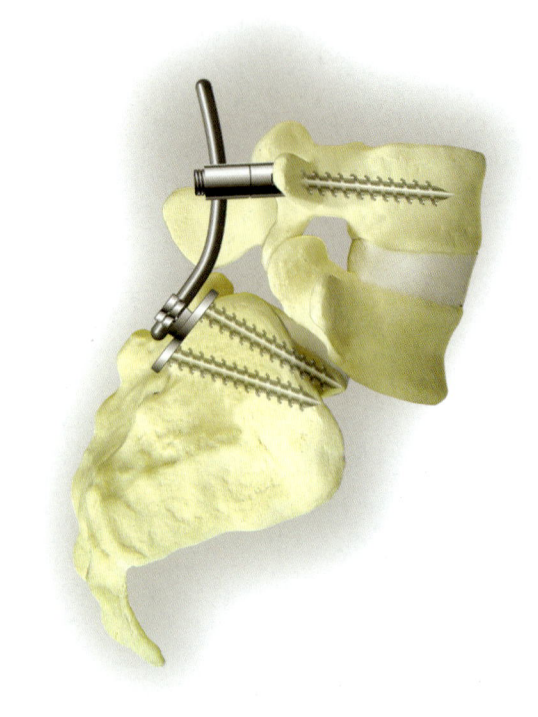

Fig. 34-4 Sacral fixation and L4 screws have been placed. The rod is then tightened securely to the sacral fixation.

CHAPTER 34 Spondylolisthesis Reduction   283

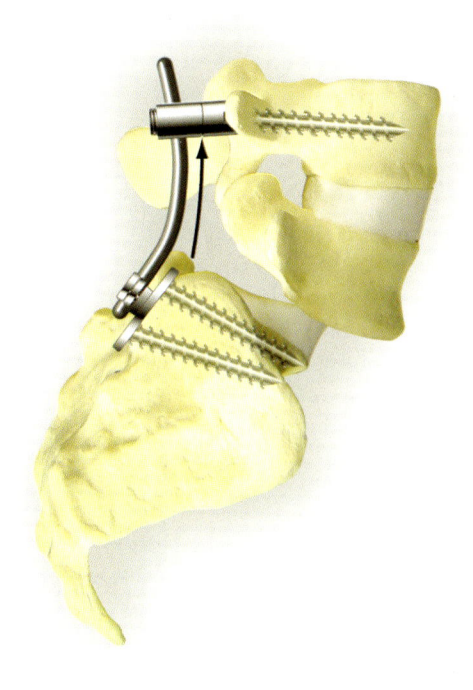

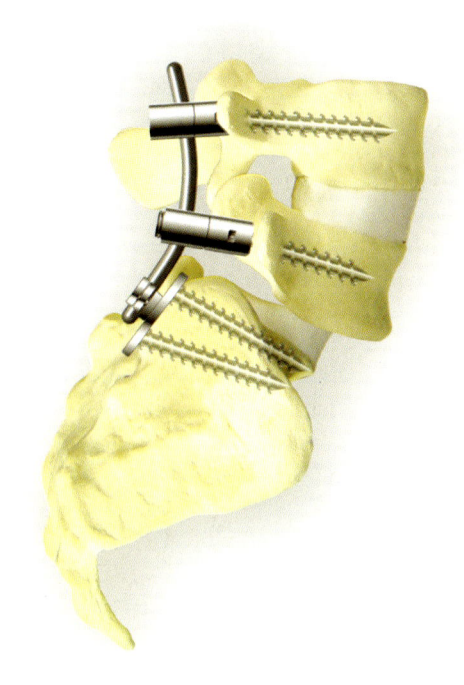

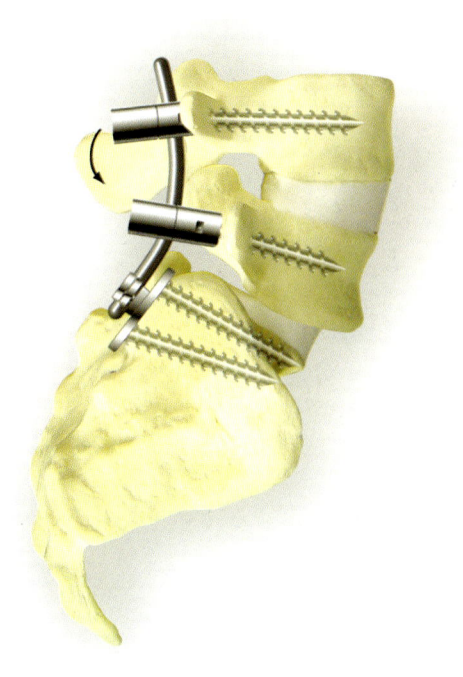

Fig. 34-5 *A,* Distraction is applied between L4 and sacral fixations. *B,* The L5 screw can be placed more easily as it comes under direct vision. *C,* Converging the L4 and L5 screws toward the sacral fixation will reduce the lumbosacral kyphosis.

the slip angle as well. At this point, if the L5 pedicle screw has not been placed, it can be placed more easily as it comes under direct vision (see Fig. 34-5B). After placement of the L5 screw, it can be attached to the rod assembly.

Further angular correction can be performed by manipulation of the L4 and L5 screws by manually converging the proximal aspect of the pedicle screws toward the sacral fixation (see Fig. 34-5C). The nerve roots should be monitored under direct vision and manually palpated to test its tension with neuromonitoring verification. Once the desired angular correction is achieved, the L4 and L5 pedicle screw can be fixed to the rod, which will translate the slipped vertebra dorsally. The screw shanks are threaded, and as the rod connectors are tightened, the screws and therefore the vertebra are translated dorsally (Fig. 34-6). Again, the nerve roots should be monitored during this translation maneuver. The angular correction is the most important reduction maneuver. The posterior translation maneuver should be stopped if there is any concern with regard to nerve root tension either under direct visualization or by neuromonitoring. Once the reduction has been completed, the screws can be tightened to the rod. Alternatively, one may opt to remove the L4 pedicle screw to maintain only L5-S1 fixation, saving the L4-L5 level.

POSTERIOR FUSION

A posterior and posterolateral fusion can be performed in the usual fashion. This entails exposure of the transverse processes of the involved vertebrae as well as the sacral ala, making sure the area is devoid of all soft tissue. A decordication of the transverse processes and the sacral ala is then followed by bone grafting in the posterolateral areas. The local autogenous bone graft from the decompression can be used in this area.

ANTERIOR FUSION

Depending on the surgeon's choice, the addition of anterior fusion will add to the stability as well as the fusion rate.[40,41] The addition of an anterior fusion can be performed via a separate approach and performance of an anterior lumbar interbody fusion. Alternatively, one can opt to perform a posterior lumbar interbody fusion or a transforaminal lumbar interbody fusion depending on the surgeon's preference (Fig. 34-7). The techniques for these are described in separate chapters of this textbook.

SPONDYLOPTOSIS

Occasionally, one is faced with a complete anterior slippage of L5 on S1, referred to as *spondyloptosis*. The authors prefer to perform the spondylectomy with an anterior approach at first. The anterior exposure is preferably performed retroperitoneally. The intraoperative radiograph verified good positioning. The L4 as well as L5 vertebral bodies are identified. A dissection is carefully taken laterally, and the L4 and L5

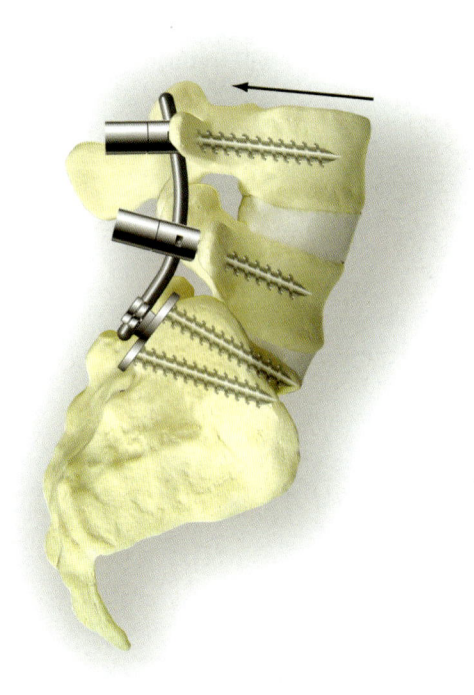

Fig. 34-6 Tightening the screws and fixation to the rod will translate the vertebral bodies dorsally.

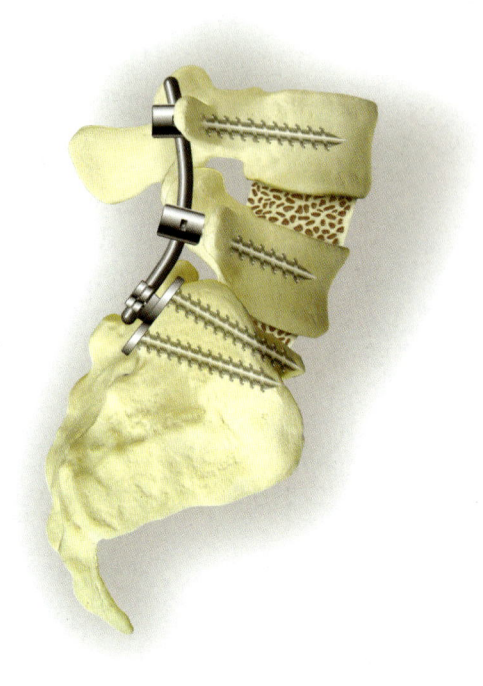

Fig. 34-7 Anterior interbody fusion can be performed via anterior or posterior approaches.

nerve roots should be identified. At this point, a L4-L5 diskectomy is performed in the usual fashion, going all of the way posterior to the posterior longitudinal ligament behind the L4-5 disk space. The disk is removed from the end plates of L4 and superior end plate of L5. The posterior longitudinal ligament is then taken down with Kerrison rongeurs. Next, a vertebrectomy of L5 is performed. This can be done in a piecemeal fashion with osteotomes and rongeuers. Once the L5 vertebrectomy has been done all the way to the spinal canal, this should allow visualization of the L5-S1 disk. The L5-S1 diskectomy is then performed with curettes removing it from the superior end plate of S1. At this point, the L4 should actually be in close proximity to the S1. The L4 and L5 nerve roots should be examined. At this point, the anterior abdominal exposure can be closed and the patient carefully turned to be prone on the operating table.

The posterior approach is performed to the L4-sacrum level. Decompression is performed with complete removal of the spinous processes and lamina of the L5 vertebra. The transverse processes are resected followed by resection of the pedicles. The inferior and superior facets of L5 are subsequently removed.

At this point, the L4 and L5 nerve roots are reidentified, and the end plates are examined for removal of all soft tissues. Bone grafting can be done via a posterior lumbar interbody fusion, by translumbar interbody fusion, or by going anteriorly again.

The instrumentation should be performed with placement of stable fixation such as previously mentioned with a sacral plate. The pedicle screws should be placed in L4. One may need to put a towel clip on the spinous process of L4 with application of a dorsally applied force to stabilize L4 as one is putting ventrally directed force with a pedicle finder to the pedicle of L4. This will help avoid instability and damage to any neural structures. Once the pedicle screws from L4 and sacral stabilization are performed, the rods and screws are tightened securely together.

References

1. Herbiniaux G: Traite sur divers accouchmements laborieux et sur les polypes de la matrice. Bruxelles, 1782.
2. Kilian H: Schilderungen neuer becken formen und ihres verhaltens in lebened. Mannheim, Verlag Von Bosserman, 1854.
3. Wiltse LL, Newman PH, Macnab I: Classification of spondylolisis and spondylolisthesis. Clin Orthop 1976;117:23–29.
4. Meyerding H: Spondylolisthesis: Surgical treatment and results. Surg Gynecol Obstet 1932;54:371–377.
5. Dubousset J: Treatment of spondylolysis and spondylolisthesis in children and adolescents. Clin Orthop 1997;337:77–85.
6. Harris IE, Weinstein SL: Long-term follow-up of patients with grade-III and IV spondylolisthesis: Treatment with and without posterior fusion. J Bone Joint Surg Am 1987;69:960–969.
7. Amuso SJ, Neff RS, Coulson DB, et al: The surgical treatment of spondylolisthesis by posterior element resection. J Bone Joint Surg Am 1970;52:529–536.
8. Bohlman HH, Cook SS: One-stage decompression and posterolateral and interbody fusion for lumbosacral spondyloptosis through a posterior approach: Report of two cases. J Bone Joint Surg Am 1982;64:415–418.
9. Bosworth DM, Fielding JW, Demarest L, et al: Spondylolisthesis; a critical review of a consecutive series of cases treated by arthrodesis. J Bone Joint Surg Am 1955;37A:767–786.
10. Burkus JK, Lonstein JE, Winter RB, et al: Long-term evaluation of adolescents treated operatively for spondylolisthesis: A comparison of in situ arthrodesis only with in situ arthrodesis and reduction followed by immobilization in a cast. J Bone Joint Surg Am 1992;74:693–704.
11. Dandy DJ, Shannon MJ: Lumbo-sacral subluxation (group 1 spondylolisthesis). J Bone Joint Surg Br 1971;53:578–595.
12. Herring JA, Bradford DS: Severe spondylolisthesis. J Pediatr Orthop 1985;5:737–739.
13. Nachemson A: Repair of the spondylolisthetic defect and intertransverse fusion for young patients. Clin Orthop 1976;117:101–105.
14. Peek RD, Wiltse LL, Reynolds JB, et al: In situ arthrodesis without decompression for Grade III or IV isthmic spondylolisthesis in adults who have severe sciatica. J Bone Joint Surg Am 1989;71:62–68.
15. Pizzutillo PD, Mirenda W, MacEwen GD: Posterolateral fusion for spondylolisthesis in adolescence. J Pediatr Orthop 1986;6:311–316.
16. Rombold C: Treatment of spondylolisthesis by posterolateral fusion, resection of the pars interarticularis, and prompt mobilization of the patient: An end-result study of seventy-three patients. J Bone Joint Surg Am 1966;48:1282–1300.
17. Sherman FC, Rosenthal RK, Hall JE: Spine fusion for spondylolysis and spondylolisthesis in children. Spine 1979;4:59–66.
18. Smith MD, Bohlman HH: Spondylolisthesis treated by a single-stage operation combining decompression with in situ posterolateral and anterior fusion: An analysis of eleven patients who had long-term follow-up. J Bone Joint Surg Am 1990;72:415–421.
19. Stanton RP, Meehan P, Lovell WW: Surgical fusion in childhood spondylolisthesis. J Pediatr Orthop 1985;5:411–415.
20. Takeda M: A newly devised "three-one" method for the surgical treatment of spondylolysis and spondylolisthesis. Clin Orthop 1980;147:228–233.
21. Turner RH, Bianco AJ Jr: Spondylolysis and spondylolisthesis in children and teen-agers. J Bone Joint Surg Am 1971;53:1298–1306.
22. Velikas EP, Blackburne JS: Surgical treatment of spondylolisthesis in children and adolescents. J Bone Joint Surg Br 1981;63B:67–70.
23. Verbiest H: The treatment of lumbar spondyloptosis or impending lumbar spondyloptosis accompanied by neurologic deficit and/or neurogenic intermittent claudication. Spine 1979;4:68–77.
24. Balderston RA, Bradford DS: Technique for achievement and maintenance of reduction for severe spondylolisthesis using spinous process traction wiring and external fixation of the pelvis. Spine 1985;10:376–382.
25. Bartolozzi P, Sandri A, Cassini M, et al: One-stage posterior decompression-stabilization and trans-sacral interbody fusion after partial reduction for severe L5-S1 spondylolisthesis. Spine 2003;28:1135–1141.
26. Bradford DS: Treatment of severe spondylolisthesis: A combined approach for reduction and stabilization. Spine 1979;4:423–429.
27. Bradford DS, Gotfried Y: Staged salvage reconstruction of grade IV and V spondylolisthesis. J Bone Joint Surg Am 1987;69:191–202.

28. DeWald RL, Faut MM, Taddonio RF, et al: Severe lumbosacral spondylolisthesis in adolescents and children: Reduction and staged circumferential fusion. J Bone Joint Surg Am 1981;63:619–626.
29. Harrington PR, Tullos HS: Spondylolisthesis in children: Observations and surgical treatment. Clin Orthop 1971;79:75–84.
30. Kaneda K, Satoh S, Nohara Y, et al: Distraction rod instrumentation with posterolateral fusion in isthmic spondylolisthesis: 53 cases followed for 18–89 months. Spine 1985;10:383–389.
31. Lance EM: Treatment of severe spondylolisthesis with neural involvement: A report of two cases. J Bone Joint Surg Am 1966;48:883–891.
32. Matthiass HH, Heine J: The surgical reduction of spondylolisthesis. Clin Orthop 1986;203:34–44.
33. McPhee IB, O'Brien JP: Reduction of severe spondylolisthesis: A preliminary report. Spine 1979;4:430–434.
34. McQueen MM, Court-Brown C, Scott JH: Stabilisation of spondylolisthesis using Dwyer instrumentation. J Bone Joint Surg Br 1986;68:185–188.
35. Roy-Camille R, Saillant G, Mazel C: Internal fixation of the lumbar spine with pedicle screw plating. Clin Orthop 1986;203:7–17.
36. Scaglietti O, Frontino G, Bartolozzi P: Technique of anatomical reduction of lumbar spondylolisthesis and its surgical stabilization. Clin Orthop 1976;117:165–175.
37. Sevastikoglou JA, Spangfort E, Aaro S: Operative treatment of spondylolisthesis in children and adolescents with tight hamstrings syndrome. Clin Orthop 1980;147:192–199.
38. Sijbrandij S: A new technique for the reduction and stabilisation of severe spondylolisthesis: A report of two cases. J Bone Joint Surg Br 1981;63B:266–271.
39. Sijbrandij S: Reduction and stabilisation of severe spondylolisthesis: A report of three cases. J Bone Joint Surg Br 1983;65:40–42.
40. Molinari RW, Bridwell KH, Lenke LG, et al: Anterior column support in surgery for high-grade, isthmic spondylolisthesis. Clin Orthop 2002;394:109–120.
41. Muschik M, Zippel H, Perka C: Surgical management of severe spondylolisthesis in children and adolescents: Anterior fusion in situ versus anterior spondylodesis with posterior transpedicular instrumentation and reduction. Spine 1997;22:2036–2042; discussion 43.
42. Boxall D, Bradford DS, Winter RB, et al: Management of severe spondylolisthesis in children and adolescents. J Bone Joint Surg Am 1979;61:479–495.
43. Seitsalo S, Osterman K, Hyvarinen H, et al: Progression of spondylolisthesis in children and adolescents: A long-term follow-up of 272 patients. Spine 1991;16:417–421.

CHAPTER 35

NITIN GOYAL

ALEXANDER R. VACCARO

MICHAEL A. PAHL

Minimal Access Exposure for Posterior Lumbar Instrumented Fusions

INTRODUCTION

MINIMAL ACCESS APPROACH

Minimal access surgical approaches to the lumbar spine were developed with the intention of safely exposing the proper procedure-related anatomy while at the same time minimizing the disadvantages of excessive soft tissue stripping, dissection, and prolonged retraction. The traditional open posterior surgical approach involves a midline longitudinal incision of sufficient length to expose the desired spinal levels, subsequent stripping of the paraspinal muscles off the posterior spinal elements, and static retraction of the superficial and deep paraspinal muscles to allow for adequate visualization and hemostasis throughout the surgical procedure. Studies have shown that prolonged soft tissue retraction and the greater the force per unit area compression on the retracted soft tissues combine to increase the degree of regional ischemia,[1] resulting in paraspinal electromyographic abnormalities[2] and decreased muscle density.[3] Muscle weakness and denervation are clearly critical consequences that may have adverse long-term side effects such as chronic pain and muscular dysfunction. It is apparent that minimizing soft tissue dissection translates into less acute postoperative pain, necessitates less narcotic pain medication, and often shortens hospital stays.

Minimally invasive surgery is not without its own set of associated difficulties. Minimally invasive endoscopic spinal procedures demand a lengthy learning curve due to the complexity of instrument manipulation in a closed space, necessitating using two-dimensional visual aids and inferred depth perception through adjacent visualized structures. Working within the boundaries of an endoscopic cannula is considered a technically challenging task, especially when working within the lateral margins of the field of view during a spinal procedure.

Minimal access procedures have been popularized in posterior cervical and lumbar spinal decompressive surgery. These procedures rely on tubular retraction following soft tissue dilation. Variations in tube design have involved wider diameter tubes with an independent fiberoptic light source to avoid the need for reliance on endoscopic visualization and tubes that dilate distally to allow greater freedom of instrument manipulation and implant delivery. The greatest challenge to the spinal surgeon is the placement of segmental spinal fixation (i.e., pedicle screws) in a minimally invasive manner.[4-13] Two methods of minimally invasive implant placement are currently in practice. One involves the use of a distally expansive tube retractor system relying on utilization of an attached light source, microscope, or endoscopic two-dimensional visualization of implant site application and fluoroscopic imaging to guide implant trajectory. Another method uses orthogonal fluoroscopic image guidance, or computer image guidance, to percutaneously place guidewires within the pedicle that subsequently guide screw placement. The placement of the longitudinal connector (rod) with this latter method is then guided by an attached spinal anchor frame that directs the rod into the spinal anchors.

MONOSEGMENTAL SPINAL ACCESS

In 1997, Foley and Smith described a minimal access tubular retractor system (MED System, Medtronic Sofamor Danek, Memphis, TN), designed to minimize traditional soft tissue dissection while preserving the ability to indirectly visualize the spinal elements through use of an endoscope.[14] The tubular access strategy described by Foley and colleagues allowed access to the spinal elements through soft tissue

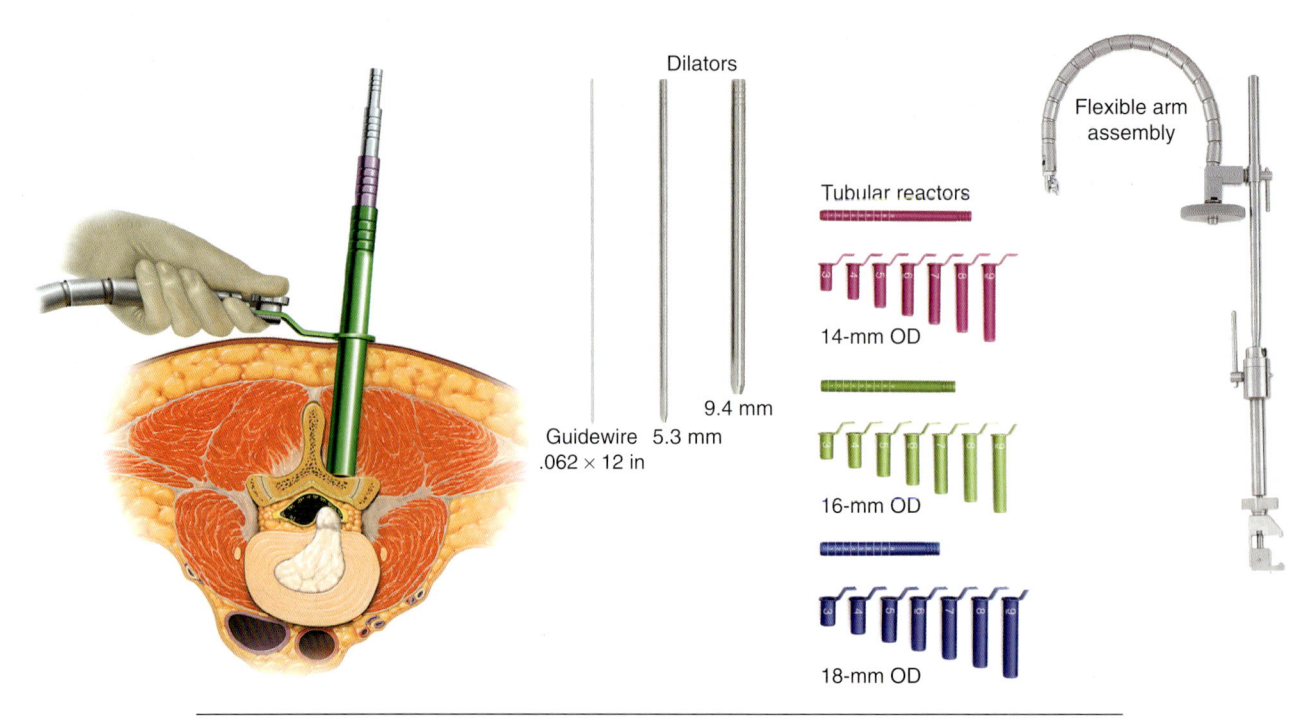

Fig. 35-1 METRx Tube Retractor System (Medtronic Sofamor Danek, Memphis, TN).

cannula dilation with the advantage of providing the surgeon with a familiar access portal similar to one in the standard posterolateral approach used in open exposures. The latest version of this system (METRx, Medtronic Sofamor Danek, Memphis, TN) employs an enlarged access portal and a fiberoptic ring light source that provides the surgeon with the option of direct visualization of the spinal elements rather than relying on an endoscope to indirectly visualize the spine (Fig. 35-1). Use of this system begins with the posterior placement of a K-wire down to the intended spinal level using fluoroscopic guidance. A small skin incision is then made around the K-wire to allow placement of a succession of increasingly larger cannulas to dilate the field of view. The surgeon can then operate through the tube system using endoscopy to indirectly visualize the spinal elements or using traditional loupe or microscope visualization with the addition of a fiberoptic ring optical light source.

The disadvantage of a rigid tube access system is the technical difficulty of working along the lateral borders of the exposure through the cannula tube. Instrument manipulation is limited by the diameter and length of the tube. To improve spinal access the surgeon often has to move the portal cannula multiple times during the procedure, resulting in obscured visualization due to soft tissue invasion under the terminal port aperture.

In response to these difficulties, the METRx X-Tube retractor system (Medtronic Sofamor Danek, Memphis, TN; Fig. 35-2) was developed; it includes an expandable tubular base that dilates from 2.5 to 4.0 cm. The distal tube dilation allows for greater freedom of instrument manipulation and the ability to place spinal anchors such as pedicle screws. The degree of visualization is improved over a solid tube system but is still somewhat constrained by the confines of a restricted proximal tubular ring. A benefit of this design is that endoscopy is no longer requisite because of the addition of a fiberoptic ring optical light source and larger tube diameters. Fluoroscopy can be used to guide implant (screw) trajectory in the sagittal plane but is not absolutely necessary for screw starting point or positioning in the coronal plane. The major limitation of a proximally constrained tubular retractor system, outside of the inability to significantly

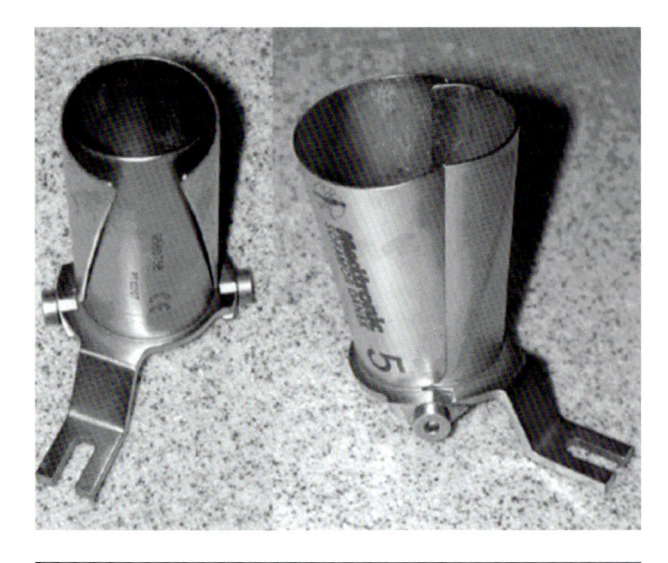

Fig. 35-2 METRx X-Tube Retractor (Medtronic Sofamor Danek, Memphis, TN).

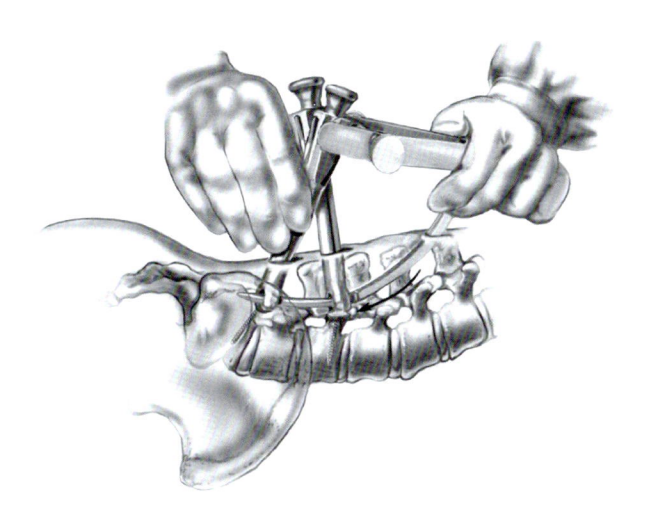

Fig. 35-3 Sextant Spinal System (Medtronic Sofamor Danek, Memphis, TN).

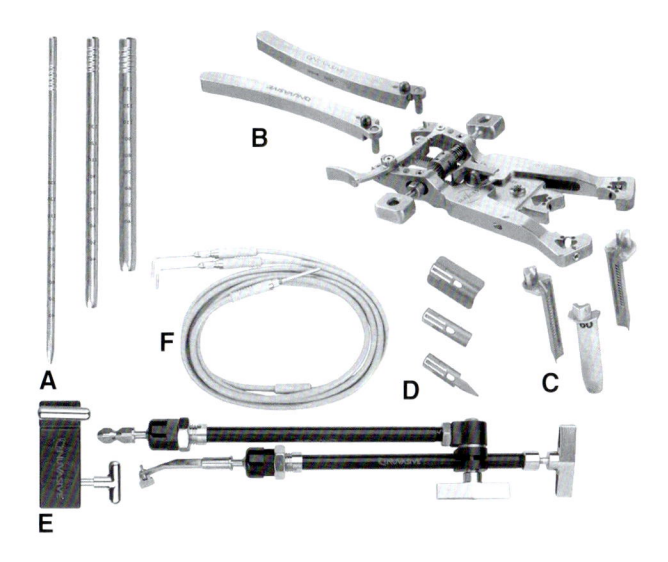

Fig. 35-4 MaXcess Retractor System. *A*, Dilators. *B*, Access driver. *C*, Blades. *D*, Shims. *E*, Articulating arm. *F*, Bifurcated light cable. (NuVasive, Inc., San Diego, CA.)

manipulate the access path of spinal instruments, is the longitudinal distance of visualization in the coronal plane and the inability to establish distal conformity with the spinal elements. This limits the ability to prevent soft tissue migration into the field of view with tube manipulation.

MULTISEGMENTAL SPINAL ACCESS— SEXTANT SPINAL SYSTEM

To improve the inherent limitations of a fixed tubular system in regard to accessing multiple spinal segments, strategies have been developed to accurately guide the delivery of a longitudinal connector (rod) into multiple spinal anchors. This has been accomplished with the aid of biplanar fluoroscopy for spinal anchor placement and an attachable guidance frame for rod delivery (Sextant Spinal System, Medtronic Sofamor Danek, Memphis, TN). The Sextant Spinal System (Fig. 35-3) uses biplanar fluoroscopy or computer-assisted image guidance to place guidewires into the pedicles of vertebral levels within the intended fusion segments. Cannulated pedicle screws are then placed over the wires using fluoroscopy to guide their depth of delivery. Long metal shaft screw extenders are attached to the proximal pedicle screws prior to their placement. The ends of the screw extenders are enjoined by a machined couple prior to their attachment to a guidance frame, which directs percutaneous rod insertion into the heads of the pedicle screws. The guidance frame is an arc-shaped (sextant) arm that swings on an axis established by the screw extenders to deliver a precut rod percutaneously into the heads of the fixed screws. A distinct feature of the Sextant system is that it allows for consistent accurate rod insertion by creating a geometrically constrained corridor through which the rod enters. Lock plugs, which are attached to the screw extenders, are then tightened to secure the rod to the pedicle screw heads. The rod inserter and screw extenders are then removed from the spinal anchors (pedicle screws).

MAXCESS AND METRX QUADRANT WILTSE-TYPE APPROACH FOR PEDICLE SCREW PLACEMENT

Many surgeons have avoided adoption of the Sextant Spinal System technique of screw delivery because of reliance on biplanar fluoroscopy and the uncertainty of accuracy of guidewire placement within the spinal pedicle. Additionally, rod length cannot be accurately adjusted to minimize rod overhang beyond the cephalad screw heads, and rod delivery may be difficult when stabilizing two spinal segments. An evolution of tubular access technology, in which the tube can expand on independent blades along its length (MaXcess modular blade retractor system, NuVasive, Inc., San Diego, CA; Fig. 35-4; and the METRx Quadrant retractor system, Medtronic Sofamor Danek, Memphis, TN; Fig. 35-5), has

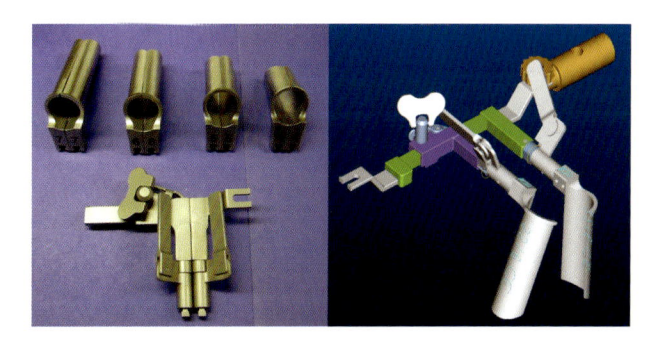

Fig. 35-5 METRx Quadrant Retractor System (Medtronic Sofamor Danek, Memphis, TN).

allowed the surgeon to directly visualize two to three spinal anchor starting points, similar to an open spinal procedure. The MaXcess and METRx Quadrant systems, similar to the static tubular systems, are designed to maximize surgical access while minimizing retraction and manipulation of the surrounding soft tissue. The MaXcess Access System is unique in its design in that it is composed of three independent blades, all adjustable in depth, which may be separated in a triangulated fashion to improve the field of view. The key differentiating characteristic of this access system is that the superior-inferior exposure can be adjusted as needed, allowing adequate visualization and screw anchor and rod placement through parallel para-midline 2-cm incisions for a two-level fusion. Medial-lateral exposure is controlled as needed with expansion of the third, independent, blade.

Current clinical uses of the MaXcess System include decompressive laminectomy, foraminotomy, diskectomy, posterolateral and interbody fusion, and multilevel (two motion segment) pedicle screw placement. This system can be tailored to individual patient girth in that the individual blades may be exchanged or modified with in situ extension shims to address variations in local anatomy (depth and width). The independent-blade design allows operative instruments to be leveraged against the incision border through openings between the blades during retractor expansion. The MaXcess System has a built-in bifurcated optical light source to assist in visualization, obviating the need for an endoscope. The ability to manipulate independent blade separation allows the surgeon to adequately decompress a spinal segment and deliver an interbody implant without the need for an endoscope, and to perform a multisegmented fusion without the need for biplanar fluoroscopy or adjunctive guidance systems for rod delivery. Lateral fluoroscopy or plain radiographs are recommended to confirm sagittal plane screw trajectory.

Although newly released, the METRx Quadrant retractor system uses the concept of independent expandable bladed technology to access the spine in a minimally invasive manner, simulating an open approach with direct visualization familiar to the average spine surgeon. The Quadrant retractor is made up of two separate expandable blades that allow for superior-inferior exposure control.

MAXCESS SYSTEM COMPONENTS

ACCESS SYSTEM

- Articulating arm
- K-wire
- Dilators: 6, 9, and 12 mm
- Access driver
- Blades: 30, 40, 50, 60, 70, 80, 90, 100, 110, 120, 130 mm
- Shims: standard, intradiscal, and wide
- Shim inserter
- Light cable
- Hex driver

OPERATIVE TECHNIQUE
Preparation and Positioning

The patient is placed in the standard prone position on a radiolucent table such as a Jackson frame. A bedrail should be present on the table to allow attachment of an articulating arm, which stabilizes the MaXcess retractor system once it is inserted into the spinal incision.

Exposure

Fluoroscopy in the lateral (adequate) or anteroposterior and lateral planes is used to locate the desired spinal level or segment. The spinous process is palpated to define midline. At the level of the desired disk space, an incision point is marked on the skin approximately 3 to 4 cm laterally from the midline (Fig. 35-6). A spinal needle or preferably a blunt trochar is introduced into the skin using fluoroscopic guidance to verify the desired spinal docking site. A 2- to 3-cm longitudinal incision is made at the site of the spinal needle or trochar entry, downward through the level of the superficial and deep fascia, to easily accommodate the spinal dilators. The path created by the spinal needle or trochar can be widened by one's finger, if desired, by removing the needle or trochar to initially widen the surgical path. The trochar or needle is then replaced and advanced carefully through the superficial and deep fascia, making sure not to unintentionally advance through the interlaminar space. Next, successively increasing dilating tubes are inserted with intermittent fluoroscopy to verify their position. The depth of the last dilator is noted, and, consequently, the corresponding retractor blades are attached to the access driver. Blades of varying

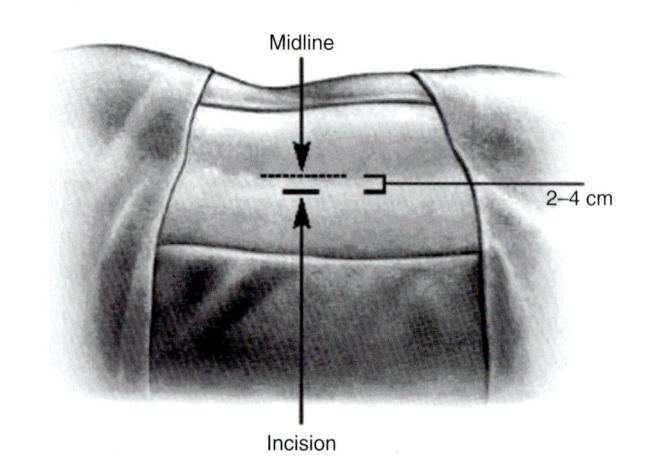

Fig. 35-6 MaXcess Access operative technique: Determine the location of the spinous process and mark the incision site 3 to 4 cm lateral to the midline, over the level of the disk space.

CHAPTER 35 Minimal Access Exposure for Posterior Lumbar Instrumented Fusions

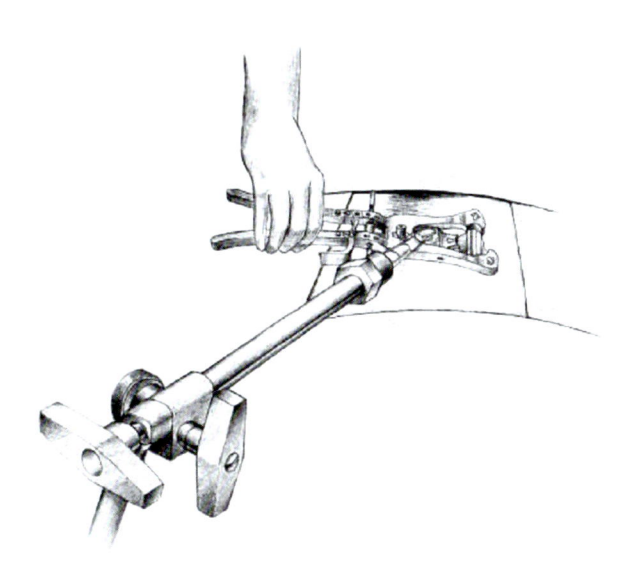

Fig. 35-7 MaXcess Access operative technique: Squeeze the handles of the access driver to expand the blades superoinferiorly. Control the medial-lateral exposure by twisting the knob on the handle toward the incision.

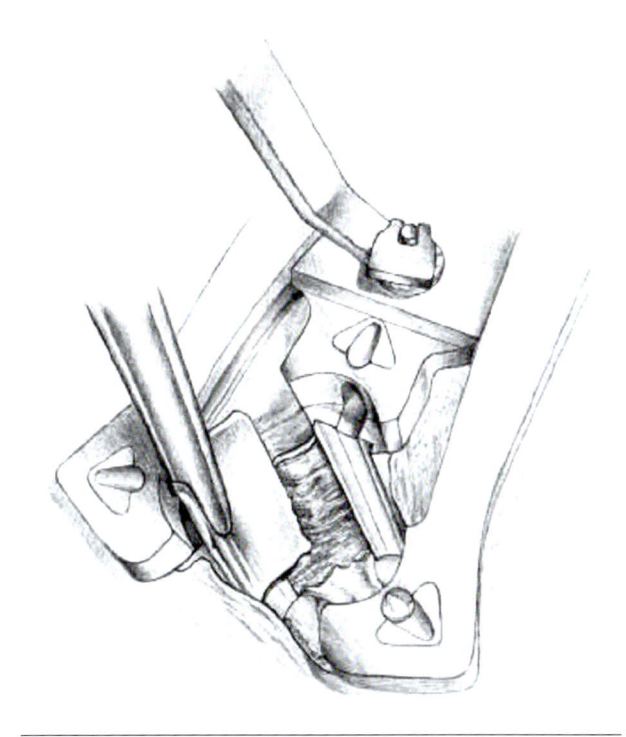

Fig. 35-8 MaXcess Access operative technique: Use the shims to expand the blades, so as to modify the exposure as needed.

length may be attached independently in order to best suit the appropriate landscape of the varying surgical anatomy. The access driver is advanced over the dilators, down to the facet joint, making sure to slant the driver obliquely toward the midline to guarantee adequate exposure. The articulating arm is attached to the contralateral bedrail and the other end is attached to the access driver. To lock the articulating arm, both T-handles are turned clockwise. The expandable handles are attached to the access driver and gently squeezed to expand the blades in a superior-inferior direction (Fig. 35-7).

The medial-lateral exposure can be adjusted independently by rotating the respective knobs on the access driver toward the incision. A xenon light source (one bifurcated light cable) may then be attached to the access driver to illuminate the operative corridor. Any soft tissue within the exposure field may now be removed by electrocautery. To limit invasion of soft tissue into the operative corridor, shims may be utilized to lengthen or widen the blades (Fig. 35-8). By loosening the articulating arm T-handles, the driver may be maneuvered to direct visualization as needed for spinal decompression or implant placement.

SPHERX PEDICLE SCREW SYSTEM

NuVasive has designed a pedicle screw system specifically for posterior lumbar minimal access procedures (SpheRx System, NuVasive, Inc., San Diego, CA). This system uses cannulated instruments and implants (drills, taps, screws, lock screws, and rods) that may be passed over a K-wire once introduced into a pedicle (Figs. 35-9 and 35-10). The spherical, cannulated end of the rod is inserted over the K-wire for simplified placement (Fig. 35-11). The spherical-end rod design provides additional rotational capability in combination with the polyaxial and fixed-angle screws. Additionally, the spherical end of the rod does not extend beyond the end of the superior screw, which makes it ideal at the superior end of a fusion in order to avoid facet impingement (Fig. 35-12). The spherical end of the rod is geometrically constrained within

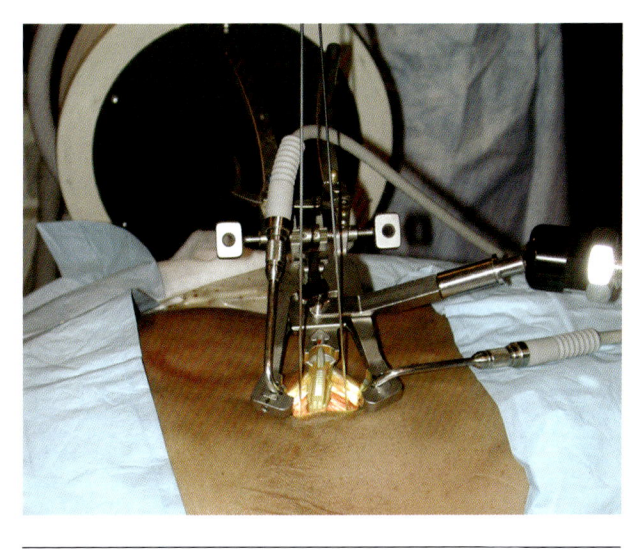

Fig. 35-9 SpheRx Pedicle Screw System: K-wire placement. (NuVasive, Inc., San Diego, CA.)

Fig. 35-10 SpheRx Pedicle Screw System: screw placement. (NuVasive, Inc., San Diego, CA.)

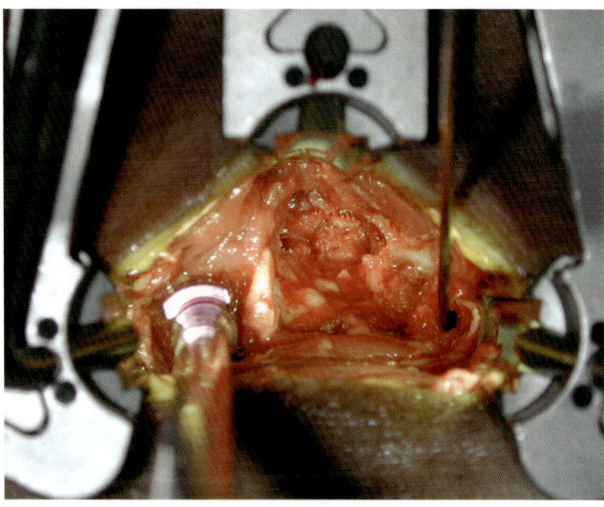

Fig. 35-12 SpheRx Pedicle Screw System: screws and rod in place. (NuVasive, Inc., San Diego, CA.)

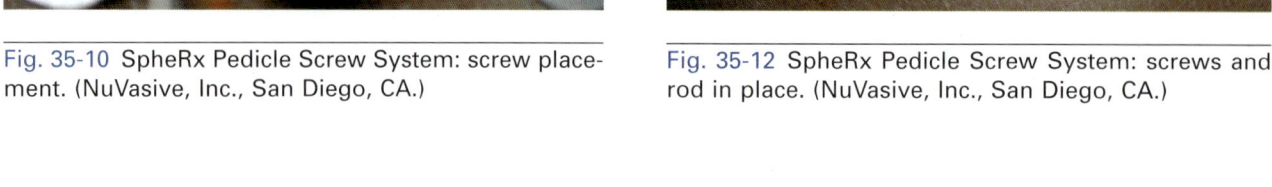

the head of the screw, simplifying compression by eliminating the need to have access to both ends of the rod with the rod compressor. Tightening following compression is necessary only at the caudal rod-screw connection. This design allows the use of a fixed-angle screw at the cephalad end of the instrumentation where the spherical end of the rod is inserted to provide a more stable, less expensive biomechanical construct.

COMPLICATIONS

Only recently has minimally invasive spinal access become commonplace in posterior lumbar degenerative spinal procedures. Therefore, published data regarding complications represent only preliminary results, and long-term follow-up is required to determine the relative risks and benefits of minimal access surgery as compared with more traditional open procedures. Complications related to the surgical exposure are rare. The major difficulty with minimal access procedures is the lack of adequate visualization for safe and reproducible neural decompression and implant placement. Systems that rely on indirect biplanar fluoroscopy for guidewire placement risk the potential for pedicle violation and implant canal intrusion with eccentric wire placement within the pedicle boundaries. Lack of clear direct visualization of the neural elements risks the potential for dural violation or stretch neuropraxia.

Published reports reveal little information regarding complications related to the Sextant or SpheRx pedicle screw systems owing to their recent introduction into clinical practice. Minimal access procedures have been shown to generate comparable results in terms of functional outcomes in the hands of experienced surgeons as compared with open procedures, but with reduced length of hospital stays and decreased blood loss, with equivalent infection rates. Minimal access paramidline exposures require significantly less soft tissue dissection and therefore carry a lower morbidity rate owing to the blunt muscle splitting approach compared with the requisite soft tissue stripping associated with an open midline procedure. Risks more pronounced with minimal access surgery are primarily related to visualization. Specific complications such as a dural tear are much more difficult to repair using a minimal access exposure. The advantage of an access approach that avoids the need for biplanar fluoroscopy or endoscopy is that it mimics the surgical skills used in open procedures. This avoids the prolonged learning curve associated with traditional minimally invasive spinal procedures.

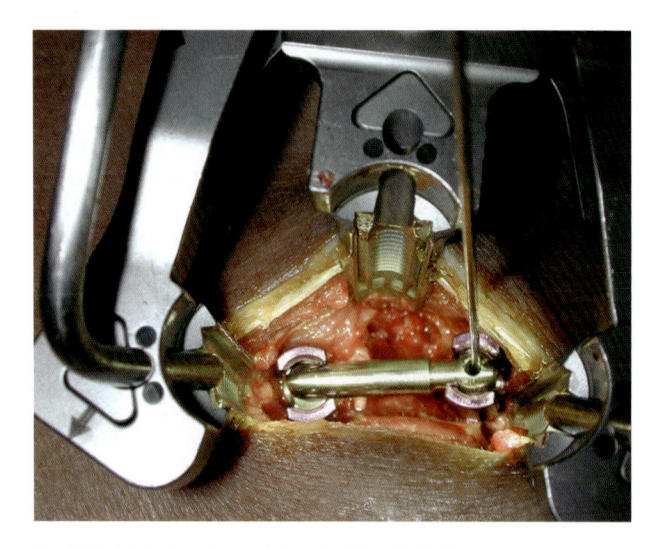

Fig. 35-11 SpheRx Pedicle Screw System: rod placement. (NuVasive, Inc., San Diego, CA.)

CHAPTER 35 Minimal Access Exposure for Posterior Lumbar Instrumented Fusions

DISCUSSION

Over the last several years, minimal access exposure of the posterior spine has become more popular as newer access tools have been developed and refined, minimizing the morbidity and shortening the learning curve of older endoscopic techniques. It has also become a popular choice for patients educated in the morbidities related to extensive soft tissue dissection and retraction commonly associated with open spinal procedures. The minimization of soft tissue dissection, the reduction of local paraspinal muscle tension and ischemia, and the reduction of intraoperative blood loss associated with minimal access surgery have led to shorter hospital stays and a more accelerated recovery time. The early experience with expandable-blade retractor systems for minimal access decompression has been extremely encouraging. The MaXcess modular blade retractor and METRx Quadrant systems are easily adjustable for customized exposure and provide superior illumination and visibility, affording the ability to perform mutisegmental pedicle screw fixation through an open direct surgical exposure, similar to open conventional procedures. The improved longitudinal and medial-lateral visibility offered by an independent blade retractor system appears to have significantly alleviated the access-related limitations experienced with static tubular systems or fluoroscopy-dependent implant-guided systems.

The Sextant "percutaneous" spinal system has demonstrated great success as a minimally invasive procedure for pedicle screw-rod placement. However, if one measures the length of the three parallel incisions required to place two ipsilateral screws and the introduction of the longitudinal connector (rod) percutaneously, it is often comparable to or even greater than the single 2-inch incision needed for successful use of an expandable blade access system (MaXcess or METRx Quadrant systems) and paramedian fixation construct placement (SpheRx Pedicle Screw System) (Figs. 35-13 and 35-14). In addition to the need for healing of three separate ipsilateral incisions, greater muscular disruption is required for rod placement with the Sextant system due to the long swing arm of the rod (see Fig. 35-3) as compared to the single smaller muscle-splitting direct Wiltse-type approach provided by the MaXcess and METRx Quadrant systems. Direct exposure of the spinal anchors using the MaXcess or METRx Quadrant systems minimizes the degree of rod protrusion beyond the end of the superior screw, potentially sparing contact disruption of the superior non-fused facet joint. This is an ongoing problem with the Sextant system, which by its design results in asymmetrical (longer) rod extension beyond the superior spinal anchor (Fig. 35-15). The MaXcess and METRx Quadrant retractor systems allow the combination of an interbody fusion procedure, such as a transforaminal lumbar interbody fusion (TLIF) and pedicle screw placement through the same incision, rather than the requisite separate incisions and tools when using the Sextant system. An adjustable retractor system provides a direct path for spinal visualization that enables ease of spinal decompression and implant delivery, all through a single incision without the need for endoscopy or biplanar fluoroscopy.

A minimally invasive one- or two-level posterior exposure of the spine is now safely attainable with the latest minimal access systems that exploit the biomechanics of an adjustable blade retractor. This is proving to be a valuable alternative operative approach to traditional open procedures. As the clinical use of these developing systems escalates, more outcomes data will become available to determine the value of these minimally invasive procedures.

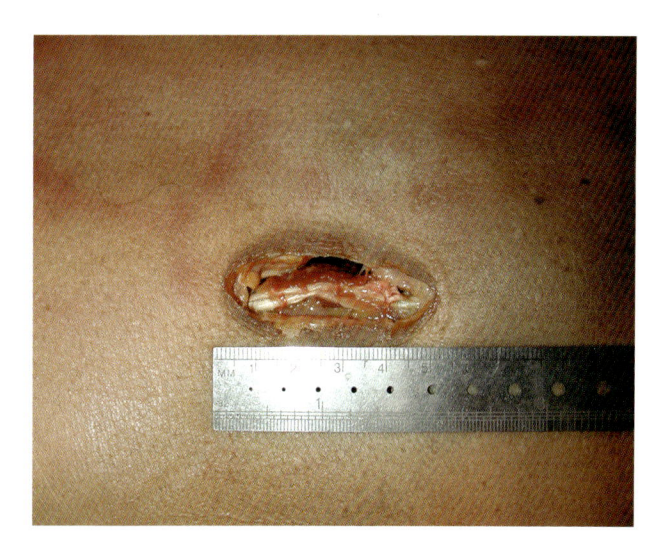

Fig. 35-13 Incision length using the SpheRx Pedicle Screw System (approximately 2 inches).

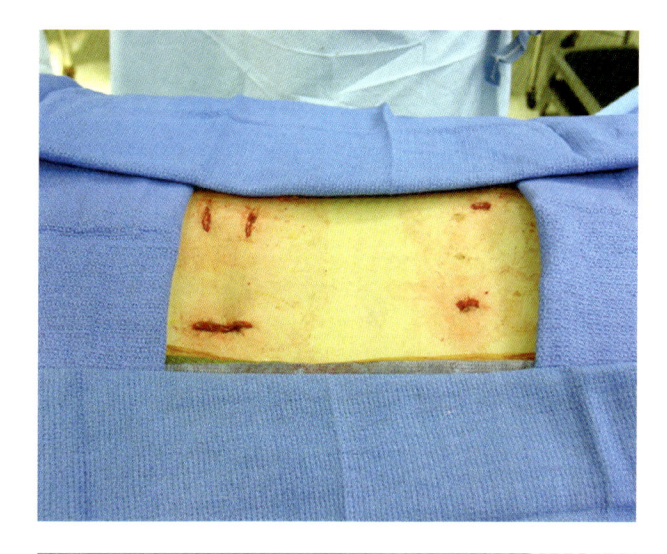

Fig. 35-14 A comparison of the incision lengths of the Sextant and SpheRx spinal systems.

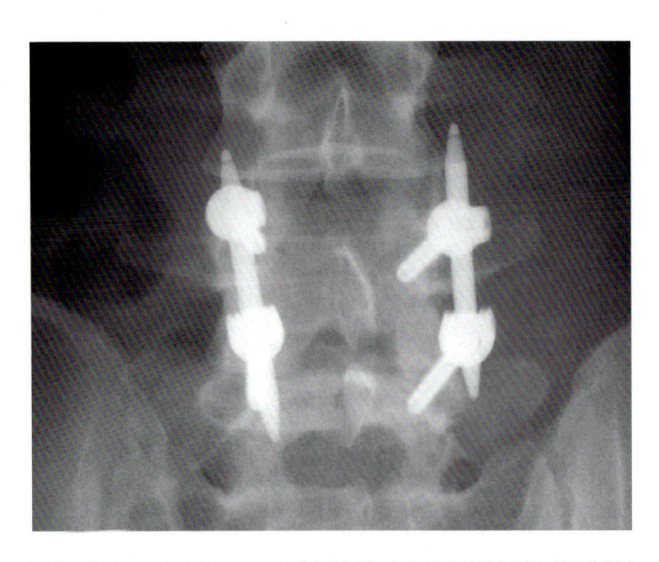

Fig. 35-15 An anteroposterior radiograph illustrating the sextant pedicle screw-rod system in place and significant rod overhang.

References

1. Styf JR, Willen J: The effects of external compression by three different retractors on pressure in the erector spine muscles during and after posterior lumbar spine surgery in humans. Spine 1998;23(3):354–358.
2. Kraft DH, Kraft GH: Electromyography in paraspinal muscles following surgery for root compression. Arch Phys Med Rehab 1975;56(2):80–83.
3. Mayer TG, Vanharanta H, Gatchel RJ, et al: Comparison of CT scan muscle measurements and isokinetic trunk strength in postoperative patients. Spine 1989;14(1):33–36.
4. Steffee AD: The variable screw placement system with posterior lumbar interbody fusion. In Lin PM, Gill K (eds): Lumbar Interbody Fusion. Rockville MD, Aspen Publishers, 1989, pp 81–93.
5. Steffee AD, Sitkowski DJ: Posterior lumbar interbody fusion and plates. Clin Orthop 1988;227:99–102.
6. Wiltse LL: Surgery for the intervertebral disc disease of the lumbar spine. Clin Orthop 1977;129:22–45.
7. Branch CL Jr: Posterior lumbar interbody fusion In Hardy RW Jr (ed): Lumbar Disc Disease, 2nd ed. New York, Raven Press, 1993, pp 187–200.
8. Brodke DS, Dick JC, Kunz DN: Posterior lumbar interbody fusion: A biomechanical comparison, including a new threaded cage. Spine 1997;22:26–31.
9. Lin PM, Cautilli RA, Joyce MF: Posterior lumbar interbody fusion. Clin Orthop 1983;180:154–168.
10. Sidhu KS, Herkowitz HN: Spinal instrumentation in the management of degenerative disorders of the lumbar spine. Clin Orthop 1997;335:39–53.
11. Khoo LT, Palmer S, Laich DT: Minimally invasive percutaneous posterior lumbar interbody fusion. Neurosurgery 2002;51(5 Suppl):166.
12. Regan, JJ, Yuan H, McAfee PC: Laparoscopic fusion of the lumbar spine: Minimally invasive spine surgery: A prospective multicenter study evaluating open and laparoscopic lumbar fusion. Spine 1999;24:402–411.
13. Zdeblick TA, David SM: A prospective comparison of surgical approach for anterior L4-L5 fusion: Laparoscopic versus mini anterior lumbar interbody fusion. Spine 2000;25:2682–2687.
14. Foley K, Smith M: Microendoscopic discectomy. Tech Neurosurg 1997;3:301–307.

SECTION III

INFLAMMATORY DISEASE

CHAPTER 36

AZADEH FARIN

K. CHARLES Y. LIU

MICHAEL Y. WANG

The Transoral Approach for Ventral Cervicomedullary Decompression in Rheumatoid Arthritis

INTRODUCTION

Rheumatoid arthritis (RA) is a chronic, progressive systemic inflammatory disease primarily affecting the synovial joints of the body. The cervical region is affected more often than any other part of the spine, with cervical synovial and facet joints diseased in 25% to 90% of RA patients. Cervical spine disease in RA involves joint inflammation and synovitis, loss of articular cartilage, ligamentous laxity, and joint and bone erosion, leading to cervical instability.

Spinal instability is caused most commonly by atlantoaxial subluxation due to loss of transverse ligament integrity and granulation formation between the C1-C2 lateral masses. This leads to anteroposterior and rotatory subluxation. In addition, cranial settling due to bony erosion of the atlantoaxial lateral masses and occipital condyles is frequently associated with atlantoaxial instability. The combination of these two processes results in rostral and posterior migration of the dens and compression of the brainstem. Furthermore, exacerbation of the synovitis at C1-C2 results in retroodontoid pannus formation. The pannus can become quite exuberant, leading to cervicomedullary compression.

DIAGNOSIS

The most common symptom in RA patients with cervical spine disease is pain in the upper cervical area, frequently associated with radiation to the mastoid or cranial regions. Radicular pain and numbness in the distribution of the greater occipital nerve can be the result of C2 nerve root compression from atlantoaxial subluxation. Less frequently, patients will complain of limb paresthesias exacerbated by neck movement, hand clumsiness, urinary retention or incontinence, involuntary leg spasms, diplopia, and vertigo.

However, the debilitating effects of advanced RA on the musculoskeletal system can make detection of even critical cervical or medullary compression difficult. In this context, diffuse hyperreflexia, spasticity, pathologic reflexes, or a Lhermitte sign with neck flexion may be the only signs on neurologic examination. Because of the potential for devastating neurologic compromise, RA patients with cervical spine pathology should be monitored closely. Early diagnosis is crucial, as advanced cases can result in sudden respiratory arrest from brainstem compression, and half of the patients diagnosed with cord compression will die within a year if left untreated.

The initial diagnostic studies for RA patients suspected of harboring cervical pathology are lateral, flexion, and extension x-rays. Odontoid erosion, atlantoaxial subluxation, atlantoaxial instability, and cranial settling can all be reliably detected with x-rays. In particular, a fixed increased atlantodental interval, excessive excursions between the anterior arch of C1 and the odontoid peg, and severe cranial settling should raise suspicions of cevicomedullary compression. Magnetic resonance imaging (MRI) provides good visualization of the neural elements as well as any periodontoid pannus. In patients unable to tolerate MRI, computed tomographic (CT) myelography should be performed when neural compression is suspected.

THE TRANSORAL APPROACH

Severe compression of the cervicomedullary region by a fixed atlantoaxial malalignment, atlantoaxial instability, or an exuberant pannus requires surgical treatment (Fig. 36-1). In select cases standalone rigid posterior fixation is adequate for treating spinal compression due solely to C1-C2 subluxation or cranial settling that can be reduced with cervical traction. In addition, a periodontoid pannus that does not cause

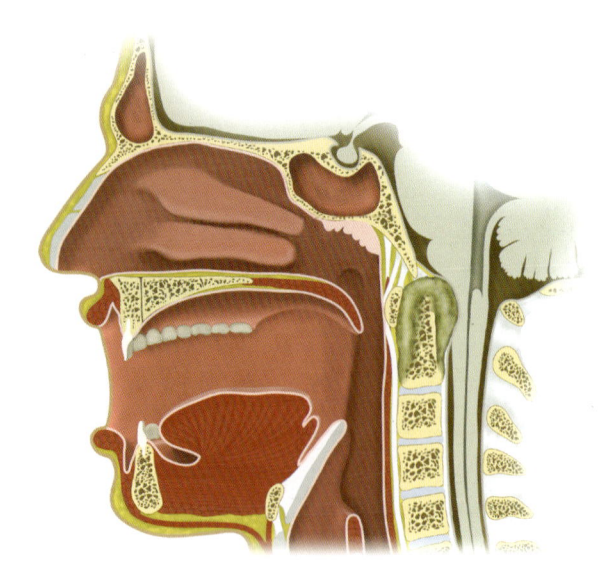

Fig. 36-1 Rheumatoid pannus formation at C1-C2 with attendant cervicomedullary compression.

critical neural compression will often be seen to involute with rigid posterior fixation of C1-C2 and can thus be addressed without direct surgical removal. However, fixed deformities or cases with a large rheumatoid pannus require direct surgical decompression. In these cases a transoral approach enables direct midline access to the pathology from the clivus to the C2-C3 disk space (Fig. 36-2). A midline maxillary osteotomy provides additional rostral exposure of the midclivus if needed. A mandibular osteotomy with midline glossotomy can be utilized if the temporomandibular joint is severely ankylosed, limiting the exposure between the upper and lower incisors.

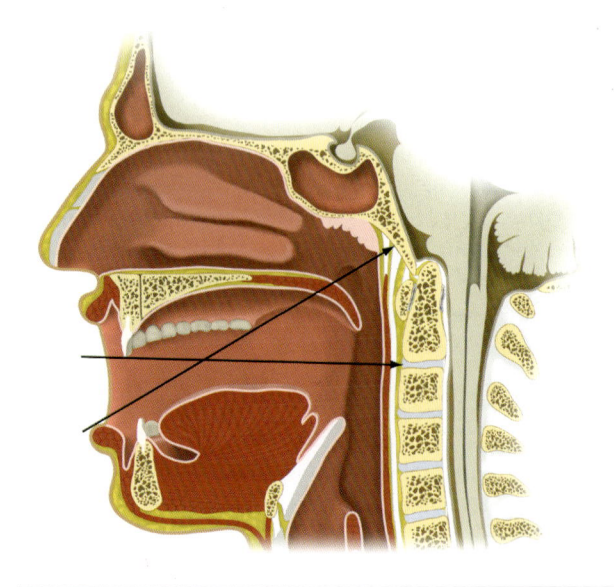

Fig. 36-2 Standard transoral exposure showing exposure from the midclivus to the C2-C3 interspace.

INDICATIONS AND CONTRAINDICATIONS

INDICATIONS

- Irreducible ventral extradural compression of the cervicomedullary junction due to cranial settling or atlantoaxial subluxation displacing the odontoid superiorly and posteriorly into the spinal canal and foramen magnum. Although critical neurologic compression is easily visualized on MRI, specific criteria have been set forth to determine thresholds for operative intervention:
  - Vertical subluxation shortening the distance between the center of the lower end plate of C2 and the palato-occipital line to less than 34 mm in men and 29 mm in women.
  - A maximal atlantodental interval of greater than 7 mm on dynamic x-rays.
  - A posterior atlantodental interval (the sagittal diameter of the spinal canal at C1-C2) of 14 mm or less.
- A large fibrous periodontoid pannus causing anterior cord compression.
- Motion-induced neck pain or sensory disturbances.
- C2 root entrapment due to atlantoaxial subluxation.
- Nonrheumatoid pathologies producing invagination of the odontoid peg into the posterior fossa such as odontoid fractures, neoplastic disease, congenital malformations, and mycobacterial lesions may also be approached in through the transoral route. Similarly, extradural clival chordomas and chondrosarcomas can be resected in this manner.
- Resection, biopsy, or débridement of the odontoid following unsuccessful attempts at needle aspiration.

RELATIVE CONTRAINDICATIONS

- The population of RA patients is frequently afflicted by multiple comorbidities, including rheumatoid lung disease, restricted chest wall movement, anemia, coagulopathies, and pharmacologic immunosuppression. For this reason the general medical status of these patients should be carefully evaluated prior to any surgical intervention.
- Synovitis of the temporomandibular joint can restrict jaw opening, reducing the height of the surgical corridor. For patients unable to open their jaw more than 3 cm, consideration must be given to the incorporation of a maxillary or mandibular splitting operation.
- The subaxial cervical spine must be investigated to ensure that intraoperative neck manipulation will not result in trauma to the spinal cord.

- Surgery should be considered only in patients with some remaining neurologic function. For patients with advanced disease resulting in quadriparesis or respirator dependence, the reduced likelihood of neurologic recovery must be weighed against surgical morbidity.
- Intradural or lesions incorporating the dura must be approached with great care. Opening of the dura through a transoral approach exposes the subarachnoid space to the nasopharyngeal flora. The risk of severe central nervous system infections is high.

OPERATIVE TECHNIQUE

PREOPERATIVE PREPARATION

- The range of motion of the temporomandibular joints should be assessed to ensure adequate oral exposure. Similarly, the degree of neck motion should be assessed to eliminate the risk of injury from intraoperative neck manipulation.
- Oropharyngeal and nasal cultures should be obtained prior to surgery for later identification of any pathogenic organisms if antibiotic treatment is necessary. Normal flora do not typically require antibiotic treatment.
- In severely debilitated patients or patients with lower cranial nerve deficits that impair swallowing and respiratory function, tracheostomy and gastrostomy tubes should be placed perioperatively.
- Any attempts at reduction of deformities with skeletal traction should be performed in the intensive care unit.
- Gross cervical instability should be identified and preparations made for an occipitocervical fusion.
- The patient's nutritional status preoperatively should be optimized.

EQUIPMENT

- Fluoroscopic C-arm
- Dingman or Spetzler transoral retractor
- Red Robinson rubber catheter
- Periosteal elevator
- Operating microscope
- High-speed drill with cutting and diamond burrs with a long extension
- Bipolar and monopolar cautery
- Long-handled pituitary rongeurs
- Long-handled ring and spoon curettes
- Hemostatic cellulose wool
- Hydrocortisone ointment, 1%
- Nasogastric tube
- Fibrin glue (optional)
- Lumbar drain (optional)
- Tracheostomy tray (optional)
- Bicortical iliac crest graft (optional)

PATIENT POSITIONING AND APPLICATION OF CERVICAL TRACTION

- The patient is positioned supine on a standard operating room table with a horseshoe headrest placed under the head. Rigid Mayfield head fixation is optional.
- For patients who have been reduced under traction, 5- to 10-lb weights in light traction are continued to maintain normal anatomic alignment of the craniovertebral junction and to place the neck in slight extension. Even in cases of seemingly irreducible lesions, placement of light traction can make ventral decompression easier.
- A lateral x-ray of the upper cervical spine is obtained to confirm proper positioning.

INTUBATION, TRACHEOSTOMY, AND PREPARATION OF ORAL CAVITY

- The patient should be intubated either awake or using fiberoptic guidance to minimize neck manipulation. Either orotracheal or nasotracheal intubation may be used. Orotracheal tubes interfere less with the exposure if the patient's jaw is not ankylosed; however, intubation may be difficult if jaw opening is restricted, and endotracheal tube may be easily kinked by the retractor. Nasotracheal intubation does not require a wide oral opening; however, the endotracheal tube will have to be swept lateral to the surgical corridor.
- In select cases a tracheostomy tube is placed.
- The oropharynx is packed with gauze to prevent excessive blood and fluid passage down the esophagus.
- A Dingman or Spetzler self-retaining retractor is placed (Fig. 36-3A and B). The superior end of the retractor is buttressed against the four upper incisors with a thin rubber guard used to prevent chipping of the teeth. The inferior arm of the retractor is used to depress the tongue and orotracheal tube, spreading the oral cavity open. Tongue retraction should be released every 20 minutes to prevent lingual congestion.
- The oral cavity is cleaned with 10% povidone iodine, then hydrogen peroxide, before being rinsed with saline.
- Somatosensory and motor evoked potential monitoring is routinely employed.

PALATE INCISION AND RETROPHARYNGEAL EXPOSURE

- The posterior pharyngeal wall is visualized in the depth of the oral cavity with the soft palate and uvula in the midline.
- If the uvula is the only obstructing structure a red Robinson catheter should be passed through one nostril into the oropharynx. The tip of the catheter should then be stitched to the tip of the uvula. Tension of the proximal catheter should then retract the uvula superiorly and

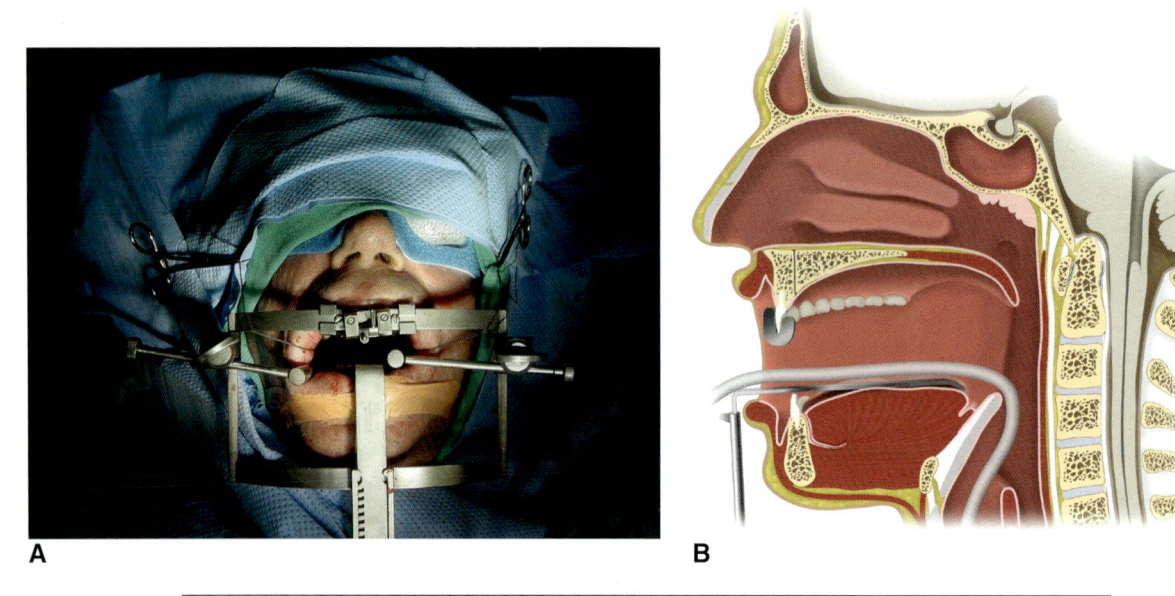

Fig. 36-3 Placement of the Dingman retractor: intraoperative (A) and sagittal (B) views.

out of view. The catheter can then be secured to the surgical drapes.
- If the soft palate is also obstructing the surgical corridor, then it must be divided (Fig. 36-4). Lidocaine with epinephrine is first injected into the midline soft palate for its vasoconstrictive effects. A scalpel is then used to make an incision starting at the hard palate midline and extending to the uvula base laterally, leaving the entire uvula attached to one side of the soft palate. No electrocautery is used, sparing the palatine artery and nerve, which supply the lateral aspect of the soft palate before terminating midline. This minimizes bleeding and optimizes healing postoperatively.
- Lateral arms are attached to the retractor system to spread the soft palate open. If necessary, stay sutures can also be placed to assist in lateral exposure.
- If adequate rostral caudal exposure is not possible after these maneuvers, then consideration must be given to splitting the maxilla or mandible.

EXPOSURE OF THE ANTERIOR LONGITUDINAL AND ATLANTO-OCCIPITAL LIGAMENTS

- Identification of the midline, which is determined through palpation of the anterior tubercle of the atlas, is critical for proper orientation. Lateral deviation can lead to an incomplete, off-centered decompression or vascular injury.
- The body of the axis and base of the clivus can also be palpated through the posterior pharyngeal wall.
- The soft tissues in the midline of the posterior pharyngeal wall are injected using lidocaine with epinephrine to promote vasoconstriction. This maneuver as well as strict attention to opening in the midline will prevent bleeding.
- A sharp incision is made through the posterior pharynx and retropharyngeal musculature, exposing the anterior longitudinal ligament and the atlanto-occipital ligament (Fig. 36-5). Once again, electrocautery is minimized to prevent retraction of these tissues, which will be primarily closed later.
- For lesions requiring greater lateral exposure an "H"-shaped incision will provide a rectangular opening as compared to the ellipsoid exposure produced with a vertical linear opening (Fig. 36-6). This "H" can also be extended superiorly and inferiorly without difficulty. Drawbacks include increased soft tissue bleeding and more complicated closure.

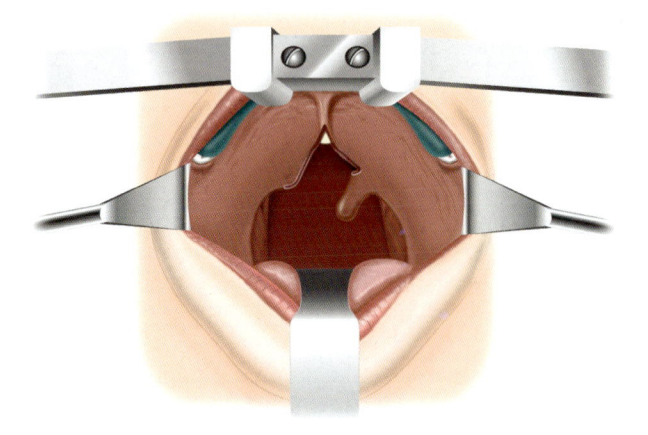

Fig. 36-4 Splitting of the soft palate in the midline with preservation of the uvula.

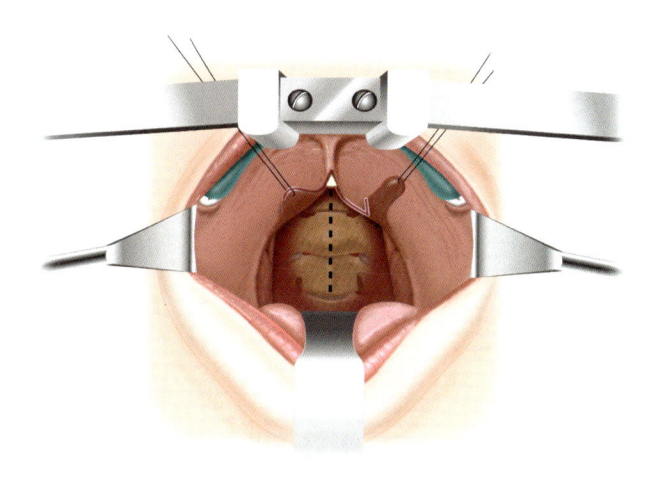

CHAPTER 36 The Transoral Approach for Ventral Cervicomedullary Decompression

Fig. 36-5 Linear incision of the posterior oropharynx.

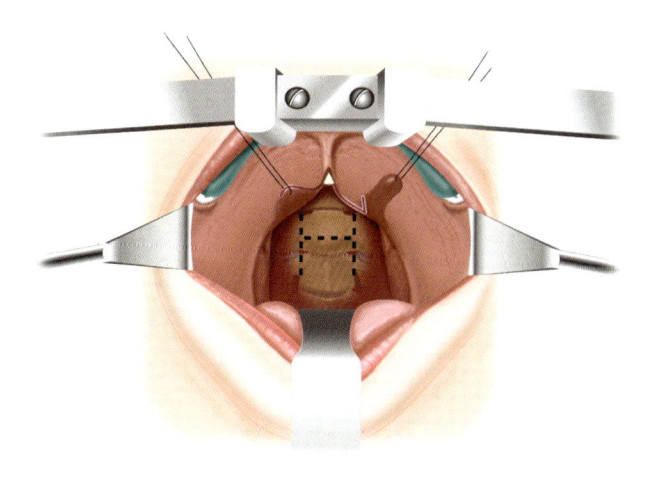

Fig. 36-6 H-shaped incision of the posterior oropharynx.

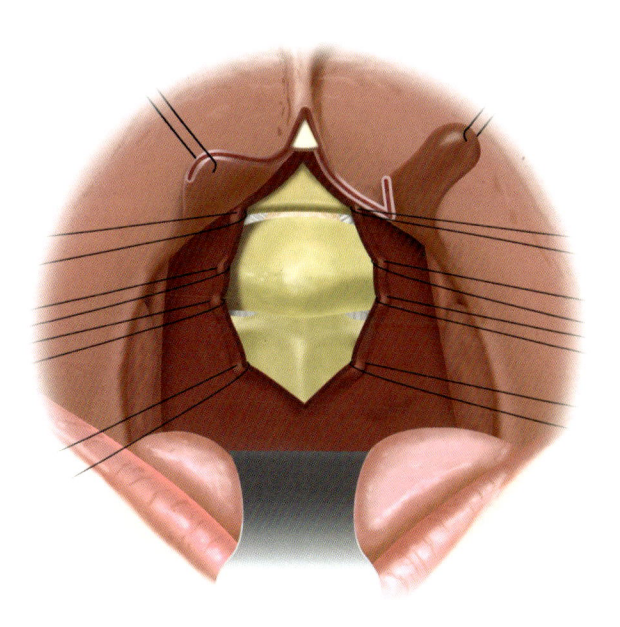

Fig. 36-7 Exposure of the anterior aspect of the atlantoaxial complex.

- The anterior aspect of the atlantoaxial joint is disarticulated. A high-speed drill with a cutting burr is used to remove the anterior arch of the atlas, exposing the odontoid peg (Fig. 36-8).
- The apical and alar ligaments attaching the odontoid to the caudal clivus are removed.
- Extreme odontoid invagination requires resection of the caudal clivus. To avoid an inadvertent dural tear and

- The retropharyngeal musculature is retracted laterally (or vertically with the "H" incision) with stay sutures or the lateral arms of the self-retaining retractor.

RESECTION OF THE ANTERIOR ARCH OF THE ATLAS, CAUDAL CLIVUS, ODONTOID, AND PANNUS

- The prevertebral fascia and longus colli muscles are dissected away with monopolar cautery exposing the anterior longitudinal ligament combining with the atlantooccipital ligament. These are opened with monopolar coagulation.
- A periosteal elevator is used to expose the body of the axis, anterior arch of the atlas, and caudal clivus (Fig. 36-7). Lateral exposure of up to 2 cm to either side of the midline is acceptable before there is a risk of entering the eustachian tube orifice, hypoglossal nerve, or vertebral artery.

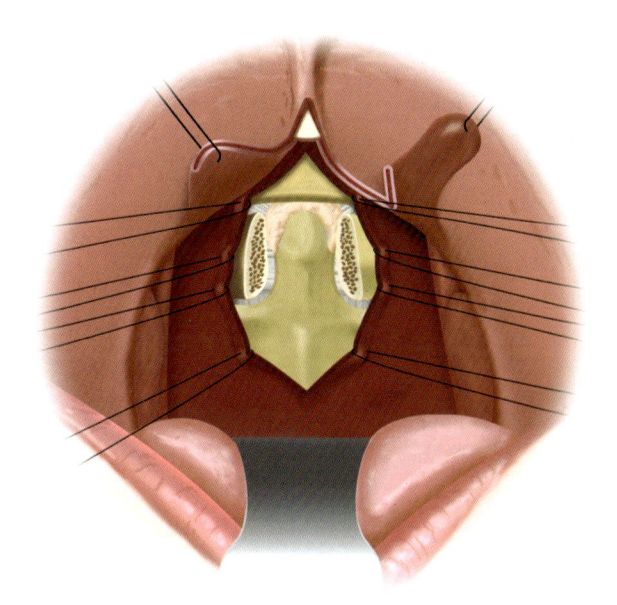

Fig. 36-8 Removal of the anterior C1 arch, revealing the odontoid in its entirety.

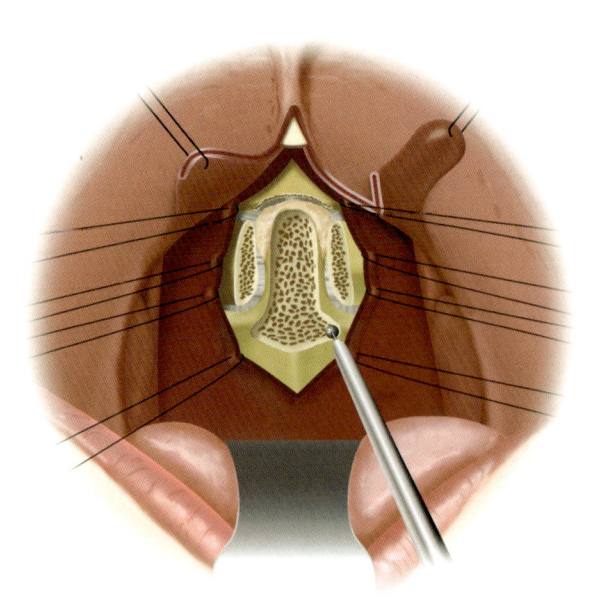

Fig. 36-9 Coring out of the odontoid with a high-speed drill.

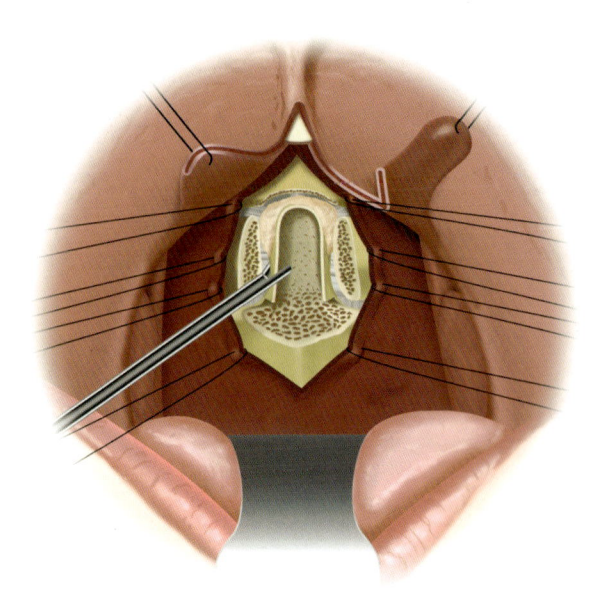

Fig. 36-10 Extraction of the shelled-out odontoid peg in a single maneuver to ensure complete removal.

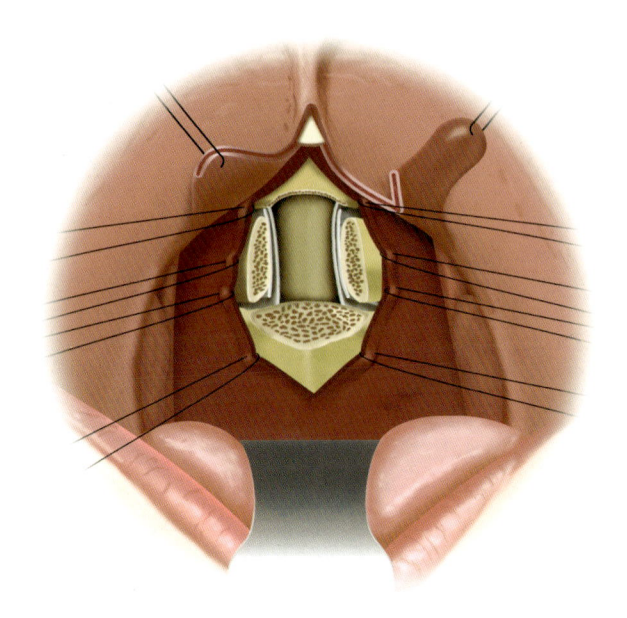

Fig. 36-11 Complete pannus, ligament, and bone removal to expose the cervicomedullary dura.

subsequent hemorrhage from the marginal sinus, the clivus must first be properly separated from posterior tissues with blunt dissection. If the clivus is foreshortened, then the soft palate is divided, the hard palate is exposed, and the posterior 10 mm is resected, enabling high nasopharyngeal exposure without splitting the mandible or median glossotomy.

- Ligamentous tissue is dissected away from the odontoid process with rongeurs, and the distal tip is identified. A cutting burr is used to remove most of the odontoid and the body of the axis in a rostral to caudal direction (Fig. 36-9). Switching to a diamond burr, the odontoid tip and posterior shell are carefully drilled away, avoiding injuring the posterior neural tissues. The anterior and posterior shell can be left attached to the C2 body to prevent migration away from the drill bit. This thin shell of bone can then be fractured away from the C2 body, removing the remaining peg in a single maneuver (Fig. 36-10). The remaining ligamentous tissues composed of the degenerated cruciate ligaments and tectorial membrane lie anterior to the dura. If the tissues are pulsatile then the dura has been adequately decompressed. A lack of pulsations suggests firm redundant ligament or residual pathologic tissue superiorly, and the remaining ligamentous tissue should be removed to expose the underlying dura (Fig. 36-11).
- Complete pannus resection is not universally necessary, particularly if supplemental posterior fixation is used, and overly aggressive removal may violate the dura and subarachnoid space.
- Any residual epidural or sinus bleeding is stopped by packing the area with cellulose wool.
- In select cases direct anterior grafting to fuse the clivus to C3 can be performed prior to closure. Careful carpentry of a bicortical iliac crest graft to accommodate the lower lip of the clivus and a notch in the C3 body must be performed. Vertical distraction of the cranium then allows wedging of this graft securely into place (Fig. 36-12).

CLOSURE

- The longus colli muscles are reapproximated in the midline and the posterior pharyngeal musculature and mucosa are

CHAPTER 36 The Transoral Approach for Ventral Cervicomedullary Decompression

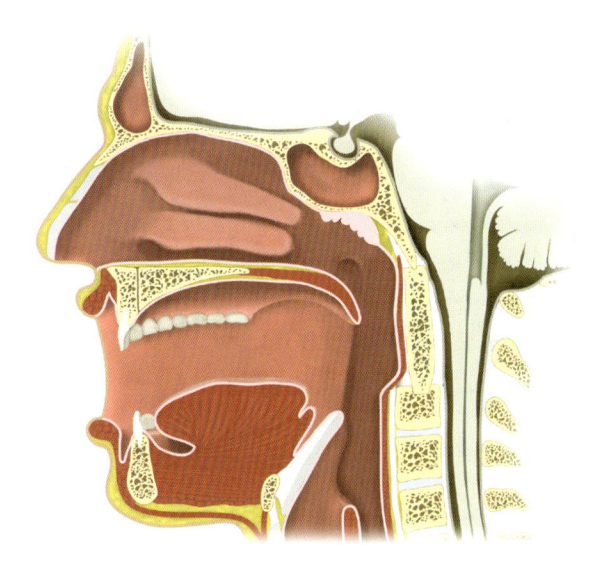

Fig. 36-12 Anterior strut grafting with iliac crest bone to span from the clivus to C3.

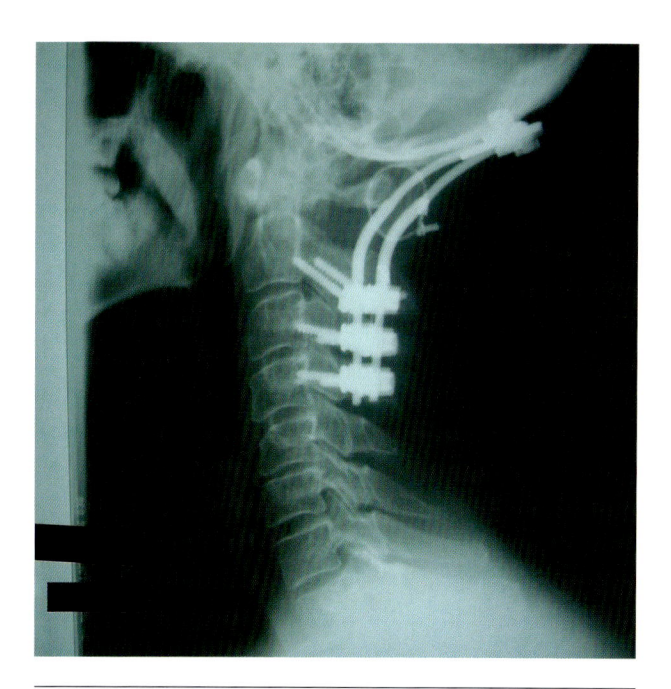

Fig. 36-13 Occiput to C4 fusion.

closed with interrupted 3-0 absorbable sutures in two layers.
- The gauze is removed from the pharynx and a nasogastric tube is placed under direct visualization and carefully secured for postoperative alimentation.
- The soft palate is carefully reapproximated with interrupted sutures.
- Hydrocortisone ointment 1% is rubbed onto the glottis to minimize swelling.

POSTERIOR RIGID FIXATION

- In cases in which spinal instability is suspected postoperatively, the patient should undergo occiput to cervical fixation. This can be performed under the same anesthesia or in a delayed fashion (Fig. 36-13).
- The choice of how many levels of the cervical spine to incorporate depends on the extent of instability, the degree of osteoporosis, and the presence of any subaxial instability.
- Contemporary techniques utilizing prebent rod-plate constructs attached to the occiput and spine with screw fixation yield the strongest biomechanical constructs.

POSTOPERATIVE CARE

- The patient is maintained in a Philadelphia collar and mobilized as soon as possible.
- In routine cases the patient can be extubated immediately. Patients with medical debility or severe respiratory disease who undergo prolonged surgery should remain on mechanical ventilation for 24 to 48 hours.
- Standard intravenous antibiotics are given for 24 hours.
- The patient should be kept NPO (nothing by mouth) for at least 7 days. Initial hydration is maintained with intravenous fluids, and once bowel sounds are present, tube feeding may commence. Examination of the soft palate and oral pharynx should be performed prior to oral feeding, which is advanced slowly from clear liquid to solids.
- A sign should be placed above the patient's bed specifying that the nasogastric tube is not to be manipulated.

COMPLICATIONS

- Small dural tears are closed primarily and then covered with fibrin glue. Large tears are covered with a patch of fascia, muscle, or commercially avaiable dural substitute. This is tacked into place with interrupted sutures, as a watertight suture line may not be possible. The patch is then reinforced with fibrin glue. A lumbar drain is used to keep pressure off the durotomy for 4 to 10 days.
- Meningitis may occur secondary to an untreated retropharyngeal abscess or cerebrospinal fluid leakage. In cases of suspected meningitis a local wound culture and lumbar puncture should be performed first. An aggressive full spectrum intravenous triple antibiotic regimen must then be started without delay until a definitive organism can be isolated. This regimen typically must be administered for at least 6 weeks. Large abscesses will also need to be surgically drained and can be identified through direct inspection or CT scans with contrast material.
- Vertebral and carotid artery injuries are uncommon but serious complications. If a large artery injury is suspected, the hemorrhage can usually be controlled with local packing and pressure. After hemostasis has been secured the patient should be taken to the angiography suite to

identify any vascular dissection or occlusions. Patients with a Klippel-Feil syndrome, RA patients with severe upward migration of the dens, and patients with complete destruction of the C1 lateral mass are especially at risk for vertebral artery injury.
- Lingual swelling can be prevented by occasionally releasing the tongue retractor, administering intravenous steroids, and local hydrocortisone appplication.
- Palatal or pharyngeal wound dehiscence may result from early feeding or suboptimal wound closure. Dehiscence within the first week should be treated with primary closure. An abscess or other infection should be considered if the dehiscence occurs at greater than 2 weeks postoperatively or later.
- Velopalatine incompetence may result from soft palate and nasopharynx contracture, requiring pharyngeal retraining for swallowing, palatal prosthesis, or pharyngeal flap.
- Chronic pharyngeal fistula requires either a vascularized muscle flap or rotation flap with the septal mucosa and posterior nasal cavity mucoperiosteum.
- In select cases a gastrostomy tube may need to be placed to protect the oropharyngeal incision. This should be done only with great care, using an endoscope, as there is some risk of perforation of the posterior pharynx. A truly percutaneous radiographically guided technique is preferred.

CONCLUSION

Ventral cervicomedullary decompression through the transoral approach can produce excellent clinical recovery. This technique provides for direct removal of the offending mass. Meticulous attention to patient preparation, surgical technique, and postoperative care will reduce the complication rate to less than 5%.

CHAPTER 37

MAURICE L. GOINS
MATTHEW D. EICHENBAUM
ALAN S. HILIBRAND

Ankylosing Spondylitis— Posterior Approaches (Osteotomy) to the Cervical and Lumbar Spine in the Management of a Fixed Sagittal Plane Deformity

OSTEOTOMY FOR CORRECTION OF KYPHOTIC DEFORMITY OF ANKYLOSING SPONDYLITIS

INDICATIONS

The involvement of the cervical spine in patients with AS is often overlooked because lumbar spine and appendicular sequelae may appear more obvious. Cervical kyphosis may slowly progress in an insidious fashion until a chin-on-chest deformity is manifested. When cervical kyphosis progresses to the point of causing difficulty with function and hygiene, a corrective cervical osteotomy is indicated. Functional diffi-

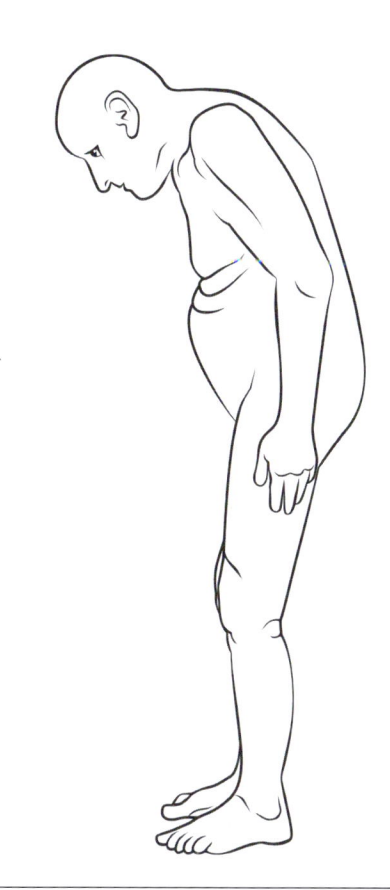

Fig. 37-1 A patient with ankylosing spondylitis.

INTRODUCTION

Ankylosing spondylitis (AS) is a chronic inflammatory disease of unknown etiology that affects approximately 197 people per 100,000 per year in the United States. An idiopathic seronegative spondyloarthropathy, AS is strongly associated with the class I antigen HLA-B27. The sacroiliac joints and the axial skeleton are most commonly affected by AS, but clinically significant peripheral joint involvement may also occur. The chronic inflammatory nature of the condition causes stiffness and loss of lordosis or increased kyphosis of the spine through destruction and autofusion of the vertebral motion segments. This can ultimately lead to a dramatic imbalance of sagittal alignment, causing severe deformities throughout the cervical, thoracic, and lumbosacral spine (Fig. 37-1).

culty may present as dysphagia or inability to lift the head to allow forward gaze. The alterations in forward gaze inhibit activities of daily living that involve forward ambulation as well as ascending and descending stairs. Also, difficulty swallowing solids may cause patients to be malnourished. In addition to the cervical spine, the thoracic spine and lumbar spine may contribute to the kyphotic deformity.

The kyphosis that develops in the ankylosed thoracic spine usually does not reach significant enough proportions to require surgical intervention. Increased kyphosis of the thoracic spine, when it occurs in ankylosing spondylitis, is often unnoticed owing to the naturally occurring kyphosis in this region of the spine. In addition, the small spinal canal and degree of naturally occurring kyphosis in this region of the spine place the spinal cord at higher risk of traction or ischemic injury with osteotomy.

Ankylosing spondylitis presents in the lumbar spine as low back pain for greater than 3 months, stiffness, diminished range of motion, and hypolordosis. Osteotomy is the procedure of choice to address severe fixed kyphotic deformities in the lumbar spine due to AS. The midportion of the lumbar spine is the safest area for correction, below the termination of the spinal cord (i.e., the conus medullaris at the L1-L2 level). Correction of kyphotic deformity of the lumbar spine via osteotomy may be safer than in the cervical spine because of the absence of the spinal cord at the preferred osteotomy level of L3. In cases of coexisting deformities of the cervical and lumbar spine, osteotomy of the lumbar spine is generally preferred for reasons of safety as well as the ability to correct forward gaze with correction of lumbar kyphosis.

CONTRAINDICATIONS

Extra-articular manifestations of AS include aortic incompetence, cardiac conduction defects, fibrotic lung disease, and renal amyloidosis. These extraskeletal expressions of AS can present a significant risk for serious perioperative complications, including cardiopulmonary compromise and renal insufficiency. In some instances, the severity of these concomitant medical conditions may pose too high a level of morbidity for the patient to withstand such a surgical procedure.

Appendicular skeletal manifestation of AS, such as hip flexion contractures and osteoarthritis, may exaggerate kyphotic spinal deformity by causing the patient to tip forward. Correction of hip pathology in AS is safe and efficacious and should be addressed prior to spinal management.

POSTERIOR CERVICAL OSTEOTOMY FOR CORRECTION OF KYPHOTIC DEFORMITY OF ANKYLOSING SPONDYLITIS

ADVANTAGES

- High degree of correction
- Single level surgery for correction
- Availability of segmental internal fixation for precise control and maintenance of osteotomy correction

DISADVANTAGES

- Neurologic injury (infrequent)
- Vascular injury
- Technically demanding
- Inability to correct concomitant lumbar deformities

PREOPERATIVE EVALUATION

Preoperative evaluation begins with a thorough history and physical evaluation. The past medical history should focus on premorbid conditions that may compromise surgical treatment and recovery. In addition to evaluating the entire spinal column, the musculoskeletal examination should also evaluate the hip joints, which are often affected by osteoarthritis in AS. As a result, the loss of the normal "chin-brow to vertical angle" either occurs due to flexion deformity throughout the spine or through fixed hip flexion contractures (Fig. 37-2). Surgical correction should be planned for the area of the major deformity after conducting a thorough medical evaluation.

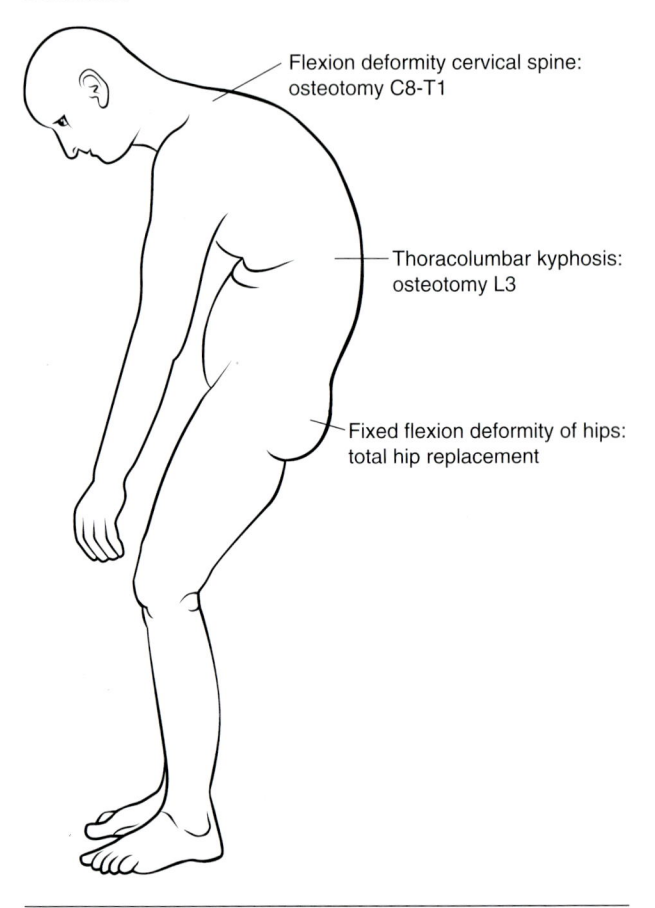

Fig. 37-2 Anatomic sites of deformity in ankylosing spondylitis and their surgical correction.

CHAPTER 37 Ankylosing Spondylitis 307

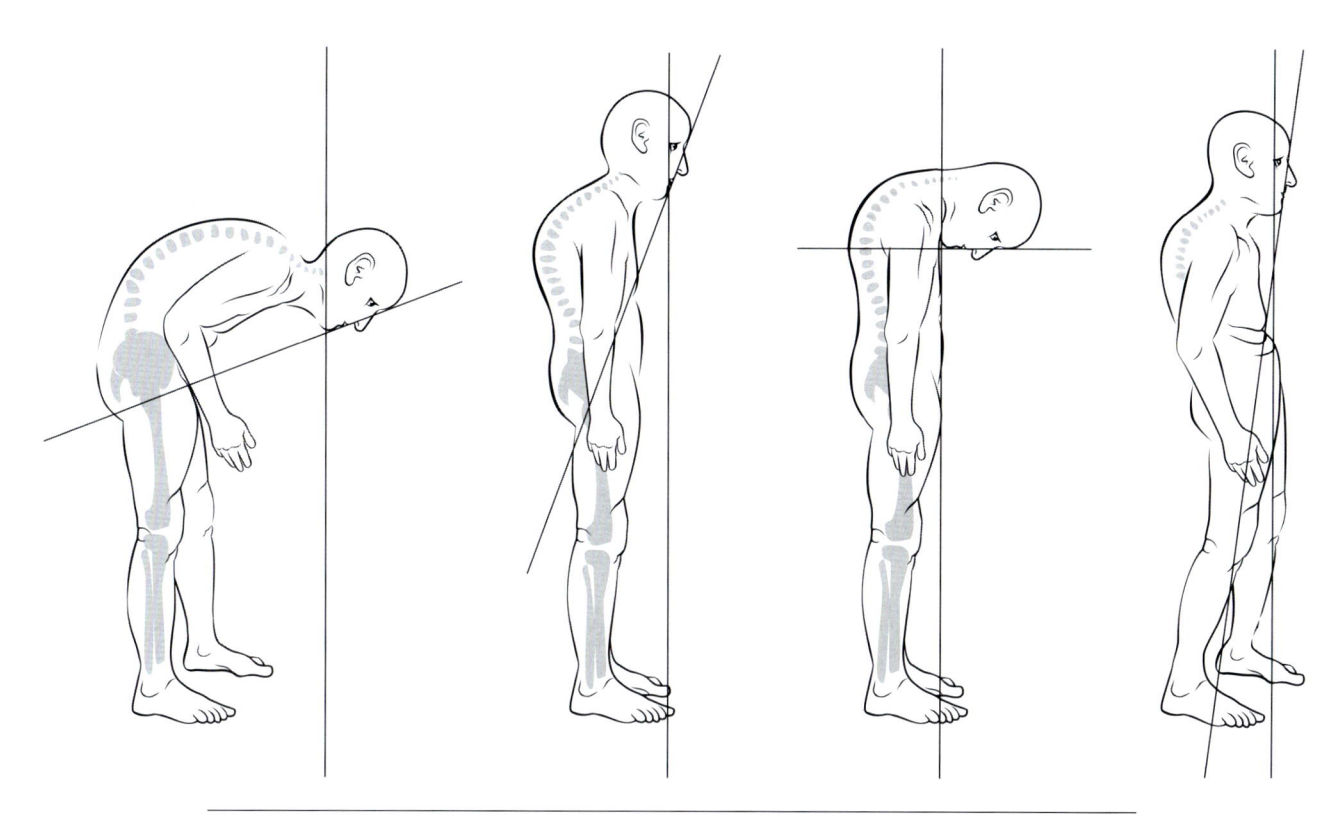

Fig. 37-3 Measurement of sagittal-vertical and chin-brow angles in preparation of ankylosing spondylitis deformity correction surgery.

Measurement of the chin-brow and sagittal vertical angles is necessary for preoperative planning of the degree of correction needed from the osteotomy (Fig. 37-3). In addition, the inion-wall angle can also be helpful in preoperative planning. It is measured by standing the patient against the wall and measuring the distance between the inion at the base of the skull and the wall. This provides an additional useful tool for monitoring the progression of cervical kyphosis.

Once the chin-brow angle has been determined, one can determine the angle necessary to bring the face to within 10 degrees of horizontal gaze. The goal is to provide a reasonably safe correction with respect to postoperative function for forward gaze and activities of daily living (grooming, eating, reading, ambulation, etc.). Correction beyond neutral (overcorrection) is not recommended, as a fixed gaze above the horizon creates significant difficulty for the patient with straightforward ambulation and stair descent.

To view the entire spine and assist with determining the level for corrective osteotomy, lateral radiographs of the entire cervical, thoracic, and lumbar spine on a 36-inch cassette are necessary. A sketch of the spinal osteotomy can be drawn on the tracing paper along with the surgical algorithm. Alternatively, the osteotomy and operative plan can be written on the radiographs with a wax pen (Fig. 37-4).

One day prior to surgery, the patient should be admitted to the hospital. This allows for the application of a halo cast with a contoured plaster jacket. After the halo cast is applied, the patient is placed in a seated position to evaluate for potential areas of undue pressure that will be placed on the patient intraoperatively. Once defined, these pressure points are trimmed and padded.

The restrictive nature of their kyphotic posture causes many patients with AS to have a protuberant abdomen that affects their breathing (Fig. 37-5). The abdominal portion of the contoured body cast must be modified to prevent abdominal compression that may inhibit respiratory function. The cast is also modified posteriorly to allow access to the cervical and upper thoracic spine. Preadmission also allows for the establishment of central venous access, which will be needed to assist with intraoperative hemodynamic monitoring by anesthesiology. Completing these procedures preoperatively maximizes patient safety and surgical efficiency upon arriving in the operating room for surgery.

INTRAOPERATIVE TECHNIQUE

1. The patient should be placed in a beach chair position after awake fiberoptic intubation and anesthesia induction have been performed.
2. It is imperative to have the appropriate neurophysiologic monitoring available throughout the entire procedure including, if available, transcranial evoked motor potentials, somatosensory evoked potentials, and C8 dermatomal evoked potentials.

308 SECTION III INFLAMMATORY DISEASE

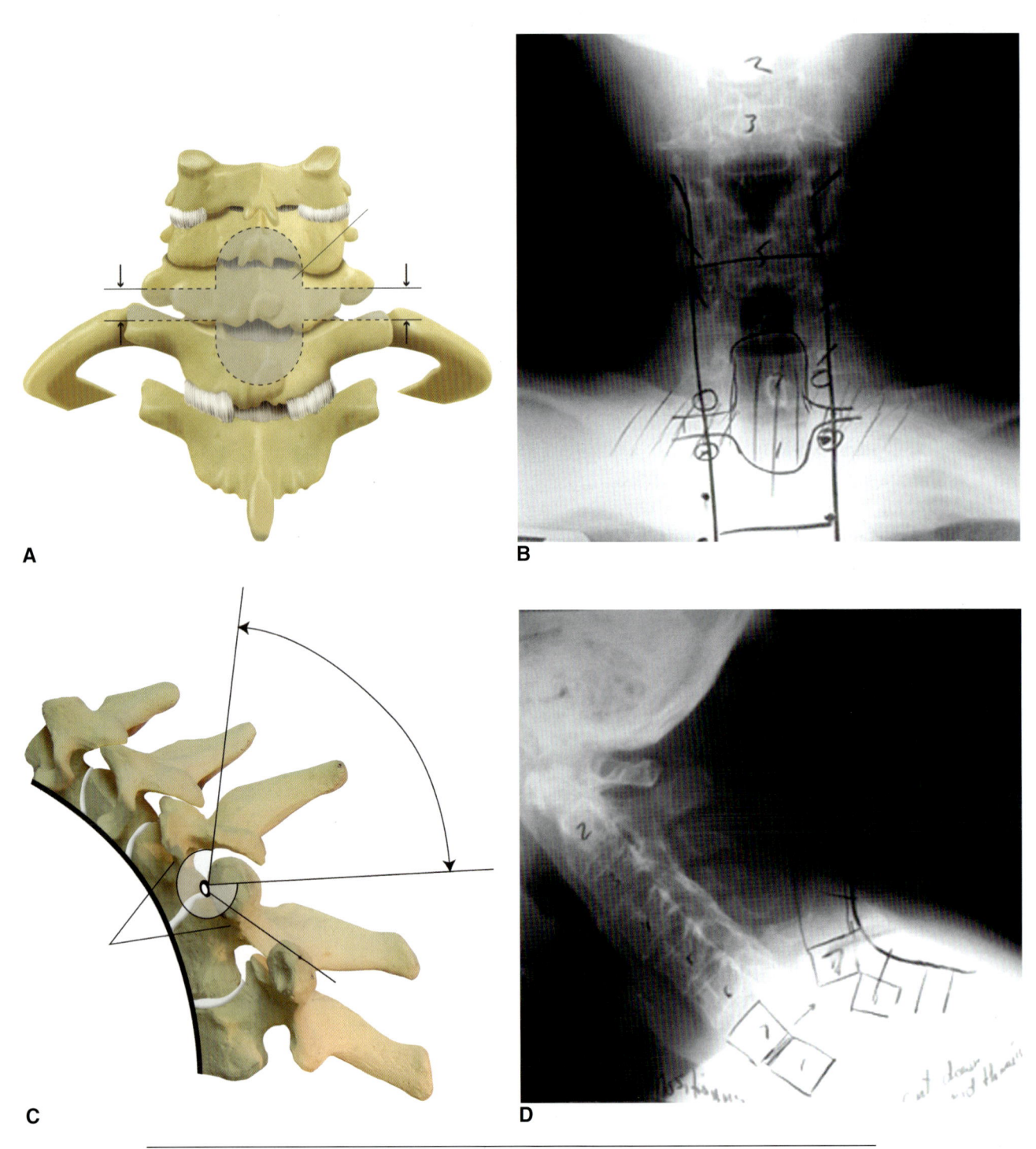

Fig. 37-4 *A,* Anteroposterior schematic of preoperative planning for posterior cervical osteotomy. *B,* Anteroposterior radiograph showing preoperative planning for posterior cervical osteotomy. *C,* Lateral schematic of preoperative planning for posterior cervical osteotomy. *D,* Lateral radiograph showing preoperative planning for posterior cervical osteotomy.

CHAPTER **37** Ankylosing Spondylitis 309

3. If neurophysiologic monitoring is unavailable, the procedure should be performed under local anesthesia.
4. The patient is positioned on the operating room table in the seated position, and the halo cast is secured to the operating room table. Cervical traction is then applied to the halo to stabilize the head and cervical spine (Fig. 37-6). The posterior support bars of the halo may be removed if they hinder the approach to the cervical spine.
5. Following the induction of general anesthesia, transesophageal echocardiographic monitoring should be established to assist with detection of a possible air embolus, which may occur secondary to the patient's upright position. Air can be removed via central venous pressure line if necessary.
6. The posterior cervical spine is approached through a standard midline incision. Gelpi retractors are used to provide exposure. Meticulous hemostasis is essential. Subperiosteal dissection should widely expose lamina, facets, and transverse processes.
7. The C7-T1 interval is identified with intraoperative radiographs. Performing the osteotomy at the cervicothoracic junction minimizes the risk of vertebral artery injury, because the transverse foramina is entered initially at the C6 level in the majority of patients (Fig. 37-7).
8. The incision should be extended long enough to allow placement of fixation in four spinal segments proximally and distally to the level of osteotomy.

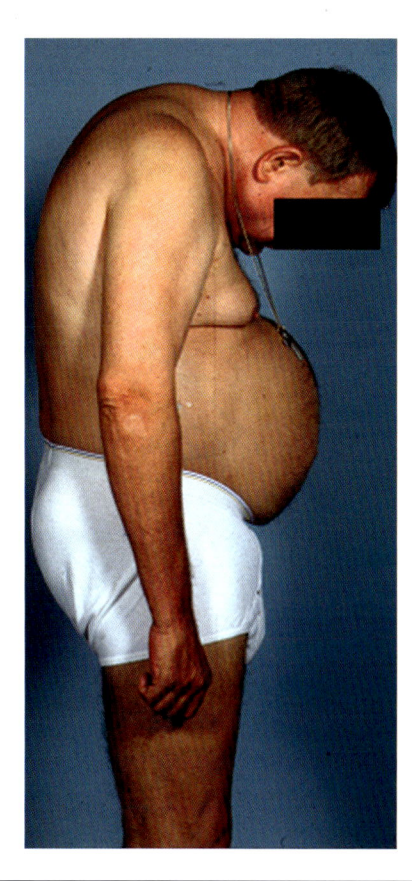

Fig. 37-5 Ankylosing spondylitis patient with protuberant abdomen secondary to pulmonary restriction.

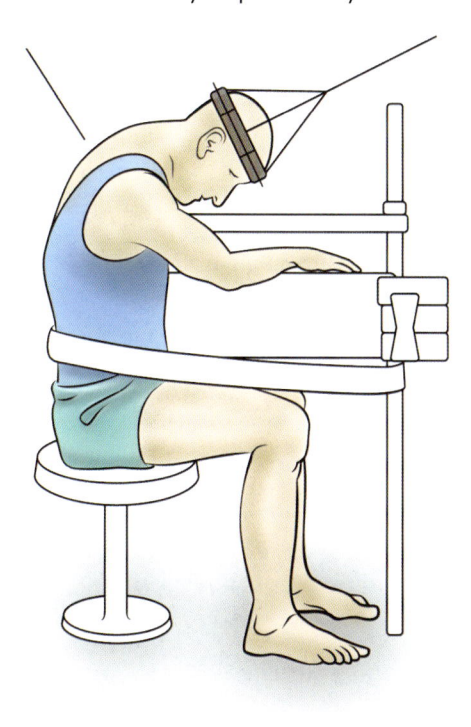

Fig. 37-6 Ankylosing spondylitis patient in upright position and cervical traction in preparation for posterior cervical osteotomy.

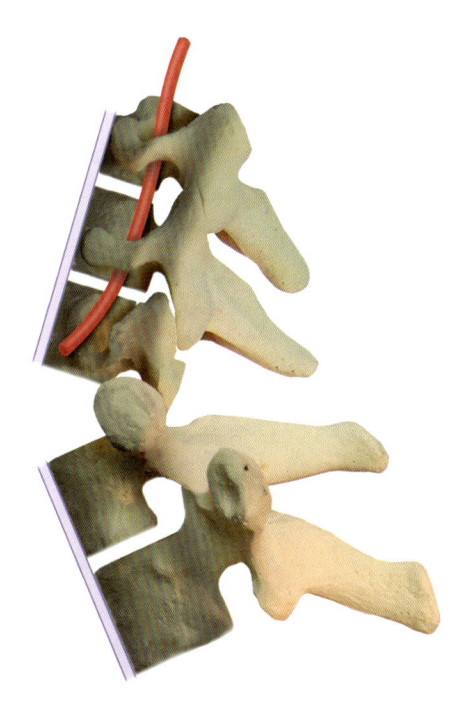

Fig. 37-7 Schematics showing the location of the prominent vasculature in the cervical spine relative to posterior cervical osteotomy site.

9. Internal fixation points should be established prior to the bony resection and osteotomy, in order to minimize the amount of time the osteotomy will be vulnerable to manipulation. Segmental instrumentation, with lateral mass screw placement at C3, C4, and C5, and pedicle screw placement distal to the osteotomy site (typically at T2-T4), is usually placed.
10. A wide laminectomy of C7 should be performed. A partial laminectomy of C6 and T1 should also be performed. This will prevent cord compression that may occur after closing the osteotomy owing to impingement by the lamina of the adjacent levels (Fig. 37-8).
11. After performing the laminectomy, remove the C7 pedicles with a combination of rongeurs and motorized burrs. This should be performed very carefully so as not to cause an iatrogenic nerve injury to C8 or C7.
12. Next, any remaining soft tissue or bone contacting the C7 and C8 nerve roots should be resected (Fig. 37-9).
13. Osteoclasis is now performed with extreme caution by gradually extending the head from its kyphotic posture. It is imperative that neurophysiologic monitoring be performed prior to, during, and after osteoclasis. Special attention must be paid to avoiding anterior or posterior translation of C7 on T1, which may lead to spinal cord compression.
14. The head should be positioned in such a way that the horizontal gaze will be directed approximately 10 degrees downward from the standing horizontal gaze when the correction is complete. This will minimize the risk of overcorrection. Having the patient upright in the seated position provides for easy assessment of the patient's horizontal gaze.
15. When approaching the desired amount of correction, the spinous processes of C6 and T1 should approximate each other, yielding adequate bony apposition of the remaining transverse processes of C7 and T1. At this time, readjust and secure the halo in position to stabilize the cervical spine.
16. Internal fixation points should now be connected via longitudinal rods.
17. After closing the osteotomy and securing it in position with instrumentation, bone graft from resection of the posterior elements may be used to supplement the arthrodesis (Fig. 37-10).
18. Closure of the wounds is often difficult. We recommend interrupted fascial closure and meticulous skin closure using interrupted vertical mattress sutures. Retention sutures may also be needed to assist with approximation of wound edges.
19. The posterior aspect of the halo vest may be replaced to provide further mechanical support.

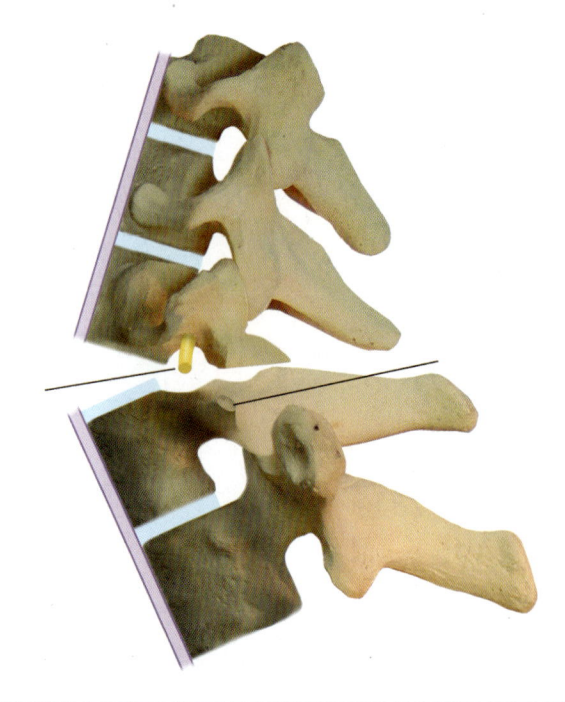

Fig. 37-9 Lateral cervical schematic following removal of tethering bone and soft tissue near C8 nerve root following osteotomy and osteoclasis.

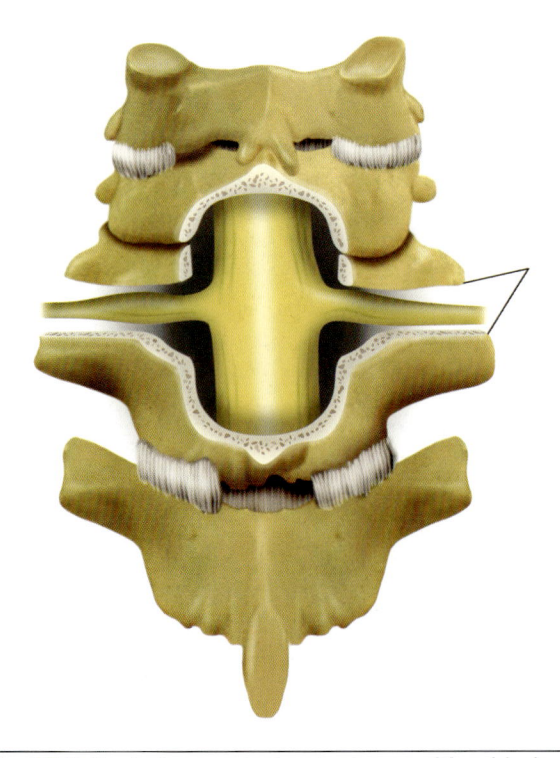

Fig. 37-8 Posterior cervical osteotomy with wide laminectomy of C7 and partial laminectomy of C6 and T1.

POSTOPERATIVE MANAGEMENT

The sudden change in cervical positioning may cause formation of a retropharyngeal hematoma, which can potentially lead to airway compromise. There are also dramatic fluid shifts that occur postoperatively as these patients go from an upright operative position to a supine postoperative

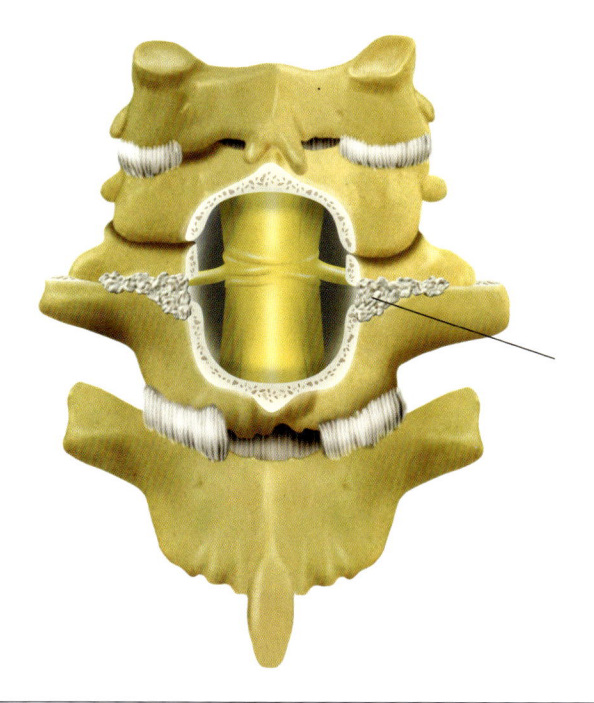

Fig. 37-10 Closed posterior osteotomy with local bone graft supplementation.

position. In addition, many of these patients have underlying pulmonary compromise due to restrictive lung disease. Large fluid shifts create an environment for patients with restrictive lung disease to develop congestive heart failure. As a result, we recommend that these patients remain intubated in an intensive care unit until the airway and cardiopulmonary function have stabilized.

Because the fulcrum of rotation for the osteotomy is along the posterior vertebral cortex, the anterior column of the spine is lengthened. Structures anterior to the spine, therefore, are very vulnerable to stretch/traction injury, including the esophagus. This often leads to postoperative dysphagia and may necessitate a period of parenteral nutrition. For prolonged dysphagia, we recommend placement of a feeding tube. In addition, we also recommend that the surgical team keep a cast saw at the patient's bedside in the event that the patient requires rapid removal of the halo vest. Postoperative immobilization in a halo vest is mandatory for 6 to 12 weeks. After this, the patient is placed in a standard Philadelphia collar for another 6 to 8 weeks. Radiographs are taken at 1-, 3-, and 6-month intervals to evaluate fusion healing and graft incorporation.

COMPLICATIONS

Significant neurovascular complications may occur following cervical osteotomies, including spinal cord compression or traction causing paraparesis or paraplegia, vascular injury to the spinal cord causing an anterior spinal cord ischemic injury, and nerve-root impingement resulting in radiculopathy. Performing the operative procedure in the seated position also brings the additional risk of air entering the low-pressure venous system, causing an air embolus. If this occurs the wound should be immediately filled with irrigant and moist sponges to prevent air from entering the low-pressure venous system.

Additional complications such as infection, loss of fixation, nonunion, malunion, dysphagia, halo-pin infection or loosening, and loss of fixation with recurrence of kyphotic deformity may potentially occur in the postoperative period.

INDICATIONS AND CONTRAINDICATIONS FOR PEDICLE SUBTRACTION OSTEOTOMY FOR KYPHOTIC DEFORMITY OF THE THORACOLUMBAR SPINE

ADVANTAGES

- Achieves posterior correction via a single osteotomy
- Avoids anterior approach
- Avoids creation of an anterior gap that occurs with Smith-Peterson technique
- Eliminates need for multiple osteotomies
- Reduces distraction/stretch on abdominal structures
- May improve forward gaze and avoid or delay need for correction of cervical kyphosis in patients with deformities of both regions

DISADVANTAGES

- Potential for excessive blood loss
- Neurologic injury

PREOPERATIVE EVALUATION

Localize the level of the deformity: cervical, thoracic, or lumbar.
1. Full-length radiographs to review spinal alignment
2. Specialized views to assess for correction
   - Traction
   - Hyperextension
3. Radiographic assessment
   - Sagittal vertical axis
   - Regional assessment of lordosis and kyphosis
   - Chin-brow angle
   - Trace deformity and plan corrective osteotomy site
   - Plan hardware insertion

LOCATION OF OSTEOTOMY

Osteotomies performed in the lumbar spine in patients with ankylosing spondylitis often provide sufficient correction such that additional osteotomies in the cervical or thoracic spine are usually not needed. Ideally, the level for a lumbar osteotomy is at or below L2. This places the osteotomy below the level of the conus medullaris and the rib cage, and above the level of the aortic bifurcation, which minimizes surgical complications.

OPERATIVE TECHNIQUE

EQUIPMENT

- Fluoroscopic/x-ray-compatible table
- Fluoroscopy
- Straight and angled curettes
- Kerrison punches
- Rongeurs
- Stille Horsley bone cutting forceps
- Impactor
- Bechman Adson retractor
- Adson cerebellar retractor
- Gelpi retractors
- Osteotomes
- Scoville nerve root retractor
- Pedicle screw fixation system
- Cell saver
- Neurophyisiologic monitoring

PATIENT POSITIONING

Once intubation, general anesthesia induction, and placement of the appropriate hemodynamic and neurophysiologic monitors are complete, the patient is carefully turned onto the operating table to the prone position. Proper surgical positioning for a patient with a severe kyphotic deformity is challenging, but not impossible. We recommend using a radiolucent table which flexes to accommodate the patient's posture. Extension of the table will assist with reduction after completion of the osteotomy (Fig. 37-11). It is critical to meticulously pad all bony prominences and assure that no undue pressure is exerted on the ocular region. In addition to evaluating these areas at regular intervals, they must also be evaluated after a change in table position from a flexed to an extended posture.

Alternatively, to accommodate the kyphotic posture, the patient's trunk could be placed on a four-poster frame, omitting the thigh supports (Fig. 37-12). This will assist with positioning by allowing the hips to flex and the knees to touch the table at the level of the kidney rest. Elevation of the kidney rest later in the procedure will assist with reduction of the patient's deformity. Pillows should also be used to maintain knee flexion. This will decrease the amount of tension placed on the sciatic nerve when the reduction maneuver is eventually performed.

Another option is to perform the procedure on a Jackson lordosing table. The head may be suspended with cranial tongs to prevent undue pressure on the face. On this table, the patient's pelvis and iliac crests may be suspended above the bed, but will be reduced down toward the hip bolsters

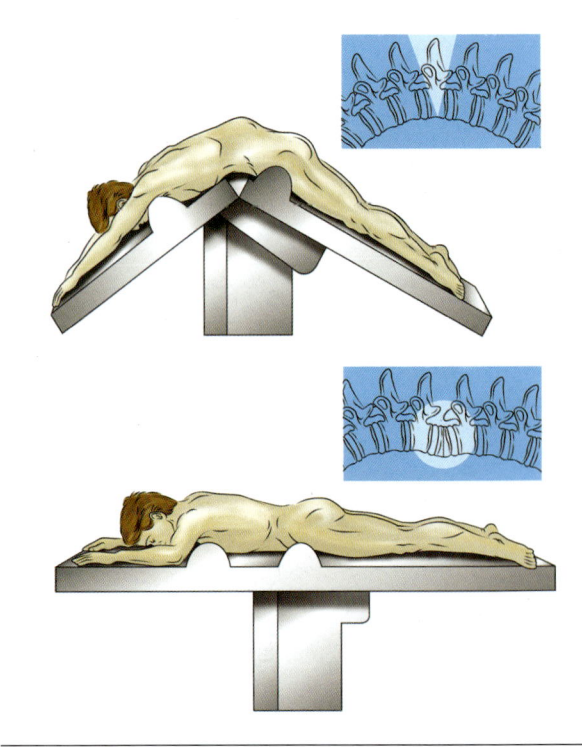

Fig. 37-11 Patient positioning for lumbar pedicle subtraction osteotomy showing table extension to close osteotomy site.

once the correction is performed. The lordotic nature of the frame will provide the reduction force to reduce the osteotomy.

LOCATION OF INCISION

The spine should be exposed through a midline posterior approach centering over the level of the osteotomy, which is

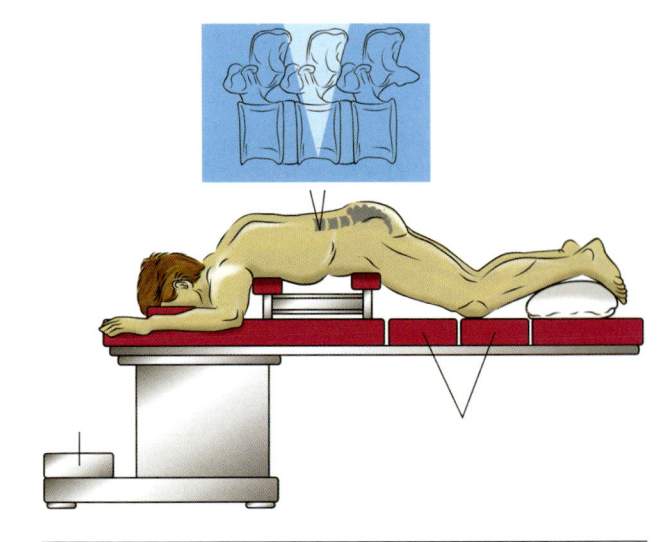

Fig. 37-12 Alternative patient positioning for lumbar pedicle subtraction osteotomy to accommodate kyphotic posture with hip flexion and kidney rest supports.

usually done at the center of the lumbar lordosis (L3-L4). The skin incision is marked in a longitudinal fashion allowing exposure from T12 to the sacrum.

INTRAOPERATIVE TECHNIQUE

After the skin incision is marked, the surgical area is cleaned and draped in the usual sterile fashion. The area is widely prepped, including the iliac crest, for possible autograft bone harvesting if local bone graft is insufficient.

1. Incision is made and soft tissue dissection is done.
2. The lumbar spine is exposed through a standard posterior midline approach.
3. The incision is taken down through the subcutaneous tissues to the fascia, which is incised over the spinous processes.
4. The paraspinal muscles are dissected off the spinous processes and lamina subperiosteally with a combination of bovie cauterization and a Cobb periosteal elevator.
5. Sponges are packed into the wound to assist with dissection of soft tissue and also to provide hemostasis.
6. Elevation of the paraspinal muscles and soft tissue should continue laterally over the facets and out to the tips of the transverse processes.
7. If needed, large Gelpi retractors replace cerebellar retractors at this point to provide a wider, deeper exposure.
8. Intraoperative radiographs or fluoroscopy are used at this point to assure that the osteotomy will be performed at the correct level.
9. Pedicle screws should be placed prior to performance of the bony resection and osteotomy. If the procedure is performed on a Jackson table, a provisional rod should be placed as laterally as possible connecting fixation points above and below the osteotomy at this time.
10. For an L3 osteotomy, a complete resection of the posterior elements of L3 along with the caudal half of the lamina of L2 and the cephalad half of the lamina of L4 will need to be performed. It is imperative that portions of L2 and L4 be resected to prevent a pincer effect in which the correction maneuver causes the laminae of L2 and L4 to compress the thecal sac.
11. A Horsley bone rongeur is used to remove the spinous processes of L2-L4 and a Leksell rongeur is used to thin the lamina.
12. A large curette may be used to resect the ligamentum flavum from the lamina, allowing entrance into the spinal canal.
13. Kerrison punches are used to perform a wide laminectomy of L3 out to the pedicles. Caution should be used when resecting the lamina in fixed kyphotic deformities because the dura may have adhered to the lamina. A Penfield elevator is useful to free adherent dura from the lamina.
14. Using a combination of Leksell rongeurs and Kerrison punches, the resection of the posterior elements should continue to include the pars interarticularis, superior and inferior facets, and the transverse processes of L3. At this point the pedicles are the only remaining posterior elements of the L3 vertebrae.
15. The inferior facets of L2 and the superior facets of L4 must also be resected.
16. Curettes are used to remove the cancellous bone from within the pedicles and to begin decancellation of the L3 vertebral body.
17. The lateral aspect of the pedicle can be removed with Kerrison punches and rongeurs to allow curettes to be advanced into the posterior portion of the vertebral body to remove the cancellous bone.
18. The posterior vertebral wall cortex is left in position while the cancellous bone is removed. Leaving the posterior vertebral wall intact provides a bony barrier protecting the thecal sac, which lies intimately along the posterior vertebral wall.
19. Once the cancellous bone has been removed from the posterior two thirds of the vertebral body, the thecal sac along with the nerve root is retracted toward the contralateral side. This will allow access to the posterior wall of the vertebrae, which is now cut using a $\frac{1}{4}$-inch osteotome.
20. Bone tamps are used to implode the posterior wall into the defect of the vertebral body created by the previously removed cancellous bone (Fig. 37-13).
21. The osteotomized posterior cortical wall is removed with pituitary rongeurs and Kerrison punches.
22. The bony resection creates a large surface area of exposed cancellous bone that may hemorrhage tremendously. Hemostatic agents such as Gelfoam and Flo-seal should be readily available to place onto bleeding surfaces.

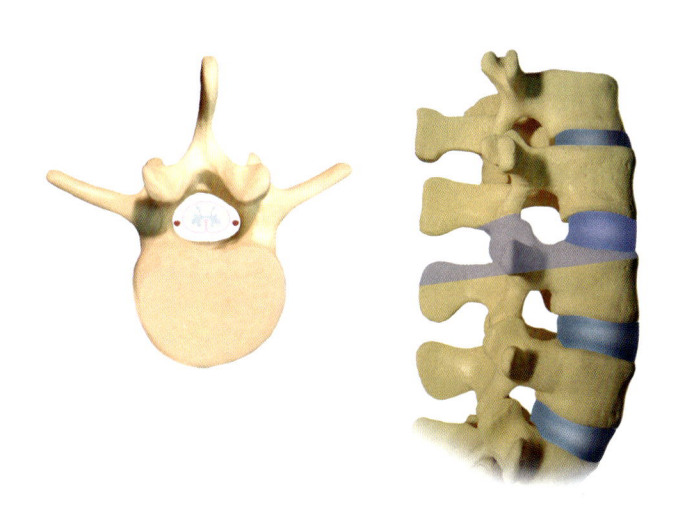

Fig. 37-13 "Eggshell" procedure for removal of lumbar vertebral body in closing wedge osteotomy.

23. Once the hemorrhage is controlled, any excess hemostatic agent should be removed because it may be extruded into the canal during reduction of the osteotomy and may cause neurologic compression.
24. The previously flexed table is now gradually brought into extension, thereby closing the osteotomy. If a Jackson table is used, the provisional rod is loosened and the connecting fixation points are allowed to approach one another in order to close down the posterior bony resection.
25. Rods are contoured and placed into the previously placed pedicle screws to secure the reduction of the osteotomy.
26. The osteotomy edges are brought in closer contact by compressing across the pedicle screws. Careful neurologic monitoring should be performed while closing the osteotomy site. If there are any changes in neurologic monitoring, the osteotomy site should be reopened.
27. The canal should be inspected carefully for sites of impingement by extruded bony fragments or hemostatic agent. After this inspection, the osteotomy site should be closed and secured into position by the previously placed fixation construct.
28. The bony surfaces should be decorticated and local bone graft placed. The wound is then closed in layers over a drain.

POSTOPERATIVE CARE

Postoperatively, the patient is placed in a custom TLSO until the osteotomy site is healed, which is approximately 3 months. Radiographs are taken at monthly intervals to evaluate fusion healing.

COMPLICATIONS

As noted earlier, the complications of thoracolumbar pedicle subtraction osteotomy are principally neurologic and vascular. Translation across the osteotomy site may cause severe compression of the cauda equina, resulting in paraparesis and bowel and bladder dysfunction. Another possible cause of postoperative paresis may be due to decreased blood flow to the thoracic spinal cord itself due to hemodynamic instability, causing an anterior spinal cord injury due to ischemia. Blood loss with this procedure can be quite high (typically over 2 L), and anesthesia personnel must be prepared for the potential need for rapid infusion of blood products and crystalloid to maintain spinal cord perfusion pressures. In addition, the blood replacement may also require concomitant replacement of clotting factors.

Although the risks of abdominal stretch and the potential for superior mesenteric artery syndrome are lower with this procedure than the traditional Smith-Peterson osteotomy, the patient's abdomen must be carefully evaluated for signs of an extended postoperative ileus. Large fluid shifts may occur in the first 3 days after surgery such that the patient's hemodynamic status must be carefully monitored. Other postoperative complications may include loss of correction and nonunion as well as wound infection.

CONCLUSION

Patients who have kyphotic deformities as a result of ankylosing spondylitis are often extremely disabled. They have difficulty with activities of daily living due to an inability to sustain a forward gaze to view the horizon. This poses a unique challenge for the patient and also for the treating spine surgeon. The fixed kyphosis of the cervical spine is further complicated by profound osteopenia. Serious complications or unsatisfactory results in the past have often made patients as well as doctors hesitant to choose surgery in the treatment of AS. Although the techniques for correction of fixed flexion deformity remain demanding, advancements in surgical techniques, instrumentation, neurophysiologic monitoring, and medical management have minimized the risk of intraoperative complications and have made surgical treatment of kyphotic deformities of the ankylotic spine a safer option. In all such patients, the goals of surgical management remain the correction of forward gaze to the horizon and improvement of gait and ambulation by restoring the C7 plumb line over the sacrum.

SECTION IV

SPINAL TRAUMA

SECTION A
Craniovertebral and Cervical Spine

CHAPTER 38

IMAN FEIZ-ERFAN
JEFFREY D. KLOPFENSTEIN
VASSILIOS I. VOUGIOUKAS
CURTIS A. DICKMAN

Surgical Therapy for Fractures and Dislocations of the Craniocervical Junction and Upper Cervical Spine

INTRODUCTION

This chapter describes operative techniques used to fixate and fuse traumatic injuries of the craniocervical junction, atlas, and axis.

TRAUMATIC CRANIOCERVICAL AND ATLANTOAXIAL INSTABILITY

Occipitocervical dislocation can be purely ligamentous, or it can involve associated fractures. This injury is highly unstable and few victims survive.[1] It is most commonly associated with high-velocity trauma and is especially prone to occur in children because of the laxity of their muscles and ligaments. Three forms of occipitocervical dislocation are described: anterior dislocation of the occiput to C1, posterior dislocation, and vertical dislocation. After undergoing initial resuscitation, patients should be immobilized using sand bags placed around the neck and head. A halo vest is required for immediate immobilization. Collars are not recommended because they increase the distraction deformity associated with the injury. Because these injuries are highly unstable, the goal is to treat these patients immediately with internal fixation. If not already present, devastating neurologic deficits can occur.

Atlantoaxial instability is present once the transverse ligament is disrupted, the odontoid process is fractured, or both. Unless the transverse ligament is avulsed with its bony base, there is little chance of healing with external immobilization alone.[2] Therefore, internal fixation is often necessary to treat atlantoaxial instability. Depending on the type of odontoid fracture, surgical fixation may be indicated to achieve fusion.[3,4] Atlantoaxial instability can also result from vertical distraction that damages the atlantoaxial joint and capsule. If the injury is severe, internal fixation and fusion may be necessary.[5]

OPERATIVE TECHNIQUE FOR OCCIPITOCERVICAL FIXATION

The patient is log-rolled into a prone position. Somatosensory evoked potentials (SSEPs) can be monitored to achieve safe positioning. The halo ring is attached to the Jackson table. After the suboccipital portion of the head is shaved, the craniocervical junction area and skin over the iliac crest on either side are prepared and draped in a sterile fashion.

Next, an incision is made from the external occipital protuberance to C4-C5. The lower extent of the incision depends on the patient's local anatomy and the desired level of fusion or fixation. After positioning and before the surgery begins, a fluoroscopic image should be obtained to verify that cervical alignment is maintained. The intent is to place the patient in a neutral head position, if possible.

After the skin has been incised, dissection proceeds to the spinous process of C2-C3, or further if necessary. Subperiosteal dissection is performed using monopolar cauterization. Because this segment is very unstable, periosteal elevators should be applied with care. Too much pressure exerted on the posterior bony elements can cause motion at the subluxed level.

After the spinous process, lamina, and posterior arch of C1 are exposed, gentle dissection continues laterally over the facet joints of C2-C3 and C3-C4 and, if necessary, other levels. Injury to the vertebral artery, especially at the C1-C2 complex and overlying the arterial sulcus of C1, should be avoided. At this point, gentle subperiosteal dissection and bipolar cauterization is preferred over monopolar cauterization. If brisk venous bleeding is encountered, it is usually a warning sign that the vertebral artery is near. After the bony structures are exposed, several methods of fixation are possible.

THREADED STEINMANN PIN FIXATION

A threaded titanium Steinmann pin can be bent and shaped for craniocervical fixation. The BendMeister (Sofamor Danek, Memphis, TN) is used to create a "U" bend in the Steinmann pin. A second bend is then made to fit the construct as flush as possible over the craniovertebral junction.

The ligamentum flavum of C1 and C2, and, if necessary, C3, are detached from the laminae using curettes. Each lamina is undercut with Kerrison rongeurs on each side to facilitate passing the sublaminar wires or cables. With the blunt end of a curved needle, vicryl suture (2-0 or 0-0) is passed under the lamina of C1 and C2, and, if necessary, C3. A small suboccipital craniectomy can be performed with drills and Kerrison rongeurs (Fig. 38-1A). Using the burr, three to four holes are drilled in the suboccipital bone for wires. A suture is passed through the holes. Braided cables or wires are attached to the sutures, and the stitch is pulled with countertraction on the cables or wires (see Fig. 38-1B) so that the cables or wires are passed beneath the lamina and suboccipital bone. The wires and cables must be passed near the midline of the occiput where the bone is thickest to decrease the risk of the wire-cable cutting through the bone.

The wires or cables are passed on each side of C1-C2, all other levels that need to be fused, and the occiput. The prebent Steinmann pin is laid over the cranio-occipital junction and is then trimmed to the appropriate length. After the pin has been inserted, the wires or cables are secured with crimps. The cable tension is adjusted between 20 to 40 Nm, depending on the patient's age and bone quality. For children, we prefer to palpate the torque on the cables manually. Finally, the cables are crimped.

A cable cutter is used to cut the end of the cable flush with the crimp. A burr is used to decorticate the cortical layer of remaining suboccipital bone, lamina, C1, C2, and, if necessary, further. At this point, either structural autograft harvested from the iliac crest or ribs (or calvarium in younger children) can be sutured or wired on the sides of the decorticated lamina and suboccipital bone using drill holes placed through spinous processes and into the autograft. Additional onlay autograft can be placed over the decorticated areas (see Fig. 38-1C). We prefer for the autograft to be compressed snug against all fusion surfaces.

Other instrumentation, which is similar to the Steinmann pin technique, is available: the Hartshill rectangle (see Fig. 38-1D), Ransford loop (see Fig. 38-1E), titanium frame (see Fig. 38-1F), and Cotrel-Dubousset rod-screw plate (see Fig. 38-1G). The techniques are similar to insertion of a Steinmann pin, but the contour of the rods differ slightly. We prefer threaded titanium rods because they offer more stability for the construct. If the posterior elements are fractured, sublaminar wire-cable techniques cannot be used. Alternative methods using plate and screws or rod and screws must be used.

C1-C2 LATERAL MASS–PARS INTER-ARTICULARIS SCREW FIXATION

If screw fixation of the craniocervical junction is desired, screws can be placed in the lateral mass of C1 and in the pars inter-articularis of C2. If necessary, screws can be placed into the lateral masses on the subaxial spine. Placing screws into the lateral masses of the subaxial spine is reviewed elsewhere in this book. This section reviews placement of screws into the C1 lateral mass and pars inter-articularis of C2.

After the C1 posterior arch is exposed completely, an air drill is used to drill the pilot hole for the screw within the underside of the lamina of C1 where it joins the C1 lateral mass (Fig. 38-2A). A drill is used to drill a pilot hole into the C1 lateral mass under fluoroscopic guidance. The lateral mass screw has a slight medial and superior angulation (less than 10 degrees, see Fig. 38-2B and C). Care is taken to avoid injuring the vertebral artery. The No. 4 Penfield dissector is inserted along the medial aspect of the C1 lateral mass to delineate its medial border.

Under direct lateral fluoroscopic visualization of the medial border, the sagittal angle is identified. Unicortical purchase is desired. Bicortical purchase, which can injure structures anterior to the spine, should not be attempted.

The length of the screw is measured. The diameter of the screw depends on the local anatomy. Again, the medial border of the occiput of the C1 junction is palpated with a No. 4 Penfield dissector to ensure that the cortex is not violated.

Next, the venous plexus around the medial and superior side of the C2 pars interarticularis is cauterized with the bipolar device, cut with microscissors, and compressed with Nu-Knit (Johnson & Johnson, Arlington, TX) or Gelfoam (Upjohn, Kalamazoo, MI) and cottonoids. A pilot hole is drilled in the inferior side of the lateral mass of C2 at the midportion of the C2-C3 facet joint.

The pilot hole is drilled into the C2 pars interarticularis, which has been exposed to the junction of the C1-C2 articulation. To visualize the trajectory of the screw, the C2 nerve root is retracted rostrally with a No. 4 Penfield dissector. A 10- to 15-degree medial angulation is used for the pars inter-articularis screw (Fig. 38-3A). The sagittal trajectory misses the C1-C2 joint (see Fig. 38-3B). Lateral fluoroscopy is also used to guide the drilling. Usually, the C2 pars interarticularis screw is short, measuring less than 12 mm.

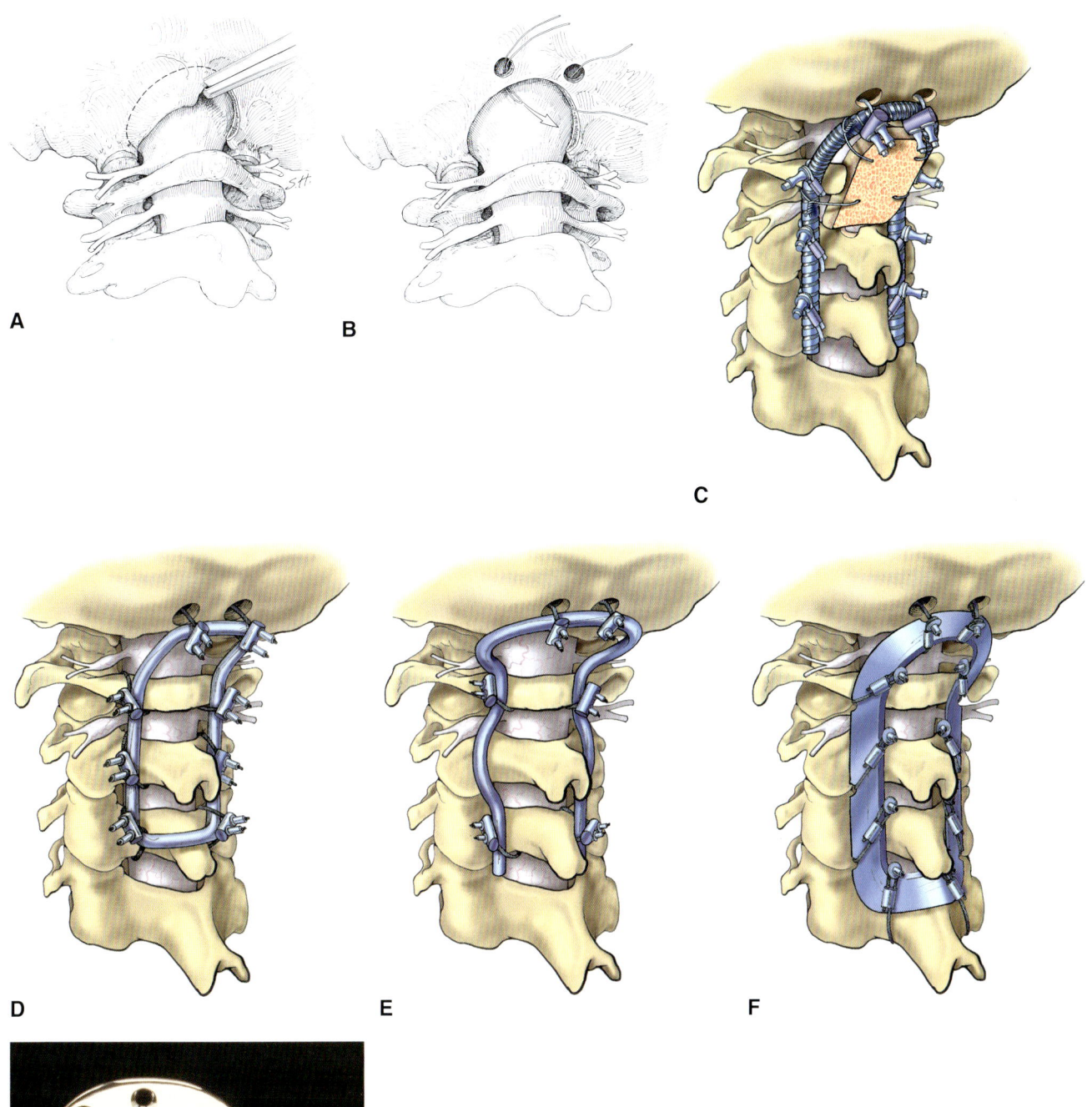

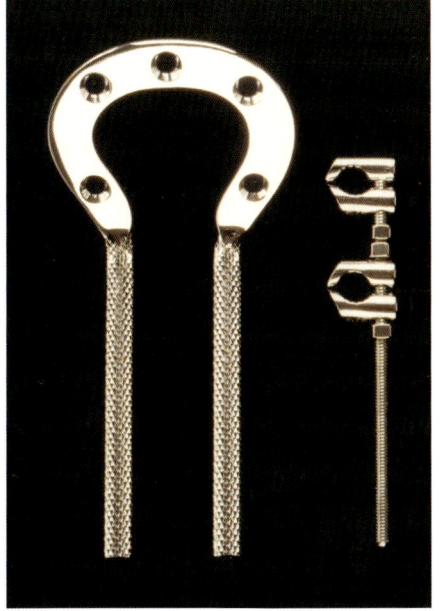

Fig. 38-1 *A,* The foramen magnum can be enlarged by removing its posterior rim with a rongeur. *B,* After a series of holes is drilled in the suboccipital bone, wires or cables are passed epidurally from the drill hole to the foramen magnum. *C,* A contoured and bent threaded Steinmann pin is placed and wired to the craniocervical junction. A piece of autograft is wedged and wired between the occiput and axis to promote fusion. Other examples of wired occipitocervical fixation devices include the Hartshill rectangle (*D*), the Ransford loop (*E*), the titanium frame (*F*), and the Cotrel-Dubousset rod-screw plate system with cross-link (*G*). (*A–F* used with permission from Barrow Neurological Institute. *G* from Dickman CA: Occipitocervical screw plates. In Dickman CA, Spetzler RF, Sonntag VKH (eds): Surgery of the Craniovertebral Junction. New York, Thieme, 1998, p 764.)

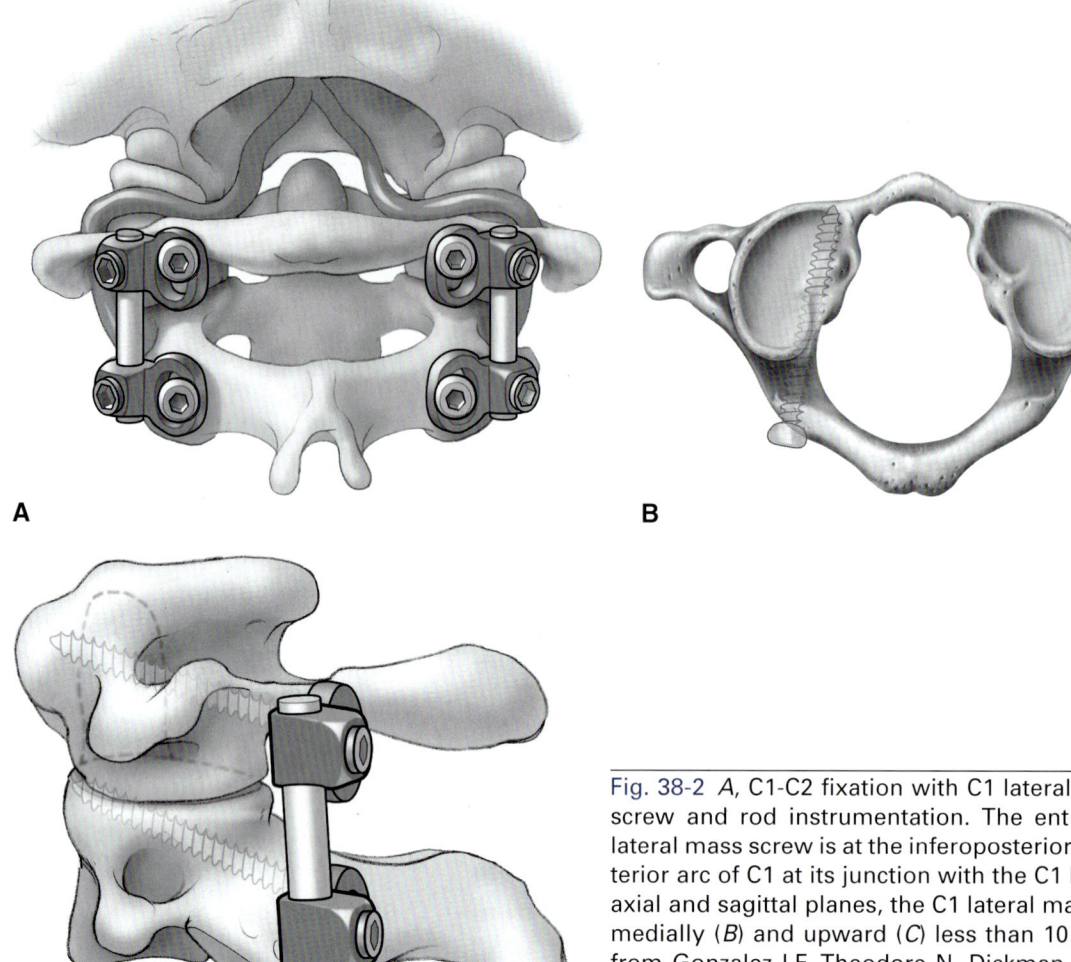

Fig. 38-2 *A*, C1-C2 fixation with C1 lateral mass and C2 pars screw and rod instrumentation. The entry point of the C1 lateral mass screw is at the inferoposterior surface of the posterior arc of C1 at its junction with the C1 lateral mass. In the axial and sagittal planes, the C1 lateral mass screw is angled medially (*B*) and upward (*C*) less than 10 degrees. (*A* and *C* from Gonzalez LF, Theodore N, Dickman CA, Sonntag VKH: Occipitoatlantal and atlantoaxial dislocation. Operative Techniques Neurosurg 2004;7(1):16–21. *B* Used with permission from Barrow Neurological Institute.)

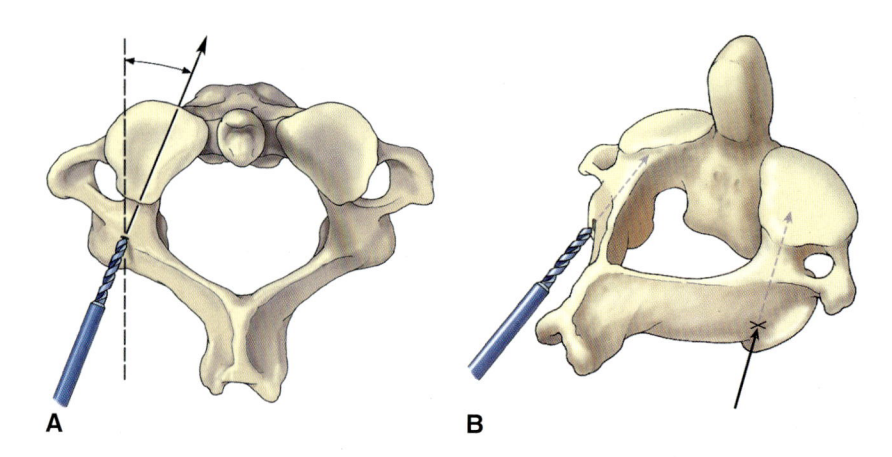

Fig. 38-3 *A*, The C2 pars screw is angled medially 10 to 15 degrees. *B*, The sagittal trajectory of the C2 pars screw is angled slightly upward to follow the trajectory of the dissected pars interarticularis of the axis. The sagittal trajectory misses the C1-C2 joint. (Used with permission from Barrow Neurological Institute.)

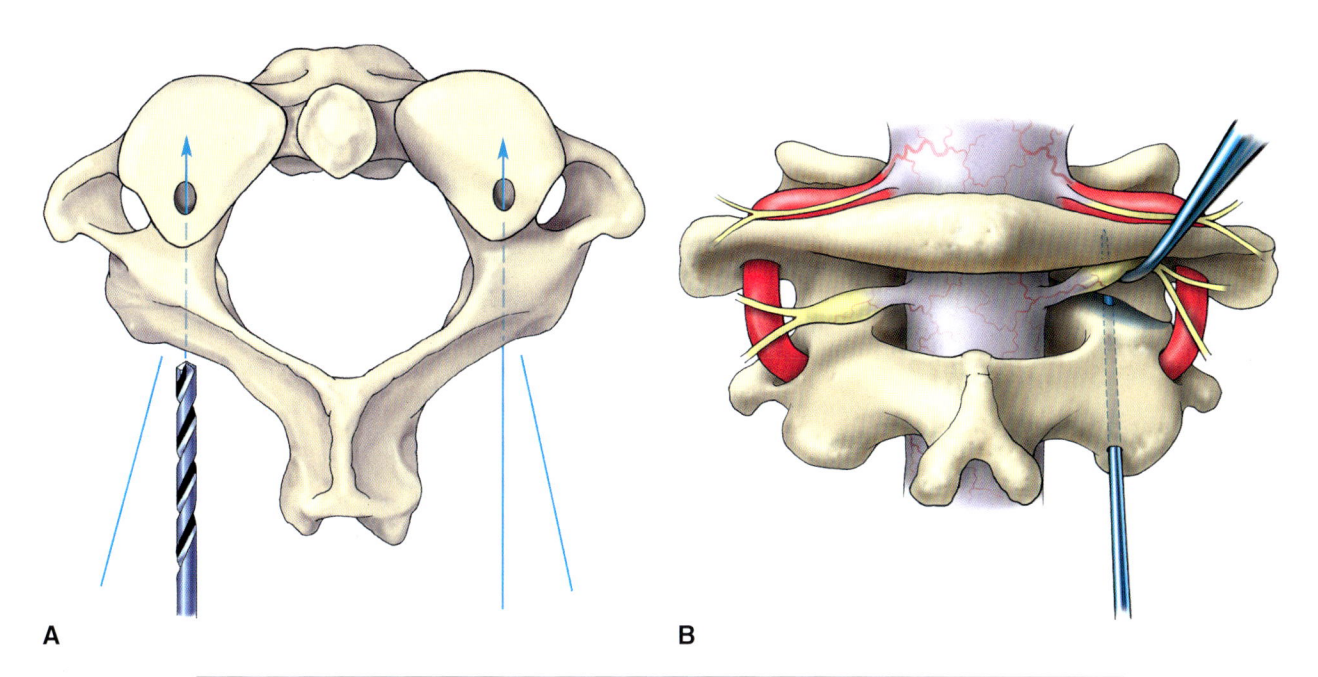

CHAPTER 38 Surgical Therapy for Fractures and Dislocations

Fig. 38-4 *A*, The entry point for a C1-C2 transarticular screw (as pointed out by the drill) is slightly medial to the entry point for a C2 pars screw (as depicted by the line lateral to the drill). *B*, There is almost no medial or lateral angulation of the C1-C2 transarticular screw in the coronal plane. The screw is aimed across the C1-C2 joint. (*A* from Marcotte P, Dickman CA, Sonntag VK, et al: Posterior atlantoaxial facet screw fixation. J Neurosurg 1993;79(2):234–237. *B* Used with permission from Barrow Neurological Institute.)

ATLANTOAXIAL TRANSARTICULAR FIXATION

After the path is tapped, the screw is inserted. If a C1-C2 transarticular screw is required, the screw is angled toward the anterior tubercle of C1 using a slightly more medial pilot hole as used for the C2 pars interarticularis screw (Fig. 38-4*A*). However, there is almost no medial angulation of the screw, and the trajectory is straight up into the C1 lateral mass (see Fig. 38-4*B*). The pars interarticularis of C1 and the C1-C2 articulation are dissected as described for placement of a C2 pars interarticularis screw. The length, which is usually about 40 mm, is again measured using the K-wire method. If a lag effect is desired, an end-threaded screw can be used instead of a fully threaded screw.

OCCIPITOCERVICAL FIXATION WITH SCREWS, RODS, AND PLATES

If occipitocervical fusion is desired, different systems using rod-plate and occipitocervical screw constructs are available. The rod is inserted over the C1-C2 screws. If necessary, it can be extended caudally to the subaxial spine. Using bending tools, the plate is contoured to the suboccipital bone and bent to achieve a curve that allows the occiput to be fixated with suboccipital or keel screws. The plate is continued into or connected to the rod, which is attached to the upper cervical spine with screws (Fig. 38-5*A* and *B*).

Different systems are available for incorporating a C1-C2 transarticular screw or a C1 lateral mass and C2 pars interarticularis screw into the construct. If necessary, a C1 lateral mass screw can be omitted and fixation can be achieved at C2 and further into the subaxial spine. To insert the suboccipital screws, a drill is used. The suboccipital bone is drilled down to the dura. Care should be taken not to violate the dura to prevent leakage of cerebrospinal fluid. A tap is inserted and tapped. The screws can usually be measured with a measuring device to determine the thickness of the suboccipital bone.

A malleable endotracheal stylet can be used to prebend the plate-rod construct to align the hardware to the desired contour. The model is used to bend the actual rod-plate construct. If the occipitocervical plate (Fig. 38-6) is chosen instead of a plate-rod construct, the screws are placed in a similar fashion. A plate can be bent in a similar fashion to achieve rigid fixation. Again, fusion is performed with sutured or onlay autograft.

322 SECTION IV SPINAL TRAUMA

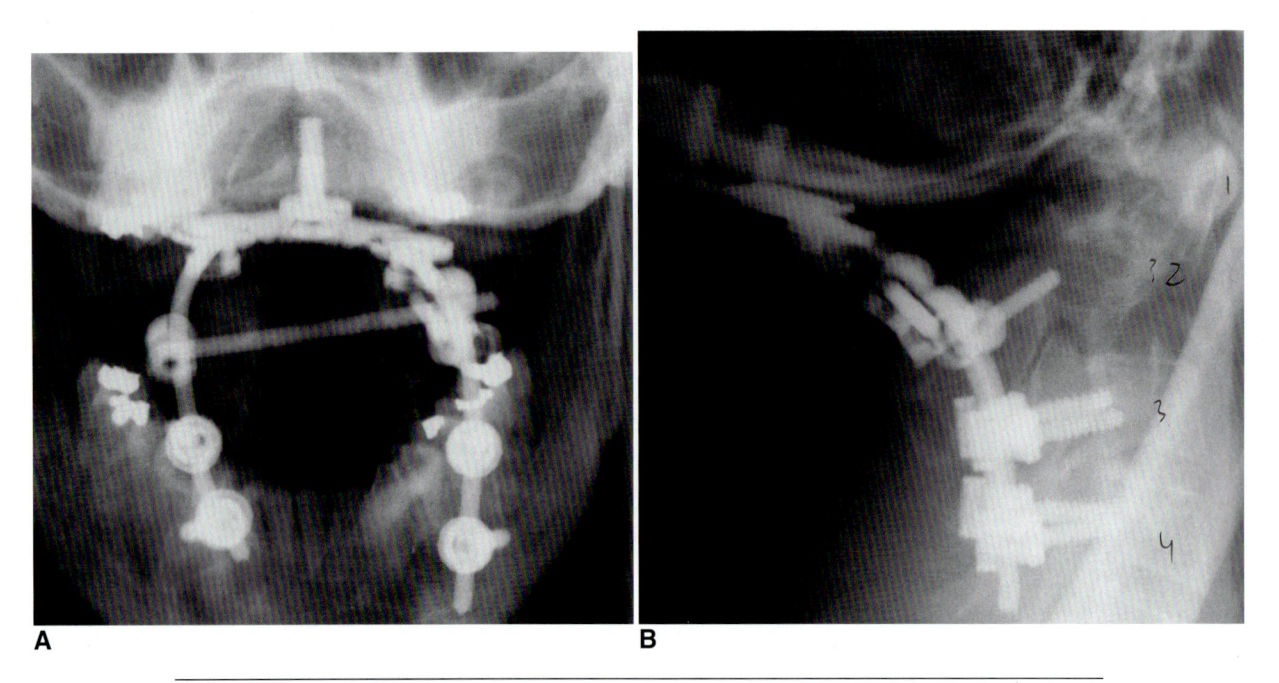

Fig. 38-5 Frontal (*A*) and lateral (*B*) radiographic views of occipitocervical fixation with an occipital plate connected to cervical rods. Rods are fixated to the cervical spine via C2 pars interarticularis screws and subaxial lateral mass screws.

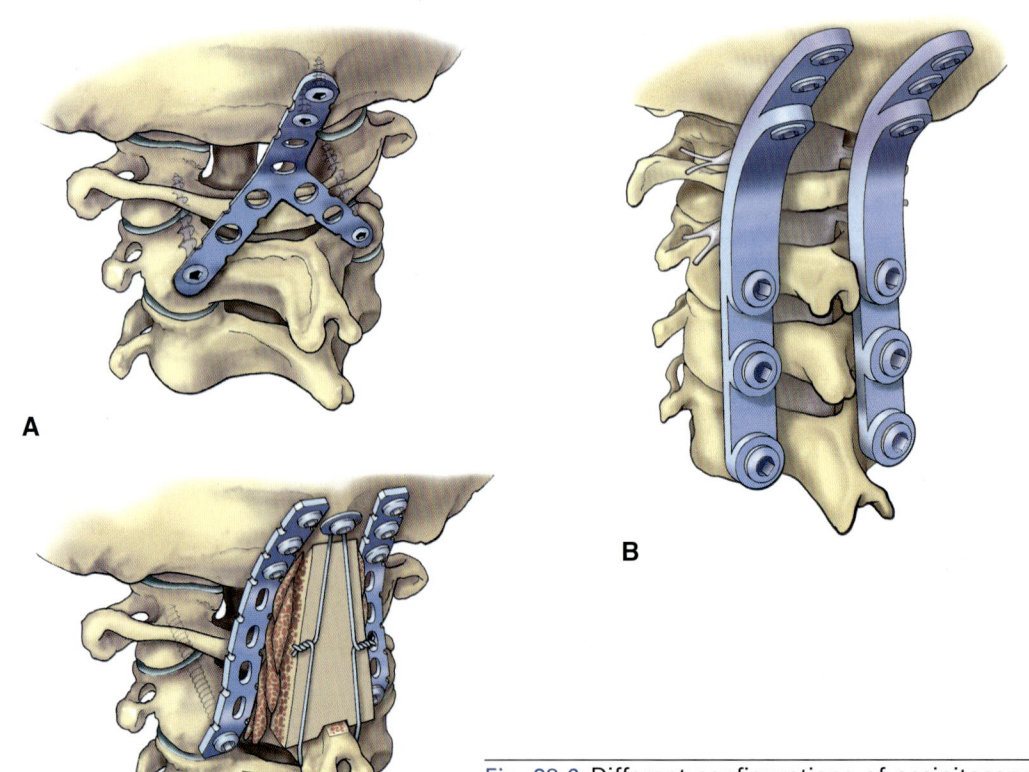

Fig. 38-6 Different configurations of occipitocervical plate-screw fixation systems. *A*, The Grob "Y" plate; *B*, Roy-Camille plate; and *C*, Magerl technique. (Used with permission from Barrow Neurological Institute.)

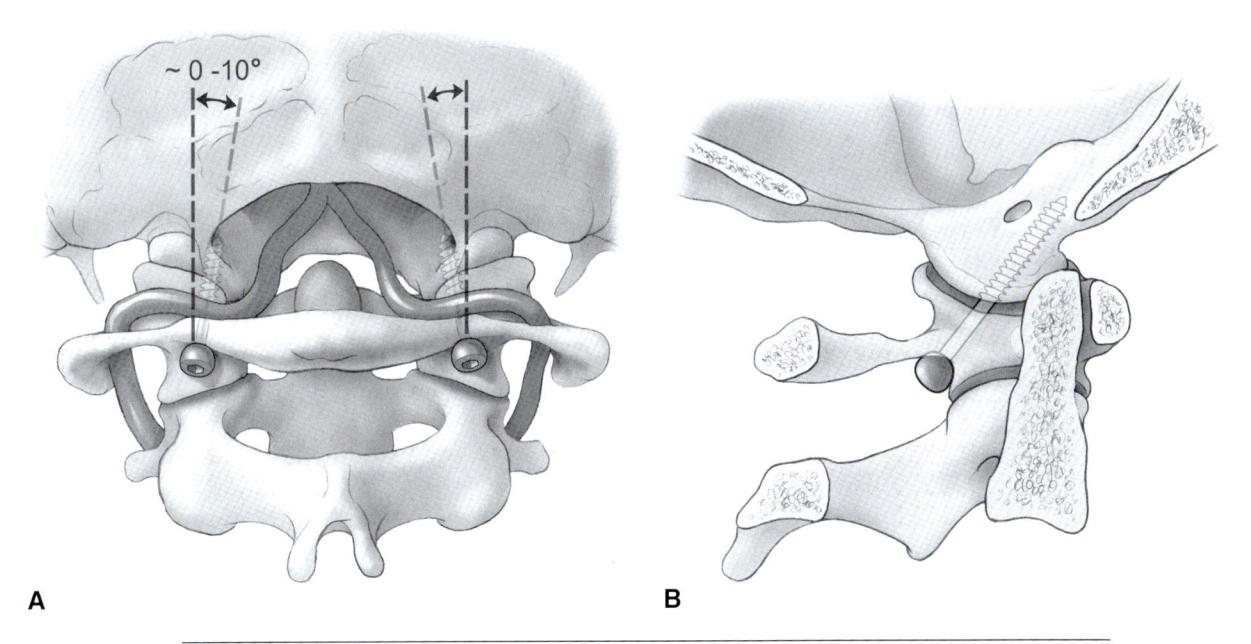

Fig. 38-7 *A*, The entry point for the atlantocondylar transarticular screw is under the C1 lamina at its junction with the C1 lateral mass. Less than 10 degrees medial angulation is required in the coronal plane. *B*, The sagittal trajectory of the atlantocondylar transarticular screw is aimed toward the tip of the clivus to miss the hypoglossal foramen. (From Gonzalez LF, Theodore N, Dickman CA, Sonntag VKH: Occipitoatlantal and atlantoaxial dislocation. Operative Techniques Neurosurg 2004;7(1):16–21.)

ATLANTO-OCCIPITAL FIXATION

Several options are available using a plate and short rod system with a suboccipital plate and a C1 lateral mass screw. This procedure is performed in a similar fashion to that for occipitocervical fusion with plates, rods, and screws. However, a novel technique is available to place transarticular atlantocondylar screws.[6,7] The entry point for this screw is under the C1 lamina at its junction with the C1 lateral mass where a pilot hole is drilled (Fig. 38-7*A*).

A drill guide is inserted using long K-wires and lateral fluoroscopy. The K-wires are drilled into the C1 condyle complex under lateral fluoroscopic guidance aimed toward the tip of the clivus (see Fig. 38-7*B*). There is less than 10 degrees of medial angulation, and the trajectory of the screws is almost straight up (see Fig. 38-7*A*). Veins are dissected from the medial aspect of the condylar-atlantal junction, which is probed with No. 4 Penfield dissectors to avoid medial breakout. The screw is measured as in the K-wire method. The path is tapped. An end-threaded screw can be inserted to achieve a lag effect. Care needs to be exerted to avoid damage to the hypoglossal nerve.

If C1 and C2 need to be incorporated into an occipitocervical fusion, a C1-C2 transarticular screw alone can be placed to achieve pure fixation of the occipitocervical junction. Rods or plates are unnecessary (Fig. 38-8).

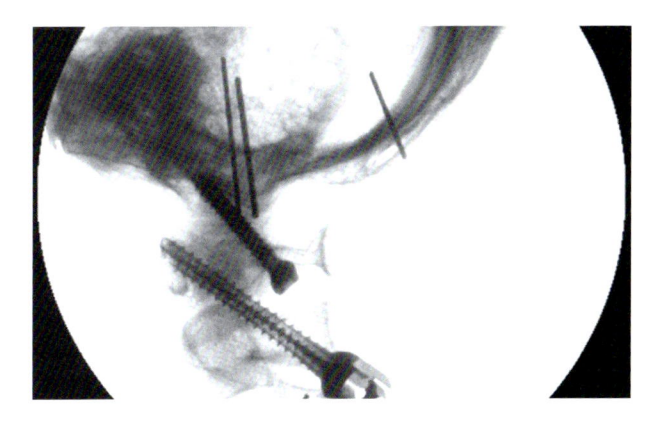

Fig. 38-8 Occipitocervical fixation using only occipitoatlantal and atlantoaxial transarticular screws. (From Gonzalez LF, Crawford NR, Chamberlain RH, et al: Craniovertebral junction fixation with transarticular screws: Biomechanical analysis of a novel technique. J Neurosurg (Spine 2) 2003;98:204.)

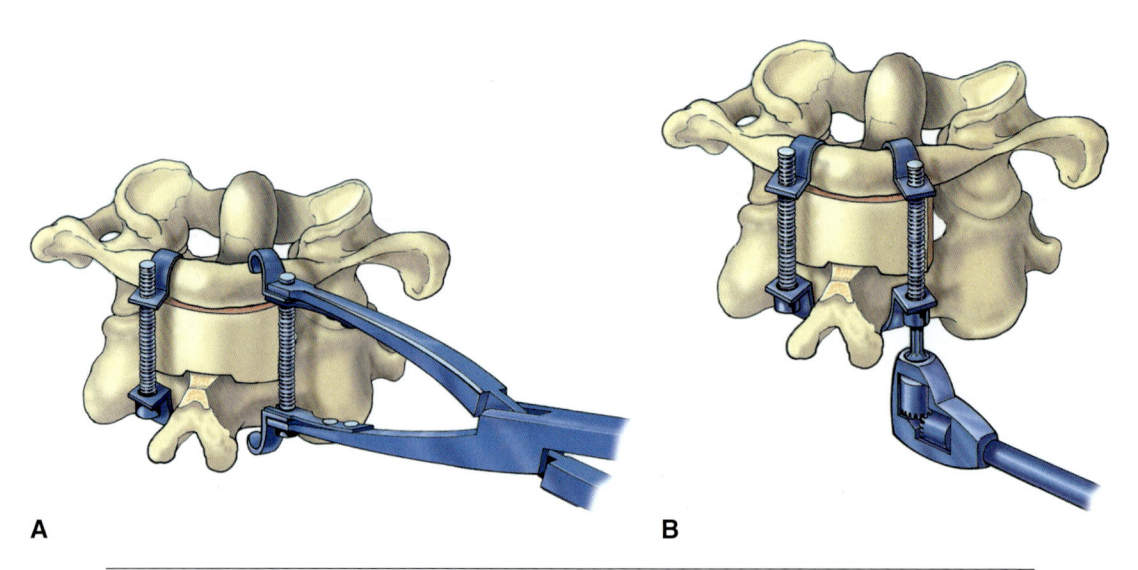

Fig. 38-9 *A*, Halifax clamps are positioned and applied. *B*, A right-angled screwdriver is used to tighten the clamp. (Used with permission from Barrow Neurological Institute.)

HALIFAX CLAMP FIXATION

Halifax clamps (Codman, Raynham, MA) are designed to immobilize a single motion segment and are indicated to replace a lost posterior tension band. Therefore, the anterior and middle columns need to be intact to apply rigid fixation with Halifax clamps. At the craniocervical area, Halifax clamps have been inserted to provide fixation between C1 and C2 for instability. However, they do not afford a more rigid construct than screw fixation for this area and therefore are rarely applied. Furthermore, Halifax clamps require intact bony structures, which can be compromised from fracture in a trauma case or from a laminectomy performed for decompression. The laminae at C1 and C2 is freed from ligamentous tissue, and the epidural space is dissected. A bone strut is fitted between C1 and C2, and the bony surfaces are decorticated with a drill. Special clamp pliers are used to insert the clamps on each side of C1 and C2 (Fig. 38-9*A*). The wires are clamped, and the screw is tightened between the two clamps using a right-angle screwdriver (see Fig. 38-9*B*). A bone strut is essential in the biomechanical construct created by Halifax clamps. Otherwise, the clamps would loosen when the neck was extended. Because better techniques for internal screw fixation have been developed, Halifax clamps are now seldom applied to treat C1-C2 instability from trauma.

ATLANTOAXIAL WIRING TECHNIQUES

Atlantoaxial wiring techniques are often applied in conjunction with atlantoaxial screw fixation to add stability to a construct, especially during flexion, and to provide fusion. Wiring without screw fixation, however, can be applied. Halo immobilization is recommended until bony fusion is achieved.

INTERSPINOUS FUSION

After bony exposure of C1-C2 is achieved posteriorly, the posterior occipitoatlantal membrane is removed. A high-speed drill is used to decorticate bony contact surfaces from the superior edge of the C2 spinous process and laminae and from the inferior edge of the C1 ring (Fig. 38-10*A*). Kerrison rongeurs are used to make bilateral notches on the inferior surface of the C2 lamina to seat the wires (see Fig. 38-10*B*). A autologous iliac crest bone graft, usually about 4 cm long and 3 cm high, must be obtained for the posterior iliac crest. A vicryl suture is passed beneath the lamina. Braided cables or wires (20-gauge monofilament wire or double-strand 24-gauge wire) is looped and passed beneath the lamina of C1 (see Fig. 38-10*C*). The upper cortical edge is removed, creating a bicortical autograft, which is wedged between C1 and C2 (see Fig. 38-10*D*). The autograft is inserted on top, and the loop of wire is passed over the autograft to notch under the spinous process of C2. Doing so compresses the autograft between C1 and C2 (see Fig. 38-10*E*).

GALLIE FUSION

For this fusion technique, a unicortical piece of autologous bone, usually 5 to 8 mm thick, is harvested from the iliac crest. After decortication, the cable wire is looped and passed under the lamina of C1 and looped over the spinous process of C2 (Fig. 38-11*A*). The graft is placed and the free ends of

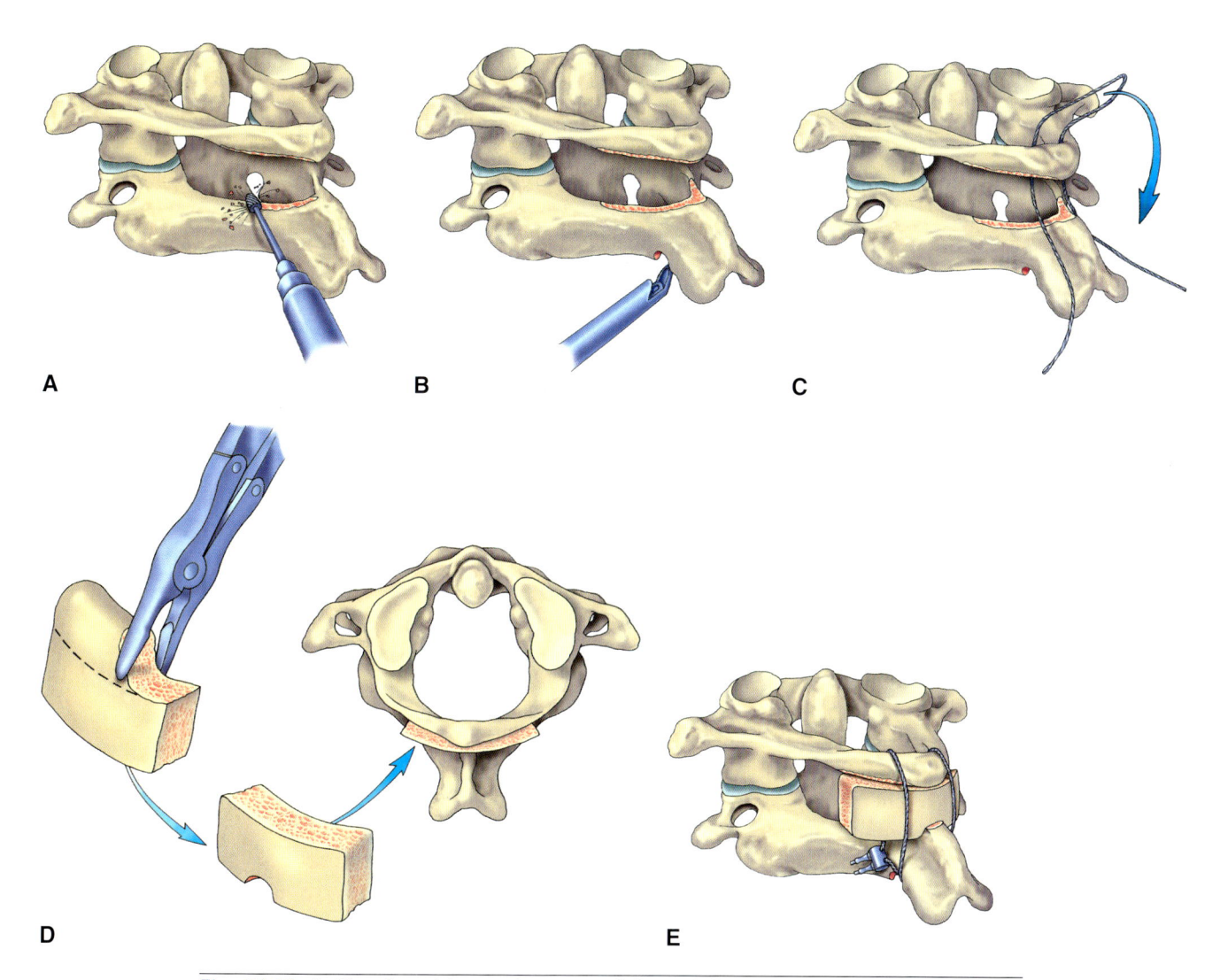

Fig. 38-10 A, The dorsal bony elements of C1 and C2 are decorticated with a high-speed drill to promote fusion. B, A notch is created in the caudal surface of the C2 spinous process to tighten the wire or cable after fusion. C, A cable is looped under C1 and over the spinous process of C2. D, A tricortical iliac crest autograft is decorticated to obtain a bicortical graft. A small wedge of bone is removed from the side facing C2 so that the upper part of the C2 spinous process can be inserted into the notch created in the graft to enhance stability of the construct. E, Final construct after the autograft has been wedged between C1-C2 and wired into place. (Used with permission from Barrow Neurological Institute.)

the wire are wrapped around the autograft and tightened (see Fig. 38-11B and C).

BROOKS FUSION

In this wiring technique, two wires are passed sublaminarly beneath C1 and C2 (Fig. 38-12A). The dura is visualized to avoid dural lacerations. Two cortical pieces of cancellous autograft are wedged on each side of the lamina of C1 and C2. The two loops of wires are placed circumferentially around the lamina of C1 and C2 on each side to engulf the bone grafts and are then tightened in place (see Fig. 38-12B).

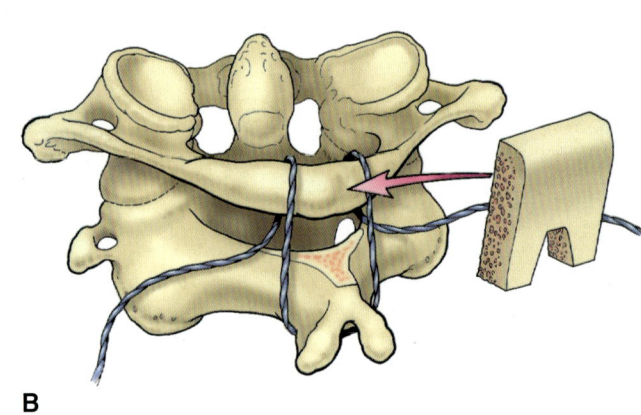

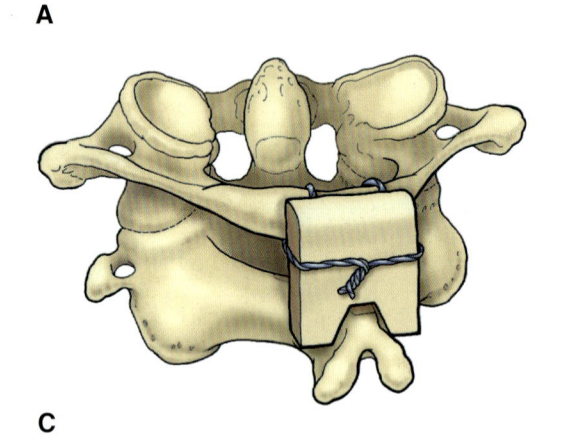

Fig. 38-11 *A,* A wire is looped under the C1 lamina and over the C2 spinous process. *B,* Autograft is notched to fit the C2 spinous process. *C,* The autograft is secured with the free ends of the wire to complete the Gallie fusion construct. (Used with permission from Barrow Neurological Institute.)

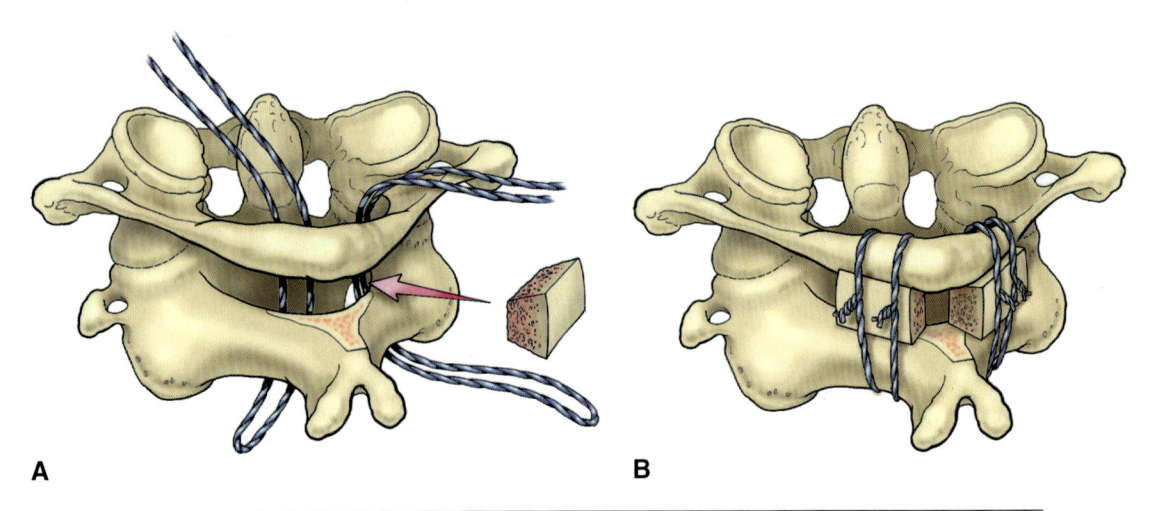

Fig. 38-12 *A,* Two loops of wire are passed from the top to underneath the laminae of C1 and C2 bilaterally, and the two pieces of iliac crest autograft are wired to C1 and C2 on each side. *B,* In the final construct of the Brooks fusion, wires are wrapped around the C1 and C2 laminae and twisted over the bone graft to secure the graft. (Used with permission from Barrow Neurological Institute.)

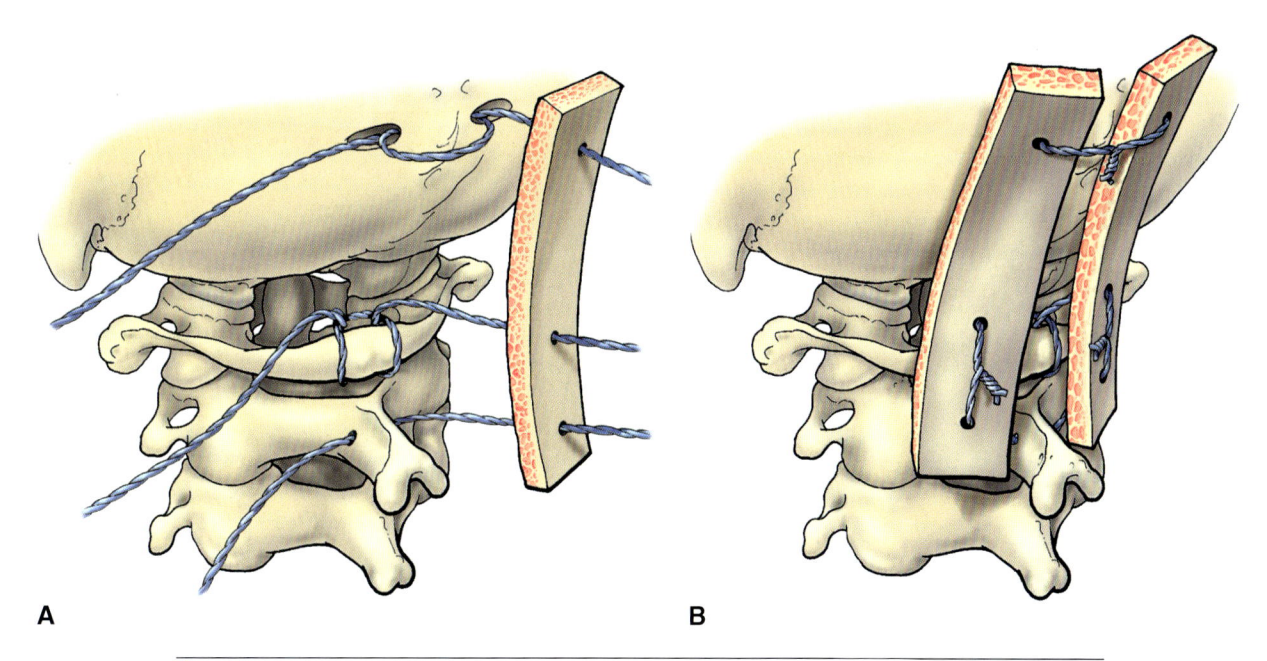

Fig. 38-13 *A*, For a Wertheim-Bohlman craniocervical wired fusion, a strut of autograft is wired from the occiput to C2. Wires are passed over the lamina of C1 and through drill holes at the occiput, C2, and strut graft. *B*, Final appearance of the Wertheim-Bohlman fusion construct. (Used with permission from Barrow Neurological Institute.)

OCCIPITOCERVICAL WIRE FIXATION

The occipitocervical junction can be fused and fixated with wiring techniques. Exposure of the bony occipitocervical junction is obtained as described. The occiput should be wired as close as possible to the midline crest where the bone is thickest. Burr holes placed about 5 mm away from the rim of the foramen magnum can be thinned with Kerrison rongeurs and widened. The dura, which must not be injured, should be separated by blunt dissection from the overlying occipital bone. Wires can be passed between each burr hole and the foramen magnum. Alternatively, the occiput can be wired at the midline by placing burr holes on each side of the crest and passing wires from hole to hole, or holes can be drilled tangentially to the midline crest to avoid an epidural exposure. Wires are passed around the lamina of C1 and C2 and, if necessary, around the subaxial spine. The many methods of wire fixation, including facet and spinous process wiring, are reviewed elsewhere in this book.

Bone struts, either ribs or curved iliac crest struts, are wired directly to the decorticated bony structures of the occipitocervical area. Holes are drilled through the struts to accommodate the wire as it is passed through. The wires are twisted to obtain rigid compression of the autograft to the craniocervical bone.

Different techniques have been described. The Wertheim-Bohlman technique uses midline occiput wires along with wires across the C1 lamina and across the base of the C2 spinous process (Fig. 38-13*A*). The pair of bone struts is tightly pressed against the occipitocervical area (see Fig. 38-13*B*). The Brattström technique uses wires with occipital screws placed on each side paramedian to the occiput. The occipital screws are used to anchor the bone graft with wires against the occipital bone. The wires also wrap beneath the spinous process of the axis and trap the bone graft against the decorticated bony surfaces of C1 and C2 (Fig. 38-14). Wire and bone graft techniques are seldom used. When possible, additional internal fixation enhances stability of the construct in a trauma setting and therefore is always preferred to wire and bone grafts alone.

INDICATIONS FOR POSTERIOR FIXATION AND FUSION OF THE CRANIOCERVICAL JUNCTION AND UPPER CERVICAL SPINE

Occipitocervical dislocation is the indication for occipitocervical fusion. Very rarely, a conservative nonoperative treatment with only an external arthrosis can be used. This procedure has been successful in the very young pediatric population in whom internal fixation devices are difficult to insert.[8] During open reduction, however, internal fixation is indicated for most patients with this diagnosis.

Fixation of C1 and C2 is indicated for traumatic injury involving vertical distraction between C1 and C2. However, the level at which conservative management fails is unclear.

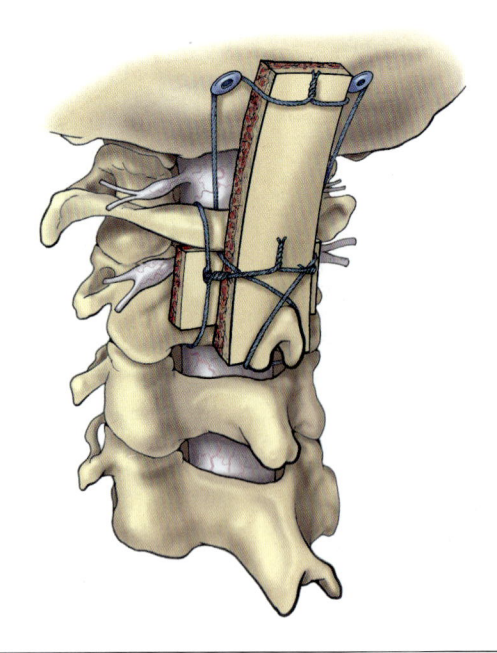

Fig. 38-14 A modified Brattström technique is another alternative for a wired craniocervical fusion. (Used with permission from Barrow Neurological Institute.)

If significant distraction is evident on computed tomography, magnetic resonance imaging, or both, surgical fixation and fusion can be performed safely to provide immediate stabilization of the unstable segment.[5] If the transverse ligament is insufficient or disrupted without avulsion of its bony insertion, as is sometimes associated with type II odontoid fractures, C1 needs to be fixated to C2 internally.[2,9] Either C1-C2 transarticular screws or lateral mass–pars interarticularis screws can be used, based on the surgeon's preference. The C2 pars interarticularis can be fixated for certain hangman's fractures.[10,11]

ANTERIOR APPROACHES FOR CRANIOCERVICAL AND UPPER CERVICAL SPINE INSTABILITY AFTER TRAUMA

INDICATIONS AND TECHNIQUES

The most common indications for anterior fixation for craniocervical instability associated with trauma consist of type II odontoid fractures and failure of fusion after rigid external orthosis. If a type II odontoid fracture is encountered with comminution at its base or with a dislocation more than 6 mm, the chances of fusion occurring with halo immobilization are less than with open reduction and internal fixation.[3,4]

Odontoid screw fixation is achieved as follows. A transverse incision is made in the neck crease at C5. The approach is usually performed from the right side, but a left-sided approach can be performed if preferred. The platysma is divided, and dissection proceeds along the medial aspect of the sternocleidomastoid muscle medial to the sheath of the carotid artery. The dissection remains lateral to the trachea and esophagus. The prevertebral fascia, which is reached at C5-C6, is bluntly dissected upward with gentle strokes of sponges held in a hemostat clamp. After the C2-C3 disk space is identified, the midline is dissected and identified. Usually, the anterior rim of the inferior end plate of C2 can be drilled with an air drill. A minimal anterior diskectomy at C2-C3 may be needed to place the drill guide under the end plate of C2 in a midline position as defined by anteroposterior and lateral biplanar fluoroscopy. The sagittal trajectory of the odontoid screw is verified with lateral fluoroscopy. Under biplanar fluoroscopy, the long K-wire is drilled with a powered hand drill across the fracture into the odontoid process.

The screw length is measured using the K-wire method. A cannulated end-threaded screw is placed over the K-wire into the odontoid process across the fracture site, and the K-wire is removed (Fig. 38-15A). A lag effect is created to capture and reduce the dislocated fracture (see Fig. 38-15B). Placement of a single screw is sufficient to obtain adequate fixation.

ANTERIOR ATLANTOAXIAL FACET SCREW FIXATION

This technique is rarely applied. Its major indication is failed posterior atlantoaxial fusion and instability with destruction of posterior elements of C1 and C2. A transverse skin incision is usually made on the right side in the neck crease over the C5-C6 interspace. Soft tissue dissection proceeds in the usual manner through the prevertebral fascia, which is scraped rostrally to the atlantoaxial facet joint. The atlantoaxial joints are decorticated on both sides with curettes. The groove between the superior facet and the body of the axis are localized anatomically. A bone awl is used to penetrate the bone at the point where the screw will be inserted. Next, the pilot holes are tapped. The angle must not be directed too far laterally to avoid potential injury the vertebral artery. The joint space should be crossed in a 90-degree angle in the coronal plane (Fig. 38-16). The diameter of screws ranges from 3.5 to 4 mm. The screws are typically 22 to 25 mm long. This technique is not recommended for osteoporotic patients or in patients with a fracture of the superior articular facets, vertebral body of C2, or lateral mass of C1. The afferent course of the vertebral artery must be verified.

CONCLUSION

Diverse techniques of fixation and fusion of the occipitocervical junction and upper cervical spine were outlined. For most instances of traumatic instability in this region, open reduction and internal fixation are the preferred management techniques. Newer rod-screw constructs are applied posteriorly and have become more popular than wiring techniques

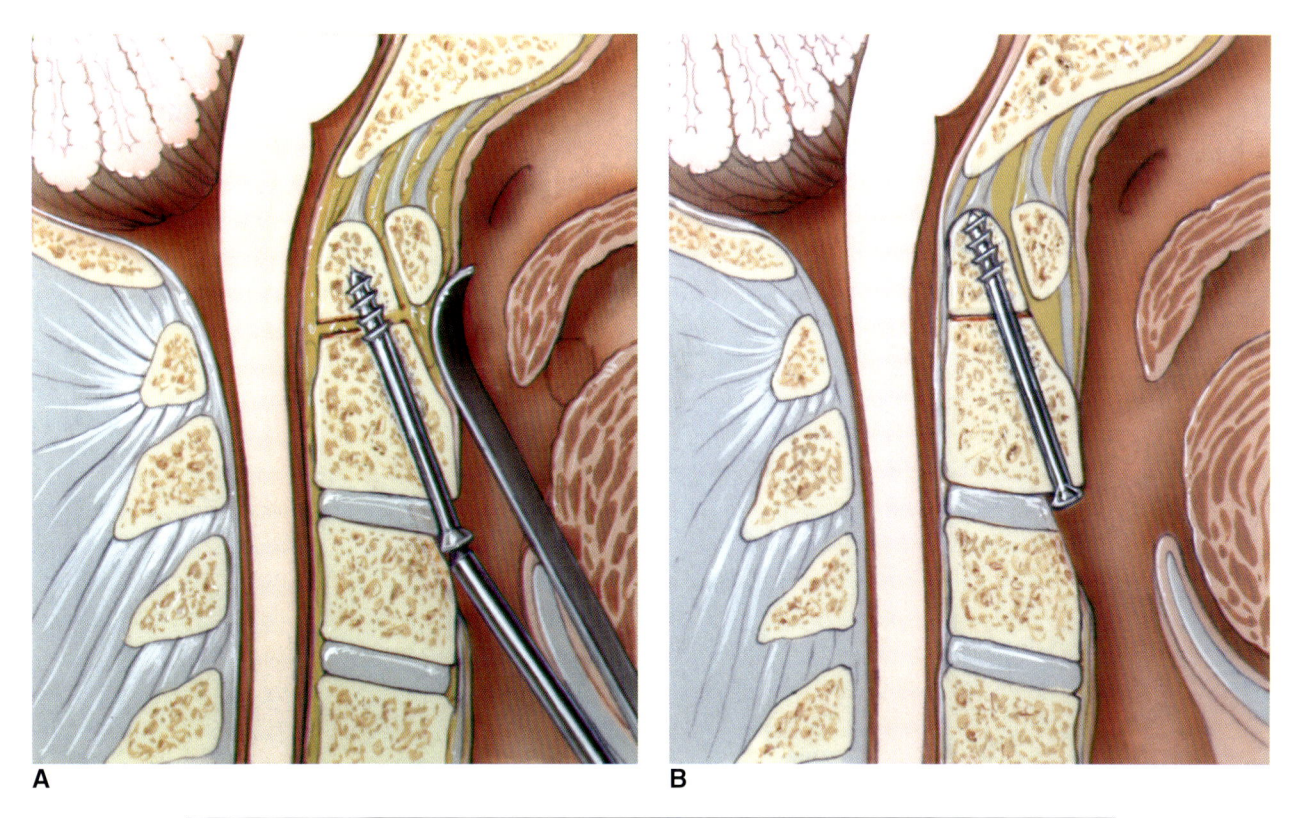

CHAPTER 38 Surgical Therapy for Fractures and Dislocations

Fig. 38-15 *A*, A lag screw is placed across the odontoid fracture. *B*, The lag effect created by the end-threaded screw pulls the fractured fragment down to reapproximate the fracture line. (Illustrations provided courtesy of Aesculap, Inc., San Francisco, CA. Reproduced with permission from the American Association of Neurological Surgeons, 5550 Meadowbrook Drive, Rolling Meadows, IL, 60008.)

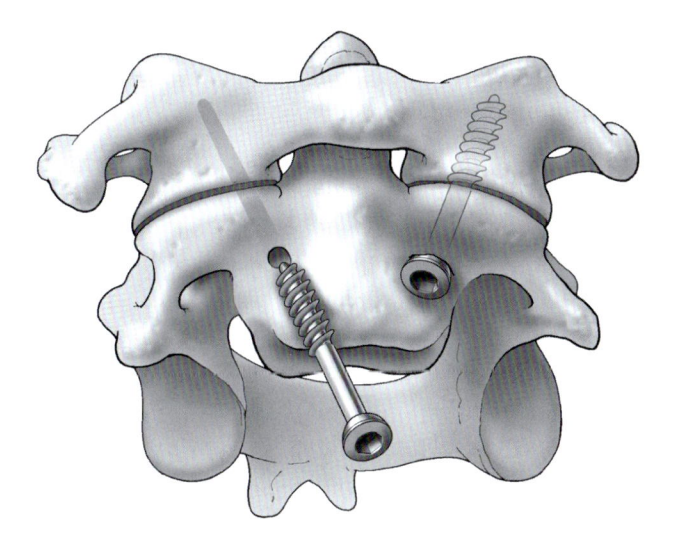

Fig. 38-16 Anterior atlantoaxial facet screw placement requires 90-degree angulation of the screw in the coronal plane to avoid injuring neurovascular structures. (Used with permission from Barrow Neurological Institute.)

alone because they offer immediate stability. New constructs for occipitocervical fixation, especially for occipitoatlantal fixation, are now available. In trauma patients, the placement of internal fixation devices is sometimes aided by the use of neuronavigation. However, detailed knowledge of anatomy and local pathology is imperative for successful implantation of hardware in this territory.

Compared to external immobilization, internal fixation has become a safe and highly effective method for facilitating fusion and for preventing future posttraumatic deformity. Consequently, it has gained widespread acceptance and application for the management of unstable traumatic injuries of the craniocervical junction and upper cervical spine.

REFERENCES

1. Dickman CA, Papadopoulos SM, Sonntag VK, et al: Traumatic occipitoatlantal dislocations. J Spinal Disord 1993;6(4):300–313.
2. Hadley MN, Dickman CA, Browner CM, Sonntag VK: Acute traumatic atlas fractures: Management and long term outcome. Neurosurgery 1988;23(1):31–35.
3. Hadley MN, Browner C, Sonntag VK: Axis fractures: A comprehensive review of management and treatment in 107 cases. Neurosurgery 1985;17(2):281–290.

4. Hadley MN, Browner CM, Liu SS, Sonntag VK: New subtype of acute odontoid fractures (type IIA). Neurosurgery 1988;22(1 Pt 1):67–71.
5. Gonzalez LF, Fiorella D, Crawford NR, et al: Vertical atlantoaxial distraction injuries: Radiological criteria and clinical implications. J Neurosurg Spine 2004;1(3):273–280.
6. Grob D: Transarticular screw fixation for atlanto-occipital dislocation. Spine 2001;26(6):703–707.
7. Feiz-Erfan I, Gonzalez LF, Dickman CA: Atlantooccipital transarticular screw fixation for the treatment of traumatic occipitoatlantal dislocation. J Neurosurg Spine 2005;2(3):381–385.
8. Ghatan S, Newell DW, Grady MS, et al: Severe posttraumatic craniocervical instability in a very young patient: Report of three cases. J Neurosurg (Pediatrics 1) 2004;101:102–107.
9. Management of combination fractures of the atlas and axis in adults. Neurosurgery 2002;50(3 Suppl):S140–S147.
10. Bristol RE, Henn JS, Dickman CA: Pars screw fixation of a hangman's fracture: Technical case report. Neurosurgery 2005;56(1 Suppl):E204; discussion E204.
11. Verheggen R, Jansen J: Hangman's fracture: arguments in favor of surgical therapy for type II and III according to Edwards and Levine. Surg Neurol 1998;49(3):253–261.

CHAPTER 39

MAX C. LEE
DANIEL H. KIM

Burst Fractures of the Cervical Spine

INTRODUCTION

Subaxial cervical spine trauma can be divided into two groups. The first group includes facet dislocations, while the second group does not. The topic of facet dislocations and reductions is discussed in Chapter 40. This chapter focuses on subaxial cervical spine trauma excluding facet dislocation.

Burst fractures and compression fractures of the cervical spine present after a mechanical axial load is exerted.[1] This has also been demonstrated with mathematical modeling.[2] The spectrum of burst fractures is diverse. Variations may include diastatic fractures associated with posterior column injury, small teardrop fractures, and complete vertebral burst.

Complications from vertebral body fractures include mechanical and neurologic instability. Combined with bilateral facet dislocations, burst fractures of the cervical spine are a significant risk factor for neurologic and spinal cord injury.[3] Neurologic instability can be attributed to direct spinal cord compression or nerve root compression, as burst fractures may lead to retropulsed bone and disk. This initial neurologic function and outcome are dependent on spinal canal diameter.[4] On the other hand, the measurement of the spinal canal diameter may underestimate the amount of transient spinal canal compromise.[5–7] Therefore, one goal of surgery is decompression.[8]

In addition to neurologic instability, mechanical instability is a state whereby the cervical spine is no longer able to tolerate normal physiologic loads. Unfortunately, mechanical stability is not dependent on degree of fracture—with teardrop fractures demonstrating more ligamentous damage from extreme flexion.[9] Thus, the surgical management will include neural decompression and restoration of mechanical stability. Finally, the importance of restoring sagittal balance cannot be underemphasized.

Although anterior cervical decompression has been demonstrated to be safe,[10] decompression for complete spinal cord injuries continues to be debated. Justification for surgical decompression continues to include improved neurologic outcome and mechanical stability. Improved neurologic outcome may be demonstrated in a comparison to those treated conservatively—by demonstrating preserved nerve root function.[11]

The conservative management of a cervical burst fracture has been described. Although this may be a viable alternative, depending on the extent of fracture and medical condition of the patient, long-term follow-up demonstrates a worse outcome. In a comparison between anterior decompression and conservative management, surgical fixation led to improved neurologic outcome, less narrowing of the spinal canal, and less kyphosis.[12–14] In addition, 5% of patients treated with external immobilization demonstrated continued instability. This contrasts with those with either an anterior or posterior stabilization in whom near complete fusion was demonstrated. Unfortunately, no standards or guidelines exist for the management of burst fractures of the cervical spine. The only options suggest reduction and internal or external fixation.[15]

SURGERY

The surgical correction for burst fractures of the cervical spine must incorporate the extent of the fracture and neural compression, presence of posterior column injury, associated soft tissue injury, and loss of sagittal balance. In addition, other associated injuries must be addressed. Such injuries may include esophageal perforation[16] and vertebral artery occlusion/dissection.[17] Thus, although various approaches can be taken, the approach must incorporate the multiple variables associated with these fractures.

After the decision has been made for decompression, even before induction of general anesthesia, several decisions must be made. Namely, the method of induction, use of intraoperative monitoring, and type of exposure must be assessed. With severe compression (radiographic or based on subjective/objective findings), the head and neck must be kept in a neutral position. Thus, intubation may have to be performed with fiberoptics or awake. In addition, intraoperative monitoring can assist with positioning and surgery. Lastly, the location of the burst fracture has to be considered in the preoperative management. Burst fractures within the cervicothoracic junction may require a modified/full sternotomy for anterior exposure.[18]

The cervical spine can be maintained in a neutral position by placing the head in a horseshoe or doughnut rest. This may be facilitated with the placement of a shoulder roll. Depending on concomitant injuries to the upper extremities, the shoulders may be fixated to the operating table with tape. In addition, a slight shoulder pull may provide for increased radiographic visualization of the level involved.

After the patient is prepared, the patient is draped in the standard surgical fashion including the fluoroscopic C-arm. A linear incision is made overlying the involved segment. The platysma muscle is split and undermined. As with an anterior cervical diskectomy/corpectomy, dissection is then accomplished anterior to the sternocleidomastoid muscle. While lateral to the trachea, dissection of the anterior belly of the omohyoid muscle is accomplished. For injuries above the sixth cervical vertebra, dissection can continue above the omohyoid. For dissection caudal to that level, this muscle may be split in order to enhance exposure of the involved segments.

Palpation of the carotid sheath and its contents is done; and dissection in continued medial to this complex. Within this plane of dissection, lateral to the esophagus and trachea, dissection is continued until the anterior longitudinal ligament and the ventral surface of the involved level is appreciated. In order to facilitate later work, the level above and below the fracture is also dissected. The longus coli muscles are undermined on both sides and a self-retaining retractor is placed (centered on the level involved) (Fig. 39-1).

Then, the ventral surface of the involved level and two adjacent levels are prepared for the future ventral plate. Careful removal of ventral osteophytes may easily be accomplished with a high-speed drill. Distraction screws are placed in the vertebral body above and below the fracture (Fig. 39-2). In addition to distracting the involved segment, distraction pins may be used to assist in the correction of sagittal balance. By placing divergent screws cervical lordosis is accomplished as the screws are distracted to a parallel position.

An intraoperative microscope is brought into the field. With a No. 15 blade scalpel, the annulus of the disk above and below the fracture are incised (Fig. 39-3), and a diskectomy is performed at both levels (Figs. 39-4 and 39-5). Because of the future stress that the adjacent vertebral bodies will experience after the graft insertion, careful attention is paid to maintain the end plates on both sides.

Once the diskectomies are accomplished, a corpectomy can be done with a high-speed drill and rongeurs (Fig. 39-6). The bone harvested may be incorporated into the future graft. Careful attention is paid not to apply any downward

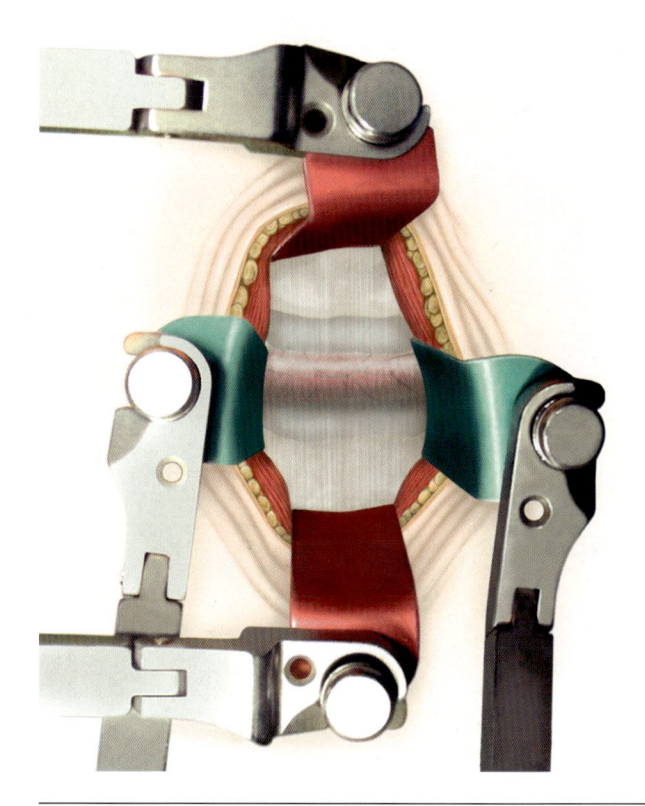

Fig. 39-1 The longus colli muscles are undermined on both sides, and a self-retaining retractor is placed (centered on the level involved).

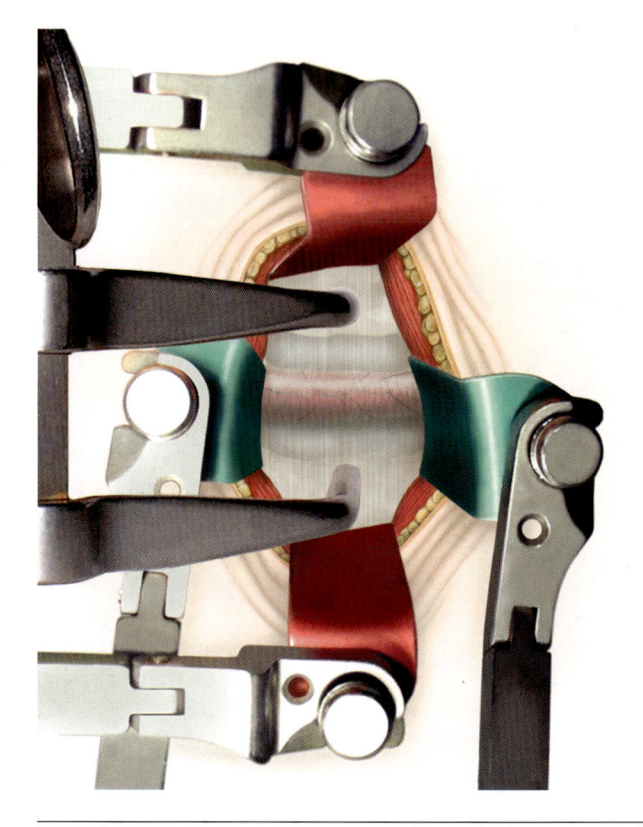

Fig. 39-2 Distraction screws are placed in the vertebral body above and below the fracture.

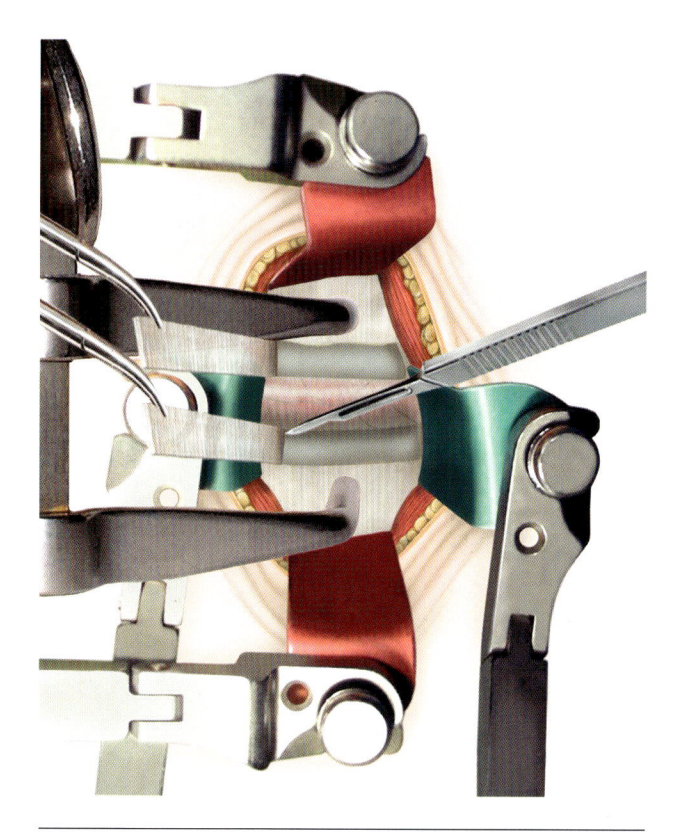

CHAPTER 39 Burst Fractures of the Cervical Spine 333

Fig. 39-3 With a No. 15 blade scalpel, the annulus of the disk above and below the fracture are incised.

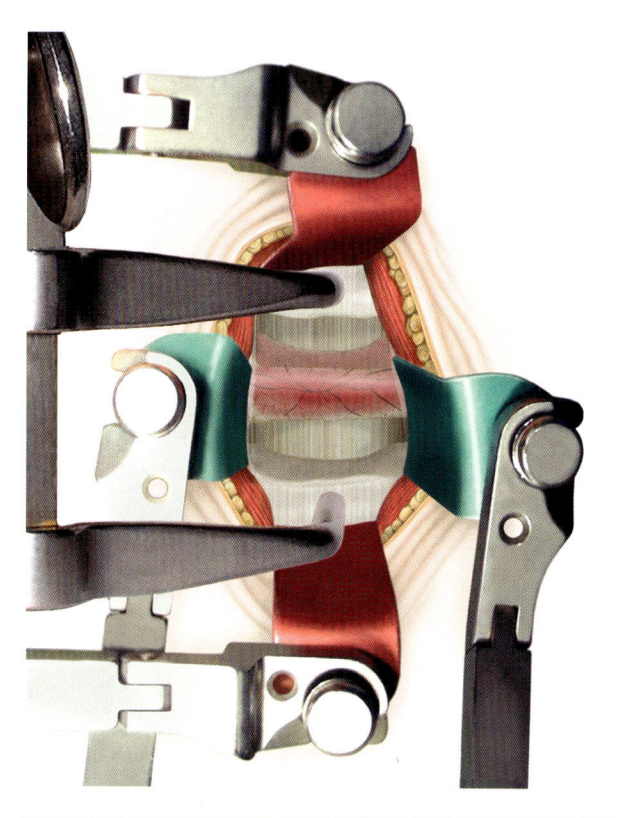

Fig. 39-5 Diskectomy performed at both levels.

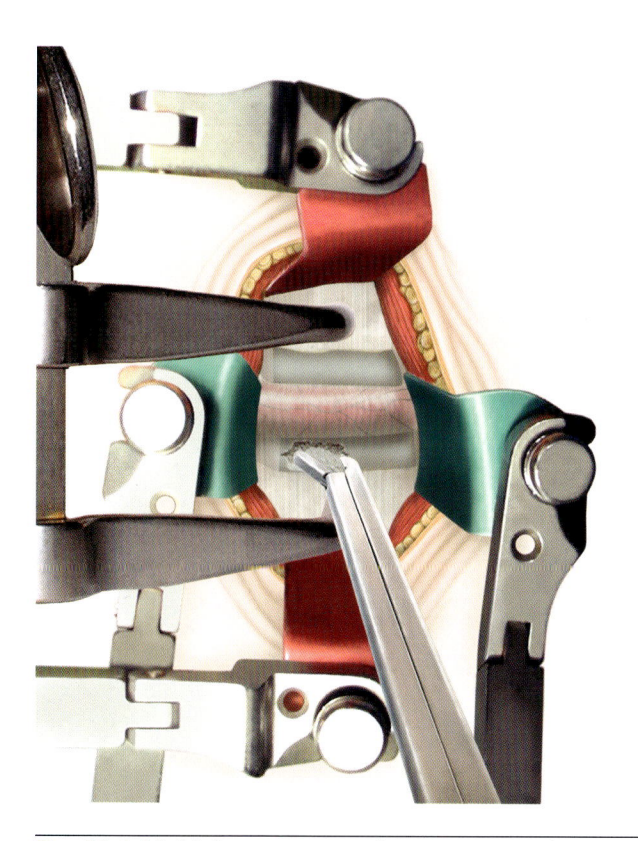

Fig. 39-4 Multiple curettes and rongeurs used to perform a diskectomy.

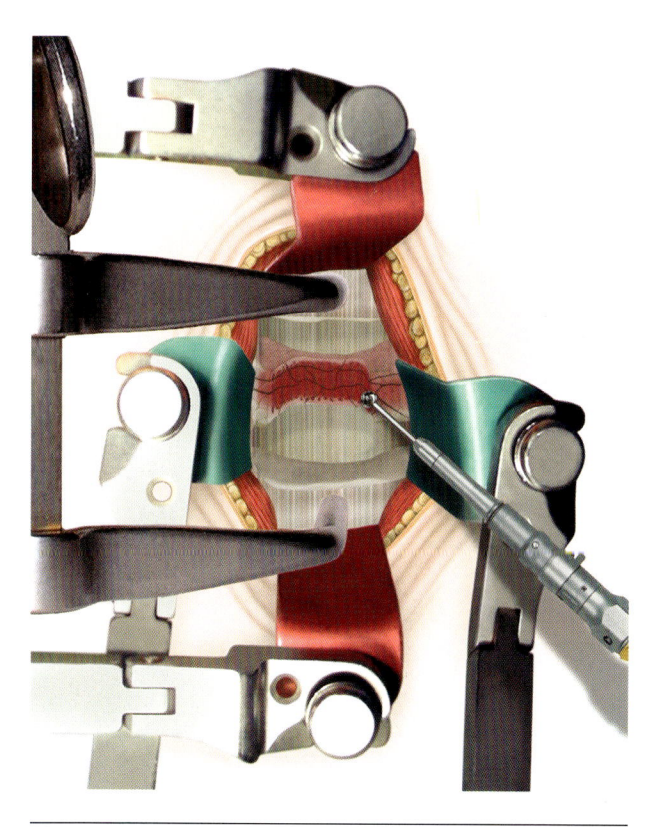

Fig. 39-6 Next, perform a corpectomy with a high-speed drill and rongeurs.

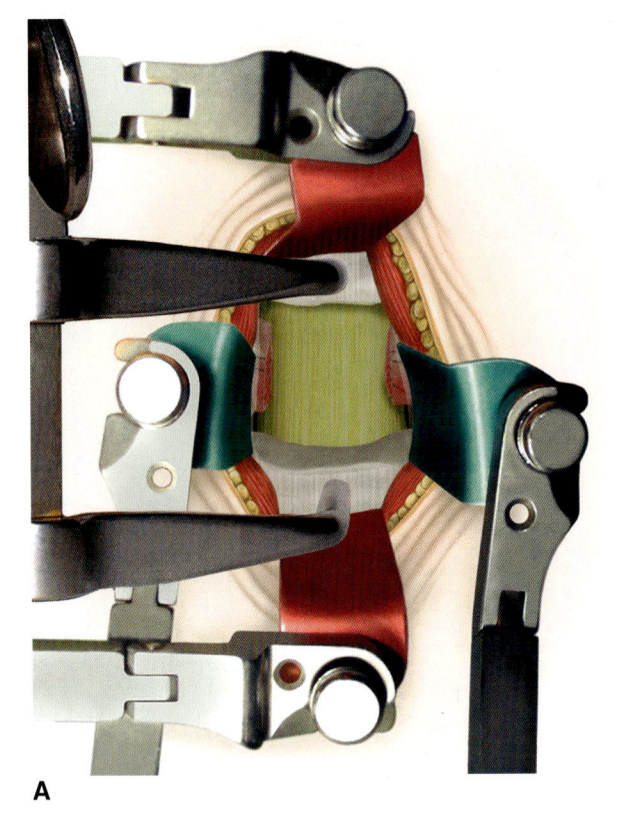

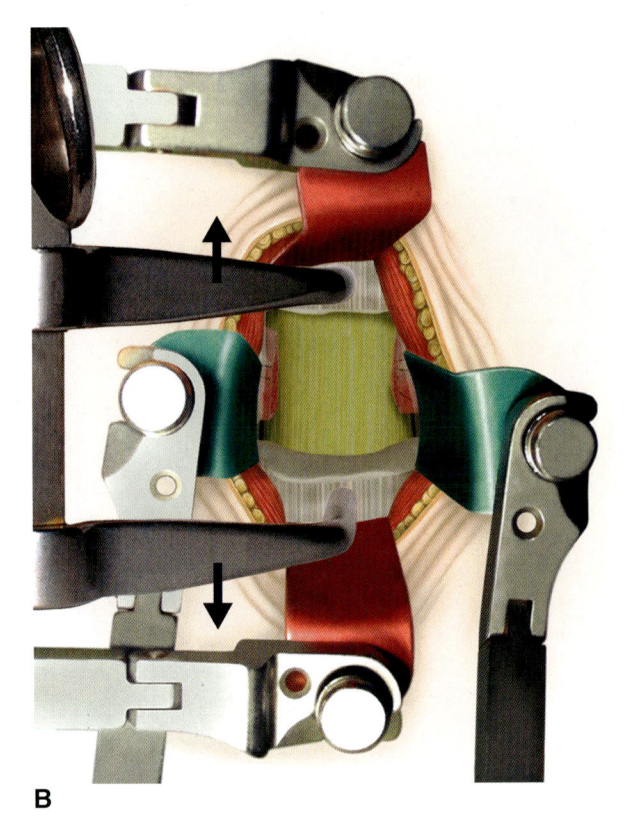

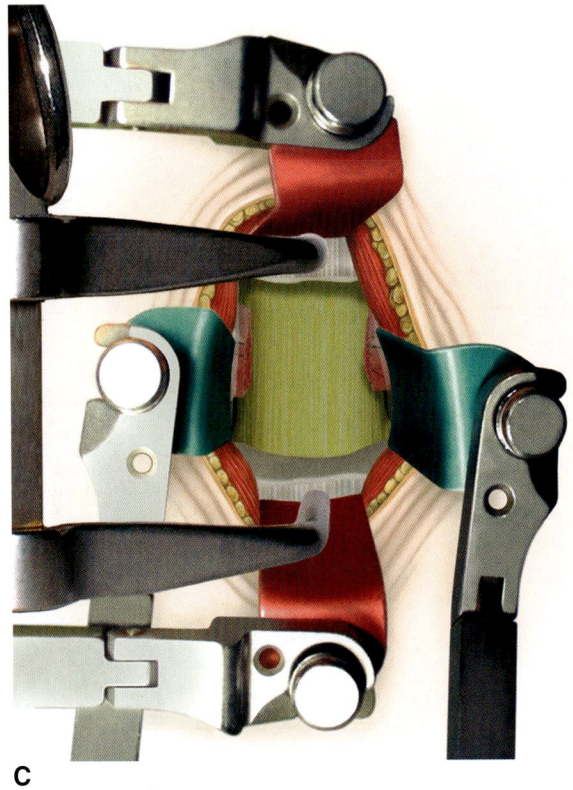

Fig. 39-7 *A*, If suspicious for herniated bone or disk material, the posterior longitudinal ligament is removed with the use of microinstruments, curettes, and Kerrison rongeurs. *B* and *C*, If needed, further distraction can be accomplished to restore sagittal balance and vertebral body height.

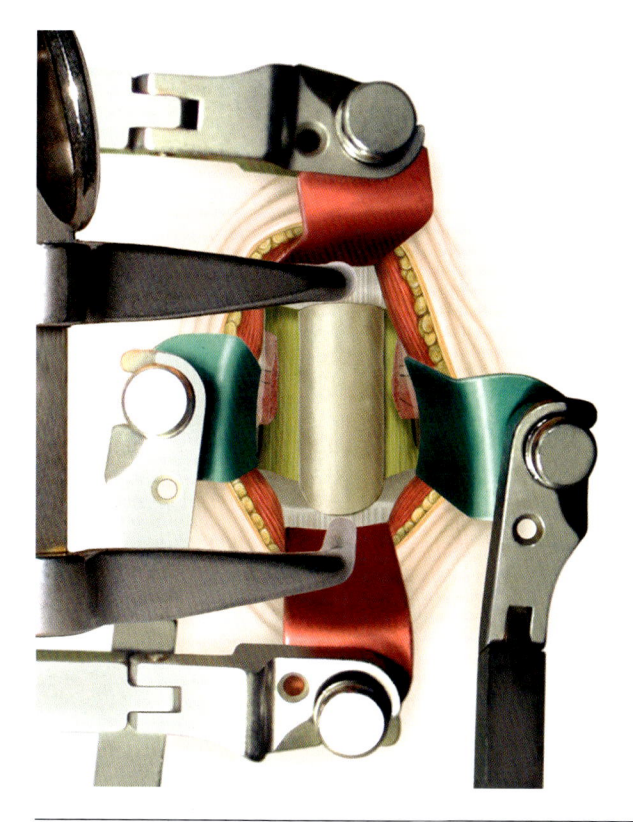

Fig. 39-8 A decision on the graft is dependent not on availability, but on each individual situation.

pressure on the thecal sac or spinal cord. The extent of dissection is dependent on the preoperative imaging and symptoms. Although some may advocate leaving a cortical edge posteriorly, this does not add to any biomechanical benefit. Thus, the corpectomy is completed. If suspicious for herniated bone or disk material, the posterior longitudinal ligament is removed with use of microinstruments, curettes, and Kerrison rongeurs (Fig. 39-7A). If needed, further distraction can be accomplished to restore sagittal balance and vertebral body height (see Fig. 39-7B and C). Once adequate decompression is accomplished, the graft site is prepared. We prefer to drill parts of the end plate above and below to maximize both structural strength and future fusion surface area.

The choice of graft is controversial. From autograft, allograft, titanium alloy cage, and polyetheretherketone cages (PEEK), a variety of grafts exist. Many of these grafts have been proved to be efficacious, but the choice of graft is dependent on availability but on each individual situation (Fig. 39-8). In addition, the ventral graft is supplemented with a screw-plate construct. Although several plate systems exist, in the setting of trauma, we continue to use fixed, angled screws with a translational, restricted backout plate.

Depending on the severity of the injury, additional fixation can be accomplished. Bicortical screw purchase for the ventral plate screw construct may add additional strength. With burst fractures associated with a posterior column bone or ligamentous injury, supplementation of the anterior construct with posterior instrumentation is plausible. Posterior instrumentation includes interspinous wiring, lateral mass screws, and sublaminar wiring. Unicortical screw purchase, in a ventral screw-plate construct, can provide sufficient biomechanical strength in the biomechanical laboratory; however, posterior instrumentation adds significant strength.[19–21]

DISCUSSION

The spectrum of burst fractures is large. In addition, they may be associated with other visceral injuries, herniated disks, and posterior column fractures. The management of burst fractures must encompass these other injuries. Nonetheless, the goals for surgery will continue to include neurologic decompression and restoration of mechanical stability.

References

1. Koo DW, Fish WW: Spinal cord injury and snowboarding—The British Columbia experience. J Spinal Cord Med 1999;22:246–251.
2. Bozic KJ, Keyak JH, Skinner HB, et al: Three-dimensional finite element modeling of a cervical vertebra: An investigation of burst fracture mechanism. J Spinal Disord 1994;7:102–110.
3. Coelho DG, Brasil AV, Ferreira NP: Risk factors of neurological lesions in low cervical spine fractures and dislocations. Arq Neuropsiquiatr 2000;58:1030–1034.
4. Sapkas G, Korres D, Babis GC, et al: Correlation of spinal canal post-traumatic encroachment and neurological deficit in burst fractures of the lower cervical spine (C3-7). Eur Spine J 1995;4:39–44.
5. Carter JW, Mirza SK, Tencer AF, et al: Canal geometry changes associated with axial compressive cervical spine fracture. Spine 2000;25:46–54.
6. Chang DG, Tencer AF, Ching RP, et al: Geometric changes in the cervical spinal canal during impact. Spine 1994;19:973–980.
7. Ching RP, Watson NA, Carter JW, et al: The effect of post-injury spinal position on canal occlusion in a cervical spine burst fracture model. Spine 1997;22:1710–1715.
8. Schweighofer F, Fellinger M, Schippinger G, et al: Complications after an unusual procedure in the treatment of a cervical spine burst fracture. A case report. Langenbecks Arch Chir 1992;377:235–236.
9. Scher AT: 'Tear-drop' fractures of the cervical spine—Radiological features. S Afr Med J 1982;61:355–356.
10. Aebi M, Zuber K, Marchesi D: Treatment of cervical spine injuries with anterior plating: Indications, techniques, and results. Spine 1991;16:S38–S45.
11. Yablon IG, Palumbo M, Spatz E, et al: Nerve root recovery in complete injuries of the cervical spine. Spine 1991;16:S518–S521.
12. Evans DL, Bethem D: Cervical spine injuries in children. J Pediatr Orthop 1989;9:563–568.
13. Stauffer ES, Rhoades ME: Surgical stabilization of the cervical spine after trauma. Arch Surg 1976;111:652–657.
14. Koivikko MP, Myllynen P, Karjalainen M, et al: Conservative and operative treatment in cervical burst fractures. Arch Orthop Trauma Surg 2000;120:448–451.

15. Management of acute central cervical spinal cord injuries. Neurosurgery 2002;50:S166–S172.
16. Tomaszek DE, Rosner MJ: Occult esophageal perforation associated with cervical spine fracture. Neurosurgery 1984;14:492–494.
17. Handa Y, Hayashi M, Kawano H, et al: Vertebral artery thrombosis accompanied by burst fracture of the lower cervical spine: Case report. Neurosurgery 1985;17:955–957.
18. Knoller SM, Brethner L: Surgical treatment of the spine at the cervicothoracic junction: An illustrated review of a modified sternotomy approach with the description of tricks and pitfalls. Arch Orthop Trauma Surg 2002;122:365–368.
19. Adams MS, Crawford NR, Chamberlain RH, et al: Biomechanical comparison of anterior cervical plating and combined anterior/lateral mass plating. Spine J 2001;1:166–170.
20. Do Koh Y, Lim TH, Won You J, et al: A biomechanical comparison of modern anterior and posterior plate fixation of the cervical spine. Spine 2001;26:15–21.
21. Fehlings MG, Cooper PR, Errico TJ: Posterior plates in the management of cervical instability: Long-term results in 44 patients. J Neurosurg 1994;81:341–349.

CHAPTER 40

MAX C. LEE
DANIEL H. KIM

Subaxial Cervical Spinal Injuries and Facet Dislocation Injuries

INTRODUCTION

This chapter will focus on the surgical management facet dislocation (unilateral or bilateral) via open reduction and fixation. Facet dislocations account for one half of all cervical injuries.[1] The mechanism of injury is generally attributed to a distractive flexion injury.[2] In this injury, a unilateral facet dislocation occurs to the opposite side of the rotation.[3] On the other hand, this has been difficult to reproduce in a cadaveric model.[4]

Injuries to the facet joint, surrounding capsule, and superspinous and interspinous ligaments occur in both unilateral and bilateral facet dislocations. Meanwhile, the posterior longitudinal ligament is generally spared in unilateral facet dislocations (Figs. 40-1 and 40-2). On the other hand, bilateral facet dislocation involves a greater ligamentous injury. In addition to the injury of the joint capsule and interspinous ligament, bilateral facet dislocations are associated with injury to the posterior longitudinal ligament[5,6] (Fig. 40-3).

PRESENTATION

Patients who present with acute injury from facet dislocations are a heterogenous group—from neurologically intact to complete spinal cord injury. With a unilateral facet dislocation, one quarter will present with a nerve root injury and another quarter will present with an incomplete spinal cord injury.[7] With bilateral facet dislocations, approximately two thirds of patients will have a complete spinal cord injury and one third will have a combination of an incomplete spinal cord injury or nerve root injury.

RADIOGRAPHIC EVALUATION

Plain films continue to be the mainstay of radiographic evaluation of cervical spine trauma. Anteroposterior (AP) and lateral x-rays provide an abundance of information on the subaxial cervical spine. Alignment of the vertebral bodies, pedicles, facet complexes, and spinous processes is essential. In addition to demonstration of the facet dislocation, x-rays also may demonstrate other lesions adjacent to or distant to the dislocation.

Unilateral facet dislocation is associated with a vertebral body dislocation less than half of the anteroposterior distance of one vertebral body whereas bilateral facet dislocation is generally associated with a larger disruption. Dislocation of the rostral vertebral body anterior to the inferior vertebral body occurs with this flexion distraction injury.

Computed tomography (CT) is frequently used to provide more information regarding a facet dislocation. Sim-

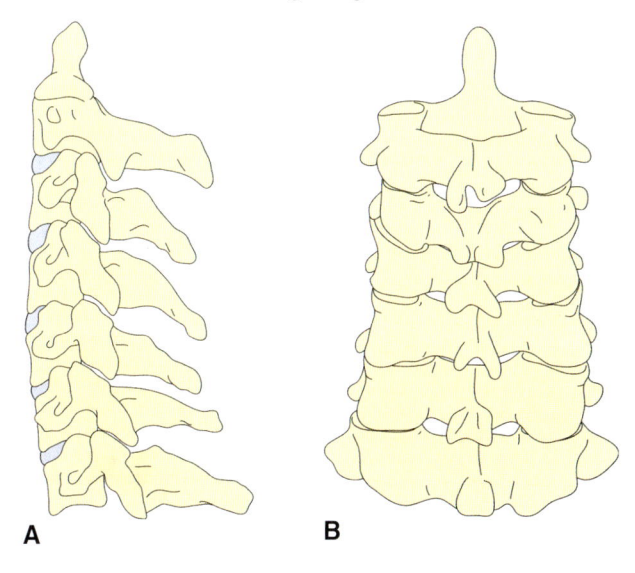

Fig. 40-1 Lateral (A) and posterior (B) views of the cervical spine with normal alignment.

337

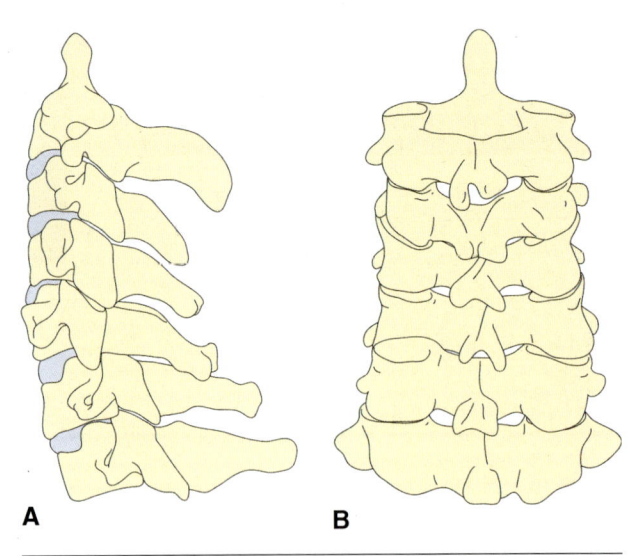

Fig. 40-2 Lateral (A) and posterior (B) views of the cervical spine with left, unilateral C5-C6 facet dislocation.

ilarly, CT may be of particular benefit in clarifying injuries to the posterior elements and facet complexes.[8] On axial imaging, the dislocated facets are seen with this dislocation, as the inferior facet of the vertebra above dislocates over the superior facet of the vertebra below. In addition, axial imaging provides further definition of the osseous structures of the cervical spine, as facet dislocations may be associated with fractures of the superior or inferior facet. Other fractures of the cervical spine may be appreciated. For instance, fractures of the lamina, pedicle, involved vertebral bodies, or fractures distant to the involved dislocation may be appreciated.

Magnetic resonance imaging (MRI) continues to be the mainstay in the evaluation of the soft tissue and disks of the cervical spine. Controversy continues in regard to obtaining further information about the disks before reduction. Thus, in addition to the information obtained via CT, MRI demonstrated changes in adjacent verterbral bodies, disks, and spinal cord.

TREATMENT AND OUTCOME

In the past, conservative measures have been attempted. Although a unilateral facet dislocation may be stable immediately after the injury on dynamic radiographs, progressive deformity and future instability have been appreciated afterward. Instability has also been appreciated in half of the patients treated without surgery. Even with the management with a halo vest, further instability has been appreciated in 37.5% of patients with a facet dislocation.[7] As with these patients treated without halo stabilization, there is a high rate of postimmobilization kyphotic deformity. This high rate of instability has been attributed to the large ligamentous disruption in both unilateral and bilateral facet dislocations. In addition, closed reduction without internal fixation has been associated with resubluxation and progressive cervical spine deformities. Subluxations have been seen after closed reduction, both with and without halo immobilization.

Neurologic improvement after reduction is mixed. Appreciating neurologic improvement after reduction may be difficult.[5,9,10] Spinal cord injury, with facet dislocation, may be permanent. Even with complete spinal myelopathy, nerve root recovery may occur with reduction. On the other hand, neurologic recovery after a spinal cord/nerve root injury does not encompass all the benefits from early reduction and stabilization. Reduction and stabilization may prevent further spinal deformity, disrupt the sagittal balance, and cause further neurologic compromise.

Treatment options have been summarized in the American Association of Neurological Surgeons Guidelines for the Management of Acute Cervical Spine and Spinal Cord Injuries in the March 2002 supplement of *Neurosurgery*.[11] There are no standards or guidelines. Options include the following:

- Closed reduction versus open reduction
- Anterior versus posterior reduction
- Anterior versus posterior fixation
- External immobilization
- Prolonged bed rest in traction

Owing to the high rate of failure after closed reduction and external fixation, we advocate internal fixation with closed or open reduction. In the event that closed reduction is not possible, open reduction and fusion have been demonstrated to be effective.[12]

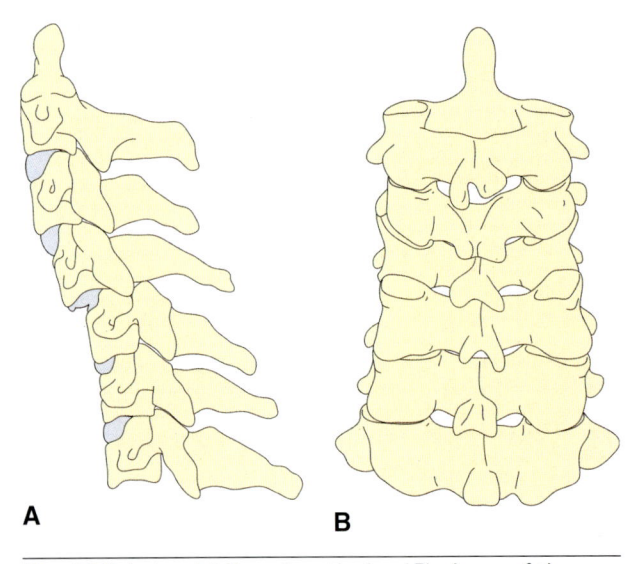

Fig. 40-3 Lateral (A) and posterior (B) views of the cervical spine with bilateral C4-C5 facet dislocation.

OPERATIVE TECHNIQUE

Operative technique can be divided into three groups—anterior, posterior, and both. Surgical reduction can be achieved via each direction. We will review operative techniques for both an anterior and posterior reduction. Finally, we will recap on the fixation techniques mentioned in other chapters.

POSTERIOR REDUCTION

Although both anterior and posterior approaches have accomplished the reduction of facet dislocations, we prefer a posterior reduction for numerous reasons.[13] Placing a patient with a cervical spine injury in a prone position can be a challenge in itself. Three-point skull fixation is achieved with Mayfield pins, and the patient is carefully placed prone on chest bolsters. Intraoperative monitoring is frequently used before, during, and after positioning. Once the patient has been placed in a prone position, closed reduction can be attempted once more with monitoring and fluoroscopic guidance. With the aid of general anesthesia, frequently reduction can be achieved with distractive loads of less than what was previously used with closed reduction. If reduction is achieved, Mayfield fixation is achieved, and posterior fixation is done.

If reduction is not achieved, open reduction may be accomplished. Exposure is obtained through a midline vertical incision and subperiosteal dissection. The soft tissue is retracted laterally using a self-retaining retractor. The facet dislocation is dissected and manual reduction is attempted. Several mechanisms may achieve reduction. Although a facet dislocation is a distractive, flexion injury, intraoperative open reduction can be achieved with minimal direct distraction (Fig. 40-4). Direct manipulation of the facets can generally correct this dislocation.

If reduction cannot be achieved via distraction, reduction can be obtained via drilling off of the superior facet of the lower involved segment (Fig. 40-5). If reduction is still not achieved, reduction can be accomplished by placing a gentle downward force on the caudal segment or can be accomplished with the assistance of instrumentation with a screw-rod system.

In addition, a posterior approach may be used in the stabilization of patients in whom closed reduction is obtained. Posterior stabilization procedures include lateral mass screw-rod systems, lateral mass screw-plate systems, facet wiring techniques, laminar clamps, and interspinous wiring.

POSTERIOR STABILIZATION

Interspinous wiring has been found to be safe and effective.[14] This procedure requires intact posterior elements. Although wiring may limit the degree of flexion and extension, it offers little rotational stability.[15] With that said, this method may add as a supplement to other posterior techniques.

After a periosteal dissection is accomplished, reduction is achieved with radiographic verification of the correct level. A right-angled drill is used to make a hole in the rostral aspect of the base of the spinous process above and the caudal aspect of the spinous process below. Then, the drill is used to roughen the spinous processes and lamina in the area of interest. A Sanger cable is passed from one of the aforementioned holes to the other and tightened. During this process, allograft/autograft may be placed between the cable and posterior elements to supplement this fusion process.

Laminar Clamps

Similar to spinous process wiring, laminar clamps require intact posterior elements. As the name implies, laminar clamps consist of two clamps. One clamp is secured over the rostral lamina, while the other clamp is secured below the caudal lamina. These two clamps are secured with a screw that will sequentially approximate these two clamps. Clamp application is accomplished bilaterally. As with interspinous wiring, laminar clamps provide little rotational stability.

Facet Wiring

Facet wiring was initially described in the stabilization of the cervical spine after a laminectomy.[16] After a hole is placed within the inferior facet of the vertebra above, a wire is placed through the facet process. Then, a bone strut is secured to the wire. In addition, facet wiring may be combined with interspinous wiring. Bilateral facet to spinous process fusion has been described by Cahill and colleagues.[15] Double-braided wire is passed through the inferior facet of the superior vertebra and through the spinous process of the inferior vertebra.

Lateral Mass Screw-Rods and Screw-Plates

The technique for the placement of lateral mass screws has been exhaustively reviewed. After exposure of the lateral mass is accomplished in the prone position, a high-speed drill is used to place a hole in the exact center of the lateral mass. Then, with a drill and tap, the starter hole is lengthened to the future screw length. Previously, we used a screw-plate technique, as designed by Roy-Camille. Currently, the screw-plate technique has been replaced by a screw-rod technique.

Thus, after drilling and tapping, polyaxial screws may be placed within the lateral mass of each level. Similar polyaxial screws can also be placed within the pedicles of the affected levels. Then, a prebent rod may be placed on the top-loading system and secured with screw caps.

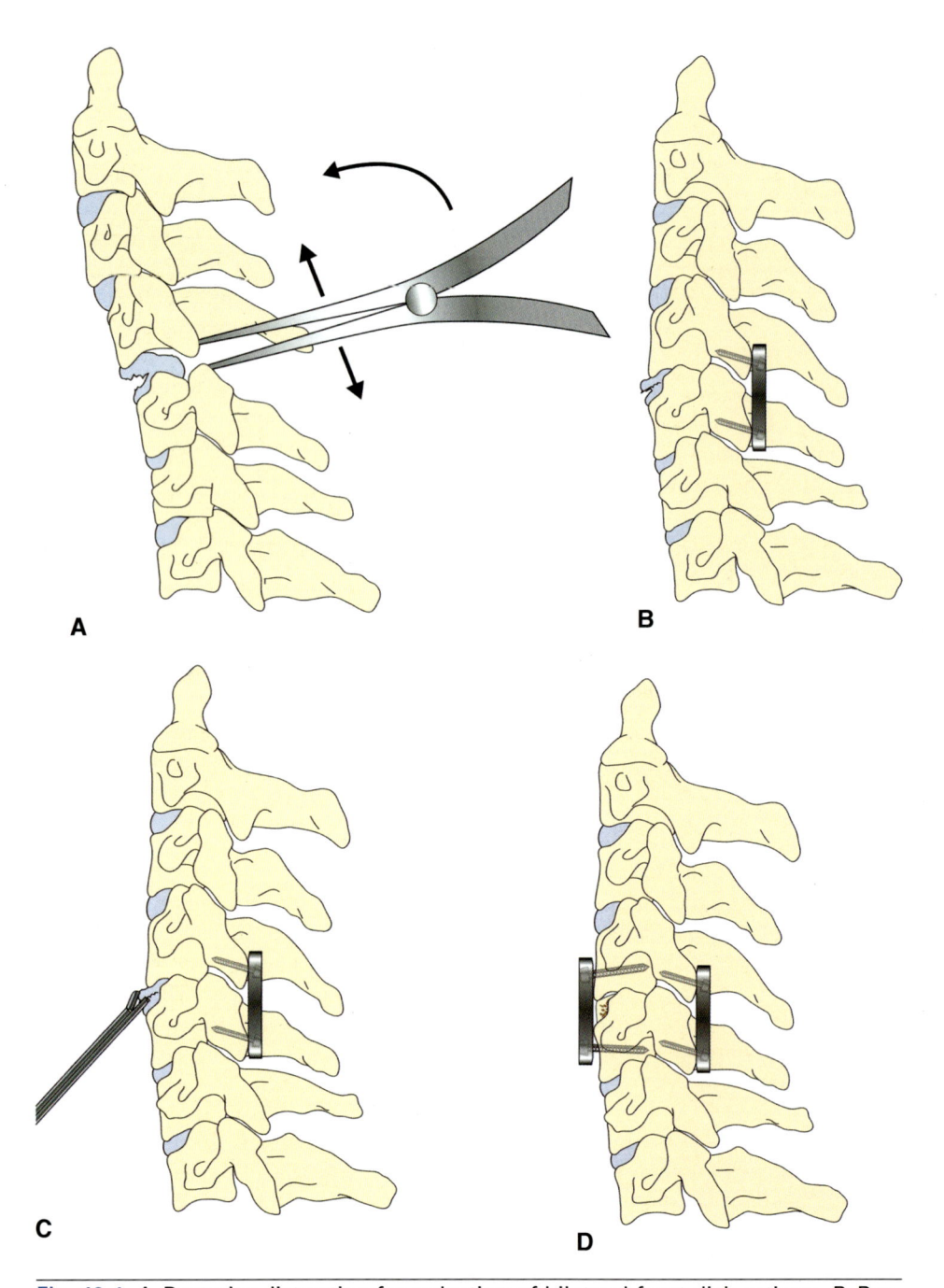

Fig. 40-4 A, Posterior distraction for reduction of bilateral facet dislocations. B, Posterior stabilization with a lateral mass screw-plate assembly. C, Anterior diskectomy at C4-C5. D, Anterior C4-C5 stabilization with an interbody graft and anterior screw-plate assembly.

ANTERIOR APPROACH

An anterior approach can be attempted for reduction and fixation. Although disk herniations are uncommon with facet dislocations, reduction of a facet dislocation with associated disk herniations is considered an indication for anterior reduction and stabilization. Associated herniated disks occur less than 5% of the time.[17]

As with a posterior approach, with intraoperative monitoring and fluoroscopy, reduction may frequently be obtained under general anesthesia with minimal distraction.

As with the posterior approach, descriptions of anterior reduction have been mentioned via distraction. Distraction can be accomplished via several different mechanisms. Distraction posts can be placed the involved levels (Fig. 40-6), or external distractor can be placed after a diskectomy is

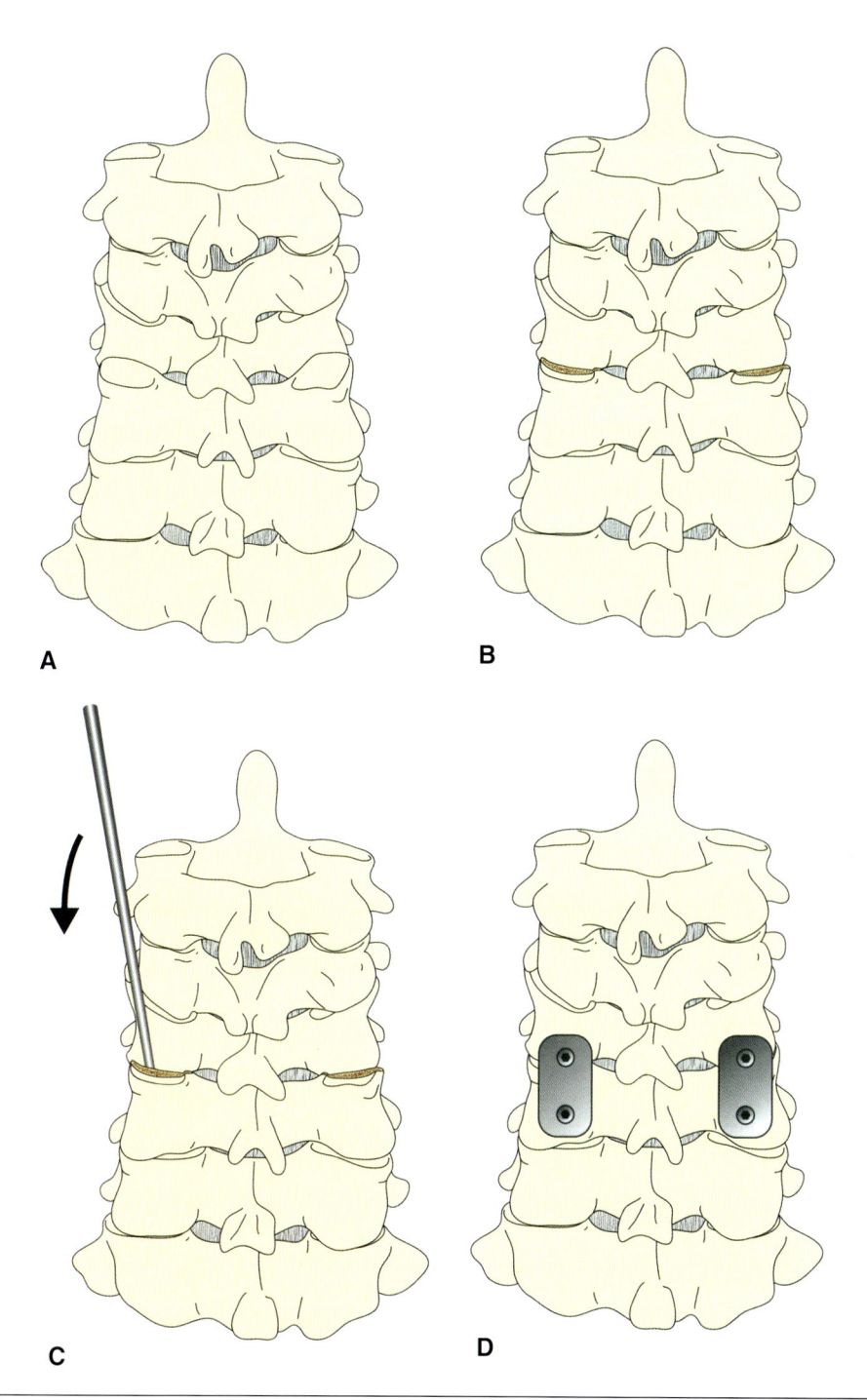

CHAPTER 40 Subaxial Cervical Spinal Injuries and Facet Dislocation Injuries

Fig. 40-5 *A*, Posterior view of C4-C5 bilateral facet dislocation. *B*, With difficulty in reduction, the superior facets of C5 are drilled bilaterally. *C*, With minimal distraction, the dislocation is reduced. *D*, Posterior stabilization is continued with a screw-plate system depicted.

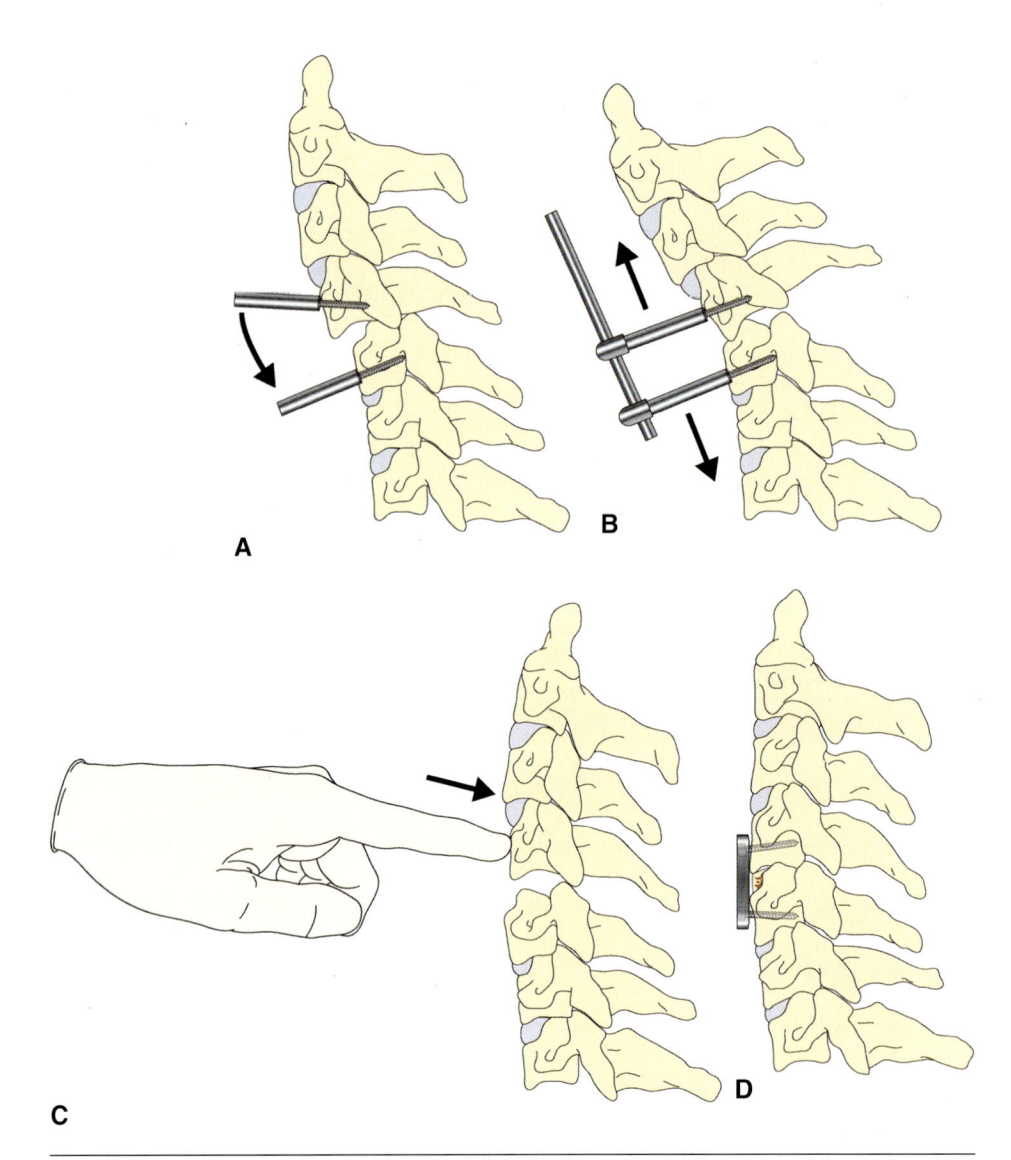

Fig. 40-6 *A*, Lateral view of a bilateral facet dislocation with distraction pins placed within C4 and C5. *B*, With distraction, reduction may be achieved. *C*, If reduction is not achieved with distraction, downward pressure may be applied to assist with this reduction process. *D*, Stabilization is accomplished with an interbody graft and screw-plate construct.

performed. In addition, a vertebral spreader may accomplish a similar task (Fig. 40-7).

POSTOPERATIVE CARE

With internal fixation (whether anterior, posterior, or both), we continue to use a hard collar for external bracing. Otherwise, management is dependent on the level of spinal cord injury, the extent of injury (neurologic and mechanical), other comorbidities, and associated injuries.

CONCLUSION

The management of facet dislocations has two goals: retaining/restoring neurologic function while maintaining mechanical stability. Both anterior and posterior approaches have been demonstrated to be effective in reduction of unilateral and bilateral facet dislocation. In addition, both anterior and posterior approaches for spinal fixation have been demonstrated to be adequate. With this said, the surgical approach in the management of patients with a facet dislocation has to be individualized to each patient.

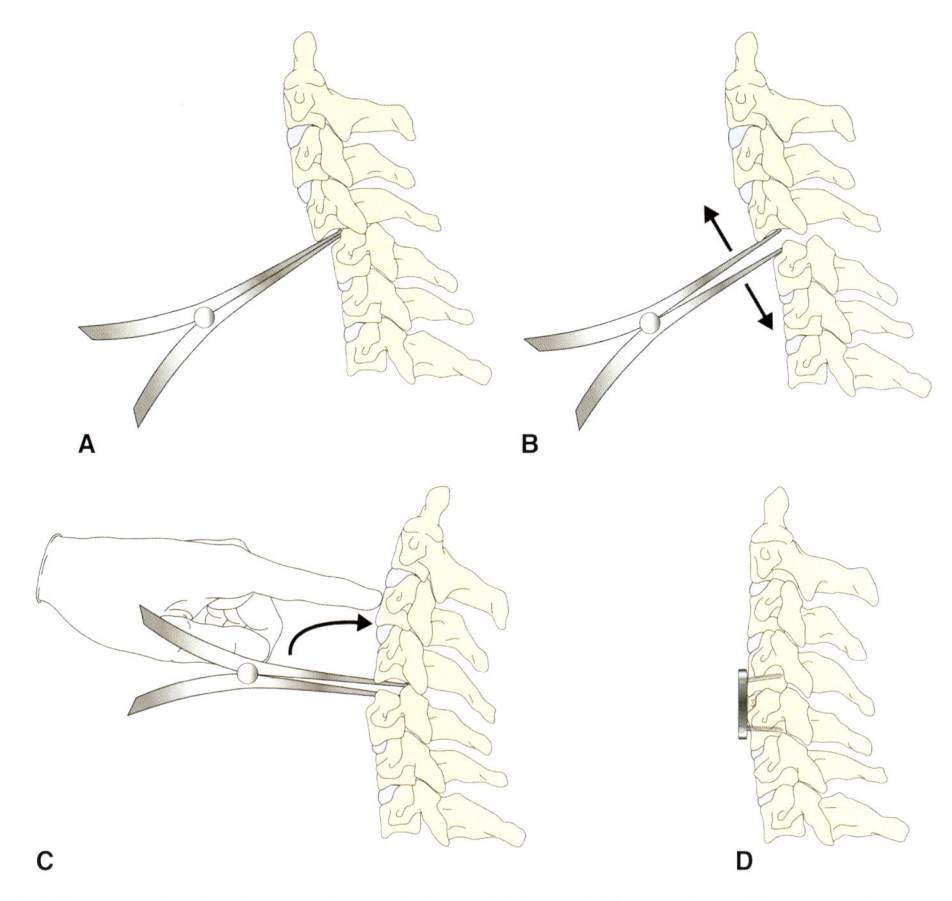

Fig. 40-7 *A,* Lateral view of a bilateral facet dislocation at C4-C5. *B,* Distraction is applied to the affected level. *C,* Minimal downward pressure is applied, rostral to the dislocation. *D,* Anterior fixation with a graft and screw-plate construct.

References

1. Bedbrook GM: Spinal injuries with tetraplegia and paraplegia. J Bone Joint Surg Br 1979;61-B:267–284.
2. Allen BL Jr, Ferguson RL, Lehmann TR, et al: A mechanistic classification of closed, indirect fractures and dislocations of the lower cervical spine. Spine 1982;7:1–27.
3. Argenson C, Lovet J, Sanouiller JL, et al: Traumatic rotatory displacement of the lower cervical spine. Spine 1988;13:767–773.
4. Maiman DJ, Sances A Jr, Myklebust JB, et al: Compression injuries of the cervical spine: A biomechanical analysis. Neurosurgery 1983;13:254–260.
5. Maiman DJ, Barolat G, Larson SJ: Management of bilateral locked facets of the cervical spine. Neurosurgery 1986;18:542–547.
6. Norrell H: The treatment of unstable spinal fractures and dislocations. Clin Neurosurg 1978;25:193–208.
7. O'Brien PJ, Schweigel JF, Thompson WJ: Dislocations of the lower cervical spine. J Trauma 1982;22:710–714.
8. Clark CR, Igram CM, el-Khoury GY, et al: Radiographic evaluation of cervical spine injuries. Spine 1988;13:742–747.
9. Lind B, Sihlbom H, Nordwall A: Halo-vest treatment of unstable traumatic cervical spine injuries. Spine 1988;13:425–432.
10. Stauffer ES: Neurologic recovery following injuries to the cervical spinal cord and nerve roots. Spine 1984;9:532–534.
11. Management of acute central cervical spinal cord injuries. Neurosurgery 2002;50:S166–S172.
12. Stauffer ES, Rhoades ME: Surgical stabilization of the cervical spine after trauma. Arch Surg 1976;111:652–657.
13. Roy-Camille R, Saillant G, Mazel C, et al: The surgical treatment of post-traumatic vertebral deformities. Ital J Orthop Traumatol 1986;12:419–426.
14. Benzel EC, Kesterson L: Posterior cervical interspinous compression wiring and fusion for mid to low cervical spinal injuries. J Neurosurg 1989;70:893–899.
15. Cahill DW, Bellegarrigue R, Ducker TB: Bilateral facet to spinous process fusion: A new technique for posterior spinal fusion after trauma. Neurosurgery 1983;13:1–4.
16. Callahan RA, Johnson RM, Margolis RN, et al: Cervical facet fusion for control of instability following laminectomy. J Bone Joint Surg Am 1977;59:991–1002.
17. Harrington JF, Likavec MJ, Smith AS: Disc herniation in cervical fracture subluxation. Neurosurgery 1991;29:374–379.

CHAPTER 41

HOANG N. LE
DANIEL H. KIM

Cervicothoracic Junction Fractures

INTRODUCTION

Approximately 9% of traumatic cervical fractures will occur at the cervicothoracic junction and can be missed unless adequate films are obtained. This junction is an inherently unstable area, as it represents a transition zone both anatomically and biomechanically. Stabilization of cervicothoracic instabilities should favor an aggressive approach, for the demands on the fixation construct are high. Anterior stabilization procedures alone will have a failure rate of 50%. Posterior fixation is biomechanically superior over that of a standalone anterior procedure, but the posterior construct should span multiple segments to minimize the risk of hardware failure. Often, neural decompression, anterior column reconstruction, and stabilization can all be achieved from a posterior approach. With complete destruction of all three spinal columns and its associated ligamentous complex, a 360-degree approach will yield the greatest stability. In this chapter, we describe our surgical techniques for treating fractures of the cervicothoracic junction causing instability.

CLASSIFICATION OF CERVICOTHORACIC JUNCTION FRACTURES

Although there are no accepted classification schemes specific for spinal fractures of the cervicothoracic junction, classification schemes based on mechanism of injury applied for lower cervical fractures can be extrapolated to the cervicothoracic junction. Despite a lack of a universally accepted system, the one described by Ducker appears to be the simplest. This system does not include gunshot and penetrating injuries.

FLEXION DISLOCATION INJURIES (Fig. 41-1)

These injuries represent more than 50% of all cervical injuries and are potentially the most unstable. Included in this group are the unilateral and bilateral jumped facets. Forces may be translational, rotational, or distractive. Posterior ligamentous disruption is significant with minimal damage to the anterior column.

Unilateral Facet Subluxation

The mechanism of injury is hyperflexion and rotation. The superior facet overrides the inferior facet and the corresponding interspinous ligament, and the joint capsule of the affected facet is completely ruptured.

Bilateral Facet Subluxation

The mechanism of injury is predominantly hyperflexion with some distraction. All the ligaments, including the interspinous, facet capsules, posterior longitudinal ligament (PLL), and annulus are ruptured. The anterior longitudinal ligament (ALL) may be spared. Subluxation is greater than 50% of the anteroposterior (AP) dimension of the vertebral body and is associated with a high rate of spinal cord injury.

FLEXION COMPRESSION INJURIES (Fig. 41-2)

Wedge Compression

The mechanism of injury is hyperflexion, causing compression of the anterior aspect of the vertebral body. Posterior elements are intact.

Teardrop Flexion Fracture

Less than 50% of the height of the vertebral body is lost. ALL is usually intact, with the teardrop fragment attached to it. Posterior ligamentous structures, including PLL, are usually affected. Extension helps to reduce the deformity. Compression of less than one third of vertebral body height with no additional ligamentous instability can be managed in a soft collar and is considered stable. Greater than 50% anterior compression is considered unstable. Stabilization is best achieved from behind.

CHAPTER 41 Cervicothoracic Junction Fractures

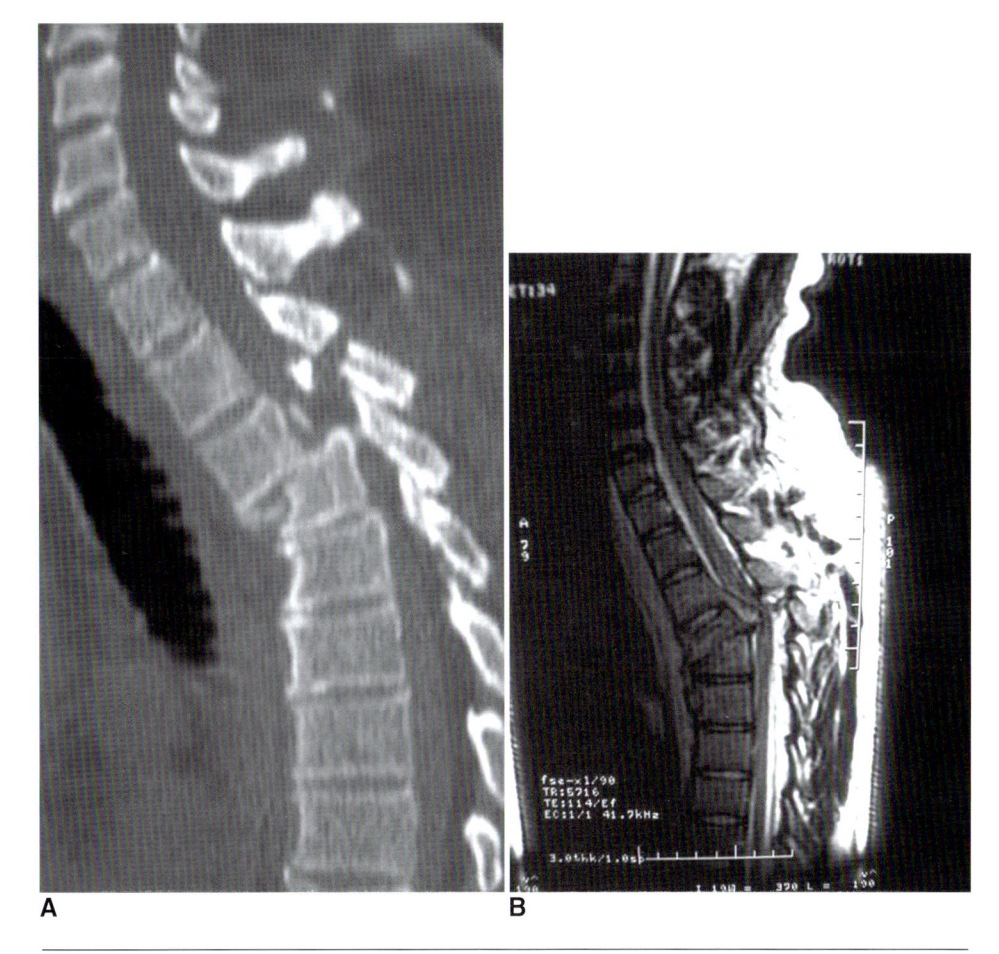

Fig. 41-1 Flexion dislocation injuries. *A*, Sagittal computed tomograph of reconstruction in a patient with bilateral jumped facets. *B*, Magnetic resonance image in same patient with severe cord compression.

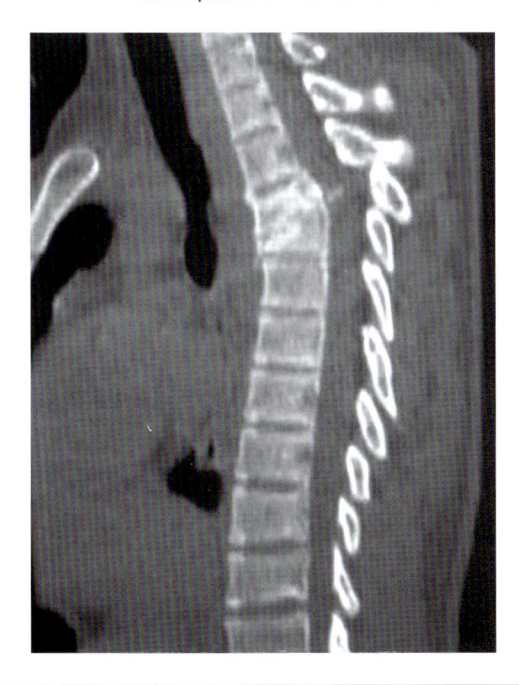

Fig. 41-2 Flexion compression injury, computed tomograph of sagittal reconstruction.

COMPRESSION BURST FRACTURES

Compression burst fractures are axial loading injuries to a spine held in neutral/slightly flexed position. The force is absorbed by the vertebral body, which bursts. These injuries range from a simple sagittal fracture through the body to significant comminution of vertebral body fractures with continuation into the neural arch structures. Retropulsion of the fragments into the spinal canal can cause spinal cord injury. The injury, however, is often incomplete.

EXTENSION INJURIES

Extension injuries may occur with distraction or compression. Minor distraction-extension injuries result in the failure of the ALL with an associated chip fracture of the injured vertebral body. In severe cases, PLL may be injured, with resultant retrolisthesis of the superior vertebrae. Compression extension injuries usually result in fracture of the posterior elements. The majority of these patients are neurologically intact.

SURGICAL INDICATIONS

- Inability to obtain reduction
- Inability to maintain reduction
- Fragments in spinal canal with incomplete spinal cord injury (SCI)
- Progressive neurologic deficit from spinal instability
- Persistent compression causing neurologic symptoms
- Chronic progressive deformity

CERVICOTHORACIC JUNCTION ANATOMIC CONSIDERATIONS

Anatomic understanding of the cervicothoracic junction is required for accurate screw placement and choosing the appropriate fixation technique. Because the cervicothoracic junction represents a transition zone, significant anatomic variations are common. The lower cervical laminae are thinner and weaker compared to upper thoracic vertebrae. This, together with a narrow spinal canal, often limits the use of hook and rod stabilization at the cervicothoracic junction. Use of lateral mass screws should take into consideration the location of the vertebral artery and the spinal nerves. Compared to T1, the C7 vertebrae have a closer anatomic relationship with the vertebral artery. The vertebral artery will be at risk of injury if a lateral mass screw is too long or directed less than 14 degrees laterally from the midpoint of the lateral mass of C7. These neurovascular relationships may change with significant kyphotic/scoliotic deformity of the spine and can subject them to greater risk of injury with posterior screw fixation. Aiming too caudal with the lateral mass screws may lead to spinal nerve injury. Furthermore, the C6 and C7 lateral masses are the thinnest in the cervical spine, as they are in transition into becoming transverse processes. A gentle touch will be needed to obtain adequate screw purchase of the lateral masses at C6 and C7.

Although in the midcervical spine, the facet/lateral mass forms a substantial complex into which a screw may be securely anchored, this complex frequently provides inadequate screw purchase at C7 and below. Traditional techniques of lateral mass plating may not produce a biomechanically stable construct at the cervicothoracic junction. Pedicle screw constructs, however, have shown excellent biomechanical stability in this region.

A number of careful anatomic studies of the cervicothoracic pedicles have been conducted to assess the feasibility and safety of placing cervicothoracic pedicle screws. The mean pedicle width increases on average from 5 mm at C5 to 8 mm at T1 and then decreases to 4.5 mm at T5. Although the pedicles at C7, T1, and T2 are frequently large enough to permit placement of a 3.5-mm screw, those above and below were usually significantly smaller. T3 to T5 will often have small narrow pedicles that prevent their screw placement. Incorporating this area will often require the use of thoracic hooks. The pedicle angle also decreases from 50 degrees medially at C5 to 11 degrees medially at T5 vertebrae. However, the pedicle length increases gradually from C5 to T5 vertebrae without any significant differences between adjacent vertebral levels. The mean distance of the spinal nerve to the superior and inferior pedicles ranged between 0.8 and 2.3 mm, with greater separation between the nerve and the superior pedicle. Thus, pedicle screw violation of the superior cortex may place the nerve at higher risk of injury than inferior cortex violation.

SURGICAL TECHNIQUES

A growing number of options for posterior cervicothoracic instrumentation now exist (Fig. 41-3). They range from the application of a simple tension band to complex hook, rod, and screw constructs. The application of tension bands effectively resists flexion and distraction. In cases of pure ligamentous disruption, a tension band may be the only intervention required. Tension bands usually take the form of interspinous wiring, which, when given the long lever arm from the instantaneous axis of rotation, can exert tremendous resistive forces. This simple technique is safe, fast, and a useful adjunct to other techniques.

As the cervicothoracic junction is under significant biomechanical stress, surgical fixation should incorporate several segments above and below the injured site. For the most part, current stabilization techniques of the cervicothoracic junction will require experience with cervical lateral mass or pedicle screws placement and with upper and lower thoracic pedicle screws placement as well as the use thoracic transverse, pedicle, and laminar hooks (Fig. 41-4). Sublaminar wiring techniques can add to construct stability when cross-links are used and the lamina is intact. This will be especially useful in the cervical area, as there will be a tendency for cervical screw pullout. By using two cross-links as part of a screw-rod construct, quadrilateral stability can also be achieved (Fig. 41-5).

Cervical lateral mass screws placement—general guidelines:

- Starting at the midpoint of the lateral mass, aim approximately 30 degrees cephalad and 30 degrees lateral.
- The lateral angle will be less of an issue if shorter screws are used.
- We generally use 14-mm screws for the average male and 12-mm screws for the average female. At these screw lengths, injury to the vertebral artery is unlikely.
- A handheld power drill is preferred for drilling out the pilot hole, followed by tapping to the full length of the screw.
- The C7 lateral mass may be small and thin and can fracture during screw placement. A pedicle screw at this site is preferable. If T1 and T2 pedicle screws are placed, one may skip C7 because these screws may "run" into each other.

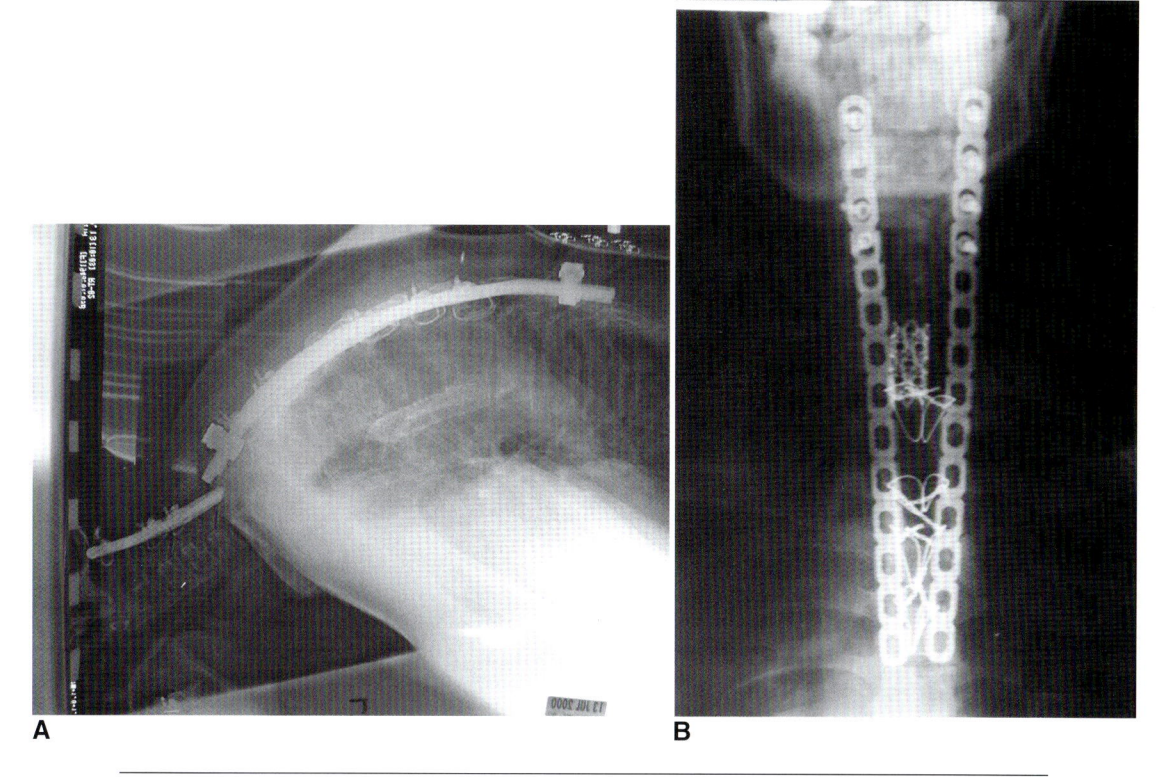

CHAPTER 41 Cervicothoracic Junction Fractures   347

Fig. 41-3 Traditional ways of cervicothoracic stabilization. *A*, Sublaminar wiring with Luque rods. Interlinking the thoracic area with cervical area was difficult. *B*, Cervicothoracic plates. Holes were constrained and thoracic stabilization methods were suboptimal.

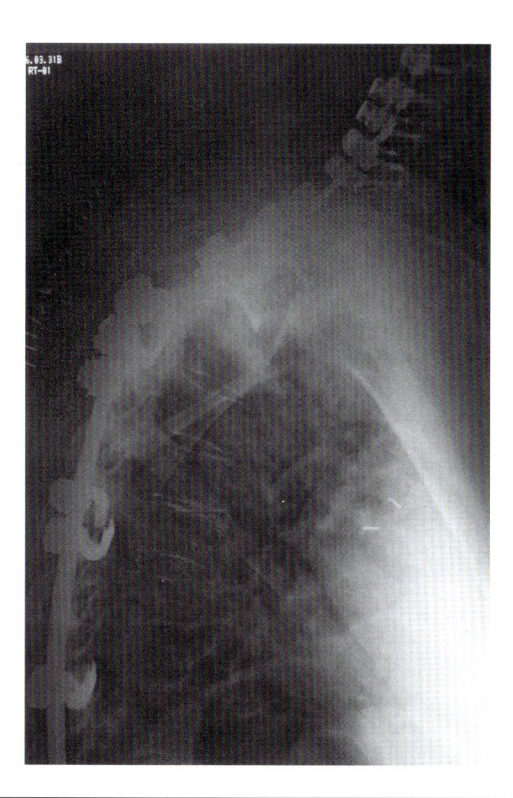

Fig. 41-4 Note the use of cervical lateral mass screws, upper thoracic pedicle screws, and midthoracic hooks. Dual diameter rods and interlinking systems were not yet available.

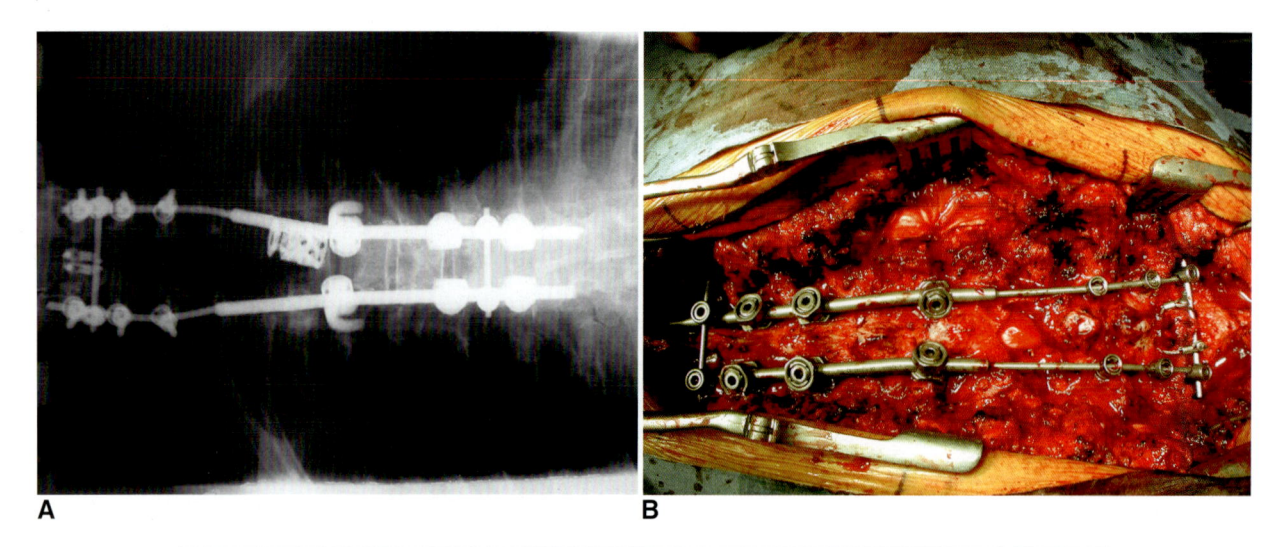

Fig. 41-5 Quadrilateral stability. *A,* Anteroposterior cervicothoracic x-ray. Note the use of transition rods and cervical and thoracic cross-links to achieve quadrilateral stability. Cervical lateral mass screws are used in combination with thoracic hooks. Cage placement was performed through a costotransversectomy approach. *B,* Intraoperative photograph. Note the double cross-link use, thoracic hooks, cervical lateral mass screws, and a cervical sublaminar wire secured to the top cross-link.

C7, T1, T2 pedicle screws placement (Fig. 41-6):
- The most reliable technique involves making a small laminotomy and palpating for the pedicle.
- Superior, medial, and inferior borders of the pedicle should be palpated.
- Screw trajectory should hug the medial wall.
- Use of a handheld power drill is preferable, followed by tapping (Fig. 41-7).
- Usually, 3.5-mm-width 20- to 22-mm screw should be of adequate length.
- Posterior stabilization of the cervicothoracic junction should incorporate these screws whenever possible.

Thoracic hooks (Fig. 41-8):
- Transverse hooks in combination with pedicle-facet hooks are preferable to laminar hooks.
- Transverse hooks are usually downgoing, and pedicle-facet hooks are upgoing.
- In placing pedicle-facet hooks, the inferior aspect of the superior articulating facet should be drilled out to expose the facet joint.

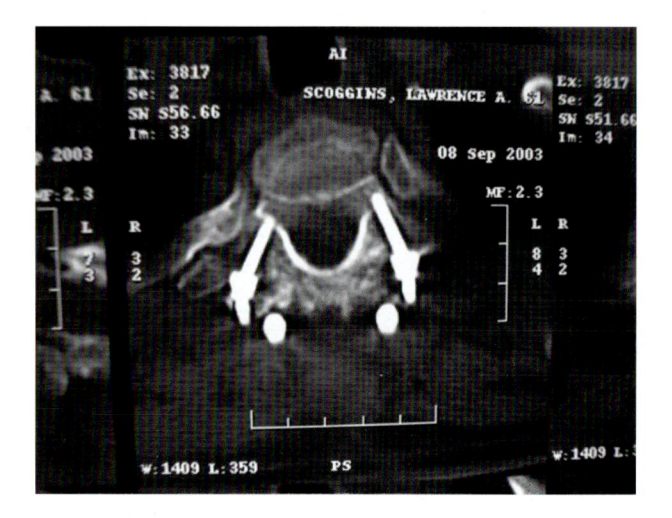

Fig. 41-6 Axial computed tomograph of a T1 pedicle screw.

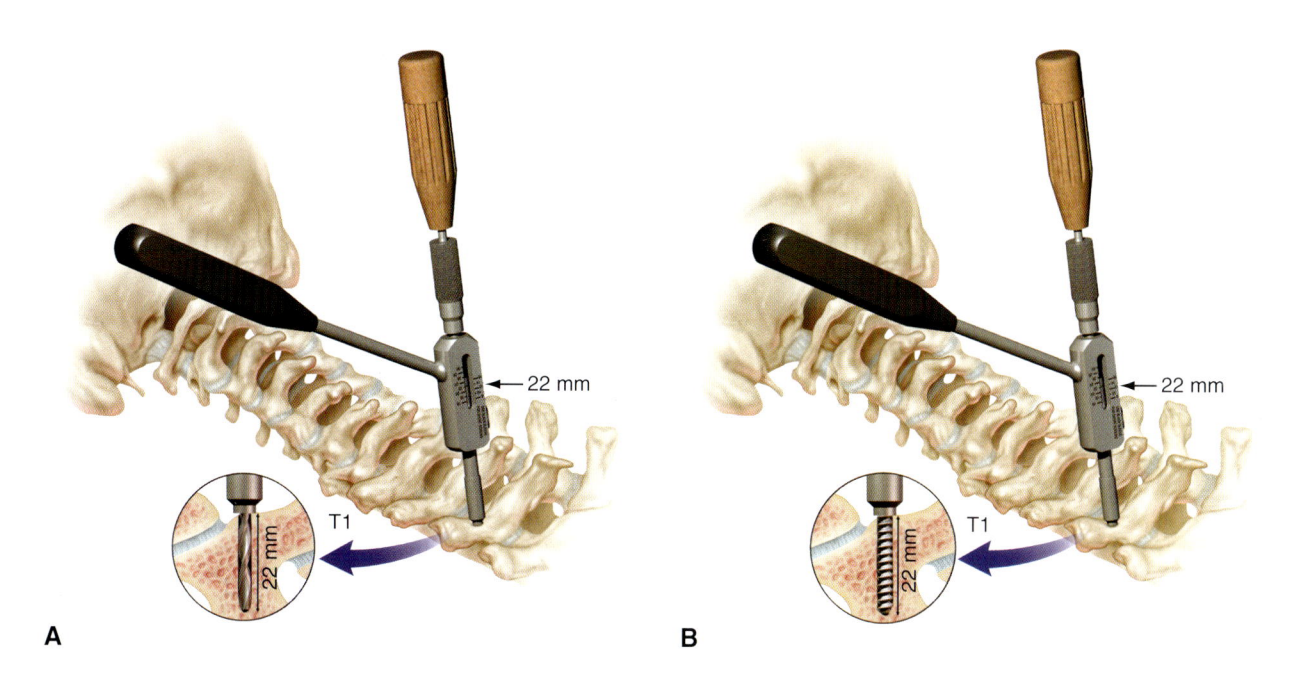

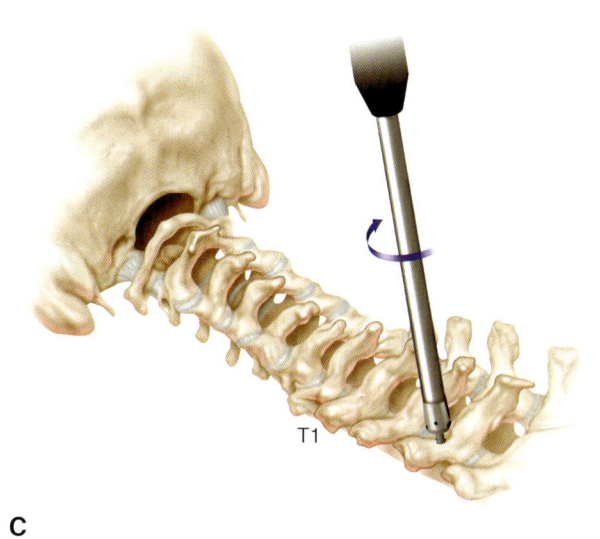

Fig. 41-7 Placement of a T1 pedicle screw. *A,* Pedicle is drilled. *B,* Drilled hole is tapped. *C,* Screw is placed into final position at depth of 20 to 22 mm.

Fig. 41-8 Note the placement of downgoing transverse hooks and upgoing pedicle hooks.

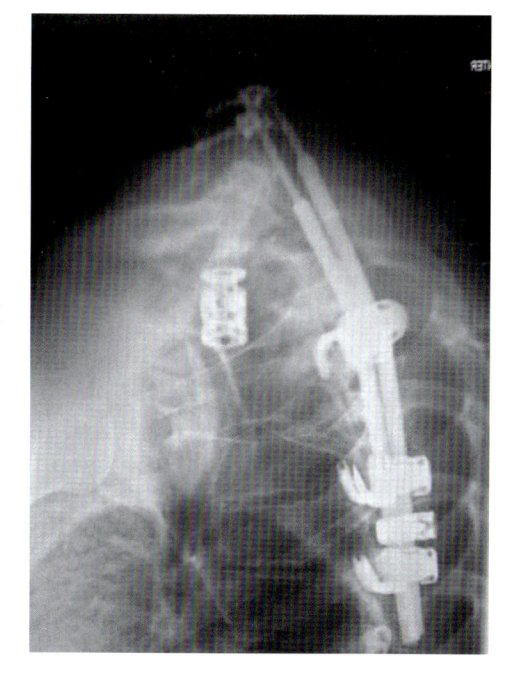

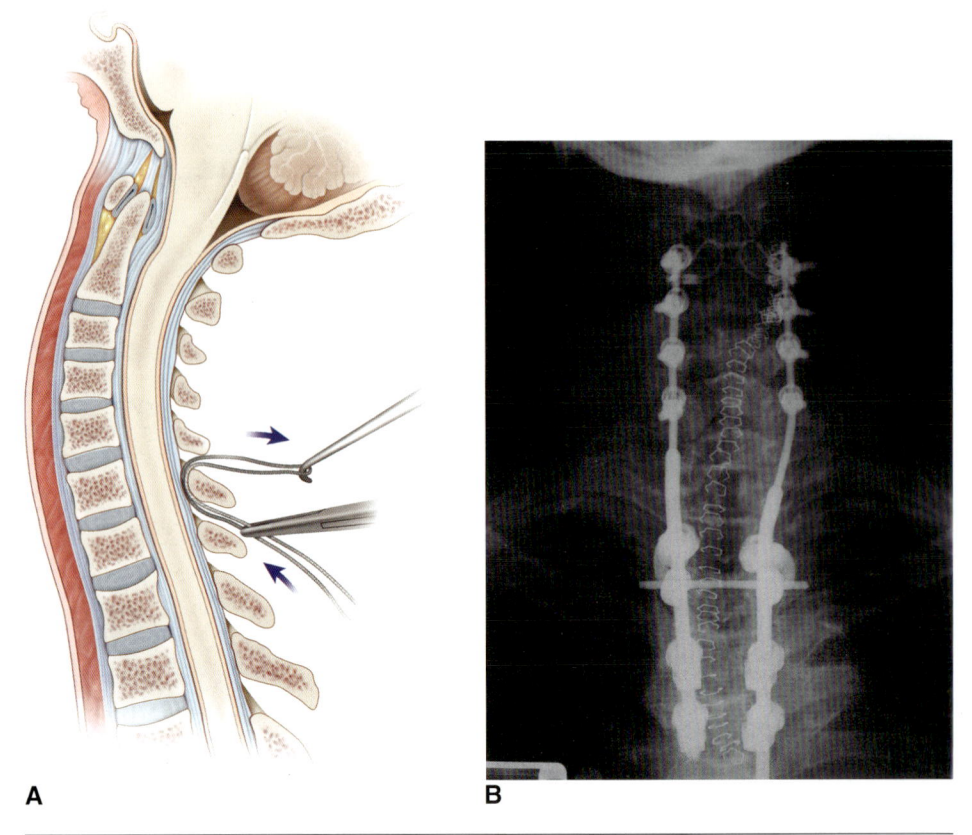

Fig. 41-9 *A*, Placement of a sublaminar Songer cable. *B*, Sublaminar wiring with loops around the cross-link in the cervical area will prevent upper screw pullout.

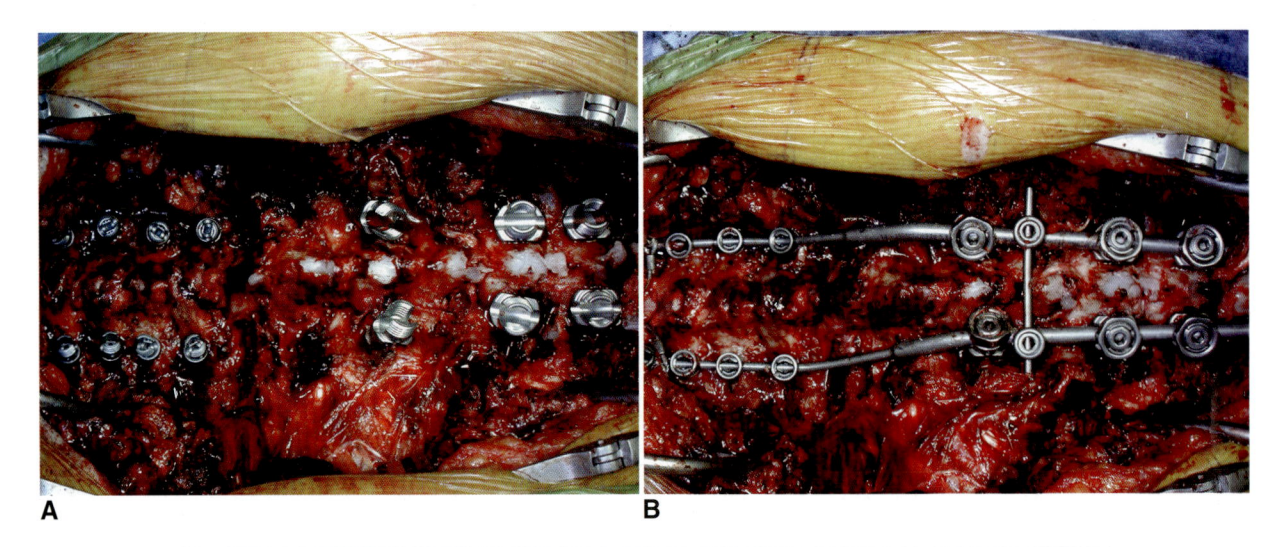

Fig. 41-10 Intraoperative photograph. *A*, Cervical lateral mass screws and thoracic hooks are placed prior to final rod placement. *B*, Final construct with transition rods: A sublaminar wire is placed at the top.

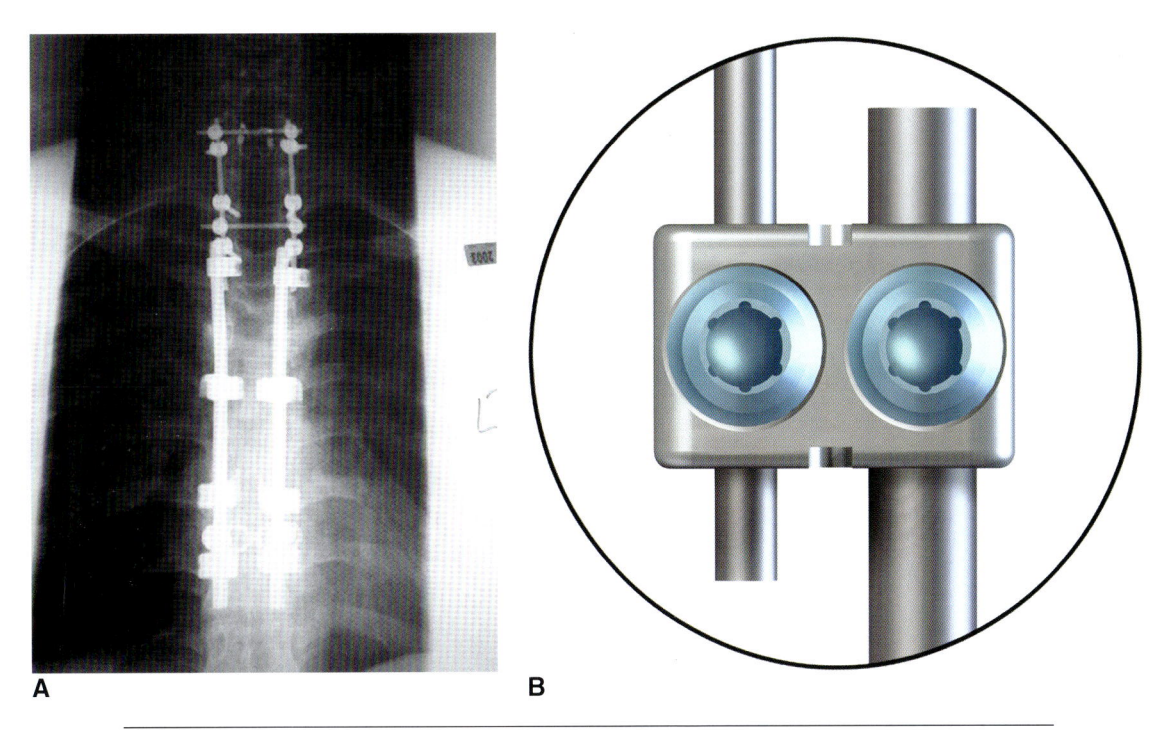

Fig. 41-11 Dual diameter rods and connectors. *A*, X-ray showing the use of dual diameter rods and linking connectors. Cross-links in cervical and thoracic area creates quadrilateral stability in both areas. *B*, Sample connector for the dual diameter rod.

- The pedicle-facet hook will "hook" underneath the superior articulating facet toward the direction of the pedicle.

Sublaminar wiring (Fig. 41-9*A*):
- Songer cables are ideal.
- Sublaminar wiring with loops around the cross-link in the cervical area will prevent upper screw pullout (see Fig. 41-9*B*). Alternatively, a C2 pedicle screw can be placed.

Rods specialized for the cervicothoracic junction:
- Transition rods (Fig. 41-10).
- Dual diameter rods with linking connectors (Fig. 41-11).

CHAPTER 42

ISSADA THONGTRANGAN
HOANG N. LE
JON PARK
DANIEL H. KIM

Thoracic and Thoracolumbar Fractures

INTRODUCTION

Thoracolumbar spine is the transitional zone between the stiff thoracic cage and the mobile lumbar spine. Therefore, it is a vulnerable region for injury, including fracture and dislocation.

Classification for the thoracolumbar injury is still controversial. Currently, there are several classifications for thoracolumbar burst fracture in order to predict the prognosis and also guide the treatment options. Moreover, proper surgical procedure for the thoracolumbar area is still debatable. Nevertheless, multifactorial factors should be considered to dictate the appropriate treatment for the patients.

The posterior procedures have a long history and have been popularized among spinal surgeons. In the remote past, laminectomy had been advocated for spinal injuries, unfortunately the outcomes were poor secondary to postoperative instability and deterioration of the neurologic status.[1] Therefore, laminectomy only has been abandoned and is not an acceptable procedure at the thoracolumabr junction, particularly in the treatment of burst fractures. Posterior stabilization with instrumentation, which was a hook-rod system, had been popularized for spinal deformities by Harrington.[2] It was used for reduction, correction of the deformity, and stabilization of thoracolumbar fractures before the pedicle screw era.

Recently, the anterior procedure has been advocated for direct decompression of the retropulsed fragment as well as stabilization with instrumentation. There have been many anterior stabilization systems developed in the past decade. Several published reports also support the anterior procedure rather than the posterior procedure.

The purposes of the chapter are to review the appropriate indications for surgical treatment of thoracolumbar fractures and to review the surgical technique via anterior approach.

CLASSIFICATION

There are several classifications for thoracolumbar fractures based on presumed mechanisms of injury, anatomic pattern of disruption, and radiographic measures of the severity of structural deformity. Unfortunately, there is no universal and ideal classification yet; for example, none of the currently used classification systems incorporates neurologic status.

ANATOMIC CLASSIFICATION

Holdsworth[3] first developed a "two-column" concept, assessing anterior and posterior column to determine "instability." The anterior column consists of the vertebral body, disk, the anterior longitudinal ligament (ALL), and the posterior longitudinal ligament (PLL). It transmits the compressive load. The posterior column consists of the neural arch and the interspinous ligament. Disruption of more than one column defines instability.

Denis[3-5] modified Holdsworth's work and popularized the three-column concept. In this classification the anterior column consists of the anterior two thirds of the vertebral body, disk, and the ALL. The middle column consists of the posterior third of the vertebral body, disk, and PLL. The posterior column includes the pedicle, neural arch, spinous process, facet joint, transverse process, and the interspinous ligament. Instability was defined as a failure of two of the three columns.

MECHANISM OF INJURY

Holdsworth[3] was the first to describe four common mechanisms of injury: flexion, flexion with rotation, extension, and compression. This classification was well accepted until Ferguson and Allen further modified the classification based on the six degrees of freedom of spinal motion in three

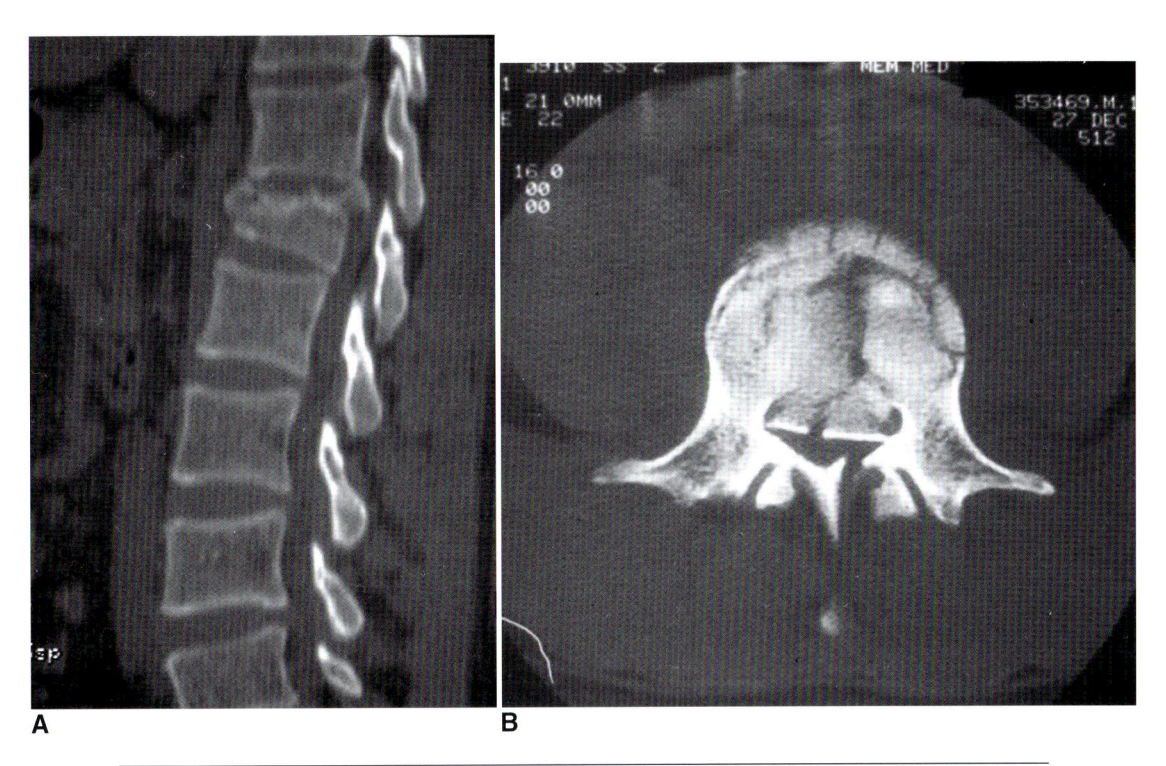

Fig. 42-1 Sagittal (A) and axial (B) computed tomographic scan of the thoracolumbar spine demonstrating burst fracture with significant retropulsion fragment and associated laminar fracture.

distinguished axes: axial compression, distraction, flexion, extension, rotation, and shear.[6,7]

Axial Compression

The anterior column fails under compression, causing fracture, and if the load continues, the vertebral body explodes, the pedicles are driven apart, and the middle column retropulses posteriorly, resulting in a "burst" fracture (Fig. 42-1).

Some authors defined "stable" burst as a burst fracture with intact posterior ligaments, whereas several authors maintain that "stable" burst does not exist.[8]

Flexion-Compression

This type of injury accounted for nearly 50% of the thoracolumbar fractures. It causes tensile stresses of the posterior ligamentous complex in addition to a "burst" of the vertebral body. Classic characteristics include failure of the end plate under nucleus, anterior vertebral body compression, middle column retropulsion, facet-joint capsule disruption, and interspinous ligament failure. Disruption of the posterior ligament leads to progressive kyphosis, pain, and neurologic deterioration.

Distraction

Characteristics of this fracture depend on the location of the center of rotation at the time of injury. When the axis of rotation is in the anterior vertebral body, the result is a compression fracture of the anterior vertebral body associated with posterior ligament disruption and unilateral or bilateral facet joint disruption or dislocation.

When the axis of rotation is anterior to the anterior vertebral column, all three columns are failed under distraction force. This can occur either through the bone or soft tissue. Type I is a classic "chance" fracture (Fig. 42-2), in which the spinous process fails first and the distraction force passes through all bony elements and emerges in a variable position within the vertebral body. In type 2 the force enters the interspinous ligament, whereas type 3 is complicated by rotational force. Because this severe injury is associated with the "deceleration" phase, associated life-threatening vascular injuries are possible.

Rotation

The facet joints and annulus are the primary restraint against rotational forces. One facet joint may fracture and dislocate anteriorly, whereas the other side fails under tension with disruption of the joint capsule. With further rotational force

354   SECTION IV   SPINAL TRAUMA

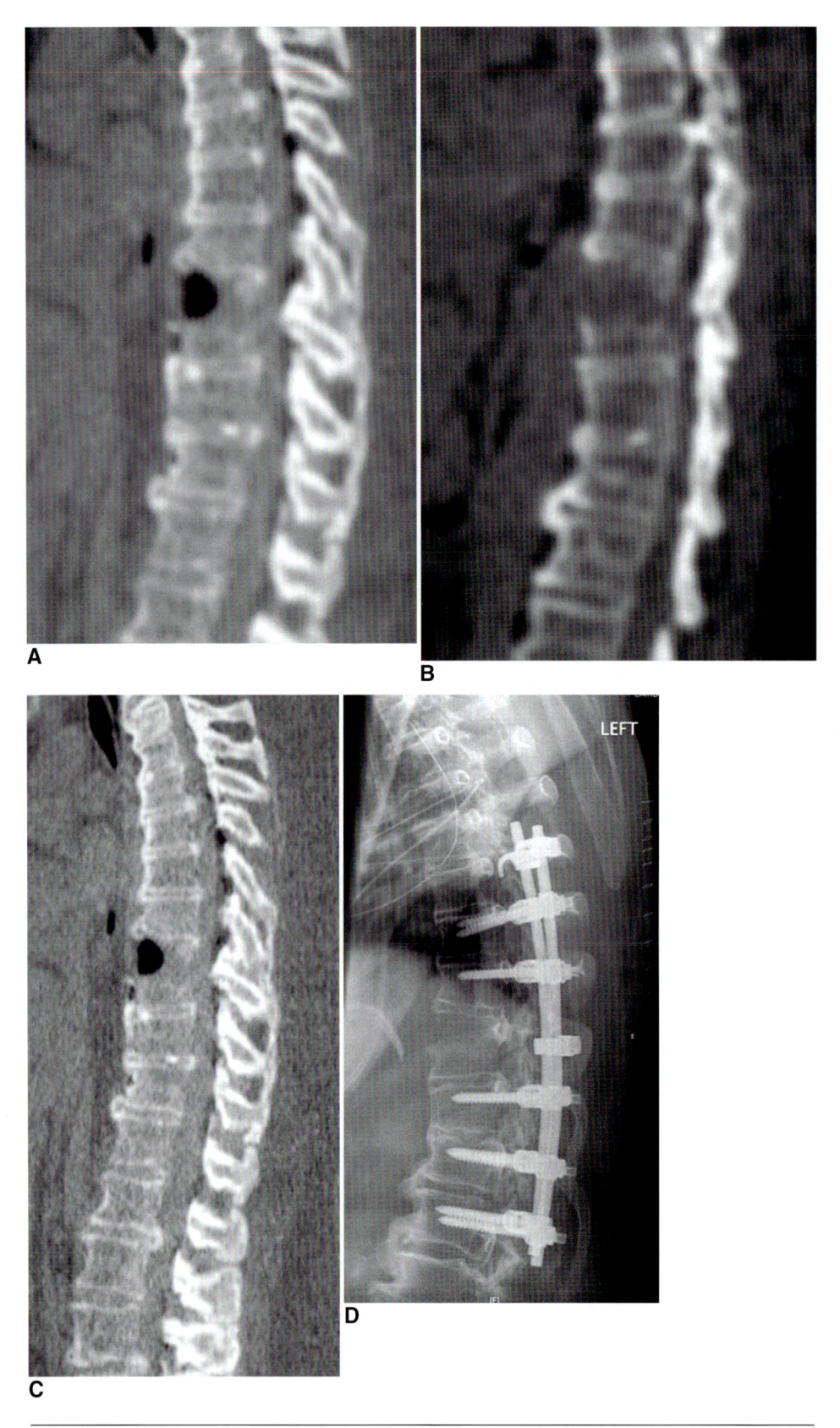

Fig. 42-2 *A* to *C*, Reformatted sagittal computed tomograph of the thoracic spine showing a "chance" fracture of T9 with air entrapped into the fracture site. This patient also suffered from associated bilateral hemopneumothorax. *D*, Postoperative x-ray showing posterior reduction, fusion, and instrumentation in T9 chance fracture.

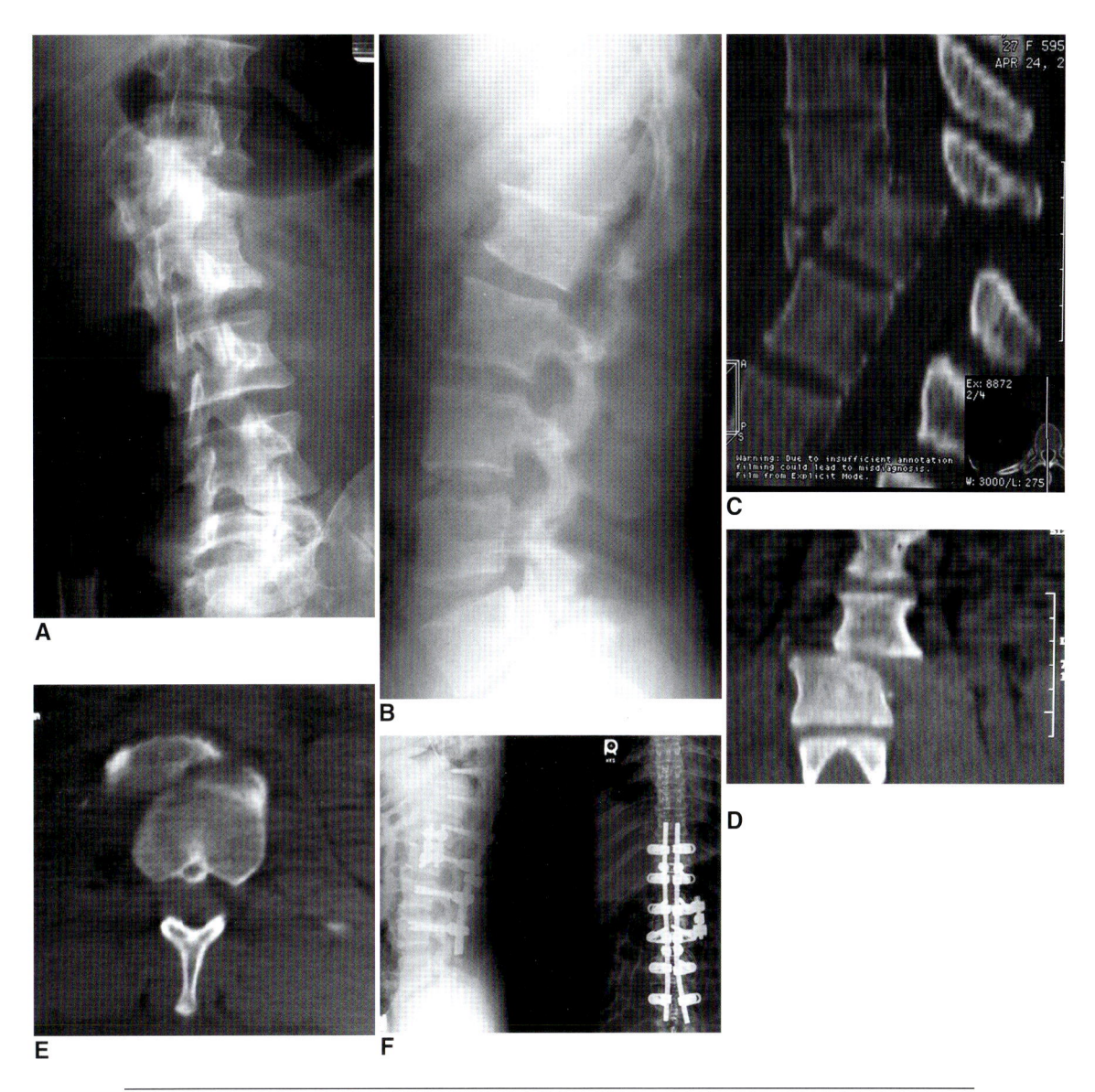

CHAPTER 42 Thoracic and Thoracolumbar Fractures   355

Fig. 42-3 Anteroposterior (A) and lateral (B) radiographic images showing a fracture dislocation at the thoracolumbar junction with severe displacement. Reformatted sagittal (C) and coronal (D) computed tomographs demonstrating a fracture dislocation of the thoracolumbar region with severe displacement. E, Axial computed tomograph shows double shadow of the vertebral body in the same image which can be seen only in the fracture dislocation injury. F, Postoperative x-rays showing a combined posterior and anterior reconstruction. The alignment is nicely maintained.

anteriorly, the superior vertebral body may fail and cause significant instability. Neurologic deterioration is known to be associated with this type of injury.

Extension

Extension is a rare mechanism of injury, caused by a direct force with relative hyperextension occurring within the upper spine. The ALL is disrupted, with variable injury of the anterior annulus. The posterior compressive forces generated may fracture the posterior elements, with pushing fragments ventrally into the spinal canal.

Shear

Shear is the most destabilizing mechanism and carries a relatively high risk for neurologic compromise. The classic characteristic is "fracture-dislocation," which may occur through the facet joints, allowing the vertebral body to translate with failure of the ALL, PLL, and annulus (Fig. 42-3).

Magerl Classification

Magerl classification is another system, more popularized in Europe, which is based on mechanism of injury.[9] Fracture is categorized from A to C: A is compression, B is distraction, and C is multidirectional injuries with translation. Each type is subdivided into three groups (1 to 3) based on the injury mechanisms. The classification arranges fractures in order of increasing severity of instability of the spinal column. Thus, A1 is the most stable and C3 is the least stable according to this classification.

RADIOGRAPHIC CLASSIFICATION

This mechanism was proposed by McCormack and associates,[10] who characterized it as a "load-sharing" classification based on their experiences of short-segment posterior stabilization. They emphasized three characteristics of the fracture: amount of vertebral body comminution, apposition of the fracture fragments at the fracture site, and the amount of correction of kyphotic deformity on preoperative and postoperative radiographs. They subdivided each of these factors into three grades of severity and assigned point values of 1, 2, or 3 to the increasing severity grades. Failure of the short-segment posterior stabilization correlated with 7 points or higher. Unfortunately, this classification did not address the ligamentous injury. Furthermore, it appears to lack reproducibility.

NEUROLOGIC CLASSIFICATION

The American Spinal Injury Association (ASIA) classification appears to be a consistent and reproducible classification.[11–14] Muscle function is reproducible between observers and institutions. Motor scores are valuable in comparing treatment efficacy and predicting outcome in patients with neurologic injury. A patient's neurologic status can be classified as A to E:

- A: Absent motor and sensory function below level of injury
- B: Absent motor function below level of injury, sensation intact
- C: Very weak (grade 1/5 to 2/5) motor function below level of injury; sensation intact
- D: Weak (grade 3/5 to 4/5) motor function below level of injury; sensation intact
- E: Normal motor and sensory function

A complete cord injury defined as a persistent of neurologic deficit without any improvements after the period of spinal shock. The prognosis for a functional neurologic recovery is poor.

Recovery of incomplete cord injury can be predicted using this classification. In general, most patients within grade A and B will not recover. Up to 11% of these patients may show some nonfunctional improvement.[15–18] Frankel C and D patients are expected to improve at least one motor grade with or without treatment.[19]

RADIOGRAPHIC EVALUATION

Plain radiographs of the entire spine in anteroposterior and lateral view should be obtained in all high-energy trauma to rule out the noncontiguous injuries. The radiographic images should be reviewed thoroughly and carefully, including the pre- and paravertebral soft tissue shadows; the bony landmarks; and the distance between the bony landmarks, such as interpedicular distance and the interspinous distance. Interpedicular distance widening is one of the characteristics of burst fracture. Widening of the interspinous distance may suggest disruption of posterior ligaments. However, plain radiographs may miss 25% of burst fractures, which often are misdiagnosed as stable wedge fractures.

Computed tomography (CT) scanning is generally the next step. Sagittal reconstruction and axial thin cuts are helpful for determining fracture patterns and degree of spinal canal involvement. This can be quantified in percentages or ratios. One study showed that the ratio of the sagittal to the transverse canal diameter correlated with the neurologic deficit.[20]

The role of magnetic resonance imaging (MRI) is still controversial. In the absence of neurologic injury, MRI usually is not required for assessing thoracolumbar injuries in the acute setting. It can be helpful for identifying a ligamentous injury that is suspected but not confirmed on plain x-rays or CT scan. MRI is recommended in a patient who presents with a neurologic deficit to identify any ongoing spinal cord compression and to evaluate spinal cord anatomy, intensity signal changes in the spinal cord, and the uncommon epidural hematoma.

TREATMENT

THORACIC SPINE INJURY

Spinal stability in the upper thoracic region is augmented by the ribs, sternum, and costotransverse ligaments. Injury to this region, therefore, usually requires high-energy trauma and is less common than injury elsewhere in the spine. Upper thoracic fractures are usually stable injuries unless accompanied by sternal and rib injuries, in which case they may be unstable and progress to late collapse and kyphotic deformity. Other evidence of potential unstable fracture includes posterior ligamentous disruption detected on MRI and more than 50% of anterior height loss.

Most compression fractures are relatively stable injuries conducive to nonoperative treatment in thoracolumbar orthosis for approximately 12 weeks.[21] For thoracic fractures above T7, a cervical extension to the orthosis often is required for proper immobilization. Close radiographic follow-up is mandatory, as progressive loss of sagittal alignment or neurologic deterioration is often managed with surgical reduction, decompression, and stabilization. One critical pitfall is inappropriate brace selection; for above T6 or T7,

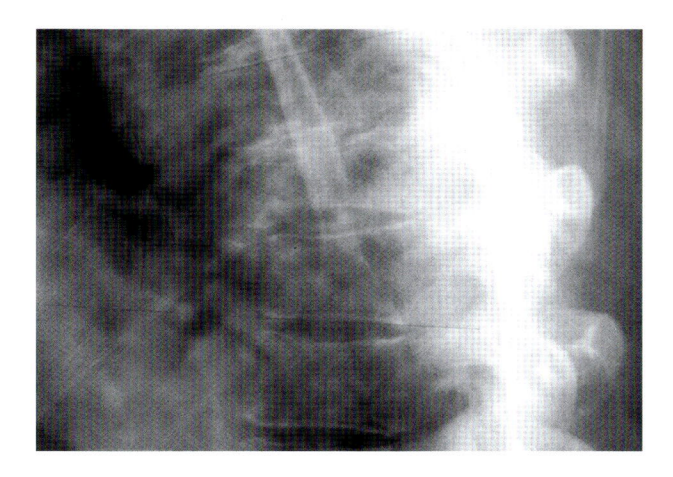

Fig. 42-4 Compression fracture of T7 spine with anterior height loss less than 50% and intact both middle and posterior columns.

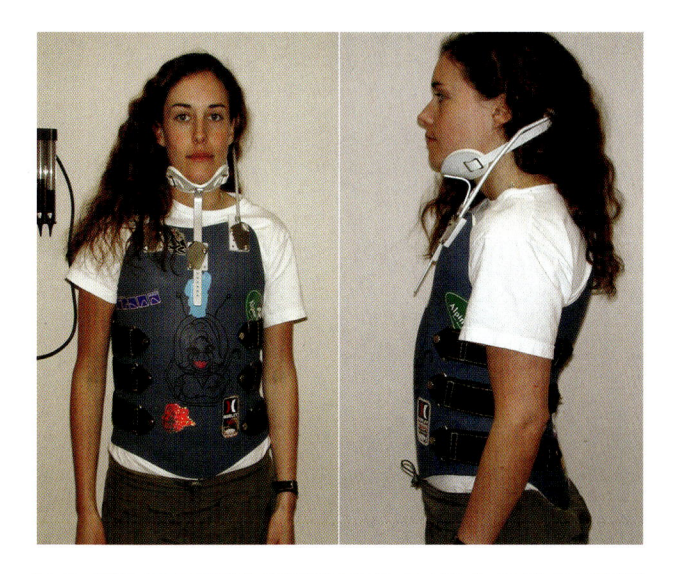

Fig. 42-5 Orthosis with chin extension is mandatory for fracture at T7 or above.

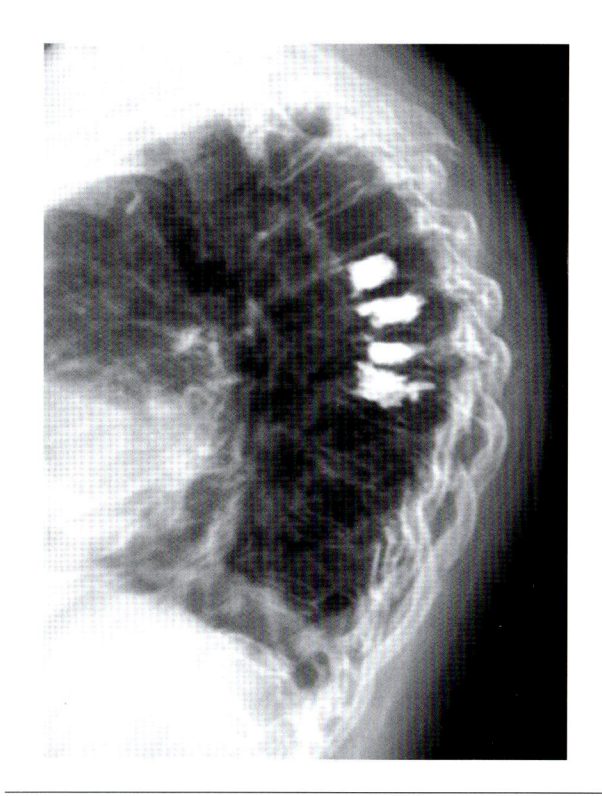

Fig. 42-6 Osteoporotic compression fracture of the thoracic spine without neurologic deficit can be successfully treated with kyphoplasty.

we recommend TLSO orthosis with chin extension (Figs. 42-4 and 42-5).

Nonoperative treatment is generally recommended for low-energy osteoporotic compression and burst fractures. Vertebroplasty and kyphoplasty (Fig. 42-6) are two techniques that show good potential in terms of decreasing pain and improving function in this subset of patients. Early reports demonstrate these techniques to be highly effective with good pain relief and relatively few complications. However, long-term results are not yet available, and the indications for these techniques are still evolving.

THORACOLUMBAR SPINE INJURY

Burst fracture is the most common injury in this region. Usually, the retropulsed fragment was pushed into the spinal canal, and the fracture may or may not be associated with neurologic deficit. Overall, the factors to be considered when deciding on treatment for patients with a thoracolumbar spine fracture are neurologic status, spinal stability, degree of deformity, and associated injuries.

INDICATIONS FOR SURGERY

In general, the indications for surgery are neurologic instability and mechanical instability. Neurologic instability includes neurologic deficit; progressive neurologic deficit; and compromise of the spinal canal, especially if the decrease in cross-sectional area of the spinal canal is more than 30% at T11-T12, 40% or more at L1, and 50% or more at L2.

Mechanical instability includes burst fracture associated with posterior element disruption, kyphosis of 20 degrees or more, vertebral height loss of 50% or more, and CT scan demonstrating free bony fragment.

TIMING OF SURGERY

The issue of greatest concern is the neurologic recovery; however, the appropriate timing of surgery following spinal cord injury is the subject of considerable controversy, with conflicting information from animal and clinical studies. Although animal models have suggested that early decompression may improve neurologic recovery, the window of opportunity appears to be very small. In addition, the prospective randomized published data fail to demonstrate this issue.[22] Nevertheless, we still recommend early but not emergent decompression of the spinal canal.

SURGICAL APPROACHES

Anterior, posterior, or circumferential fusion is chosen, depending on the level of injury and degree of neurologic and osteoligmentous instability.

POSTERIOR APPROACH

The posterior approach is used most often. In a neurologically intact patient, a three- or four-point fixation bending moment strategy using cantilever forces to restore sagittal alignment is often used. Moreover, the intact posterior annulus is believed to be the crucial structure for indirect reduction method to decompress the retropulsed fragment. Care must be taken to avoid retropulsion of vertebral bone fragments into the spinal canal, and distraction should be minimized in the setting of posterior column disruption to avoid tension on the neural elements. Intaoperative monitoring is also helpful but not mandatory. This indirect decompression technique may be less effective when surgery is performed after 3 days or more than 67% of the canal is compromised.[23-27]

Indications

Parker and associates[28] used the "load-sharing" classification system and reported a high failure rate of short-segment posterior stabilization in patients with scores higher than 7. Therefore, they suggested that the candidates for short-segment posterior fusion and stabilization are patients who suffer flexion-distraction injuries, "mild" burst fractures, or score less than 6 according to "load-sharing" classification.

Long-segment posterior fusion and stabilization is appropriate for patients with fracture-dislocation injuries who are unable to tolerate 3 to 4 months of postoperative bracing or patients who are unable to tolerate a two-stage dorsal-ventral procedure because of medical problems, including severe cardiopulmonary status.

Decompression during the posterior procedure can be done via the transpedicle technique.

Patient Positioning

- The patient is placed in the prone position on radiolucent operating table, the Wilson frame, or the bolsters.
- Care must be taken to avoid more kyphotic deformity if placement is done on the Wilson frame. Prominent bones, eyes, genital area, and upper extremities are checked, padded, and placed properly to avoid complications.
- Intraoperative monitoring can be used but is not mandatory or routine.
- Intraoperative C-arm is required for pedicle screw placement.

Incision

- The incision is carried along the midline of the spine, spanning at least two to three levels above and below the fractured level.
- Meticulous hemostasis and dissection are performed in the soft tissue, fascia, and paraspinal muscles from the spinous process.
- Continue dissection on to the lamina and laterally toward the facet joints into the transverse process to identify the entry points for pedicle screw placements.
- Care must be taken to avoid bleeding from facet artery and to avoid injury to the nerve roots underneath the intertransverse fascia/ligament.
- Preoperative CT scan should be meticulously read because associated fracture of the lamina is not uncommon and accidentally plunging into the epidural space may occur.
- At this point, intraoperative C-arm is brought in to confirm the level.

Posterior Fusion and Instrumentation

- Internal fixation devices are only temporary and will ultimately fail unless the adequate fusion occurs.
- Standard instrumentation in the thoracolumbar junction is a pedicle screw-rod-hook system. The thoracic pedicle screw must be placed very carefully with full understanding of the anatomy, particularly in the neurologically intact patient. Intraoperative monitoring may play an important role in this part.
- How many levels should be fused is still questionable, but several factors (as mentioned previously) should be considered. It is our practice that at least two levels above and two levels below should be included.
- There is also no difference in outcome and rate of fusion between use of monoaxial and polyaxial pedicle screws; the choice depends on the surgeon's familiarity.
- Autograft or allograft remains controversial, and several papers support both. Nevertheless, key of fusion is the surface area of the fusion and the proper biologic environment. Therefore, we recommend that the bony surface should be decorticated and bone graft should be carefully packed to the transverse process.

Posterolateral Decompression

- Posterolateral decompression is indicated if there is significant residual compression fragment after indirect reduction with posterior instrumentation. This technique is described originally for thoracolumbar fractures treated with Harrington rod distraction device, but it can be performed with any posterior instrumentation based on the same anatomic landmark.
- Preoperative CT is performed to determine the size of the fragment and the proper side to remove the bony fragment.

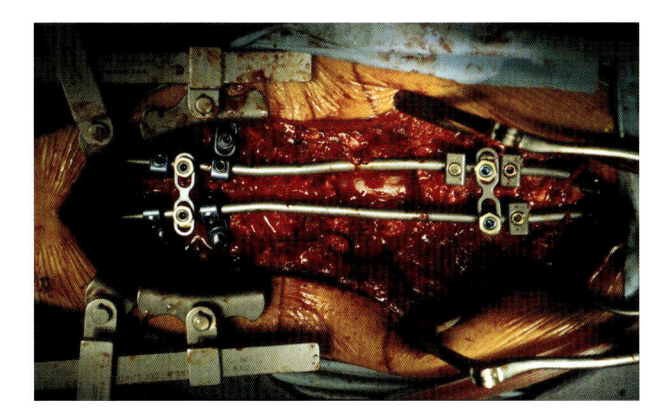

Fig. 42-7 Intraoperative pictures showing posterior decompression via posterolateral (pedicle) bilaterally combined with posterior fusion and instrumentation in T12 burst fracture. The spinal canal and thecal sac are well decompressed.

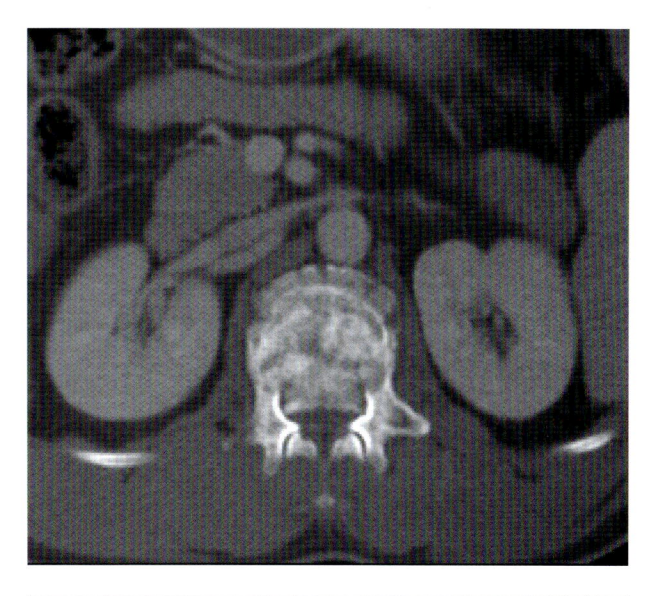

Fig. 42-8 Axial computed tomograph of the L1 showing residual canal compromise nearly 50% after unsuccessful of indirect decompression via distraction through the posterior construct which will require second stage of anterior procedure.

- A laminotomy is performed at the site of the maximal neural compression.
- Carefully identify the pedicle and medial wall of the pedicle by gradually removing bone from the lamina.
- Then the pedicle is carefully drilled, taking care not to violate the wall or exiting nerve root.
- Carefully identify the bony fragment and posterior vertebral body; then, a reverse angle curette can be used to isolate the bony fragment from the ventral surface of the dura and finally to push down toward the vertebral body.
- The small bony fragment can be directly removed safely.
- Care is taken not to agressively retract the thecal sac.
- If the fragment is considered "big," a similar approach can be done on the other side. Figure 42-7 demonstrates decompression via the posterior approach with fusion and instrumentation at the same setting.

In conclusion, this technique allows removal of the paramedian fragments. By avoiding the anterior approach, which will require transpleural or transdiaphragmatic dissection, the surgeon can perform both decompression and stabilization in one setting. The disadvantage is further destabilizing the spine by removal of lamina and pedicle at the injured segment. Nevertheless, several authors showed satisfactory outcomes using this approach.[19,29]

ANTERIOR APPROACH

The advantage of this approach is direct decompression of the spinal canal, reconstruction the anterior column, and stabilization in one setting.[30–37] However, the complex anatomy of the pleura, diaphragm, and retroperitoneal space, which will require division of the diaphragm and entering the pleural cavity, makes this approach less attractive. Another issue is a potentially higher complication rate that is associated with the surgeon's unfamiliarity.

Indications
- The anterior approach is indicated for acute severe canal compromise (more than 67%) because the published data demonstrate that the posterior annulus usually disrupted and is no longer effective for a ligamentotaxis effect (Fig. 42-8).
- It is also indicated if there is a residual significant retropulsed fragment (canal compromised more than 35%) after the posterior procedure has been performed.
- Another indication is correction of the kyphotic deformity when malunion or failure of the posterior instrumentation occurs.

Patient Positioning
- Double lumen endotracheal tube is needed if the pleural cavity is entered.
- Patient is placed in the lateral decubitus position with left side up on the radiolucent operating table or beanbag.
- All the prominent bones are checked and padded.
- Intraoperative monitoring can be used in cases of severe deformity but is not mandatory.
- Intraoperative fluoroscope is helpful to confirm the injured level and to determine the anterior construct.

Incision
- In general, a left-sided approach is preferred in order to avoid the inferior vena cava and liver. The tenth or eleventh rib can be removed to get access to L1 burst fracture.[38–40]

- Subperiosteal resection of the selected rib is performed. Then the pleural cavity is carefully entered and the rib spreader can be used to further widen this space.
- The diaphragm is identified and the parietal pleura on its top surface is mobilized using blunt dissection.[38–40]
- Next, the peritoneal sac is identified and bluntly mobilized from the undersurface of the diaphragm.
- The retroperitoneal space is entering using blunt dissection. The diaphragm is now divided at the peripheral margin.
- The arcuate ligament and crus of the diaphragm are also divided. Sutures should be placed along the border of the divided diaphragm in order to accurately repair the diaphragm during closure.
- A self-retaining retractor system is brought in at this time to maintain the exposure during the procedure.
- The injured vertebral body can be identified at this point. It is necessary that the surgeon can expose the disk above and below the injured vertebral body as well as the body above and below for anterior instrumentation.

Decompression

- The psoas muscle must be mobilized carefully without injury to the genitofemoral nerve or the segmental vessels overlying the middle of the vertebral body.
- Continue dissection until one can easily identify T12 and L2 vertebral bodies. The segmental vessels are ligated using a hemoclip. The pedicle and neural foramen are the critical landmarks for direct decompression.
- Next, the T12-L1 and L1-L2 disk spaces are identified and then removed using a combination of curette, osteotome, and ronguer. As mentioned earlier, the pedicle and neural foramen of L1 are identified as a posterior landmark. The ALL will serve as an anterior landmark for corpectomy.
- The goal of decompression is to perform subtotal corpectomy, removing the significant bony fragment while preserving 5 mm to 8 mm of bone anteriorly and posteriorly to protect the aorta and spinal canal, respectively.
- The fractured vertebral body L1 is quickly removed using a combination of osteotome, curette, and ronguer. The removed bone should be used as a source of bone graft for fusion (Fig. 42-9).
- One critical point is not to penetrate into the spinal canal or the contralateral cortex of the vertebral body when performing a subtotal corpectomy.
- Penetrating or breaking of the contralateral cortex may injure the inferior vena cava.
- We then focus on decompressing the ventral dura by using a combination of curette and high-speed drill to remove the posterior wall of the vertebral body.
- We recommend that the direction of the instrument is aiming away from the spinal canal toward the corpectomy site.
- Adequate decompression is defined as pedicle-to-pedicle decompression. The surgeon must perform an adequate decompression to ensure that no bony fragment is left behind.

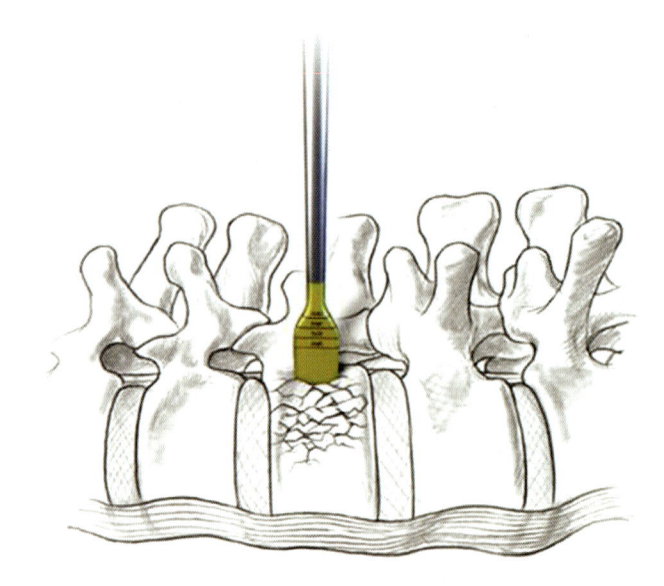

Fig. 42-9 Anterior decompression of the spinal canal can be done by using combination of curette, drill, and osteotome. The osteotome must be directed away from the spinal cord.

Stabilization

Goals of reconstruction are to replace the anterior column, fuse the injured segment, correct the deformity, and maintain the alignment. Several options are available to replace the anterior column, such as iliac crest autograft, fibula strut graft, rib graft, femoral ring allograft, tibial graft, titanium mesh cage, carbon-fiber cage, and expandable cage (Fig. 42-10). However, structural bone graft still appears to be the gold standard (Fig. 42-11).

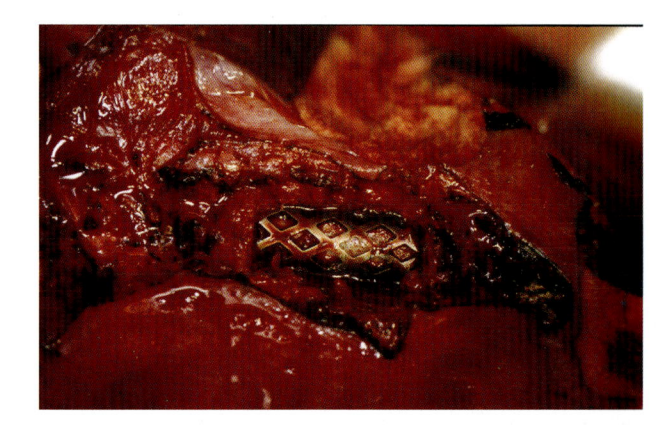

Fig. 42-10 Intraoperative pictures demonstrating placement of the titanium cage after successful canal decompression.

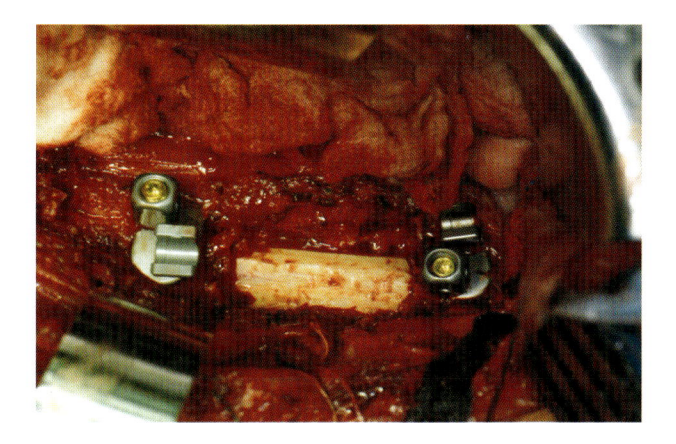

Fig. 42-11 Structural bone graft can also be used for reconstruction of the anterior column followed by anterior instrumentation.

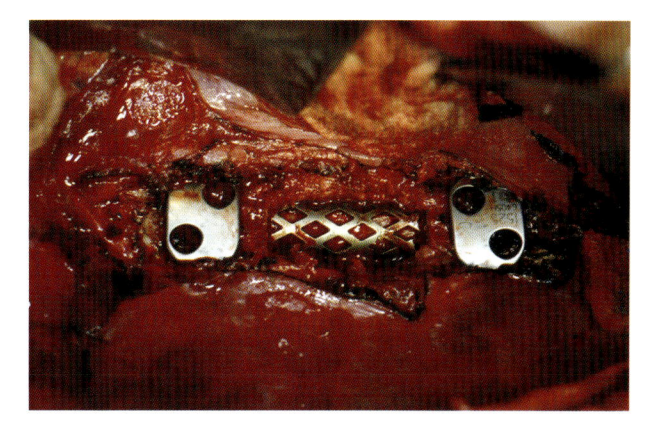

Fig. 42-12 Staple should be placed appropriately in order to allow proper placement of the anterior construct.

The main requirements of an anterior device, however, are a low profile and superior mechanical stabilization. Several anterior constructs are available, depending on the surgeon's preference, but in general they are classified into two groups: plate-screw construct or rod-screw construct. Anterior rod-screw construct, such as the Kaneda device, has been popularized and the outcomes are promising. Our preference is also a rod-screw construct because of its superiority in terms of biomechanics. The following is a review of the anterior construct technique.

1. Determine screw length
   - Anterior screw length should be determined at this point.
   - Using the depth gauge, measure the width of the vertebral bodies above and below the corpectomy site. The distance measured can be used as a guide to select the correct screw length to achieve bicortical fixation. As a general rule, anterior screws are typically 5 mm shorter than posterior screws.
   - Alternatively, preoperative MRI and CT scans can be used to determine the width of the vertebral body.
2. Staple selection
   - Using the provided staple templates, determine the appropriate size of vertebral body staple.
   - The proper staple is selected by identifying the size that maximizes the coverage of the lateral aspect of the vertebral body without violating the adjacent disk space.
3. Staple placement
   - Attach the selected staple to the dual hole staple; once it is secured to the instrument, the staple can be rotated via the central spike into the proper position on the vertebral body. The center spike allows the surgeon to fine-tune the staple location before impacting it into the bone.
   - A mallet is used to impact the staple (Fig. 42-12).
4. Staple positioning
   - When placed, the staples should be oriented on the spine so that the anterior screw holes are further apart than the posterior screw holes. All staples are marked "A" for anterior and "P" for posterior to facilitate proper implantation.
   - Arrows etched on the rostral/caudal staples should be pointing into the corpectomy site.
   - The awl will create a 15-mm-deep channel into the bone to guide the tap and screw.
5. Screw insertion
   - Screws should be inserted until the underside of the screw head comes into contact with the staple. Screw openings should be parallel to the spine to allow for insertion of the rods (Fig. 42-13).
6. Fracture reduction
   - If necessary, the distractor can be secured to the screw heads using the set screws.
   - Reduce the fracture until the anterior longitudinal ligament (if intact) is taut.

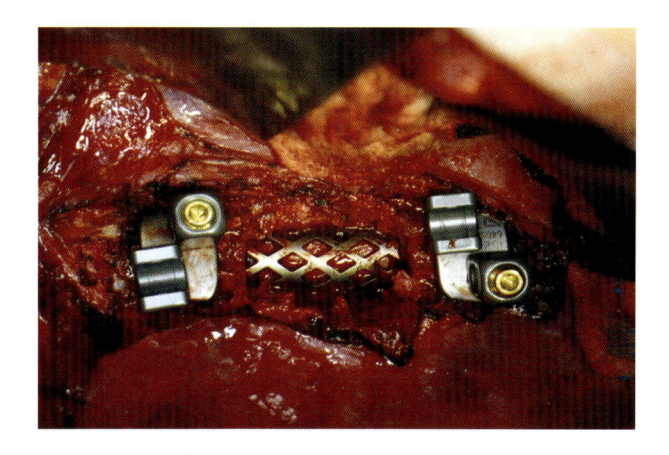

Fig. 42-13 Screws are placed on top of the staples.

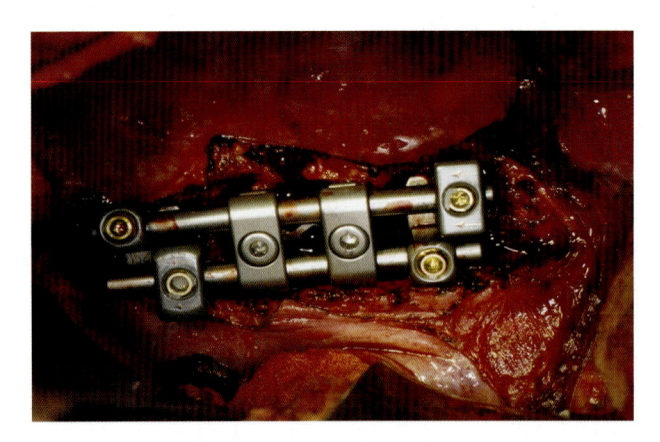

Fig. 42-14 Intraoperative pictures of the final construct of the Kaneda device after anterior decompression in T12 burst fracture.

- Insert the selected vertebral body replacement, depending on the surgeon's preference.
- Release the distractor and remove it from the screws.
- Intraoperative C-arm can be used at this point to check the overall alignment and the position of the construct.

7. Rod placement
   - Using the graft measuring caliper or rod template, measure the length of the rods required for the construct.
   - Insert the rods using the rod holder and lock down the rostral screws with the rod stabilizer and X25 final tightening torque wrench. All set screws are torqued to 80 inch-pounds.
   - Caudal set screws remain loose for compression of the construct.

8. Compression and final tightening
   - Compress caudal screws on both the posterior and anterior rods.
   - Lock caudal set screws using the stabilizer and X25 final tightener.
   - All set screws are tightened to 80 inch-pounds.

9. Cross connector application
   - Using the measuring templates, determine the appropriate size of cross connector to apply to the rods.
   - Apply cross connectors and tighten set screws to 80 inch-pounds.
   - Two cross connectors are recommended for each construct.
   - More cancellous bone graft may be placed around the cage or interbody spacer anteriorly. Figure 42-14 demonstrates the final construct.

POSTOPERATIVE CARE

- Pain is controlled either by standard pain protocol or pain management consultants.
- Chest tube is removed within 48 hours followed by chest x-ray to ensure that no residual pleural cavity related complications are not detected.
- Early mobilization is strongly encouraged.
- The patient should be placed in TLSO brace for at least 8 to 12 weeks.
- The patient should be followed up closely with radiographs and neurologic status assessment at 6 weeks, 3 months, 6 months, and annually for 2 years to ensure fusion is successful.

CONCLUSION

The transitional anatomy of this area renders it vulnerable to the high-energy deceleration trauma associated with instability and neurologic compromise. Understanding the mechanisms of injury as well as the complex anatomy in this area is crucial to proper management. Several issues remain controversial, including timing of surgery, surgical approaches, and choices of instrumentation. Overall, short-segment posterior stabilization is not an option for burst fracture in this area because of the high failure rate. Long posterior stabilization in selected case provides good results. An anterior approach also has the advantage of direct decompression as well as stabilization performed in one setting and the outcomes in the literature are promising.

References

1. Morgan TH WG, Austin GN: The results of laminectomy in patients with incomplete spinal cord injury. Paraplegia 1971;9: 14–22.
2. Harrington PR: Treatment of scoliosis. Correction and internal fixation by spine instrumentation. Am J Orthop 1962;44-A:591–610.
3. Holdsworth F: Fractures, dislocations, and fracture-dislocations of the spine. J Bone Joint Surg Am 1970;52:1534–1551.
4. Denis F: Spinal instability as defined by the three-column spine concept in acute spinal trauma. Clin Orthop 1984;189:65–76.
5. Denis F: The three column spine and its significance in the classification of acute thoracolumbar spinal injuries. Spine 1983;8: 817–831.
6. Allen BL Jr, Ferguson RL, Lehmann TR, et al: A mechanistic classification of closed, indirect fractures and dislocations of the lower cervical spine. Spine 1982;7:1–27.
7. Ferguson RL, Allen BL Jr: A mechanistic classification of thoracolumbar spine fractures. Clin Orthop 1984;189:77–88.
8. McAfee PC, Yuan HA, Lasda NA: The unstable burst fracture. Spine 1982;7:365–373.
9. Magerl F, Aebi M, Gertzbein SD, et al: A comprehensive classification of thoracic and lumbar injuries. Eur Spine J 1994;3: 184–201.
10. McCormack T, Karaikovic E, Gaines RW: The load sharing classification of spine fractures. Spine 1994;19:1741–1744.
11. Barneschi G, D'Andrea M, Pratelli R, et al: Neurologic evaluation in thoracolumbar vertebral fractures. Chir Organi Mov 2000; 85:101–119.
12. Donovan WH, Brown DJ, Ditunno JF Jr, et al: Neurological issues. Spinal Cord 1997;35:275–281.
13. Marino RJ, Ditunno JF Jr, Donovan WH, et al: Neurologic recovery after traumatic spinal cord injury: Data from the Model Spinal Cord Injury Systems. Arch Phys Med Rehabil 1999;80:1391–1396.

14. Priebe MM, Waring WP: The interobserver reliability of the revised American Spinal Injury Association standards for neurological classification of spinal injury patients. Am J Phys Med Rehabil 1991;70:268–270.
15. Ducker TB, Russo GL, Bellegarrique R, et al: Complete sensorimotor paralysis after cord injury: Mortality, recovery, and therapeutic implications. J Trauma 1979;19:837–840.
16. Ducker TB, Salcman M, Daniell HB: Experimental spinal cord trauma, III: Therapeutic effect of immobilization and pharmacologic agents. Surg Neurol 1978;10:71–76.
17. Ducker TB, Salcman M, Lucas JT, et al: Experimental spinal cord trauma, II: Blood flow, tissue oxygen, evoked potentials in both paretic and plegic monkeys. Surg Neurol 1978;10:64–70.
18. Ducker TB, Salcman M, Perot PL Jr, et al: Experimental spinal cord trauma, I: Correlation of blood flow, tissue oxygen and neurologic status in the dog. Surg Neurol 1978;10:60–63.
19. Hardaker WT Jr, Cook WA Jr, Friedman AH, et al: Bilateral transpedicular decompression and Harrington rod stabilization in the management of severe thoracolumbar burst fractures. Spine 1992;17:162–171.
20. Vaccaro AR, Nachwalter RS, Klein GR, et al: The significance of thoracolumbar spinal canal size in spinal cord injury patients. Spine 2001;26:371–376.
21. Vanichkachorn JS, Vaccaro AR: Nonoperative treatment of thoracolumbar fractures. Orthopedics 1997;20:948–953; quiz 954–945.
22. Vaccaro AR, Daugherty RJ, Sheehan TP, et al: Neurologic outcome of early versus late surgery for cervical spinal cord injury. Spine 1997;22:2609–2613.
23. Crutcher JP Jr, Anderson PA, King HA, et al: Indirect spinal canal decompression in patients with thoracolumbar burst fractures treated by posterior distraction rods. J Spinal Disord 1991;4:39–48.
24. Dai L, Jia L, Zhao D, et al: [Remodelling of the spinal canal after thoracolumbar burst fractures: Significance of nonoperative management.] Zhonghua Wai Ke Za Zhi 2000;38:610–612.
25. Dai LY: Remodeling of the spinal canal after thoracolumbar burst fractures. Clin Orthop 2001;382:119–123.
26. Gertzbein SD, Court-Brown CM: Rationale for the management of flexion-distraction injuries of the thoracolumbar spine based on a new classification. J Spinal Disord 1989;2:176–183.
27. McAfee PC, Yuan HA, Fredrickson BE, et al: The value of computed tomography in thoracolumbar fractures: An analysis of one hundred consecutive cases and a new classification. J Bone Joint Surg Am 1983;65:461–473.
28. Parker JW, Lane JR, Karaikovic EE, et al: Successful short-segment instrumentation and fusion for thoracolumbar spine fractures: A consecutive $4^1/_2$-year series. Spine 2000;25:1157–1170.
29. Eismont FJ, Green BA, Berkowitz BM, et al: The role of intraoperative ultrasonography in the treatment of thoracic and lumbar spine fractures. Spine 1984;9:782–787.
30. Been HD, Bouma GJ: Comparison of two types of surgery for thoraco-lumbar burst fractures: Combined anterior and posterior stabilisation vs. posterior instrumentation only. Acta Neurochir (Wien) 1999;141:349–357.
31. Carl AL, Tranmer BI, Sachs BL: Anterolateral dynamized instrumentation and fusion for unstable thoracolumbar and lumbar burst fractures. Spine 1997;22:686–690.
32. Dimar JR 2nd, Wilde PH, Glassman SD, et al: Thoracolumbar burst fractures treated with combined anterior and posterior surgery. Am J Orthop 1996;25:159–165.
33. Harris MB: The role of anterior stabilization with instrumentation in the treatment of thoracolumbar burst fractures. Orthopedics 1992;15:347–350.
34. Kaneda K, Abumi K, Fujiya M: Burst fractures with neurologic deficits of the thoracolumbar-lumbar spine: Results of anterior decompression and stabilization with anterior instrumentation. Spine 1984;9:788–795.
35. Kaneda K, Taneichi H, Abumi K, et al: Anterior decompression and stabilization with the Kaneda device for thoracolumbar burst fractures associated with neurological deficits. J Bone Joint Surg Am 1997;79:69–83.
36. Kirkpatrick JS: Thoracolumbar fracture management: Anterior approach. J Am Acad Orthop Surg 2003;11:355–363.
37. Kirkpatrick JS, Wilber RG, Likavec M, et al: Anterior stabilization of thoracolumbar burst fractures using the Kaneda device: A preliminary report. Orthopedics 1995;18:673–678.
38. Dulchavsky SA, Diebel LN: Retroperitoneal approach to first lumbar vertebral body. J Am Coll Surg 1995;180:495–496.
39. Kim M, Nolan P, Finkelstein JA: Evaluation of 11th rib extrapleural-retroperitoneal approach to the thoracolumbar junction: Technical note. J Neurosurg 2000;93:168–174.
40. Mirbaha MM: Anterior approach to the thoraco-lumbar junction of the spine by a retroperitoneal-extrapleural technic. Clin Orthop 1973;91:41–47.

SECTION C
Lumbar and Sacral Spine

CHAPTER 43

HO-YEOL ZHANG

DANIEL H. KIM

Lumbar and Sacral Fractures

INTRODUCTION

Fractures in the lower lumbar spine (levels L3 through L5) account for less than 4% of all spinal fractures.[1,2] Although a great deal of literature currently exists about the treatment of thoracolumbar fractures, little information is available about low lumbar spine fractures.

Treatment of injuries to the lumbar spine and sacrum requires the consideration of a number of additional factors beyond those relevant to injuries of the thoracic and thoracolumbar spine. These considerations are related to the anatomic complexity of the sacrum and the posterior elements of the lumbar spine, as well as to the lordosis and increased normal mobility of the lumbosacral junction.

In the lumbar spine, anatomic and motion considerations make instrumentation more difficult in this area than in other regions of the spine. Injuries to the lumbar spine and upper sacrum disrupt the normal lordotic alignment of the spine, and restoration of that lordotic alignment is critical to overall vertebral mechanics and spinal alignment in the sagittal plane. Failure to maintain or restore the normal sagittal alignment in the lower lumbar spine after either elective fusions or fractures have led to degenerative changes and symptoms in long-term follow-up. The lumbosacral junction in particular must resist a number of large forces, but must also permit a significant amount of motion.[3]

There are many classification systems for lumbar and sacral spine fractures. The classification allows the physician to determine the stability of the spine and, thus, determine the need for conservative treatment, reduction, and decompression and the type of stabilization. The system used plays a key role in determining whether operative or nonoperative treatment is initiated.

CLASSIFICATION OF LUMBAR AND SACRAL FRACTURES

LUMBAR SPINE FRACTURES
Denis Classification[4]

- Compression fracture
- Burst fractures
  - Type I: Both end plates of the vertebra are fractured.
  - Type II: The superior end plate of the vertebra is fractured (most common).
  - Type III: The inferior end plate of the vertebra is fractured.
  - Type IV: A burst fracture with rotation is present.
  - Type V: A burst facture with lateral flexion is present.
- Seatbelt injury
- Fracture-dislocation

McAfee Classification[5]

- Wedge compression fracture
- Stable burst fracture
- Unstable burst fracture
- Chance-type fracture
- Flexion-distraction injury
- Translational injury

Load-Shearing Classification System by McCormack[6]

Three factors are independently graded from 1 to 3 depending on severity of the fracture: (1) the amount of comminution, (2) the apposition of the fragments, and (3) the amount of deformity that is to be corrected. Points are assigned for each of three quantities, and the final score indicates ability of the fracture to share the load. The lowest score is 3 and the highest score is 9.

In a study of short-segment pedicle screw instrumentation, no screw breakage was noted in patients with scores of 6 or less.[6] Patients with scores higher than 6 need some type of anterior support, because the ability of the anterior structures to share the load transmitted across the injured vertebra is compromised.

This classification system does not assess amount of soft tissue and ligamentous injury, which plays a key role in assessing overall stability of the spine, and therefore is not useful to base the decision for operative or nonoperative treatment. However, it helps to direct the proper approach and surgical instrumentation of those fractures that are taken to surgery.

SACRAL FRACTURES
Denis Classification

The most comprehensive analysis of sacral fractures has been reported by Denis and colleagues; it consists of 235 sacral fractures in a series of 776 patients with pelvic injuries. To assist in the analysis of their data, these authors also performed anatomic cadaveric studies of the sacral roots and foramina.

This classification system is based on identifying three vertical zones through the sacrum (Fig. 43-1).[7]
- Zone 1 is in the region of the sacral foramina.
- Zone 2 encompasses the region of the foramina.
- Zone 3 encompasses the region of the central sacral canal.

Injuries are assigned to the highest zone that the fracture line transgresses. Therefore, a fracture that passes through all three zones would be classified as a zone 3 injury.
- Zone 1 injuries ranged from minor avulsion fractures to unstable vertical shear mechanisms with fractures lateral to the sacral foramina. These injuries rarely presented with neurologic deficit (6%) and were limited to either sciatic nerve or L5 root involvement.
- Zone 2 fractures passed through one or more foramina and carried a 28% incidence of neurologic injury. Because these fractures were usually unilateral and did not involve the central canal, bowel and bladder deficits were not expected. The L5 root may, however, be involved by entrapment in the alar fracture, leading to a "traumatic far out syndrome."
- Zone 3 fractures, by definition, transgressed the central canal and carried an overall 57% incidence of neurologic injury; 76% of patents presented with bowel, bladder, and sexual function deficit.

Roy-Camille Classification

Transverse fractures were initially classified into three groups by Roy-Camille and coworkers[8] and then modified to add a fourth group by others.[9] Roy-Camille and colleagues reviewed 13 cases of transverse sacral fractures and also conducted cadaveric experiments to study the fracture mechanism. They noted that 11 of 13 cases resulted from suicide jumps, implicating axial loading as the predominant force of injury. From their clinical and biomechanical data, four distinct fracture types were described (Fig. 43-2).
- Type 1 injuries are flexion injuries without significant displacement or deformity.[8,9]
- Type 2 fractures are flexion injuries with posterior displacement of the cephalad fragment.[8,9]
- Type 3 fractures are caused by an extension moment with anterior displacement of the cephalad fragment.[8,9]
- Type 4 injuires are neutral position fractures with total comminution of the upper sacrum without displacement from the lower fragment.[9]

Classification by the Direction of Fracture Line

Fractures of the sacrum can be classified in a number of different ways. One of the most common is according to the direction of the fracture line within the sacrum. Therefore, fractures can either be vertical, oblique, or transverse (Fig. 43-3) and can occur at any level in the sacrum.
- Vertical fractures may occur in the ala or through the foramina.
- Oblique fractures can occur at any location.
- Transverse fractures are less common and more frequently occur at the apex of the sacral kyphosis between S2 and S3, but they may occur as a high transverse fracture at S1 or S2.[10]

The L5-S1 articulation can be disrupted by an oblique fracture of the sacrum. Extra-articular fracture of the base of the superior S1 facet may cause instability and listhesis at that level, or alternatively the fracture may disrupt the joint integrity directly.

MANAGEMENT

The treatment goals for spine trauma in general are (1) anatomic reduction of the injury, (2) rigid fixation of the fracture, and, when necessary, (3) decompression of the neural

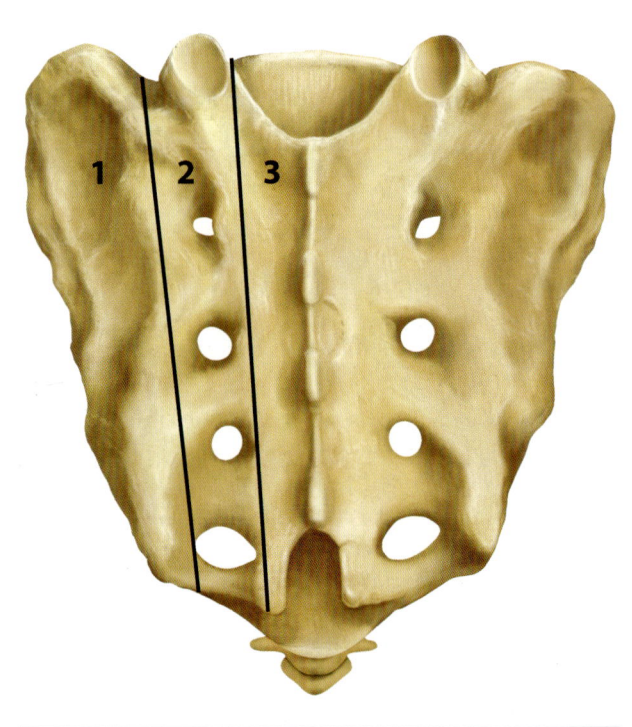

Fig. 43-1 Denis classification of sacral fractures. Zone 1 is the sacral ala fracture; zone 2 is through the neural foramina; and zone 3 is through the central canal.

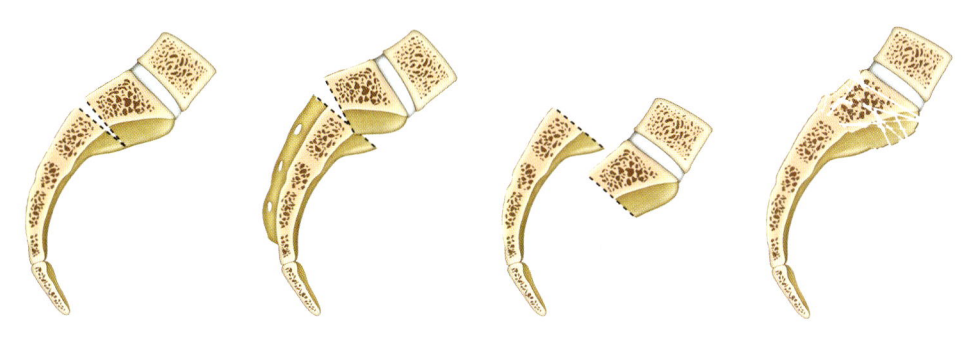

Fig. 43-2 From left to right, Roy-Camille classification type 1, type 2, and type 3; and at far right, Strange-Vognsen classification type 4. Type 1: flexion fracture with an anterior simple bending of the upper sacrum. Type 2: flexion fracture with a posterior displacement of the cephalad fragment that becomes more or less horizontal and settles with its anterior surface on the fractured surface of the lower fragment. Type 3: extension fracture with an anterior displacement of the cephalad fragment, more or less vertical, that slips down in front of the caudad fragment. Type 4: neutral position fracture with total comminution of the upper sacrum without displacement from the lower fragment.

elements. For the treatment of the lumbar and sacral spine, the goals also include (4) maintenance of sagittal alignment, (5) conservation of motion segments, and (6) prevention of frequent complications.[11]

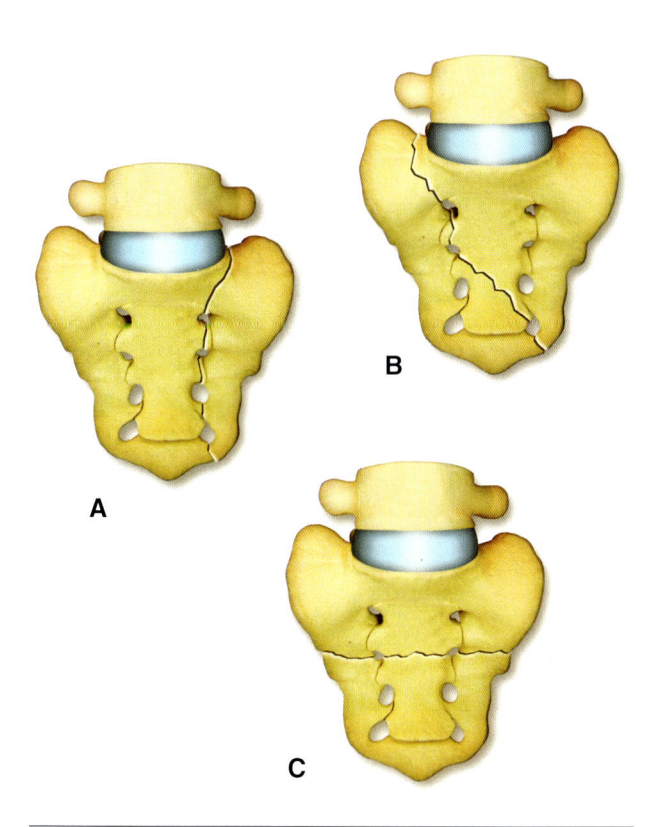

Fig. 43-3 Classification according to the direction of the fracture line of sacrum. Fractures can be vertical (A), oblique (B), or transverse (C).

INDICATIONS

1. Instability
   - Severe posterior ligamentous complex disruptions from a flexion or flexion-distraction injury.
   - Gross ligamentous instability, such as bilateral facet dislocations with complete disruption of the posterior ligamentous complex and the disk, will result in continued loss of sagittal alignment.
   - Shear injuries with circumferential disruption.
   - Burst injuries with significant canal compromise, disruption of the anterior and posterior portions of the vertebral body, and laminar fractures.
   - Vertical sacral fractures with other pelvic ring fractures.
   - Proximal transverse fractures of the sacrum with translational instability.
2. Neurologic deficit
   - Direct neural decompression:
     - A larger degree of canal compromise (50%), accompanied by high-grade neurologic compromise (cauda equina syndrome).
     - Specific root involvement with localized compression of the root.
     - Patients with sagittal spinous process fractures, neurologic deficit, and dural tears with roots outside the dural sac.
   - In the small group of patients with high transverse sacral fractures with kyphosis and neurologic deficit.
   - Other neurologic injuries that accompany fractures of the sacrum are less likely to respond to direct operative intervention. A significant portion of these are root avulsions and the remainders are neurapraxia, which frequently respond to conservative treatment.
3. Disruption of axial or sagittal spinal alignment.

TREATMENT GOALS

The major goals of treatment of lumbar spine and sacral injuries are (1) anatomic reduction of the injury deformity, (2) rigid fixation, (3) neural decompression (when indicated), (4) maintenance of sagittal alignment, (5) minimization of fixation length, and (6) reduction of the incidence of complications. The time from injury must also be considered, because the efficacy of various methods changes with the time course.

OPERATIVE TECHNIQUES FOR LUMBAR SPINE FRACTURE

POSTERIOR APPROACH WITH INSTRUMENTATION

Advantages

- The approach may provide lumbar lordotic curvature and distraction force.
- This technique may restore anatomic lordosis and vertebral body height, and it provides the most canal clearance through indirect reduction of fracture fragments.
- Pedicle screw instrumentation systems are the treatment method of choice for operative treatment of low lumbar spine fractures. They provide a stable, rigid construct that has the ability to withstand the loads placed on the lumbar spine.
- It may allow for the shortest possible fusion length and preservation of the critical lumbar motion segments.
- Usually, this approach allows placement of pedicle screws into the injured segment, which increases the stability of the construct.
- Most pedicle screw systems allow the variable positioning of the screws to gain purchase in the structurally sound portion of the vertebral body.

Operation Technique

- The patient is positioned by log-rolling and moving the spine as one unit. The patient is placed on bolsters to allow the abdomen to hang free to prevent venous congestion, and the spine is placed in the neutral position. A radiolucent table is used to allow for plain radiographs and fluoroscopy for the assessment of reduction, restoration of normal alignment, and direct visualization of the pedicles.
- The injured segment (as well as one level above and one level below) is exposed with a standard posterior approach. A lateral radiograph is used to confirm that the level is appropriate.
- A careful examination of the injury radiographs should concentrate on fracture or disruption of posterior lamina and bony structures.
- To avoid injury to the dura, carefully expose the fractured lamina without any downward pressure. Normal levels with intact posterior elements to be included in the fusion should be exposed first to establish some normal anatomic relationships, which facilitate exposure of the fractured elements.
- Do not disturb facet joints of the levels that are not to be fused to prevent late instability or degenerative changes in these important motion segments.
- Identify pedicles using the available anatomic landmarks (Fig. 43-4). The proper orientation for angling the screw superior or inferior can be determined by looking at the angle of the pedicle in a cross table, lateral radiograph that was used for localizing the appropriate level. The screw must also be angled medially approximately 5 to 10 degrees to assure that it follows the pedicle into the vertebral body.
- In the fractured segment, the screw may be angled to ensure that the screw has the best bone purchase. Once the posterior entry point has been defined for the pedicle, use a burr to decorticate the posterior cortex.
- Place the Steinmann pin into the path. These pins can then be visualized by plain radiograph or under fluoroscopy to assure they are in the pedicles. This pedicle may then be tapped, and a pedicle "feeler" may be used to feel the grooves for the threads of the screw along the circumference of the pedicle pathway.

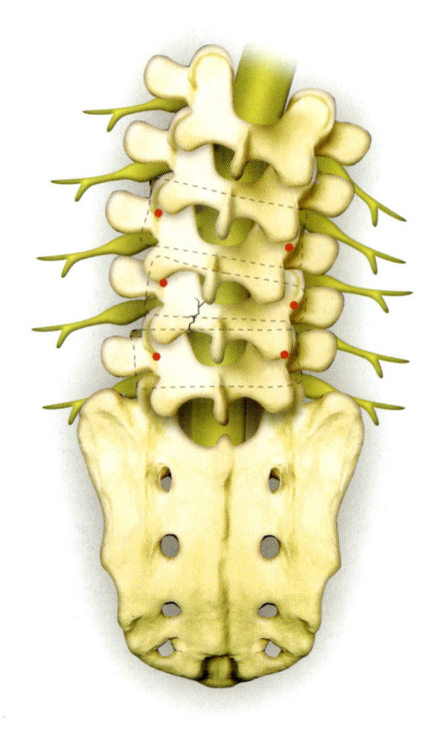

Fig. 43-4 Pedicles are identified and the proper orientation for angling the screw superior or inferior can be determined by looking at the angle of the pedicle in a cross table, lateral radiograph that was used for localizing the appropriate level. The screw must also be angled medially approximately 5 to 10 degrees to assure it follows the pedicle into the vertebral body.

- An appropriate screw length is then inserted into the anterior portion of the vertebral body, being careful not to penetrate the anterior cortex (Fig. 43-5). Indirect reduction is next performed by distracting the spine along rods contoured for the normal amount of anatomic lordosis in the lumbar spine (Fig. 43-6). Extension or lordosis of the screws may be added if the system allows for the independent positioning of the screws in relation to the contoured rods.
- For low lumbar spine fractures, which usually do not have a large amount of loss of vertebral body height or kyphotic deformity, indirect reduction using ligamentotaxis performed within 48 hours may suffice for reduction of canal encroachment.[2]
- Fragments encroaching on the spinal canal must be examined carefully. In cases in which indirect decompression is inadequate, a laminectomy with direct removal of the encroaching fragments is necessary.
- A laminectomy may be performed, and the anterior fragments may be impacted by placing an impacter underneath the dura directly on the posterior bony fragments. If the fragment appears rotated, patency of the posterior longitudinal ligament may be compromised and the fragment does not reduce by ligamentotaxis.
- If the fracture has been present for more than 4 to 6 days, the fracture may have already consolidated to the point where indirect reduction may not suffice.

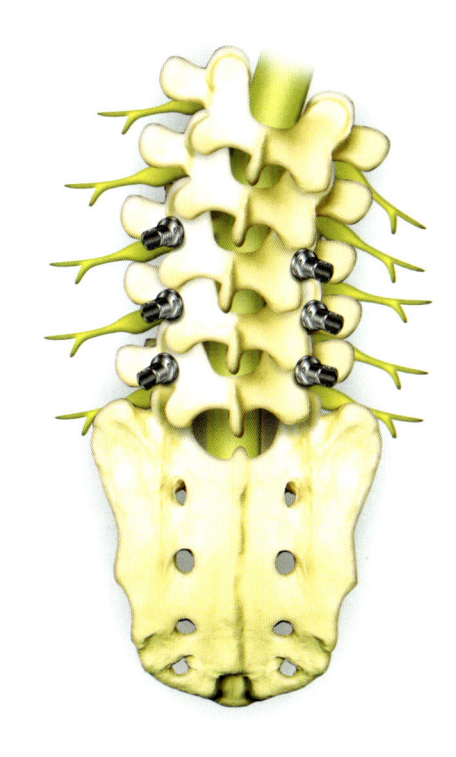

Fig. 43-5 After confirmation of proper position of Steinmann pins, these pins are removed. Pedicle screws are placed on the pedicle with appropriate length.

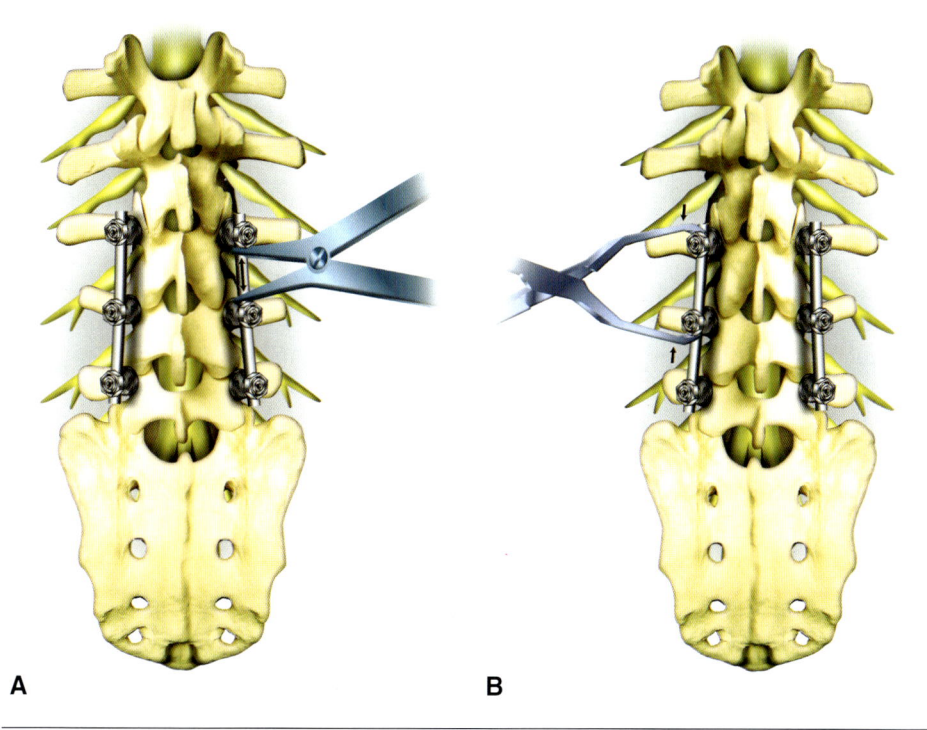

Fig. 43-6 *A* and *B*, Indirect reduction can be performed by distracting or compressing the spine along rods contoured for the normal amount of anatomic lordosis in the lumbar spine.

- Adequate reduction of the bony fragments may be assessed by palpating the fragments underneath the dura. If the fragments cannot be reduced by an indirect method, a direct posterior decompression may be performed by a laminectomy or transpedicle decompression.[12]
- Care must be taken in those patients with lamina fractures because they may have dural tears. In some cases with lamina fractures, the dura is torn and the nerve roots are protruding through the lamina fracture. The neural elements must not be injured during the exposure of the fracture, and the dural tears must be carefully repaired.
- The area involved in the fusion must be properly decorticated to form a proper bed for the bone graft. Iliac crest bone graft is then taken and placed posterolaterally for an intertransverse process fusion.
- Postoperatively, the patient is placed into a custom-molded thoracolumbosacral orthosis (TLSO). The patient is allowed to ambulate in the brace as soon as possible.
- Radiographs are checked when the patient first ambulates to assure that the position of the construct has not changed. Serial radiographs are taken, and the fusion is usually solid in 3 to 6 months.
- Occasionally, an anterior decompression is needed to supplement posterior surgery.

ANTERIOR SURGERY WITH INSTRUMENTATION

Anterior surgery requires more expertise and is less commonly used for fractures of the low lumbar spine. In the more common thoracolumbar spine fractures, anterior decompression and instrumentation provide an optimal environment for neural decompression and recovery. Its use is limited in the less common low lumbar spine fractures, however, and there are no long-term studies to support its general use over posterior instrumentation in low lumbar fractures.

Advantages

- It allows direct decompression of the spinal canal.
- It provides more canal decompression than posterior indirect decompression.
- Immediate stability can be achieved.
- Another theoretic advantage is the load sharing aspect of an anterior reconstruction.
- The load sharing classification system described earlier in this chapter can help recognize which fractures are poorly controlled with posterior fixation and which require some type of anterior support.
- In a biomechanical study on unstable burst fractures, anterior reconstruction with grafting and instrumentation was found to be more stable than posterior devices.[13] The constructs were tested in axial compression, rotation, and flexion-extension, and in all cases, the anterior instrumentation surpassed the posterior devices. This makes sense when one remembers that unstable burst fractures disable the anterior and middle columns, which can be directly reconstructed by anterior strut grafting and solid instrumentation.
- Anterior instrumentation allows for fusion of only one level above and below the fracture. This preserves motion segments in the low lumbar spine, where each segment is valuable.

Indications for Anterior or Combined Surgery

- Posterior indirect reduction of the fracture fragments is inadequate.
- Anterior supplemental grafting is needed in fractures that have required a significant amount of anterior bone removal for the decompression.
- Grossly unstable fractures are not sufficiently stabilized by posterior instrumentation alone.[14]

Techniques

- Anterior surgery should be performed by more experienced surgeons. In many institutions, general surgeons collaborate with the spine surgeon for the approach.
- The retroperitoneal approach is commonly used and has been shown to provide excellent access to the low lumbar levels.
- The patient is placed in a right lateral decubitus position. The table may be tilted in the lumbar region and a kidney rest provided, enlarging the distance between the costal arch and the iliac crest. To stabilize the position, the patient's right leg is flexed at the hip and knee, while the left leg remains relatively extended. To avoid pressure sores, a cushion is placed between the legs, and the patient is secured with straps (Fig. 43-7).
- If access to L4 is required, a subcostal flank incision is used. The skin incision begins near the midline at the level of spinous process L1 and continues first beneath the twelfth rib, before running obliquely and anteriorly toward the vicinity of the rectus sheath. Depending on the exposure desired, the incision may be extended caudally lateral to the rectus sheath.
- The retroperitoneal tissue over the lumbar spine is divided in the longitudinal direction, with the sympathetic trunk being left in place laterally. Following the mandatory radiographic identification of the operating level (L4), the segmental vessels of L3, L4, and L5 vertebrae are exposed in the usual way, and are ligated and transected as far medially as possible (Fig. 43-8).
- Decompression is performed under direct visualization, and strut grafting is commonly used. The grafting that is used must reconstruct anterior and middle columns and withstand the axial loads place on the spine to achieve immediate stability.
- Commonly used grafts include iliac crest bone graft or fibular graft. Allograft with iliac crest bone graft placed inside the allograft ring may also be used. These grafting techniques provide for load sharing of the anterior portion

CHAPTER 43 Lumbar and Sacral Fractures

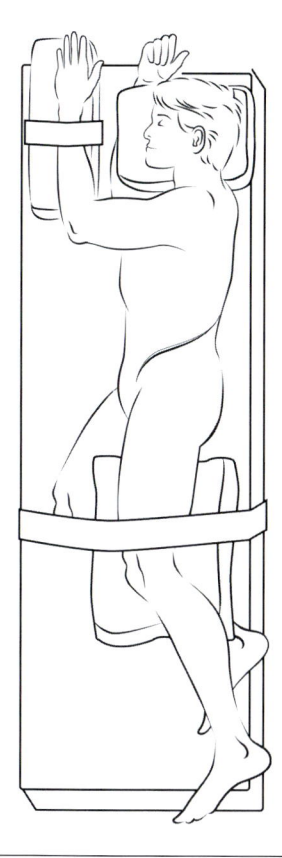

Fig. 43-7 The patient is placed in a right lateral decubitus position.

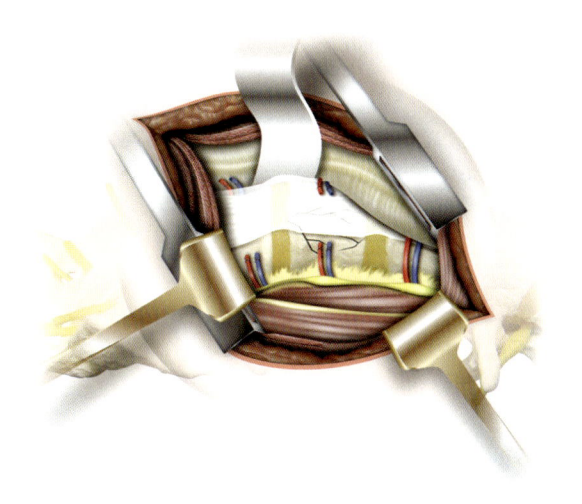

Fig. 43-8 Exposure of fractured L4 vertebra.

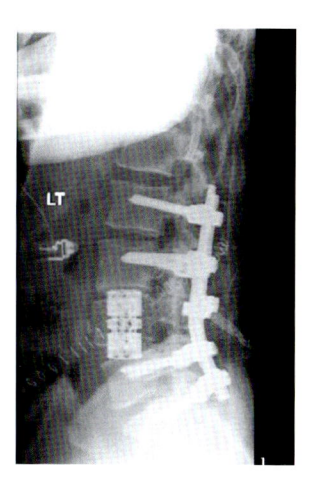

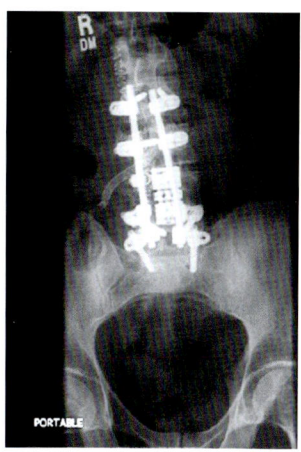

Fig. 43-9 Postoperative x-rays of L4 burst fracture. Anterior direct decompression and expandable cage graft and posterolateral fusion was done.

of the lumbar spine. Metal cages with bone graft placed inside are also commonly used (Fig. 43-9).
- If anterior instrumentation is necessary, many forms of anterior plating systems are available. Instrumentation placed in the anterior portion of the low lumbar spine approximates several important structures such as the aorta or iliac veins. The complications of anterior instrumentation could prove disastrous if the hardware is prominent and erodes into these vital structures.

OPERATIVE TECHNIQUES FOR SACRAL SPINE FRACTURES

For most sacral fractures, treatment decisions are based on three factors of the classification schema: (1) it is important to know whether the sacral injury is isolated or is accompanied by a pelvic injury; (2) the fracture line must be identified as either vertical or transverse; and (3) if the fracture is oblique, it is important to ascertain whether it involves the L5-S1 articulation.

The three principal goals in managing sacral fractures are (1) reestablishment of stability of the pelvic ring and lumbosacral junction; (2) correction and prevention of angular (kyphotic) and translational (shear) deformities of both the pelvic ring-sacrum and lumbosacral junction; and (3) prevention of further neural deficit and treatment of existing neurologic injury with appropriate decompressive and stabilizing procedures.

TREATMENT PROTOCOL

- The goal is a stable, pain-free pelvis ring and the preservation of neural function.
- Conservative care—This treatment approach is for patients with intact neurologic function and minimally displaced or angulated fractures (e.g., stable zone 1 and 2 injuries). Care requires a short period of bed rest followed by progressive mobilization in a cast or brace and then ambulatory status as tolerated. During this period, neurologic functions are monitored, and fractures are assessed with

serial radiographs. Because the site is typically well vascularized, these injuries should be fully united by 3 months.
- External fixator—Unstable pelvic injuries should be treated with emergent application of an external fixator. If vertical displacement is present, then skeletal traction should be added.
- Operation—For vertical fractures, especially in zones 1 and 2 (with or without other pelvic involvement), fixation with horizontal compression across the posterior aspect of the ilium and sacrum seems to provide adequate fixation. Although this can be done using sacral bars, the point of compression is posterior to the fracture line, and the potential exists for an opening on the anterior portion of the sacrum unless anterior fixation is also used. In addition, for zone 2 injuries through the region of the foramen, compression is not desirable.
- The sacral bar technique depends on compression for fixation and thus may compress the comminuted bone in the region of the foramen. Direct screw fixation can be done with little or no compression. Recent biomechanical studies evaluating fixation for transforaminal fractures has shown little difference between one or two iliosacral screws in combination with posterior tension bands or posterior transiliac bar devices. Sacral bars have also been compared with a new plate devised for fixation of these fractures.

ILIOSACRAL SCREW FIXATION

- The technique of iliosacral screw placement, in both prone and supine operative positions, has been well described.[10] Likewise, the verification of reduction and screw placement can be done with either image intensification or computed tomography (CT) scan guidance.
- Whether the patient is in a prone or supine position, the operation must be done on a radiolucent table. The image intensifier is placed on the opposite side from the surgeon. Initial calibration of the angles is performed, which is necessary to obtain simulated inlet (40 degrees caudad) and outlet (40 degrees cephalad) views for monitoring the screw insertion (Fig. 43-10).
- Next, perform anatomic reduction by positioning or traction with fluoroscopic confirmation. The position of the starting hole is the most critical feature in obtaining adequate screw position. A number of different techniques exist for determining the starting hole, but most are based on the intersection of a line from the sciatic notch and one from the posterior superior iliac crest. Ideally, the screw should be perpendicular to the ilium and should cross the sacroiliac joint and remain within the sacral ala, proximal to the S1 foramen and distal to the L5-S1 disk, entering the vertebral body of S1.
- The screw penetration needs to be at least to the midline for zone 1 injuries and across the midline for zone 2 injuries. Penetration should cross the midline into the contralateral ala for zone 3 fractures with an oblique or vertical component.
- It is preferable to use a 6.5-mm fully threaded cannulated cancellous screw. This prevents further compression across the comminuted fracture site, which decreases the chance for impingement of roots in transforaminal fractures. Screw length generally averages between 60 and 90 mm, but as much as 130 mm may be required to reach the contralateral ala. Use of the calibrated direct measurement on the image intensifier makes choice of screw length easier. Washers should be used to prevent penetration of the screw head into the ilium.

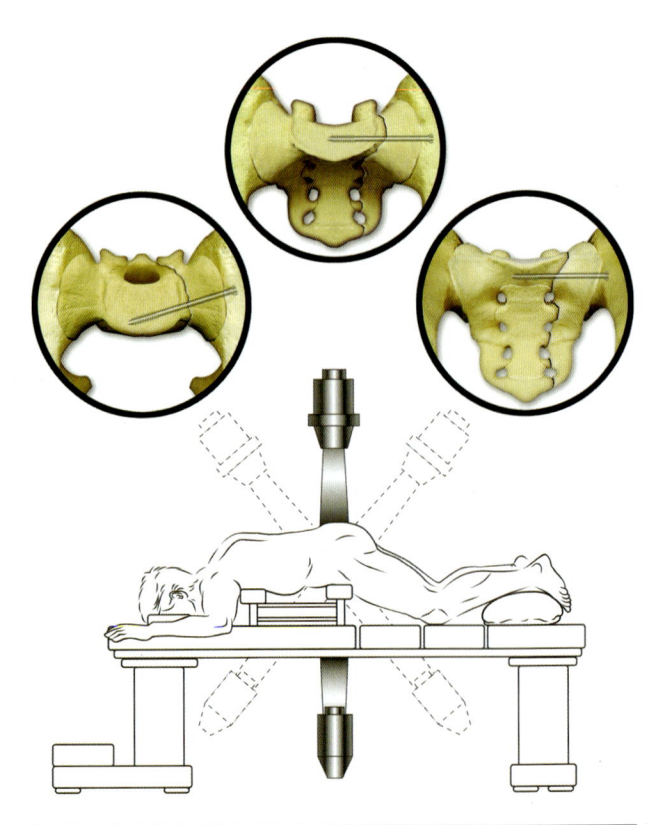

Fig. 43-10 Iliosacral screw fixation. To be certain that iliosacral screw fixation into the sacrum is accurate, some type of monitoring is necessary. The image must be placed so that 40 degrees caudal and 40 degrees cephalad views can be obtained. Screws can be used for fractures in zone 1 (partially threaded screw) and in zone 2 (transforaminal) fractures (fully threaded screw).

BILATERAL PLATING

- For patients with either isolated oblique or transverse fractures of the sacrum, with or without involvement of the lumbosacral junction, the technique of bilateral plating of the posterior surface of the sacrum is applicable.[10] It is also applicable to fractures that are unstable and have significant deformity and to patients with neurologic deficit.

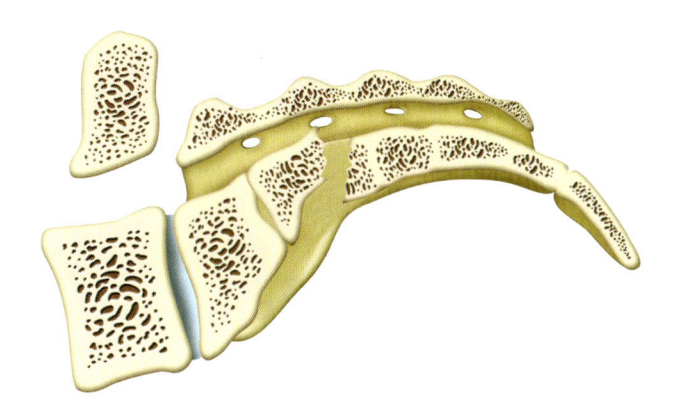

Fig. 43-11 Lateral view of the transverse sacral fracture with kyphotic deformity. Exposure from L5 to S4 is needed.

- Situate the patient in a prone position, with slight flexion of the table in its midportion; use a radiolucent operating table with image.
- The exposure should be a wide exposure of the spine from L5 down to S4 through the midline (Fig. 43-11).
- During the posterior dissection in the area of the fracture line, care must be taken to avoid motion of the comminuted fragments to prevent further damage of the compromised roots.
- The dissection is carried out laterally beyond the dorsal foramen at all levels from S1 to S4. The L5-S1 facet joint capsules are preserved if there is no involvement at L5-S1. Otherwise, the L5-S1 facet joint capsules can be removed. Plate placement is generally in a line directly over the dorsal foramina. The posterior aspect of the fracture line can be fully identified after exposure of the posterior aspect of the sacrum.
- Perform a sacral laminectomy to identify the sacral roots and the area of maximal deformity and compression. The lateral decompression must extend laterally enough to identify the take-off point of the ventral root sleeves and the bone of the vestigial sacral pedicles. Once the deformity is identified and the laminectomy is completed to enable direct visualization of the roots, attention is turned to reduction of the fracture. Little attempt is made at this time to decompress the roots, as reduction of the kyphosis often accomplishes much of this. Care should be taken, however, to ascertain that the ventral surface of the roots at the level of the maximal fracture angulation is not trapped in the fracture site.
- Because the sacral roots are freely visible after the decompression, a Cobb elevator can be safely placed within the fracture to lever the fragments, or bone clamps may be used to apply corrective translational forces to reduce the fracture.
- Intraoperative use of the image intensifier is often helpful at this stage. Complex multiplanar fractures would be reduced in similar fashion, with the possible addition of intraoperative skeletal traction to reduce the vertical shear.
- For fractures that are predominantly transverse, the fracture line can be identified in the region of S2-S3 and the dissection carried laterally to allow complete exposure of that fracture line. Using a small curette, the fracture line is identified, as is the obliquity of the fracture line, with care taken to remove as little of the crushed cancellous bone as possible in the process.
- A Cobb elevator can then be placed within the fracture on both sides so that the kyphosis of the fracture may be corrected manually.
- The direction of application of leverage of the fracture line is based on the direction of displacement. If the proximal fragment is lying posterior to the distal fragment, then an attempt will be made to pass the Cobb elevators over the superoanterior aspect of the distal fragment, after which the proximal fragment is gently levered into a less kyphotic configuration and is translated anteriorly.
- If the reduction can then be maintained using a single Cobb elevator, instrumentation can be initiated. For more oblique fracture lines that may pass through the central canal at anywhere from a 20- to 45-degree angle, some foreshortening of the sacrum may occur. Length can be regained temporarily by placing bicortical screws through the sacral ala and then using a pelvic reduction clamp to slightly distract the screws to disimpact the fracture line and achieve length for correction of angulatory deformity.
- If a large fragment of the floor of the sacral canal continues to compress the dural sac, even after initial temporary reduction, consideration is given to the excavation of the sacral ala just lateral to the canal, so that the fragments that are impinging the canal can be removed through an oblique lateral exposure. This may require bilateral excavations at the level of the fracture or simply unilateral excavation.
- No attempt should be made to tamp the fragments into place. Rather, the fragments should be removed using a pituitary rongeur. Care is taken not to damage the roots during removal of the fragments. Fragments should be put aside for subsequent bone grafting.
- At this point, internal fixation can be accomplished. Commonly, pelvic reconstruction plates are used to achieve stabilization. This may require either a 3.5- or 4.5-mm plate. The characteristics on which the choice of this hardware is based are its malleability over the posterior contours of the sacrum and the correlation of hole spacing with the proper fixation points on the sacrum.
- For transverse or transverse/oblique fractures within the body of the sacrum, a minimum of two sets of screws proximal and distal to the fracture line is preferable. Because bone stock and screw fixation points are limited in the sacrum, reduction should never be attempted using the instrumentation to avoid screw pullout while levering on the plate. If the fracture configuration permits, we prefer

to insert both medial and lateral screws into the sacrum at S1, thereby achieving optimal fixation into the superior fragment.
- The most proximal screw, at the lateral border of the S1 superior facet, is directed approximately 30 degrees medially into the S1 body through the pedicle, aiming at the sacral promontory. The next screw, at the inferior edge of the S1 facet, is directed 35 degrees laterally into the sacral ala and parallel to the sacral end plate. In the remainder of the levels, a single or double screw traversing the pedicle laterally and parallel to the sacroiliac joint is preferred.
- The average proximal screw inserted at the level of the medial border of the S1 facet is usually directed about 30 degrees medially, entering into the S1 body; screw length generally averages 35 to 45 mm. The next screw is inserted below the inferior edge of the S1 facet and is directed laterally approximately 35 degrees into the sacral ala and parallel into the plane of the sacroiliac joint. The proximal screws average approximately 30 to 45 mm in length. The screws at S2, S3, and S4 are shorter (approximately 20 mm at the most distal point). Trajectory is between 20 and 35 degrees laterally.
- If the fracture line is more oblique than transverse, and involves the L5-S1 articulation, the most proximal end of the construct needs to be extended to the L5 pedicle. This is sufficient if there is minimal translation (less than 20% of the body width). However, the construct may need to be extended even more proximally to L4 to achieve adequate purchase on the distal portion of the spine if 50% or more displacement is present at the L5-S1 level.
- After fixation is complete, the canal is reassessed. Reconfirmation of sacral roots decompression by gentle retraction of the roots toward the midline. If any residual impinging bone is remained, it is removed with a curette or pituitary rongeur. Tamping the fragments down into the sacrum is much less effective.
- The contralateral side is also checked and if reduction was incomplete, decompression is still possible by resecting the residual bone of the displaced portion of the floor of the canal. Decompression should not be attempted without stabilization, as shifting of the fracture alignment can easily cause compression to recur.
- If the reduction is incomplete and some translational deformity still exists, but the fracture is in a stable position, additional excavation of the floor of the canal will be undertaken to remove any bone that may be pressing on the ventral surface of the sacral roots.
- Cancellous grafting is usually not necessary for fractures contained totally within the sacrum, although any residual graft can be used to fill in the defects. However, for those that traverse the L5-S1 articulation, standard transverse process sacral alar grafting should be done with autologous cancellous bone. Reapproximation of the paraspinous musculature over the hardware and fracture is critical.
- Postoperatively, the patients are placed into a custom-molded total-contact orthosis, with one thigh incorporated into the brace. Once in the brace, the patient progresses to ambulation as tolerated. Bracing is typically continued on a full-time basis for 10 to 12 weeks. We do not advocate routine removal of the plates unless they are causing soft tissue irritation.

ILIAC FIXATION WITH FOUR SCREW FOUNDATION

For patients with either isolated oblique or vertical fractures of the sacrum, with or without involvement of the lumbosacral junction, the technique of iliac fixation with four screw foundation is applicable.
- Proximal anchor site preparation (lumbar and sacral pedicle screw)—Lumbar and sacral pedicles are prepared with awls, pedicle probes, ball tip feelers, and bone taps. Appropriate insertion of lumbar and S1 pedicle screws is completed (Fig. 43-12).
- Distal anchor site preparation (inferior and superior iliac screws)—The iliac screw entry points are identified and prepared by resecting the posterior superior iliac spine with a curved osteotome. The resection should be flush with the sacrum to prevent entry into the sacroiliac joint. This will also place the iliac foundation more anteriorly, improving the soft tissue coverage over the ilium. This resection results in a flat and oval cancellous starting point for both the superior and inferior iliac screws.

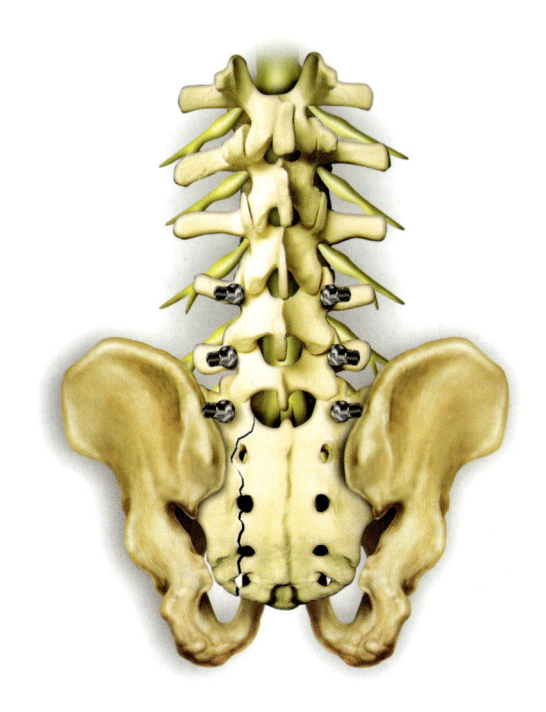

Fig. 43-12 Proximal anchor site preparation and proper insertion of lumbar and S1 pedicle screw.

- Inferior iliac screw—With the fingertip of the opposite hand in the sciatic notch, the ISOLA iliac starter probe is inserted into the inferior portion of the oval cancellous window and worked between the two cortical plates of the ilium. The standard ISOLA iliac probe is then inserted and advanced to just above the sciatic notch. The surgeon should palpate the lateral wall of the ilium when advancing the ISOLA iliac probe. When the desired depth is reached, a plain anteroposterior radiograph may be obtained with the probe in place. Fluoroscopy can be used at the surgeon's discretion. A ball tip feeler is inserted into the prepared channel to confirm that the path has not perforated the pelvis.
- The inferior iliac screw size is determined. Inferior screw is recommended to use a large diameter and long length screw. A 10-mm ISOLA closed iliac screw is recommended for this use. The screw's large diameter is intended to purchase both iliac cortices for maximum fixation. The average length is 70 mm, but some patients will accept up to a 100-mm screw.
- The inferior iliac screw path is tapped and a closed ISOLA iliac screw is inserted into the inferior ilium. Some key points to remember include the following: (1) the iliac screw should be placed as perpendicular to the coronal plane of the spine as possible, (2) the inferior screw should not be inserted at an angle like a traditional Galveston position, (3) screw position is critical for ease of construct assembly, (4) minimal convergence of the iliac screws is optimal as this allows the contoured rod to pass easily through the screw heads, and (5) the opening of the screw faces cephalad/caudal.
- Superior iliac screw—The second iliac screw insertion site is the superior end of the oval cancellous window. The ISOLA iliac starter probe is inserted into the superior end of the oval cancellous window with a direction of slight cephalad inclination. The standard ISOLA iliac probe is then inserted to widen the path in the ilium. The surgeon palpates the outer upper ilium to help guide the probe placement. It is recommended that the probe is inserted to a depth of 45 to 55 mm.
- The superior iliac screw path is tapped and a closed ISOLA iliac screw is inserted into the superior ilium. The opening of the superior iliac screw faces cephalad/caudal. The recommended insertion depth of the superior iliac screw is 45 to 55 mm. A 10-mm screw can be used in most patients; however, a 7.75-mm screw can also be used. The screw is inserted with a slight cephalad inclination and will not be perpendicular to the resection site as seen with the inferior screw.
- Distal anchor rod sizing and trial—The distal anchor site preparation procedure is repeated for the opposite side of the pelvis. Rods are measured, cut, and contoured followed by provisional placement through the openings of the closed screws to verify fit (Fig. 43-13). Rods are then removed and rodded connectors added. The assemblies are placed into the closed screws. (*Note:* Unobstructed passage of the rod through the screws should be confirmed.)
- Interconnection of proximal and distal anchors—The proximal and distal anchors are interconnected using 6.35-mm rod connectors and standard ISOLA slotted connectors. This creates independent proximal and distal foundations from which the ilium and sacrum can be manipulated to achieve correction. All nuts on the pedicle screws are provisionally tightened to provide stability to the construct during corrective maneuvers. Four rodded connectors are required to interconnect the lumbar, sacral, and iliac anchors to one another. The first pair of rodded connectors (cephalad/caudal), running from the ilium into the sacrum and up into the lumbar region, are used to correct the displaced ilium/sacrum. The second pair of rodded connectors (medial/lateral), spanning across the sacrum, will be used to reduce the fracture.
- Proximal foundation manipulation and correction of displaced sacrum ad ilium—Using distraction between L5 and S1, the displaced sacrum/ilium is brought back into proper anatomic alignment. Set screws are locked.
- Distal foundation manipulation and reduction of fracture—Using compression between the transverse rodded connector and the side-by-side dual rod connector, the fracture is reduced. Set screws are locked.

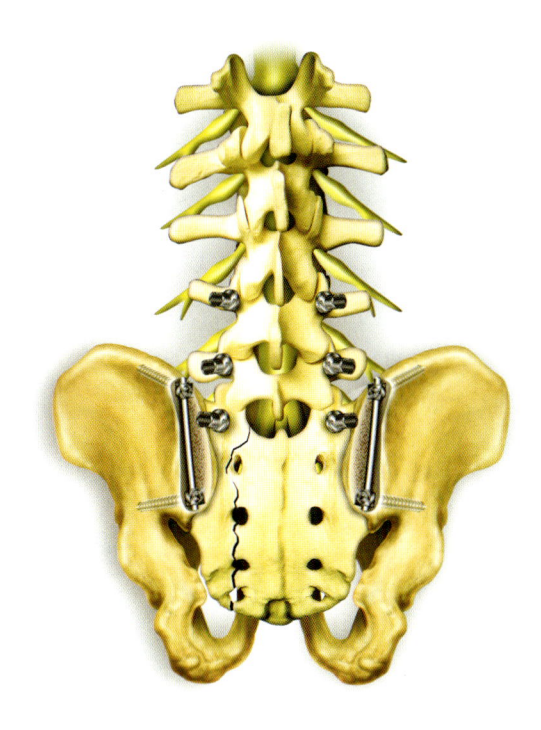

Fig. 43-13 The distal anchor site preparation procedure is repeated for the opposite side of the pelvis. Rods are measured, cut, and contoured followed by provisional placement through the openings of the closed screws to verify fit.

A

B

Fig. 43-14 *A* and *B*, Iliosacral screw plus tension band plate across the ilium.

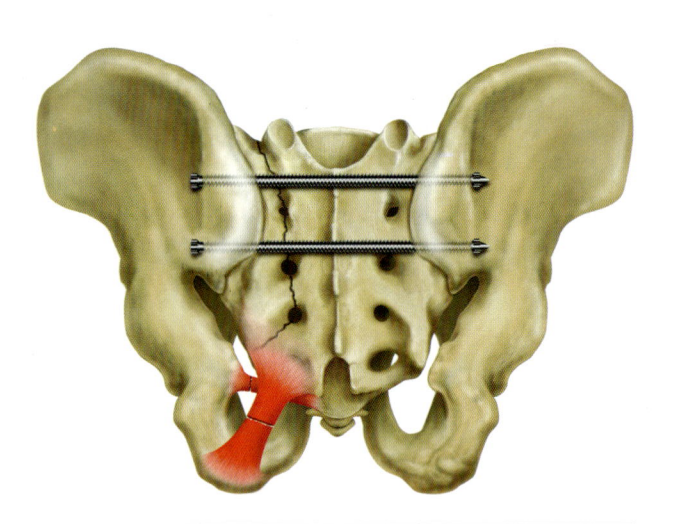

Fig. 43-15 Transiliac screw.

- Final tightening—The set screws on the slotted/rodded connectors and closed screws are tightened to 60 inch-pounds followed by final tightening of the $5/16$-inch hex nut on the pedicle screws to 100 inch-pounds. A cross connector is added at the desired level.

OTHER TECHNIQUES

Other variable techniques are available. Sacroiliac plating, sacral bar techniques, and tension band across the ilium, transiliac screw, and their combinations have been developed. Some of these are shown in Figures 43-14 and 43-15.

COMPLICATIONS

Complications may include neurologic deterioration, hardware dislodgement, nonunion, and loss of correction.

References

1. An HS, Vaccaro A, Cotler JM, Lin S: Low lumbar burst fractures: Comparison among body cast Harrington rod, Luque rod, and Steffee plate. Spine 1991;16(8 Suppl):S440–S444.
2. Levine AM, Edwards CC: Low lumbar burst fractures: reduction and stabilization using the modular spine fixation system. Orthopedics 1988;11(10):1420–1432.
3. Levine AM: Lumbar and sacral spine trauma. In Browner BD, Jupiter JB, Levine AM, Trafton PG (eds): Skeletal Trauma–Fractures, Dislocations, Ligamentous Injuries. Philadelphia, WB Saunders, 1998, pp 1035–1093.
4. Denis F: Updated classification of thoracolumbar fractures. Orthop Trans 1982;6:8.
5. McAfee PC, Yuan HA, Frederickson BE, Lubicky JP: The value of computed tomography in thoracolumbar fractures. J Bone Joint Surg Am 1983;65A:461–473.
6. McCormack T, Karaikovic E, Gaines R: The load sharing classification of spine fractures. Spine 1994;19:1741–1744.
7. Denis F, Davis S, Comfort T: Sacral fractures: An important problem: Retrospective analysis of 236 cases. Clin Orthop 1988; 227:67–81.
8. Roy-Camille R, Saillant G, Gagna G, et al: Transverse fracture of the upper sacrum. Spine 1985;10:838–845.
9. Strange-Vognsen HH, Lebech A: An unusual type of fracture in the upper sacrum. J Orthop Trauma 1991;5:200–203.
10. Levine AM, Curcin A: Fractures of the sacrum. In Levine AM, Eismont FJ, Garfin SR, Zigler JE (eds): Spine Trauma. Philadelphia, WB Saunders, 1998, pp 506–524.
11. Levine AM: Low lumbar spine trauma. In Levine AM, Eismont FJ, Garfin SR, Zigler JE (eds): Spine Trauma. Philadelphia, WB Saunders, 1998, pp 452–495.
12. Hardaker WT Jr, Cook WA Jr, Friedman AM, Fitch RD: Bilateral transpedicular decompression and Harrington rod stabilization in the management of severe thoracolumbar burst fractures. Spine 1992;18:692–699.
13. Maiman DJ, Pintar F, Yoganadan N, Reinartz J: Effects of anterior vertebral grafting on the traumatized lumbar spine after pedicle screw plate fixation. Spine 1993;18(15)2423–2430.
14. Wang J, Delamarter RB: Lumbar fractures of the spine. In Capen AC, Haye W (eds): Comprehensive Management of Spine Trauma. St. Louis, Mosby, 1998, pp 214–234.

SECTION V

SPINAL DEFORMITY

CHAPTER 44

DANIEL J. SUCATO

Anterior Release and Fusion Techniques for Thoracic Scoliosis

INTRODUCTION

The anterior approach to the thoracic spine is used in surgery for spinal deformity to achieve an anterior release for larger curves, to achieve anterior fusion (and to avoid the crankshaft phenomenon), and to achieve anterior fusion and correction of scoliosis using instrumentation. For anterior fusion and anterior release without instrumentation, the indications have changed throughout the years as the result of a better understanding of spinal growth and how it relates to the crankshaft phenomenon as well as the availability of more powerful posterior segmental fixation methods. The indications for these techniques are dependent on the type of approach used (open versus thoracoscopic), the training of the surgeon, the goals of the surgery, and the type of posterior implant system and technique that is used. For anterior instrumentation and fusion for spinal deformity, many proposed advantages for thoracic curve patterns have led to a greater use of this technique over the past 15 years. With a better understanding of correction mechanics and improved minimally invasive techniques (thoracoscopy), the indications for an anterior procedure in thoracic scoliosis continue to expand. These are certainly weighed against the continually evolving posterior techniques and implant systems that are also available. As in any technique, anterior surgery of the thoracic spine requires intimate knowledge of the anatomy to safely and effectively perform surgery of the anterior thoracic spine. This chapter will discuss the anterior approach to spine deformity in the pediatric and adolescent population.

INDICATIONS

The three main indications for anterior surgery for spinal deformity in the thoracic spine are (1) anterior release for severe spine deformity, (2) anterior release and fusion for skeletal immaturity, and (3) anterior fusion and instrumentation for spinal deformity. The first two indications require a posterior procedure, which almost always includes posterior instrumentation. The third indication is an isolated anterior procedure to achieve correction as well as maintenance of correction over time.

There is a higher threshold today for performing an anterior release and fusion because of greater correction mechanics posteriorly, and greater use of posterior segmental pedicle screw fixation. It is generally recommended that an anterior release be performed for scoliotic curve magnitudes greater than 80 degrees in which the curve fails to bend to less than 50 to 60 degrees on a supine best bend radiograph. The indications to perform an anterior fusion include the skeletally immature patient who is a Risser stage 0 and has open triradiate cartilage. Performing an anterior fusion becomes more difficult when the patient is a Risser stage 0 and the triradiate cartilage is closed because the peak growth velocity has passed. In these cases, other factors may lead one to decide to do an anterior fusion, including young age (girls ≤10 years or male patients ≤12 years), premenarchal status, and documentation of peak growth. Each surgeon must recognize these factors as well as the goal of surgery to determine whether anterior surgery is necessary when combined with posterior instrumentation and fusion. Variables that also affect decision making for these indications include whether the anterior surgery will be performed thoracoscopically or using an open thoracotomy approach. Certainly, a more minimally invasive approach with smaller incisions may lower the threshold to perform an anterior release in those cases in which decisions are more difficult. Finally, if an anterior release can be performed with the patient in the prone position without requiring single lung ventilation or needing to reposition the patient for the posterior aspect of the procedure, the decision may be made more easily.[1–3]

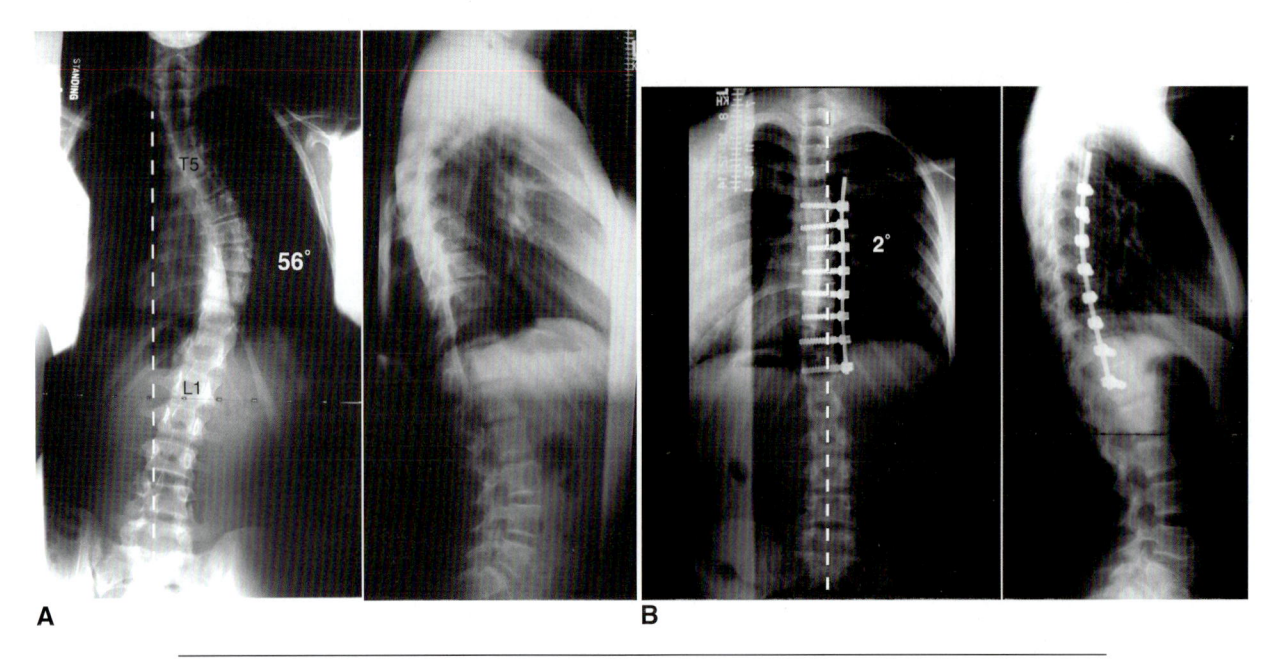

Fig. 44-1 *A,* Preoperative posteroanterior and lateral radiographs of a 12-year-old female with a Lenke 1A curve pattern who underwent a T5 to T12 anterior thoracoscopic instrumentation and fusion with excellent radiographic and clinical results. *B,* The 2-year postoperative radiographs demonstrating excellent correction in the coronal and sagittal planes.

The ideal indications for an anterior instrumentation and fusion for spinal deformity are patients who have single thoracic curve patterns (Lenke 1), who are relatively thin, have good bone quality to obtain good screw purchase, have good pulmonary function (greater than 70% predicted for forced expiratory volume and forced vital capacity), and no thoracic kyphosis (T5-T12 kyphosis less than 30 degrees). The Lenke 1 curve patterns are the most common and appropriate curve patterns for anterior instrumentation and fusion. The specific curve pattern that appears to yield excellent results in anterior instrumentation and fusion are the Lenke 1A curves in which the distal fusion levels are saved, especially when the distal end vertebra (distal fusion level for anterior instrumentation and fusion) is significantly deviated from the center sacral line (Fig. 44-1). The Lenke 1B and 1C patterns also result in excellent correction while maintaining overall coronal balance and may have a better result when compared to a posterior fusion and instrumentation[4] (Fig. 44-2). This is due, in part, to the lowest instrumented vertebra being the distal end vertebra of the thoracic curve, thus avoiding instrumentation into the lumbar curve and risking decompensation.

CONTRAINDICATIONS

Anterior surgery is contraindicated for those patients who will have a difficult time tolerating anterior surgery and the postoperative course primarily because of the impact on pulmonary function with this technique. Pulmonary function is adversely affected with any anterior surgery and requires patients to have preoperative pulmonary function tests greater than 70% of predicted.[5,6] It is generally felt that thoracoscopic approaches to the spine have less adverse effects on the patient's postoperative pulmonary function and may allow the surgeon to perform anterior thoracic surgery. The contraindications to anterior instrumentation and fusion are larger patients (greater than 70 kg), larger curve patterns (greater than 70 degrees), curves with less flexibility index (less than 50%), and thoracic kyphosis greater than 30 degrees. The thoracoscopic approach to the spine is technically more difficult than an open thoracotomy technique and is most challenging in patients who have had a previous thoracotomy approach with postoperative adhesions. Although this is not an absolute contraindication to thoracoscopy, it makes surgical treatment more difficult. The thoracoscopic anterior instrumentation and fusion in the thoracoscopic technique requires single lung ventilation, which may not be tolerated by some patients.

SURGICAL TECHNIQUE

ANTERIOR RELEASE AND FUSION

Understanding the thoracic anatomy is important when performing anterior surgery on the thoracic spine. Both the spine and its relationship to the ribs and other structures are important, as well as understanding the anatomy of the soft tissues surrounding the spine. These soft tissue structures

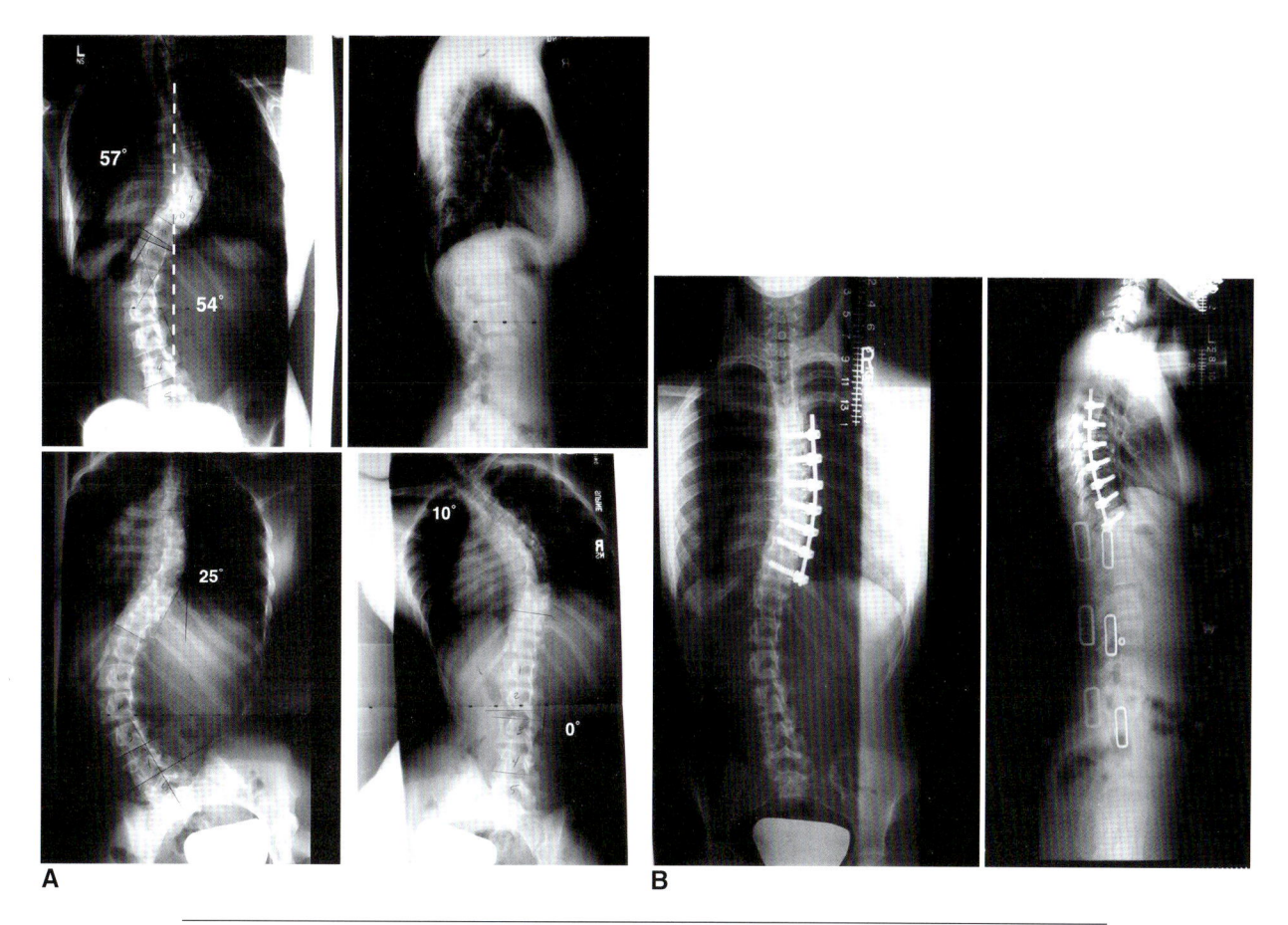

Fig. 44-2 *A,* Preoperative posteroanterior and lateral radiographs and supine bend radiographs of a 13-year-old female with a Lenke 1C curve pattern. Although there is a trunk shift to the left, the lumbar curve bends to 0 degrees. *B,* The 2-year postoperative radiographs following a thoracoscopic anterior fusion and instrumentation demonstrating intentional undercorrection of the thoracic curve with excellent response of the lumbar curve and a well-balanced patient. Note that the distal level of the anterior fusion stopped at the end vertebra, limiting the influence on the lumbar spine.

include the position of the great vessels (aorta and vena cava), the lungs, the thoracic duct, and the heart, and in the proximal thoracic spine the esophagus and trachea are in proximity (Fig. 44-3). Sucato and Duchene analyzed the position of the thoracic aorta in right thoracic idiopathic scoliosis and demonstrated that it was on the posterolateral aspect of the vertebral bodies on the concavity of the curve.[7] This is important to understand when performing any anterior surgery in the thoracic spine because long vertebral body screws that protrude beyond the contralateral cortex are at risk for proximity to the aorta.[8] The thoracic duct is most concerning when operating on the right lower thoracic spine because the cisterna chylae coalesce into the thoracic duct at the T11 and T12 areas. Penetration into the thoracic duct will yield chylothorax, which can be very challenging to treat.

For an open anterior approach to the thoracic spine, an incision is made over the rib, usually the rib of the most proximal planned level (i.e., fifth rib for a T5 to T12 anterior procedure). Additional thoracotomies can be made through the same incision that is used for the initial incision to gain better access to more distal levels. A variety of methods can be used to position the portal incisions for a thoracoscopic surgery. Generally, for an anterior release procedure, four incisions are placed in the anterior axillary line so that excellent access anteriorly, posteriorly, and in the midline can be achieved (Fig. 44-4*A* and *B*). Once access into the chest is achieved, the parietal pleura is incised in a longitudinal fashion in the midvertebral body, and it is then teased and bluntly dissected anteriorly to give good visualization of the anterior longitudinal ligament and contralateral annulus, as well as posteriorly to unveil the rib heads as they attach into the vertebral bodies (see Fig. 44-4*C*). Understanding the insertion point of the rib heads onto the spine is important when performing an anterior release as this serves as a reference for the

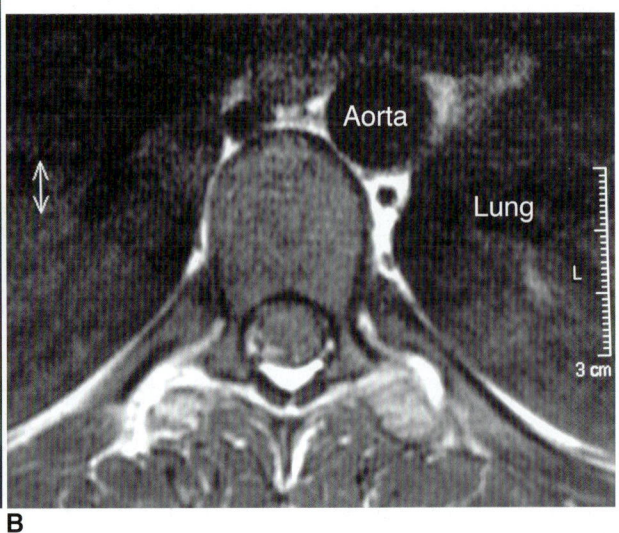

Fig. 44-3 *A* and *B*, Axial magnetic resonance image in the midthoracic spine demonstrating the position of the aorta and the lung fields.

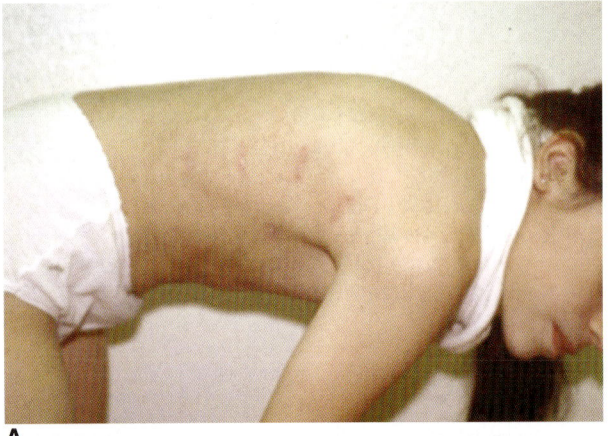

Fig. 44-4 *A,* Clinical photograph of a patient who underwent a thoracoscopic anterior spinal fusion and instrumentation. The four posterolateral portals and the single anterior portal are seen. For a thoracosopic release/fusion only, four portals would be placed in the anterior axillary line. *B,* An intraoperative photograph during a thoracoscopic procedure, prior to pleural incision. The segmental blood vessels and the sympathetic chain can be seen as well as the rib heads. Excellent visualization of the spine is accomplished with the thoracoscopic technique. *C,* Following longitudinal pleural incision with preservation of the segmental blood vessels. The disk is easily accessed with retraction of the pleura anteriorly.

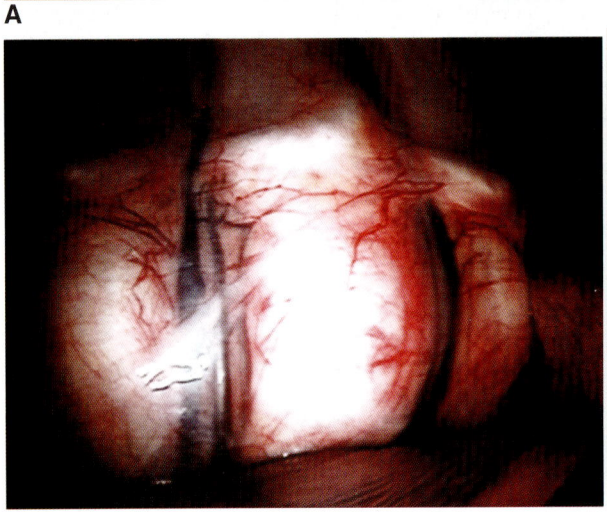

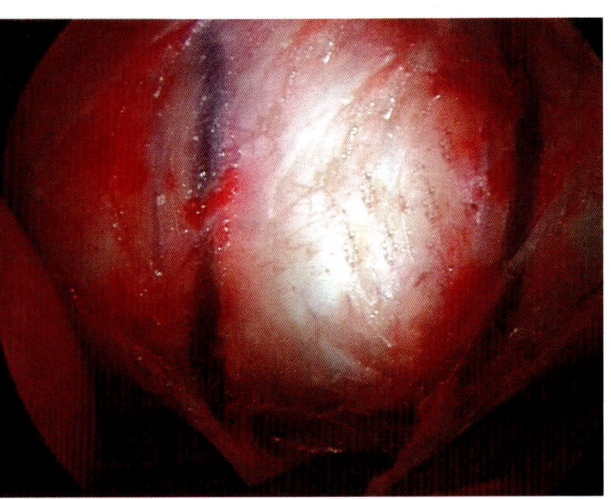

location of the spinal canal. The rib head inserts more anteriorly in the proximal thoracic spine and gradually moves more posteriorly in the distal thoracic spine.[9] Approximately 30% of the posterior vertebral body is obscured by the rib head at T5 and necessitates partial rib head excision to obtain complete access to the disk, which also assists in gaining release of the spine. The position of the rib changes in the distal thoracic spine with a more posterior postion and, therefore, does not obscure the disk space at T12.

Once the disk material is removed, a hemostatic agent is placed in the disk space to prevent excessive end plate bleeding. Access to the T12-L1 disk is possible with partial dissection of the diaphragm. The diskectomy should be complete from rib head to rib head, and this can be better visualized by viewing each end plate, recognizing that they are spherical in nature. Each anterior release should be tailored to the goal of surgery. Segmental vessel ligation is not necessary when performing an anterior release because a good anterior release can be performed thoracoscopically and preservation of spinal cord perfusion is maintained.[10] Certainly, hypotensive anesthesia should not be performed when anterior segmental blood vessels are ligated.

Pleural closure should be performed in all cases, whether done as an open thoracotomy or thoracoscopically (Fig. 44-5). This may be important to maintain the bone graft in the disk space, decrease chest tube output, decrease postoperative adhesion formation, and potentially improve pulmonary function.

Following pleural closure, the chest is reapproximated when using the open thoracotomy approach, and a chest tube is placed. Thoracoscopic access to the spine allows for closure of the portals relatively quickly and placement of the chest tube using the inferior portal incision and tunneling the tube into the next-to-last portal chest entry.

ANTERIOR INSTRUMENTATION AND FUSION

For anterior instrumentation and fusion using an open thoracotomy approach, the most proximal rib is the rib associated with the most proximal fusion level. For example, T5-T12 fusion requires resection of the fifth rib. Often, long fusions require a double thoracotomy through the same incision in which two ribs are harvested. The diskectomy is performed in the same fashion as an anterior release or fusion; however, segmental blood vessels are ligated. The surgeon may choose to temporarily ligate vessels and monitor somatosensory evoked potentials and motor evoked potentials for 20 minutes following temporary ligation.

Upon completion of the diskectomies, screws are placed. Screws are often initially placed at the apex of the curve and are placed as posterior as possible without entrance into the spinal canal (Fig. 44-6A and B). The rib head again is used as a landmark, and the screw starting point is just anterior to the rib heads (see Fig. 44-6C and D). At the apex of the curve, because of the rotational aspect of the spine deformity, screws are oriented in an anterior direction so that they are in the midaxial plane of the vertebral body. At the more proximal and distal vertebrae, the screws are started slightly more anteriorly and their direction may be across the vertebral body oriented horizontally to the patient because of less rotation of the vertebral bodies. Although bicortical screw purchase has been recommended for many years, it does carry risk for penetration across the vertebral body adjacent to the aorta when instrumenting right thoracic curves.[7,11] The most proximal screws are more at risk for screw plow or pullout and must be placed in the midvertebral body. It is necessary to remove the rib heads at T5, T6, and T7 to ensure that the screws are in the midvertebral body (Fig. 44-7). The most proximal screws can be directed slightly obliquely from proximal to distal because proximal screw plow often occurs during correction of the spine owing to smaller vertebral bodies and low bone mineral density in many of these patients. Following completion of screw placement, inspection of the screws should be performed using fluoroscopy to ensure that adjacent screws are at similar height so that rod placement is easy (Fig. 44-8).

Correction mechanics for anterior instrumentation and fusion include compression and cantilever. The rod is placed without any contour and can be initially placed proximally, distally, or in the middle of the construct and seated in two to four screws, depending on the magnitude of deformity. Compression is performed across those levels to gain correction (Fig. 44-9). Cantilever of the rod down to the remaining screws is performed, and compression is completed. With a flexible rod and correctly oriented screws, thoracic kyphosis is restored owing to the compressive forces applied, with excellent coronal plane correction as well as axial plane

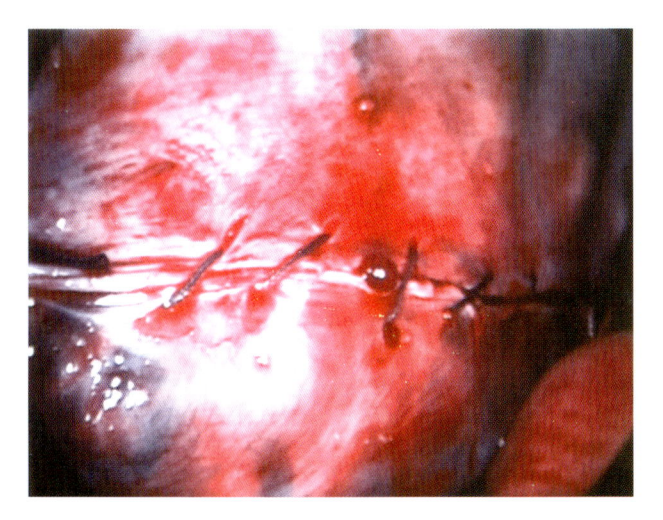

Fig. 44-5 Pleural closure following an anterior release and fusion procedure without instrumentation performed using thoracoscopic techniques.

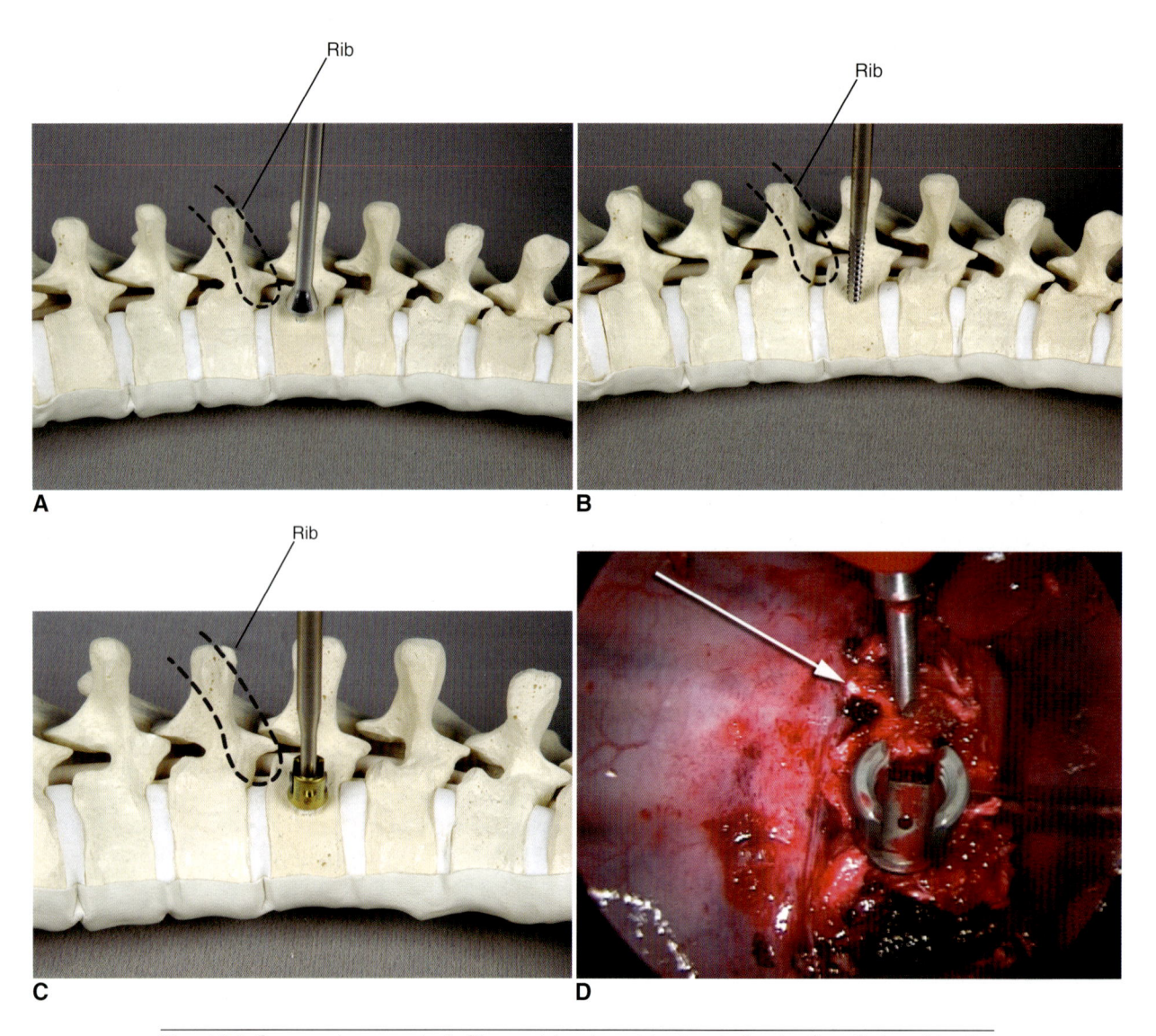

Fig. 44-6 Screw placement. *A,* The awl is placed just anterior to the rib head in the midthoracic spine. *B,* The tap is placed. *C,* Placement of the screw. *D,* Intraoperative photograph demonstrating the position of the screw just anterior to the rib head (*arrow*).

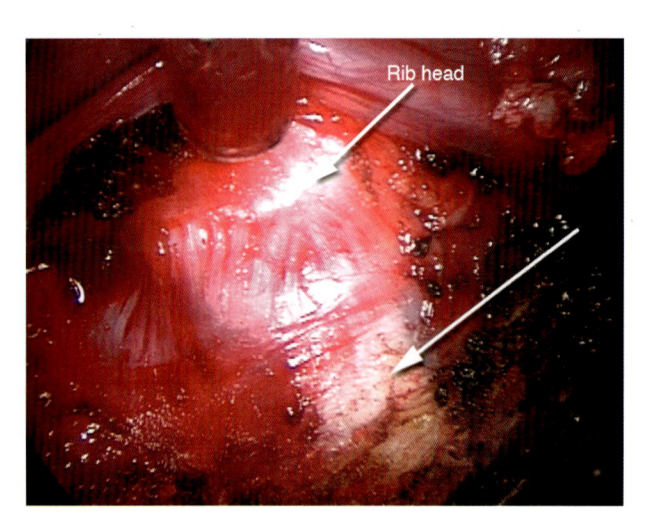

Fig. 44-7 Intraoperative photograph during a thoracoscopic anterior instrumentation at the T5-T6 disk level (*arrow*). Note the rib head of T6 is anterior on the vertebral body, obscuring the location for screw placement. The rib head is usually removed at the T4 to T7 levels to adequately place the screws because the rib head lies far anterior on the vertebral body, as shown here.

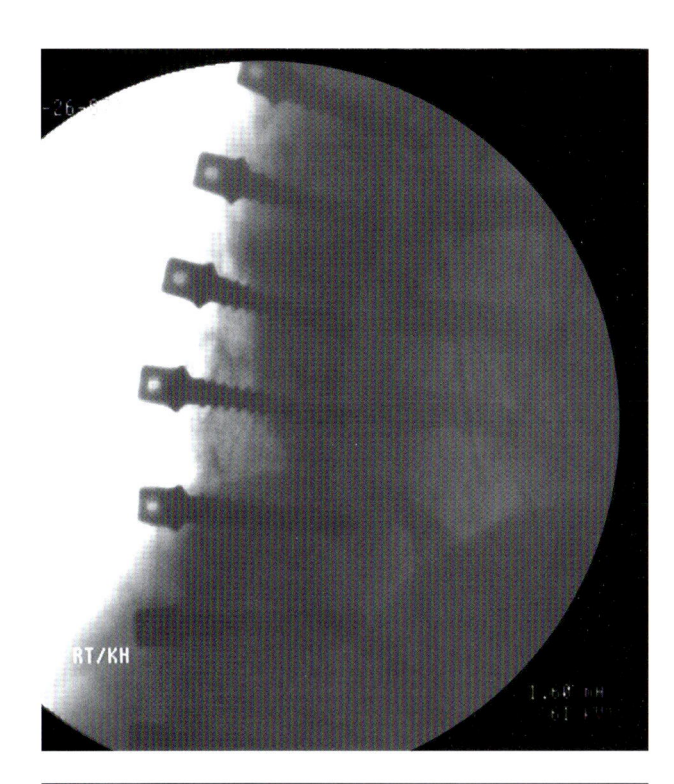

Fig. 44-8 Intraoperative fluoroscopy image following placement of all screws. The level of the screw heads is the same and will allow easy placement of the rod.

correction. Thoracic kyphosis may be prebent into the rod prior to placing the rod, and then rod rotation may be performed. This is less commonly used today and cannot be performed thoracoscopically. Prior to rod placement, bone graft material is placed. For open procedures this utilizes the rib that has been harvested for the approach, and for thoracoscopic instrumentation and fusion, small segments of rib or iliac crest bone graft have been utilized. Bone graft substitutes as a standalone bone grafting material is to be strictly avoided.

After correction of the spine we recommend pleural closure over the instrumentation to help contain bone graft, decrease the chest tube drainage, and prevent intrathoracic adhesion development and loss of pulmonary capacity (Fig. 44-10). Pleural closure is facilitated by teasing the pleura both anteriorly and posteriorly during the surgery so that it can easily be placed over the instrumentation at the completion of the surgery, allowing closure without excess tension.

Several unique steps are required when performing a thoracoscopic anterior instrumentation and fusion. Single lung ventilation is used to allow complete access to the spine and requires specialized training by the anesthesiologist because placement of a double lumen endotracheal tube and maintenance of single lung ventilation can be challenging. Portal placement is crucial for thoracoscopic anterior instrumentation and fusion to allow for complete diskectomy and to accurately place the intravertebral body screws. Portal placement is varied, especially with respect to the utilization of anterior portals; however, it is critical that the posterolateral portals are placed directly over the vertebral bodies, erring on being more posterior (over the rib heads) to allow for safe and easy screw placement. We generally recommend a single anterior portal (placed in the anterior axillary line) and three or four posterolateral portals (see Fig. 44-4A). The anterior portal is used to place the thoracoscope and is used extensively to gain excellent access to the anterior spine to remove the anterior longitudinal ligament as well as the contralateral annulus. The most proximal posterolateral portal is always the most difficult and challenging to place, partly because of the close position of the scapula, which tends to push this portal anterior and distal. This should be kept in mind when placing this portal to ensure adequate placement over the most proximal intended fusion level, especially because this screw is most at risk for screw plow and pullout.

Using guidewires prior to skin incisions for these posterolateral portals may ensure adequate and accurate placement (Fig. 44-11). Screws can be placed over a guidewire or directly following placement of the awl and tap (Fig. 44-12A and B). The guidewire allows for fine-tuning of the starting hole; however, it must be used with great care because cannulated instruments over the guidewire risk advancing the guidewire to the opposite side of the chest, potentially causing significant injury to soft tissue structures.[12] Alternatively, a combination awl and removable circular staple can be initially introduced and then followed by the tap and screw (see Fig. 44-12C). This seems to enable faster placement of screws while utilizing less fluoroscopy, but it requires exact screw starting hole position.

RESULTS

Anterior release and fusion to prevent the crankshaft phenomenon has been successful in several reports using either an open thoracotomy or thoracoscopic approach.[13-16] Although more recent studies indicate that posterior segmental fixation may help in preventing the crankshaft phenomenon without an anterior procedure,[17,18] we would continue to recommend anterior fusion of the apical levels when there is an open triradiate cartilage in the young patient who has not reached their peak growth velocity. This recommendation is especially strong when the surgery can be done using thoracoscopic techniques with the patient in the prone position, which precludes the use of single lung ventilation and avoids repositioning of the patient for the posterior aspect of the surgery.[1] The anterior approach appears to achieve an excellent release of the anterior structures and to allow for excellent correction of the deformity using posterior implants and correction maneuvers. The amount of release of the anterior structures and the resultant biomechanical flexibility appear to be similar, whether using an open thoracotomy approach or a thoracoscopic

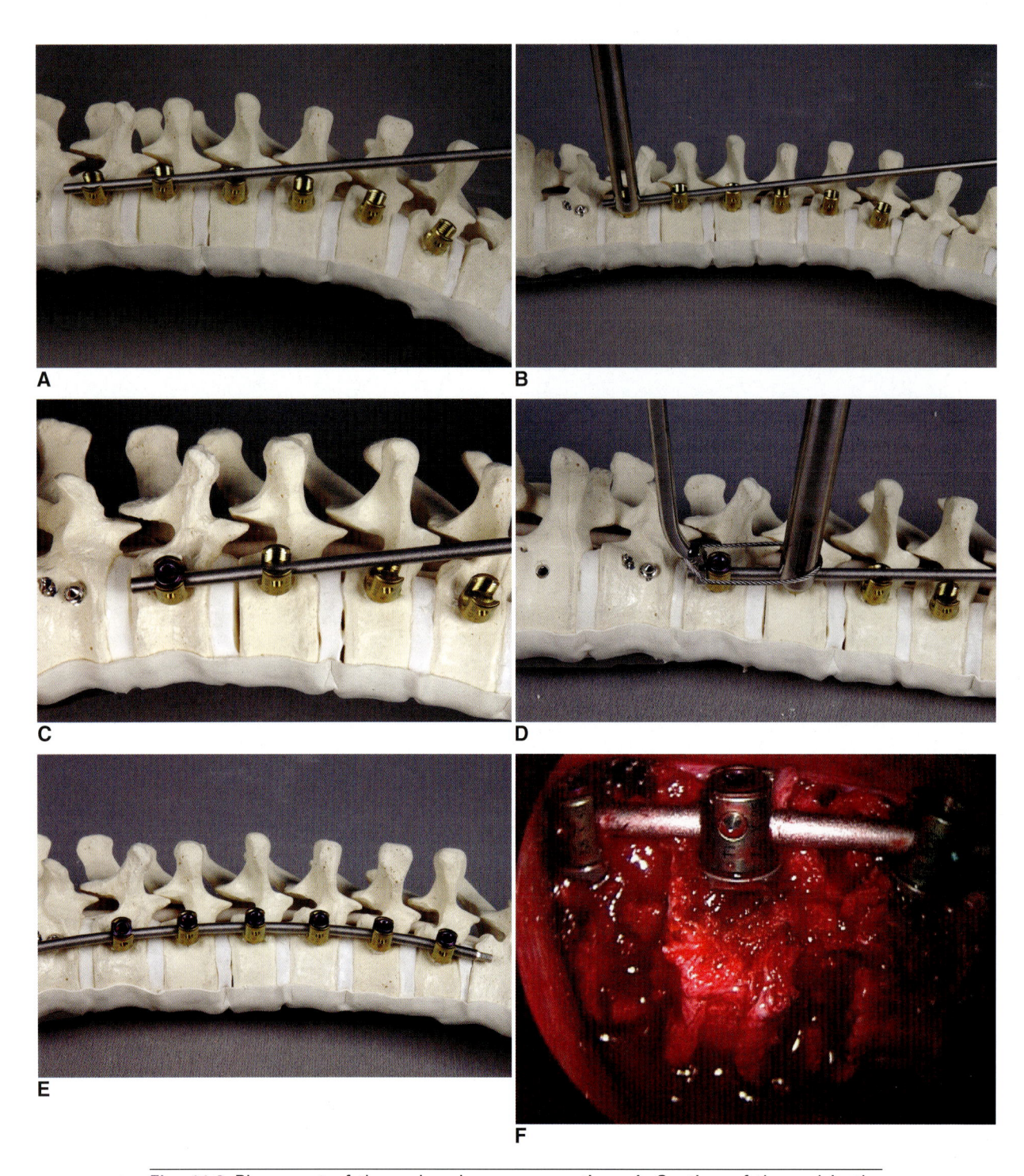

Fig. 44-9 Placement of the rod and curve correction. *A*, Seating of the rod in the distalmost screw. *B*, Placement of the set screw in the distal screw. *C*, Following set screw placement. *D*, Compression of the distal motion segment. *E*, Final implant construct. *F*, Intraoperative photograph following thoracoscopic anterior fusion and instrumentation.

CHAPTER 44   Anterior Release and Fusion Techniques for Thoracic Scoliosis 387

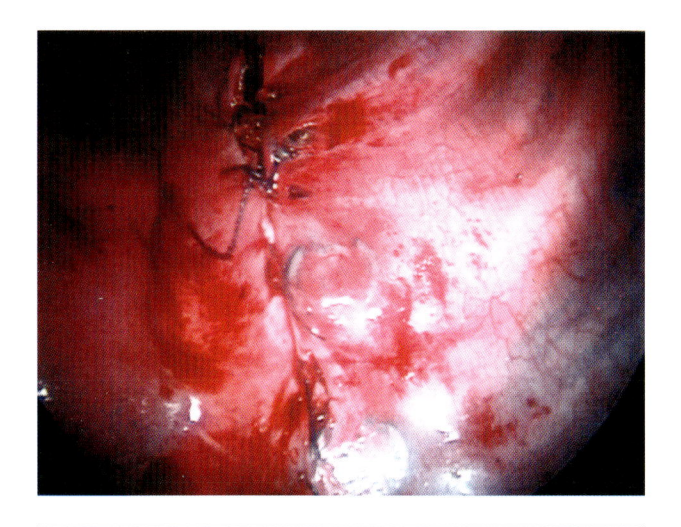

Fig. 44-10 Intraoperative photograph following thoracoscopic anterior fusion and instrumentation and pleural closure over the instrumentation, which can be seen under the relatively thin parietal pleura.

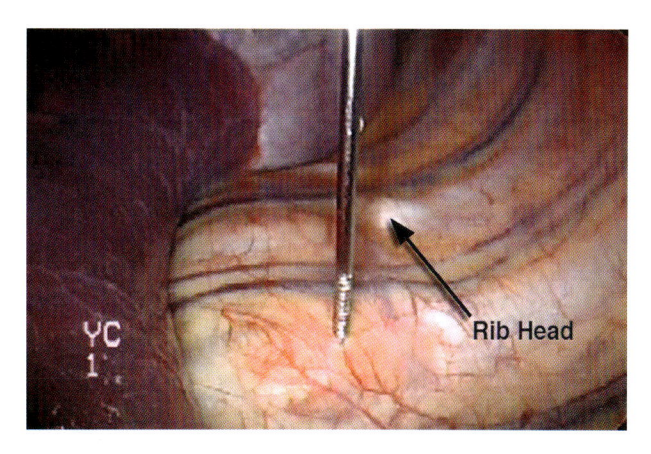

Fig. 44-11 Guidewire placed percutaneously and viewed using the thoracoscope to assist in locating the correct position of the posterior portal. Note that the wire is oriented vertically and is located just anterior to the rib head—a perfect location for posterolateral portal location for a thoracoscopic anterior fusion and instrumentation.

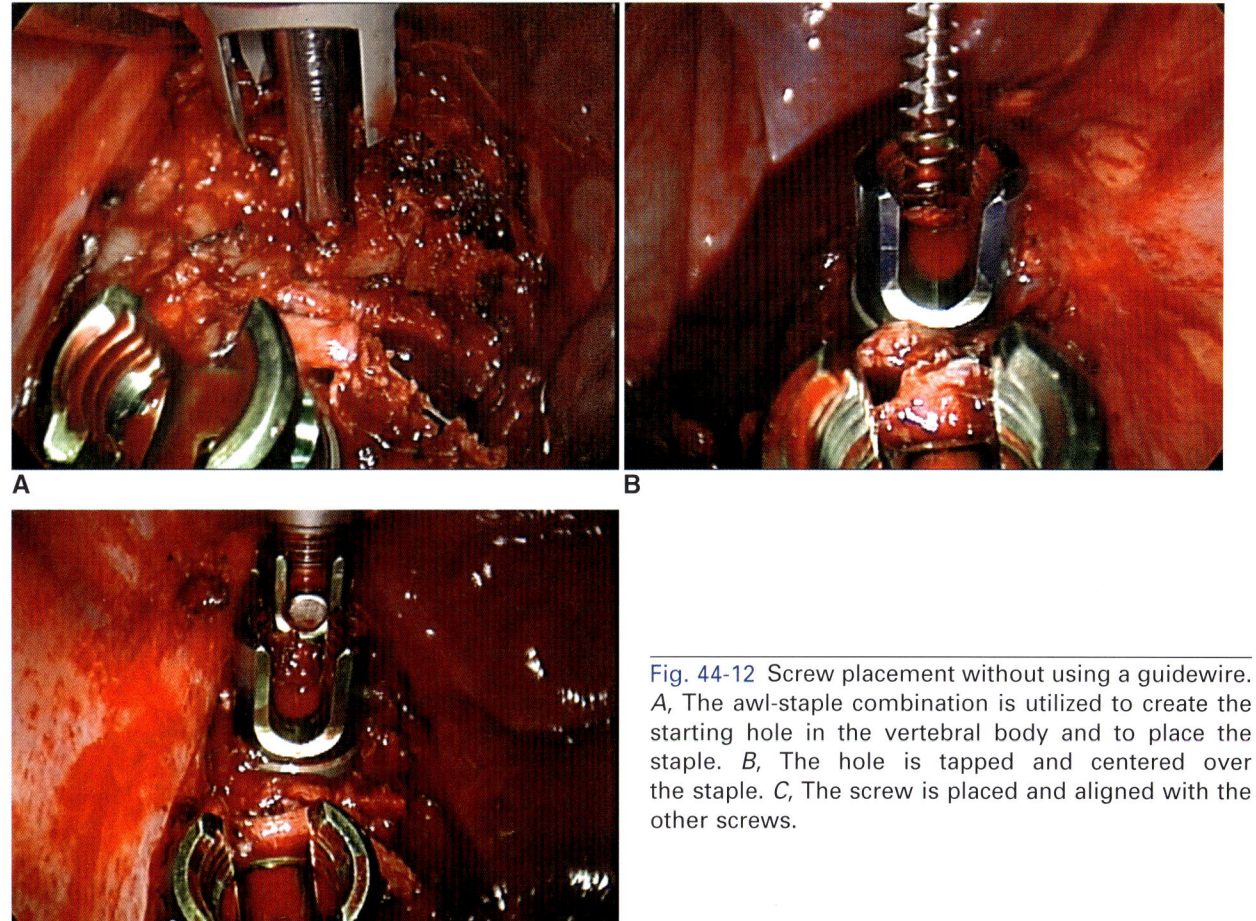

Fig. 44-12 Screw placement without using a guidewire. *A*, The awl-staple combination is utilized to create the starting hole in the vertebral body and to place the staple. *B*, The hole is tapped and centered over the staple. *C*, The screw is placed and aligned with the other screws.

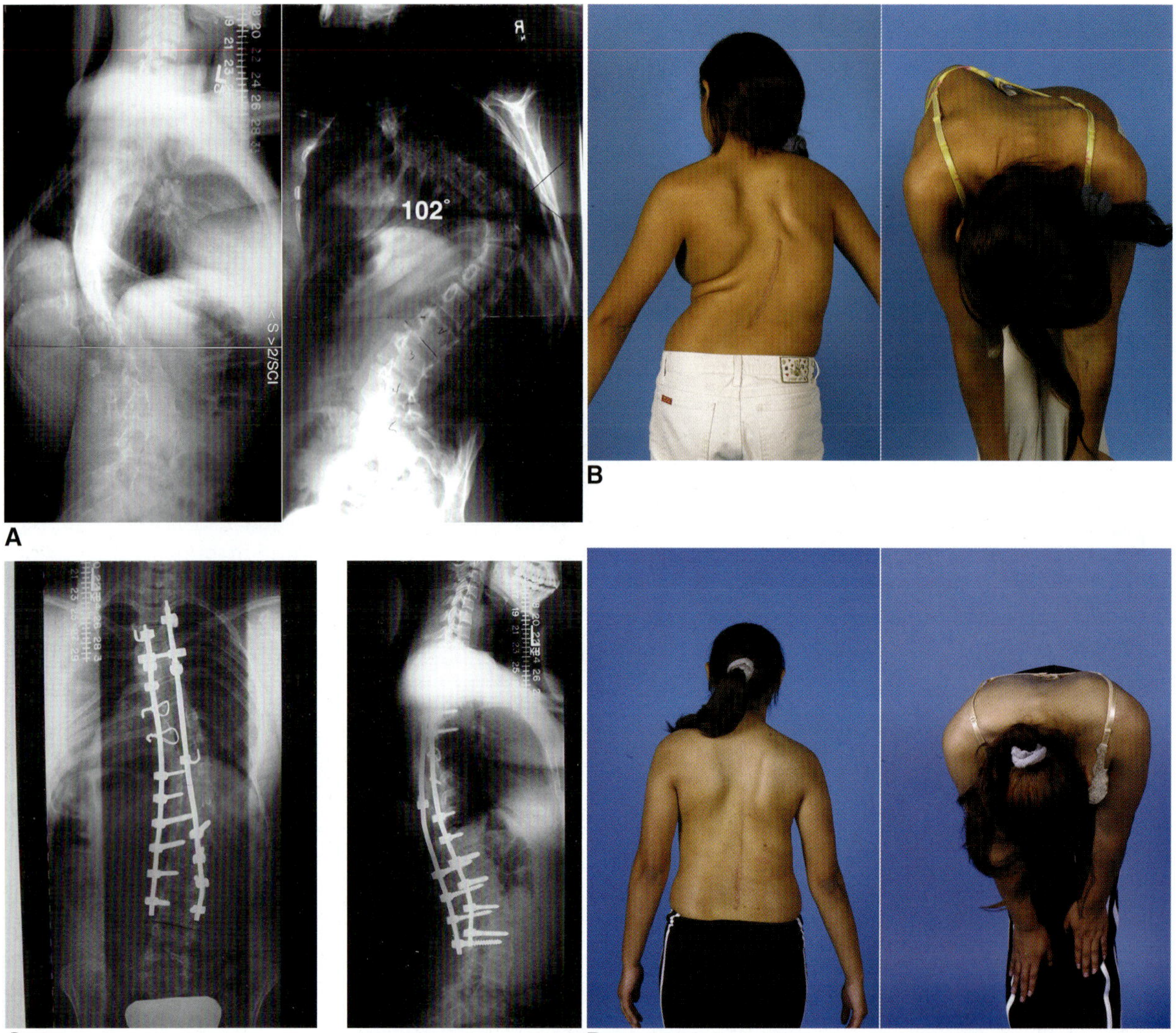

Fig. 44-13 A 14-year-old girl with a previous history of decompression of a large syringomyelia from T9 to L2 who developed a large deformity measuring over 100 degrees requiring surgical treatment. *A,* The preoperative posteroanterior and lateral radiographs. Note the large rib deformity on the lateral radiograph. *B,* The preoperativel clinical photographs. *C,* The 2-year postoperative radiographs following thoracoscopic anterior release from T6 to L1 and posterior spinal fusion and instrumentation from T4 to L3, all performed in the prone position. *D,* The 2-year postoperative clinical pictures demonstrating excellent coronal and sagittal plane correction.

procedure.[19-24] Clinically, excellent results are seen for patients with severe deformity who undergo a thorough anterior release followed by a posterior instrumentation and fusion (Fig. 44-13).

Anterior instrumentation and fusion for thoracic scoliosis achieves excellent correction in the coronal, axial, and sagittal planes and relies on a complete diskectomy and safe screw placement (Fig. 44-14). The anterior thoracic approach often saves distal motion segments because fusion always ends at the distal end vertebra, which is uncommon when performing a posterior instrumentation and fusion, even with modern segmental pedicle screw fixation. Betz and associates compared the anterior and posterior approaches for thoracic curves and demonstrated similar correction in the coronal plane, although restoration of thoracic kyphosis and the ability to save distal fusion levels was greater in the anterior group.[25] The thoracoscopic anterior approach appears to compare favorably to the posterior approach in recent series with reported coronal plane correction of 67% and 62% at 2 years, respectively.[26] Blood loss was greater in the posterior group, and surgical time was greater in the thoracoscopic group.

CHAPTER 44   Anterior Release and Fusion Techniques for Thoracic Scoliosis   389

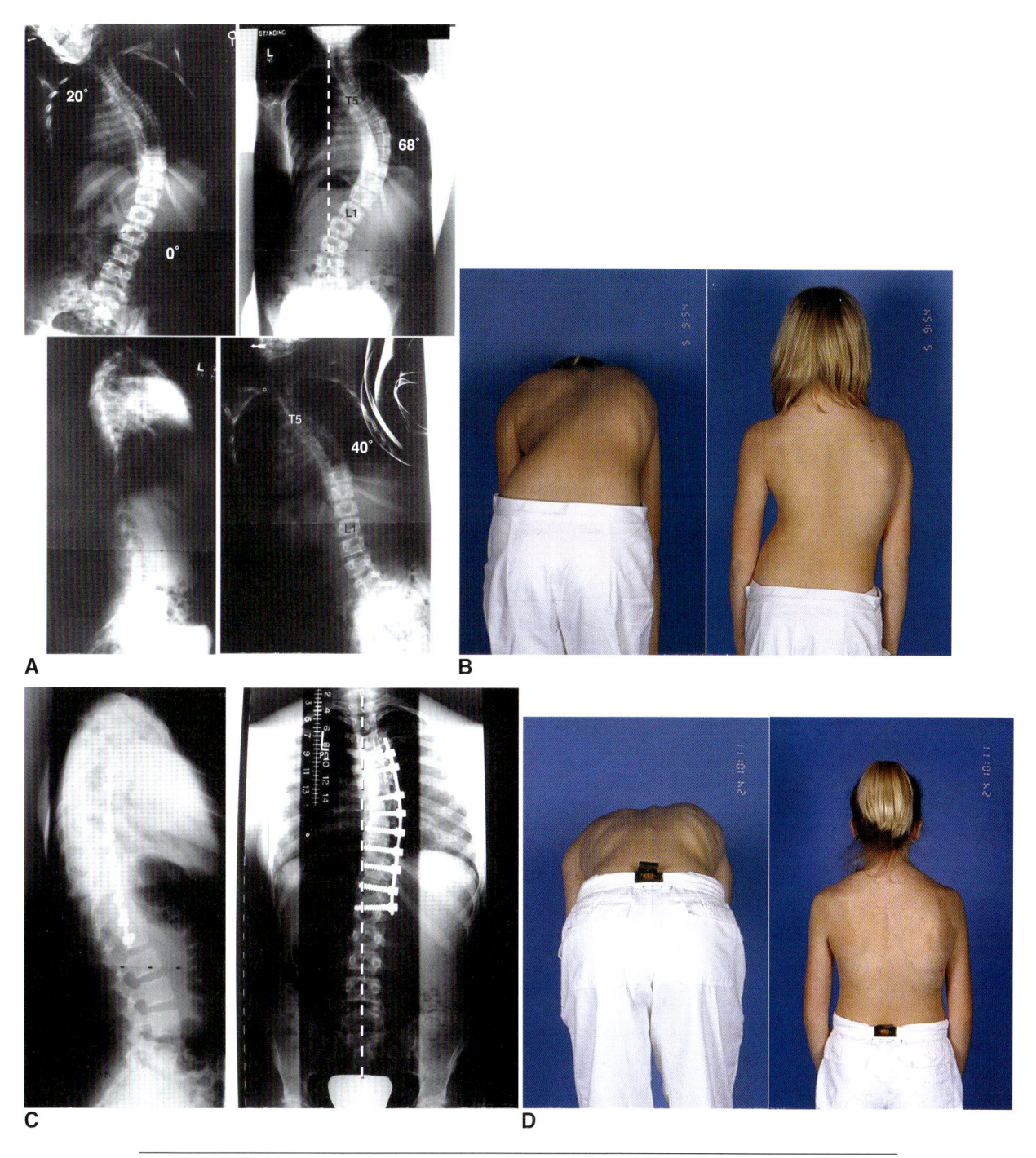

Fig. 44-14 An 11-year-old girl with adolescent idiopathic scoliosis. *A*, Preoperative posteroanterior and lateral radiographs demonstrating a 68-degree thoracic curve and the supine bend radiographs demonstrating a relatively flexible curve. *B*, The preoperative clinical photos. *C*, The 2-year posteroanterior and lateral radiographs following a thoracoscopic anterior fusion and instrumentation from T4 to L1 with excellent correction. The screw at T7 was cut out of the vertebral body and was removed uneventfully. *D*, The 2-year postoperative clinical pictures demonstrating excellent coronal and sagittal plane correction.

The anterior approach, however, leads to greater compromise of pulmonary function within the first year following surgery when compared to a posterior approach and should be taken into consideration when deciding on the surgical approach, especially for the patient with previous pulmonary issues.[5,6,27] The thoracoscopic approach appears to produce less detrimental effect on postoperative pulmonary function when compared to an open thoracotomy approach, which may be due to less chest cage disruption and postoperative pain.[28,29]

COMPLICATIONS

The incidence and type of complications related to anterior surgery for thoracic scoliosis can be categorized based on the type of surgery to be performed (anterior release/fusion alone or anterior instrumentation and fusion) and the approach used (open thoracotomy or thoracoscopic). An open anterior release and fusion has few complications; most are related to the impact of the open thoracotomy on postoperative pulmonary function. When performing the same procedure using thoracosocopic techniques, the learning curve of each surgeon should be taken into consideration because it is a technically challenging approach with up to 10% rate of complications.[30] These complications include excess bleeding that requires conversion to an open thoracotomy, injury to the thoracic duct with resultant chylothorax, and significant atelectasis secondary to the use of single lung ventilation.

Anterior instrumentation and fusion can be safely performed using an open thoracotomy or a thoracoscopic approach. Careful preoperative planning to exclude those types of cases that have been shown to have poor results (preoperative kyphosis greater than 30 degrees, coronal thoracic curve greater than 75 degrees, poor pulmonary function, patient weight above 70 kg)[31,32] will improve outcome, and careful surgical technique will decrease the incidence of intraoperative problems (screw pullout, guidewire migration, segmental vessel injury with excess bleeding).[11,12,33-36]

REFERENCES

1. Sucato DJ, Elerson E: A comparison between the prone and lateral position for performing a thoracoscopic anterior release and fusion for pediatric spinal deformity. Spine 2003;28:2176–2180.
2. Lieberman IH, Salo PT, Orr RD, Kraetschmer B: Prone position endoscopic transthoracic release with simultaneous posterior instrumentation for spinal deformity: A description of the technique. Spine 2000;25:2251–2257.
3. King AG, Mills TE, Loe WA, et al: Video-assisted thoracoscopic surgery in the prone position. Spine 2000;25:2403–2406.
4. Lenke LG, Betz RR, Bridwell KH, et al: Spontaneous lumbar curve coronal correction after selective anterior or posterior thoracic fusion in adolescent idiopathic scoliosis. Spine 1999;24:1663–1671.
5. Graham EJ, Lenke LG, Lowe TG, et al: Prospective pulmonary function evaluation following open thoracotomy for anterior spinal fusion in adolescent idiopathic scoliosis. Spine 2000;25:2319–2325.
6. Vedantam R, Lenke LG, Bridwell KH, et al: A prospective evaluation of pulmonary function in patients with adolescent idiopathic scoliosis relative to the surgical approach used for spinal arthrodesis. Spine 2000;25:82–90.
7. Sucato DJ, Duchene C: The position of the aorta relative to the spine: A comparison of patients with and without idiopathic scoliosis. J Bone Joint Surg Am 2003;85A:1461–1469.
8. Sucato D, Kassab F, Dempsey M: Thoracoscopic anterior spinal instrumentation and fusion for idiopathic scoliosis: A CT analysis of screw placement and completeness of discectomy. Scoliosis Research Society. Cleveland, Ohio, 2001.
9. Zhang H, Sucato DJ: Regional differences in anatomical landmarks for placing anterior instrumentation in the thoracic spine. 39th Annual Meeting of the Scoliosis Research Society. Buenos Aires, Argentina, 2004.
10. Sucato DJ, Welch RD, Pierce B, et al: Thoracoscopic discectomy and fusion in an animal model: Safe and effective when segmental blood vessels are spared. Spine 2002;27:880–886.
11. Sucato DJ, Kassab F, Dempsey M: Analysis of screw placement relative to the aorta and spinal canal following anterior instrumentation for thoracic idiopathic scoliosis. Spine 2004;29:554–559; discussion 559.
12. Roush TF, Crawford AH, Berlin RE, Wolf RK: Tension pneumothorax as a complication of video-assisted thoracoscopic surgery for anterior correction of idiopathic scoliosis in an adolescent female. Spine 2001;26:448–450.
13. Dohin B, Dubousset JF: Prevention of the crankshaft phenomenon with anterior spinal epiphysiodesis in surgical treatment of severe scoliosis of the younger patient. Eur Spine J 1994;3:165–168.
14. Shufflebarger HL, Clark CE: Prevention of the crankshaft phenomenon. Spine 1991;16:S409–S411.
15. Lapinksy AS, Richards BS: Preventing the crankshaft phenomenon by combining anterior fusion with posterior instrumentation: Does it work? Spine 1995;20:1392–1398.
16. Gonzalez Barrios I, Fuentes Caparras S, Avila Jurado MM: Anterior thoracoscopic epiphysiodesis in the treatment of a crankshaft phenomenon. Eur Spine J 1995;4:343–346.
17. Burton DC, Asher MA, Lai SM: Scoliosis correction maintenance in skeletally immature patients with idiopathic scoliosis. Is anterior fusion really necessary? Spine 2000;25:61–68.
18. Kioschos HC, Asher MA, Lark RG, Harner EJ: Overpowering the crankshaft mechanism. The effect of posterior spinal fusion with and without stiff transpedicular fixation on anterior spinal column growth in immature canines. Spine 1996;21:1168–1173.
19. Birnbaum K, Pieper S, Prescher A, et al: Thoracoscopically assisted ligamentous release of the thoracic spine: A cadaver study. Surg Radiol Anat 2000;22:143–150.
20. Wall EJ, Bylski-Austrow DI, Shelton FS, et al: Endoscopic discectomy increases thoracic spine flexibility as effectively as open discectomy: A mechanical study in a porcine model. Spine 1998;23:9–15: discussion 15–16.
21. Huntington CF, Murrell WD, Betz RR, et al: Comparison of thoracoscopic and open thoracic discectomy in a live ovine model for anterior spinal fusion. Spine 1998;23:1699–1702.
22. Huang EY, Acosta JM, Gardocki RJ, et al: Thoracoscopic anterior spinal release and fusion: Evolution of a faster, improved approach. J Pediatr Surg 2002;37:1732–1735.
23. Connolly PJ, Ordway NR, Sacks T, et al: Video-assisted thoracic diskectomy and anterior release: A biomechanical analysis of an endoscopic technique. Orthopedics 1999;22:923–926.
24. Newton PO, Cardelia JM, Farnsworth CL, et al: A biomechanical comparison of open and thoracoscopic anterior spinal release in a goat model. Spine 1998;23:530–535; discussion 536.

25. Betz RR, Harms J, Clements DH, et al: Comparison of anterior and posterior instrumentation for correction of adolescent thoracic idiopathic scoliosis. Spine 1999;24:225–239.
26. Wong D, Baker CJ: Pain in children: Comparison of assessment scales. Pediatr Nurs 1988;14:9–17.
27. Kim Y, Lenke LG, Bridwell KH, et al: Prospective evaluation of pulmonary function in adolescent idiopathic scoliosis relative to the surgical approach: Minimum 5 year follow-up. Annual Scoliosis Research Society Meeting, Seattle, WA, 2002.
28. Sucato DJ, Rathjen KE, Harris K: The effect of surgical approach on early postoperative pulmonary function in the treatment of adolescent idiopathic scoliosis. Scoliosis Research Society, 39th Annual Meeting. Buenos Aires, Argentina, 2004.
29. Newton P, Faro F, Marks M, et al: Pulmonary function in anterior scoliosis surgery: Open vs. thoracoscopic approaches. Annual Meeting of the Pediatric Orthopaedic Society of North America. St. Louis, MO, 2004.
30. Newton P, Shea K, Granlund K: Defining the pediatric spinal thoracoscopy learning curve: Sixty-five consecutive cases. Spine 2000;25:1028–1035.
31. Betz R: Anterior instrumentation for thoracic adolescent idiopathic scoliosis: Open and minimally invasive techniques (abstract). American Academy of Orthopedic Surgeons, 2000.
32. Sweet FA, Lenke LG, Bridwell KH, et al: Prospective radiographic and clinical outcomes and complications of single solid rod instrumented anterior spinal fusion in adolescent idiopathic scoliosis. Spine 2001;26:1966–1975.
33. Sucato DJ, Girgis M: Bilateral pneumothoraces, pneumomediastinum, pneumoperitoneum, pneumoretroperitoneum, and subcutaneous emphysema following intubation with a double-lumen endotracheal tube for thoracoscopic anterior spinal release and fusion in a patient with idiopathic scoliosis. J Spinal Disord Tech 2002;15:133–138.
34. Picetti GD 3rd, Pang D, Bueff HU: Thoracoscopic techniques for the treatment of scoliosis: Early results in procedure development. Neurosurgery 2002;51:978–984; discussion 984.
35. Newton PO, Betz R, Clements DH, et al: Anterior thoracoscopic instrumentation: A matched comparison to anterior open instrumentation and posterior open instrumentation. Paper Presentation at the 70th Annual Meeting of the American Academy of Orthopaedic Surgeons, New Orleans, LA, 2003.
36. Huang TJ, Hsu RW, Sum CW, Liu HP: Complications in thoracoscopic spinal surgery: A study of 90 consecutive patients. Surg Endosc 1999;13:346–350.

CHAPTER 45

RON EL-HAWARY

DANIEL J. SUCATO

Anterior Treatment for Thoracolumbar/Lumbar Scoliosis

INTRODUCTION

The anterior approach for thoracolumbar/lumbar idiopathic scoliosis has been successfully utilized for many years.[1-3] Although recent posterior techniques have been applied to thoracolumbar/lumbar curves with acceptable results,[4] the anterior approach continues to be the predominant method of operative treatment for these curves.[1] The advantages of the anterior approach over posterior instrumentation include limited fusion levels,[1,5,6] improved mobility of the spine due to disk and end plate removal, and considerable force application by anterior instrumentation[7,8] resulting in excellent three-dimensional correction. Advances in the treatment of thoracolumbar/lumbar curves using the anterior approach include the use of structural anterior support and the development of more rigid anterior fixation systems.[9-11] Despite these advances, the most important aspect of this surgery is to perform a complete diskectomy in order to improve the flexibility of the spine while allowing for maximum bone surface area available for fusion. Overall, excellent clinical results have been achieved when a technically adequate surgical procedure has been performed to include complete diskectomy, anterior structural support, and correct application of instrumentation.[12]

INDICATIONS

Indications for anterior surgery in the thoracolumbar and lumbar spine include (1) severe curve magnitude and deformity in which anterior release and fusion complements a posterior spinal fusion, (2) scoliosis in young patients in whom anterior fusion will limit or prevent the crankshaft phenomenon, (3) anterior fusion and instrumentation in a patient predisposed to pseudoarthrosis, and (4) anterior instrumentation and fusion for thoracolumbar and lumbar idiopathic scoliosis.

The indications for anterior fusion combined with posterior fusion and instrumentation for severe deformity are varied and depend on the goal of surgery, surgeon preferences, curve magnitude, curve flexibility, and the type of implant system to be utilized. For example, nonambulatory patients with neuromuscular conditions (i.e., cerebral palsy) may not require an anterior release and fusion because the goal of surgical treatment is to achieve a balanced patient without risk for curve progression. In this setting, an adequately performed posterior fusion and instrumentation will produce the intended goal of a well-balanced patient.[13]

The specific indications for fusion in this setting are evolving as new posterior techniques continue to be developed. For example, anterior release and fusion for larger curves in any patient may not be necessary when segmental pedicle screw fixation is performed in the thoracolumbar/lumbar spine. Despite this, it is generally accepted that curves above 75 degrees with a flexibility index less than 50% will require an anterior release.

Similarly, the indications for anterior fusion in the immature patient with a thoracolumbar/lumbar curve have changed throughout the years since the crankshaft phenomenon was first described in 1989.[14] When planning a posterior instrumentation and fusion, we recommend anterior fusion to prevent the crankshaft phenomenon in patients during the peak height velocity[15,16] and in young patients (younger than 10 years old for females and younger than 11 to 12 years old for males) who have open triradiate cartilages and Risser stage 0. Although some data suggest that pedicle screw fixation limits the crankshaft phenomenon, this has been studied only in animal models and is not well documented clinically.[17] It is necessary to adequately assess each patient's growth potential preoperatively to accurately determine whether anterior surgery is necessary. Additional factors are considered in this decision, including the type of implants to be utilized and whether a structural thoracic curve is also present.

Anterior fusion is necessary in a subset of patients with scoliosis in whom it is predictably difficult to achieve fusion through posterior methods alone. This group includes those with neurofibromatosis (especially with kyphosis greater than 50 degrees, thinning of the lamina from dural ectasia) as well as those who have questionable posterior elements, such as those with myelomeningocele and patients with postlaminectomy spine deformity.[18]

The primary indication for anterior instrumentation and fusion of the thoracolumbar/lumbar spine is for adolescent idiopathic scoliosis with a curve apex at T12 or below. These curves are mainly type 5 and a select few type 6 curves as defined by the classification of Lenke and associates.[19] One 2003 study suggests that an anterior thoracolumbar/lumbar fusion and instrumentation will be successful if its associated thoracic curve is 55 degrees or less, the thoracolumbar/lumbar : thoracic (TL/L : T) Cobb ratio is 1.25 or more, the thoracic curve bends out to 20 degrees or less, and the triradiate cartilages are closed.[12] The most common curve pattern for these patients is a thoracolumbar or lumbar curve in which four to six vertebrae are in the Cobb measurement of the curve. In the Lenke type 6 curve, the patient has coronal plane imbalance with trunk shift to the convexity of the curve and waist line asymmetry. Patients often feel that a limb-length discrepancy exists because of the perceived "higher hip" and shorter pant leg (caused by pants riding higher because of the more curved waist line on the concavity of the curve).[9] The Adam's forward bend test will reveal a flank prominence on the convexity of the curve. The anterior approach with anterior fusion and instrumentation corrects the coronal, axial, and sagittal deformity resulting in restoration of the coronal balance and improvement of the flank prominence (Fig. 45-1). Anterior instrumentation and fusion is not only useful in the adolescent age group, but has also found success in the treatment of thoracolumbar-lumbar curves in adult scoliosis.[20–22]

PREOPERATIVE PLANNING

The patient with adolescent idiopathic thoracolumbar/lumbar scoliosis should be carefully assessed with a good physical examination and a detailed analysis of the preoperative radiographs. The physical examination should include a thorough neurologic examination, assessment of trunk balance, and measurement of shoulder heights. A significant trunk shift ipsilateral to the side of the thoracolumbar/lumbar curve with level shoulders will confirm an isolated thoracolumbar/lumbar curve, but a fairly well-balanced patient with shoulder asymmetry (right elevated compared to the left) suggests that a structural thoracic curve may also be present. The Adam's forward bend test should be utilized to analyze the rotational deformities of the thoracolumbar/lumbar curve and to determine whether significant rotational deformity is present for the main thoracic or upper thoracic curve (see Fig. 45-1B). The findings of the physical examination will direct the surgeon as to the structural nature of each curve and whether inclusion in the fusion is necessary. The clinical appearance of the patient, together with a thorough evaluation of the radiographs, will determine the surgical plan.

Preoperative radiographs should include standing posteroanterior (PA) and lateral radiographs, and supine best effort bend films to the right and left (see Fig. 45-1C to F). The PA radiograph is used to assess trunk shift using Floman's method,[23] measurement of Cobb angles of all curves, assessment of leg-length discrepancies by assessment of the height of the pelvis, determination of the end vertebra for upper thoracic, main thoracic, and lumbar curves, assessment of the apical vertebral translation of the main thoracic and lumbar curves, assessment of the status of the triradiate cartilage (open or closed), and determination of the Risser stage. The lateral radiograph is utilized to measure overall sagittal balance by drawing a plumb line from C7 to the sacrum, measuring thoracic kyphosis (T5 to T12) and lumbar lordosis (L1 to S1). Junctional kyphosis at the thoracolumbar junction (T10-L2) indicates that the main thoracic curve, in addition to the thoracolumbar/lumbar curve, is structural and may require inclusion in the fusion levels. Supine bend radiographs will allow the surgeon to understand the flexibility of of all curves and confirms the radiographic curve type as described by Lenke and colleagues.[19]

If an isolated thoracolumbar/lumbar curve (Lenke type 5) is confirmed, the anterior fusion levels are identified best on the PA radiograph to include the proximal and distal end vertebrae. These end vertebrae are defined as the most tilted vertebrae both proximally and distally and are determined by assessing the obliquity of the disks at each level. For example, in a left thoracolumbar/lumbar curve, the disk space that opens into the left aspect of the curve are disks within the curve, and fusion of these levels is necessary (see Fig. 45-1C). These fusion levels have worked extremely well for anterior surgery and disregard the deviation from the midline of these end vertebras. However, some obliquity of the disk below the distal fusion level is expected when significant tilt of the distal end vertebra is present preoperatively.

Although these are the well-accepted anterior fusion levels, there are those who utilize other criteria and fuse fewer segments of the spine. Hall and Bernstein described the "short-segment" fusion of thoracolumbar/lumbar curves in which only three or four segments are fused.[24] Fusion levels are determined based on the location of the apex of the curve: When the apex is at the level of a vertebral body, fusion includes one vertebral body above and one vertebral body below the apex, resulting in fusion across two disk spaces and three vertebral bodies; when the apex is at the level of a disk space, fusion should include two vertebrae above and two vertebrae below that motion segment, resulting in a fusion of three disks and four vertebral bodies. It is recommended that these curves should be less than 60 degrees with a good

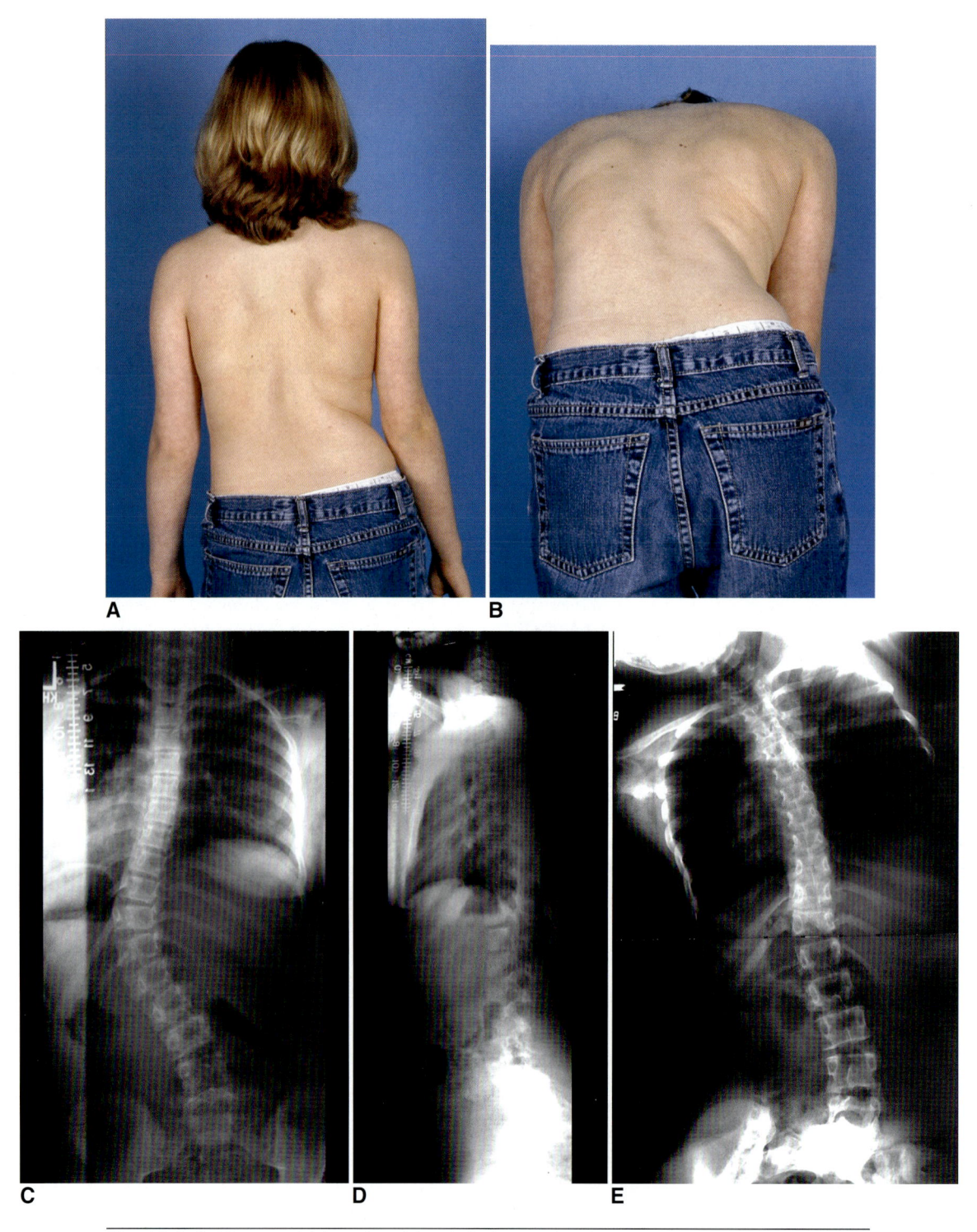

Fig. 45-1 A 12-year-old female with a left thoracolumbar adolescent idiopathic scoliosis (Lenke type 5C). *A*, Preoperative clinical photograph demonstrating a trunk shift to the left with waistline asymmetry. *B*, Preoperative photograph demonstrating a left thoracolumbar prominence. *C*, Preoperative standing posteroanterior (PA) radiograph. Left thoracolumbar curve (T9-L2) with Cobb measurement 54 degrees, small compensatory curves, and Risser stage 0. *D*, Preoperative lateral radiograph demonstrating thoracic hypokyphosis and loss of lumbar lordosis. *E*, Left supine bending film demonstrating flexibility of the thoracolumbar curve to 10 degrees.

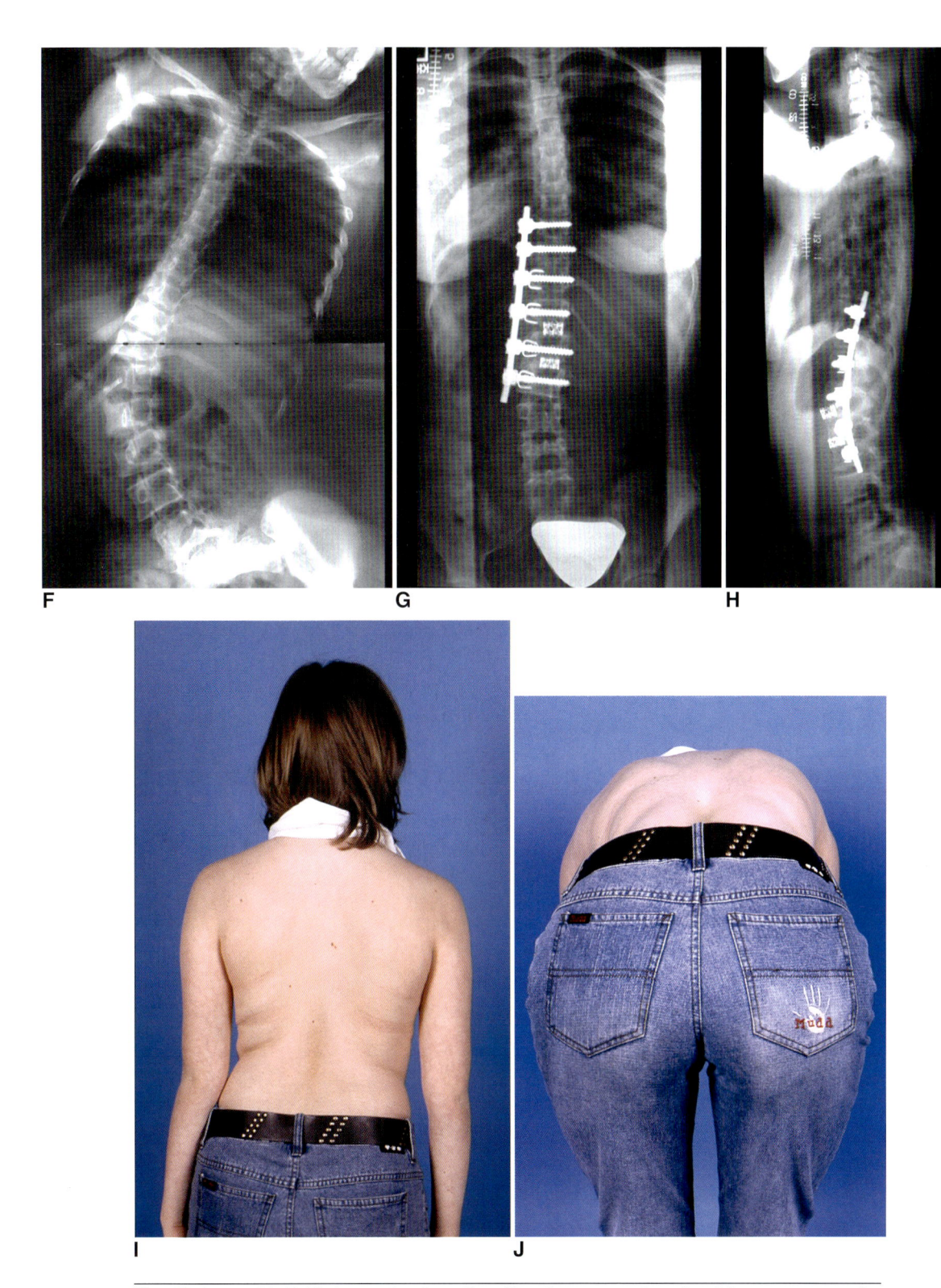

CHAPTER 45 Anterior Treatment for Thoracolumbar/Lumbar Scoliosis 395

Fig. 45-1, cont'd. *F,* Right supine bending film demonstrating that L2 centers over the mid center sacral line. *G,* Postoperative standing PA radiograph. Anterior spinal fusion and instrumentation had been performed in a left thoracoabdominal approach. A single rod construct from T9 to L2 with titanium mesh cages at the T12-L1 and L1-L2 was used with excellent coronal plane correction. *H,* Postoperative lateral radiograph demonstrates restoration of sagittal plane alignment. *I,* Postoperative photograph reveals significant improvement on the trunk shift. *J,* Postoperative photograph of forward bend demonstrating symmetry.

flexibility index, and it is mandatory to achieve overcorrection of the instrumented levels for success. More recently, others have described short-segment fusion with bone-on-bone correction of the thoracolumbar/lumbar curves; however, long-term studies are necessary to ensure maintenance of correction at the instrumented levels and, more important, the response of the curves proximal and distal to the fusion.[25]

PATIENT PREPARATION AND PATIENT COUNSELING

Preoperatively, it is necessary to discuss with the patient and the family the indications for surgery as well as the surgical approach utilized. Patients should anticipate a flank incision on the convex side of the curve and they may note slight dimpling of the skin over the absent rib which was harvested during the approach. Because the psoas muscle requires retraction posteriorly to obtain exposure of the anterior vertebral bodies and disks, mild weakness of hip flexion may be experienced early in the postoperative period. Finally, the sympathetic chain is often dissected off the spine and can result in asymmetric temperature of the legs with the affected side being warmer than the nonoperative side and resolution between 3 and 6 months after surgery.

Preoperative assessment of respiratory function is appropriate because an anterior thoracolumbar approach to the spine results in decreased postoperative pulmonary function in the initial postoperative period.[26–28] Although pulmonary function is restored to baseline by 1 year postoperatively, we avoid anterior surgery when the preoperative predicted forced vital capacity (FVC) or forced expiratory volume (FEV_1) is below 70%.

SURGICAL APPROACH

For an anterior approach to a thoracolumbar/lumbar curve, patients are placed in the lateral decubitus position with the convex aspect of the spine up. Following selection of fusion levels, the most common approach is through the rib just proximal to the upper instrumented vertebra (i.e., the tenth rib is harvested for a T11-L3 fusion). This allows for excellent access to the most proximal disk and vertebra in order to achieve a complete diskectomy and to accurately place the intervertebral body screws. This incision is directed over the rib and then travels down anteriorly just lateral to the umbilicus. The incision is then carried down to the periosteum of the rib, which is then subperiosteally dissected.

Anteromedially, the costochondral junction is incised in a longitudinal fashion (as seen by the retroperitoneal fat), resulting in easy entrance into the retroperitoneal space and is most easily accessible at the T10 level (Fig. 45-2). Once the entrance into the retroperitoneal space is achieved, blunt dissection is carried out to dissect the abdominal contents and peritoneum from the inferior aspect of the diaphragm and the lateral aspect of the abdominal wall (Fig. 45-3). The diaphragm can be incised one fingerbreadth proximal to its insertion in order to protect the phrenic nerve as well as to help facilitate closure.

As the dissection and incision of the diaphragm is carried out medially and posteriorly, this takes the surgeon down to the level of the spine (Fig. 45-4). The pleura can now be incised both proximally and distally while leaving the segmental blood vessels intact on the first pass (Fig. 45-5). At this point, a general assessment of spine levels should be performed by palpation of the ribs, identification of the inser-

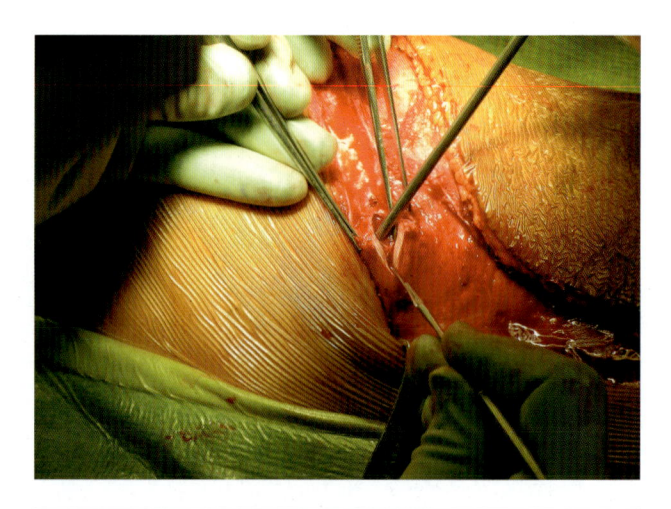

Fig. 45-2 The skin and subcutaneous incision is performed, and the muscle layers are divided to the level of the rib to be removed. This rib is circumferentially exposed using subperiosteal technique; the rib is disengaged at the costochondral junction, which is incised as shown. The retroperitoneal space can then be entered with blunt dissection.

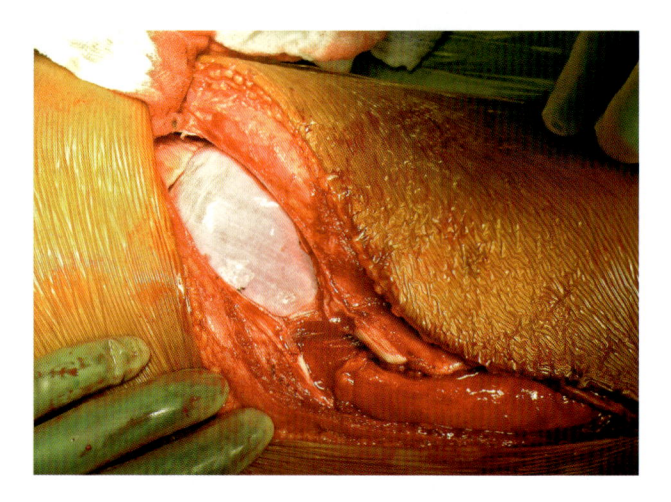

Fig. 45-3 The diaphragm is visualized and will be incised 1 to 2 cm from its peripheral margin to allow reattachment at the completion of the surgery.

CHAPTER 45 Anterior Treatment for Thoracolumbar/Lumbar Scoliosis

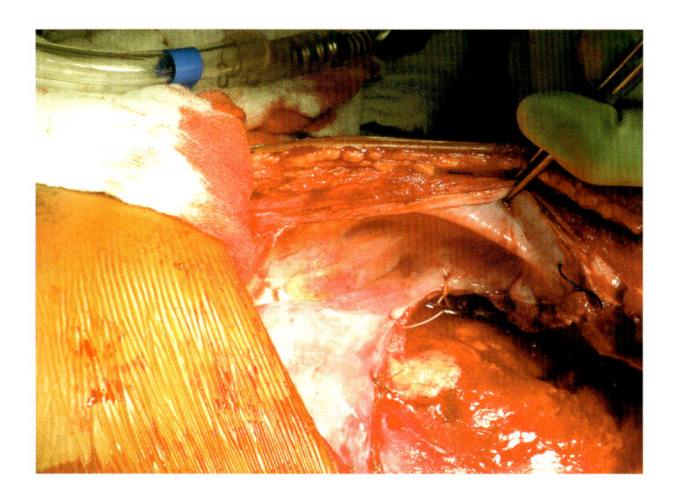

Fig. 45-4 Marking sutures have been placed in the diaphragm to facilitate accurate closure.

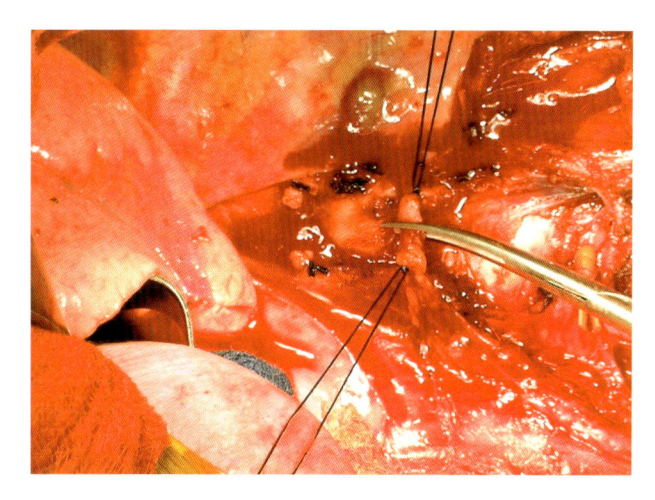

Fig. 45-6 The segmental vessels are isolated and divided at the level of the midvertebral body. The segmental vessels are easily located over the vertebral bodies. They should be ligated with suture and then incised in the midvertebral body.

tion of the crus of the diaphragm (T12 and L1), as well as identification of the proximal insertion of the iliopsoas muscle (L1). It is always recommended that radiographic identification with a spinal needle in a disk space be performed prior to final preparation of the spine. The incised pleura should be dissected both anteriorly and posteriorly and the segmental blood vessels should be ligated in the midvertebral bodies (Fig. 45-6).

To prevent spinal cord ischemia, some recommend temporary ligation of each segmental vessel with observation of spinal cord monitoring for 20 minutes prior to permanent ligation.[29] It is also important that the anesthesiologist avoid hypotensive anesthesia during these anterior surgeries because segmental blood vessels are ligated, which may partially compromise spinal cord perfusion. The ligated segmental vessels can be retracted so that blunt and sharp dissection deep to them can be carried out all the way anteriorly to the contralateral side so that the surgeon can adequately palpate when placing screws. This wide exposure will also provide good access for diskectomy. On the ipsilateral side, the dissection should be carried out posteriorly to the level of the rib heads at the thoracic levels and to the level of the pedicles in the lumbar spine.

Diskectomies are performed to include the excision of the ipsilateral annulus to the posterior longitudinal ligament (PLL), excision of the anterior longitudinal ligament, and thinning of the contralateral annulus. The annulus is incised with a sharp knife in a box figuration which is removed with a large Leksell rongeur (Figs. 45-7 and 45-8). A Cobb elevator can then be used to disengage the cartilaginous end plate

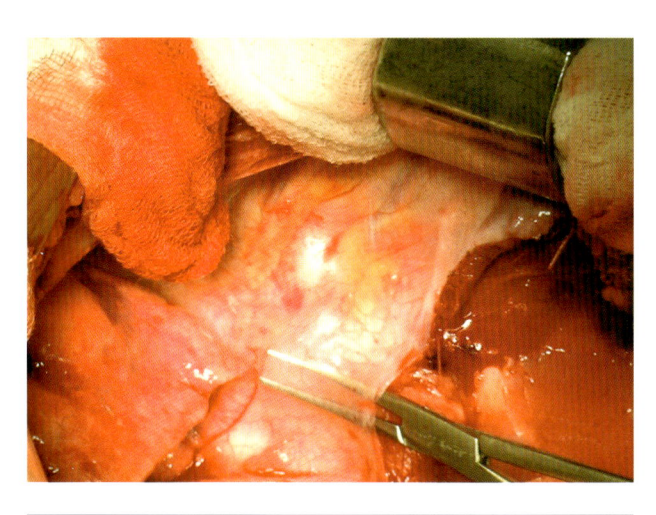

Fig. 45-5 The parietal pleura is elevated with a right-angled hemostat and incised in the midvertebral body.

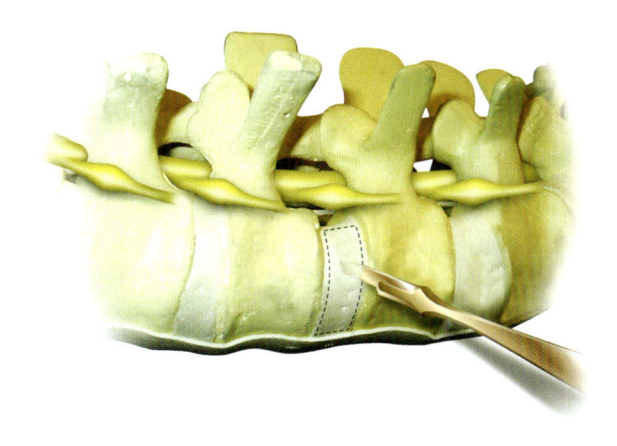

Fig. 45-7 The disk space is initially entered with a No. 15 blade. A box-cut is made through the ipsilateral annulus fibrosis and nucleus pulposus. Anatomic landmarks are utilized to safely incise the disk.

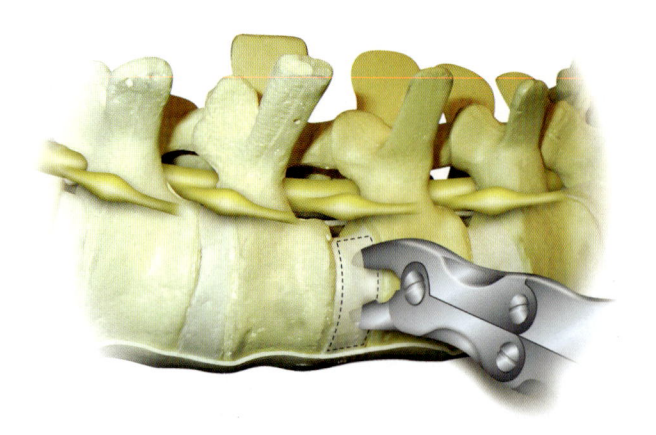

Fig. 45-8 A Leksell rongeur is used to remove the nucleus pulposus, leaving only the annulus fibrosis.

from the vertebral end plate and is then taken down along the edge of the vertebra (Fig. 45-9), resulting in a clean dissection of the entire cartilaginous end plate without bleeding (Fig. 45-10). Resection of the PLL is not routinely necessary for the typical adolescent idiopathic scoliosis curve; however, in patients with larger stiffer curves (greater than 75 degrees), resection of the PLL can be performed. Once the posterior annulus is resected, the PLL is easily identified and penetrated with a nerve hook and Kerrison rongeurs can then be used to resect this ligament. Following each diskectomy, Surgicel or Gelfoam can be placed into the disk space to limit end plate bleeding.

ANTERIOR INSTRUMENTATION

The many instrumentation systems available today fall into two major categories—single rod and dual rod constructs. Regardless of the type of implant used, screws should be placed parallel to the end plate and should obtain bicortical purchase to maximize stiffness of the construct as well as to allow maximal curve correction. We recommend orientation of the proximal and distal screws toward the center of the construct to accommodate some plow of these screws during correction. When using a single rod construct, we recommend screw placement beginning at the apex of the curve in which the screws are placed in the mid to posterior vertebral body (Figs. 45-11 to 45-13). The apical screw should be oriented in a slightly posterior-to-anterior direction to account for the rotational deformity of the spine. As the surgeon places screws away from the apex, these screws are oriented more horizontal to the axis of the patient because rotation of the vertebral bodies lessens. When dual screws are used, a similar pattern of implant placement is performed; however, less room is available to move the position the staple on the vertebral body. Contouring of the rod(s) should provide the desired lordosis in the lumbar spine with a neutral thoracolumbar junction. The desired coronal plane correction should be placed in the rod and may include some undercorrection of the proximal thoracolumbar curve to leave residual tilt of the upper end vertebra when a larger compensatory thoracic curve is present.

When using a single rod construct, the rod is seated into all implants (Fig. 45-14), and the 90-degree rod rotation

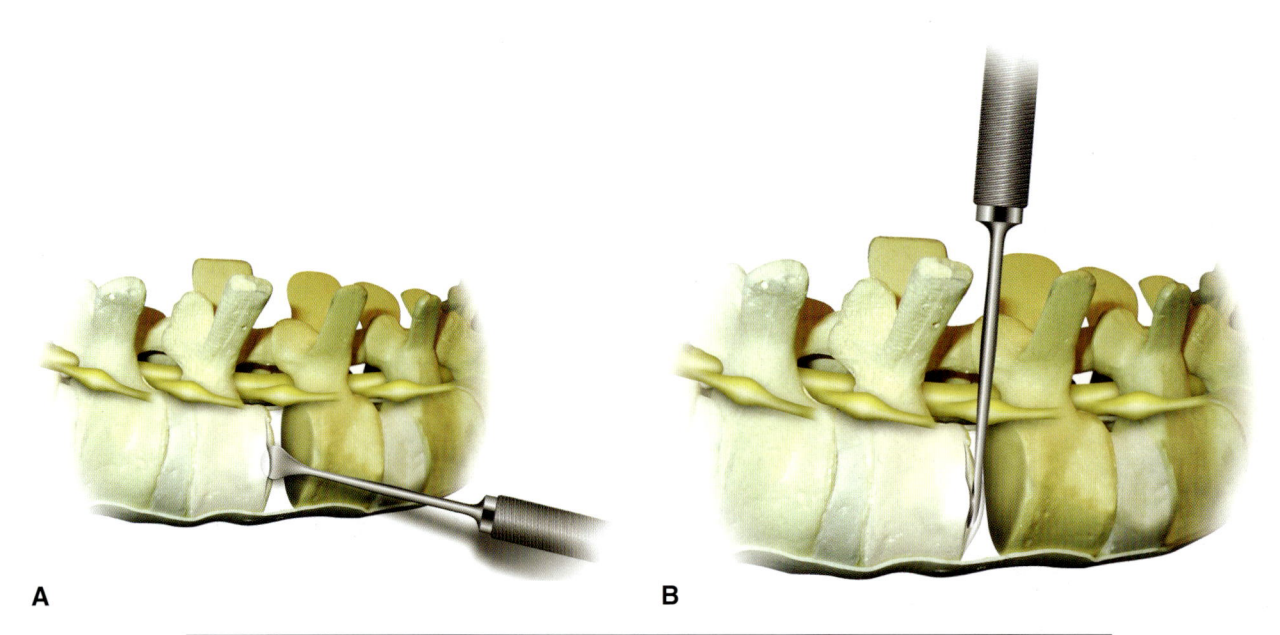

Fig. 45-9 *A,* The cartilaginous end plates are identified with subperiosteal dissection and are then "popped-off" with a Cobb elevator. *B,* The Cobb elevator is turned 180 degrees in order to remove the cartilaginous end plate and disk material by sliding down the edge of the vertebral body, freeing off the end plate.

CHAPTER 45 Anterior Treatment for Thoracolumbar/Lumbar Scoliosis

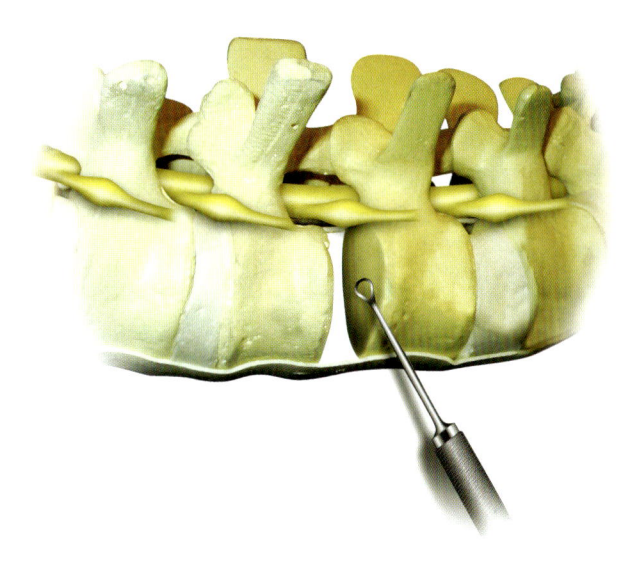

Fig. 45-10 A curette ensures that all disk material and cartilage is adequately removed and that a bleeding cancellous surface is left to facilitate fusion.

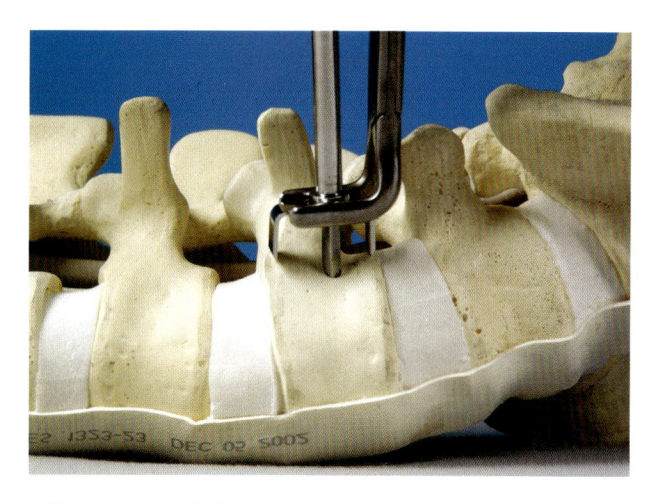

Fig. 45-12 Insertion of a screw-staple. The prongs of the staple should be placed so that they engage the vertebral body. The screw-staple combination improved tangential pullout when compared to a screw alone.

maneuver is performed to correct the coronal plane deformity while restoring or maintaining lumbar lordosis (Fig. 45-15). The rod can then be fully tightened to the screws at this point. The dual rod system can be utilized in a similar fashion with posterior rod rotation followed by seating of the anterior rod. Conversely, placement of multiple screwdrivers in the anterior screws followed by anterior rotation of the spine and placement of the posterior rod is an alternative technique.

Anterior structural support should be used for all cases of anterior instrumentation of thoracolumbar/lumbar curves to stiffen the construct, and to create and maintain lordosis. Anterior structural support can include allograft rings or metal ring cages in which morselized autologous bone is placed.[30–32] These should be placed in the anterior aspect of the intervertebral disk space and on the concavity of the curve following rod rotation and correction of the spine using the rods and screws (Fig. 45-16). The structural support is gen-

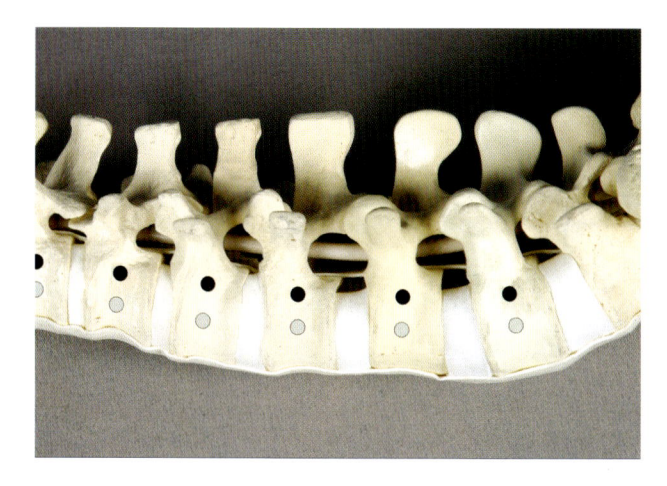

Fig. 45-11 Dark circles represent screw entry sites for a single rod construct. These screws enter the vertebral bodies just anterior to the junction between pedicle and vertebral body (posterior one third of the body) and are centered in the cranial-caudal direction. When a dual rod construct is used, the staple should be placed in the midvertebral body, allowing safe placement of two screws in the vertebral body.

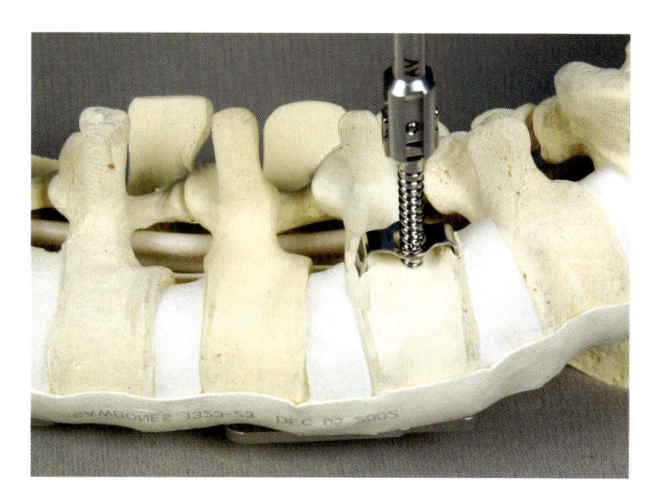

Fig. 45-13 With the staple positioned, a screw is inserted to a depth to allow its tip to penetrate the contralateral cortex. This length can be determined with a depth gauge or can be directly palpated. Appropriate screw length achieves bicortical purchase and improves screw fixation without being excessively long and risking injury to soft tissue structures.

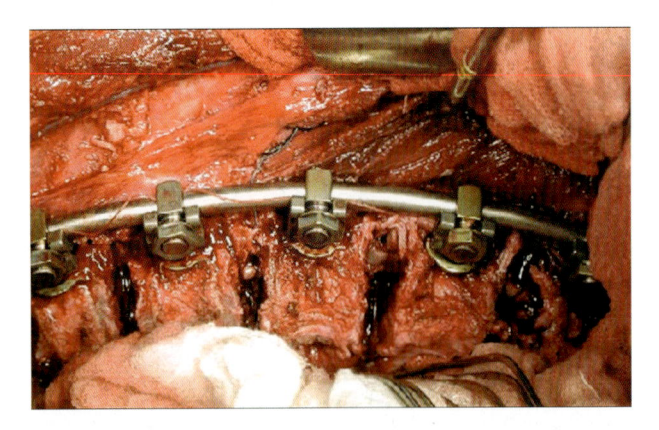

Fig. 45-14 The single rod has been contoured into lordosis. With all screws in correct position, the rod is provisionally secured with eyebolts. Following complete diskectomy and placement of screws a ¼-inch rod is contoured with the appropriate degree of lordosis and seated. In this case the lumbar spine has fairly significant kyphosis and scoliosis and the rod is seated to accommodate this deformity.

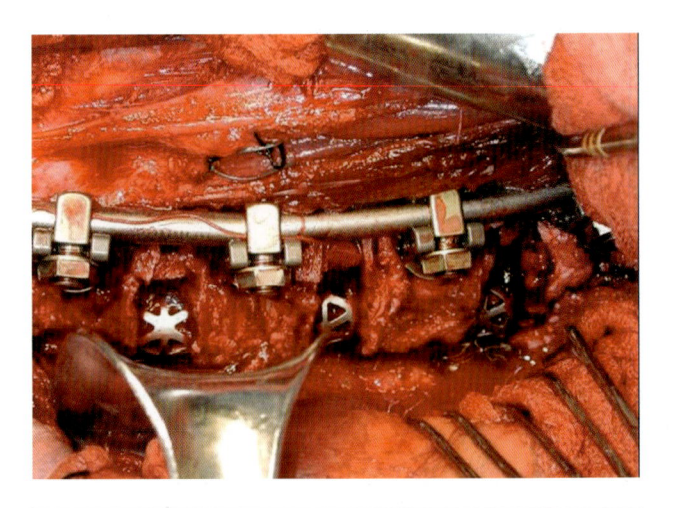

Fig. 45-16 Titanium mesh cages are placed anteriorly and to the concave side and are filled with autograft bone from the harvested rib.

erally placed at all levels distal to T12 to provide correction and maintenance of lumbar lordosis. Anterior structural support can be placed proximal to T12; however, these supports should be relatively small so that lordosis is not created in these normally neutral or kyphotic segments. Prior to placement of the anterior structural support, autologous rib graft is placed posteriorly to augment the support and to increase the fusion rate. The anterior structural support can then be placed by distraction at each level to allow placement followed by gentle compression (Fig. 45-17).

The pleura is closed over the instrumentation with running, absorbable suture (Fig. 45-18), and the diaphragm is repaired with interrupted sutures. Repair of the costochondral junction is performed and is followed by reapprox-

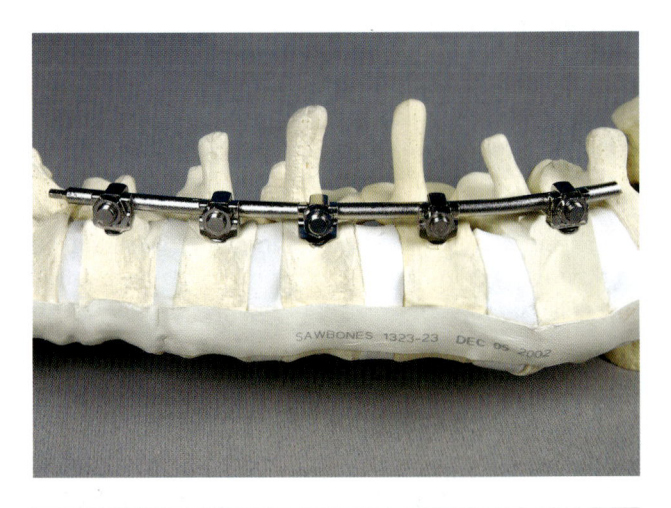

Fig. 45-17 Final single rod construct in a foam spine model. Gentle compression is used to seat the cages prior to final tightening of the nuts and eyebolts.

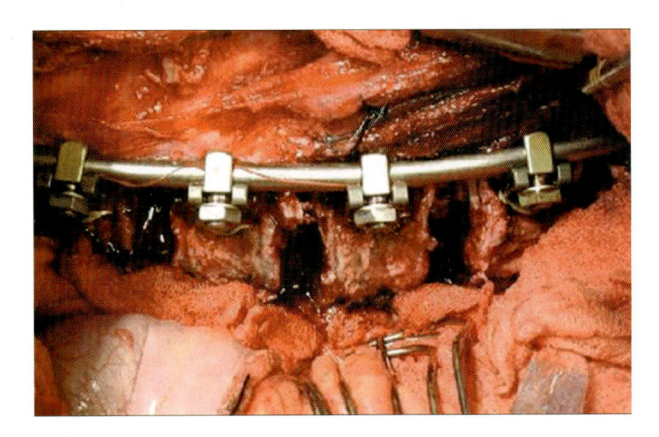

Fig. 45-15 A 90-degree rod rotation maneuver is used to correct the coronal plane deformity while placing lordosis. This increased lordosis has created anterior disk space opening.

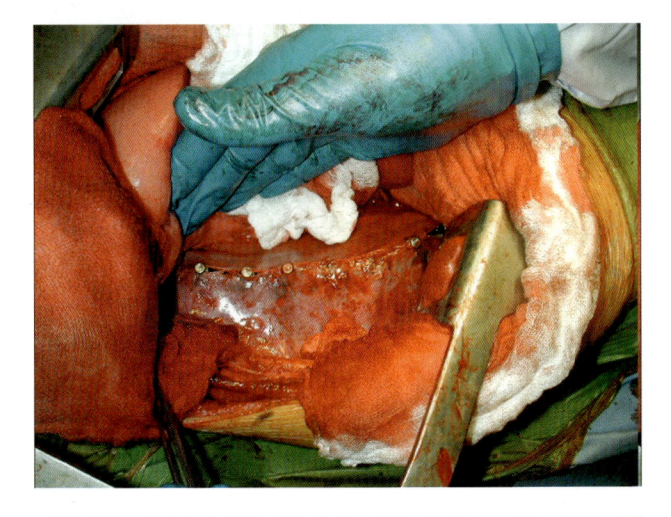

Fig. 45-18 The pleura is closed over the instrumentation with a running absorbable suture.

imation of the ribs and closure of the rib periosteum, muscle layers, subcutaneous layers, and the skin. A large chest tube is placed for postoperative drainage and is connected to wall suction for 48 to 72 hours. It is generally removed when the drainage is serous and is below 80 mL per 8-hour shift. The patient is mobilized relatively quickly, and no postoperative immobilization is required.

RESULTS

The Dwyer instrumentation was the initial anterior system used for the treatment of thoracolumbar/lumbar scoliosis.[33] Because it utilized wires, screws, and cables, it had limited rigidity and frequently resulted in pseudarthrosis and loss of correction.[8,34,35] It also relied on ventral compressive forces without derotation, which induced kyphosis with loss of the normal physiologic lumbar lordosis.[8,34] Zielke developed a new system that followed Dwyer's original principle of anterior compression, but added a derotation maneuver designed to convert the frontal plane deformity into the sagittal plane.[36,37] By applying a 3-mm threaded compression rod, the Zielke system was more stable than Dwyer's construct; however, pseudarthrosis, loss of correction, and kyphosis continued to be problems.[2,20,21,38]

These early results led to the development of newer systems with improvements to include a larger diameter single rod (¼ inch or 6.35 mm) developed at Texas Scottish Rite Hospital (TSRH) with good early results.[9,39] The initial experience using this implant and morselized rib graft demonstrated some loss of coronal plane correction and subsequent kyphosis.[39] Rib strut grafts placed in the disk space have also been utilized,[5] resulting in a decrease in the pseudarthrosis rate[10] (Fig. 45-19).

The use of anterior structural support with the single rod constructs has improved the overall stiffness of the construct, especially in flexion-extension testing, thus improving fusion rates and the ability to restore and maintain lumbar lordosis.[32,40] The advent of anterior support to augment the single rod instrumentation system has resulted in improved results when compared to patients who did not have anterior support.[31,32,41]

Sweet and associates reviewed 20 consecutive patients who had a single rod anterior instrumentation with structural titanium mesh cages and concluded that coronal plane correction and preservation of lordosis 2 years after surgery was achieved without any evidence of pseudarthrosis[32] (see Fig. 45-1G to J).

Spiegel and associates have performed biomechanical studies in a bovine model that examined the effects of augmenting anterior solid rod constructs with multilevel, threaded cortical bone dowels.[31,41] They determined that these grafts increased construct stiffness in lateral bending and in axial compression as compared to both the intact situation and to a rib grafting technique.[41] In a prior study, he had previously determined that cortical bone dowels improved the construct stiffness when compared to posterior instrumentation techniques. This improved rigidity should translate into improved rates of arthrodesis and maintenance of alignment.[31]

The single rod construct has been utilized for many years, is easy to use, provides excellent biomechanical stiffness when combined with anterior structural support, is less expensive, and has a lower profile than the newer dual rod implant systems. The dual rod implants offer greater versatility, are stiffer in flexion-extension testing, and provide two fixation points to each vertebra when compared to the single rod constructs without anterior support.[40]

Dual rod–dual screw systems have been utilized in the treatment of thoracolumbar and lumbar adolescent idiopathic scoliosis curves, offering greater versatility and greater stiffness when compared to single rod systems.[42] Biomechanical studies analyzing single and dual rod systems[40,43,44] demonstrate greater stiffness in torsion and in flexion-extension loading than single rod constructs; however, with the addition of interbody support, the stiffness in flexion for the single rod systems was similar in the two systems.[40] It is also apparent that increasing the number of rods or structural interbody support did not have a significant effect on lateral bending.[40,43] The preliminary results using the Kaneda system demonstrated excellent correction with rigid rotational stability and maintenance of lumbar lordosis.[42] More recently, dual rod instrumentation has demonstrated 60% coronal plane correction, 52% improvement in axial plane correction, and significant improvement in the sagittal plane, especially when preoperative lumbar kyphosis was present[45] (Fig. 45-20).

COMPLICATIONS

Complications can be divided into early and late postoperative complications following anterior instrumentation and fusion for thoracolumbar and lumbar scoliosis. The early complications, which include prolonged chest tube drainage, atelectasis, wound infection, and loss of fixation, are rare. The more common late complications include pseudarthrosis at one or more fusion levels, loss of coronal plane correction, and loss of lordosis. With improved surgical technique (more complete diskectomy and bone grafting) and implant design, the incidence of these complications continues to decline. The use of single large rod instrumentation without anterior support can result in an incidence of pseudarthrosis approaching 30% in some series.[6,10,39] The use of anterior structural support with single rods and the use of dual rod constructs has resulted in a decline in the incidence of pseudarthrosis to acceptable levels.[30,32,42,45] Risk factors for pseudarthrosis with anterior thoracolumbar/lumbar techniques appear to be a history of smoking and patients who weigh greater than 70 kg.[46] Despite radiographic evidence of a pseudarthrosis, many patients are clinically asymptomatic and do not necessarily require reoperation. Patients with a

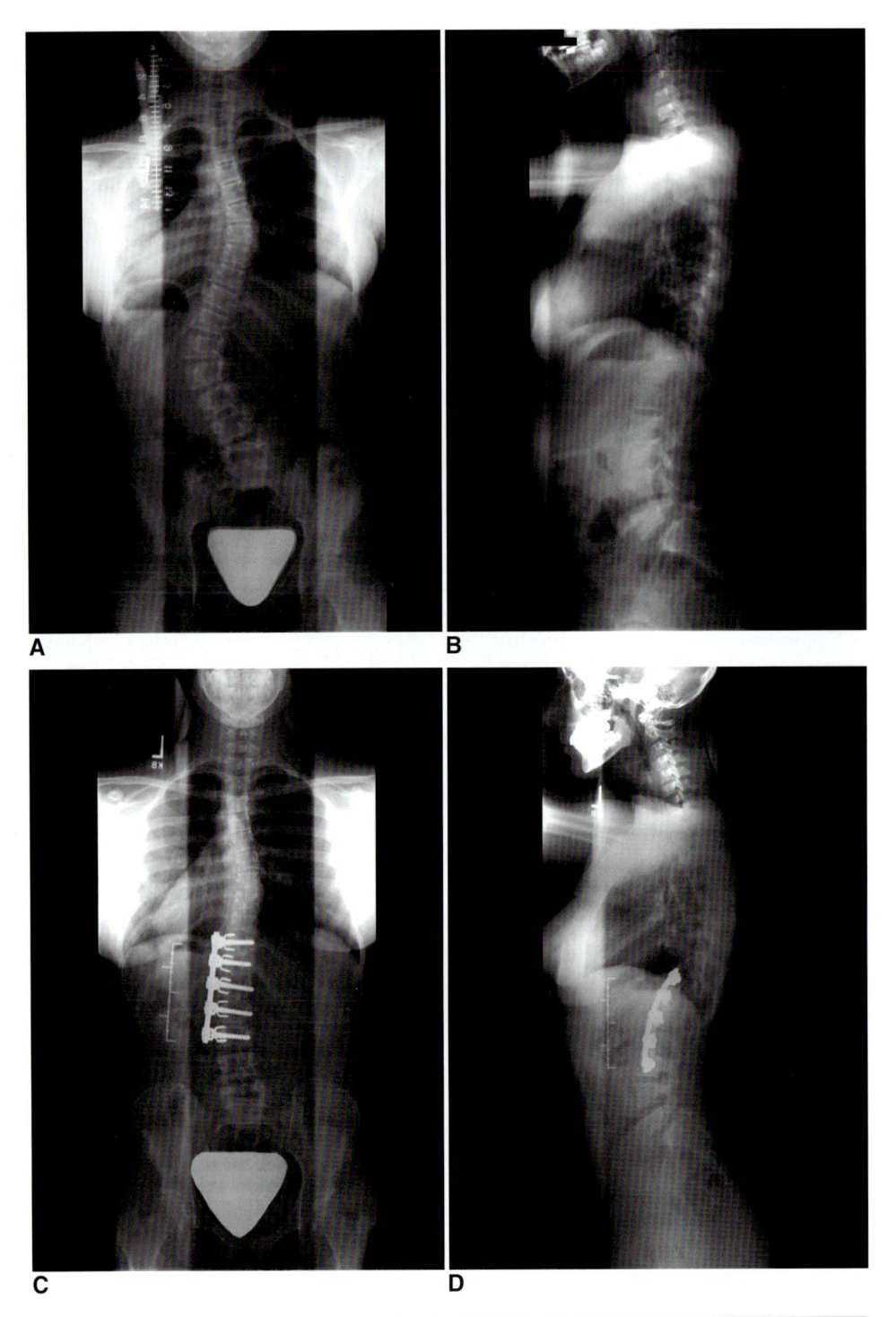

Fig. 45-19 A 13-year-old female with a left lumbar adolescent idiopathic scoliosis (Lenke type 5C). *A,* Preoperative standing posteroanterior (PA) radiograph. Left thoracolumbar curve (T11-L3) with a coronal Cobb measurement at 52 degrees, a compensatory main thoracic curve of 37 degrees, and Risser stage 3. *B,* Preoperative lateral radiograph demonstrating thoracic hypokyphosis and loss of physiologic lumbar lordosis. An incidental grade I spondylolisthesis was diagnosed at the L5-S1 level. *C,* Two-year postoperative standing PA radiograph. Anterior spinal fusion and instrumentation had been performed with a left thoracoabdominal approach through the tenth rib. A single rod construct from T11-L3 was performed with anterior rib strut grafts placed at all levels. *D,* Two-year postoperative lateral radiograph demonstrating restoration of sagittal plane alignment. There has not been progression of the L5-S1 spondylolisthesis.

CHAPTER 45   Anterior Treatment for Thoracolumbar/Lumbar Scoliosis   403

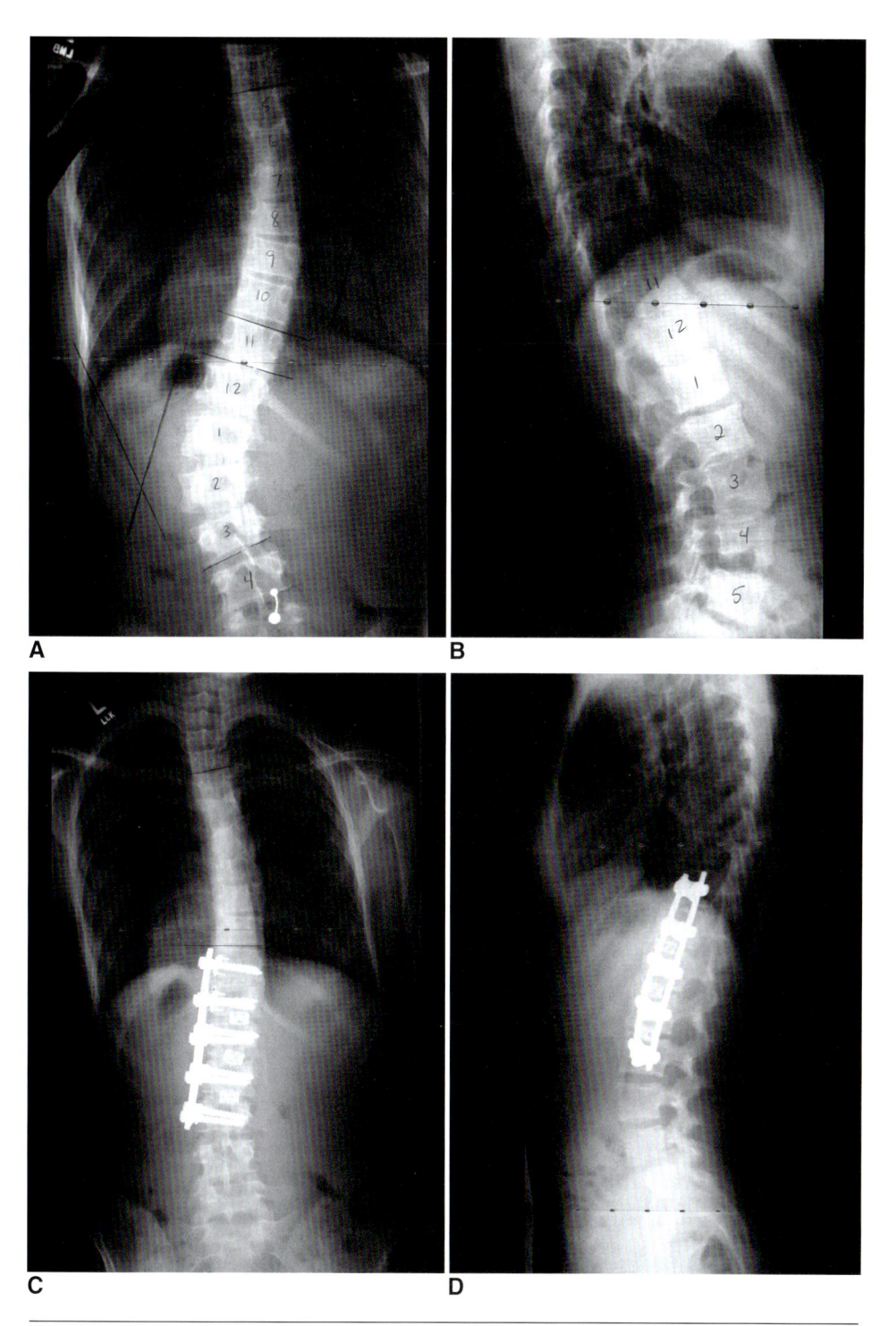

Fig. 45-20 A 13-year-old female with left thoracolumbar/lumbar adolescent idiopathic scoliosis (Lenke type 5C). *A*, Preoperative standing posteroanterior (PA) radiograph. Left thoracolumbar curve (T11-L3) with Cobb measurement 46 degrees, and small compensatory right main thoracic curve. *B*, Preoperative lateral radiograph demonstrating loss of lumbar lordosis. *C*, Two-year postoperative standing PA radiograph. Anterior spinal fusion and instrumentation has been performed through a left thoracoabdominal approach through the tenth rib. A double rod construct from T11-L3 with titanium mesh cages at the T12-L1, L1-L2, and L2-L3 levels have been placed. *D*, Two-year postoperative lateral radiograph demonstrates improved lumbar lordosis.

symptomatic pseudarthorisis are successfully managed with surgical treatment to include posterior fusion and instrumentation of the affected levels.

Loss of coronal plane correction is mild in these patients; however, loss of kyphosis can be problematic, leading to significant symptoms. This can be avoided with resoration of lumbar lordosis and maintenance utilizing anterior structural support, usually in the form of metal cages or allograft rings. Loss of lordosis, which becomes symptomatic, is a challenging problem, especially when solid fusion has occurred. This will require removal of anterior implants with posterior osteotomies and instrumentation.

CONCLUSION

Anterior fusion and instrumentation continues to be the main approach used in the surgical treatment of thoracolumbar-lumbar scoliosis. The indications for its use are well described, but continue to evolve as newer techniques are developed. Despite the complications associated with early generations of anterior implant systems, including pseudarthrosis and kyphosis, more modern surgical techniques and instrumentation have provided excellent clinical results. Current generation implants, with large diameter one- and two-rod constructs, provide sufficient rigidity to maintain sagittal plane alignment and to ensure a complete fusion. Despite these advances, the most important step of anterior surgery is to perform a complete diskectomy, which provides the flexibility necessary for deformity correction as well as adequate surface area for arthrodesis.

REFERENCES

1. Burton DC, Asher MA, Lai SM: Patient-based outcomes analysis of patients with single torsion thoracolumbar-lumbar scoliosis treated with anterior or posterior instrumentation: An average 5- to 9-year follow-up study. Spine 2002;27:2363–2367.
2. Lowe TG, Peters JD: Anterior spinal fusion with Zielke instrumentation for idiopathic scoliosis: A frontal and sagittal curve analysis in 36 patients. Spine 1993;18:423–426.
3. Roaf R: The basic anatomy of scoliosis. J Bone Joint Surg Br 1966;48:786–792.
4. Shufflebarger HL, Geck MJ, Clark CE: The posterior approach for lumbar and thoracolumbar adolescent idiopathic scoliosis: Posterior shortening and pedicle screws. Spine 2004;29:269–276.
5. Lowe TG, Betz R, Lenke L, et al: Anterior single-rod instrumentation of the thoracic and lumbar spine: Saving levels. Spine 2003;28:S208–S216.
6. Bitan FD, Neuwirth MG, Kuflik PL, et al: The use of short and rigid anterior instrumentation in the treatment of idiopathic thoracolumbar scoliosis: A retrospective review of 24 cases. Spine 2002;27:1553–1557.
7. Ogilvie JW: Anterior spine fusion with Zielke instrumentation for idiopathic scoliosis in adolescents. Orthop Clin North Am 1988;19:313–317.
8. Hsu LC, Zucherman J, Tang SC, Leong JC: Dwyer instrumentation in the treatment of adolescent idiopathic scoliosis. J Bone Joint Surg Br 1982;64:536–541.
9. Shen J, Qiu G, Weng X, et al: Anterior spinal fusion with TSRH instrumentation for scoliosis. Chin Med Sci J 2003;18:41–45.
10. Ouellet JA, Johnston CE: Effect of grafting technique on the maintenance of coronal and sagittal correction in anterior treatment of scoliosis. Spine 2002;27:2129–2135; discussion 2135–2136.
11. Kaneda K, Shono Y, Satoh S, Abumi K: Anterior correction of thoracic scoliosis with Kaneda anterior spinal system: A preliminary report. Spine 1997;22:1358–1368.
12. Sanders AE, Baumann R, Brown H, et al: Selective anterior fusion of thoracolumbar/lumbar curves in adolescents: When can the associated thoracic curve be left unfused? Spine 2003;28:706–713.
13. Richards BS: The importance of pelvic fixation in posterior spinal fusion for cerebral palsy. Scoliosis Research Society Annual Meeting, Quebec City, Canada, 2003.
14. Dubousset J, Herring JA, Shufflebarger H: The crankshaft phenomenon. J Pediatr Orthop 1989;9:541–550.
15. Song KM, Little DG: Peak height velocity as a maturity indicator for males with idiopathic scoliosis. J Pediatr Orthop 2000;20:286–288.
16. Little DG, Song KM, Katz D, Herring JA: Relationship of peak height velocity to other maturity indicators in idiopathic scoliosis in girls. J Bone Joint Surg Am 2000;82:685–693.
17. Burton DC, Asher MA, Lai SM: Scoliosis correction maintenance in skeletally immature patients with idiopathic scoliosis: Is anterior fusion really necessary? Spine 2000;25:61–68.
18. Winter RB, Moe JH, Bradford DS, et al: Spine deformity in neurofibromatosis. A review of one hundred and two patients. J Bone Joint Surg Am 1979;61:677–694.
19. Lenke LG, Betz RR, Harms J, et al: Adolescent idiopathic scoliosis: A new classification to determine extent of spinal arthrodesis. J Bone Joint Surg Am 2001;83-A:1169–1181.
20. Trammell TR, Benedict F, Reed D: Anterior spine fusion using Zielke instrumentation for adult thoracolumbar and lumbar scoliosis. Spine 1991;16:307–316.
21. Kostuik JP, Carl A, Ferron S: Anterior Zielke instrumentation for spinal deformity in adults. J Bone Joint Surg Am 1989;71:898–912.
22. Smith JA, Deviren V, Berven S, Bradford DS: Does instrumented anterior scoliosis surgery lead to kyphosis, pseudarthrosis, or inadequate correction in adults? Spine 2002;27:529–534.
23. Floman Y, Penny JN, Micheli LJ, et al: Osteotomy of the fusion mass in scoliosis. J Bone Joint Surg Am 1982;64:1307–1316.
24. Bernstein RM, Hall JE: Solid rod short segment anterior fusion in thoracolumbar scoliosis. J Pediatr Orthop Part B 1998;7:124–131.
25. Brodner W, Mun Yue W, Maller HB, et al: Short segment bone-on-bone instrumentation for single curve idiopathic scoliosis. Spine 2003;28:S224–S233.
26. Graham EJ, Lenke LG, Lowe TG, et al: Prospective pulmonary function evaluation following open thoracotomy for anterior spinal fusion in adolescent idiopathic scoliosis. Spine 2000;25:2319–2325.
27. Sucato DJ, Rathjen KE, Harris K: The effect of surgical approach on early postoperative pulmonary function in the treatment of adolescent idiopathic scoliosis. Scoliosis Research Society, 39th Annual Meeting. Buenos Aires, Argentina, 2004.
28. Kim Y, Lenke LG, Bridwell KH, et al: Prospective evaluation of pulmonary function in adolescent idiopathic scoliosis relative to the surgical approach: Minimum 5 year follow-up. Annual Scoliosis Research Society Meeting, Seattle, WA, 2002.
29. Bassett G, Johnson C, Stanley P: Comparison of preoperative selective spinal angiography and somatosensory-evoked potential monitoring with temporary occlusion of segmental vessels during anterior spinal surgery. Spine 1996;21:1996–1999; discussion 2000.
30. Lenke LG, Bridwell KH: Mesh cages in idiopathic scoliosis in adolescents. Clin Orthop 2002;(394):98–108.

31. Spiegel DA, Drummond DS, Cunningham BW, et al: Augmentation of an anterior solid rod construct with threaded cortical bone dowels: A biomechanical study. Spine 1999;24:2300–2306.
32. Sweet FA, Lenke LG, Bridwell KH, Blanke KM: Maintaining lumbar lordosis with anterior single solid-rod instrumentation in thoracolumbar and lumbar adolescent idiopathic scoliosis. Spine 1999;24:24:1655–1662.
33. Dwyer AF, Newton NC, Sherwood AA: An anterior approach to scoliosis: A preliminary report. Clin Orthop 1969;62:192–202.
34. Kohler R, Galland O, Mechin H, et al: The Dwyer procedure in the treatment of idiopathic scoliosis: A 10-year follow-up review of 21 patients. Spine 1990;15:75–80.
35. Hall JE: Dwyer Instrumentation in anterior fusion of the spine. J Bone Joint Surg Am 1981;63:1188–1190.
36. Zielke K, Berthet A: [VDS—ventral derotation spondylodesis—Preliminary report on 58 cases.] Beitrage Orthopad Traumatol 1978;25:85–103.
37. Zielke K, Stunkat R, Beaujean F: [Ventrale derotations-spondylodesis (author's transl).] Arch Orthopad Unfall-Chirurg 1976;85:257–277.
38. Hammerberg KW, Rodts MF, DeWald RL: Zielke instrumentation. Orthopedics 1988;11:1365–1371.
39. Turi M, Johnston CE 2nd, Richards BS: Anterior correction of idiopathic scoliosis using TSRH instrumentation. Spine 1993;18:417–422.
40. Fricka KB, Mahar AT, Newton PO: Biomechanical analysis of anterior scoliosis instrumentation: Differences between single and dual rod systems with and without interbody structural support. Spine 2002;27:702–706.
41. Spiegel DA, Cunningham BW, Oda I, et al: Anterior vertebral screw strain with and without solid interspace support. Spine 2000;25:2755–2761.
42. Kaneda K, Shono Y, Satoh S, Abumi K: New anterior instrumentation for the management of thoracolumbar and lumbar scoliosis: Application of the Kaneda two-rod system. Spine 1996;21:1250–1261.
43. Shimamoto N, Kotani Y, Shono Y, et al: Static and dynamic analysis of five anterior instrumentation systems for thoracolumbar scoliosis. Spine 2003;28:1678–1685.
44. Shono Y, Kaneda K, Yamamoto I: A biomechanical analysis of Zielke, Kaneda, and Cotrel-Dubousset instrumentations in thoracolumbar scoliosis: A calf spine model. Spine 1991;16:1305–1311.
45. Bullmann V, Halm HF, Niemeyer T, et al: Dual-rod correction and instrumentation of idiopathic scoliosis with the Halm-Zielke instrumentation. Spine 2003;28:1306–1313.
46. Sweet FA, Lenke LG, Bridwell KH, et al: Prospective radiographic and clinical outcomes and complications of single solid rod instrumented anterior spinal fusion in adolescent idiopathic scoliosis. Spine 2001;26:1956–1965.

CHAPTER 46

FERNANDO E. SILVA

LAWRENCE G. LENKE

Surgical Treatment of Adolescent Idiopathic Scoliosis: Lenke Curve Types 1 to 6

INTRODUCTION

Lenke and associates recently designed a new classification system of adolescent idiopathic scoliosis (AIS) that is universal for all curve patterns, two-dimensional, and more reliable than the previous system of King and associates[1,2] (Fig. 46-1). This three-tiered system consists of a curve type (1 through 6), a lumbar spine modifier (A, B, C), and a sagittal thoracic modifier (−, N, +). The Lenke curve classification combines one component of each of these three features to produce a complete curve classification (e.g., 1A−).

Curve types 1 to 6 (Fig. 46-2) are determined following assessment of the upright coronal, lateral, and right and left side bending radiographs (Fig. 46-3A). Each of the three regions of the spine—the proximal thoracic (PT), main thoracic (MT), and thoracolumbar/lumbar (TL/L)—are designated as the major curve (largest Cobb measurement) or as a minor structural or nonstructural curve. Criteria for a structural minor curve include inflexibility on side-bending (≥25 degrees), hyperkyphosis in the PT region (T2-T5 ≥ +20 degrees), or thoracolumbar junction (T10-L2 ≥ +20 degrees). Thus, a schema of six curve types may be created whether the MT or the TL/L regions are the major curve, and whether the other two regions are minor structural or nonstructural curves (see Fig. 46-1, Table 46-1).

The lumbar spine modifier (A, B, or C) is then added based on the position of the apex of the lumbar spine to the center sacral vertical line (CSVL). The CSVL is the vertical line drawn parallel to the radiograph edge and perpendicular to the floor from the geometric center of S1 that depicts the coronal position of the lumbar spine in relation to the pelvis. When the CSVL falls between the pedicles up to the stable vertebra, then a lumbar modifier A is assigned. When the CSVL touches the apical pedicles, then a lumbar modifier B is assigned. When the apex of the lumbar spine is completely off the CSVL, then a lumbar modifier C is assigned (see Fig. 46-3B).

Finally, a sagittal thoracic modifier (−, N, or +) is assigned based on the T5-T12 thoracic sagittal alignment. When sagittal kyphosis is less than +10 degrees, a − hypokyphotic sagittal modifier is assigned; +10 to +40 degrees is N, or normal; and greater than +40 degrees is assigned a + hyperkyphotic modifier. The use of this new classification system, leading to successful surgical treatment of AIS, will be highlighted in the six curve types presented (see Fig. 46-3C).

INDICATIONS FOR SURGICAL TREATMENT OF ADOLESCENT IDIOPATHIC SCOLIOSIS[3,4]

- Failure of bracing
- Curve progression
- Cosmesis
- Curves of 45 degrees or greater in the coronal plane after skeletal immaturity, and of 40 degrees or more in skeletally immature patients
- Pain (rare)

OPERATIVE TECHNIQUE[5,6]

BASIC EQUIPMENT

- Jackson frame (four poster)
- Headlight system
- Nerve monitoring system
- Deep muscle retractors
- Osteotomes, Kerrison punches, curettes

CURVE TYPE

Type	Proximal Thoracic	Main Thoracic	Thoracolumbar/Lumbar	Description
1	Nonstructural	Structural (major)*	Nonstructural	Main Thoracic (MT)
2	Structural	Structural (major)*	Nonstructural	Double Thoracic (DT)
3	Nonstructural	Structural (major)*	Structural	Double Major (DM)
4	Structural	Structural (major)*	Structural	Triple Major (TM)**
5	Nonstructural	Nonstructural	Structural (major)*	Thoracolumbar/ Lumbar (TL/L)
6	Nonstructural	Structural	Structural (major)*	Thoracolumbar/ Lumbar-Main Thoracic (TL/L-MT)

*Major= Largest Cobb measurement, always structural.
Minor= All other curves with structural criteria applied.
**Type 4 - MT or TL/L can be major curve.

STRUCTURAL CRITERIA (Minor Curves)

Proximal Thoracic	Side-Bending Cobb ≥ 25° T2-T5 Kyphosis > +20°
Main Thoracic	Side-Bending Cobb ≥ 25° T10-L2 Kyphosis > +20°
Thoracolumbar/Lumbar	Side-Bending Cobb ≥ 25° T10-L2 Kyphosis > +20°

LOCATION OF APEX (SRS Definition)

Curve	Apex
Thoracic	T2-T11/12 Disc
Thoracolumbar	T12-L1
Thoracolumbar/Lumbar	L1/2 Disc-L4

LUMBAR SPINE MODIFIERS

Lumbar Spine Modifier	CSVL to Lumbar Apex
A	Between Pedicles
B	Touches Pedicles
C	Medial to Pedicles

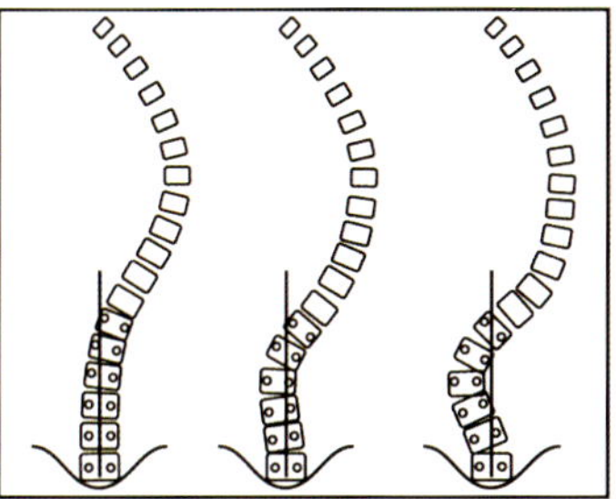

THORACIC SAGITTAL MODIFIERS

Thoracic Sagittal Profile T5-T12	
- (Hypo)	<10°
N (Normal)	10°–40°
+ (Hyper)	>40°

Curve Type (1-6) + Lumbar Spine Modifier (A, B, C) + Thoracic Sagittal Modifier (-, N, +) = Classification (e.g., 1B+)

Fig. 46-1 Lenke classification scheme. (Modified from Lenke LG, Betz RR, Harms J, et al: Adolescent idiopathic scoliosis: A new classification to determine extent of spinal arthrodesis. J Bone Surg Am 2001:83-A:1169–1181.)

TABLE 46-1 Lenke Curve Patterns*

CURVE TYPE	DESCRIPTION	PROXIMAL THORACIC	MAIN THORACIC	THORACOLUMBAR/ LUMBAR	STRUCTURAL REGION OF EACH CURVE TYPE
1	Main thoracic	Nonstructural	Structural (major)	Nonstructural	Main thoracic
2	Double thoracic	Structural	Structural (major)	Nonstructural	Proximal thoracic, main thoracic
3	Double major	Nonstructural	Structural (major)	Structural	Main thoracic, thoracolumbar/lumbar
4	Triple major	Structural	Structural (major[†])	Structural (major[†])	Proximal thoracic, main thoracic, thoracolumbar/lumbar
5	Thoracolumbar/lumbar	Nonstructural	Nonstructural	Structural (major)	Thoracolumbar/lumbar
6	Thoracolumbar/lumbar-main thoracic	Nonstructural	Structural	Structural (major)	Thoracolumbar/lumbar, main thoracic

*A structural proximal thoracic curve has a Cobb angle of 25 degrees or more on side-benidng radiographs and/or kyphosis between the second and the fifth thoracic levels of at least +20 degrees. A structural main thoracic curve has a Cobb angle of 25 degrees or more on side-bending radiographs and/or kyphosis between the tenth thoracic and the second lumbar level of at least +20 degrees. A structural thoracolumbar/lumbar curve has a Cobb angle of 25 degrees or more on side-bending radiographs and/or kyphosis between the tenth thoracic and the second lumbar level of at lest +20 degrees.
[†]Either the main thoracic or the thoracolumbar/lumbar curve can be the major curve.

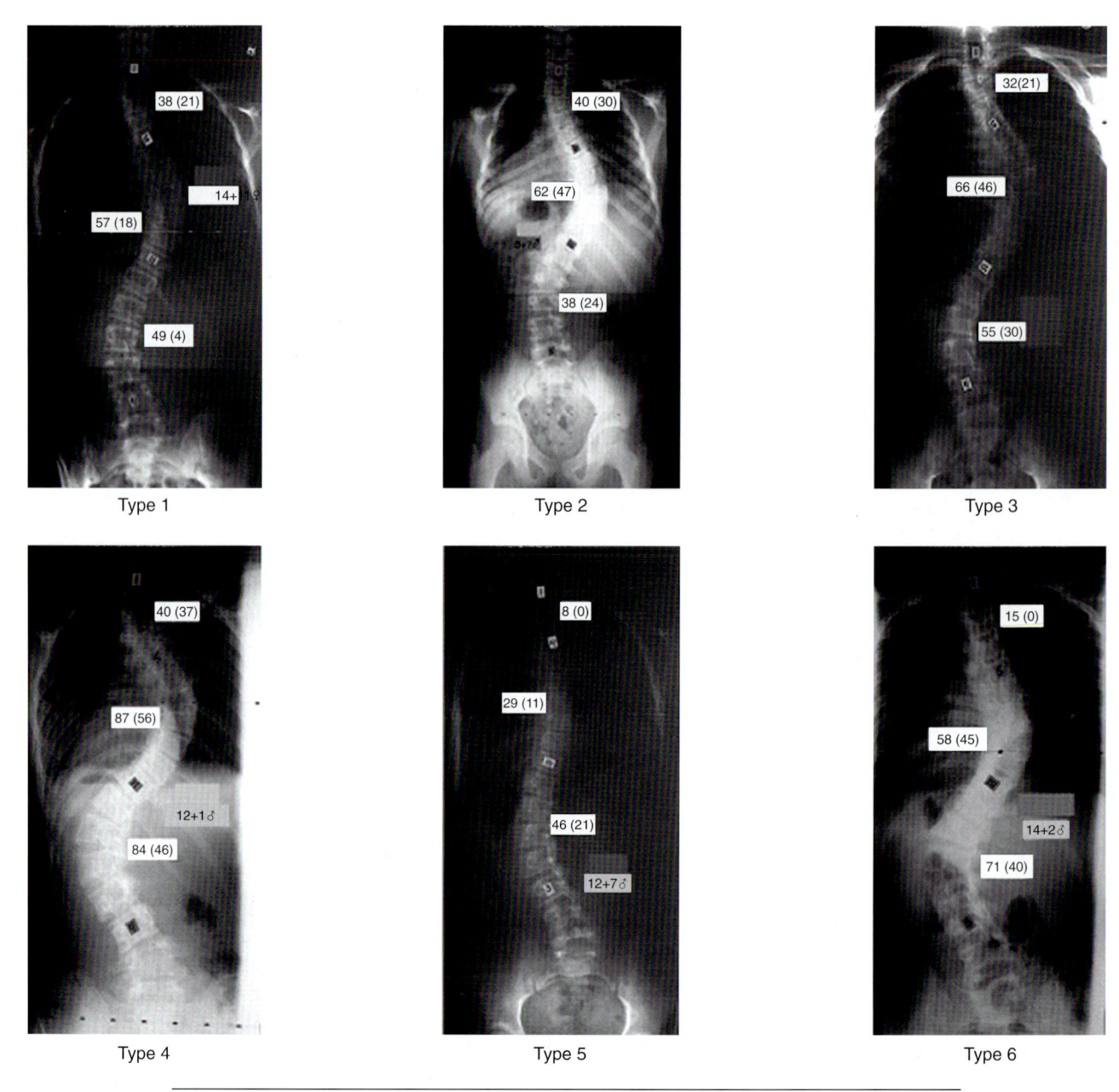

Fig. 46-2 Lenke curve types (side-bending Cobb measures).

- Lenke pedicle probe
- Segmental pedicle screw instrumentation system
- Coronal and sagittal benders
- Apical derotation set
- Bone graft source

PATIENT POSITIONING[7]

- Patient undergoes induction of general anesthesia and endotracheal intubation.
- All neurologic monitoring equipment is placed.
- The patient is gently placed in the prone position.
- Jackson frame pads are strategically placed over the chest, anterior superior iliac spines, and anterior thighs. The arms are placed in the 90-90 position and all pressure points are attended to with adequate padding.

PREPARATION AND DRAPING

- The incision is marked based on the theoretical midline and not over the curvature; except for severe curves, in such cases the incision is slightly curved along the curve.

CHAPTER 46 Surgical Treatment of Adolescent Idiopathic Scoliosis 409

A

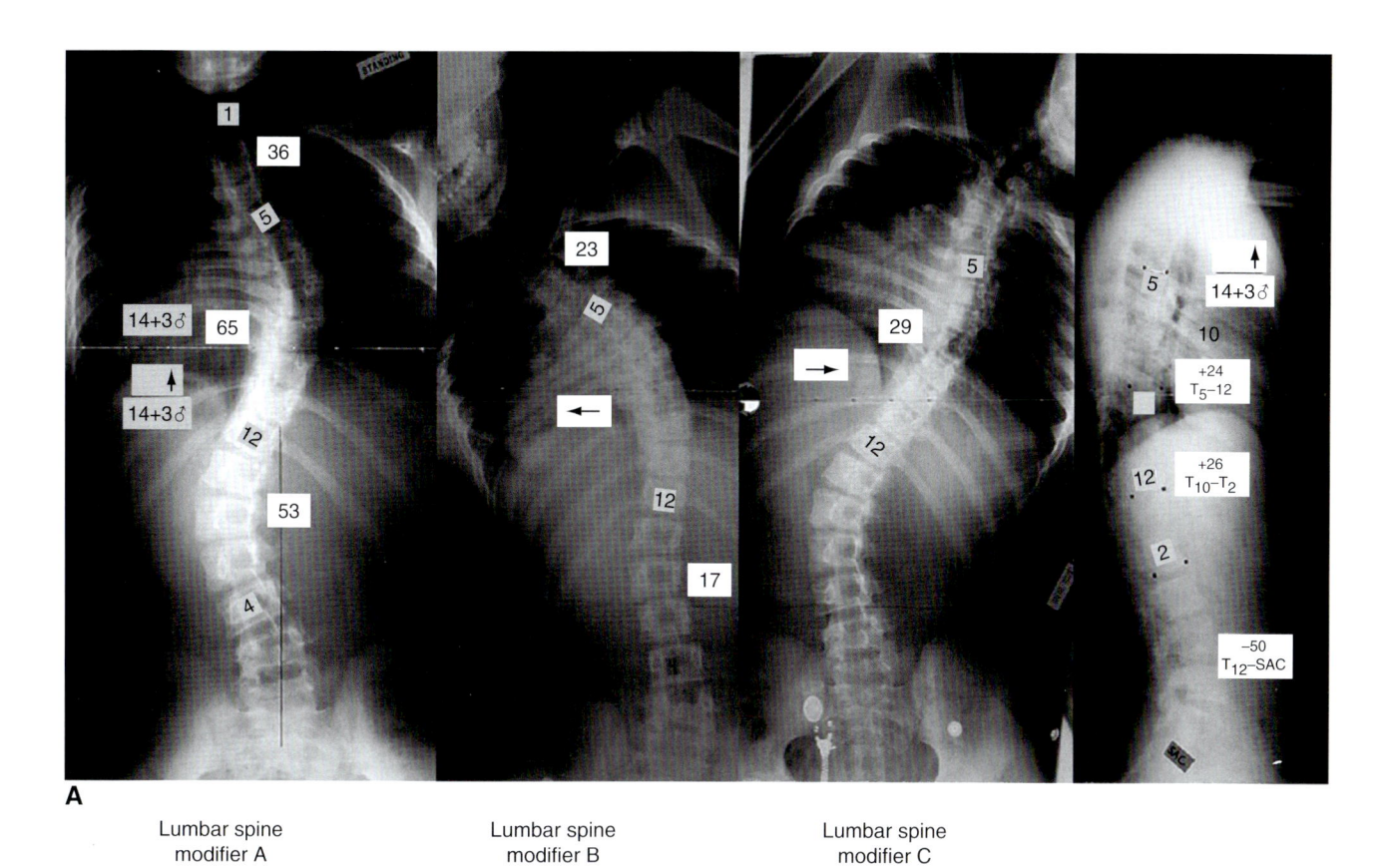

Lumbar spine
modifier A

Lumbar spine
modifier B

Lumbar spine
modifier C

B

Fig. 46-3 Radiographic assessment for Lenke classification. Lumbar modifier A has the CSVL between the pedicles, lumbar modifier B has the CSVL touch the pedicles, and lumbar modifier C has the CSVL fall medial to the pedicles.

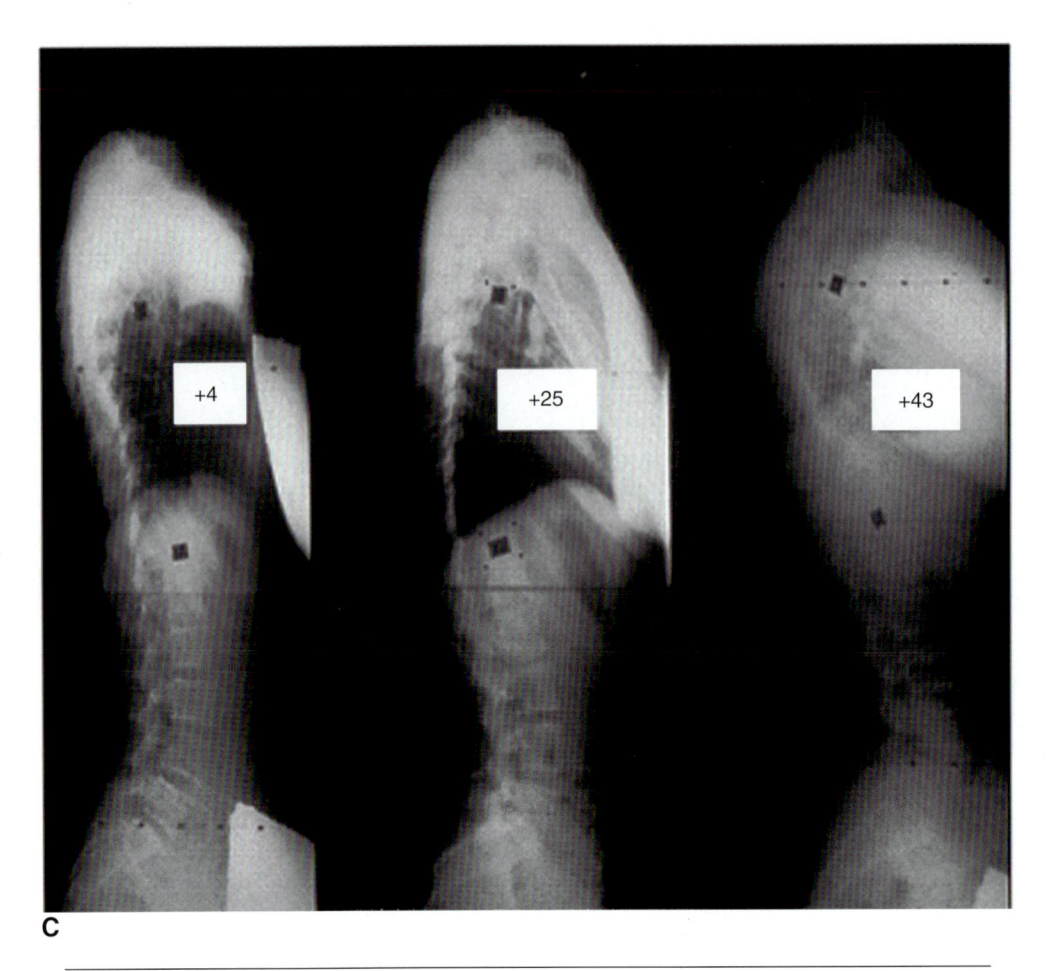

Fig. 46-3, cont'd. For legend see p. 409.

- Starting at the cervicothoracic junction, the entire spine is sterilely prepped down to the pelvis, including the intended area for bone graft harvesting.

FREE HAND PLACEMENT OF PEDICLE SCREWS[5]

- Technique is equivalent for lumbar and thoracic screws.
- Each step is repeated sequentially at each level to be instrumented.

Incision and Exposure (Fig. 46-4A)

- Posteroanterior and lateral localization radiographs are obtained soon after the exposure is begun.
- Meticulous subperiosteal exposure of the posterior elements is performed from the planned upper to the lower end instrumented vertebrae extending out to the transverse process tips bilaterally.
- Disruption of proximal and distal facet capsule, supraspinous ligaments, and ligamentum flavum is avoided.

Facetectomy (see Fig. 46-4B)

- Except for the lowermost instrumented vertebrae, the inferior 3 to 5 mm of the inferior facet and cartilage of the superior facet are removed.
- It imperative to clearly expose the base of the superior facet for imaginary location of the ventral pedicle.
- Starting points for pedicle screw placement can now be consistently localized anatomically without intraoperative radiography, fluoroscopy, or other image guidance.

Starting Point (see Fig. 46-4C)

- The supine preoperative films are studied to best find the ideal starting point.
- The starting point is slightly variable for each thoracic pedicle.
- Always start from neutrally rotated and distal vertebrae, working in a proximal direction.
- The pedicles move in a cephalad and medial direction as one moves from T12 to the midthoracic region (T7-T9).

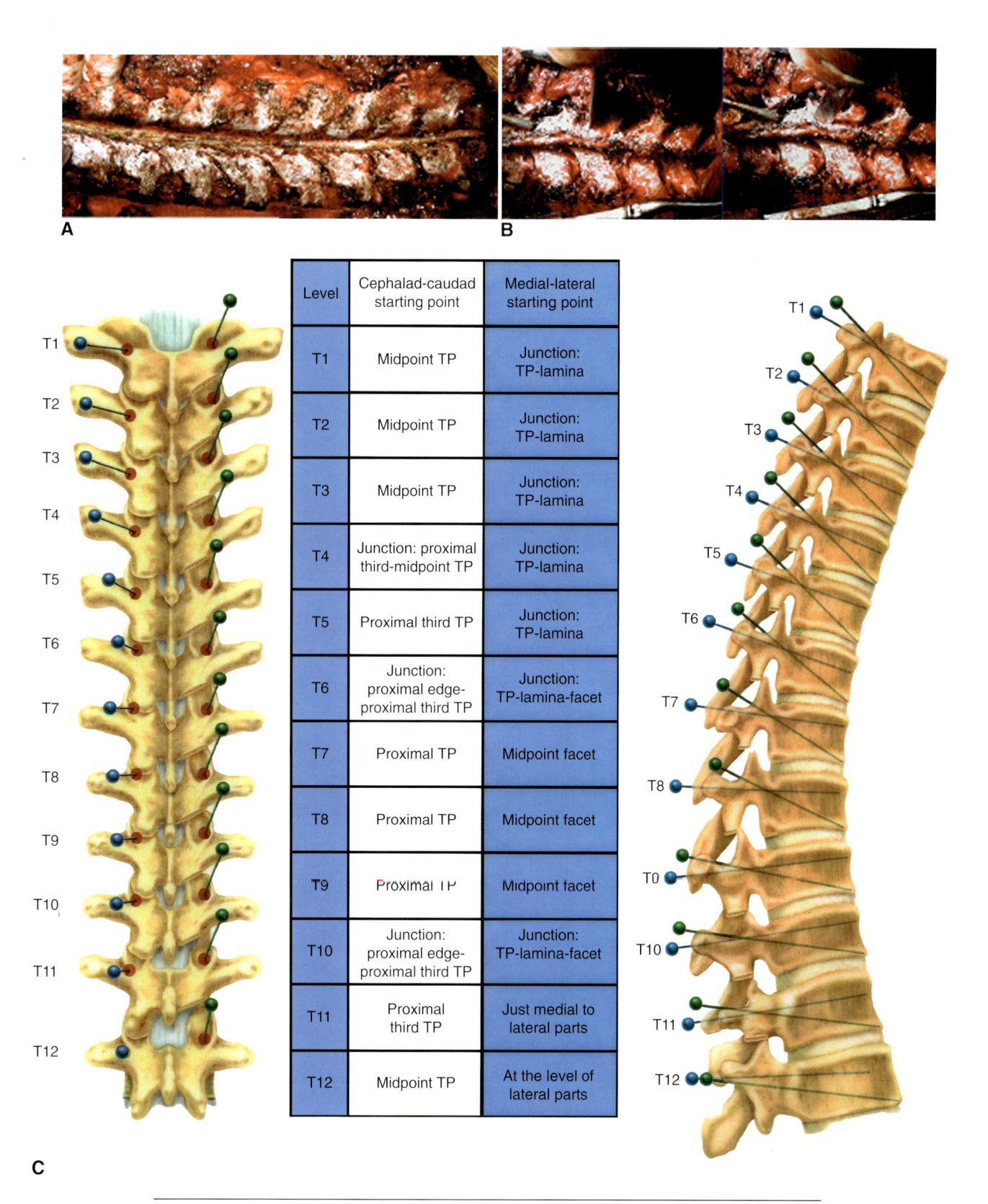

CHAPTER 46   Surgical Treatment of Adolescent Idiopathic Scoliosis   411

Level	Cephalad-caudad starting point	Medial-lateral starting point
T1	Midpoint TP	Junction: TP-lamina
T2	Midpoint TP	Junction: TP-lamina
T3	Midpoint TP	Junction: TP-lamina
T4	Junction: proximal third-midpoint TP	Junction: TP-lamina
T5	Proximal third TP	Junction: TP-lamina
T6	Junction: proximal edge-proximal third TP	Junction: TP-lamina-facet
T7	Proximal TP	Midpoint facet
T8	Proximal TP	Midpoint facet
T9	Proximal TP	Midpoint facet
T10	Junction: proximal edge-proximal third TP	Junction: TP-lamina-facet
T11	Proximal third TP	Just medial to lateral parts
T12	Midpoint TP	At the level of lateral parts

Fig. 46-4 Freehand technique of pedicle screw placement. *A*, Step 1: Complete exposure of the bony anatomy. *B*, Step 2: Facetectomy. *C*, Step 3: Use fixed angle or multiaxial screws for the straightforward approach (blue pins). Use multiaxial screws only for the anatomic approach (green pins). (TP, thoracic pedicle.)

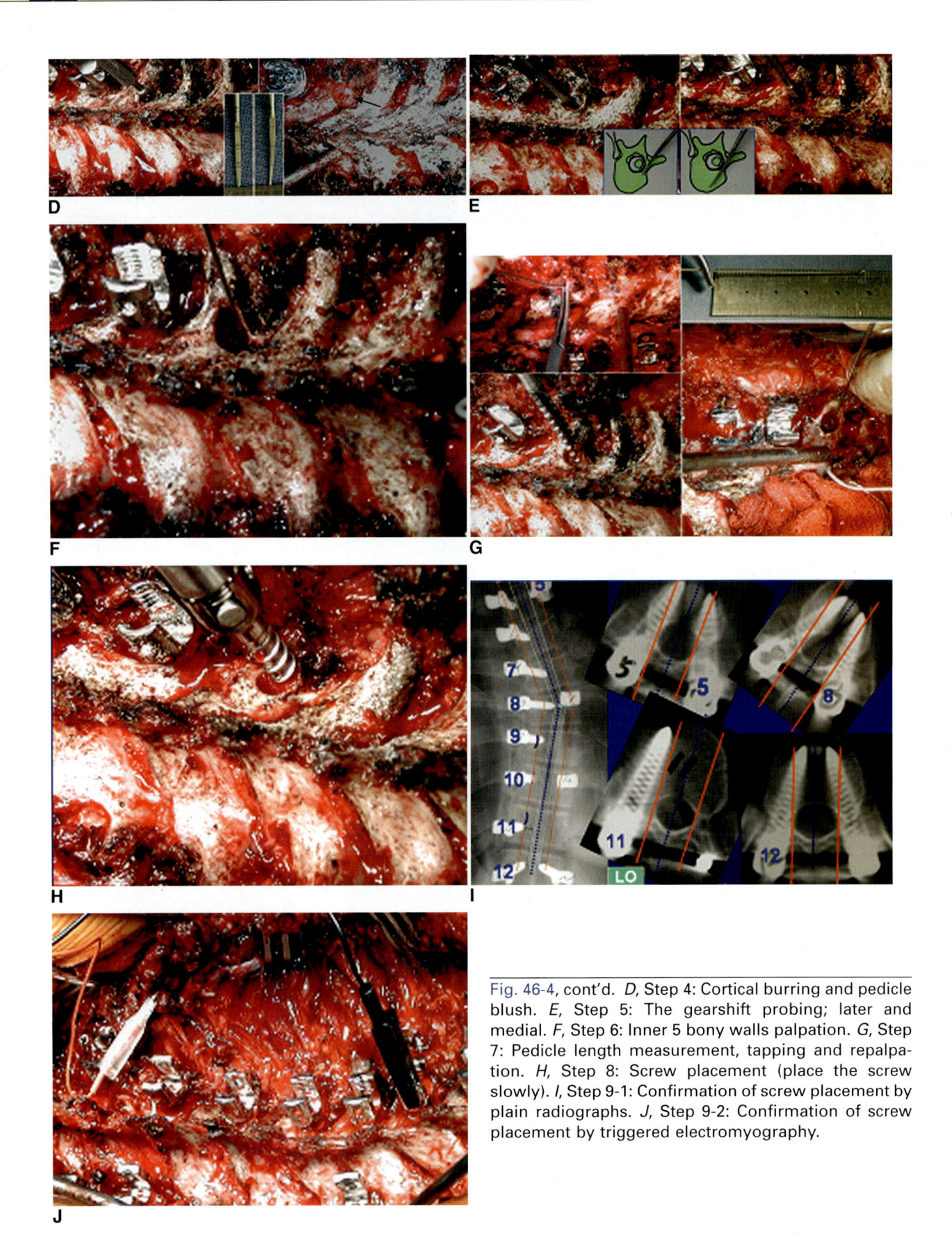

Fig. 46-4, cont'd. *D,* Step 4: Cortical burring and pedicle blush. ***E,*** Step 5: The gearshift probing; later and medial. ***F,*** Step 6: Inner 5 bony walls palpation. ***G,*** Step 7: Pedicle length measurement, tapping and repalpation. ***H,*** Step 8: Screw placement (place the screw slowly). ***I,*** Step 9-1: Confirmation of screw placement by plain radiographs. ***J,*** Step 9-2: Confirmation of screw placement by triggered electromyography.

- The starting point then moves in a caudal and lateral direction as one moves toward T1.
- Finding the starting point is anatomically based on the transverse process, lateral portion of the pars interarticularis, and base of the superior articular process.
- There should be a smooth transition between each screw in order to facilitate rod placement.

Cortical Burring (see Fig. 46-4D)

- A 3- to 5-mm cutting drill bit is employed to breach the posterior cortical aspect of the pedicle to a depth of about 5 mm or when the pedicle blush is encountered.
- When the pedicle blush is not encountered, as in very small apical concave pedicles, the Lenke probe is slowly used to expand the pedicle.

Gearshift Probing (see Fig. 46-4E)

- Initially pointed laterally as a safety measure, the Lenke probe is gently advanced with appropriate ventral pressure searching for the pedicular cancellous bone.
- After inserting the tip of the probe about 12 to 20 mm, the length of the pedicle, the probe is removed and reinserted facing medially into the base of the previous probed hole. The probe is then advanced to an adequate depth.
- Avoid penetration of the anterior cortex as there is no significant strength in the anterior vertebral body, which would risk vascular and visceral damage.
- The Lenke probe is rotated 180 degrees once the optimal depth is encountered to make room for the screw.

Palpation (see Fig. 46-4F)

- Gross inspection of the created tract must reveal only blood and no cerebrospinal fluid present.
- Using a pedicle sounder, the floor, medial, lateral, superior, and inferior walls of the pedicle tract are inspected for possible breaches.
- The junction of the middle and upper portions of the tract must be specially and very carefully inspected, as these regions correlate with the location of the spinal canal and isthmus.
- If the medial wall is breached, the Lenke probe is reangled to a more appropriate lateral trajectory.
- If a wall other than the medial pedicle wall has been breached, the pedicle may be salvaged as the screw is placed into an appropriated direction.

Pedicle Length Measurement, Tapping, and Repalpation (see Fig. 46-4G)

- The length of the anticipated pedicle tract is measured after ensuring that all five bony walls are intact.
- If the length is short, the Lenke probe is carefully reinserted to an appropriate length.
- The pedicle is undertapped 1 mm less than the intended pedicle screw diameter, and a smaller tap is used if it is difficult to pass this initial tap.
- A K-wire is placed when the pedicle is very small or more than one pass has been made with the Lenke probe. *The bony floor of the pedicle tract must be intact*; if there is *any* question as to it not being intact, a K-wire should *never* be used as cardiac tamponade can ensue from cardiac injury, such as injury to a coronary artery.
- The screw diameter is determined by using the internal diameter of a neutrally rotated pedicle as a reference diameter and also by tap tightness. We are able to insert screws if the internal pedicular diameter is 3 mm or more; additionally, a technique for placing screws in noncancellous pedicles has been developed by Lenke.
- The ideal screw diameter is 80% of the pedicle isthmus, but given the plasticity of the pediatric pedicular cortex, screws up to 115% of the pedicle diameter may be inserted without losing significant screw holding power.
- A second palpation of all five osseous walls is carried out after tapping and feeling the tapped bony ridges and remeasuring the pedicular length. This final measurement is compared with the chosen pedicle screw length as another safety check to ensure no pedicular tract violation and appropriate screw length.

Screw Placement (see Fig. 46-4H)

- The screw is slowly placed into the pedicle and down the vertebral body in the same alignment, allowing viscoelastic expansion of the pedicle.
- Screw diameters and lengths from 4.0 to 7.0 mm, in 0.5-mm increments, and 25 mm to 55 mm, respectively, can be inserted.
- Screws are placed at every segment on the correction side of the deformity. On the holding side, screws can be placed on every other vertebra, but only after two screws above and below the construct on this side have been placed. Additionally, screws must be placed bilaterally at the apex if one plans to carry out an apical derotation maneuver.
- Electromyography (EMG) stimulations are carried out with real-time stimulation of the thoracic nerve roots and recording from the rectus abdominus musculature.
- Given the fact that the origin of innervation of the rectus abdominis is T6-T12, such pedicular assessment is appropriate for these levels.
- If the EMG threshold is less than 6 mA or less than 65% of the mean of all other screws from T6-T12, that screw is removed, the tract repalpated, and the findings evaluated in the context of pedicle palpation and screw position on the radiograph.

Confirmation of Intraosseous Screws[8] (see Fig. 46-4I and J)

- Intraosseous placement is documented by fluoroscopy or radiography or both.
- The coronal plane must reveal harmonious position of all screws. Screws crossing the imaginary midline raise the suspicion of a medial breach and those not crossing the medial

pedicle cortical wall raise the suspicion of a medial wall breach.
- The lateral plane must reveal screws parallel to the superior vertebral end plate and never past the anterior border of the vertebral body.

ROD CONTOURING

- The rods are measured and contoured in the coronal and sagittal planes. The cut end of the rod is oriented vertically so as to serve as a reference point while contouring in the other direction. This is particularly useful given the fact that rods tend to rotate with three-dimensional contouring.
- The rod is secured with two clamps over the wound during contouring to allow visualization.

DEFORMITY CORRECTION[5] (FIG. 46-5)

- For hypokyphotic or normokyphotic curves, the correction is carried out on the concavity. Conversely, the convex side is corrected first when hyperkyphosis is present.
- In addition, the correction is carried out in the concavity when an apical derotation maneuver is not performed.
- While the set screws are loose, or locked at one end, coronal benders are used to reduce the scoliosis by placing the benders on either side of each pedicle screw. This is accomplished with several passes so as to take advantage of the viscoelastic properties of the spine.
- Careful attention must be paid at all times to the bone-screw interface, assessing any signs of screw plowing or loosening, which would indicate purchase failure, loss of correction, and possible neural element compromise.
- The holding rod is placed; posteroanterior and lateral radiographs are obtained.
- While monitoring neurogenic motor and somatosensory evoked potentials to detect slow progressions of neurologic deficits, iliac bone graft is harvested.
- All screws are again evaluated on the films to ensure that no changes have occurred. The tilt of the end vertebrae and overall balance are also assessed.
- Set plugs are sheared, posterior elements are decorticated, and the bone graft is placed.
- Morselized autogenous graft is used for adolescent idiopathic scoliosis patients and allograft for neuromuscular scoliosis patients.
- Cross-links are placed, and the wound is débrided and closed with deep and superficial drains over the lumbodorsal fascia.

BILATERAL APICAL VERTEBRAL DEROTATION MANEUVER[9] (Fig. 46-6)

- The bilateral apical vertebral derotation (BAVD) maneuver is performed if screw placement is adequate, the tho-

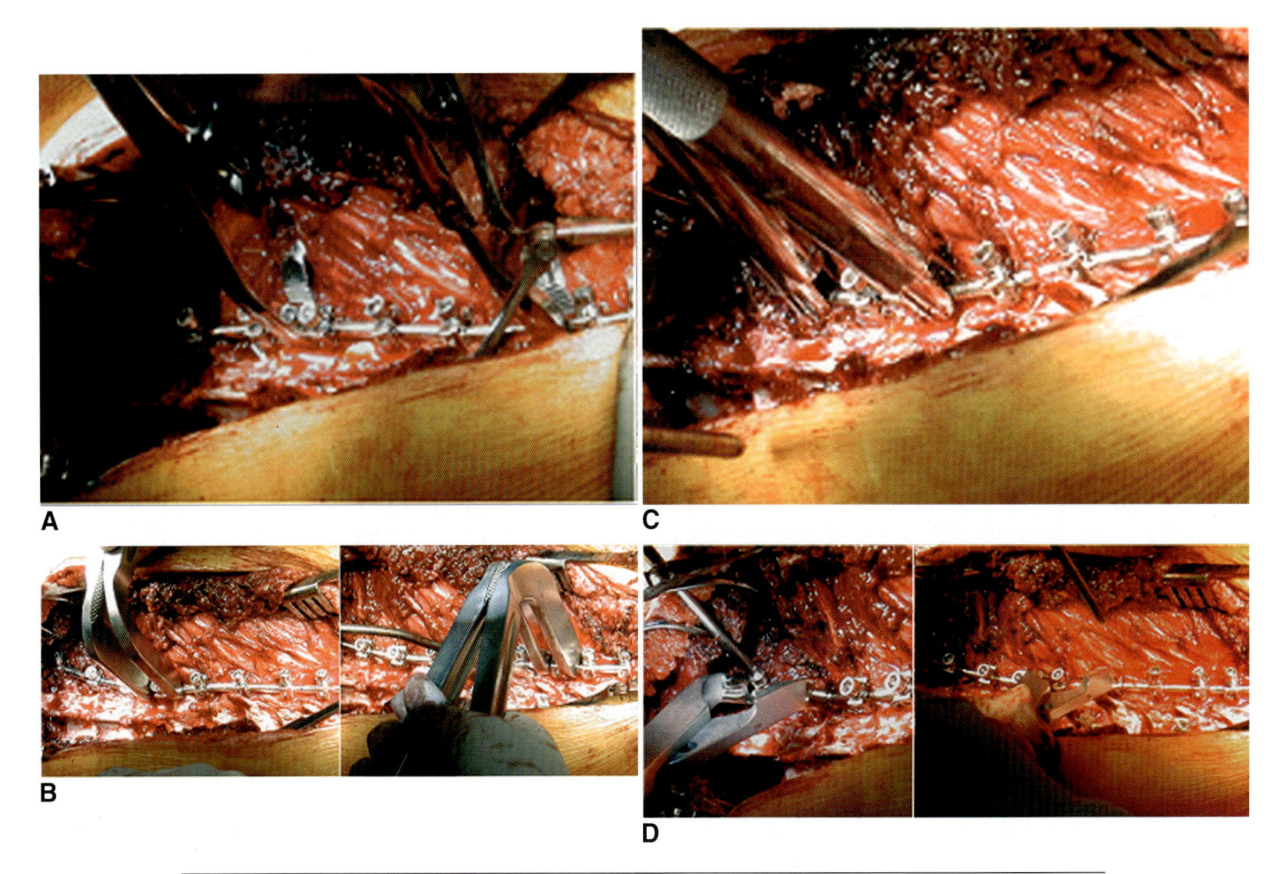

Fig. 46-5 Deformity reduction technique. *A*, Rod derotation. *B*, Translation. *C*, Direct apical vertebral derotation. *D*, Compression and distraction.

Fig. 46-6 Apical vertebral derotation maneuver. *A*, Step 1: Initial pedicle screw insertion and periapical post placement. *B*, Step 2: Periaplica screws derotation and concave rod placement. *C*, Step 3: Concave rod translation by in situ bending technique and loosening of periapical set screws. *D*, Step 4: Second derotation around the concave rod. *E*, Step 5: After fixation of the concave rod, fix the convex rod.

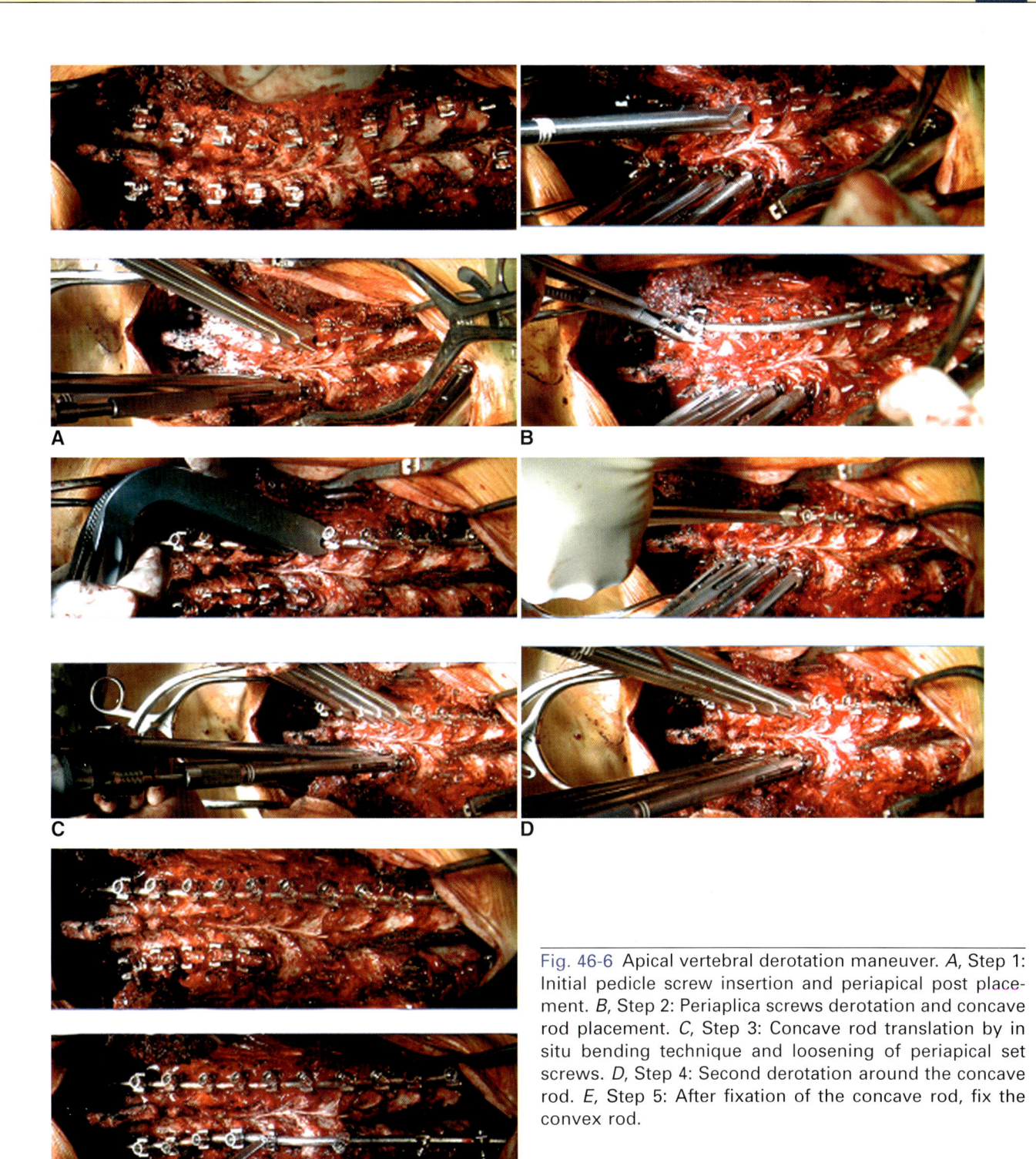

racic spine is not overly kyphotic, and there is thoracic or lumbar prominence.
- When a (+) sagittal modifier according to the Lenke classification is present at high levels of the thoracic spine, BAVD is avoided, as such degree of kyphosis places considerable strain on the proximal screws. In these patients, the coronal and sagittal deformity is addressed by "convex rod" instrumentation first.

- BAVD steps:
  - Four threaded screwdrivers used in the placement of pedicle screws are placed on the convexity so as to enhance correction. Nonthreaded tube attachments are placed on the concavity, allowing for tightening of the set screws through these posts.
  - The first BAVD maneuver is carried out by placing derotation and downward pressure over the apex with the aid

of the convex-side screws. Ventral pressure is simultaneously placed on the convex rib prominence.
- If the concavity is on the side of the correcting rod, the posts on the concavity are removed while maintaining the correction with the posts on the convexity.
- A previously contoured rod is placed, and all set screws are inserted. With the exception of the four apical set screws and an additional level above and below, all set screws are tightened. In situ benders are employed to carry out coronal and sagittal correction.
- A second BAVD maneuver is carried out as previously described by first placing again the concave posts and then tightening the concave set screws through the hollow posts. Further correction can be carried out with the in situ benders as well as appropriate compression/distraction as needed.
- The holding rod is placed. Although no additional correction is performed in this step, appropriate compression/distraction is carried out on this rod to maximize correction.

POSTOPERATIVE MANAGEMENT

- After 1 to 2 days in the pediatric intensive care unit, patients are transferred to the floor.
- Patient-controlled anesthesia is changed to oral narcotics once patients resume their oral intake.
- Patients commonly sit and briefly stand with assistance on the first postoperative day and progressively ambulate. Later, mild trunk range-of-motion exercises are started, based on the patients' comfort.
- The Foley catheter is removed once the patients are ambulatory, and perioperative antibiotics are discontinued once all drains and Foley catheter are removed.
- No bracing is instituted and standing posteroanterior/lateral films are obtained once the patients become ambulatory in the hallways.
- Once discharged from the hospital and if the wound is healing well, showering is allowed.

SURGICAL TREATMENT BASED ON THE LENKE CLASSIFICATION CURVE TYPES

The Lenke classification system (see Figs. 46-1 and 46-2 and Table 46-1) enables the scoliosis surgeon to plan treatment based on the curve types analyzed with this three-tiered system as previously described.[3,4]

LENKE TYPE 1—MAIN THORACIC CURVES (FIG. 46-7)

- MT region, major curve.
- PT and TL/L regions, nonstructural minor curves.
- Lumbar modifier may be A, B, or C; and sagittal modifier may be −, N, or +.
- Surgical treatment involves treating only the MT curves posteriorly, anteriorly, or circumferentially.
- All curves can be treated with posterior instrumentation and fusion if so desired.
- Curves with Cobb measurements between 40 and 70 degrees, especially those that have a minus (−) or a hypokyphotic sagittal modifier may be better treated with endoscopic or open anterior instrumentation and fusion.
- Rarely, extremely large or stiff curves and those with severe sagittal plane malalignment may be treated with open or endoscopic releases followed by posterior instrumentation and fusion. Fusion levels normally are proximal starting at T3-T5, and distally ending at the last vertebra touched in part by the CSVL (when utilizing pedicle screw instrumentation). Anterior instrumentation extends from the upper end vertebra to the lower end vertebra (Cobb levels).
- Posterior instrumentation, concave rods placed for − or N sagittal modifiers, convex rods placed first for + or hyperkyphotic sagittal planes.
- Corrective maneuvers include a combination of: cantilever, compression/distraction, in situ contouring, bilateral apical vertebral derotation (BAVD), and rod rotation maneuvers.
- Posterior implants include hooks, wires, or (more commonly utilized at our institution) screws.
- Anterior instrumentation consists of a dual rod system, vertebral body staples, screws, and cross-links.

LENKE TYPE 2—DOUBLE THORACIC CURVES

- MT region, major curve.
- PT is structural; TL/L is nonstructural.
- Besides the aforementioned structural criteria, a positive T1 tilt, and/or left shoulder elevation (for a right MT curve) also renders the PT curve structural.
- Lumbar modifier A, B, or C and sagittal modifier −, N, or + can apply.
- Surgical treatment involves treating both the PT and MT curves either posteriorly or circumferentially (MT only).
- The instrumentation sequence depends on the sagittal profile of each curve.
- The goals are coronal and sagittal malalignment correction, level shoulders, and the best possible lumbar spine position.

LENKE TYPE 3—DOUBLE MAJOR CURVES (Fig. 46-8)

- MT region major curve.
- TL/L is structural; PT is nonstructural.
- Similar thoracic to lumbar structural characteristics.
- Regardless of structural criteria of the TL/L curves, if thoracolumbar junction kyphosis exists, then consider the curve double major.
- Lumbar modifier A, B, or C and sagittal modifier −, N, or + can apply.

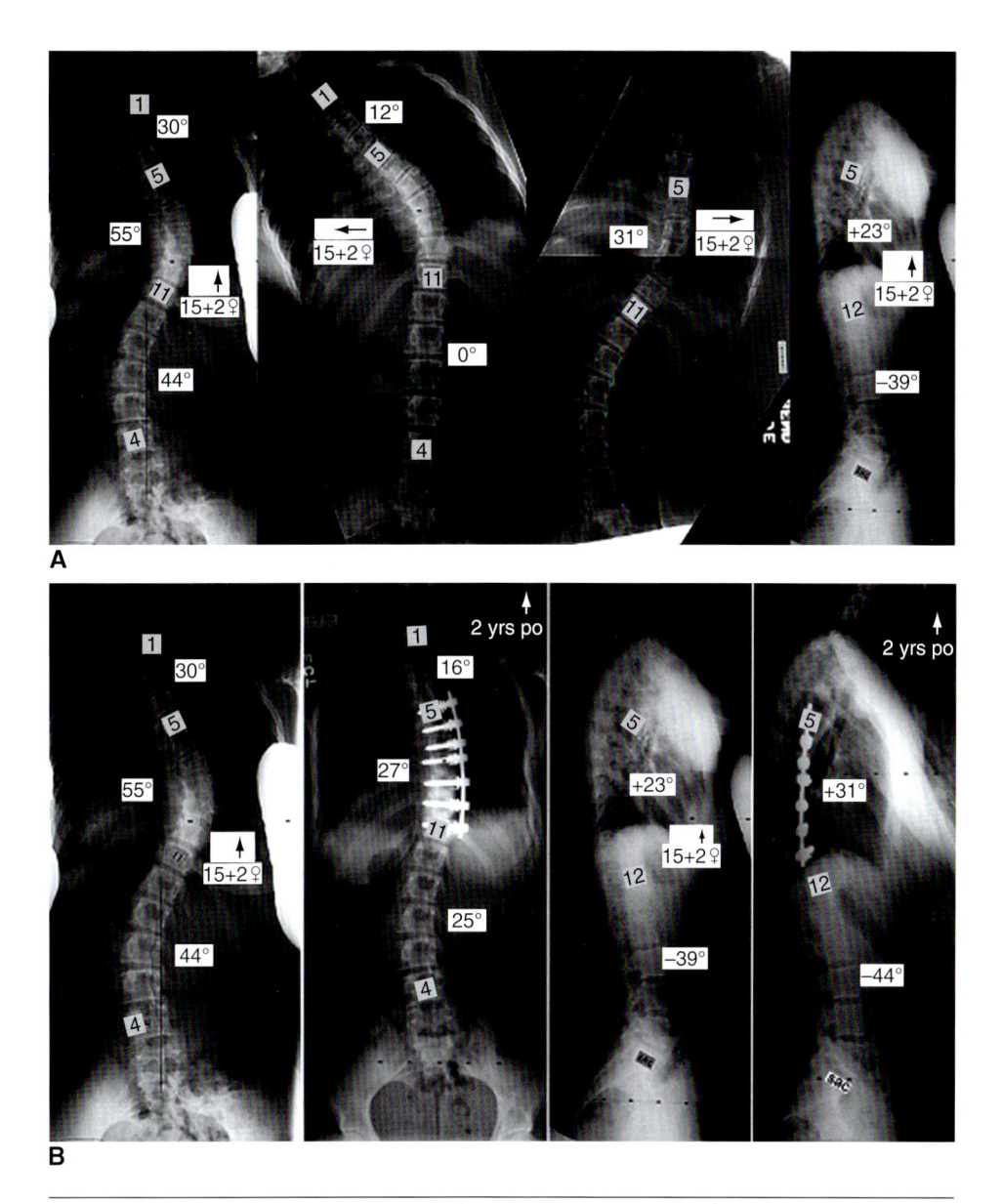

Fig. 46-7 Type 1 BN curve—endoscopic instrumentation and fusion. *A,* Preoperative radiograph of a Lenke 1 BN curve. *B,* Preoperative and 2-year postoperative radiographs.

- Clinically, these reveal the least deformity as both curves offset each other; however, on Adams forward test, thoracic and lumbar prominences are separately noted.
- The thoracic sagittal plane modifier dictates which instrumentation sequence to perform first in the thoracic region.

LENKE TYPE 4–TRIPLE MAJOR CURVES

- MT region is usually major, although TL/L is occasionally larger.
- PT, MT, and TL/L are structural.
- Type 4 curves are rare.
- All curves require posterior fusion and instrumentation.
- Anterior release and fusion of MT or TL/L if curve is greater than 100 degrees, more than 80 degrees residual on side-bending, and hyperkyphosis in the thoracic, thoracolumbar, or lumbar planes. However, with current pedicle screw instrumentation and techniques, this is at times not necessary.

LENKE TYPE 5–THORACOLUMBAR/LUMBAR CURVES[10] (Fig. 46-9)

- TL/L is the major curve: thoracolumbar if the apex is between bodies of T12 and L1; lumbar if the apex is between L1-L2 disk and the L4 body.
- PT and MT are nonstructural.
- Essentially, all these curves have a lumbar type C modifier.
- Surgical treatment involves an anterior or posterior approach to the TL/L region.

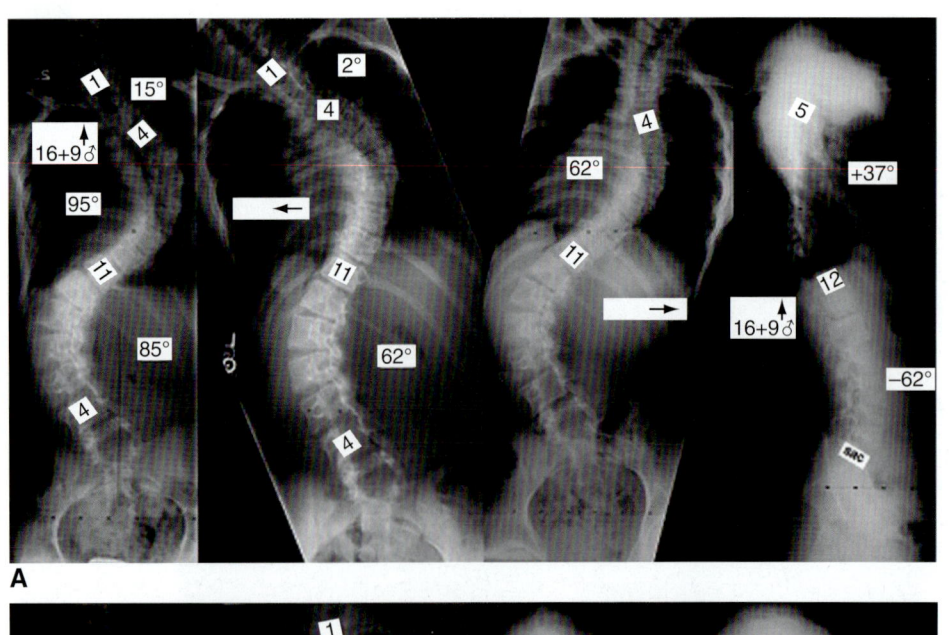

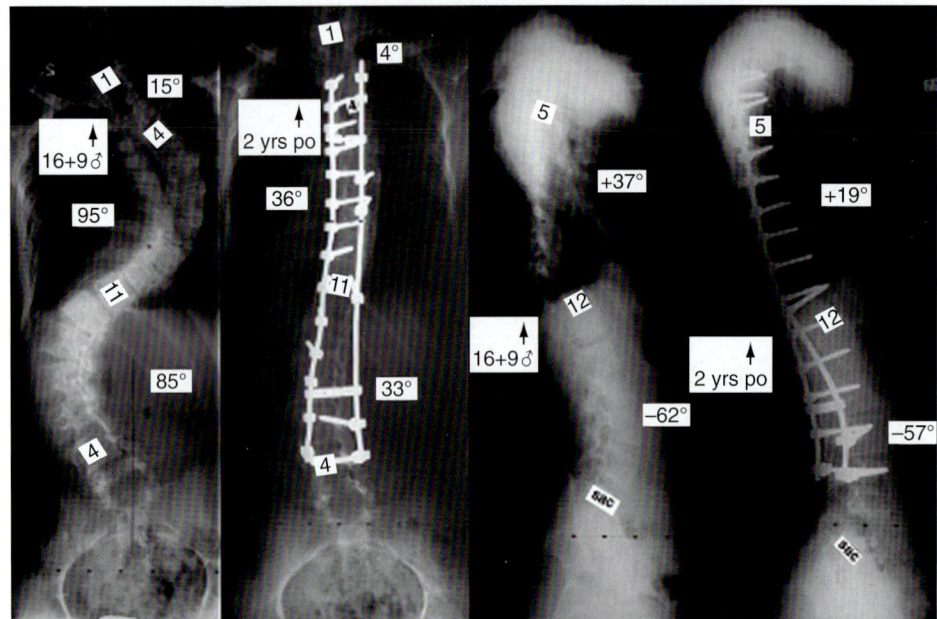

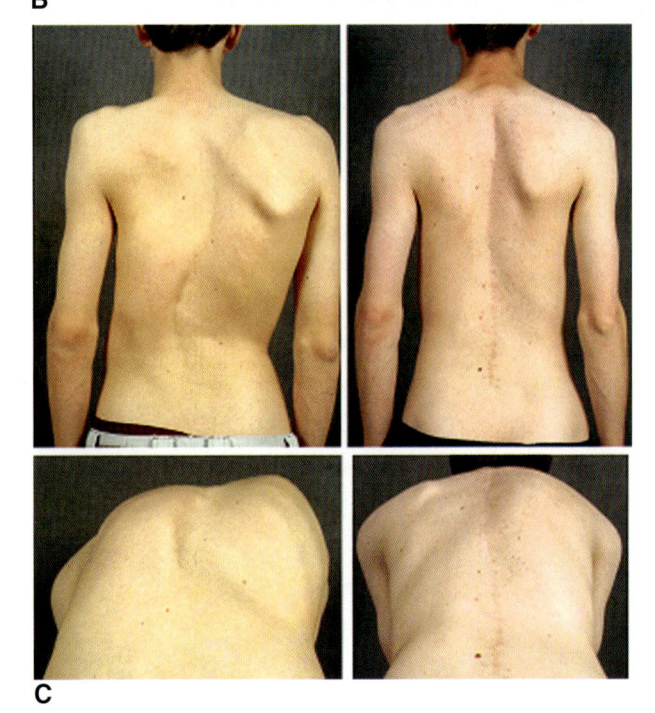

Fig. 46-8 Type 3 CN curve—posterior instrumentation and fusion. *A,* Preoperative radiographs of a Lenke 3 CN curve. *B,* Preoperative and 2-year postoperative radiographs. *C,* Preoperative and postoperative clinical photographs.

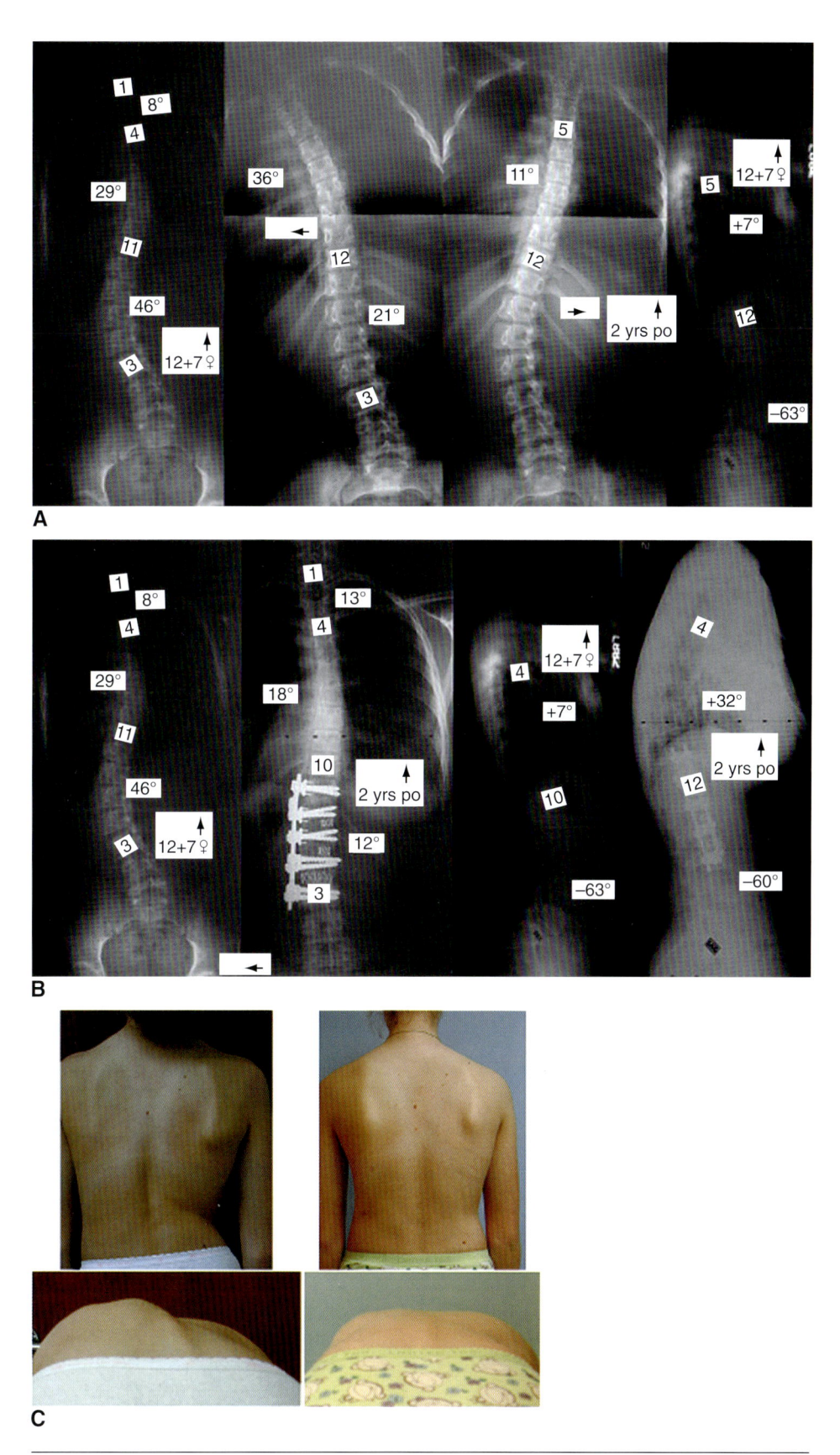

CHAPTER 46   Surgical Treatment of Adolescent Idiopathic Scoliosis   419

Fig. 46-9 Type 5 C curve—anterior instrumentation and fusion. *A,* Preoperative radiographs of a Lenke 5 C curve. *B,* Preoperative and postoperative radiographs. *C,* Preoperative and postoperative clinical photographs.

- With an anterior approach, the fusion and dual rod instrumentation of the TL/L curve covers the measured Cobb angle.
- Cages are placed anteriorly, holding the anterior part of the disk in segmental lordosis. Cantilever, rotation, and compression forces are then applied on the convexity of the curve to complete the coronal correction. At the end of the correction, the end-instrumented vertebra should be derotated and horizontal in the coronal plane, and sagittal alignment achieved.
- Using a posterior approach, the lowest level of instrumentation is usually one more distal than with anterior techniques. However, with current posterior derotation maneuvers, this more distal level can often be spared. Usually, correction is carried out at the convexity of the curve.

LENKE TYPE 6–THORACOLUMBAR/LUMBAR AND MAIN THORACIC CURVES

- TL/L is the major curve and MT is structural.
- PT is nonstructural.
- Surgical management is posterior fusion and instrumentation, similar to type 3 curves.
- Anterior release is sometimes necessary for the TL/L component based on the curve magnitude, kyphosis, rigidity, or risk of crankshaft phenomenon in skeletally immature patients.

COMPLICATIONS

Complications are all fairly rare. They include:
- Acute and delayed neurologic deficits
- Pseudarthrosis
- Early and late implant failure
- Coronal or sagittal imbalance
- Late onset spinal pain
- Infection
- Superior mesentery artery syndrome

CONCLUSIONS

The Lenke classification for adolescent idiopathic scoliosis, and for thoracic and lumbar pedicle instrumentation has significantly improved the management of this patient population. Such classification is a significant improvement of previous classifications as it is comprehensive, emphasizes sagittal plane analysis, objectively assesses curve flexibility for selective fusions, demonstrates good-to-excellent inter- and intraobserver reliability, and clearly recommends a treatment plan. Additionally, pedicle screw instrumentation coupled with bilateral apical derotation maneuvers, as described by Lenke and associates, have revolutionized and significantly improved correction of both scoliotic and kyphotic deformities. Given the power of such techniques, the need to perform anterior releases and fusions, as well as thoracoplasty, is now seldom necessary. Such techniques are not only powerful but also safe as they minimize complications from implant failure or dislodgement noted with other instrumentation techniques. Finally, these current techniques often allow for distal fusion levels to be saved proximal to the stable vertebra.

Note: The authors wish to thank Yongjung Kim, MD, for providing intraoperative photographs for this chapter.

References

1. Lenke LG, Betz RR, Harms J, et al: Adolescent idiopathic scoliosis: A new classification to determine extent of spinal arthrodesis. J Bone Joint Surg Am 2001;83:1169–1181.
2. King HA, Moe JH, Bradford DS, et al: The selection of fusion levels in thoracic idiopathic scoliosis. J Bone Joint Surg Am 1983; 65:1302–1313.
3. Lenke LG: Cotrel-Dubousset spinal instrumentation. In Weinstein, SL (ed): Pediatric Spine Surgery, 2nd ed. Philadelphia, Lippincott Williams & Wilkins, 2001, pp 367–416.
4. Bess RS, Lenke LG: The Lenke classification system of adolescent idiopathic scoliosis. In Heary RF, Albert TJ (eds): Spinal Deformities: The Essentials. New York: Thieme Medical Publishers (in press).
5. Lenke LG, Rinella AS, Kim YJ: Freehand thoracic pedicle screw placement. Semin Spine Surg 2002;14:48–57.
6. Lenke LG, Kim YJ, Rinella AS: Treatment of spinal deformity utilizing thoracic pedicle screws. Semin Spine Surg 2002;14:66–87.
7. Lenke LG: Posterior and posterolateral approaches to the spine. In Bridwell KH, DeWald RL (eds): The Textbook of Spinal Surgery. Philadelphia, Lippincott-Raven, 1997, pp 193–215.
8. Kim YJ, Lenke LG, Cheh G, Riew KD: Evaluation of Pedicle Screw Placement in the Deformed Spine Using Intraoperative Plan Radiographs: A comparison with CT scans. (Paper #78). Scoliosis Research Society 39th Annual Meeting, September 7, 2004.
9. Lenke LG: Posterior Spinal Instrumentation Techniques for Spinal Deformities. Presented at the 7th Annual International Course On Global Spine: Surgical Principles and the Latest Techniques, Dana Point, CA, June, 2003.
10. Bridwell KH: Limits of anterior scoliosis surgery: When is the posterior approach the better option? In Lenke, LG, Betz RR, Harms J (eds): Modern Anterior Scoliosis Surgery. St. Louis, Quality Medical Publishing, 2004, pp 259–269.

CHAPTER 47

TIMOTHY R. KUKLO
BENJAMIN K. POTTER

Surgical Management of Flatback Syndrome

INTRODUCTION

Flatback syndrome, or fixed sagittal imbalance, is a fixed forward inclination of the trunk, which is most commonly recognized following the use of Harrington distraction instrumentation into the lower lumbar spine or sacrum.[1-7] However, it has also been recognized following the use of anterior compression instrumentation without structural interbody support,[8] secondary to pseudarthrosis after posterior spinal fusion (PSF),[3] with adjacent segment decompensation above or below a fusion mass,[9-11] secondary to post-traumatic kyphosis,[12] and after iatrogenic loss of lumbar lordosis caused by the placement of other rigid instrumentation that failed to restore normal lordosis.[13,14]

The clinical presentation is often quite similar, as patients present with symptomatic loss of lumbar lordosis, forward inclination of the trunk, inability to stand erect with the knees extended, and pain (Fig. 47-1). A history of multiple previous operations is often noted. Patients commonly attempt to compensate for the fixed sagittal imbalance by flexing the knees and hips, and hyperextending the cervical spine and other remaining mobile segments in the thoracic and lumbar spine. Pain frequently ensues secondary to muscle fatigue.[9,15] Radiographic evaluation requires standing anteroposterior (AP) or posteroanterior (PA) and lateral full-length radiographs with the knees extended. Occasionally, a supine hyperextension lateral radiograph or a push-prone radiograph will help determine the rigidity of the deformity. Sagittal balance is determined by dropping a plumb line from the center of C7 to determine its relative position in reference to the posterior-superior corner of S1 on the lateral radiograph (Fig. 47-2). Positive sagittal balance, or imbalance, is considered to be present when the plumb line falls at least 2 to 3 cm anterior to S1.[16] When standing radiographs are taken, the patient's arms should be positioned in 30 to 45 degrees of forward flexion to reduce an inaccurate posterior shift of the sagittal vertical axis (SVA).[17]

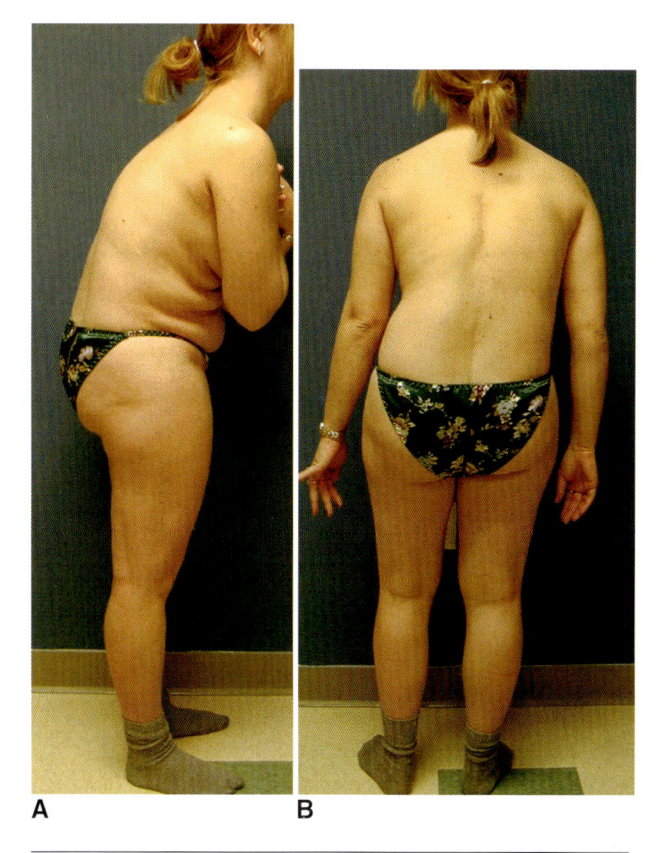

Fig. 47-1 *A*, Lateral clinical photograph of patient with flatback syndrome. Note the loss of lumbar lordosis and forward inclination of the trunk. *B*, Posterior clinical photograph of patient with flatback syndrome. Again flattening of the lumbar region with evidence of residual kyphoscoliosis are appreciated. The patient's surgical scar is also seen in this view from her previous posterior spinal fusion with Harrington distraction instrumentation.

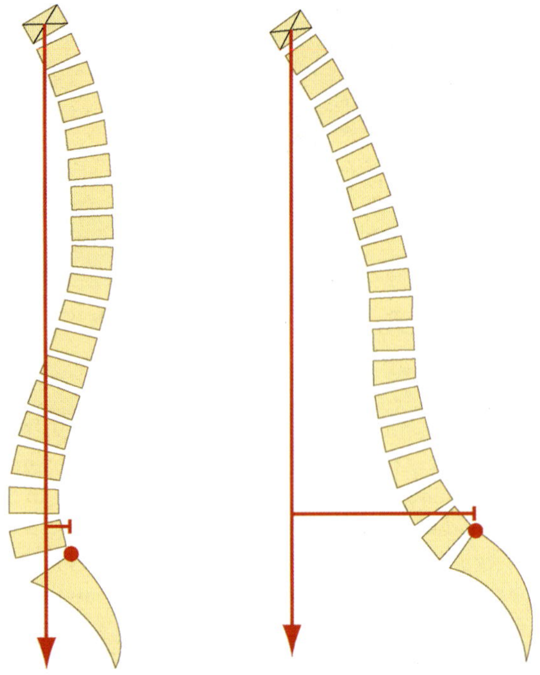

Fig. 47-2 Diagram of the sagittal vertical axis (SVA), assessed by measuring the distance from a C7 plumb line to the posterior-superior corner of the sacral end plate. The left specimen is within normal limits of approximately 3 cm of the sacral end plate. The specimen shown at right has lost lumbar lordosis, resulting in fixed sagittal imbalance reflected by the grossly positive SVA.

Various techniques have been identified for the surgical management of flatback syndrome. These techniques include Smith-Petersen,[3,9,10,12,18–20] various pedicle subtraction, transpedicular or three-column osteotomies (including the eggshell procedure),[11–14,21–26] vertebral column resection,[27–29] and multiple level anterior interbody fusions with posterior spinal compression instrumentation.[12,30] This chapter will review the two primary procedures most commonly performed for flatback syndrome, specifically the Smith-Petersen osteotomy (SPO) and the pedicle subtraction osteotomy (PSO). Regardless of the osteotomy, the general rule of thumb is to perform the osteotomy at the deformity apex, or most kyphotic segments, if possible.

The SPO is a posterior column shortening procedure, which hinges on the middle column and lengthens the anterior column. Correction of approximately 5 degrees, but up to 15 degrees, can often be achieved with each osteotomy, and therefore, multiple SPOs are frequently performed. As a rule of thumb, this is about 1 degree of correction per millimeter of resected posterior bone in the thoracic and lumbar spine.[3,9,10,12] However, one prerequisite is that the anterior longitudinal ligament cannot be contracted or ossified, and the disk height should be at least 5 mm, or significant correction cannot be achieved. Additionally, various authors recommend releasing or grafting the anterior column with this procedure.[10,13,20,31–33]

In contrast, the PSO is a posterior and middle column shortening procedure, which hinges on the anterior column. Correction of up to 30 to 35 degrees can be expected with each PSO.[9,11,14] It is most commonly, and safely, performed in the lumbar spine at L2 or L3, but can be performed in the thoracic spine as well. More proximal PSO may increase the risk of conus medularis or spinal cord injury, while more a caudal PSO limits the number of fixation points available distal to the osteotomy.[9]

SMITH-PETERSEN OSTEOTOMY

INDICATIONS AND CONTRAINDICATIONS
Indications

- Fixed sagittal or coronal imbalance/flatback syndrome
- Posttraumatic kyphosis
- Scheuermann's kyphosis
- Congenital scoliosis

Relative Contraindications

- Foraminal stenosis
- Coronal or rotational deformity where symmetric osteotomies may further decompensate the spine (this would require asymmetric osteotomies)
- Calcification of the great vessels
- Anterior instrumentation across the planned SPO site
- Severe, localized kyphosis greater than can be corrected with SPO
- Posterior wound infection or active bacterial infection elsewhere
- Medical and nutritional status not optimized preoperatively

OPERATIVE TECHNIQUE
Equipment

- X-ray-compatible operating table and frame permitting patient positioning with hips in extension (Some surgeons prefer jackknifing the table for severely kyphotic deformities for resection, with flattening of the table for correction and instrumentation.) (Fig. 47-3)
- Fluoroscopy or portable radiographs
- Headlight system
- Lumbar retractor system
- Bovie electrocautery (unipolar and bipolar)
- Cobb elevators
- Pituitary, Stille-Horsley, Leksell, and Kerrison rongeurs
- Spinal decompression instruments (surgeon dependent)
- Straight and curved osteotomes
- Segmental instrumentation system; pedicle screw-rod instrumentation (preferred) with possible iliac fixation when fusing to the sacrum

CHAPTER 47 Surgical Management of Flatback Syndrome

- Supplemental bone graft source (autologous bone graft preferred, but can complicate instrumenting to the pelvis/iliac wings when iliac fixation is planned)
- Neuromonitoring (authors' preference for somatosensory and motor evoked potential monitoring, as well as pedicle screw stimulation)
- Cell saver

Patient Positioning and Preparation

- The patient is positioned in the prone position with axillary rolls, prominences and extremities appropriately padded, or on an open Jackson table with two pads on the chest and four pads on the thighs to permit maximum lordosis with gravity. Additional padding or pillows may be placed under the extended thighs just prior to closing the osteotomies to assist with closure (Fig. 47-4).
- Trial positioning in the operating room may be required before the day of surgery.
- If the severity of the fixed sagittal imbalance prevents hip extension during preoperative positioning, alternate positioning supplementation may be required.
- Hip extension on the table is mandatory to assess restoration of sagittal balance and lumbar lordosis. Additionally, gradual extension of the table may assist in "reducing" or closing the osteotomy site in controlled fashion. For this reason, positioning the patient's hips and pelvis to be centered over a break in the table is often recommended, or extending the hips intraoperatively with pads and pillows.

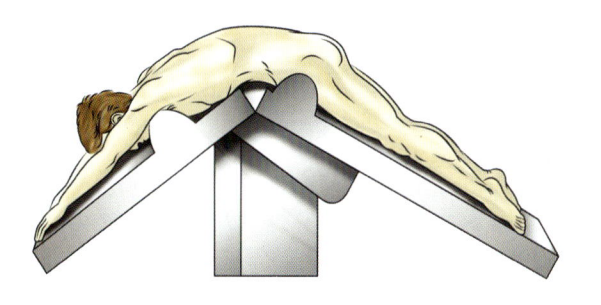

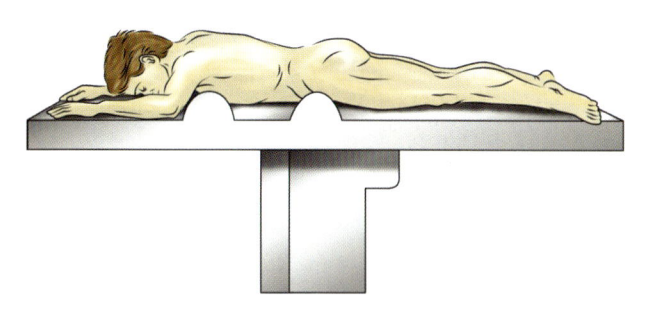

Fig. 47-3 Schematic of an operating room table jack-knifed to facilitate surgical positioning for the procedure (A) and then extended for deformity correction and final instrumentation following corrective osteotomy (B).

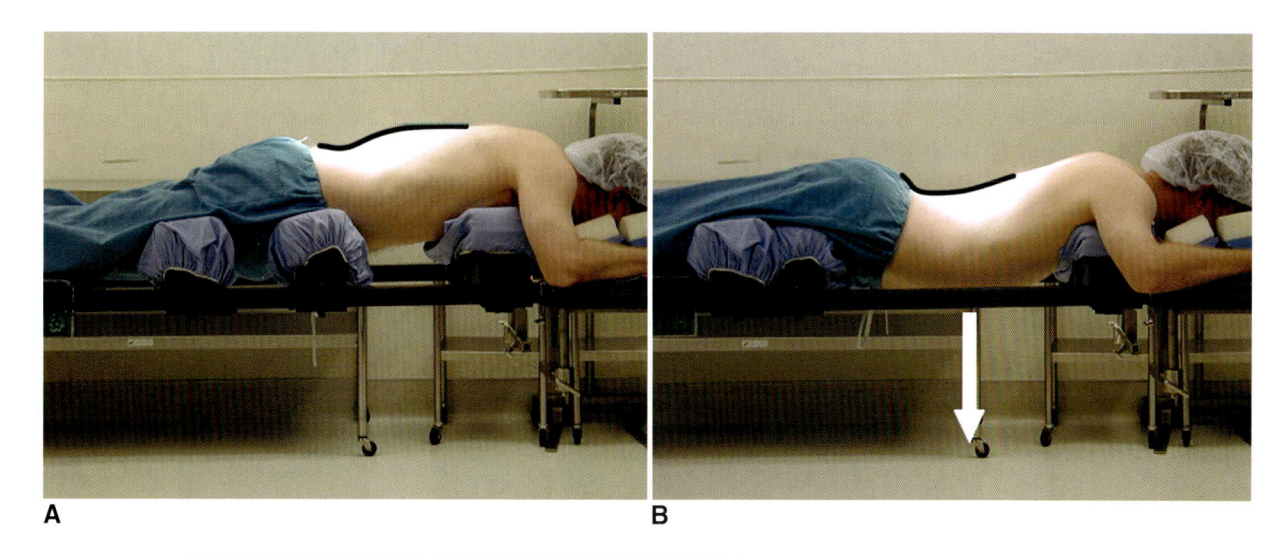

Fig. 47-4 Photographs of volunteer "patient" in the operating suite on a Wilson frame (OSI, Union City, CA). Note the flattened lumbar region of the patient in the preoperative position (A), followed by the restoration of lumbar lordosis following surgical correction and removal of the central sacropelvic support pillow for a gravity-assisted osteotomy closure (B).

- General endotracheal anesthesia should be utilized for maximal airway control.
- The incision is marked and the skin prepared in standard sterile fashion.
- Standard draping is utilized. It is recommended to prep and drape the entire posterior trunk and pelvis from the shoulders to the buttocks crease. This will permit adequate exposure for the planned instrumentation, as well as for possible iliac crest bone graft site harvesting, and an appreciation of any sagittal and coronal balance before and after correction.
- If fluoroscopy is utilized, the C-arm is draped and sits above the operating field toward the patient's head when not in use. A Mayo stand cover is frequently used to drape the boom in the lateral position.

Dissection/Approach/Anatomic Landmarks

- The rostral and caudal extent of the dissection varies greatly based on the levels of the hypolordotic or kyphotic pathology, previous instrumentation or pseudarthrosis, and overall sagittal and coronal balance.
- Local anesthetic may be injected at the incision site.
- A straight, midline posterior approach to the thoracolumbar or lumbar spine is used.
- Fluoroscopy may be useful to confirm levels prior to making the incision.
- At least two levels above and below the planned osteotomy(ies) should be exposed for instrumentation. Greater exposure may be required based on the status and compatibility of the previous instrumentation.
- A longitudinal incision is then made, extending to the depth of the supraspinous ligament and spinous processes with blunt dissection and electrocautery.
- Bilateral subperiosteal dissection with a Cobb elevator is utilized to reflect the erector spinae and the short rotators along the posterior elements out to the lamina, facet joints, and laterally to the tips of the transverse processes. Care should be taken to avoid injury to the facet capsules until radiographic confirmation of fusion levels. Electrocautery should be used liberally to maintain adequate hemostasis and visualization.

Instrumentation and Operative Technique

- Following exposure of the posterior elements, the supraspinous and interspinous ligaments are removed.
- The "overhang" of the spinous processes above and below the planned osteotomies are resected by means of a Stille-Horsley rongeur, morselized and saved for later use as local bone graft.
- The superior articular facet is then removed with a $1/4$- or $1/2$-inch osteotome, and a curette is used to remove the articular cartilage.
- Segmental pedicle screw instrumentation is then placed at all levels of the planned instrumentation. The authors prefer the freehand technique for both lumbar and thoracic pedicle screws. Pedicle start points vary by level, but are easily identified anatomically (Fig. 47-5). After placement of all pedicle screws, pedicle screw stimulation is performed, and anteroposterior (AP) and lateral radiographs or fluoroscopic images are obtained to verify proper pedicle screw positioning.
- Segmental instrumentation is generally recommended at least two levels above and below each osteotomy in order to ensure adequate construct rigidity and stability.
- The ligamentum flavum is then removed from the midline to expose the epidural fat.
- A 45-degree Kerrison rongeur is used to resect the remaining ligamentum flavum laterally to the facet joints. In addition, the inferior margin of the lamina of the superior vertebra and the superior lamina of the inferior vertebra are also resected. This is completed laterally to the inferior articular process. This appears as a V in the coronal plane (Fig. 47-6).
- Following resection of the lamina, the foramina are inspected visually and manually with a curved probe to ensure adequate space for the nerve roots following osteotomy closure (Fig. 47-7). Undercutting of the adjacent lamina and remaining facet joints may be required to ensure adequate space for the nerve roots and dura.
- The dura is closely inspected for inadvertent injury; a sustained Valsalva maneuver with the assistance of the anesthesia provider is useful in this regard.
- Epidural hemostasis is achieved by means of powdered thrombin or thrombin-soaked Gelfoam if needed; however, bleeding is usually well controlled.
- After completion of all planned osteotomies, rods are contoured and placed, and the site is then closed gradually utilizing cantilever forces (Fig. 47-8). Hip extension may also be helpful. After all instrumentation is placed, compression across the osteotomy site(s) is performed.
- Sudden, intraoperative cardiovascular decompensation should alert the surgeon to a possible traction injury to the great vessels, and emergent vascular surgery consultation with arteriography or exploration may be warranted.
- Adequate correction of sagittal imbalance is ensured through visual inspection, fluoroscopy, or lateral radiographs.
- Bone wax is discouraged to avoid inhibition of the fusion mass.
- Bone graft, bone graft substitute, and biomedical bone graft augmentation (bone morphogenic protein, concentrated platelets) are applied medially over the closed osteotomy site and lateral to the instrumentation.
- Closed suction drains are placed (controversial if biomedical supplementation is used), and the wound is closed in sequential layers.

CHAPTER 47 Surgical Management of Flatback Syndrome

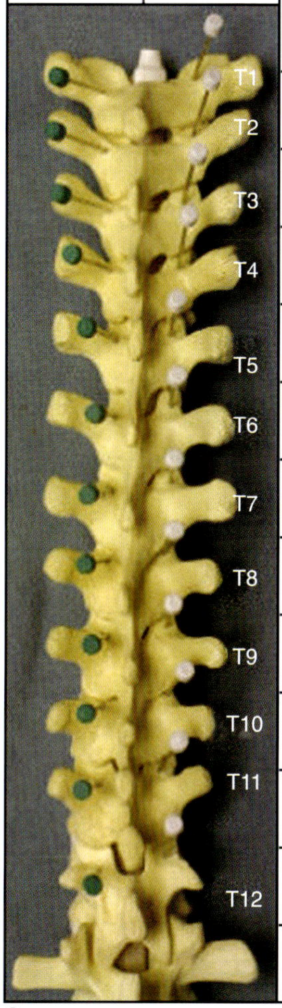

		Thoracic pedicle screw starting points—anatomic trajectory	
Straight-forward	Anatomic		
Green	White		
		Level	Cephalocaudal starting point	Medial-lateral starting point
		T1	Inferior 1/3 facet	Midpoint facet
		T2	Inferior 1/3 facet	Midpoint facet
		T3	Inferior 1/3 facet	Midpoint facet
		T4	Inferior 1/3 facet	Midpoint facet
		T5	Midpoint facet	Midpoint facet
		T6	Midpoint facet	Midpoint facet
		T7	Midpoint facet	Midpoint facet
		T8	Midpoint facet	Midpoint facet
		T9	Midpoint facet	Midpoint facet
		T10	Midpoint facet	Midpoint facet
		T11	Midpoint facet	Midpoint facet
		T12	Midpoint facet	Midpoint facet

A

Fig. 47-5 Posterior (*A*) and lateral (*B*) views of the thoracic spine with guide pins placed at the appropriate pedicle screw start points at each level for both the straight-forward and the anatomic trajectories.

- Sterile dressings are applied and the patient is rolled to the gurney, extubated, and transferred to the postanesthesia care unit.

Complications
- Nerve root injury/paraparesis
- Dural tear
- Great vessel injury or rupture
- Instrumentation failure, inadequate correction or loss of correction
- Pseudarthrosis
- Postoperative infection
- Exacerbation of preoperative coronal imbalance
- Deep venous thrombosis, pulmonary embolus, and death

PEDICLE SUBTRACTION OSTEOTOMY

INDICATIONS AND CONTRINDICATIONS
Indications
- Coronal or sagittal imbalance (any etiology)
- Ankylosing spondylitis
- Posttraumatic kyphosis

Relative Contraindications
- Anterior pseudarthrosis
- Posterior wound infection or active bacterial infection elsewhere

Straight-forward	Anatomic	Thoracic pedicle screw starting points—anatomic trajectory	
Green	White		
		Level	Cephalocaudal starting point	Medial-lateral starting point
		T1	Inferior 1/3 facet	Midpoint facet
		T2	Inferior 1/3 facet	Midpoint facet
		T3	Inferior 1/3 facet	Midpoint facet
		T4	Inferior 1/3 facet	Midpoint facet
		T5	Midpoint facet	Midpoint facet
		T6	Midpoint facet	Midpoint facet
		T7	Midpoint facet	Midpoint facet
		T8	Midpoint facet	Midpoint facet
		T9	Midpoint facet	Midpoint facet
		T10	Midpoint facet	Midpoint facet
		T11	Midpoint facet	Midpoint facet
		T12	Midpoint facet	Midpoint facet

B

Fig. 47-5, cont'd. For legend see p. 425.

- Medical and nutritional status not optimized preoperatively
- Anterior instrumentation across planned site (absolute contraindication)

Equipment

The equipment is the same as that used for the Smith-Petersen osteotomy, discussed earlier.

Patient Positioning and Preparation

- Patient positioning and preparation are the same as for the Smith-Petersen osteotomy. However, more attention is given to flexing the operative table in the jackknife position and to extending the hips with pads or pillows prior to osteotomy closure.

- Ankylosing spondylitis patients should be evaluated preoperatively by the anesthesia provider to ensure that adequate cervical positioning is possible; otherwise, fiberoptic, nasotracheal, or awake intubation may be required.

Dissection/Approach/Anatomic Landmarks

- Dissection varies greatly based on the levels of the hypolordotic or kyphotic pathology, previous instrumentation, and pseudarthrosis.
- Local anesthetic may be injected at the incision site.
- Straight, midline posterior approach to the thoracolumbar or lumbar spine is recommended. If the patient has had a previous paracentral, muscle-splitting approach, use of the same surgical incision is desirable when practicable.

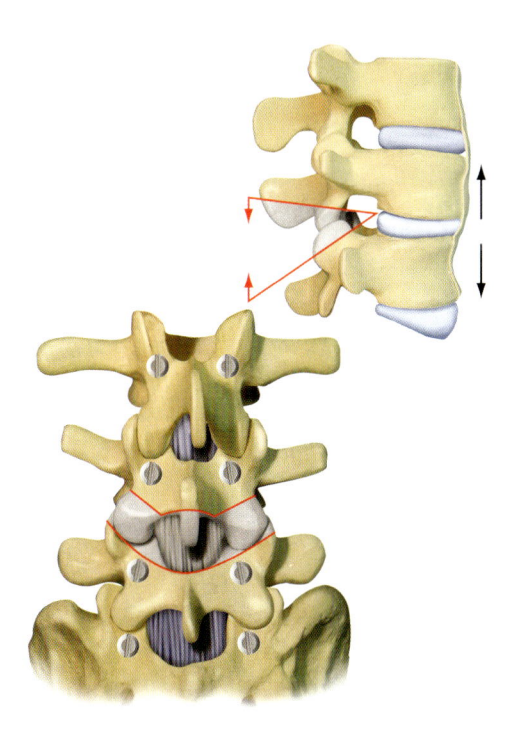

CHAPTER 47 Surgical Management of Flatback Syndrome

Fig. 47-6 Posterior and lateral schematics of the lumbar spine with the area of the lower lumbar segments exposed; the area of bone resection for the Smith-Petersen osteotomy is shaded in both images.

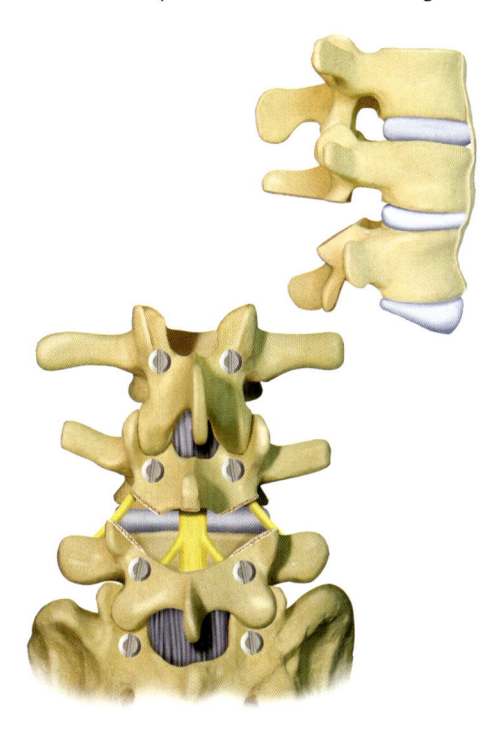

Fig. 47-7 Posterior diagram of Smith-Petersen osteotomy following resection of the articular facets and portions of the adjacent laminae. It is critical at this point to assess the anticipated space available for the neural elements in both the central canal and the foramen prior to osteotomy closure.

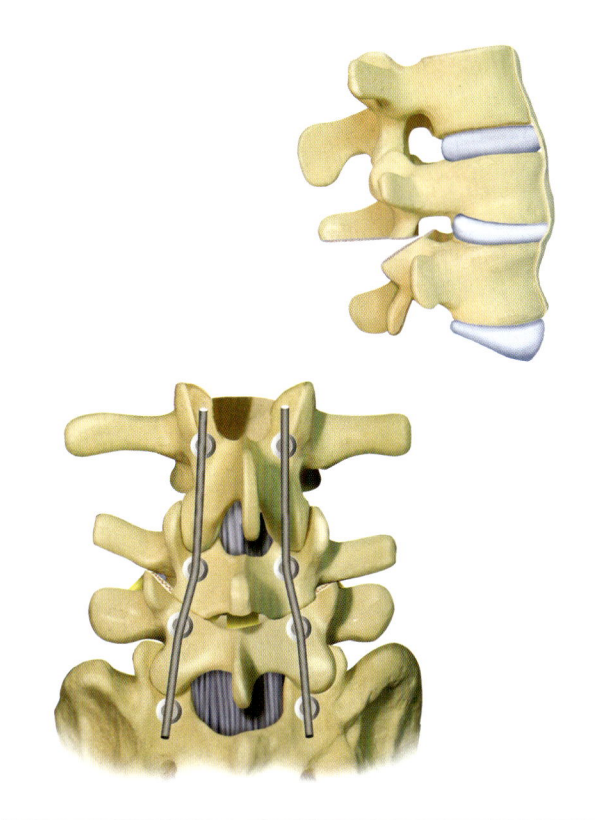

Fig. 47-8 Posterior and lateral schematics of a Smith-Petersen osteotomy following closure of the osteotomy and final instrumentation. In general, 1 degree of correction per millimeter of bone resection can be expected; however, as can be appreciated on the lateral schematic, disk stiffness and the limitations of anterior osteoclasis tend to be the limiting factors with regard to the quantity of correction achieved at each level.

- Fluoroscopy may be useful to confirm levels prior to making the incision.
- At least two levels above and below the planned osteotomy(ies) should be exposed; however, in older patients, six fixation points above and below the osteotomy site are often preferred. Greater exposure may be required based on the status and compatibility of the previous instrumentation. If previous anterior instrumentation is present at the osteotomy site, this should be removed prior to this step. If a fusion is present without instrumentation, a fusion mass osteotomy may be performed in essentially the same manner as described here.
- A longitudinal incision is then made, extending to the depth of the supraspinous ligament and spinous processes with blunt dissection and electrocautery.
- Subperiosteal dissection with a Cobb elevator is then utilized to reflect the erector spinae and the short rotators down along the posterior elements, and laterally to the lamina, facet joints, and tips of the transverse processes. Facet joint capsules should not be resected until proper levels are confirmed. Electrocautery should be used liberally to maintain adequate hemostasis and visualization.

Instrumentation and Operative Technique

- Following exposure of the posterior elements, the supraspinous and interspinous ligaments are removed, and the spinous processes above and below the planned osteotomy are resected.
- All bone removed during the procedure is stripped of soft tissue, morselized, and saved for later use as local bone graft.
- Segmental pedicle screw instrumentation is then placed and confirmed with biplanar fluoroscopy or intraoperative radiographs (Fig. 47-9). Pedicle screw stimulation is also preferred at our institution (see SPO discussion).
- The extent of the osteotomy is then confirmed on the posterior lamina, remembering that approximately 1 mm of resected bone posteriorly will result in 1 degree of correction. The lamina is then resected manually, or alternatively thinned with an air drill, then resected. The ligamentum flavum is encountered and removed to the lateral facets.
- The facet joints are removed bilaterally at the planned level of the osteotomy using rongeurs or osteotomes.
- The pedicles are circumferentially isolated and the lateral pedicles removed with rongeurs, followed by removal of the transverse processes (Fig. 47-10). If the transverse processes are detached, they do not necessarily need to be completely removed. Care should be taken to avoid the segmental arteries.

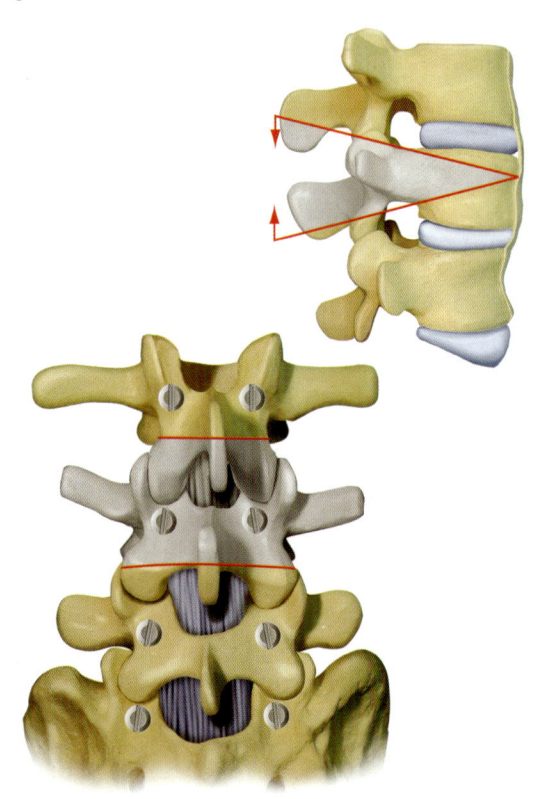

Fig. 47-9 Posterior and lateral schematics of the lumbar spine with the posterior elements exposed; the area of bone resection for a pedicle subtraction osteotomy is shaded in both images.

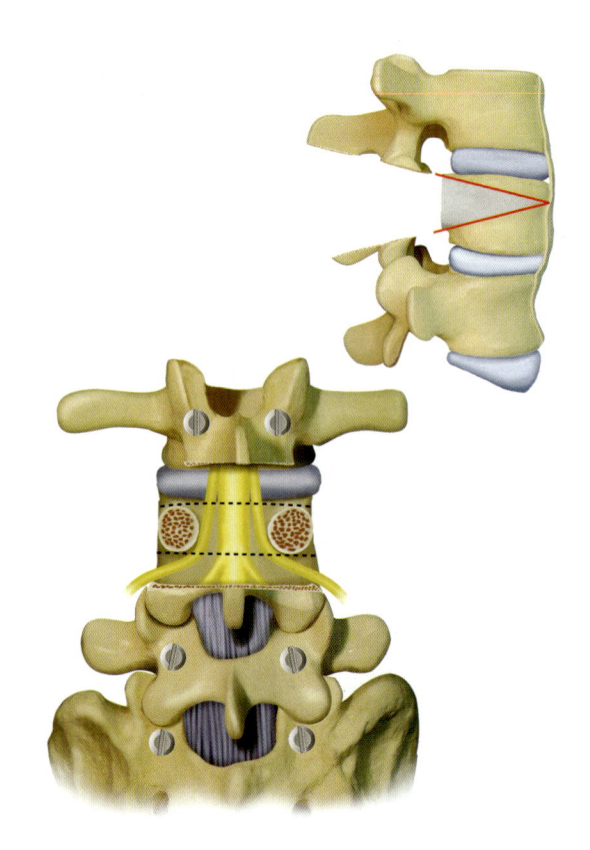

Fig. 47-10 Posterior schematic of a pedicle subtraction osteotomy following removal of the lamina and facet joints. In general, the medial wall of the pedicles is left intact until near the end of the procedure to protect the neural elements. The area of vertebral body decancellation and ultimately vertebral wall resection is demonstrated by the dotted line.

- The dura is gently retracted and any clearly visualized veins are cauterized with bipolar electrocautery. If there are no obvious veins and instead the epidurals are a diffuse coalescence, then packing with powdered thrombin or thrombin-soaked Gelfoam and cottonoids is preferred.
- The cancellous pedicle bases are then curetted into the main vertebral body, preserving the medial pedicle wall at this juncture to protect the neural elements and dura.
- Utilizing progressively larger and angled curettes, a hollow cavity is created within the vertebral body behind the posterior body wall, again saving all bone for further use as bone graft.
- This is continued until the anterior body wall is reached and the left and right cavities communicate easily. A Woodson No. 3 is an effective instrument for feeling across the undersurface of the spinal canal. Attention to maintaining a V in the sagittal plane is critical for proper correction and closure of the osteotomy site.
- The medial pedicle walls are then removed with a Leksell, using caution while retracting the dura and the exiting nerve root.

- The posterior vertebral body wall should be a thin, cortical shell, which is then resected gradually with various rongeurs. Adequate posterior wall resection is critical so that this will not limit the correction achievable. This resection may alternatively be completed last, or imploded into the vertebral body with a down-pushing curette.
- Using care to protect the foraminal segmental vessels, the lateral vertebral body wall is then slowly resected. Be sure that the resection is symmetric (or appropriately asymmetric if desired for simultaneous coronal plane correction) prior to completing the osteotomy.
- The osteotomy may start to close spontaneously if provisional fixation with rods is not used; however, epidural hemostasis, the absence of dural injury, and sufficient space in the newly created combined foramina for both exiting nerve roots bilaterally must be ensured prior to osteotomy closure and compression.
- The dura is closely inspected for inadvertent injury; a Valsalva maneuver with the assistance of the anesthesia provider is useful in this regard.
- Epidural hemostasis is achieved by means of thrombin-soaked Gelfoam.
- Inspect the exiting nerve roots for adequate space; rarely, undercutting of the pedicle above may also be required for adequate decompression. Occasionally, additional undercutting of the inferior margin of the superior lamina and the superior margin of the inferior margin is needed to prevent dural buckling.
- The osteotomy site is then closed gradually with contoured rods utilizing compression of the instrumentation or extension of the patient's hips and lumbar spine on the operating table (Fig. 47-11). Two large spanning compressors are useful to control for symmetric closure.
- Adequate correction of sagittal imbalance is ensured through visual inspection, fluoroscopy, or lateral radiographs.
- Bone wax is discouraged to avoid inhibition of the fusion mass.
- Bone graft, bone graft substitute, or biomedical bone graft augmentation is applied medially over the closed osteotomy site and lateral to the instrumentation.
- Closed suction drains are placed (controversial if biomedical supplementation is used), and the wound is closed in sequential layers.
- During closure, an on-table Stagnara wake-up test is advisable.
- Sterile dressing is applied and the patient is rolled to the gurney and extubated prior to transfer to the postanesthesia care unit.

Complications

- Nerve root injury/paraparesis
- Dural tear

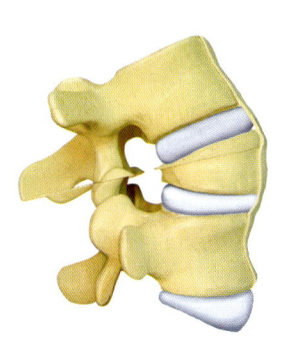

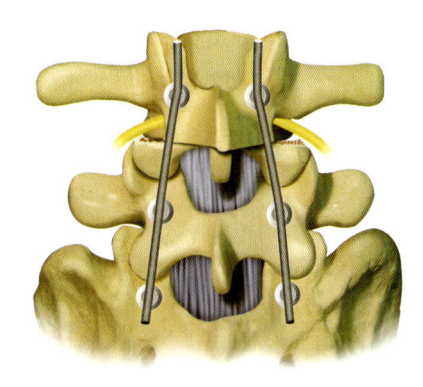

Fig. 47-11 Posterior and lateral schematics of a pedicle subtraction osteotomy following closure of the osteotomy site and final instrumentation. Note the large amount of cancellous bone contact after osteotomy closure, which offers excellent healing potential. Asymmetric lateral vertebral wall resection and body decancellation can be used for the simultaneous correction of coronal plane deformities.

- Significant blood loss with disseminated intravascular coagulation or other coagulopathies; compounded by heavy cancellous bone bleeding
- Great vessel injury or rupture (reported more commonly with SPO)
- Instrumentation failure, inadequate correction, or loss of correction
- Pseudarthrosis
- Postoperative infection
- Deep venous thrombosis, pulmonary embolus, and death

Postoperative Care and Rehabilitation

- Postoperative orders are written for frequent neurologic examinations.
- Early ambulation is encouraged, beginning on postoperative day 1 and twice daily thereafter under physical therapist supervision. Aggressive pulmonary toilette is mandatory.
- Based on patient status, bone quality, and construct rigidity, thoracolumbar or thoracolumbosacral bracing

may be utilized to encourage fusion mass development and to prevent catastrophic construct failure. There is little evidence to support this, however; we frequently recommend a postoperative thoracolumbar spinal orthosis to discourage forward bending in the early postoperative period (12 weeks). This helps "protect" the instrumentation from significant pullout forces, especially at the distal instrumentation, present with forward bending.

- Postoperative pain control includes patient-controlled analgesia for the early postoperative period, usually transitioning to long-acting narcotics with supplementation as needed thereafter, based on patient tolerance and dietary status.
- Short-term muscle relaxant augmentation of the pain regimen (diazepam) may be helpful.
- Nonsteroidal anti-inflammatory drugs may inhibit fusion mass development and should be avoided. If they are required as part of a complex, multiagent pain control regimen, then newer generation, cyclooxygenase-2 selective inhibitors are recommended.
- Diet can be advanced as tolerated, generally beginning with clears on the first postoperative day and advancing based on patient tolerance, and the passage of bowel gas and stool.
- Prolonged ileus (common) or superior mesenteric artery syndrome (rare) can occur postoperatively, particularly following significant sagittal correction at multiple levels with the anterior column-lengthening SPO. Both generally resolve with bowel rest and hyperalimentation or tube feeds beyond the site of obstruction. However, if the latter is suspected, appropriate upper gastrointestinal series and general surgical consultation are warranted.
- Dressings are changed daily beginning on postoperative day 2 and continue until the wound is completely dry.
- Surgical drains are removed at the bedside on or about postoperative day 2 or when the output falls below 100 mL for a 24-hour period or 30 mL over an 8-hour shift.
- Standing, full-length/long cassette anteroposterior and lateral radiographs are obtained prior to discharge to assess hardware placement and sagittal and coronal alignment.
- The patient is discharged on or about postoperative day 5 if there were no complications and the patient is afebrile, tolerating adequate oral intake and pain medications, and can safely ambulate with or without assistive devices.

References

1. Aaro S, Ohlen G: The effect of Harrington instrumentation on sagittal configuration and mobility of the spine in scoliosis. Spine 1983;8:570–575.
2. Casey MP, Archer MA, Jacobs RR, et al: The effects of Harrington rod contouring on lumbar lordosis. Spine 1987;12:750–753.
3. LaGrone MO, Bradford DS, Moe JH, et al: Treatment of symptomatic flatback after spinal fusion. J Bone Joint Surg Am 1988;70:569–580.
4. LaGrone MO: Loss of lumbar lordosis: A complication of spinal fusion for scoliosis. Orthop Clin North Am 1988;19:383–393.
5. Swank SM, Mauri TM, Brown JC: The lumbar lordosis below Harrington instrumentation for scoliosis. Spine 1990;15:181–186.
6. Swank S, Lonstein JE, Moe JH, et al: Surgical treatment of adult scoliosis. J Bone Joint Surg Am 1981;63:268–287.
7. van Dam BE, Bradford DS, Lonstein JE, et al: Adult idiopathic scoliosis treated by posterior spinal fusion and Harrington instrumentation. Spine 1987;12:32–36.
8. DeWald RL: Revision surgery for spinal deformity. Adult Spinal Deformity, American Academy of Orthopaedic Surgeons, Instructional Course Lecture 105, San Francisco, CA, 1993.
9. Bridwell KH, Lenke LG, Lewis SJ: Treatment of spinal stenosis and fixed sagittal imbalance. Clin Orthop 2001;384:35–44.
10. Kostuik JP, Maurais GR, Richardson WJ, et al: Combined single stage anterior and posterior osteotomy for correction of iatrogenic lumbar kyphosis. Spine 1983;13:257–266.
11. Berven SH, Deviren V, Smith JA, et al: Management of fixed sagittal plane deformity results of the transpedicular wedge resection osteotomy. Spine 2001;26:2036–2043.
12. Booth KC, Bridwell KH, Lenke LG, et al: Complications and predictive factors for the successful treatment of flatback deformity (fixed sagittal imbalance). Spine 1999;24:1712–1720.
13. Farcy J-PC, Schwab FJ: Management of flatback and related kyphotic decompensation syndromes. Spine 1997;22:2452–2457.
14. Noun Z, Lapresle P, Missenard G: Posterior lumbar osteotomy for flatback in adults. J Spinal Disord 2001;14:311–316.
15. Tveit P, Daggfeldt K, Hetland S, et al: Erector spinae lever arm length variations with changes in spinal curvature. Spine 1994;19:199–204.
16. Gelb DE, Lenke LG, Bridwell KH, et al: An analysis of sagittal spinal alignment in 100 asymptomatic middle and older-aged volunteers. Spine 1995;20:1351–1358.
17. Vedantam R, Lenke LG, Bridwell KH, et al: The effect of variation in arm position on sagittal spinal alignment. Spine 2000;25:2204–2209.
18. Smith-Peterson MN, Larson CB, Aufranc OE: Osteotomy of the spine for correction of flexion deformity in rheumatoid arthritis. J Bone Joint Surg Am 1945;27:1–11.
19. Law WA: Osteotomy of the spine. Clin Orthop 1969;66:70–74.
20. Chang K-W: Oligosegmental correction of post-traumatic thoracolumbar angular kyphosis. Spine 1993;18:1909–1915.
21. Thomasen E: Vertebral osteotomy for correction of kyphosis in ankylosing spondylitis. Clin Orthop 1985;194:142–152.
22. Leong JCY, Ma A, Yau AC: Spinal osteotomy for fixed flexion deformity. Orthop Trans 1978;2:271.
23. Heinig CA: Eggshell procedure. In Luque ER (ed): Segmental Spinal Instrumentation. Thorofare, NJ: Slack, 1984, pp 221–230.
24. Burton DC, Asher MA, Amundson GM: The Heinig "egg-shell" procedure for the treatment of thoracic and lumbar kyphosis. Paper #68 presented at the Scoliosis Research Society, San Diego, CA, Sept. 23–25, 1999.
25. Murrey DB, Brigham CD, Kiebzak GM, et al: Transpedicular decompression and pedicle subtraction osteotomy (eggshell procedure): A retrospective review of 59 patients. Spine 2002;27:2338–2345.
26. Bridwell KH: "Pedicle subtraction" (three column) osteotomy. In McCarthy RE (ed): Spinal Instrumentation Techniques Manual, Vol 2. Rosemont, IL, Scoliosis Research Society, 1998, Section 11, pp 1–9.
27. Bradford DS, Tribus CB: Vertebral column resection for the treatment of rigid coronal decompensation. Spine 1997;22:1590–1599.

28. Boachie-Adjei O, Bradford DS: Vertebral resection and arthrodesis for complex deformities. J Spinal Disord 1991;4:193–202.
29. Bradford DS: Vertebral column resection: Orthopaedic transaction. J Bone Joint Surg Am 1985;9:130.
30. Boachie-Adjei O, Dendrinos GK, Ogilvie JW, et al: Management of adult spinal deformity with combined anterior-posterior arthrodesis and Luque-Galveston Instrumentation. J Spinal Disord 1991;4:131–141.
31. Farcy J-PC, Schwab FJ: Posterior osteotomies and pedicle subtraction for flatback and associated syndromes: Technique and results of prospective study. Bull Hosp Joint Dis 2000;59:11–16.
32. LaChapelle EH: Osteotomy of the lumbar spine for correction of kyphosis in a case of ankylosing spondylo-arthritis. J Bone Joint Surg Am 1946;28:851–858.
33. Herbert J-J: Vertebral osteotomy: Technique, indications, and results. J Bone Joint Surg Am 1948;30:680–689.

CHAPTER 48

KIRKHAM B. WOOD

The Surgical Management of Scheuermann's Kyphosis

INTRODUCTION

The posterior approach to the thoracic spine for the correction of Scheuermann's kyphosis is designed to correct the structural deformity, achieve appropriate sagittal balance, provide rigid fixation to promote a successful fusion, and if pain is present, reduce the pain associated with the developmental abnormality. The procedure involves the placing of hooks or pedicle screws throughout the kyphotic thoracic spine, connected by two longitudinal rods, bent to a more physiologic sagittal curve, which force the spine into a more normal profile (Fig. 48-1). This maneuver is always accompanied by fusion of the posterolateral elements in order to maintain the correction. Depending on surgeon preference, either autologous or allograft bone may be used. On occasion, the curve will be severe enough, or rigid enough, that a preliminary anterior approach may be necessary. This aims to release rigid connections allowing greater correction as well as promoting bony fusion. This can be performed either thoracoscopically, or via a more traditional transthoracic approach.[1]

INDICATIONS AND CONTRAINDICATIONS

INDICATIONS

- Progressive deformity
- Deformity associated with painful Scheuermann's end plate pathology
- Cosmetic deformity

RELATIVE CONTRAINDICATIONS

- Spinal infection
- Hypokyphosis (thoracic kyphosis less than 40 degrees)
- Pregnancy
- Metal sensitivity

OPERATIVE TECHNIQUE

EQUIPMENT

- X-ray-compatible operating table
- Fluoroscopy (pedicle screws)
- Headlight system (optional)
- Retractor system
- Bone graft source
- Posterior instrumentation (implants)
  - Longitudinal rods
  - Sublaminar, pedicle, transverse process hooks
  - Sublaminar wires (optional)
  - Pedicle screws
  - Cross-link connectors
- Kerrison punches, 1 to 4 mm
- Bone cutter
- Hall drill
- Hemovac drains
- Jackson table or Relton-Hall frame
- Transverse rolled blankets
- Spinal cord monitoring with somatosensory evoked potential (SSEP) with or without motor evoked potential (MEP).
- Cell-saver autotransfusion system

PATIENT POSITIONING

- The patient is placed in the prone position on the appropriate frame.
- With severe cases the operating table may be flexed slightly, so that returning to the horizontal position aids in the reduction maneuver.
- Placing the bed in slight reverse Trendelenburg position aids in visualization of the upper thoracic spine.

CHAPTER 48 The Surgical Management of Scheuermann's Kyphosis

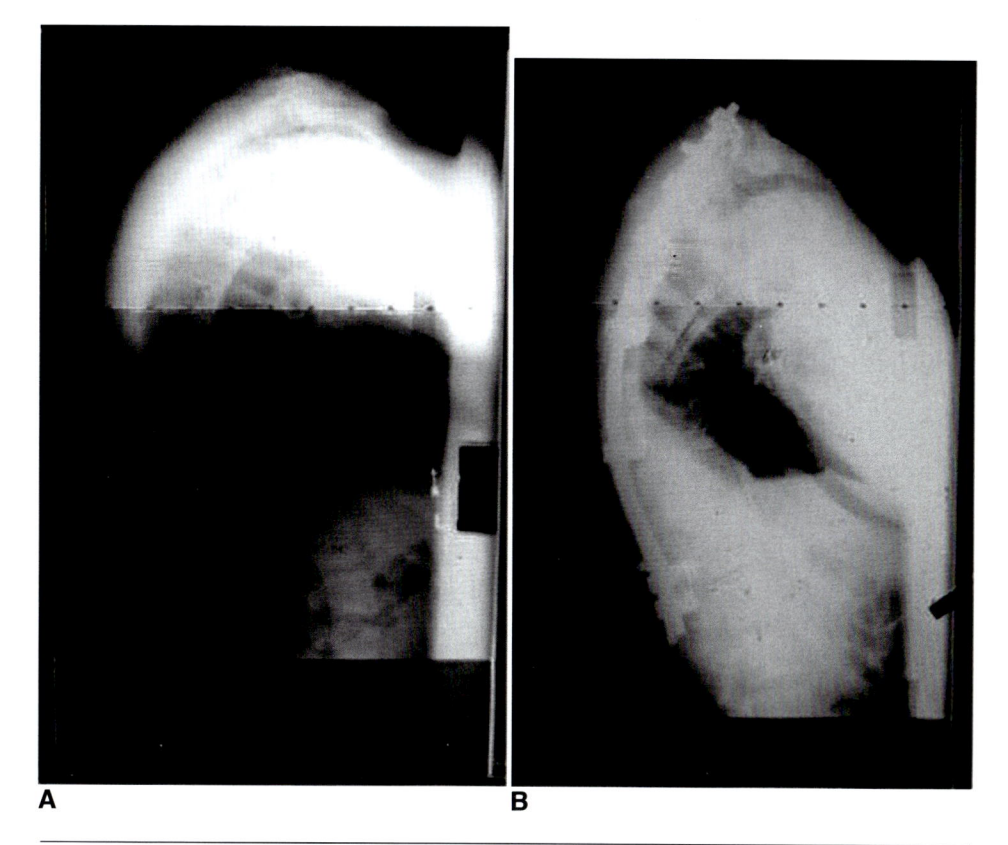

Fig. 48-1 Preoperative (A) and postoperative (B) lateral radiographs of an 18-year-old boy with 92 degrees of kyphosis corrected to 68 degrees with the use of a posterior spinal instrumentation.

- General endotracheal anaesthesia is used.
- Arms are placed in no more than 90 degrees abduction with the elbows well padded and the shoulders well supported.
- The entire back is prepped from the hairline to the buttocks and to the midaxillary lines.

LOCATION OF INCISION

- The incision extends from approximately just distal to the C7 spinous process to the upper lumbar spine in the midline.
- With severe upper thoracic kyphosis, the proximal incision may have to extend superior to the C7 spinous process to aid in pedicle screw entry.
- Local anesthetic may be injected subcutaneously along the injection site.

INCISION AND SOFT TISSUE DISSECTION

- The subcutaneous layer is divided and hemostasis obtained.
- The deep fascia is divided in the midline along its connection to the spinous processes.

EXPOSURE OF THE VERTEBRAE

- Using a Cobb elevator and electrocautery, the longitudinal muscles are exposed and stripped laterally and held with retractors.
- An 18-gauge needle or a Kocher clamp may be fixed to a spinous process so that either fluoroscopy or lateral radiography can be used to localize the desired level.
- Retractor placement:
  - Attention to the midline is important during the dissection so as to minimize bleeding.
  - Self-retaining retractors are placed within the wound at the most proximal and distal aspects and are used to hold back the longitudinal musculature.
  - Usually four retractors are necessary: Two angled, short retractors are used at the ends of the incision, and two longer straight retractors are introduced over the end retractors and extend into the body of the wound.
  - The retractors should retain the longitudinal musculature laterally so as to be able to visualize the transverse processes—on both sides—out to their most distal (lateral) aspect from the top to the bottom of the fusion mass.
- Using Cobb elevators and electrocautery, the soft tissue (longitudinal muscle) must be removed throughout the exposed spine.

- The spine to be exposed for fusion should include all vertebrae within the upper and lower Cobb levels of the kyphosis plus the first lordotic level distally.
- Take care to preserve the interspinous ligaments in the interspace superior to the most cephalad vertebra and inferior to the most caudal vertebra so as to help prevent junctional kyphosis.
- Currettes or electrocautery may be used to remove the joint capsule at the facet level bilaterally.
- A 1/4-inch osteotome may be used to remove the inferior aspect of each facet joint, exposing the cartilage of the superior facet below.
- The cartilage of the superior facet is removed exposing bleeding cancellous bone.
- The spinous processes from all the vertebrae except the most proximal and distal are removed and can be used for bone graft.
- Hemostasis from the exposed cancellous bone of the removed spinous processes can be achieved with Gelfoam squares.

INSTRUMENTATION

- Instrumentation is used to assist in manipulating spinal sagittal plane alignment in order to shorten the posterior column.
- If anterior surgery is performed, it involves diskectomy, release of the anterior longitudinal ligament, and fusion (lengthening of the anterior column).
- Instrumentation (and subsequent fusion) should extend from T2 or T3 proximally to include the first lordotic disk in the thoracolumbar region (typically L1 or L2) as seen on standing lateral radiographs.
- Either hooks in a claw configuration or pedicle screws can be placed proximally.
- Pedicle screws are the preferred means of distal fixation.
- Hooks *may* be used distally; however, the transverse processes of T10 to T12 are usually insufficient for adequate purchase.
- The hook-claw construct may be either intra- or intersegmental (i.e., either the hooks are used on the same vertebrae or span one or more vertebrae).
- The distal pedicle screws can be protected by up-going, off-set sublaminar hooks on the distal vertebral body.
- A minimum of three sets of claw hooks, or pedicle screws, proximally and three pedicle screws on each side distally is the preferred fixation scheme (Fig. 48-2).
- The implants may be staggered from side to side to increase segmental exposure and decortication for fusion.

CORRECTION

- Long 1/4-inch rods are used for the correction.
- One method is to contour the rods to reflect a more normal sagittal contour, and introduce them first into the proximal claw foundations.

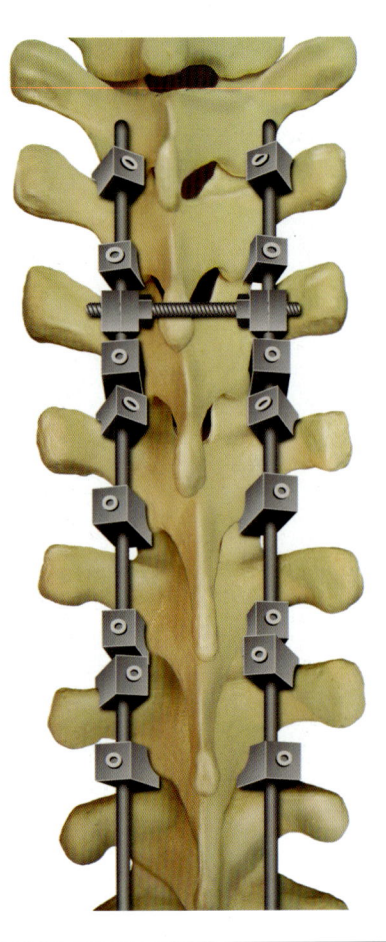

Fig. 48-2 Middle hook claw constructs in the superior thoracic spine.

- Compression is applied to each claw construct followed by locking of the set screws thus securing the proximal hooks to the rod (Fig. 48-3).
- Via cantilever introduction, the rods are then delivered sequentially distally into the hooks and more caudal pedicle screws (Fig. 48-4).
- Sublaminar wire can be used to aid in the rod introduction in the setting of larger, more rigid, curves.
- Once the rods are seated, intersegmental compression toward the apex of the curve is then used to shorten the posterior column and gain further kyphosis correction.
- Transverse rod connectors may then be placed to further stiffen the construct, especially for constructs extending into the lumbar spine.
- Another method of rod introduction may be more applicable for larger, more rigid curves.
- This involves the placement of two rods fixed proximally, and two more fixed distally. These two sets of rods are then cantilevered toward each other at the kyphotic apex until they can be connected to each other via side-to-side connectors (Fig. 48-5).
- At least two transverse connectors at each end of the fusion should be used.

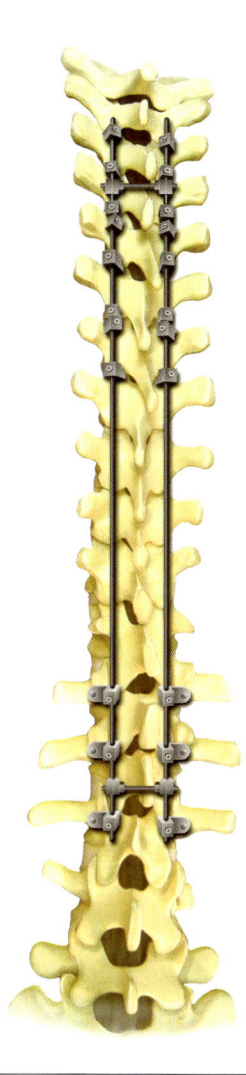

Fig. 48-3 The longitudinal rods are seen tightened down within each of the claw constructs.

- This two-rod technique helps prevent against bone-metal interface failure in the setting of these large anteriorly directed forces, especially in osteopenic bone.

BONE GRAFT

- A separate incision is made over the posterior iliac crest.
- The fascial attachment to the crest is divided in line with the ilium.
- The gluteal muscles are elevated subperiosteally from the outer surface of the ilium.
- Care is taken to prevent injury to structures in the sciatic notch.
- Cortical and cancellous bone are removed from the outer table of the ilium down to the inner cortical wall.
- Gelfoam squares may be used to control hemostasis.
- A hemovac drain is placed in the deep tissue.
- The fascia is reapproximated with watertight closure.

- The subcutaneous and subcuticular closures are done in the usual fashion.
- The bone graft can be morselized and placed about the decorticated posterolateral surface of the instrumented spine.

CLOSURE

- A wake-up test at the end of the procedure is advisable if electrophysiologic monitoring is unavailable.
- A watertight closure of the deep fascia is essential.
- A 1/4-inch hemovac drain is placed into either the deep subfascial compartment or the subcutaneous compartment.
- The subcutaneous and subcuticular layers are closed separately.

POSTOPERATIVE CARE

- A thoracolumbosacral orthosis may be used for 2 to 4 months postoperatively, depending on the rigidity of the fixation, or if the bone is osteopenic.
- A Jewett hyperextension brace may also be used when there is less concern regarding three-dimensional control.
- A lumbosacral orthosis (low back brace) is to be discouraged as the fusion mass pivots at the cephalad edge of the orthosis, risking the development of sagittal plane imbalance.
- Patients should be out of bed and walking on the second postoperative day.
- For the first 2 months, the patients are on a walking program, and then placed into light aerobic exercises (jogging, swimming, bicycling).
- As the fusion mass is not usually complete for at least 1 year, full contact sports participation is normally withheld until then.

COMPLICATIONS[2-4]

- Proximal junctional kyphosis may be seen if fusion stops short of the upper end vertebrae. It may also occur with overcorrection of the deformity, as the sagittal balance is shifted too far posteriorly. As a general rule, correction should not exceed more than 50% of the preoperative standing lateral Cobb measurement.
- Distal junctional kyphosis similarly may occur if the distal fusion does not include the first lordotic segment of the upper lumbar spine. It may also occur with overcorrection.
- Infection incidence ranges from 1% to 3%.
- Implant-bone failure is frequently seen with overcorrection or in osteopenic bone. Insufficient numbers of distal fixation sites may also lead to instrumentation-bone failure. Hook dislodgment in the distal spine is not uncommon.
- Implant failure.
- Pseudarthrosis can be as high as 20% in posterior-only surgery. With combined anterior and posterior approaches, the incidence ranges from 5% to 10%.

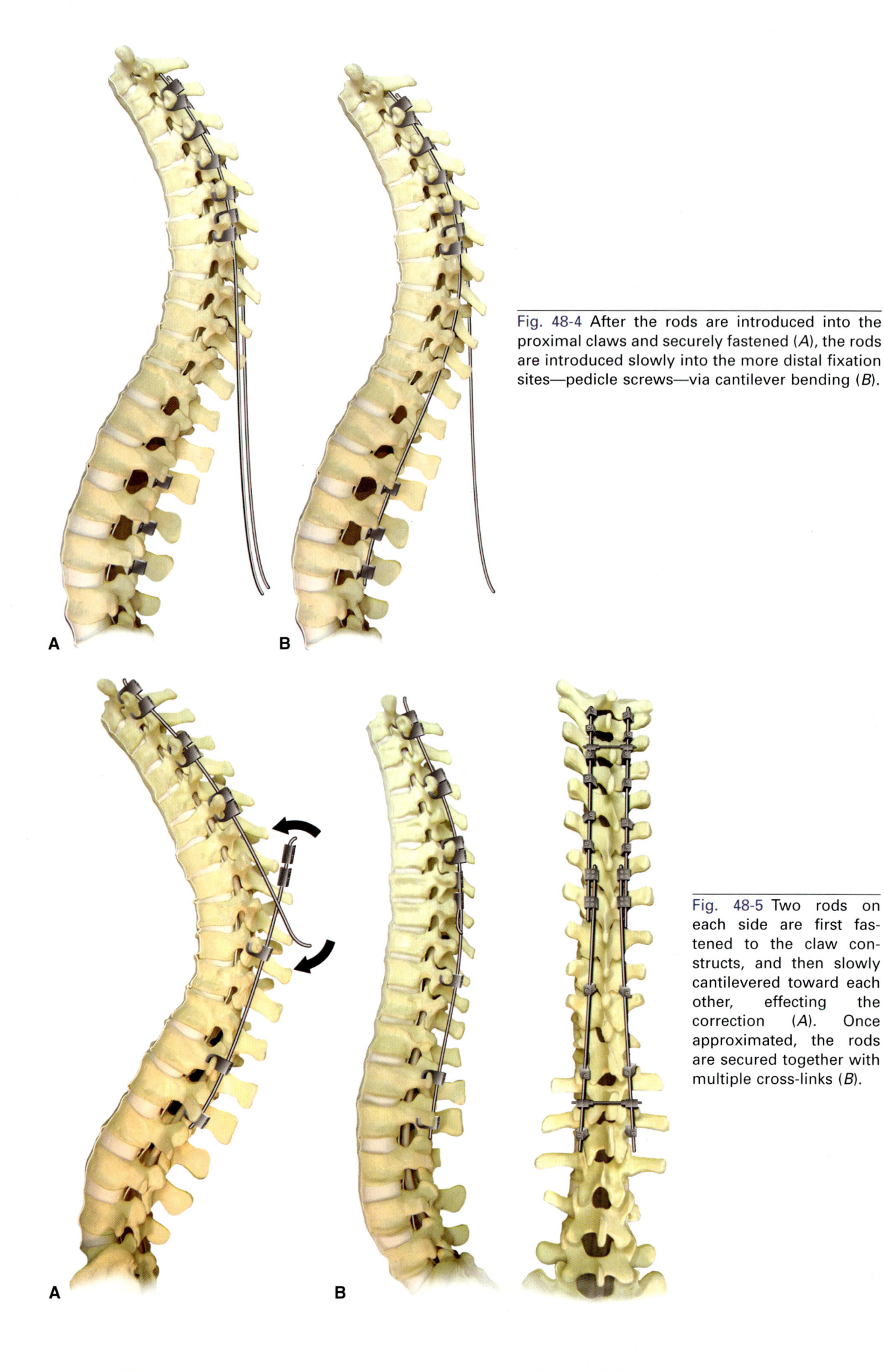

Fig. 48-4 After the rods are introduced into the proximal claws and securely fastened (A), the rods are introduced slowly into the more distal fixation sites—pedicle screws—via cantilever bending (B).

Fig. 48-5 Two rods on each side are first fastened to the claw constructs, and then slowly cantilevered toward each other, effecting the correction (A). Once approximated, the rods are secured together with multiple cross-links (B).

- Loss of correction.
- Hemothorax.
- Pneumothorax.
- Pulmonary embolism.
- Neurologic deficit: An increase in latency in motor or sensory evoked potentials of more than 10% or an amplitude drop of more than 50% is an indication to stop the procedure and perform an immediate wake-up test. If the patient fails the wake-up test, and or the evoked potentials do not correct, the instrumentation should be removed. If postoperatively the patient develops a motor deficit, consideration for immediate instrumentation removal should occur followed by emergency magnetic resonance imaging.
- Death.

References

1. Lowe TG: Current concepts review: Scheuermann disease. J Bone Joint Surg Am 1990;72:940–945.
2. Bradford DS, Moe JH, Montalvo F, et al. Scheuermann's kyphosis: Results of surgical treatment by posterior spine arthrodesis in twenty-two patients. J Bone Joint Surg Am 1975;57:439–448.
3. Bradford DS, Khalid BA, Moe JH: Scheuermann's kyphosis: Results of surgical treatment by combined anterior-posterior spine arthrodesis in twenty-four patients. J Bone Joint Surg Am 1980;62:705–712.
4. Lowe, TG, Kasten MD: An analysis of sagittal curves and balance after Cotrel-Dubousset instrumentation for kyphosis secondary to Scheuermann's disease: A review of 32 patients. Spine 1994;19:1680–1685.

SECTION VI

SPINAL TUMOR

CHAPTER 49

DEAN CHOU

CURTIS A. DICKMAN

Primary Malignant and Benign Tumors of the Vertebral Column

MALIGNANT TUMORS

CHORDOMAS

Chordomas arise from notochordal remnants of the vertebral column. They are rare, with an incidence of 0.08 per 100,000 population in the United States.[1] They occur more frequently in males than females and less often in African Americans than in other ethnic groups. A familial pattern has not yet been established.

Approximately 30% to 50% of cases occur in the sacrococcygeal region, and 30% to 40% occur in the clivus. The remainder of cases occurs through the rest of the axial skeleton. The vertebral body is usually affected, the disks are affected less often, and the posterior elements are usually spared.[2-4]

The most common presenting symptom is pain, and patients often state that it occurs at night. Pathologic fractures can manifest with the acute, sudden onset of pain.

In the sacral region, the sensation of rectal fullness may be experienced. If nerve root compression is present, radiculopathy also may be noted, although pain typically precedes radiculopathy. If spinal cord compression is involved, myelopathy may also be a presenting symptom.[5]

Histologically, chordomas can occur in sheets, and mitotic figures and nuclear pleomorphism can be found. Differentiation into mesenchymal elements such as cartilage can also occur.[6]

The radiographic evaluation for chordomas includes plain radiography, computed tomography (CT), and magnetic resonance imaging (MRI). Plain radiographs may show lytic destructive lesions and spinal alignment. CT further delineates the extent of bony destruction, and two-dimensional reconstructions provide information in the sagittal plane that may not be visible on plain radiographs. MRI is useful for defining tumor extensions, soft tissue involvement, and the degree of spinal cord compression.

The mainstay of therapy is surgical removal. In the M.D. Anderson sacral chordoma experience, tumors recurred in patients who underwent aggressive resection a mean of 2.27 years after surgery compared to a mean of 8 months after surgery in patients who underwent a subtotal resection.[7] Total spondylectomy may offer patients with large sacral chordomas the best chance for a cure and the longest survival time.[8] Intraoperatively, care must be taken to prevent the spread of tumor cells through the resection cavity. If possible, en bloc resection should be attempted to prevent spillage of residual cells. Radiation therapy has a limited role in the treatment of these radioresistant tumors, but it is used adjunctively and for palliative care.

McMaster and associates reviewed chordoma survival rates in the United States from 1973 to 1995 using data from the National Cancer Institute Surveillance, Epidemiology, and End Results. They found that the median length of survival was 6.29 years and that the 5-year survival rate was 67.6%.[1]

OSTEOSARCOMAS

Osteosarcoma is a rare disease, primarily affecting the long bones of the skeleton. Its incidence is estimated at 1 per 100,000 people.[9] It usually affects people in the first 3 decades of life, with a peak incidence around 15 years.[10] Only about 3% of these lesions affect the axial skeleton, and they usually affect the vertebral bodies more than the posterior elements. The tumors can be primary or metastatic. They also may be related to the patient having undergone previous radiation or to Paget's disease. Environmental agents such as beryllium, viruses, and electrical burns are thought to contribute to the development of osteosarcomas. Syndromes such as Rothmund-Thomson, Bloom, and Li-Fraumeni also are associated with an increased risk of developing an osteosarcoma.[11]

The most common initial presenting symptom associated with osteosarcomas is pain, which can be intermittent.[12] The pain is seldom felt at night but is related to strain.[12] A history of trauma is associated with osteosarcoma, and one third of patients have a palpable mass at their initial presentation.[12] If neural elements are compressed by mass effect or a pathologic fracture is present, patients also can develop neurologic manifestations.

Radiographic imaging is important in the evaluation of osteosarcomas to determine the extent of disease and bony destruction. On plain radiographs these tumors look like lytic lesions. The periosteum also may be elevated by the bony mass (so-called Codman's triangle). CT shows the extent of bony destruction in greater detail, and two-dimensional reconstructions may delineate sagittal plane defects that may not have been visible on plain radiographs. MRI helps delineate soft tissue destructiveness. It is also sensitive for evaluating the rest of the spine for metastases or other small nodules. The yield of bone scans is variable and not much better than that of plain skeletal radiographs. However, McKillop and associates advocate bone scans as a screening tool during follow-up.[13]

Surgery is the mainstay of therapy for osteosarcomas. Chemotherapy and radiotherapy may be added as adjuvant modalities. Chemotherapy is important for the treatment of subclinical disease, and radiotherapy is important for local control. Chemotherapeutic agents include methotrexate, doxorubicin, cisplatin, and ifosfamide/etoposide. Metastases are a problem, and prognosis is usually poor if patients initially become symptomatic with metastatic disease.[14] Five-year survival rates range from 50% to 60%.[15,16] In a study performed at Memorial Sloan-Kettering, patients who presented with a metastatic osteosarcoma had a median survival of 20 months.[17] Talac and associates showed that aggressive, en bloc resection of osteosarcomas involving the spine improved survival rates. The rate of recurrence in patients with positive margins at the time of resection was five times as high as that of patients with negative margins.[18] Although conclusive data are lacking, Ozaki and associates also found that survival rates tended to be higher for patients with gross total resection.[19]

EWING SARCOMAS

Ewing sarcomas are rare pediatric tumors with an incidence ranging from 0.1 to 0.8 per 100,000 people. Most of these tumors are diagnosed in patients younger than 20 years old.[10,20] They typically involve the long bones of the skeleton but affect the axial spine 8% of the time. The sacrum is most often involved, followed in decreasing order by the thoracic, lumbar, and cervical regions.[21]

The most common presenting symptoms in the spine are pain and neurologic deficits. In descending order, the most common neurologic manifestations are motor weakness, sensory changes, bladder dysfunction, and bowel dysfunction.[21] Pain usually is the result of tumor invasion, and neurologic manifestations either result from a pathologic fracture causing compression or from direct mass effect of a tumoral extension.

Clinical evaluation includes radiographic imaging and basic laboratory studies. Alkaline phosphatase and lactic dehydrogenase levels have been elevated in laboratory serum studies.[22] On plain radiographs the lesions look like "onion skinning" caused by splitting and thickening of the cortex. They also may appear to be "moth-eaten"—mottled with extension into the soft tissue.[23] CT further delineates the extent of bony destruction, and MRI can yield information about soft tissue involvement and the degree of compression of neural elements.

Treatment of Ewing sarcoma begins with chemotherapy. Chemotherapy is usually administered before surgery to shrink the tumor cells within the primary site and to control spread to other sites. Radiotherapy has a role in local control and treatment. Surgery should be considered not only to treat the primary disease but also to alleviate neurologic compression if present. Bacci and associates demonstrated that patients who underwent surgery and radiotherapy had a higher 5-year event-free survival rate compared to those who underwent surgery alone or even radiotherapy alone.[24]

Based on earlier data, which included patients from the 1950s, the 5-year survival rate was 33%.[25] However, better detection, imaging, and treatment have improved the 5-year survival rate for Ewing's sarcoma to about 58%.[10]

CHONDROSARCOMAS

Primary chondrosarcomas of the spine are very rare. In 43 years one major American cancer center had seen only 21 patients with primary chondrosarcomas of the spine.[7] Nonetheless, they are still the third most common primary malignant bone tumor, composing 20% to 27% of all malignant osseous tumors.[26] About 10% of chondrosarcomas arise from the spine, and the highest incidence is in men in their fifth and sixth decades.[27] Their origin is mesenchymal and they are chondrogenic.[28] Like other primary tumors of the spine, pain is the initial presenting symptom. If neural elements are compressed, neurologic signs and symptoms may be present.

The radiographic evaluation of chondrosarcomas of the spine consists of plain radiography, CT, and MRI. Plain radiographs show a "ring-and-arc" chondroid matrix mineralization and scalloping. Plain radiographs may show a destructive lesion with diffuse mottled calcification.[29] CT is helpful to further delineate the degree of matrix mineralization. Because these lesions have a high water content, their signal intensity on T_2-weighted MRIs is high and low on T_1-weighted MRIs. Compared to other imaging modalities, MRI shows the degree of soft tissue extension and neural compression most accurately.[26]

A biopsy should be obtained to determine the histologic grade of a chondrosarcoma. Chondrosarcomas are graded I to IV, with dedifferentiated chondrosarcomas being the most malignant.[30] Surgical excision is the mainstay of treatment.[31] When surgical excision is impossible or too dangerous, radiation therapy may be used. It also may be used for palliative or adjuvant therapy.[32] The role of conventional chemotherapy is limited because these tumors tend to be chemoresistant.[33] Nonetheless, some cases have been controlled to some degree with chemotherapy.[34] Promising data from photon-beam therapy with a 3-year follow-up indicate the local control rate is 85%.[35]

Survival times vary, depending on the grade of the tumor and the extent of resection. Uchida and colleagues reported 5-year and 10-year survival rates of 72% and 62%, respectively.[36] The 5-year survival rate associated with low-grade chondrosarcomas ranges from 65% to 85%. Higher grades are more deadly; their 5-year survival rate is about 15%.[30] The prognosis of more malignant variant dedifferentiated chondrosarcomas is much worse. Mitchell and associates treated 22 patients with a dedifferentiated chondrosarcoma, a highly malignant variant, and their 5-year survival rate was 18%.[37] Frassica and coworkers treated 78 patients with a dedifferentiated chondrosarcoma, and their 5-year survival rate was only 11%.[38]

PLASMACYTOMAS AND MULTIPLE MYELOMAS

There is a continuum in the disease spectrum of multiple myelomas, solitary plasmacytomas, and extramedullary plasmacytomas. All are based on plasma cell neoplasms. Each year about 5 per 100,000 people develop multiple myeloma. It tends to favor males over females and blacks over whites. In people over the age of 65 years, the incidence rises to 30 per 100,000.[9] Plasmacytomas are also neoplasms of plasma B-cell lymphocytes. They are most common in the sixth decade of life, and more than half can be located in the spine.[39] Plasmacytomas usually affect the vertebral bodies, but they also can affect the posterior elements. About 50% of plasmacytomas convert to multiple myelomas.[39]

Multiple myeloma is the most common primary tumor of the spine. Because it is a disease involving bone marrow, it is usually spread diffusely through the vertebral axis. However, 5% to 10% of cases are solitary spine lesions.[40–42]

On plain radiographs, multiple myeloma appears as "punched-out," radiolucent areas. CT is useful for determining the amount of bony destruction in fine detail. MRI is extremely sensitive in detecting not only the lesions themselves but also the extent of neural compression and soft tissue involvement[43,44] (Fig. 49-1).

The mainstay of local control is radiation.[45] Systemic control is attempted with a combination of chemotherapy and autologous stem cell reinfusion. Total cure with chemotherapy alone has been reported.[46,47] Surgery may be

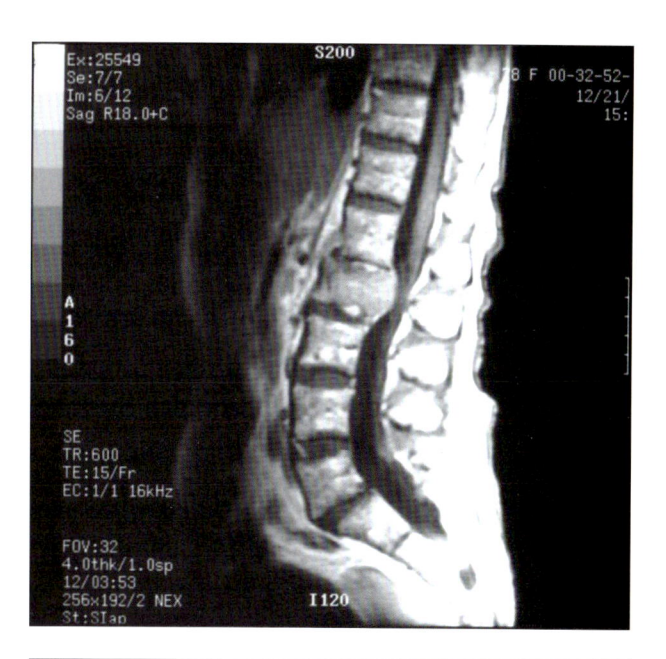

Fig. 49-1 Sagittal T_1-weighted magnetic resonance image with gadolinium demonstrating plasmacytoma.

indicated for single lesions if neural compression is involved or if a pathologic fracture is causing severe deformity or neural compression. Patients with intractable pain also may benefit from surgery. Durr and associates retrospectively analyzed 27 patients who underwent surgical intervention for multiple myeloma of the spine.[48] Postoperatively, the functional scores of 24 patients improved and pain relief improved in 26 patients (Fig. 49-2).

Despite therapeutic interventions, the prognosis of multiple myeloma remains poor. The median length of survival is 49 months, and the 5-year survival rate is about 30%.[9,49] The mean time of disease-free survival associated with solitary plasmacytomas is 81 months, and the 10-year survival rate is 85%.[39]

BENIGN TUMORS

OSTEOID OSTEOMAS AND OSTEOBLASTOMAS

Osteoid osteomas are benign tumors of bone that usually involve the long bones. They are usually less than 2 cm. About 10% to 14% of cases occur in the spine. They usually develop in young patients, and the main complaint is pain. Because these tumors are vascular, they may respond to anti-inflammatory medication. Classically, they manifest with night pain that responds to aspirin. Scoliosis may be present, and the posterior elements are usually involved.[50]

On plain radiographs, a gray bony lesion surrounded by bone may be difficult to detect. CT, however, is sensitive enough to detect and delineate these lesions, which may be associated with a periosteal sclerotic reaction. The sensitivity of MRI for detecting osteoid osteomas is somewhat limited.

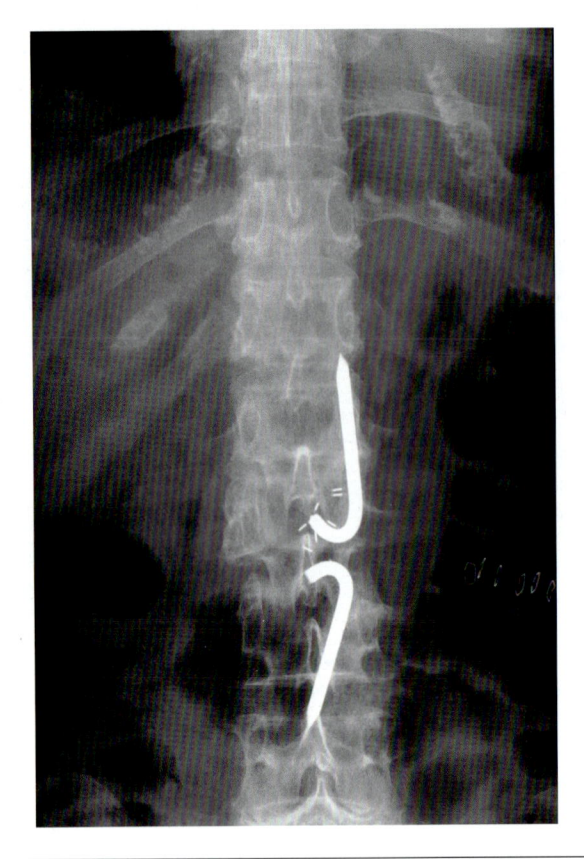

Fig. 49-2 Postoperative x-ray after plastmacytoma resection and reconstruction.

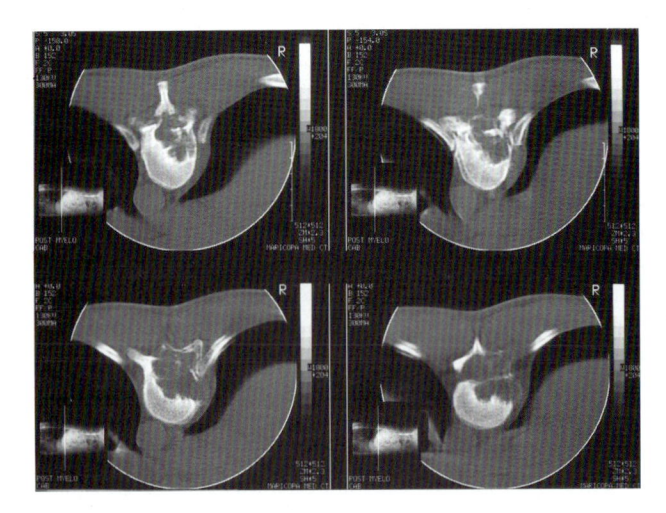

Fig. 49-3 Axial computed tomograph demonstrating osteoblastoma.

However, this modality is useful for detecting the edema that is sometimes associated with osteoid osteomas. It also may show soft tissue extensions and neural compression and may help to rule out the presence of other lesions within the spine.

Osteoid osteomas may resolve spontaneously within 2 to 4 years if treated with nonsteroidal anti-inflammatory drugs.[51] Other nonsurgical options include radiofrequency ablation. This technique involves percutaneous insertion of a needle under CT guidance. The lesion is ablated with the tip at 90° C. When treating extraspinal lesions, Rosenthal and associates found no differences in outcomes of radiofrequency ablation compared to those of surgery.[52] Hadjipavlou and associates used this technique in the spine in two patients and found symptoms were relieved 2.5 and 3 years after treatment.[53] Surgical excision of these lesions is the mainstay of therapy. Intraoperatively, it can be difficult to visualize the lesion. Two days before surgery, tetracycline can be administered (4 mg/kg four times a day) to allow the lesion to be visualized under ultraviolet light.[54]

Because the lesion is benign, it is presumed cured when resected. Aydinli and associates surgically removed osteoid osteomas in nine patients with a 27-month follow-up.[55] Pain was completely relieved in all nine patients, and there were no recurrences. Rosenthal and coworkers evaluated 263 patients with osteomas treated with radiofrequency ablation (not specifically spinal lesions): 89% to 91% of the patients initially treated experienced pain relief compared to 60% of patients with recurrent lesions.[56]

Osteoblastomas are similar to osteoid osteomas except for a few distinguishing features. The main distinguishing criterion is size: Osteoblastomas are larger than 2 cm (Figs. 49-3 to 49-5). Osteoblastomas also tend to occur in males more often than in females and tend to occur in young patients.[57] Osteoblastomas affect the posterior elements, but they seldom resolve spontaneously. They usually manifest with pain or painful scoliosis. They can also cause neurologic

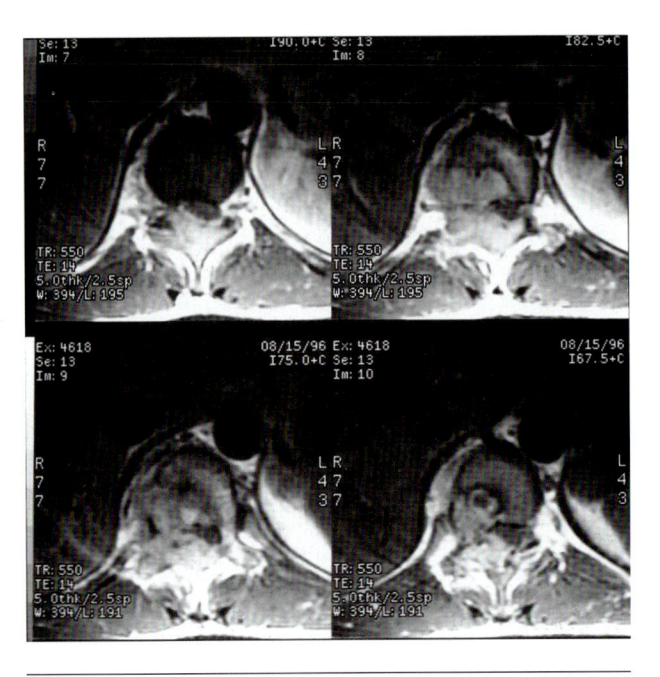

Fig. 49-4 Magnetic resonance image with gadolinium demonstrating osteoblastoma.

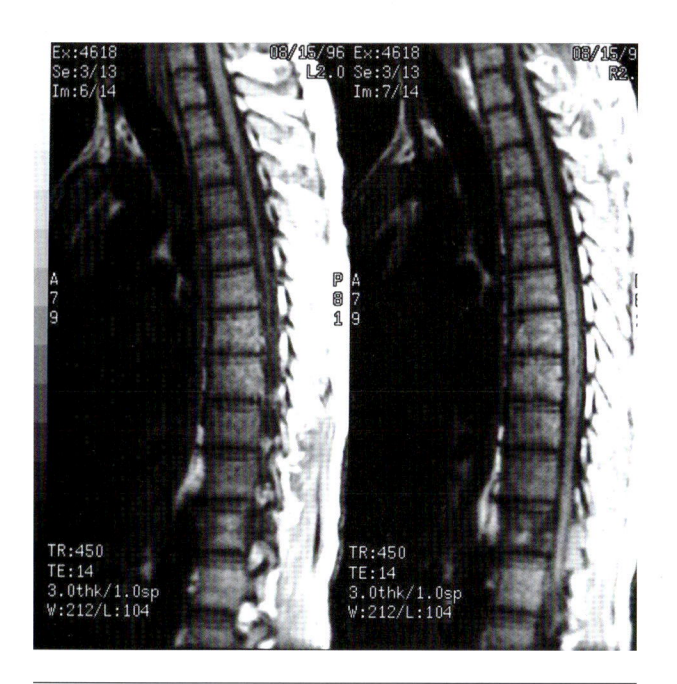

Fig. 49-5 Sagittal T$_1$-weighted magnetic resonance image demonstrating osteoblastoma.

symptoms if compression is present.[57,58] Surgery is the primary treatment, and complete cures can be attained.[58] Radiation and chemotherapy are rarely implemented except for local recurrences associated with rare malignant transformation.[59]

ANEURYSMAL BONE CYSTS

Aneurysmal bone cysts are rare, and they usually occur in young patients. They consist of expansile, vascular tissue within the bone that forms a cystic lesion. They can also occur in association with other tumors, including giant cell tumors, chondroblastomas, fibromyxomas, and nonossifying fibromas.[60] They usually involve the long bones and pelvis. When they are intraspinal, they usually involve the posterior elements and pedicles. Clinically, they manifest with pain, but they can also cause paraplegia when the vertebral bodies are involved.[61–63]

The plain radiographic appearance of aneurysmal bone cysts includes marked cortical thinning and erosion and periosteal elevation. The posterior elements are usually involved, and the pedicles may be involved. CT helps to delineate the extent of bony involvement and to confirm the diagnosis.[61] MRI is useful because of its sensitivity. On MRI these lesions are associated with intermediate signal intensity and have a "bubbly" or "honeycomb" appearance.[64]

Traditionally, the treatment of aneurysmal bone cysts has been surgical removal. Complete curettage and removal of all tumors should be the goal of surgery. Embolization helps reduce intraoperative blood loss and should be performed preoperatively, if feasible.[65] Boriani and associates obtained good results with preoperative embolization and have suggested that aneurysmal bone cysts eventually may be treated completely by embolization alone.[66] Other authors have advocated postoperative radiation as adjuvant therapy, and some cases of aneurysmal bone cysts have been completely treated with radiation alone.[67,68] However, the risk of radiation-induced sarcoma, especially in young patients who have undergone a complete resection, must be weighed.[69] Usually, radiation is reserved for lesions that cannot be completely resected or for recurrences that cannot be controlled. Feigenberg and associates irradiated nine patients, three of whom had undergone intralesional curettage. None had a recurrence at a median follow-up of 17 years.[70]

Although aneurysmal bone cysts are benign, they can recur. Papagelopoulos and coworkers evaluated 52 patients with aneurysmal bone cysts in the spine: 40 had initial primary lesions and 12 had recurrences.[71] All were treated with intralesional curettage, four with postoperative radiation, and two with preoperative embolization. The 10-year recurrence rate in patients treated for an initial primary lesions was 10% compared to 17% with recurrences after 9 years. One patient died of intraoperative bleeding, and one died of radiation-induced sarcoma.

GIANT CELL TUMORS

Giant cell tumors of the bone occur in females slightly more than in males in the fourth to sixth decades of life.[72] These expansile lytic lesions usually involve the vertebral bodies. Most giant cell tumors are found in the long bones, but as many as 9% occur in the spine. These lesions are highly aggressive and can recur locally.[73,74] Although classified as benign tumors, giant cell tumors can metastasize, and 2.6% to 5% of them do. The lung is the most common location for metastasis.[75]

The clinical presentation of grant cell tumors is axial pain, which may lead to an initial misdiagnosis. Compression of the neural elements may be associated with neurologic deficit.[76] Sanjay and associates reported that as many as half of the patients with a giant cell tumor of the spine become symptomatic with a neurologic deficit.[77] Giant cell tumors are divided into grades I, II, and III; more than 60% are grade I, and 7% are grade III. Malignant transformation has been reported in as many as 13% of cases.[78] If, however, the tumors metastasize but are histologically benign, the metastases have the potential to be cured by resection. Cheng and Johnston even described patients who had survived long term despite subtotal resection of their pulmonary nodule.[75]

On plain radiographs these lesions are expansile and lytic but may lack sclerotic margins.[79] CT further details their appearance, and two-dimensional sagittal reconstruction may help assess the extent of bony destruction. Internal septations may be present.[80] MRI helps to delineate soft tissue extensions and neural compression. Giant cell tumors are associated with heterogeneous or homogeneous intermediate signal intensity on T_1-weighted MRIs and with low to intermediate signal intensity on T_2-weighted MRIs. Fluid levels may be seen, but the finding is nonspecific.[81,82]

The treatment of giant cell tumors includes surgical removal. If possible, en bloc resection is preferred because recurrence rates are high.[83] Authors have also advocated the use of cement or phenol to help kill remaining cells after surgical removal.[83,84] Recurrence rates range from 25% to 35%.[85] Radiation has a role in the treatment of recurrent, inoperable, or malignant tumors. However, the risk of malignant transformation must be considered. The rate of malignant transformation associated with radiation can be as high as 19%.[86] Although not a standard treatment, chemotherapy has been used to treat giant cell tumors in patients with multiple metastases, inoperable lesions, or a continued recurrence, and results have been good.[87,88]

References

1. McMaster ML, Goldstein AM, Bromley CM, et al: Chordoma: Incidence and survival patterns in the United States, 1973–1995. Cancer Causes Control 2001;12(1):1–11.
2. Bergh P, Kindblom LG, Gunterberg B, et al: Prognostic factors in chordoma of the sacrum and mobile spine: A study of 39 patients. Cancer 2000;88(9):2122–2134.
3. Bjornsson J, Wold LE, Ebersold MJ, Laws ER: Chordoma of the mobile spine: A clinicopathologic analysis of 40 patients. Cancer 1993;71(3):735–740.
4. Boriani S, Chevalley F, Weinstein JN, et al: Chordoma of the spine above the sacrum: Treatment and outcome in 21 cases. Spine 1996;21(13):1569–1577.
5. Chandawarkar RY: Sacrococcygeal chordoma: Review of 50 consecutive patients. World J Surg 1996;20(6):717–719.
6. Moriki T, Takahashi T, Wada M, et al: Chondroid chordoma: Fine-needle aspiration cytology with histopathological, immunohistochemical, and ultrastructural study of two cases. Diagn Cytopathol 1999;21(5):335–339.
7. York JE, Berk RH, Fuller GN, et al: Chondrosarcoma of the spine: 1954 to 1997. J Neurosurg 1999;90(1 Suppl):73–78.
8. Marmor E, Rhines LD, Weinberg JS, Gokaslan ZL: Total en bloc lumbar spondylectomy: Case report. J Neurosurg 2001;95(2 Suppl):264–269.
9. Ries LAG, Eisner MP, Kosary CL, et al: SEER Cancer Statistics Review, 1973–1999. Web site: http://seer.cancer.gov/csr/1973_1999/, 2002. National Cancer Institute. Bethesda, 2004.
10. Ries LAG, Smith MA, Gurney JG, et al: Cancer incidence and survival among children and adolescents: United States SEER program 1975–1995. Web site: http://www.seer.ims.nci.nih.gov. National Cancer Insititute, SEER Program. NIH Pub. No. 99-4649. Bethesda, 1999.
11. Fuchs B, Pritchard DJ: Etiology of osteosarcoma. Clin Orthop 2002;397:40–52.
12. Widhe B, Widhe T: Initial symptoms and clinical features in osteosarcoma and Ewing sarcoma. J Bone Joint Surg Am 2000;82(5):667–674.
13. McKillop JH, Etcubanas E, Goris ML: The indications for and limitations of bone scintigraphy in osteogenic sarcoma: A review of 55 patients. Cancer 1981;48(5):1133–1138.
14. Ferguson WS, Goorin AM: Current treatment of osteosarcoma. Cancer Invest 2001;19(3):292–315.
15. Ogihara Y, Sudo A, Fujinami S, et al: Current management, local management, and survival statistics of high-grade osteosarcoma. Experience in Japan. Clin Orthop 1991;270:72–78.
16. Stiller CA, Craft AW, Corazziari I: Survival of children with bone sarcoma in Europe since 1978: Results from the EUROCARE study. Eur J Cancer 2001;37(6):760–766.
17. Meyers PA, Heller G, Healey JH, et al: Osteogenic sarcoma with clinically detectable metastasis at initial presentation. J Clin Oncol 1993;11(3):449–453.
18. Talac R, Yaszemski MJ, Currier BL, et al: Relationship between surgical margins and local recurrence in sarcomas of the spine. Clin Orthop 2002;397:127–132.
19. Ozaki T, Flege S, Liljenqvist U, et al: Osteosarcoma of the spine: Experience of the Cooperative Osteosarcoma Study Group. Cancer 2002;94(4):1069–1077.
20. Jurgens H, Winkler K, Gobel U: Bone tumours. In Plowman PN, Pinkerton CR (eds): Paediatric Oncology: Clinical Practice and Controversies. London and New York, Chapman & Hall Medical, 1992, pp. 325–350.
21. Venkateswaran L, Rodriguez-Galindo C, Merchant TE, et al: Primary Ewing tumor of the vertebrae: Clinical characteristics, prognostic factors, and outcome. Med Pediatr Oncol 2001;37(1):30–35.
22. Hannisdal E, Solheim OP, Theodorsen L, Host H: Alterations of blood analyses at relapse of osteosarcoma and Ewing's sarcoma. Acta Oncol 1990;29(5):585–587.
23. Eggli KD, Quiogue T, Moser RP Jr: Ewing's sarcoma. Radiol Clin North Am 1993;31(2):325–337.
24. Bacci G, Ferrari S, Longhi A, et al: Role of surgery in local treatment of Ewing's sarcoma of the extremities in patients undergoing adjuvant and neoadjuvant chemotherapy. Oncol Rep 2004;11(1):111–120.
25. Grubb MR, Currier BL, Pritchard DJ, Ebersold MJ: Primary Ewing's sarcoma of the spine. Spine 1994;19(3):309–313.
26. Murphey MD, Walker EA, Wilson AJ, et al: From the archives of the AFIP: Imaging of primary chondrosarcoma: Radiologic-pathologic correlation. Radiographics 2003;23(5):1245–1278.
27. Boriani S, De Iure F, Bandiera S, et al: Chondrosarcoma of the mobile spine: Report on 22 cases. Spine 2000;25(7):804–812.
28. Aigner T, Dertinger S, Belke J, Kirchner T: Chondrocytic cell differentiation in clear cell chondrosarcoma. Hum Pathol 1996;27(12):1301–1305.
29. Hermann G, Sacher M, Lanzieri CF, et al: Chondrosarcoma of the spine: An unusual radiographic presentation. Skeletal Radiol 1985;14(3):178–183.
30. Healey JH, Lane JM: Chondrosarcoma. Clin Orthop 1986;204:119–129.
31. Sheth DS, Yasko AW, Johnson ME, et al: Chondrosarcoma of the pelvis: Prognostic factors for 67 patients treated with definitive surgery. Cancer 1996;78(4):745–750.
32. Le A, Ball D, Pitman A, Fox R, King K: Chondrosarcoma of bone complicating Ollier's disease: Report of a favourable response to radiotherapy. Australas Radiol 2003;47(3):322–324.
33. Terek RM, Schwartz GK, Devaney K, et al: Chemotherapy and P-glycoprotein expression in chondrosarcoma. J Orthop Res 1998;16(5):585–590.
34. La Rocca RV, Morgan KW, Paris K, Baeker TR: Recurrent chondrosarcoma of the cranial base: A durable response to ifosfamide-doxorubicin chemotherapy. J Neurooncol 1999;41(3):281–283.
35. Noel G, Habrand JL, Jauffret E, et al: Radiation therapy for chordoma and chondrosarcoma of the skull base and the cervical spine: Prognostic factors and patterns of failure. Strahlenther Onkol 2003;179(4):241–248.

36. Uchida Y, Kawai A, Taguchi K, et al: Clinicopathology of chondrosarcoma. Acta Med Okayama 1996;50(4):191–196.
37. Mitchell AD, Ayoub K, Mangham DC, et al: Experience in the treatment of dedifferentiated chondrosarcoma. J Bone Joint Surg Br 2000;82(1):55–61.
38. Frassica FJ, Unni KK, Beabout JW, Sim FH: Dedifferentiated chondrosarcoma: A report of the clinicopathological features and treatment of seventy-eight cases. J Bone Joint Surg Am 1986;68(8):1197–1205.
39. Delauche-Cavallier MC, Laredo JD, Wybier M, et al: Solitary plasmacytoma of the spine: Long-term clinical course. Cancer 1988;61(8):1707–1714.
40. Bataille R, Sany J: Solitary myeloma: Clinical and prognostic features of a review of 114 cases. Cancer 1981;48(3):845–851.
41. Chak LY, Cox RS, Bostwick DG, Hoppe RT: Solitary plasmacytoma of bone: Treatment, progression, and survival. J Clin Oncol 1987;5(11):1811–1815.
42. Weinstein JN, McLain RF: Primary tumors of the spine. Spine 1987;12(9):843–851.
43. Lecouvet FE, Vande Berg BC, Malghem J, Maldague BE: Magnetic resonance and computed tomography imaging in multiple myeloma. Semin Musculoskelet Radiol 2001;5(1):43–55.
44. Ludwig H, Fruhwald F, Tscholakoff D, et al: Magnetic resonance imaging of the spine in multiple myeloma. Lancet 1987;2(8555):364–366.
45. Leigh BR, Kurtts TA, Mack CF, et al: Radiation therapy for the palliation of multiple myeloma. Int J Radiat Oncol Biol Phys 1993;25(5):801–804.
46. Notaro R, De Renzo A, De Rosa G, et al: Multiple myeloma cured by conventional chemotherapy: A report and a review. Leuk Lymphoma 2002;43(4):907–910.
47. Sonneveld P, Segeren CM: Changing concepts in multiple myeloma: From conventional chemotherapy to high-dose treatment. Eur J Cancer 2003;39(1):9–18.
48. Durr HR, Wegener B, Krodel A, et al: Multiple myeloma: Surgery of the spine: Retrospective analysis of 27 patients. Spine 2002;27(3):320–324.
49. Long-term survival in multiple myeloma: A Finnish Leukaemia Group study. Br J Haematol 1999;105(4):942–947.
50. Cohen MD, Harrington TM, Ginsburg WW: Osteoid osteoma: 95 cases and a review of the literature. Semin Arthritis Rheum 1983;12(3):265–281.
51. Kneisl JS, Simon MA: Medical management compared with operative treatment for osteoid-osteoma. J Bone Joint Surg Am 1992;74(2):179–185.
52. Rosenthal DI, Hornicek FJ, Wolfe MW, et al: Decreasing length of hospital stay in treatment of osteoid osteoma. Clin Orthop 1999;361:186–191.
53. Hadjipavlou AG, Lander PH, Marchesi D, et al: Minimally invasive surgery for ablation of osteoid osteoma of the spine. Spine 2003;28(22):E472–E477.
54. Ayala AG, Murray JA, Erling MA, Raymond AK: Osteoid-osteoma: Intraoperative tetracycline-fluorescence demonstration of the nidus. J Bone Joint Surg Am 1986;68(5):747–751.
55. Aydinli U, Ozturk C, Ersozlu S, Filiz G: Results of surgical treatment of osteoid osteoma of the spine. Acta Orthop Belg 2003;69(4):350–354.
56. Rosenthal DI, Hornicek FJ, Torriani M, et al: Osteoid osteoma: Percutaneous treatment with radiofrequency energy. Radiology 2003;229(1):171–175.
57. Nemoto O, Moser RP Jr, Van Dam BE, et al: Osteoblastoma of the spine: A review of 75 cases. Spine 1990;15(12):1272–1280.
58. Boriani S, Capanna R, Donati D, et al: Osteoblastoma of the spine. Clin Orthop 1992;278:37–45.
59. Berberoglu S, Oguz A, Aribal E, Ataoglu O: Osteoblastoma response to radiotherapy and chemotherapy. Med Pediatr Oncol 1997;28(4):305–309.
60. Marcove RC, Sheth DS, Takemoto S, Healey JH: The treatment of aneurysmal bone cyst. Clin Orthop 1995;311:157–163.
61. Chan MS, Wong YC, Yuen MK, Lam D: Spinal aneurysmal bone cyst causing acute cord compression without vertebral collapse: CT and MRI findings. Pediatr Radiol 2002;32(8):601–604.
62. Raftopoulos C, Hurrel A, Ticket L, et al: Total recuperation in a case of sudden total paraplegia due to an aneurysmal bone cyst of the thoracic spine. Childs Nerv Syst 1994;10(7):464–467.
63. Shacked I, Tadmor R, Wolpin G, Ohry A: Aneurysmal bone cyst of a vertebral body with acute paraplegia. Paraplegia 1981;19(5):294–298.
64. Asaumi J, Konouchi H, Hisatomi M, et al: MR features of aneurysmal bone cyst of the mandible and characteristics distinguishing it from other lesions. Eur J Radiol 2003;45(2):108–112.
65. Meyer S, Reinhard H, Graf N, et al: Arterial embolization of a secondary aneurysmatic bone cyst of the thoracic spine prior to surgical excision in a 15-year-old girl. Eur J Radiol 2002;43(1):79–81.
66. Boriani S, De Iure F, Campanacci L, et al: Aneurysmal bone cyst of the mobile spine: Report on 41 cases. Spine 2001;26(1):27–35.
67. Kamikonya N, Hishikawa Y, Kurisu K, et al: Aneurysmal bone cyst treated by high-energy, low-dose radiation therapy: A case report. Radiat Med 1991;9(2):54–56.
68. Shah V, Singhal NC, Udawat JP: Response of aneurysmal bone cyst to low doses of cobalt 60 gamma radiation with prolonged treatment. Br J Radiol 1978;51(608):608–612.
69. Patel SR: Radiation-induced sarcoma. Curr Treat Options Oncol 2000;1(3):258–261.
70. Feigenberg SJ, Marcus RB Jr, Zlotecki RA, et al: Megavoltage radiotherapy for aneurysmal bone cysts. Int J Radiat Oncol Biol Phys 2001;49(5):1243–1247.
71. Papagelopoulos PJ, Currier BL, Shaughnessy WJ, et al: Aneurysmal bone cyst of the spine: Management and outcome. Spine 1998;23(5):621–628.
72. Frassica FJ, Sanjay BK, Unni KK, et al: Benign giant cell tumor. Orthopedics 1993;16(10):1179–1183.
73. Dahlin DC, Cupps RE, Johnson EW Jr: Giant-cell tumor: A study of 195 cases. Cancer 1970;25(5):1061–1070.
74. Larsson SE, Lorentzon R, Boquist L: Giant-cell tumor of bone: A demographic, clinical, and histopathological study of all cases recorded in the Swedish Cancer Registry for the years 1958 through 1968. J Bone Joint Surg Am 1975;57(2):167–173.
75. Cheng JC, Johnston JO: Giant cell tumor of bone: Prognosis and treatment of pulmonary metastases. Clin Orthop 1997;338:205–214.
76. Savini R, Gherlinzoni F, Morandi M, et al: Surgical treatment of giant-cell tumor of the spine: The experience at the Istituto Ortopedico Rizzoli. J Bone Joint Surg Am 1983;65(9):1283–1289.
77. Sanjay BK, Sim FH, Unni KK, et al: Giant-cell tumours of the spine. J Bone Joint Surg Br 1993;75(1):148–154.
78. Boutou-Bredaki S, Agapios P, Papachristou G: Prognosis of giant cell tumor of bone: Histopathological analysis of 15 cases and review of the literature. Adv Clin Path 2001;5(3):71–78.
79. Manaster BJ, Doyle AJ: Giant cell tumors of bone. Radiol Clin North Am 1993;31(2):299–323.
80. Hudson TM, Schiebler M, Springfield DS, et al: Radiology of giant cell tumors of bone: Computed tomography, arthro-tomography, and scintigraphy. Skeletal Radiol 1984;11(2):85–95.

81. Tsai JC, Dalinka MK, Fallon MD, et al: Fluid-fluid level: A nonspecific finding in tumors of bone and soft tissue. Radiology 1990;175(3):779–782.
82. Waldman BJ, Zerhouni EA, Frassica FJ: Recurrence of giant cell tumor of bone: The role of MRI in diagnosis. Orthopedics 1997;20(1):67–69.
83. O'Donnell RJ, Springfield DS, Motwani HK, et al: Recurrence of giant-cell tumors of the long bones after curettage and packing with cement. J Bone Joint Surg Am 1994;76(12):1827–1833.
84. Trieb K, Bitzan P, Lang S, et al: Recurrence of curetted and bone-grafted giant-cell tumours with and without adjuvant phenol therapy. Eur J Surg Oncol 2001;27(2):200–202.
85. Haskell A, Wodowoz O, Johnston JO: Metachronous multicentric giant cell tumor: A case report and literature review. Clin Orthop 2003;412:162–168.
86. Glanzmann C, Horst W: [The place of radiation therapy in the treatment of giant cell tumors of bone (osteoclastomas): results from 32 cases (author's transl)]. Strahlentherapie 1978;154(2):81–84.
87. Stewart DJ, Belanger R, Benjamin RS: Prolonged disease-free survival following surgical debulking and high-dose cisplatin/doxorubicin in a patient with bulky metastases from giant cell tumor of bone refractory to "standard" chemotherapy. Am J Clin Oncol 1995;18(2):144–148.
88. Yamamoto M, Fukushima T, Sakamoto S, Tomonaga M: Giant cell tumor of the sphenoid bone: Long-term follow-up of two cases after chemotherapy. Surg Neurol 1998;49(5):547–552.

CHAPTER 50

DEAN CHOU
FRANK ACOSTA, JR.
DARREN B. SCHNEIDER
CURTIS A. DICKMAN

Secondary Metastatic Tumors of the Spine

RECENT DATA ON METASTATIC SPINE TUMORS

An important study, yet to be published as of this writing, was presented in abstract form at the annual meeting of the American Society of Clinical Oncology in June 2003.[1] Directed by senior author Roy Patchell, the results of this prospective, randomized, multi-institutional trial of surgery followed by radiation versus radiation alone in the treatment of spinal metastases were promising. Given the dearth of class I data in the spine literature, it represents a much-needed report that will likely be cited often and that will probably change the management paradigm for metastatic spine tumors.

The study included adults with known metastatic cancer to the spine, spinal cord compression, an MRI-demonstrated surgically accessible epidural lesion, at least one sign or symptom, and an expected survival time longer than 3 months. They excluded patients who were younger than 18 years; had previous radiation; had paraplegia longer than 48 hours; and who had primary spinal tumors, leukemia, multiple myelomas, germ cell tumors, or lymphomas. Patients were randomized to one of two arms. The surgical arm included decompression and stabilization within 24 hours of study enrollment followed by 30 Gy of radiation within 14 days of surgery. The radiation arm began within 24 hours of study enrollment and delivered 30 Gy of radiation in 10 fractionated doses. One hundred one patients were enrolled (50 in the surgery with radiation arm and 51 in the radiation alone arm).

The study was stopped at the midpoint of the trial after predetermined stopping criteria were met. In the surgical arm, the median time of ambulation was 126 days compared to 35 days in the radiation arm ($p = 0.006$). Of the 32 patients who presented as nonambulatory, 9 of 16 (56%) patients in the surgical arm regained the ability to walk compared to only 3 of 16 (19%) in the radiation alone arm ($p = 0.03$). In the surgical arm, American Spinal Injury Association (ASIA) scores and Frankel grades were maintained a median of 566 days compared to 72 days in the radiation arm ($p = 0.03$, $p = 0.01$, respectively). The median length of continence was 142 days in the surgical arm compared to 12 days in the radiation arm ($p = 0.009$). The mean daily dose of steroids (dexamethasone) was 1.6 mg in the surgical arm compared to 4.2 mg in the radiation arm ($p = 0.009$), and the mean daily morphine equivalent dose was 0.4 mg in the surgical arm and 4.8 mg in the radiation arm ($p = 0.002$). There was no statistically significant difference in length of survival, but there was a trend toward longer survival times in the surgical arm compared to the radiation arm (129 days versus 100 days, $p = 0.08$).

This report shows very promising results for role of the surgical management of metastatic spine tumors. Earlier data had questioned the benefit of surgery compared to that of radiation. However, most earlier data compared decompression via laminectomy to radiation. More recent advances in spinal instrumentation, 360-degree spinal access, and spinal reconstruction have afforded more aggressive tumor removal and better stabilization. Although these data are still preliminary, the future role of aggressive surgical intervention in extending the quality of life in patients with metastatic disease appears to be promising.

INTRODUCTION

Metastatic disease to the spine remains problematic, and its incidence in the aging population continues to challenge spine surgeons. As surgeons become more facile with spinal instrumentation in all regions of the spine and with the increased availability of neurologic monitoring and neuroanesthesia, the surgery will play an increasingly important role in the treatment of metastatic disease. Quality of life has been the main thrust for the argument of aggressive treatment of spinal metastases. Earlier reports in the literature have suggested, but not shown definitively, a benefit with surgery. However, as prospective, randomized data emerge supporting the role of surgery over radiation, the algorithm for the treatment of spinal metastases will begin to shift toward surgical treatment, depending on the tumor type. Patient selection and patient expectations are critical in deciding who should undergo surgical resection and spinal reconstruction.

INCIDENCE

Breast and prostate cancer dominate the incidence of spinal metastases. The former is the principal source in women and the latter in men. In 2000, there were an estimated 182,100 new cases of breast cancer and an estimated 180,400 new cases of prostate cancer. Lung and colorectal cancer also are significant sources of spinal metastases. In 2000 there were 164,100 new cases of lung cancer and 130,200 new cases of colorectal cancer. Although fewer renal cell cancers (31,200 new cases in 2000) occur compared to the aforementioned cancers, they still represent metastatic challenges. Thyroid and bladder cancer also can metastasize to the spine (with 18,400 and 53,200 new cases in 2000, respectively), although less often than other neoplasms. Gastric cancer, at 21,500 new cases per year, is associated with such short survival periods that symptoms from spinal metastases usually do not manifest before death.[2]

PRESENTATION

Pain is the most common symptom. Axial back pain may be insidious, and the initial differential diagnosis may not place metastatic disease high on the list. Patients may complain of pain at night. Gokaslan and associates found that 90% of patients who presented with metastatic spine disease at M.D. Anderson Cancer Center presented with pain.[3] Patients' histories may include minor trauma; however, a temporal relationship between trauma and onset of pain is not always clear. The pain is usually focal and relentless, regardless of position or activity.[4]

Neurologic manifestations can also occur. Gokaslan and associates found that 64% of patients with metastatic spine disease presented with lower extremity weakness.[3] Gilbert and associates found that 82% of patients with spinal metastases presented with motor weakness or sensory changes.[5] Bach and associates, however, reviewed 398 patients with spinal cord compression and found that 67% presented with gait disturbances and 48% with urinary retention.[4] Helweg-Larsen and Sorensen found that the neurologic manifestations were (in decreasing order of frequency) radicular pain, motor weakness, sensory dysfunction, and bladder dysfunction.[6]

CLINICAL EVALUATION

A thorough history and physical examination are essential. The onset of symptoms can provide critical information about the nature of spinal involvement. For instance, patients who present with only spinal pain may have vertebral body disease with minimal or no epidural compression. Patients who present with the sudden onset of pain and acute neurologic symptoms may have had a pathologic fracture related to bony destruction. If patients present with an insidious onset of pain, difficulty ambulating, or bowel and bladder problems, epidural compression by the tumor could be the cause of such symptoms. An acute onset of painless paraparesis also may be attributed to a vascular origin. Moreover, the timing of the onset of symptoms would guide surgical decision making.

The physical examination can yield considerable information during an evaluation for metastatic spine disease. Distribution of pain or sensory levels can indicate the spinal regions to focus radiographic studies. Motor weakness is helpful not only in diagnosing the type of compression—either spinal cord or nerve root—but also in determining whether urgent surgery is warranted. Hyperreflexia and loss of rectal tone can be indicative of a compressive spinal cord lesion. Urinary retention or high postvoid residual urine can be indicative of spinal cord dysfunction related to compression. Focal back pain to palpation also can help elucidate the level of disease. The physical examination can yield both neurologic localization of the tumor and an understanding of the neurologic dysfunction caused by the tumor.

RADIOGRAPHIC STUDIES

Radiographic evaluation begins with plain radiographs, which may or may not show a broad overview of the process. Bony destruction and spinal alignment can be seen if grossly abnormal. Moreover, they can demonstrate soft tissue involvement if the metastatic lesion is large. The cost and time needed to obtain plain x-rays are minimal. The yield can be quite significant not only in demonstrating the overall process but also in localizing where further studies should be performed.

Computed tomography (CT) is very useful in evaluating the extent of bony destruction within the vertebral bodies. CT not only can show the extent of the disease but also can guide the extent of postresection instrumentation. Two-dimensional reconstructions with CT help delineate sagittal alignment or bony destruction that may be poorly visualized on plain radiographs. CT with two-dimensional reconstructions is very useful in guiding surgery and postresection stabilization. If multiple metastases are present, CT may show the extent of bony destruction in levels in which instrumentation will be placed. Consequently, more levels that do not have bony involvement may need to be instrumented. Coupled with myelographic contrast, a myelogram-CT helps evaluate spinal cord or nerve root compression. Because CT myelography is invasive, it should be used only if magnetic resonance imaging (MRI) is precluded or yields insufficient information. Because CT demonstrates bony anatomy very well, it is a complementary examination to MRI. Colman and associates evaluated 15 patients with both MRI and CT and found that CT detected tumor in 14 of 15 patients, whereas MRI detected tumor in all 15.[7] Although CT may not be as sensitive as MRI in detecting metastases, it nonetheless plays an important role in evaluating bone integrity and damage.

MRI of the spine is invaluable, not only to detect metastases but also to show the extent of soft tissue involvement or spinal cord compression. Moreover, MRI offers tremendous sensitivity with minimal invasiveness (intravenous injection of gadolinium). Sze found that MRI was as accurate as CT-myelography in detecting the extent of tumor within the spinal canal.[8] Algra and associates found that MRI was more sensitive than bone scans by almost 50%.[9] Chadwick and associates demonstrated that MRI showed urologic metastases in 7 of 66 patients who otherwise had normal bone scans or plain radiographs.[10] Thus, because of its extreme sensitivity and its limited invasiveness, MRI should be used when trying to rule out spinal metastases.

Although bone scanning may be useful as a broad screening tool, it does have shortcomings. Mehta and associates reported a completely negative bone scan in a patient with extensive metastatic disease of the bone and bone marrow.[11] In the spine, MRI may be more useful and sensitive in detecting metastatic disease than a bone scan. Gosfield and associates evaluated 35 patients who had known metastatic disease with both bone scans and MRI within 2 months. Of 69 lesions detected by MRI, only 63 were detected by bone scan. Moreover, no patients with entirely positive bone scans were negative on MRI, but one patient who was entirely positive on MRI was negative on a bone scan.[12]

ROLE OF PERCUTANEOUS BIOPSY

Many institutions begin their evaluation of metastatic spine disease with a percutaneous needle biopsy. The yield of such procedures varies from institution to institution. Many believe that it is a reasonable first step given the limited morbidity associated with the procedure and its relative ease to perform. The published rates of diagnosis vary. Pierot and Boulin noted an 89% yield with percutaneous biopsy; Kattapuram and associates demonstrated an overall yield of 92%; and Ghelman and associates noted an 86% yield.[13-15] The yield, however, depends on the technical execution of the procedure. If insufficient material is removed or if the needle is not placed within the lesion, false-negative findings are likely. A biopsy is unnecessary for obvious known metastases or lesions causing acute symptomatic compression of the spinal cord requiring urgent surgery. Overall, however, it is reasonable to begin the diagnostic evaluation with a percutaneous biopsy to identify metastatic spine disease if no primary lesion has been established.

SURGICAL DECISION MAKING

Unlike other pathologies of the spine, metastatic cancer warrants discussion with patients and their families to delineate their expectations, the goals of surgery, the end points of rehabilitation, and overall length of survival. To date, no prospective randomized trial has demonstrated an increased survival rate associated with surgery. Patient and family expectations should be realistic. The goals of surgery, which are to treat pain, to preserve ambulation, to extend the time of bowel and bladder continence, and to prevent or correct a spinal deformity, should be emphasized. The overall prognosis of the patient also should be considered.

In patients expecting fairly long survival times, quality of life becomes an issue. Patients with breast and prostate cancer can survive quite long, and maintaining ambulation becomes a priority. Prostate and breast cancers are typical examples of tumors with fairly long survival times. Gastric cancer and sarcomas may warrant only palliative nonsurgical treatment. Discussion with the family should emphasize that surgery is not risk free and that paralysis can occur if untoward events occur intraoperatively. Moreover, preoperative functional status should be considered. Surgery in patients with many comorbidities and a poor functional status is unlikely to yield satisfactory results. Even with surgery, a complete recovery cannot be guaranteed. In a retrospective series, Rompe and associates showed that 35 of 56 patients with neurologic deficits recovered completely or partially within the first 3 months of surgery.[16] Thus, patient and family expectations must be realistic, and discussion of the goals of surgery should be emphasized.

A patient's preoperative neurologic status is an important consideration because the pretreatment status determines posttreatment status. Moreover, if patients present with a complete loss of motor and sensory function, they are seldom candidates for decompression.

EMBOLIZATION

Preoperative embolization may be useful, especially for vascular tumors. In particular, resecting metastatic renal cell cancer can lead to tremendous blood loss. Manke and associates evaluated blood loss in patients undergoing metastatic renal cell resection. Patients who had undergone preoperative embolization lost an average of 1500 mL of blood compared to the control group, which lost an average of 5000 mL.[17] In patients with vascular metastatic spine tumors, Gellad and associates found that those who underwent embolization had an average estimated blood loss of 1850 mL compared to an average of 3500 mL in those who did not.[18] Olerud and associates also found that preoperative embolization reduced blood loss.[19] Although embolization may not necessarily reduce blood loss in all cases, most authors advocate its use preoperatively if the metastatic lesion is expected to be highly vascular.

THORACIC LESIONS

When deciding whether to approach a lesion anteriorly or posteriorly, many factors must be considered. Usually, the site of disease dictates the approach, but this rule is not universally true. If an anterior approach would involve more morbidity than a posterior approach, the less morbid approach often should be undertaken if neither structural nor sagittal alignment is compromised. For instance, to perform a vertebrectomy and plating from the front for a lesion at T3 would involve a median sternotomy with dissection and retraction of the innominate vein. The same operation could be performed posteriorly via a transpedicular corpectomy. The major associated morbidity would be sacrifice of a T3 nerve root. Other considerations would be the amount of kyphotic deformity present and the loss of vertebral height. In patients with a major loss of vertebral height and a kyphotic deformity, an anterior approach usually restores more height and corrects the kyphosis at that level better than a posterior approach. The location of the great vessels and viscera also must be considered, especially in the high thoracic spine where the aorta usually sits directly over an entry approach on the left side. Sometimes anterior and posterior approaches must be combined. The factors used to decide the best approach include the number of levels destabilized, bone purchase, the potential for pseudarthrosis, sagittal balance, and compliance with external orthosis.

ANTERIOR APPROACHES

In general, anterior approaches to the thoracic spine involve a thoracotomy with possible elevation of the scapula or splitting of the diaphragm. At times, a median sternotomy or manubrial resection may be necessary. Based on body habitus, T1 is usually accessible from a standard neck incision. At T2 and T3, a median sternotomy can provide access; however, the innominate vein can be in the way and usually needs to be retracted. At T4 to T5, a thoracotomy can be used; however, the scapula usually must be elevated to access the area. From T6 to T12, a standard thoracotomy typically can be performed. To instrument onto L1 for a T12 corpectomy, however, the diaphragm may need to be split. Because of the sloping nature of the ribs, a rib two levels above is usually chosen to be removed. In the higher thoracic levels (T4-T6), a rib one level above may be removed to achieve adequate access.

In the standard thoracotomy, preoperative fluoroscopy is used to help localize the proper level. The rib two levels above the level of interest is palpated, and an incision line is drawn over that rib (Fig. 50-1). The area is prepared and draped, and an incision is made over the rib of interest (Fig. 50-2).

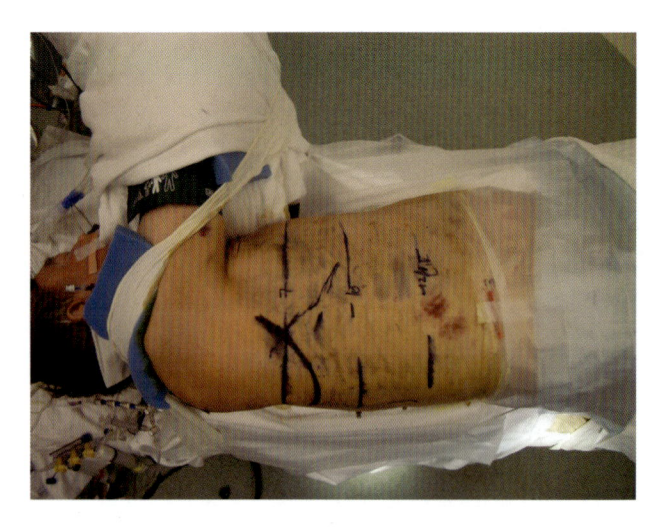

Fig. 50-1 Patient positioning for a right T5 thoracotomy. Note preoperative markings localized with fluoroscopy.

A hand may be placed underneath the scapula to palpate the second rib. Manual counting may be performed to confirm the proper level (Fig. 50-3). Once the appropriate rib is confirmed, the soft tissue and muscle are dissected using bovie cauterization. The soft tissue is dissected off the rib using the bovie device (Fig. 50-4). Extreme care is exerted to avoid violating the neurovascular bundle beneath the rib.

Once the superficial surface of the rib is exposed, the periosteum is carefully dissected off using the Alexander-Farabeuf periosteotome (Fig. 50-5). The undersurface of the rib is dissected. Circumferential dissection may be performed with the Doyen dissector (Fig. 50-6). The dissection should proceed fairly far posteriorly because most of the posterior rib must be removed to expose the spine. A general rule is to dissect the rib proximally until it becomes perpendicular to the operating table. A rib cutter is used to cut the rib at two

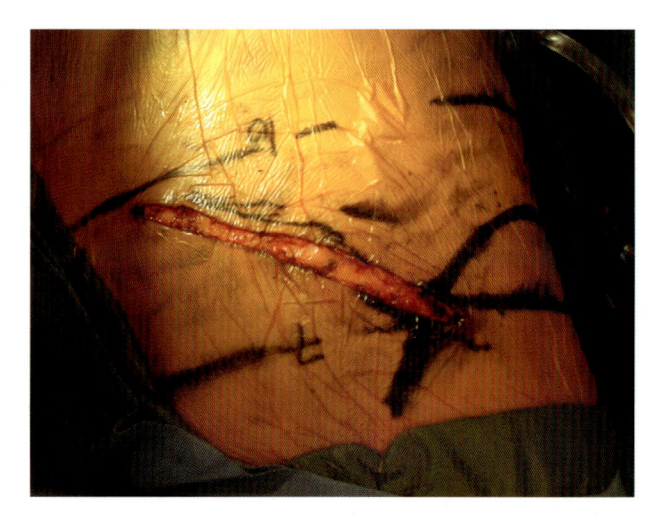

Fig. 50-2 Skin incision is made over the T5 rib.

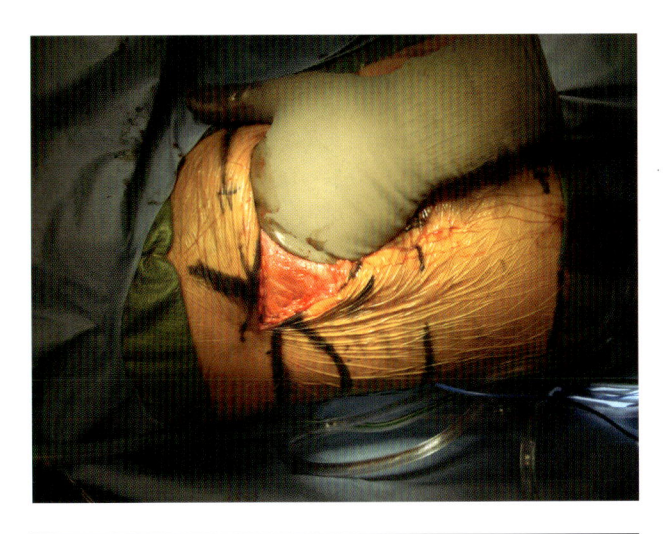

CHAPTER 50   Secondary Metastatic Tumors of the Spine

Fig. 50-3 A hand is placed underneath the scapula, and the ribs are counted from the top down. The most cephalad rib that can usually be palpated is T2.

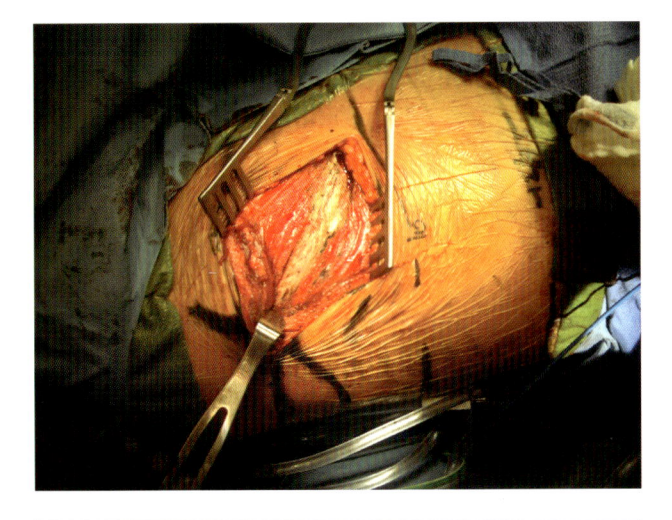

Fig. 50-4 After muscular dissection has taken place, the rib is exposed.

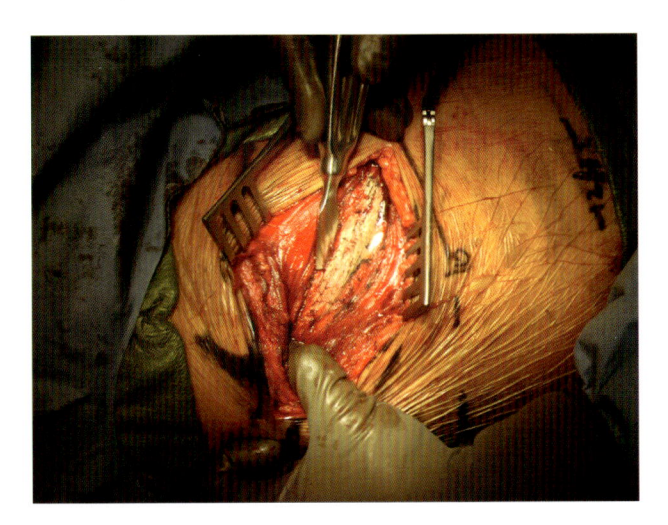

Fig. 50-5 The intercostal muscles are dissected using the Alexander periosteal dissector.

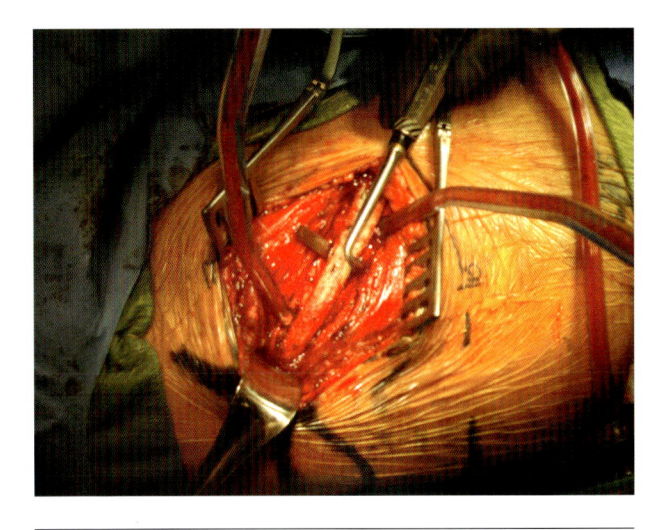

Fig. 50-6 The rib is dissected away from the parietal pleura using the Doyan dissector.

places, ensuring that the opening is wide enough for adequate exposure (Fig. 50-7). The rib is saved for arthrodesis.

The ipsilateral lung is deflated, and the parietal pleura is opened using Metzenbaum scissors (Fig. 50-8). The lung must not be damaged on entry. Adhesions may be present, especially in cancer patients who may have had a chronic inflammatory response. Adhesions should be removed, and any large pulmonary openings may be closed using 5-0 prolene. The Finochietto rib spreader is placed and spread until adequate access is obtained. Care must be taken not to break adjacent ribs, and the retractor should be opened slowly (Figs. 50-9 and 50-10).

After the lung is retracted out of the way, the parietal pleura that covers the spine needs to be dissected. In neoplastic processes, the parietal pleura may be inflamed and thickened, obscuring normal anatomy. Particularly obese

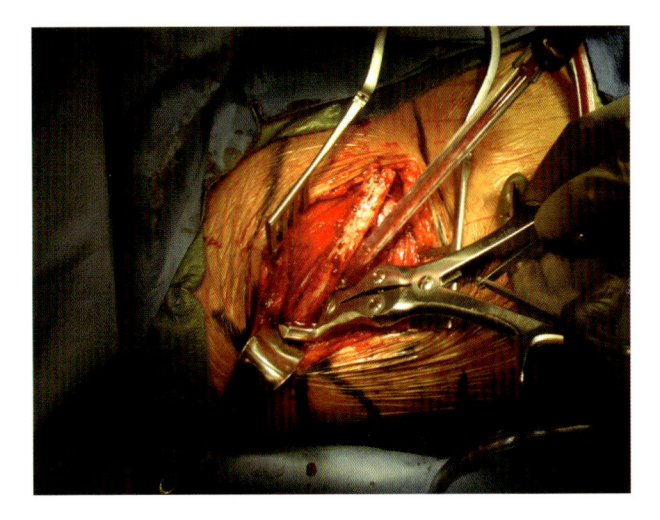

Fig. 50-7 The T5 rib is cut at both ends using a rib cutter.

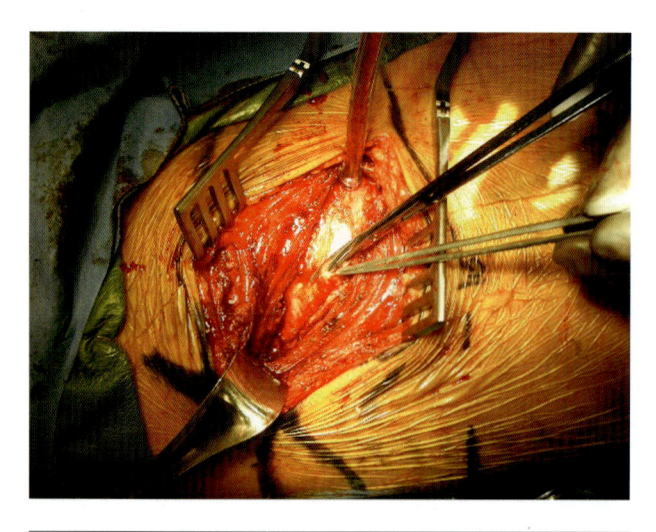

Fig. 50-8 The parietal pleura is divided using Metzenbaum scissors. Extreme care is taken to avoid the lung parenchyma, especially in cases in which pulmonary adhesions are present.

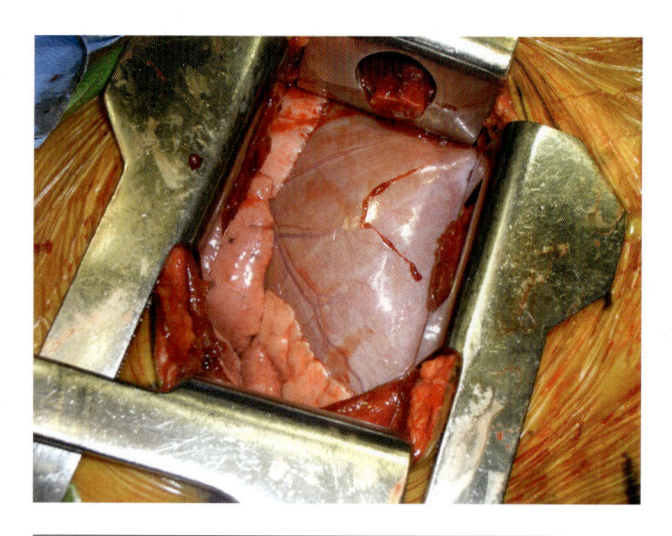

Fig. 50-10 The diaphragm is seen at the inferior aspect of the thoracotomy.

individuals also may have large layers of fat that increase the difficulty of dissection. The parietal pleura is dissected laterally. Care must be taken not to violate the segmental vessels while the parietal pleura is being dissected. After the parietal pleura is dissected laterally, it can be held out of the way with hooks or sutures (Fig. 50-11).

The segmental vessels are identified at the level of the lesion and at the vertebral bodies above and below. The segmental vessels can be clipped or ligated using silk suture and subsequently transected. Ligating the segmental vessel in the middle of the vertebral body rather than closer to the foramen increases collateral blood flow. Theoretically, the incidence of spinal cord ischemia will thereby decrease. The segmental vessels in the vertebral bodies above and below are also ligated in similar fashion.

Once the vertebral body's segmental vessels have been ligated, the next critical step is to identify the head of the rib (Figs. 50-12 and 50-13). Once identified, it usually defines the disk interspace and pedicle. For instance, a T7 rib articulates with the T6-T7 interspace and T7 pedicle. The head of the rib is identified and resected with rongeurs, a drill, or a bone cutter to reveal the pedicle. Once the pedicle is identified, it can be traced to the neural foramen, which is directly underneath the pedicle. A small, blunt dissector such as a

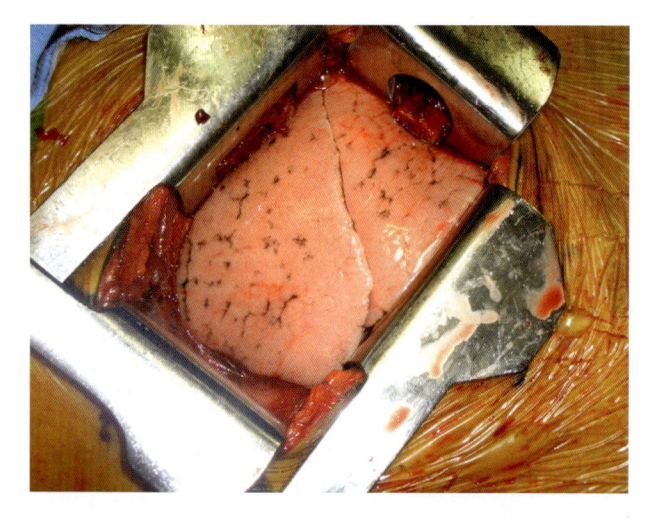

Fig. 50-9 After the parietal pleura is dissected, the lung comes into view. The Finochietto thoracotomy retractor is placed to retract the ribs. In this case, two Finochietto retractors are used for maximal exposure.

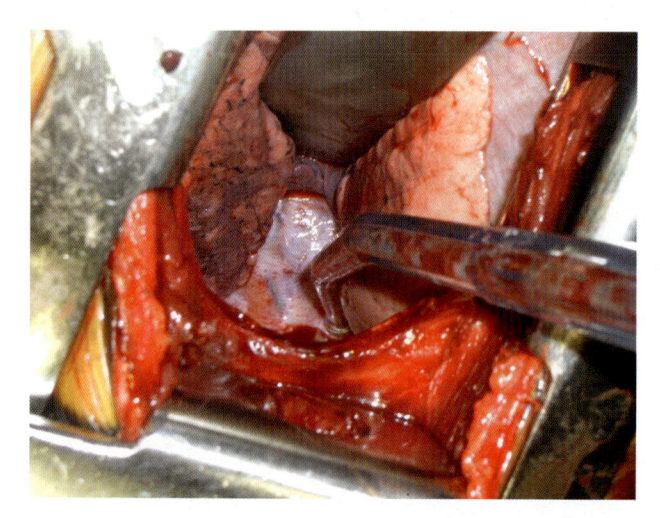

Fig. 50-11 After the ipsilateral lung is deflated via the dual-lumen endotracheal tube, the lung and diaphragm can be gently retracted using a malleable retractor. The retractor can be held in place to the Finochietto by a Kocher or other clamp.

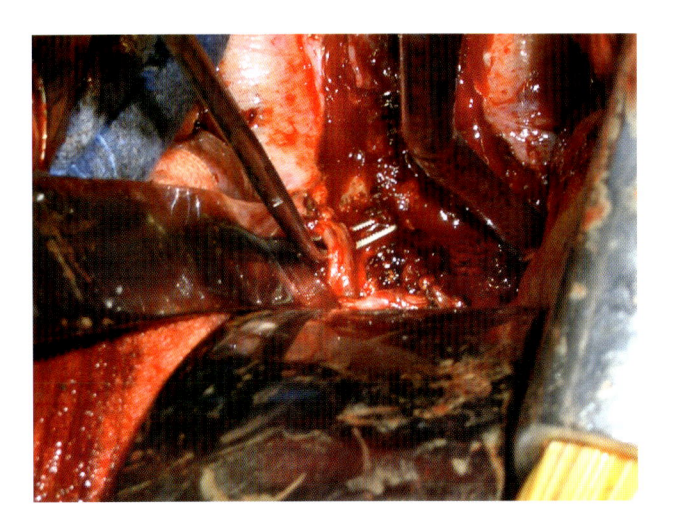

CHAPTER 50 Secondary Metastatic Tumors of the Spine

Fig. 50-12 The segmental vessels are identified and dissected away from the vertebral bodies.

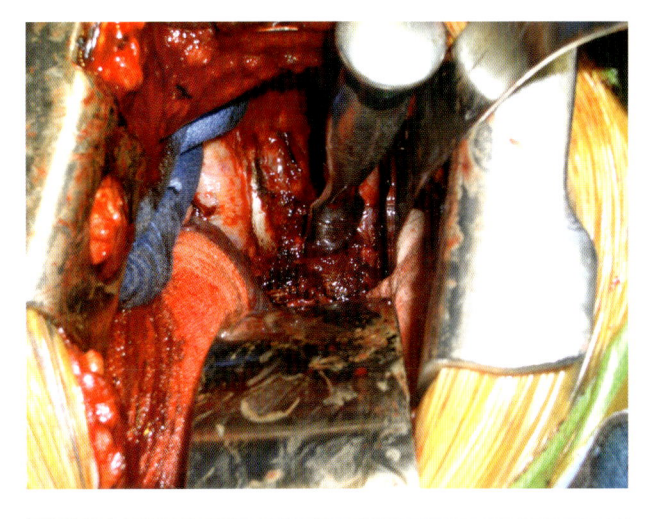

Fig. 50-14 The corpectomy is performed using a combination of osteotomes and high-speed burrs. Here is shown an osteotome in the vertebral body of T6 to begin the corpectomy.

Penfield No. 4 can be used to palpate the neural foramen. Once identified, the foramen can be used as a landmark for the spinal canal before the corpectomy is begun. Because the spinal canal is curved, the foramen can be slightly posterior to the anterior aspect of the spinal cord. The surgeon should be cognizant of this configuration while removing the posterior cortex of the vertebral body. Using monopolar cauterization, the superior and inferior end plates of the vertebral body also should be defined. The disk spaces and end plates of the adjacent vertebral bodies should be visualized.

Resection of the vertebral body begins with osteotomes (Fig. 50-14). Because the spinal canal has been identified, osteotomes allow large amounts of vertebral body to be resected quickly. Before cutting with the osteotomes begins, the anterior longitudinal ligament is divided away from the anterior aspect of the vertebral body using monopolar cauterization. The surgeon must remain directly on the bone without violating the soft tissue adjacent to the aorta. This maneuver separates the aortic tissue from the spine. Another option is to remove the disks before or after the corpectomy. Some surgeons find it easier to remove the vertebral body after the disks have been removed, and some find that the disks provide cushions for drilling the vertebral end plate.

Next, the osteotome is used to divide much of the anterior vertebral body from the posterior cortex. Two cuts are made cephalad and caudad (unnecessary if the disks have been removed first). A large wedge of vertebral body can be removed by gently angling the osteotome away from the spinal canal. Extreme care should be exerted to avoid violating the ligament anteriorly or contralaterally. The aorta sits anteriorly, and violation of the contralateral ligament can cause a contralateral pneumothorax, an obviously undesirable complication with one-lung ventilation. The ipsilateral lung can be inflated and retracted if necessary to maintain oxygen saturation.

After osteotomes have been used to remove large sections of the vertebral body, the remainder of the bone and neoplasm is removed with a high-speed burr. We prefer to use the Midas Rex drill with an AM8 drill bit (Medtronic Corporation, Minneapolis, MN). A diamond burr also may be used in neoplastic processes because the heat it generates has hemostatic activity. Moreover, diamond burrs tend to be safer if the drill inadvertently slips or kicks. The cutting burrs are perhaps the most dangerous drill bit because an inadvertent slip into the thecal sac or great vessels can instantly cause a devastating injury.

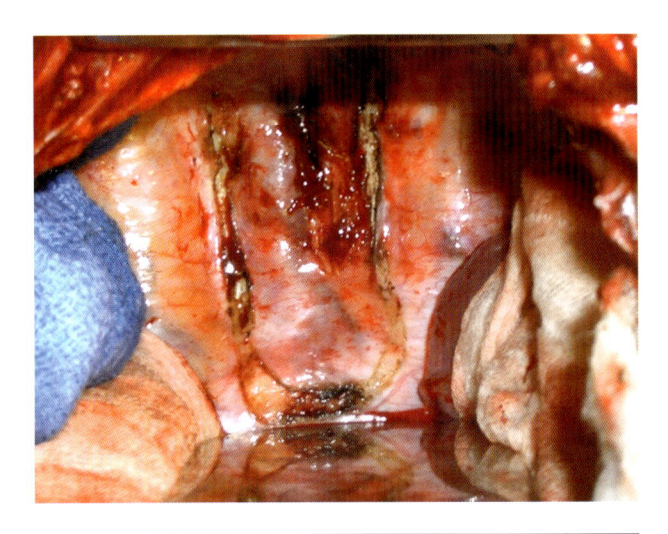

Fig. 50-13 The heads of the ribs are identified, and an intraoperative x-ray is taken to localize the level. After localization is confirmed, a small window in the parietal pleura is opened.

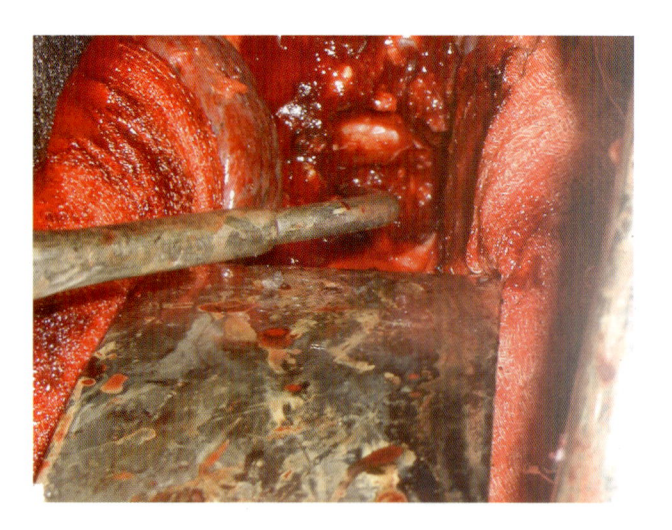

Fig. 50-15 After the corpectomy has been performed, the dura is completely decompressed and visualized.

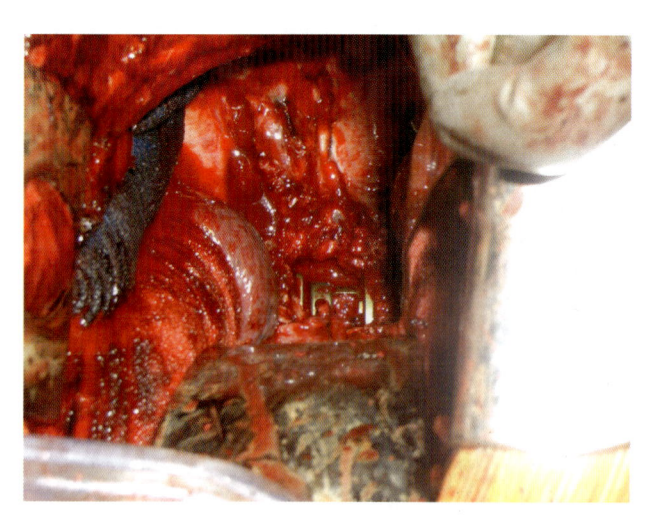

Fig. 50-16 A titanium cage or other structural graft may be placed to reconstruct the anterior column.

Because the location of the spinal canal is already known, resection can continue by drilling away the pedicle and posterior cortex of the vertebral body. Once the posterior cortex is paper thin, an up-angled curette is used to gently tease bone and tumor away from the spinal cord. The posterior longitudinal ligament also must be removed to decompress the spinal cord adequately. Because the spinal cord is usually under compression, large instruments should not be insinuated between it and the vertebral body (Fig. 50-15).

After the posterior longitudinal ligament has been removed and the spinal cord has been decompressed, the end plates must be prepared to receive the graft or cage. The cartilaginous end plates are removed using curettes. Any remnant of the superior or inferior end plate of the resected vertebral body must be drilled smooth to help accommodate the strut graft. Not too much of the end plates should be destroyed because they will provide the structural support after the graft has been placed. An appropriately sized allograft or cage can be used (Fig. 50-16). In cases with severe height loss and kyphosis, the Synex expandable cage (Synthes Spine, Paoli, PA) can be used to restore the height and to correct kyphosis. The cage can be filled with autograft from the rib removed for the thoracotomy. Given its cancerous nature, vertebrectomy bone should be sent for pathologic evaluation and not used for fusion. Intraoperative anteroposterior and lateral fluoroscopy should be obtained to assess the position of the graft. The graft or cage must not extend into the spinal canal or laterally beyond the end plate.

Once the strut graft or cage has been placed, the anterior aspects of the vertebral bodies must be prepared to accept anterior segmental instrumentation. Manual palpation of the contours of the vertebral bodies is an excellent method to determine whether the plate will sit flush. It is often necessary to remove the rib heads of the inferior vertebral body and part of the superior vertebral body with a high-speed burr or rongeurs. Osteophytic ridges at the end plates also need to be flattened to accommodate the plate. We prefer to use the Vantage anterior thoracolumbar plate (Medtronic Corporation, Minneapolis, MN) (Fig. 50-17).

To use a two-screw construct, preoperative planning is vital to determine the appropriate length of screws needed. Moreover, the shape of the vertebral bodies in the thoracic spine is ovoid to heart-shaped. Therefore, the dimensions of the vertebral bodies at the waist can differ significantly from those at the end plates. The width of the vertebral body at the level of screw placement, which usually corresponds to

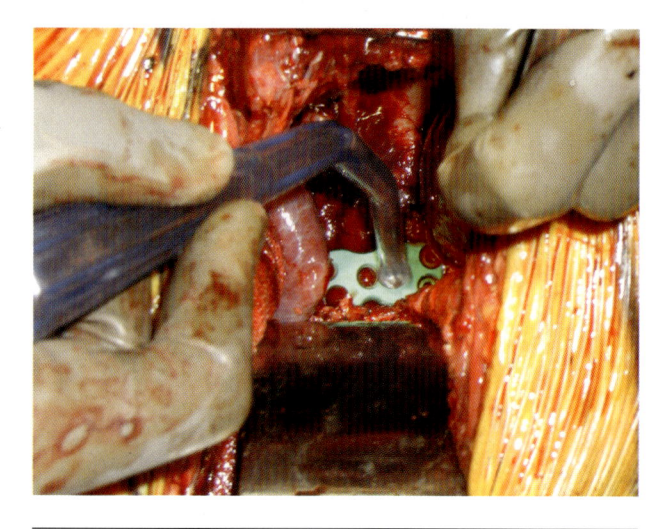

Fig. 50-17 An anterior plate or dual-rod construct may be placed for stabilization. Shown here is an anterior titanium thoracolumbar plate.

the waist of the vertebral body, should be measured carefully. If posterior pedicle screw fixation is planned at a later stage, placement of the screws below the level of the pedicle avoids creating an impediment to placement of the pedicle screw.

Once the appropriate screw length has been determined and the vertebral bodies are prepared for placement of the plate, the proximal entry points must be placed exactly parallel with the plane of the spinal canal to avoid violating the posterior cortex. The second screw is placed from an anterior entry point and angled slightly toward the spinal canal. Preoperative CT planning of the angle and length of the trajectory should afford good placement of the screw without violating the posterior cortex. After the screws have been placed, the plate may be placed with compression for load sharing with the graft. Again, intraoperative fluoroscopy should be used to assess the placement of the screws to ensure that the posterior cortex has not been violated and that the contralateral cortical protrusion is barely bicortical (if bicortical screws are used).

At this point the wound should be irrigated copiously and hemostasis obtained. The pleural flap may be used to cover the hardware to provide a smooth surface for the lung to contact. However, the pleura is often atretic and dehydrated after the procedure, and this maneuver is impractical. Chest tubes are left in the standard fashion. Usually, one chest tube can be left in the surgical bed and one at the apex of the lung. The choice, however, depends on the surgeon's preference. In the event of a durotomy during the procedure, the chest tubes should not be left to suction—only to water seal. Moreover, a lumbar drain should be placed to facilitate dural sealing in the thoracic spine. The lung is re-expanded by the anesthesiologist, and it should be observed for any obvious rents. Small tears can be closed with 5-0 prolene suture. The chest wall is closed with No. 2 interrupted Vicryl sutures. The muscles are closed in layers, usually with No. 0 Vicryl running sutures. The skin is stapled closed. The muscle closure is airtight to prevent a nonhealing pneumothorax from developing.

HIGH POSTEROLATERAL THORACOTOMY

For thoracic lesions that require a high posterolateral thoracotomy, the scapula must be elevated to access the rib. The scapula is separated from the latissimus dorsi. A plane can be developed manually between subscapularis and the chest wall. A scapula retractor is used, and a standard thoracotomy is performed.

MEDIAN STERNOTOMY/MANUBRIUMECTOMY

It is difficult to gain full access to lesions in the T1-T3 region through a posterolateral thoracotomy. A median sternotomy or manubriumectomy may have to be performed. The innominate vein needs to be retracted inferiorly. Extreme care must be exerted to prevent damage to the recurrent laryngeal nerve.

THORACOLUMBAR JUNCTION

At the thoracolumbar junction, the diaphragm becomes an important consideration. The crus of the diaphragm normally inserts on the inferior aspect of the body T12. The psoas inserts about L1-T12. Because it is sometimes necessary to span the thoracolumbar junction with instrumentation or with the corpectomy itself, the diaphragm must be split to allow access to the vertebral bodies. Usually, a T10 thoracotomy allows access for placing instrumentation at L2. We prefer to split the diaphragm completely up to the rib cage, reattaching the costal margin at the end of the procedure. Some surgeons split the diaphragm partially and leave the inferior aspect of the rib cage intact. Splitting the diaphragm requires leaving a 1- to 2-cm cuff to allow closure.

After the corpectomy and reconstruction have been performed, the diaphragm is closed using a running No. 0 prolene suture. A chest tube is typically inserted. Closure of the chest is similar to a standard thoracotomy except that the T11 and T12 ribs are floating. Therefore, tight fascial and muscle closures are critical.

POSTERIOR APPROACHES

Some thoracic metastatic lesions—usually involving the vertebral body rather than the posterior elements—can realistically be approached posteriorly. For instance, if most of the lesion is centered to one side, associated comorbidities would make a thoracotomy extremely dangerous. Lesions centered on T2-T4 would be difficult to access via a standard posterolateral thoracotomy. Such lesions would require decompression and vertebrectomy from a posterior approach.

A transpedicular corpectomy can be performed for a posterior corpectomy and subsequent reconstruction. The thoracic spine should be exposed in the standard fashion. If there is severe compression of the spinal cord, a decompressive laminectomy first should be performed over the affected levels to relieve any pressure immediately. Thoracic pedicle screws should be placed above and below the level of the corpectomy. With a high-speed burr, the pedicles on each side are drilled down into the vertebral body while tumor and bone are removed along the path. Once a cavity has been fashioned, a thoracic nerve root can be ligated and transected. The nerve root must be ligated securely to avoid cerebrospinal fluid leakage. It is usually advantageous to ligate the nerve root on the side ipsilateral to the patient's pain; this strategy addresses radicular pain. For levels lower than T1, the nerve root can be ligated with minimal morbidity (Fig. 50-18).

After the nerve root has been removed, further access into the corpectomy site is obtained. Tumor, bone, and ligament adjacent to the anterior thoracic cord can be pushed gently

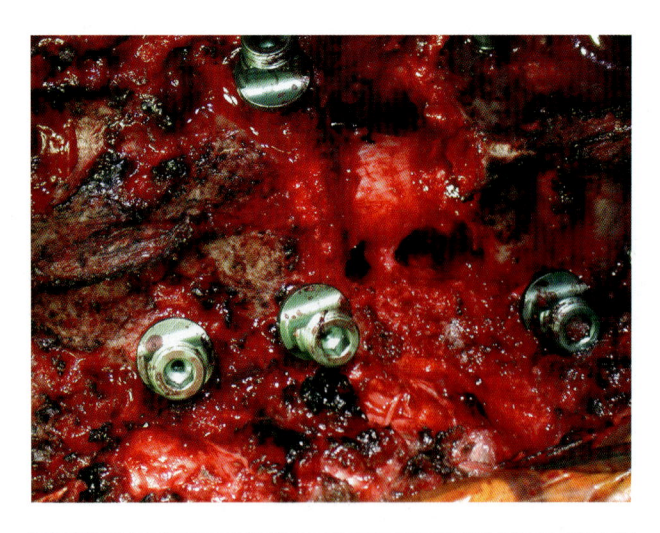

Fig. 50-18 Transpedicular corpectomy for metastatic breast cancer. Note unilateral removal of nerve root.

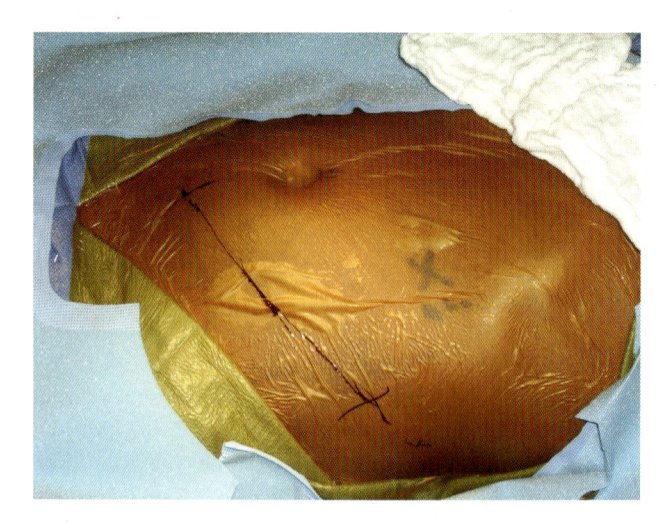

Fig. 50-19 A left-side anterior retroperitoneal approach is planned for performing corpectomies at L4-L5. A straight supine position is chosen to facilitate placement of anterior column support.

away from the spinal cord using a down-going curette into the corpectomy cavity. This maneuver allows full decompression of the spinal cord. The disks are removed using curettes to prepare either end plate. Two Steinmann pins are placed above and below into each vertebral body to secure methylmethacrylate. The pins are clamped using needle drivers, and pins are driven into the bone by gentle tapping with a mallet. With the pins in place, the methylmethacrylate is carefully poured into the corpectomy defect. No methylmethacrylate should touch the dura. Using a Penfield dissector, the surgeon can gently push away any methylmethacrylate inadvertently contacting the dura.

Once the anterior column has been reconstructed with the methylmethacrylate, the posterior rods can be placed and locked to the screws. Because the facets of the thoracic spine have been removed by laminectomy, arthrodesis is needed to transverse the corpectomy. The facets at the levels above and below should be intact, and arthrodesis can be performed there properly. The wound is closed in the standard fashion.

LUMBAR LESIONS

For lesions at L1, we prefer the aforementioned approach at the thoracolumbar junction. It not only provides access to L2, but it also provides access for the placement of the T12 screw because the rib cage is opened superiorly. For lesions at L2 to L4, a lateral retroperitoneal approach can be used. At L5, either a standard retroperitoneal approach or a paramedian retroperitoneal approach can be used. Posterior transpedicular approaches also can be used (see earlier discussion).

ANTERIOR APPROACH

The retroperitoneal dissection involves a flank incision, usually on the left side (Fig. 50-19). We prefer the left because the spleen protrudes less into the field than the liver. The external oblique, internal oblique, and transversus abdominus muscles are divided (Fig. 50-20). Retroperitoneal fat is reached posteriorly. Blunt dissection with sponge sticks is used to develop the retroperitoneal space. The peritoneum, its contents, and the ureter are swept anteriorly. Extreme care must be taken to avoid injuring the peritoneum or ureter. Peristalsis can often be seen within the ureter. Rents in the peritoneum can be repaired using a 3-0 Vicryl suture (Figs. 50-21 to 50-23).

The psoas muscle is identified, and its anterior border is dissected (Fig. 50-24). Bovie cauterization is used to dissect

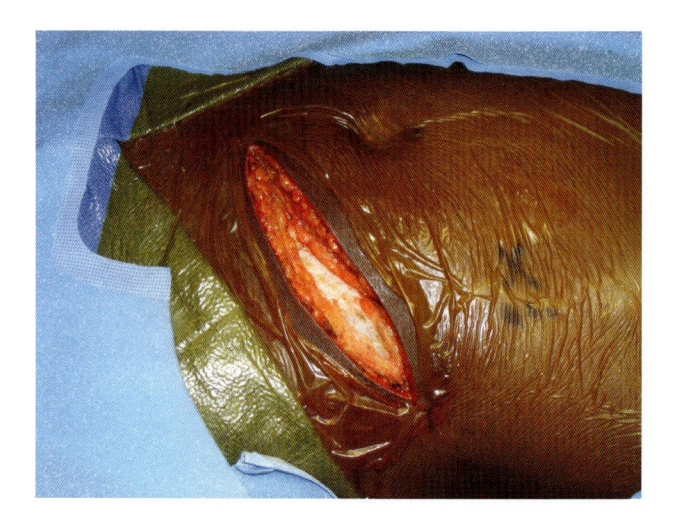

Fig. 50-20 After opening the skin, the layers of the abdominal wall are identified. External oblique, internal oblique, and transversus abdominus are identified and divided.

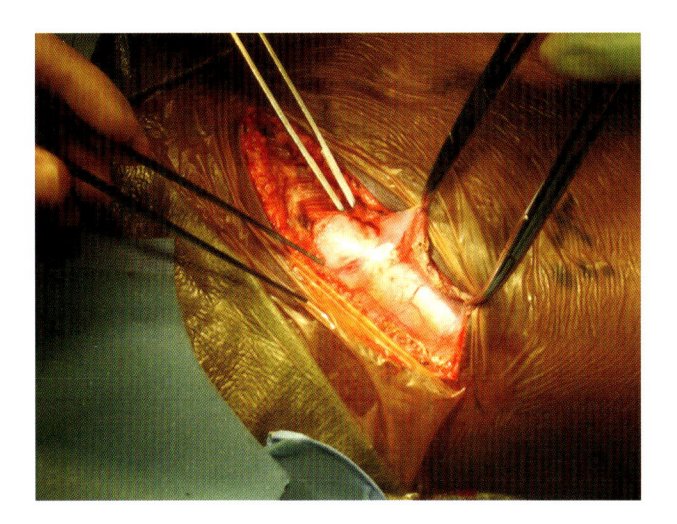

CHAPTER 50 Secondary Metastatic Tumors of the Spine

Fig. 50-21 The peritoneum is identified, and extreme care is taken not to violate it. Small rents can be repaired with 3-0 Vicryl interrupted sutures. The retroperitoneal cavity is subsequently developed using blunt dissection with sponge stick dissectors.

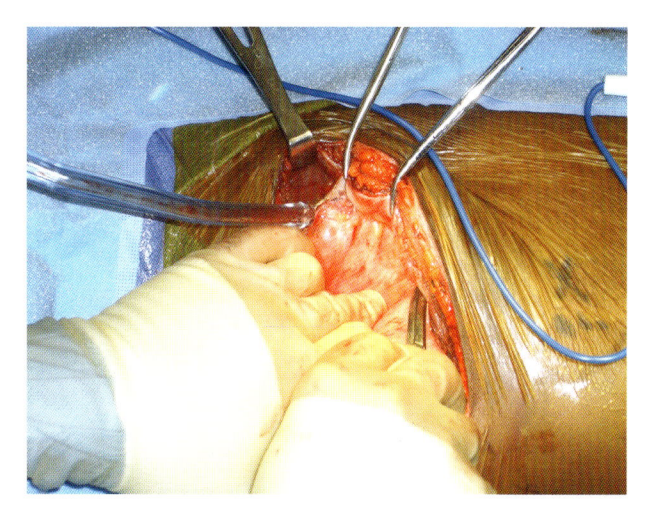

Fig. 50-23 Blunt dissection of the retroperitoneum is performed to develop the retroperitoneal cavity.

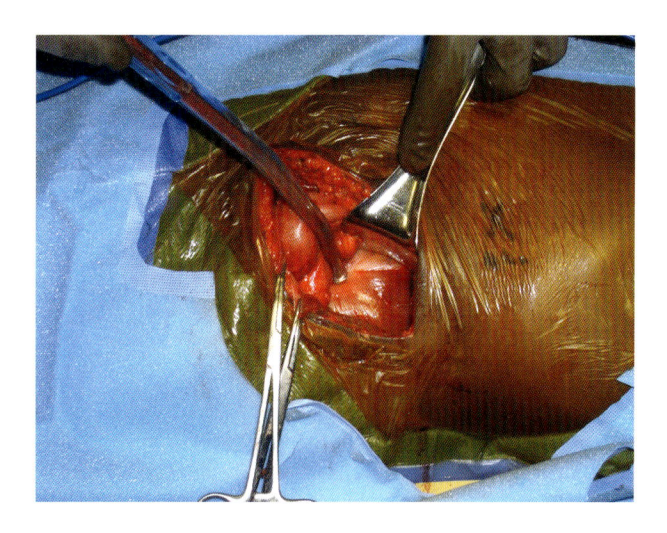

Fig. 50-24 As the peritoneum and its contents are mobilized medially, the psoas muscle is identified.

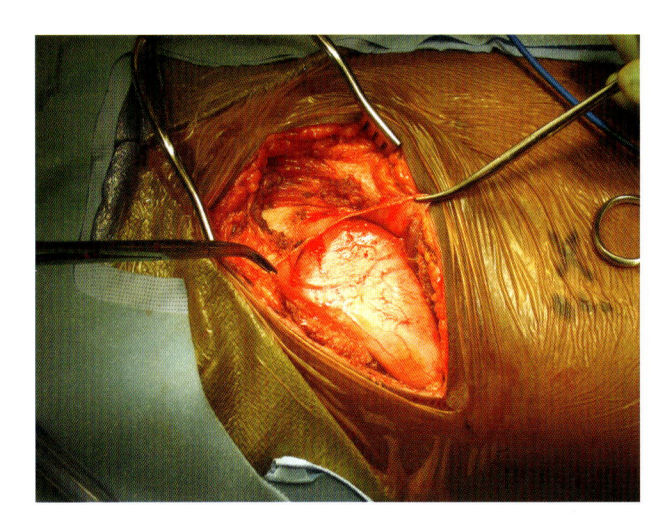

Fig. 50-22 The peritoneum is seen here separated from the transversus abdominus.

the psoas posteriorly along the bone until the pedicle is identified. The segmental vessels should not be injured during this maneuver (Fig. 50-25). Segmental bleeding can be stopped with bipolar coagulation, suture ligation, or clip placement. The spinal canal is identified using a Penfield No. 4 dissector in the neural foramen. An x-ray is obtained to confirm the level.

After the level is identified, the segmental vessels of the level above and below are dissected free, divided, and sutured or clipped. The disks are removed above and below the level of the metastatic lesion. The corpectomy is performed using a combination of osteotomes, the high-speed burr, curettes, and rongeurs. After a complete corpectomy has been performed, the end plates are prepared for reconstruction (Fig. 50-26). The vertebrectomy site can be reconstructed using a titanium cage, large structural allograft, or methylmethacrylate (Fig. 50-27). An anterior locking fixation device (plate or dual-rod construct) can be placed. Anterior instrumentation is impractical for lesions at or below L4. Such patients need to be staged for posterior fixation. The fascia is closed tightly in layers with large sutures (Fig. 50-28).

POSTERIOR APPROACH

A transpedicular corpectomy also can be performed in the lumbar spine as in the thoracic spine (see earlier discussion). In the lumbar spine, however, there are two fundamental differences. The nerve root cannot be resected, but the thecal sac can be mobilized to allow access to the corpectomy site.

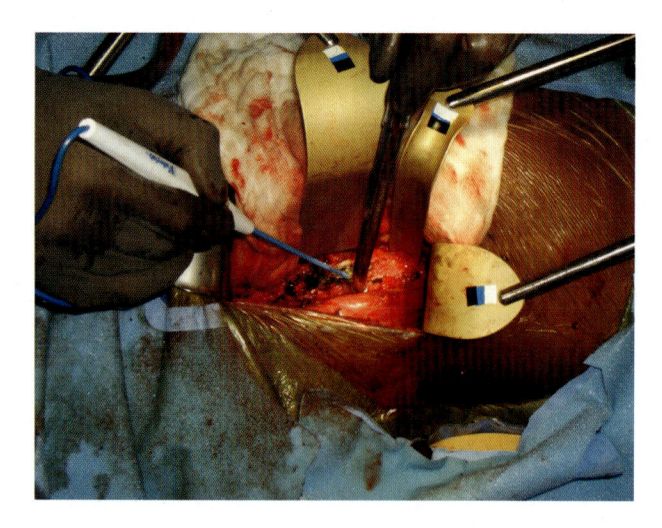

Fig. 50-25 The aorta and iliac vessels are mobilized to the contralateral side to provide exposure to the spine. Care is taken to ensure the retractors still allow blood flow distally.

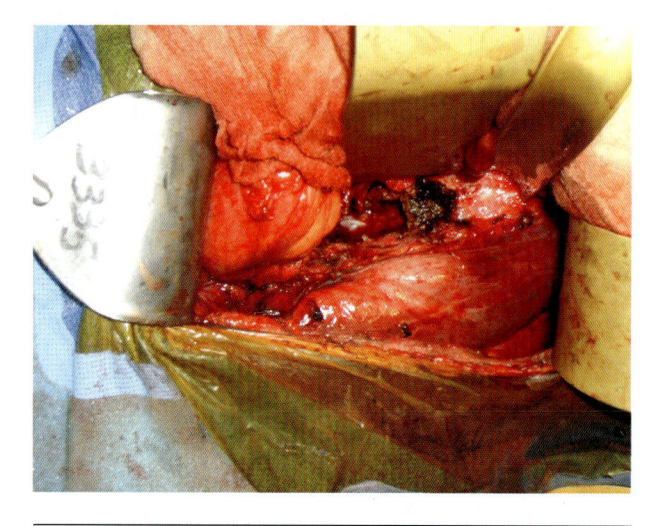

Fig. 50-26 The corpectomy is performed after dissecting the anterior longitudinal ligament. The posterior longitudinal ligament is removed to ensure excellent dural decompression.

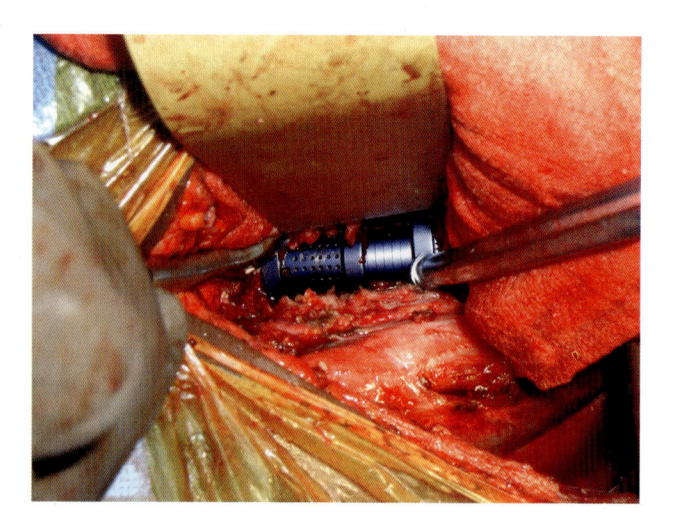

Fig. 50-27 A titanium cage or other structural graft is placed.

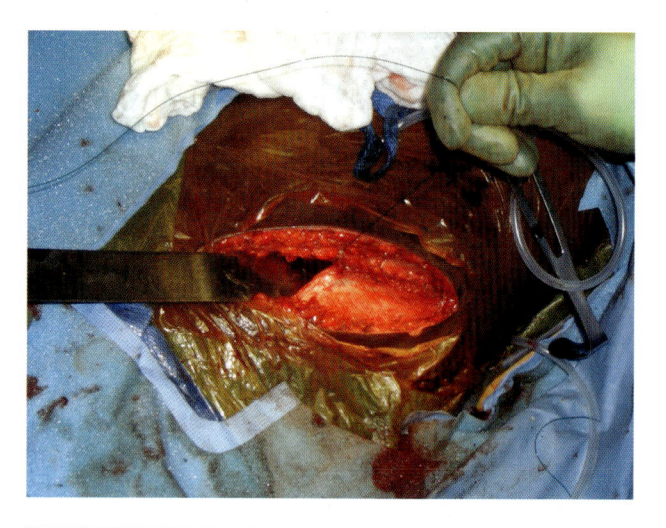

Fig. 50-28 The abdominal fascia is closed tightly with a running monofilament suture.

The transpedicular corpectomy is begun in a similar fashion to that in the thoracic spine, but the nerve roots are retracted rather than ligated. The thecal sac can be mobilized for reconstruction. Pedicle screw fixation and stabilization should follow the corpectomy.

CERVICAL LESIONS

ANTERIOR APPROACH, SUBAXIAL CERVICAL SPINE

For subaxial cervical metastases, corpectomies can be performed to decompress the spinal cord. We prefer a right-sided approach to the cervical spine. The platysma is divided and the sternocleidomastoid is identified. Dissection proceeds medially. The trachea and esophagus are mobilized medially, and the carotid and internal jugular vein are mobilized laterally. Extreme care is taken to avoid violating the tracheoesophageal groove where the recurrent laryngeal nerve lies. An intraoperative x-ray is obtained to identify the level, and the self-retaining retractors are placed. The corpectomy is begun using curettes, rongeurs, and the high-speed burr. The ligamentum flavum should be removed to ensure complete decompression of the spinal cord. The end plates are prepared using a combination of curettes and the drill. A strut graft consisting of allograft is placed, and an anterior cervical plating system is placed. The platysma is closed using 3-0 Vicryl interrupted sutures, and the skin is closed using a 4-0 subcuticular suture.

ANTERIOR APPROACH, C1-C2

Although this is a rare site for metastatic lesions to seed, this anterior approach is sometimes needed to remove lesions compressing the spinal cord and brainstem at this level. We prefer a transoral approach to such lesions. After general anesthesia is induced, the Spetzler-Sonntag transoral retractor (Aesculap Inc., Center Valley, PA) is placed. The posterior pharyngeal wall is divided using a sharp knife. The anterior ring of C1 and the body of C2 are exposed. The uvula is usually retracted with a Spetzler-Sonntag retractor. If needed, however, it may be held out of the way using a single suture. Under microscopic magnification, the anterior ring and odontoid are resected. Decompression of the spinal cord is confirmed, and the oral mucosa is closed using a 3-0 chromic suture. We prefer to pass a soft duo-tube under general anesthesia and under direct observation for postoperative feeding.

Removing the odontoid completely disrupts the alar ligaments, transverse ligament, and apical ligaments, creating severe instability. Consequently, patients must undergo posterior occipitocervical fusion.

POSTERIOR APPROACH

For decompression of the cervical spine through a posterior approach, a standard posterior cervical spine approach is performed. The paraspinous muscles are dissected using bovie cauterization. The laminae are identified, and an intraoperative x-ray is obtained to confirm the levels. The metastatic lesions are removed either via laminectomy or curettage. If facet destruction is inevitable, posterior fixation also will be needed.

CONCLUSION

Metastatic lesions to the spine present a management challenge. The patient's overall medical condition, life expectancy, and wishes must be considered. Hypervascular lesions should be embolized, and postresection stabilization should be considered.

REFERENCES

1. Patchell R, Tibbs PA, Regine WF, et al: A randomized trial of direct decompressive surgical resection in the treatment of spinal cord compression caused by metastasis. Proc Am Soc Clin Oncol 2003:22(abstract 2):1.
2. Ries LAG, Eisner MP, Hankey BF, et al: SEER cancer statistics review, 1975-2000. Web site: http://seer.cancer.gov/csr/1975_2000/. National Cancer Institute. Bethesda, MD, 2003.
3. Gokaslan ZL, York JE, Walsh GL, et al: Transthoracic vertebrectomy for metastatic spinal tumors. J Neurosurg 1998;89(4):599–609.
4. Bach F, Larsen BH, Rohde K, et al: Metastatic spinal cord compression: Occurrence, symptoms, clinical presentations and prognosis in 398 patients with spinal cord compression. Acta Neurochir (Wien) 1990;107(1–2):37–43.
5. Gilbert RW, Kim JH, Posner JB: Epidural spinal cord compression from metastatic tumor: Diagnosis and treatment. Ann Neurol 1978;3(1):40–51.
6. Helweg-Larsen S, Sorensen PS: Symptoms and signs in metastatic spinal cord compression: A study of progression from first symptom until diagnosis in 153 patients. Eur J Cancer 1994;30A(3):396–398.
7. Colman LK, Porter BA, Redmond J III, et al: Early diagnosis of spinal metastases by CT and MR studies. J Comput Assist Tomogr 1988;12(3):423–426.
8. Sze G: Magnetic resonance imaging in the evaluation of spinal tumors. Cancer 1991;67(4 Suppl):1229–1241.
9. Algra PR, Bloem JL, Tissing H, et al: Detection of vertebral metastases: Comparison between MR imaging and bone scintigraphy. Radiographics 1991;11(2):219–232.
10. Chadwick DJ, Gillatt DA, Mukerjee A, et al: Magnetic resonance imaging of spinal metastases. J R Soc Med 1991;84(4):196–200.
11. Mehta RC, Wilson MA, Perlman SB: False-negative bone scan in extensive metastatic disease: CT and MR findings. J Comput Assist Tomogr 1989;13(4):717–719.
12. Gosfield E III, Alavi A, Kneeland B: Comparison of radionuclide bone scans and magnetic resonance imaging in detecting spinal metastases. J Nucl Med 1993;34(12):2191–2198.
13. Pierot L, Boulin A: Percutaneous biopsy of the thoracic and lumbar spine: Transpedicular approach under fluoroscopic guidance. Am J Neuroradiol 1999;20(1):23–25.
14. Kattapuram SV, Khurana JS, Rosenthal DI: Percutaneous needle biopsy of the spine. Spine 1992;17(5):561–564.
15. Ghelman B, Lospinuso MF, Levine DB, et al: Percutaneous computed-tomography-guided biopsy of the thoracic and lumbar spine. Spine 1991;16(7):736–739.
16. Rompe JD, Hopf CG, Eysel P: Outcome after palliative posterior surgery for metastatic disease of the spine—Evaluation of 106 consecutive patients after decompression and stabilisation with the Cotrel-Dubousset instrumentation. Arch Orthop Trauma Surg 1999;119(7–8):394–400.
17. Manke C, Bretschneider T, Lenhart M, et al: Spinal metastases from renal cell carcinoma: Effect of preoperative particle embolization on intraoperative blood loss. Am J Neuroradiol 2001;22(5):997–1003.
18. Gellad FE, Sadato N, Numaguchi Y, Levine AM: Vascular metastatic lesions of the spine: Preoperative embolization. Radiology 1990;176(3):683–686.
19. Olerud C, Jonsson H Jr, Lofberg AM, et al: Embolization of spinal metastases reduces peroperative blood loss: 21 patients operated on for renal cell carcinoma. Acta Orthop Scand 1993;64(1):9–12.

CHAPTER 51

L. FERNANDO GONZALEZ
RANDALL W. PORTER

Surgical Technique for Resection of Intradural Tumors

INTRODUCTION

Intradural spinal lesions can either be intramedullary or extramedullary. Intradural extramedullary tumors primarily consist of schwannomas, neurofibromas, and meningiomas. In children, most intramedullary tumors are astrocytomas. Intradural intramedullary tumors are typically astrocytomas in children and ependymomas and hemangioblastomas in adults. Aneurysms, cavernous malformations, arteriovenous malformations, and dural arteriovenous fistulas are a special group of vascular entities that are beyond the scope of this review.

The surgical corridor to intradural spinal lesions should be planned based on the location of the tumor within the cervical, thoracic, or lumbar spine. The posterior approach and posterolateral approaches through a multilevel laminoplasty or laminectomy are most often used to access the cervical region. The use of anterior approaches to intradural cervical lesions is limited because multiple corpectomies are necessary. Furthermore, lateral exposure is limited with anterior approaches and stabilization is needed after resection of the tumor. In the thoracic spine, the posterior approach and the posterolateral approach with an oblique trajectory through the pedicle and transverse process (costotransversectomy) constitute the main routes for intradural lesions. Transthoracic and trans-sternal exposures are rarely used to access intradural lesions and are beyond the scope of this review. In the lumbar region, where mobilization of the spinal cord is not an issue, a posterior approach through a laminectomy or laminoplasty is the preferred method.

POSTERIOR APPROACH

The posterior approach with a laminoplasty or laminectomy is performed with the patient in the prone or sitting position. If the pathology involves the cervical spine, the head is fixated with a three-point headholder such as the Mayfield system (Codman, Inc., Raynham, MA; Fig. 51-1). Posterolateral approaches are variations of the posterior approach that include resection of the ipsilateral lamina, facet, and pedicle with dural opening around the dorsal root and posterior sectioning of the dentate ligament (Fig. 51-2).

During cervical spine surgery, we prefer the prone position to the sitting or semisitting position to reduce the risk of air embolism and hypotension. All bony prominences and

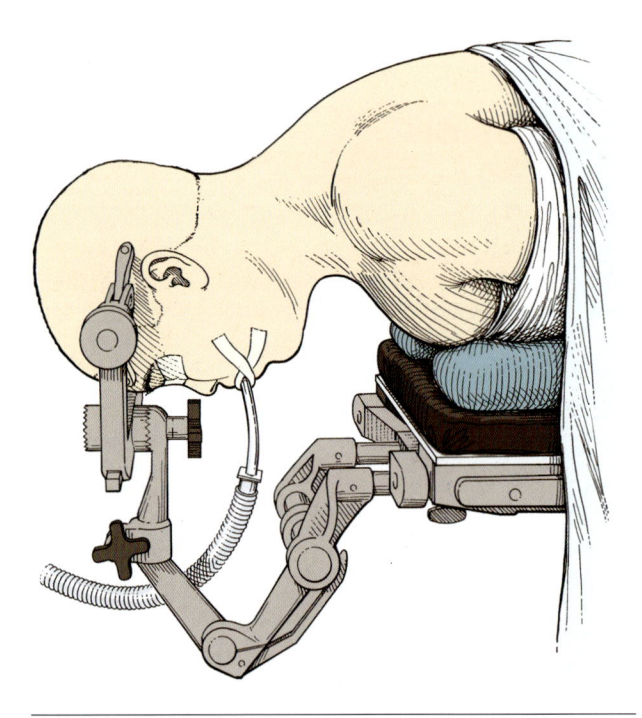

Fig. 51-1 Typical patient positioning during cervical spine surgery. The head is fixed in a Mayfield holder. Slight flexion improves visualization of the entire region. (Modified from Barrow Neurological Institute.)

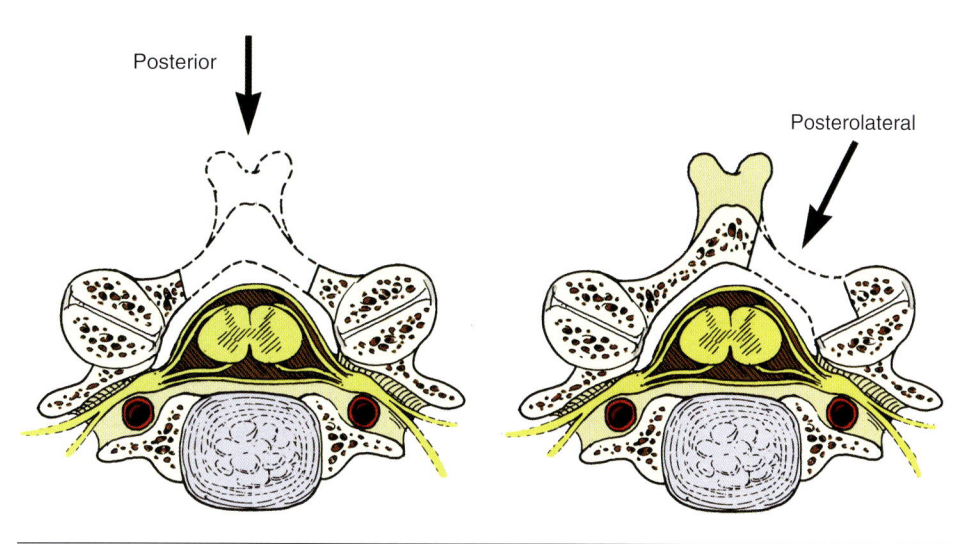

Fig. 51-2 Two approaches used to access cervical region. The posterior approach involves a standard laminectomy. The posterolateral approach is used when a laminectomy is more extensive on one side and extended into the ipsilateral facet. The latter approach is used for more laterally located lesions, and mechanical stability must be assessed. (Modified from Spetzler RF, Koos WT: Color Atlas of Microneurosurgery, 2nd ed. Vol. 3. New York, Thieme, 2000.)

pressure points are padded with gel rolls. The abdomen and thorax are left free of pressure to avoid venous hypertension and to minimize restrictions on chest expansion. Prophylactic antibiotics are administered routinely. High doses of methylprednisolone similar to those used after spinal trauma are also administered. Somatosensory evoked potentials are monitored routinely; when possible, motor evoked potentials are also monitored.

The appropriate level for the skin incision is identified with the aid of C-arm fluoroscopy and skin palpation of the spinous process. The spinous process of vertebra prominens (C7) can serve as a useful landmark. These findings are correlated with preoperative magnetic resonance images (MRIs). The level of the "localizer" cut of the MRI should be checked because the vertebral count could begin from either the sacrum or C1. The skin incision should be long enough to provide adequate access to the caudal and rostral edges of the lesion.

Subcutaneous dissection is performed with monopolar cauterization. Dissection must remain in the midline to prevent excessive bleeding and to facilitate closure once the procedure is completed. The paraspinal muscles over the lamina are dissected subperiosteally with a Cobb dissector. To avoid iatrogenic instability, especially in the cervical spine, monopolar cauterization should not be used to dissect into the facet joint. If the spine is unstable after exposure and resection of a tumor, lateral mass fixation, pedicle screw fixation, or both should be performed with posterolateral fusion.

To obtain adequate surgical exposure, the bony exposure includes one level below and one level above the lesion. We routinely use cerebellar-type retractors during dissection of the soft tissue. Once the lamina is exposed, especially in the cervical and thoracic regions, we retract the soft tissue with fishhooks attached with rubber bands to a Leyla bar. The Leyla bar is attached to the surgical table in a horizontal orientation. Fishhooks provide a low profile and excellent retraction without obstructing the surgical field.

The laminae are exposed on both sides, and the ligamentum flavum is dissected beneath the lamina with a curved curette. With a pneumatic drill and a pediatric footplate (B1 or B5, Midas Rex, Medtronic, Forth Worth, TX; Fig. 51-3), we cut the lamina starting on the caudal edge of the exposure to facilitate elevation of the laminar flap. Beginning the cut on the caudal edge is not arbitrary. It derives from the double insertion of the ligamentum flavum on the superior aspect of the caudal vertebra. The interspinous ligament is then cut caudal and rostral to the involved segment. Finally, the laminar flap is elevated (Fig. 51-4). We insist on a laminoplasty rather than a laminectomy to diminish tissue scar over the dura. Furthermore, in children a laminotomy prevents the development of a swan neck deformity, which typically follows an extensive laminectomy.

POSTEROLATERAL APPROACHES

When lesions are anterior or lateral to the spinal cord in the thoracic spine, an oblique trajectory is ideal to minimize manipulation of the spinal cord.

COSTOTRANSVERSECTOMY

A semilunar skin incision is used. Its base is oriented toward the midline, and the arc is oriented toward the side on which

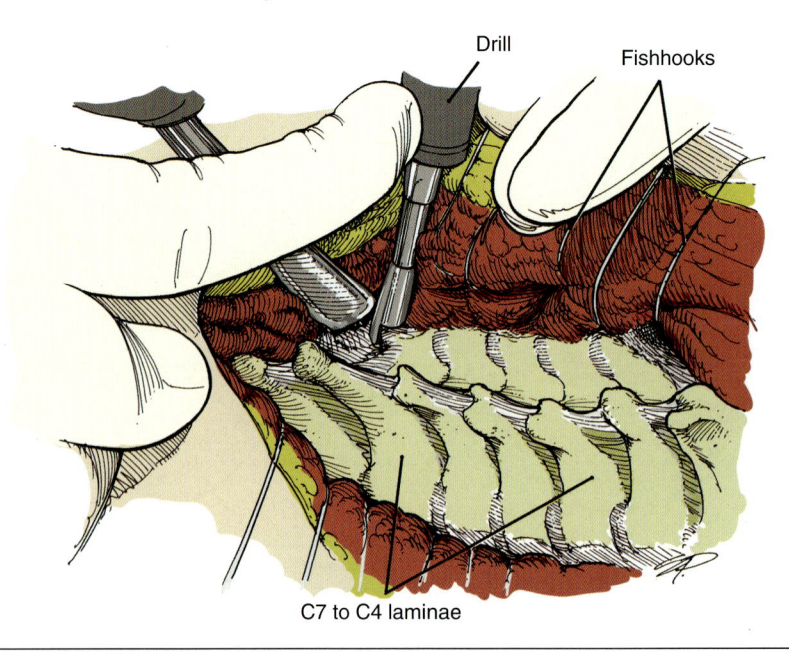

Fig. 51-3 After the soft tissue has been dissected and retracted laterally with fishhooks, the spinous processes and laminae are evident bilaterally. Just medial to the most caudal lamina, the pediatric footplate is inserted and engaged under the lamina, and the laminotomy is extended rostrally to the appropriate level. This procedure is then repeated on the other side. (Modified from Barrow Neurological Institute.)

the tumor is most evident (Fig. 51-5). The dural incision can be longitudinal in the midline or T-shaped, with the horizontal arm projecting toward the nerve root (Fig. 51-6). The surgical table is tilted 15 to 20 degrees away from the surgeon to obtain the appropriate oblique angle for exposing the anterior spine.

A costotransversectomy is often used during the resection of epidural masses, including herniated disks. For intradural lesions more than one level is usually involved and its use is limited. The surgical corridor is deeper and the site is therefore farther from the surgeon. The approach, however, offers excellent exposure of the anterior aspect of the spinal cord.

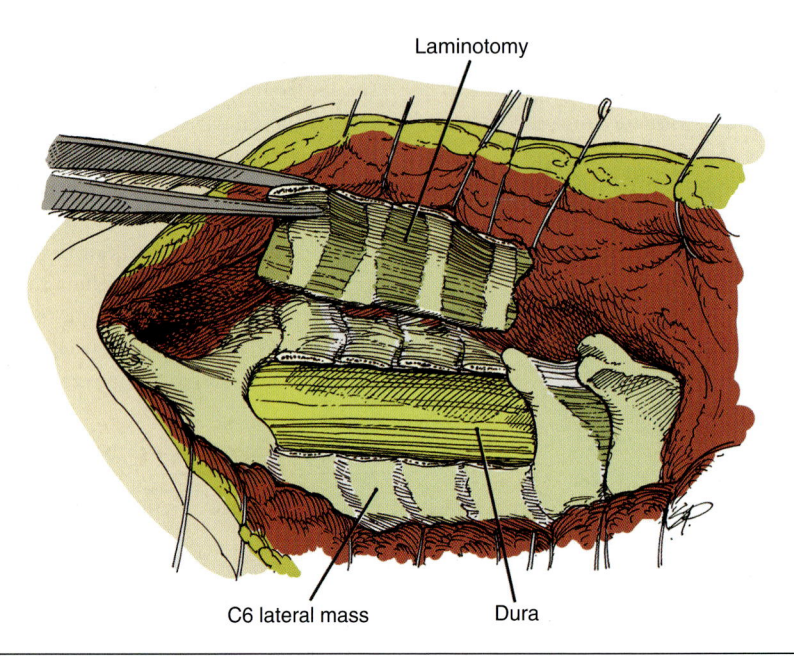

Fig. 51-4 Once the laminotomy is performed on both sides and the interspinous ligament has been sectioned caudal and rostral to the level of interest, the laminar flap is elevated. The facets are exposed and used to reattach the laminar flap with miniplates. (Modified from Barrow Neurological Institute.)

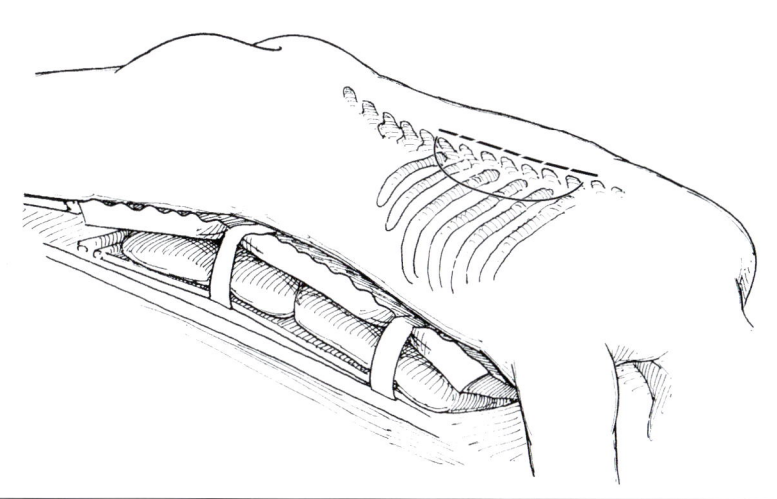

CHAPTER 51 Surgical Technique for Resection of Intradural Tumors

Fig. 51-5 To approach a posterior or posterolateral thoracic lesion, the patient is placed in the prone position, and the bony surfaces are padded. The surgical table is tilted to elevate the ipsilateral side so that an oblique trajectory can be obtained. The incision can be either longitudinal in the midline or semilunar with its base oriented toward the midline. (Modified from Spetzler RF, Koos WT: Intraspinal tumors and cysts. In Spetzler RF, Koos WT: Color Atlas of Microneurosurgery, 2nd ed. Vol. 3. New York, Thieme, 2000, p 329.)

The operating microscope is an invaluable tool to maximize visibility of the tumor and spinal cord. After significant lateral retraction, the lamina and head of the rib are exposed (Fig. 51-7).

After a unilateral hemilaminectomy, a costotransversectomy can be performed followed by transpedicular exposure (Fig. 51-8). The pedicle is drilled until it is flush with the posterior aspect of the vertebral body. The foramen is then exposed. The transverse process and head of the respective rib (Fig. 51-9) are resected to obtain the appropriate tangential angle to expose the anterior aspect of the thecal sac.

Potentially, this approach preserves the posterior tension band (unilateral approach and preservation of the interspinous ligament), thereby limiting postoperative instability. The dura usually is opened in an arc that includes the nerve root.

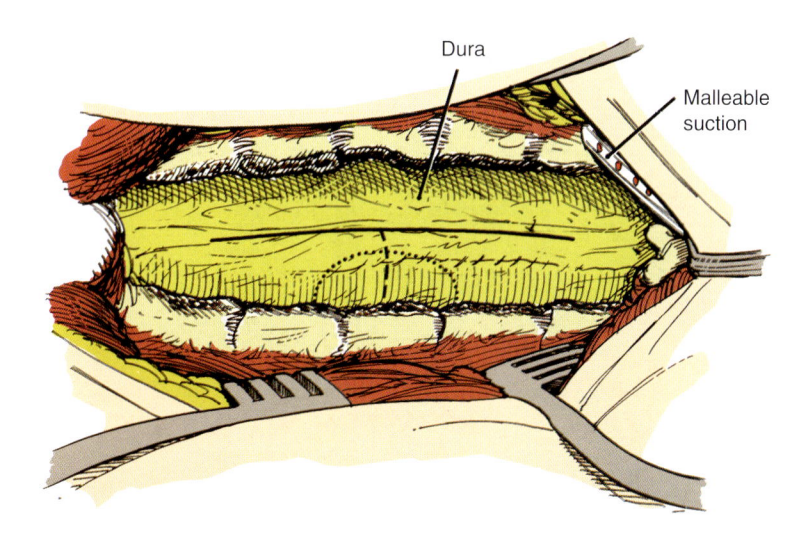

Fig. 51-6 The surgical field is ready for the dural opening. The epidural space is filled with hemostatic agents and covered with long cottonoids. A malleable suction cannula is secured to prevent epidural oozing from invading the surgical field. Two different techniques can be used to open the dura. A midline longitudinal incision can be connected with a horizontal "T," which usually runs parallel to the respective nerve root. Alternatively, a semilunar incision with its base positioned laterally will include the appropriate nerve root. (Modified from Barrow Neurological Institute.)

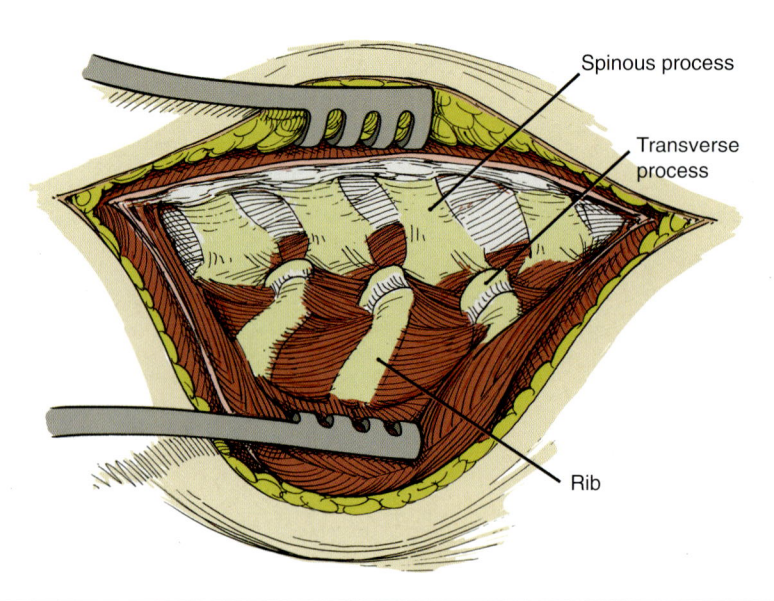

Fig. 51-7 Once the incision has been performed, the soft tissue is retracted until the respective lamina and the head of the rib are exposed. Only one side is opened. The posterior tension band is kept intact to diminish the risk of causing instability. (Modified from Barrow Neurological Institute.)

Once hemostasis is achieved with bipolar coagulation and hemostatic agents (e.g., FloSeal or Surgifoam) have been placed on the epidural space, bony edges are covered with long cottonoids. A small, plastic, malleable suction cannula is left in the epidural space to prevent continuous bleeding during the procedure (see Fig. 51-6).

The dura is raised with jeweler pick-up forceps. A small durotomy is performed carefully with a scalpel with a No. 15 blade to prevent inadvertent opening of the arachnoid layer and subsequent drainage of cerebrospinal fluid (CSF). With two jeweler pick-up forceps, one in front of the other, both edges are pulled simultaneously in opposing directions until

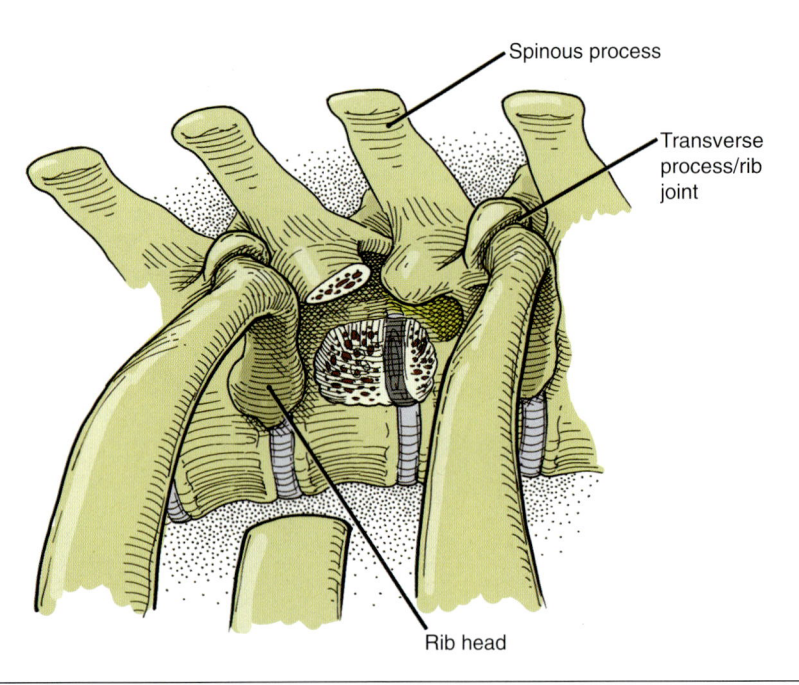

Fig. 51-8 The head of the rib and its joint with the respective transverse process have been removed. A bony wedge on the respective vertebral body is drilled to obtain the required tangential oblique exposure. (Modified from Barrow Neurological Institute.)

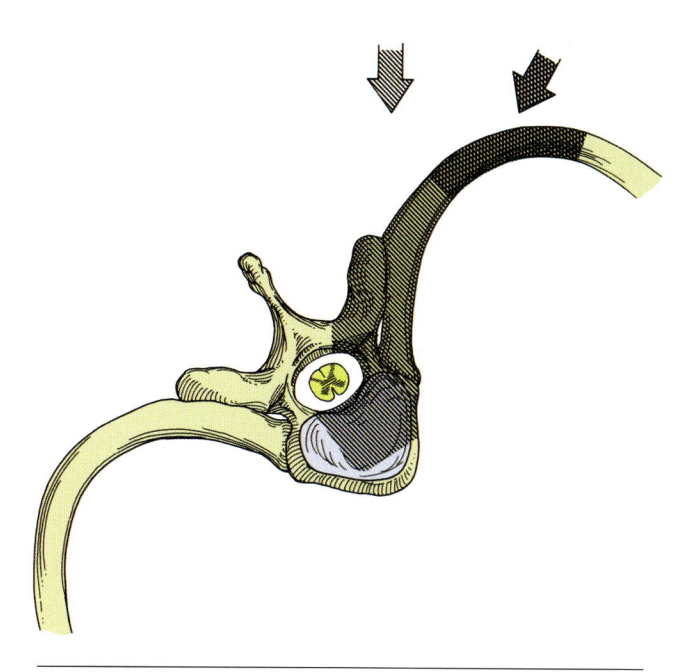

Fig. 51-9 The shaded area shows the extent of bone that is removed during a costotransversectomy. The different amounts of rib resection provide different angles of attack to the intraspinal contents. An oblique tangential angle can be obtained by tilting the surgical table. (Modified from Barrow Neurological Institute.)

the dura is torn the desired length. Dural edges are tacked up with 4-0 Nurolon suture to prevent epidural blood from entering the subarachnoid space. Once the dura is elevated, the microscope is brought into the surgical field.

Microscopic illumination and magnification are invaluable during the resection of these tumors. If the lesion is intradural extramedullary (i.e., meningiomas or schwannomas), the plane between the tumor and pia is inspected. The lesion is then removed carefully with microscissors and microsurgical dissection instruments with progressive isolation of the tumor from the spinal cord. The use of bipolar coagulation should be minimized. To improve the visibility of the tumor–spinal cord interface during dissection, it is useful to have an assistant irrigate the surgical site.

RESECTION OF INTRAMEDULLARY TUMORS

There are two routes to intramedullary tumors: through the posterior midline or through a posterolateral myelotomy through the root entry zone. The former follows the posterior median sulcus, and the spinal cord is split between the two posterior columns (Fig. 51-10). The myelotomy can be performed with a No. 11 blade, a No. 59 beaver-blade, or CO_2 laser or with a neodymium-doped yttrium aluminum garnet (Nd-YAG) contact laser. Some centers routinely use the latter during myelotomies. Compared to electrocauterization, this technique causes no artifact during electrophysiologic monitoring.

Postoperatively, patients may complain of transitory dysesthesia or of diffuse, ill-defined sensory symptoms. The symptoms are caused by microvascular damage to the posterior columns during the myelotomy. Sometimes spinal cord edema makes it difficult to identify the midline on the posterior surface of the spinal cord. The vessels usually are located off midline and do not constitute reliable markers.

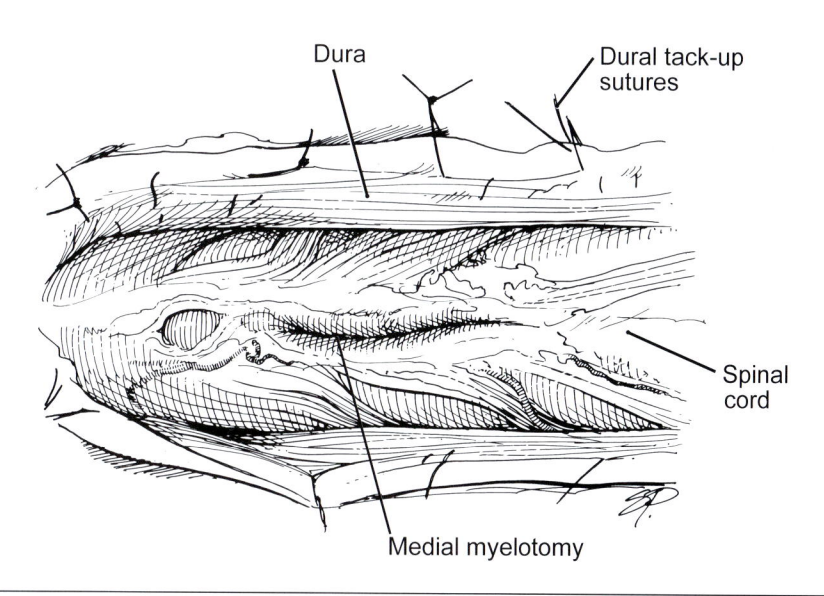

Fig. 51-10 After the dura has been opened in a longitudinal fashion, its edges are tacked to the fishhooks and the myelotomy is performed in the midline. (Modified from Spetzler RF, Koos WT: Intraspinal tumors and cysts. In Spetzler RF, Koos WT: Color Atlas of Microneurosurgery, 2nd ed. Vol. 3. New York, Thieme, 2000, p 329.)

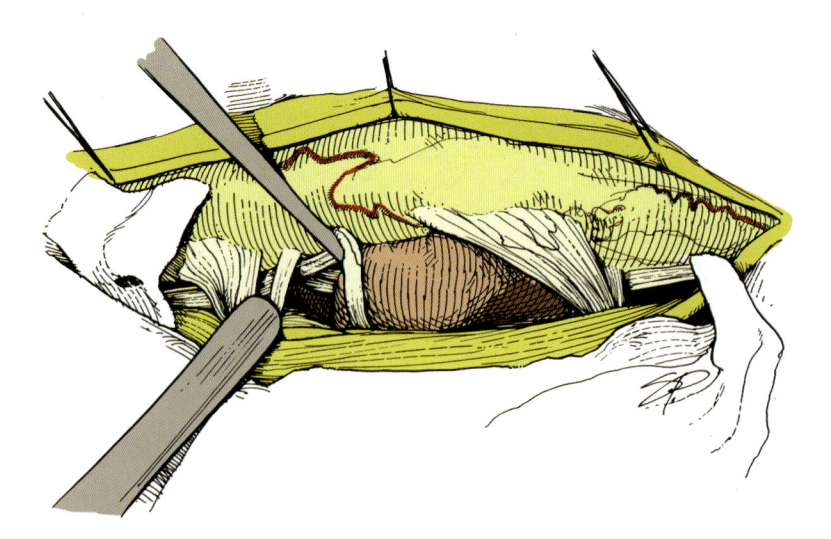

Fig. 51-11 Illustration showing the plane that separates an intradural extramedullary tumor from the spinal cord. Use of bipolar coagulation is minimized. (Modified from Spetzler RF, Koos WT: Intraspinal tumors and cysts. In Spetzler RF, Koos WT: Color Atlas of Microneurosurgery, 2nd ed. Vol. 3. New York, Thieme, 2000, p 292.)

The midpoint between the bilateral dorsal entry roots can be used to determine the site from which the myelotomy should begin.

For intradural extramedullary lesions, the surgical plane between the lesion and spinal cord is identified and followed until the lesion is removed completely (Fig. 51-11). External signs on the surface of the spinal cord may not indicate the location or extent of infiltrating lesions. To expose such lesions, the appropriate place for the myelotomy must first be determined based on the patient's MRI.

The posterolateral approach offers a lateral route where the posterior roots enter the spinal cord. The spinal cord is opened though the dorsal root entry zone (DREZ) between two or more roots. This route offers an avenue for resecting intramedullary lesions that is off midline and closer to the lateral surface of the spinal cord. A myelotomy should be chosen based on the patient's symptoms and MRI findings.

Traction sutures (6-0) have been advocated to retract the pia to keep the spinal cord open while the tumor is being removed (Fig. 51-12). The resection of intramedullary astro-

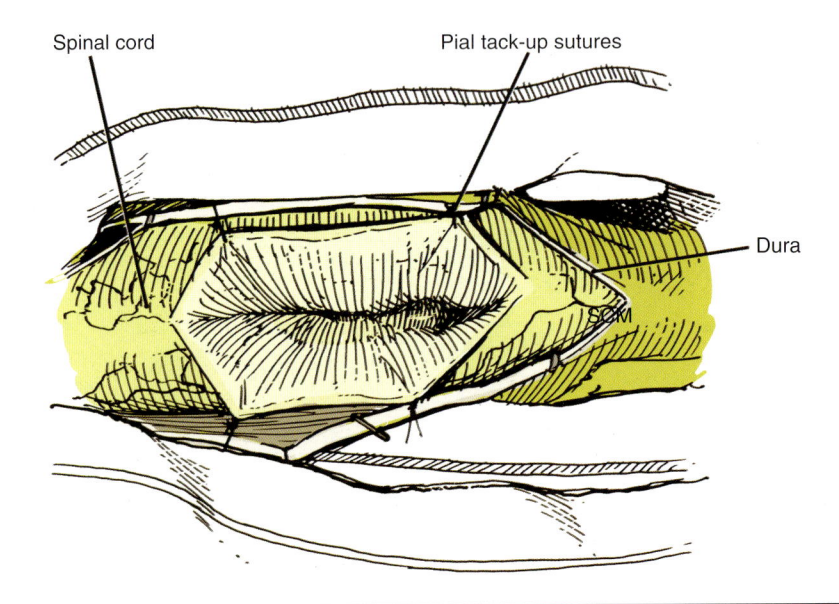

Fig. 51-12 The pia has been elevated and tacked with 6-0 sutures to keep the myelotomy open to expose the tumor while it is resected. (Modified from Spetzler RF, Koos WT: Intraspinal tumors and cysts. In Spetzler RF, Koos WT: Color Atlas of Microneurosurgery, 2nd ed. Vol. 3. New York, Thieme, 2000, p 325.)

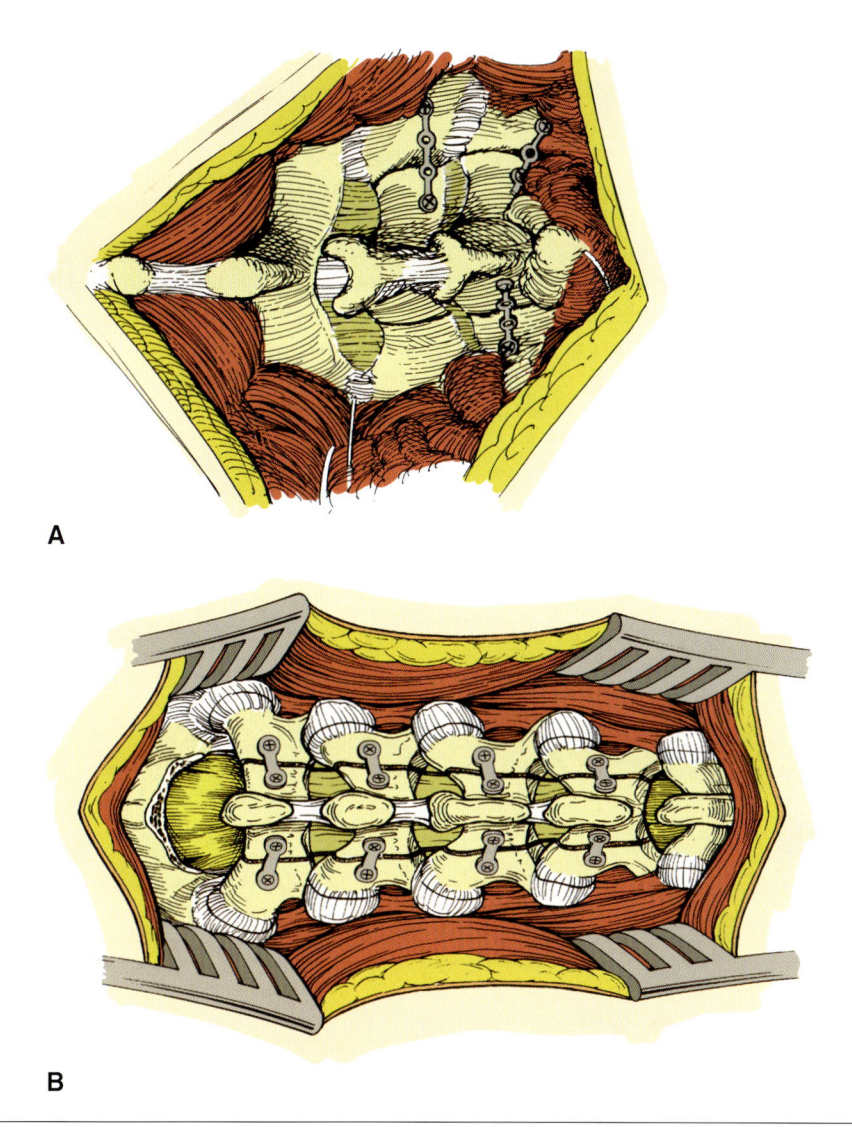

Fig. 51-13 A, In the cervical spine, the laminar flap is reapproximated with long thin titanium plates. B, In the thoracic or lumbar spine, small miniplates are used. Laminoplasty prevents scarring over the dural sac and provides a more anatomic closure that may prevent delayed instability. (A modified from Spetzler RF, Koos WT: Intraspinal tumors and cysts. In Spetzler RF, Koos WT: Color Atlas of Microneurosurgery, 2nd ed. Vol. 3. New York, Thieme, 2000, p 327. B modified from Barrow Neurological Institute.)

cytomas begins within the tumor and proceeds to the periphery (centrifugal resection) until normal tissue is reached. In contrast, ependymomas have a surrounding plane, and the tumor can be resected in a piecemeal fashion.

Once the tumor has been resected and hemostasis is obtained, the tumor bed is irrigated with normal saline solution. The use of bipolar coagulation should be limited. The pia can be reapproximated with 8-0 interrupted nylon sutures. However, we prefer to leave the pia open.

The dura is closed with 6-0 prolene running sutures in a watertight fashion. The adequacy of the dural closure can be determined with a Valsalva maneuver by increasing airway pressure to 40 mm H_2O. If part of the dura was resected with the base of the tumor (e.g., meningioma), dural patching with bovine pericardium or Gore-Tex is used to prevent postoperative scarring. This technique reduces a patient's risk of spinal cord tethering and minimizes the likelihood of recurrence, especially with meningiomas. The entire dural circumference can be replaced using fascia lata. The dural closure can be sealed with fibrin glue or Tisseel. Liberal use of a temporary (2 to 3 days) lumbar drain helps avert CSF leaks.

Once the dura is closed and hemostasis is attained, we reattach the lamina with titanium miniplates and screws (Fig. 51-13). The muscles are reapproximated with 0 Vicryl sutures. The most important step in closure is reapproximation of the fascia. Minimizing the dead space reduces the incidence of CSF leakage, hematomas, and infection. The skin is closed with a running 3-0 nylon suture.

THORACOTOMY

Anterior intradural tumors involving the thoracic spine can be approached through an open thoracotomy or through an endoscope. Both techniques use the same oblique trajectory. The head of the respective rib must be removed. Then the pedicle is approached and part of the vertebral body is resected. These procedures are not used routinely for intramedullary tumors.

The patient is placed in a lateral position (Fig. 51-14) with the surgical site elevated highest in the field. A roll is placed under the dependent arm. The ipsilateral upper extremity is supported on a holder to prevent brachial plexus injuries. The location of the incision is determined by the level of the tumor and is made above the appropriate rib. Once the thoracic cavity is entered, the relevant anatomy is identified (Fig. 51-15). After the head of the rib has been identified, the intercostal neurovascular bundle is dissected and the vessels are ligated (Fig. 51-16). The head of the rib and the appropriate pedicle are drilled with a pneumatic drill (Figs. 51-17, 51-18, and 51-19).

The best way to identify the spinal cord is to place a nerve hook into the foramen under the pedicle after the rib head has been removed. The pedicle can then be removed in a caudad-cephalad direction with a Kerrison rongeur. This maneuver exposes the nerve root, which can be followed to the dura of the spinal cord. Once the pedicle has been removed, the corpectomy can be performed safely because the surgeon knows the location of the spinal cord. The corpectomy can be performed with a configuration of drills, osteotomes, rongeurs, Kerrison rongeurs, and curettes. The microscope can be used to improve visualization, illumination, and magnification. The operating surgeon stands anteriorly, pulling fragments of the bone toward him- or herself while the assistant stands at the posterior aspect of the patient.

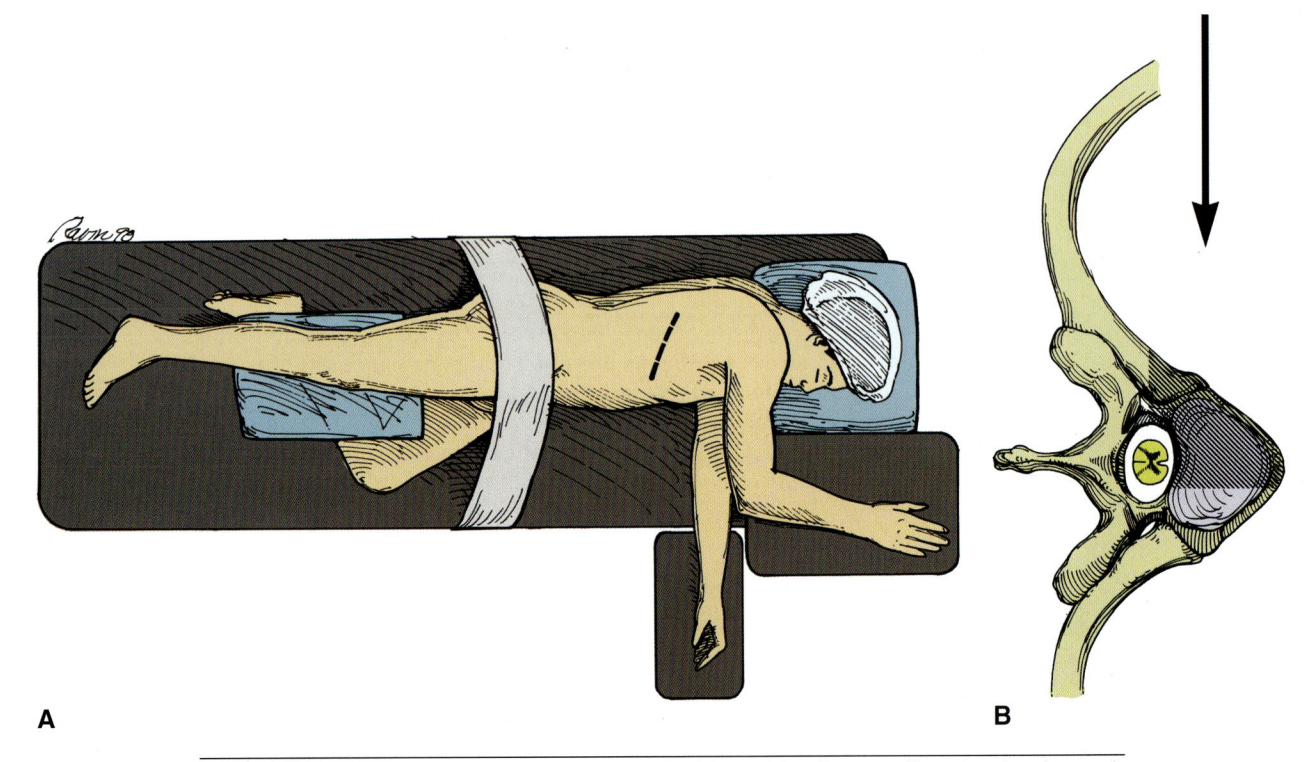

Fig. 51-14 *A*, Patients are positioned on their sides with a foam roll under the dependent arm. The upper arm is supported at the same height as the torso to prevent brachial plexus injuries. The incision is planned by using C-arm fluoroscopy to identify the appropriate rib. The incision is placed on top of the rib. *B*, The thoracic cavity is opened with a trajectory that is perpendicular to the area of interest. (*A* modified from Barrow Neurological Institute. *B* modified from Spetzler RF, Koos WT: Approaches. In Spetzler RF, Koos WT: Color Atlas of Microneurosurgery, 2nd ed. Vol. 3. New York, Thieme, 2000, p 327.)

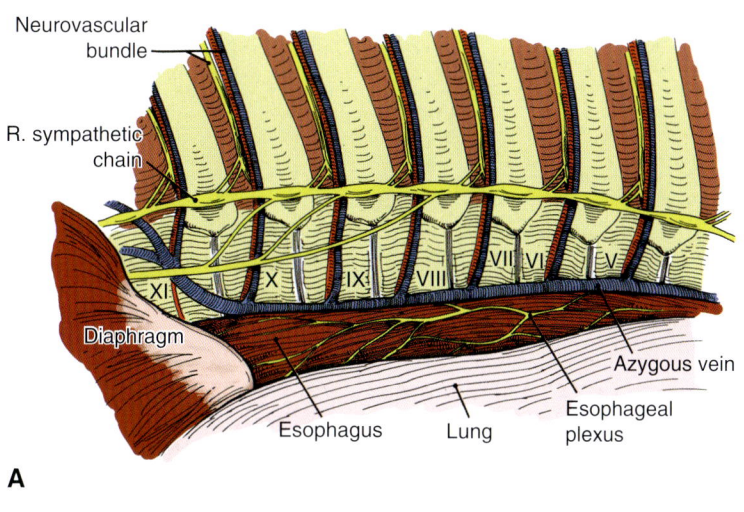

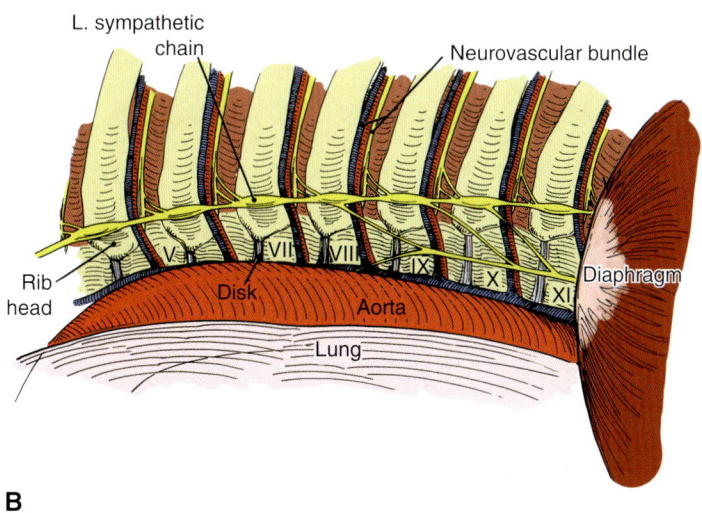

CHAPTER 51 Surgical Technique for Resection of Intradural Tumors

Fig. 51-15 The anatomic landmarks associated with the thoracic cavity differ on the left and right sides. *A,* Schematic representation of the right side showing the location of the esophagus and azygos vein. *B,* The aorta is visible on the left side. (Modified from Spetzler RF, Koos WT: Approaches. In Spetzler RF, Koos WT: Color Atlas of Microneurosurgery, 2nd ed. Vol. 3. New York, Thieme, 2000, p 92.)

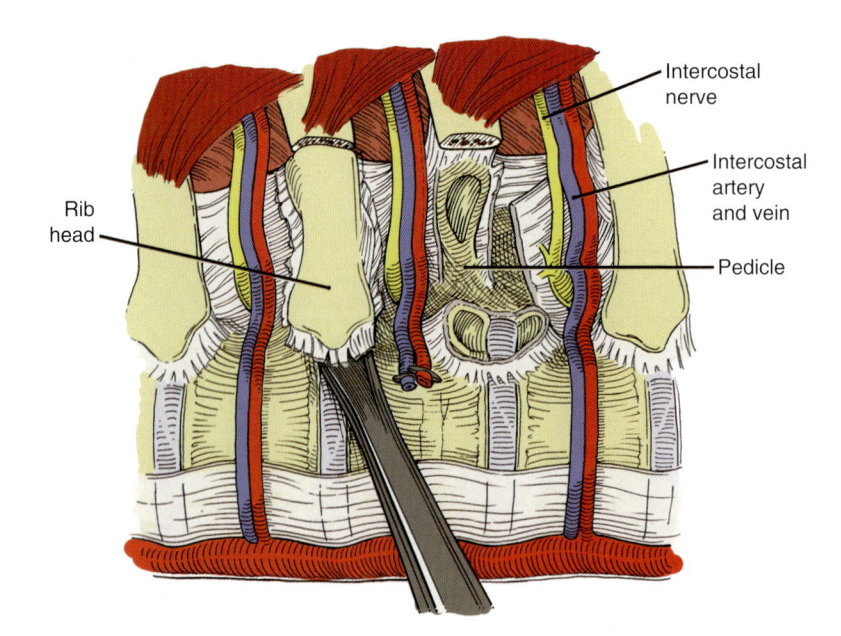

Fig. 51-16 Once the pleura has been opened, the neurovascular bundle is identified and the vessels are ligated and sectioned. The parietal pleura is dissected from the head of the rib, separated from the remaining rib, and avulsed. Once the head of the rib has been removed, the joint between the rib and the vertebral body is exposed. The respective intervertebral space can then be identified above and below the area of interest. (Modified from Barrow Neurological Institute.)

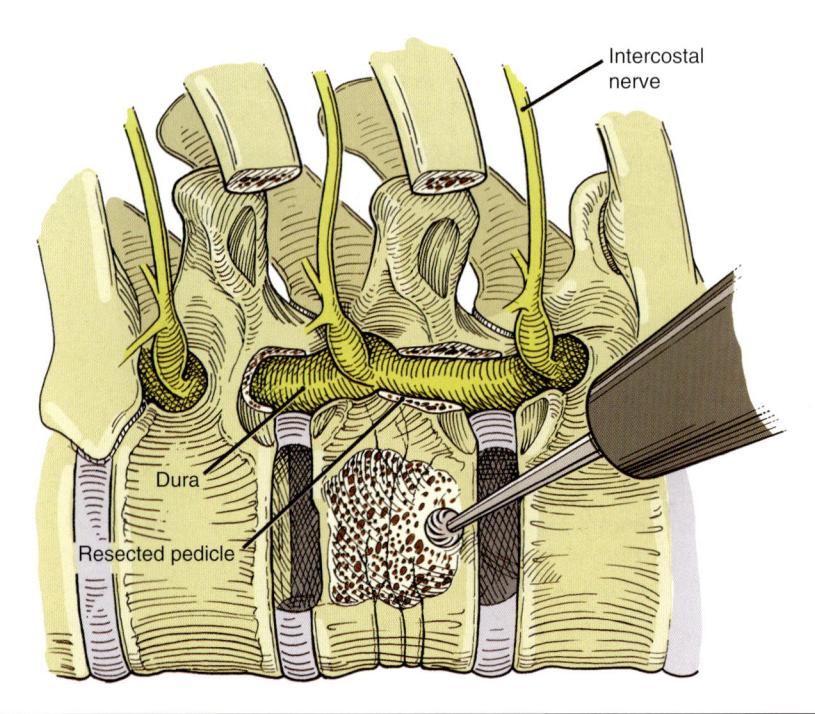

Fig. 51-17 Once the disks and the medial border of the spinal contents have been identified, a wedge of the vertebral body is resected with a pneumatic drill. (Modified from Barrow Neurological Institute.)

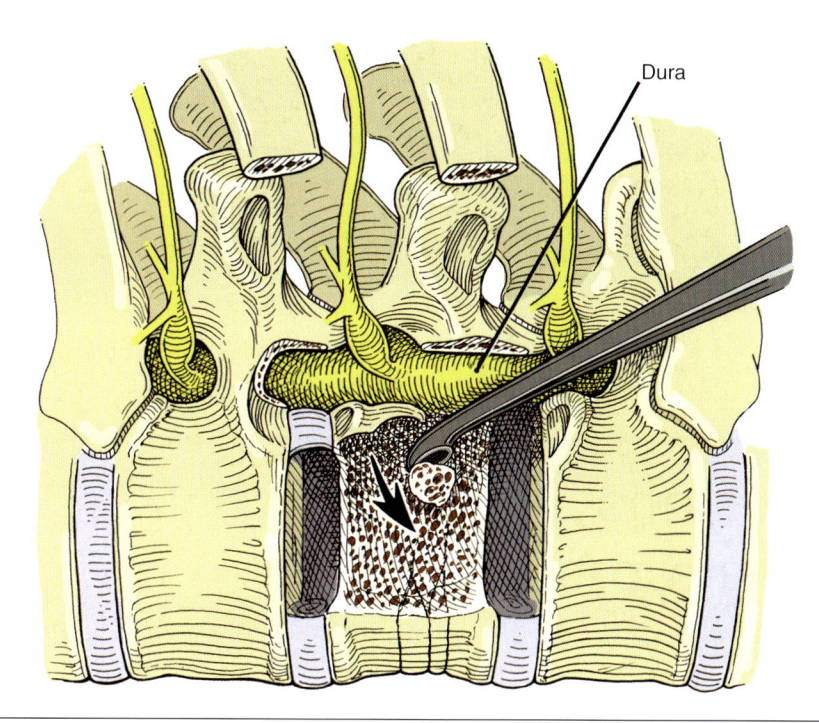

Fig. 51-18 Different sizes of curettes are used to denude the thin layer of bone and posterior longitudinal ligament that separate the thecal sac from the vertebral body. (Modified from Barrow Neurological Institute.)

CONCLUSION

Intradural tumors are mainly approached through a posterior exposure after a laminectomy or laminotomy. When the lesion is anterior or lateral to the spinal cord, especially when the cervical or thoracic region is involved, a more oblique trajectory may be desirable. Such lesions are approached through a costotransversectomy or thoracotomy, and the ipsilateral facet (and pedicle in the cervical spine) is removed. Magnification and illumination with a microscope are key during tumor resection. Within the spinal cord, the use of bipolar coagulation should be minimized.

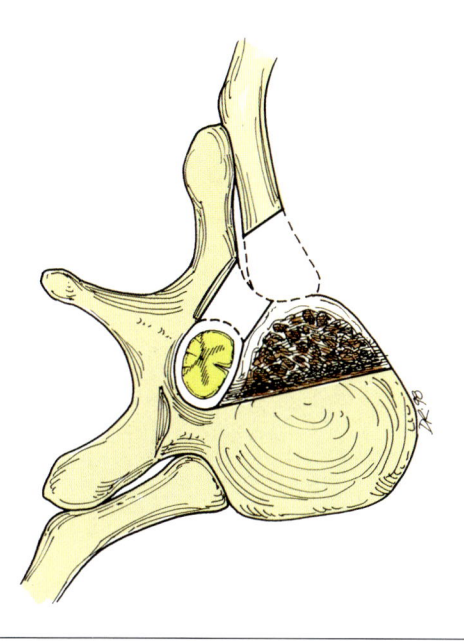

Fig. 51-19 Illustration showing the amount of bone that is removed from the vertebral body, head of the rib, and pedicle. (Modified from Spetzler RF, Koos WT: Approaches. In Spetzler RF, Koos WT: Color Atlas of Microneurosurgery, 2nd ed. Vol. 3. New York, Thieme, 2000, p 94.)

CHAPTER 52

SERGEY NECKRYSH
FADY T. CHARBEL
G. MICHAEL LEMOLE, JR.

Vascular Lesions of the Spinal Cord

INTRODUCTION

There are three classes of vascular spinal cord lesions, which will be addressed in this chapter: (1) vascular neoplastic lesions, which are represented by hemangioblastomas and cavernous malformations; (2) arteriovenous malformations and arteriovenous fistulas; and (3) spinal cord aneurysms.

HEMANGIOBLASTOMA

EPIDEMIOLOGY

Spinal cord hemangioblastomas (Figs. 52-1 and 52-2) are rare lesions that represent 1% to 3% of all intramedullary spinal cord tumors. Males are affected twice as often as females. Central nervous system (CNS) hemangioblastomas are present in 21% to 72% of patients with von Hippel–Lindau (VHL) disease, and approximately 40% of them are located in the spinal cord. Multiple lesions can be present in 25% to 33% of patients with CNS hemangioblastomas.[1] This figure may underestimate the actual incidence, as not all patients undergo a full workup for VHL disease. Spinal hemangioblastomas are intramedullary (75%) or have extramedullary-intradural extension (10% to 15%). Approximately 96% of spinal hemangioblastomas are located posterior to dentate ligament.[2] Extradural hemangioblastomas are rare and may arise from the vertebral bodies. By location, 50% of spinal hemangioblastomas occur in the thoracic cord, 40% in the cervical cord, and 6% in the lumbar region. Hemangioblastomas have also been rarely reported in the conus medullaris,[3] filum terminale,[4] nerve roots, and peripheral nerves.[5]

CLINICAL PRESENTATION AND NATURAL HISTORY

Typical age at presentation is between 40 and 50 years old in patients with sporadic hemangioblastomas (lesions are more often intracranial) and late 20 to early 30 years old in patients with VHL disease. Hemangioblastomas usually present with nonspecific signs of intramedullary mass and syrinx. Syrinx is seen in approximately 50% to 70% of patients. Initial symptoms can be divided into three major groups: (1) sensory changes in 38.9% of patients (mostly numbness and involvement of posterior columns), (2) weakness in 27.8%, and (3) pain in 33% (in these cases the tumor frequently extends into or originates from the dorsal root entry zone).[6] Patients may also present with signs of myelopathy and urinary incontinence. Surprisingly, spontaneous hemorrhage

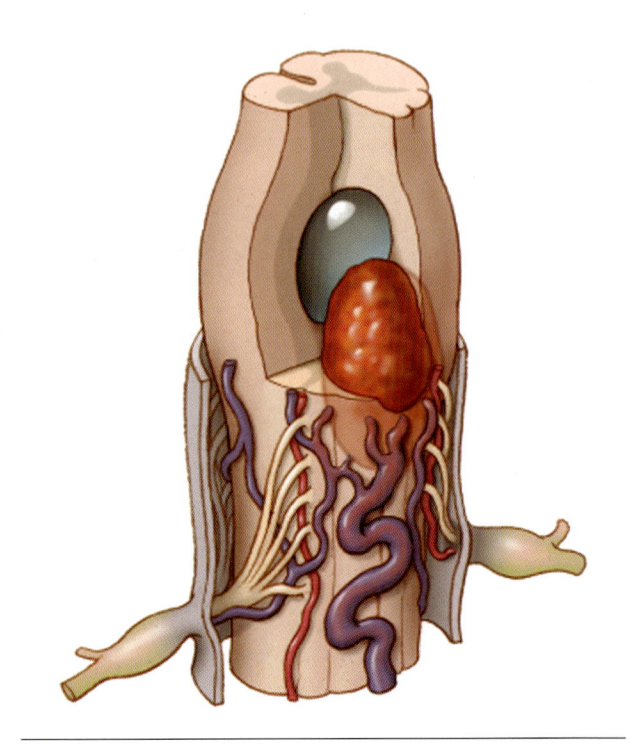

Fig. 52-1 Hemangioblastoma.

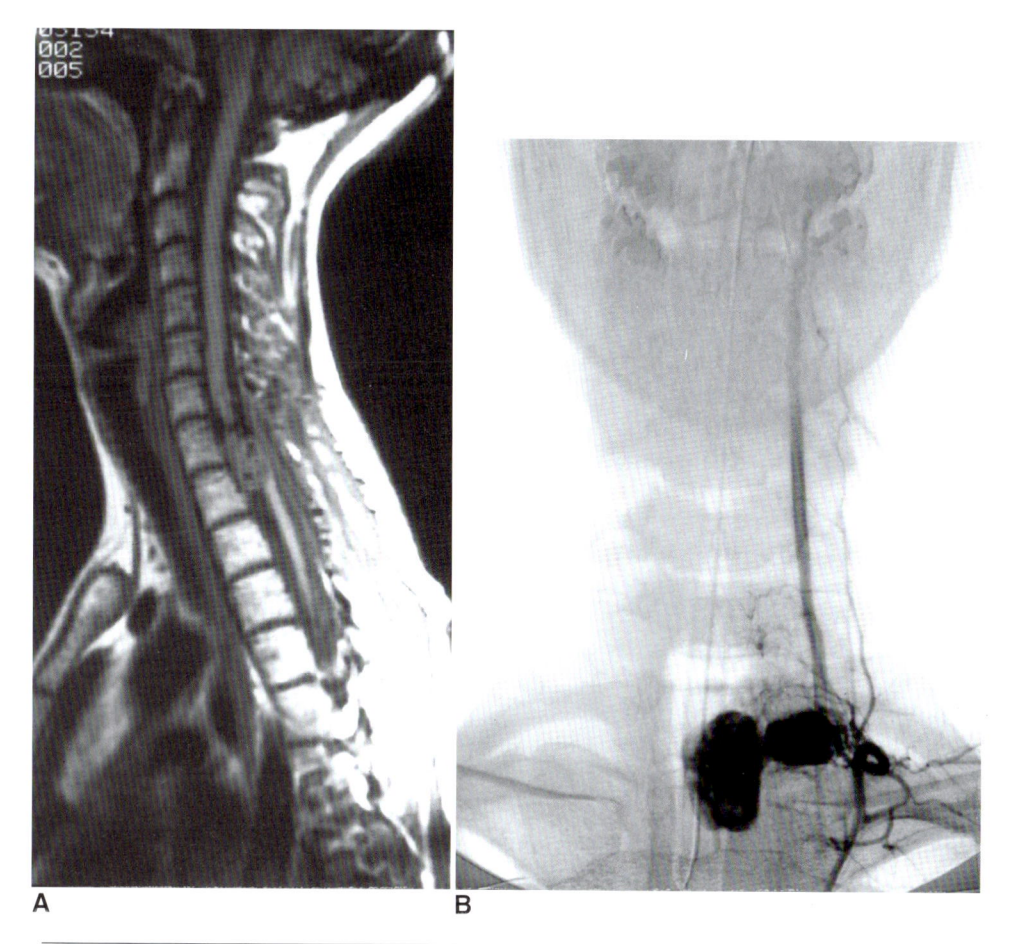

Fig. 52-2 Spinal hemangioblastoma. *A*, T$_1$-weighted sagittal magnetic resonance image demonstrating hemangioblastoma in the ventral portion of the spinal cord at the T1-T2 level. Flow voids from dilated venous plexus of the spinal cord surrounding the lesion at the corresponding levels. *B*, Selective spinal angiogram of the same patient demonstrating a lobulated highly vascular lesion, which was found to be hemangioblastoma on pathologic examination after surgical resection.

from spinal hemangioblastomas is quite rare. The majority of cases present with subarachnoid hemorrhage (SAH), and intramedullary hemorrhage was less common.[7]

PATHOLOGY

The typical spinal cord hemangioblastoma usually enlarges the cord, is well demarcated, and consists of a highly vascular nodule with an associated cyst. There are prominent leptomeningeal vessels. Histologically, these tumors are composed of an intricate vascular network of irregular and often dilated capillaries with intervening stromal cells. These stromal cells can produce erythropoietin resulting in erythrocytosis. Immunostaining for epithelial markers is negative for hemangioblastomas. These markers are important when differentiating between hemangioblastomas and metastatic renal cell carcinomas, which may also develop in patients with VHL syndrome.[8,9]

IMAGING

Dilated tortuous feeding arteries and draining pial veins can be seen on a myelogram in approximately 50% of cases. Angiography demonstrates a highly vascular mass with dense vascular blush and draining vessels, which can mimic an arteriovenous malformation (AVM). Preoperative embolization is a valid option. Magnetic resonance imaging (MRI) findings are consistent with diffuse cord expansion with high-signal intensity on T$_2$-weighted imaging with prominent foci of high-velocity signal loss. Cyst formation and syrinx are seen in 50% to 70% of cases.[1,2] There is a strong enhancement of the tumor nodule with contrast administration.

SURGICAL CONSIDERATIONS

Progressive neurologic deterioration caused by mass effect of the tumor and enlarging syrinx, or acute neurologic deficit caused by hemorrhage are indications to surgically intervene.

In patients with VHL disease, lesions can be multiple and it is very important to pinpoint the deficit to the particular symptomatic location. Ultimately, multiple surgical interventions may be needed in these patients to treat the disease over their lifetime. Hemangioblastomas are considered in the discussion of vascular spinal cord malformations because they often behave like AVMs during surgical resection.

SURGICAL TECHNIQUE

- Patient is positioned depending on the location of hemangioblastoma and appropriate approach is performed to extend one level above and one level below the margins of the tumor. Bone removal (laminectomy, laminoplasty, corpectomy) must be adequate to allow exposure of tumor margins along with associated feeding and draining vessels.
- The dura mater is incised in the midline, elevated, and retracted the entire length of the exposure with preservation of the arachnoid membrane. Sharp or blunt "tearing" techniques can be used to extend the dural opening. Cotton pads or balls are sometimes employed to protect the underlying spinal cord during dural opening. Recall that spinal dura has only one layer, unlike cranial dura. Cottonoid strips can be packed into the lateral paraspinal gutters to maintain a bloodless operative field. Dural leaflets are tacked up to adjacent muscles or drapes with 4-0 braided nylon suture.
- The microscope is brought into the operative field and arachnoid is sharply dissected from the surface of the hemangioblastoma and associated vessels. In general, the tumor is approached like an AVM with special attention to feeding and draining vessels.
- Pial vessels crossing the margin of the tumor at its junction with the pia mater are coagulated using bipolar cautery at a low setting and sharply divided to clearly expose the margin of the tumor at the pial surface. Sensory rootlets embedded into the tumor may be dissected free or interrupted if the tumor is to be completely resected.
- The plane of dissection is developed in a circumferential manner using bipolar cuatery, microscissors, and small cottonoid strips. The tumor capsule is normally prominent. It is important that dissection is performed in a completely bloodless field so that each feeding/draining vessel can be distinguished from en passant vessels and interrupted as it reaches the surface of tumor capsule. Again, surgical technique mirrors that employed for AVM resection.
- Traction on the the spinal cord or "tenting" should be avoided while reflecting the poles of the tumor.
- Bipolar electrocautery must be used judiciously and at low voltage to avoid thermal injury to adjacent neural tissue. If bleeding occurs from the tumor capsule, coagulation often makes it worse. Hemostasis can be obtained by application of a variety of hemostatic agents such as Gelfoam soaked in thrombin.
- Piecemeal resection of the tumor often causes vigorous bleeding and should not be attempted unless the tumor is large and cannot otherwise be safely removed. In this scenario meticulous coagulation and hemostasis are imperative. A portion of the tumor can be removed to afford additional exposure.
- The operative bed is directly inspected to make certain no tumor residual remains and that hemostasis is complete.
- Dural closure is performed in a watertight manner with monofilament 4-0 or 5-0 suture on a tapered needle. Some surgeons apply fibrin glue over the suture line.
- Multiple layer closure of the wound is performed in a standard fashion.

OUTCOMES

Hemangioblastomas can be safely removed without significant new postoperative deficit. Approximately 80% of the patients will remain unchanged neurologically, 10% will improve, and another 10% will worsen. A recent National Institutes of Health (NIH) study published on surgical outcomes after hemangioblastoma resection demonstrated[10]:

- Location of the tumor anterior to the dentate ligament carries higher risk of new postoperative neurologic deficit.
- Likelihood of new permanent postoperative neurologic deficit increases with lesions larger than 500 mm.[3]
- Cysts associated with hemangioblastoma diminish or resolve in almost all patients. Presence of a cyst preoperatively does not alter the surgical outcome: There is no need to perform any additional surgical manipulations on the tumor cyst during resection.[10]

SPINAL CORD CAVERNOUS MALFORMATIONS

EPIDEMIOLOGY

Cavernous malformations (Fig. 52-3) can be considered as neoplastic lesions based on their features and growth pattern. These lesions can occur sporadically or in a familial pattern and have identifiable genetic abnormality with autosomal-dominant pattern of inheritance and incomplete penetrance. Spinal cord cavernous malformations represent 5% to 12% of all spinal cord vascular malformations and 3% to 15% of all cavernous malformations occurring in the central nervous system. There is slight female predominance. The mean age at symptomatic presentation and diagnosis is usually in the fourth decade of life. Thoracic cord is affected more often than cervical. Lesions in the conus medullaris and cauda equina are rare.

CLINICAL PRESENTATION AND NATURAL HISTORY

The clinical course of spinal cord cavernous malformations is variable. Patients can develop acute symptoms attributed to hemorrhage or present with stepwise deterioration, which can mimic demyelinating disorders. Acute presentation is characterized by pain corresponding to the level of the cav-

CHAPTER 52 Vascular Lesions of the Spinal Cord

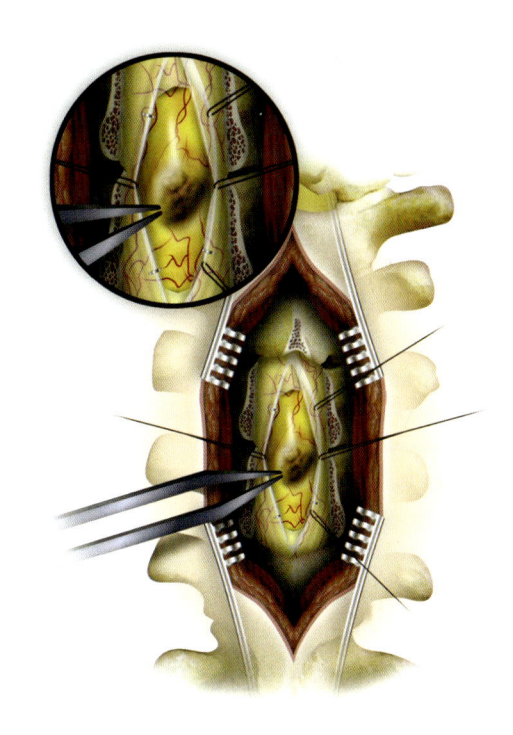

Fig. 52-3 Spinal cavernoma.

ernous malformation and neurologic deterioration, which can occur over several days. This is different from the typical hemorrhage caused by an AVM of the spinal cord, which is typically more acute and neurologic deficit is concomitant with the onset of pain. Initial hemorrhage from cavernous malformation can cause paraplegia or quadriplegia. Incomplete neurologic deficit followed by some degree of recovery, which is rarely complete, is more common. In untreated lesions repeated hemorrhages may occur months to years after the initial hemorrhage. A more subtle presentation can occur when the lesion is primarily localized on the dorsal aspect of the spinal cord, and patients will initially complain of intermittent paresthesias. Radiculopathy is more common with lesions in the dorsal root entry zone. With the widespread use of MRI, cavernous malformations are often discovered at an early symptomatic stage or even while asymptomatic.

PATHOLOGY

Spinal cord cavernous malformations are identical in appearance and histopathology to intracranial cavernous malformations. They are grossly described as soft and spongy with a dark blue to red-brown hue. Cavernous malformations are usually well circumscribed, and hemosiderin staining of the surrounding tissues caused by repeat bleeding can clearly define the plane of dissection. This discoloration is sometimes the only visual clue that a cavernous malformation may be located under the pial surface. Microscopically, cavernous malformations consist of endothelium-lined channels filled with blood with no intervening brain tissue. Vessel walls lack elastic and muscular layers. Calcifications are rare. There is usually a gliotic, often hemosiderin-laden plane around the malformation. Tongue-like extensions of the cavernous malformation can extend into the surrounding gliotic plane, and this should be kept in mind during resection of the cavernous malformation to achieve complete excision.

IMAGING

Findings on MRI include signs of hemorrhage in different stages of blood product degradation with a mixture of high- and low-intensity signal. The typical appearance of a cavernous malformation is an inhomogeneous high-intensity signal on both T_1- and T_2-weighted images with a "dark" ring of hemosiderin surrounding and appearing hypointense on T_1 and T_2 weighting. Enhancement is not typical for cavernous malformations. Unlike their intracranial counterparts, the diagnosis of spinal cord cavernous malformations with MRI is not always straightforward, especially with small lesions.[1] Classic "popcorn-like" appearance is not always seen in spinal cord cavernous malformations. In some cases spinal MRI, particularly T_2-weighted images, can be misleading for surgical planning when trying to estimate where the malformation comes closest to the pial surface. Malformations located superficially on MRI may be found to lie deeper in the spinal cord during surgical exploration. Nevertheless, MRI represents an invaluable imaging technique compared to more traditional imaging modalities, and with emergence of more powerful MR scanners, the quality of spinal cord imaging is rapidly improving. Angiography has very little value in diagnosing these angiographically occult lesions. The angiogram may demonstrate a venous anomaly associated with a cavernous malformation. The cavernous malformation, not the venous anomaly, is felt to be the source of recurrent hemorrhage. The venous anomaly represents an anatomic variant, and should be preserved during surgical resection, as it provides venous drainage to the surrounding, normal tissues. Preoperative embolization is not an option with cavernous malformations.

SURGICAL CONSIDERATIONS

The increasing experience with surgical excision of intramedullary spinal cord cavernous malformations and the high probability of neurologic deterioration if left untreated have expanded the role for surgical treatment of cavernous malformations. Studies have clearly demonstrated that progression of neurologic symptoms in patients with spinal cord cavernous malformations is the rule rather than the exception. Neurologic outcome is most dependent on the preoperative neurologic status of the patient, and best outcomes are achieved in patients with good neurologic status preoperatively. Another important consideration is that the spinal cord with its small cross-sectional area and very high eloquence is unlikely to tolerate even minor expansions from hemorrhage or cavernous malformations growth. Modern microsurgical technique can provide good outcomes with an acceptable level of postoperative morbidity in patients with spinal cord cavernous malformations. Surgery may be recommended to appropriate candidates with symptomatic lesions, especially when the cavernous malformation extends to the pial surface. This decision is, however, significantly more difficult in patients with asymptomatic or minimally symptomatic lesions or in patients with deep-seated lesions. In these cases, recommendations for radical surgical resection should be tailored to each individual case. Young patients and patients with large lesions are the most appropriate candidates in this group because they are most likely to experience long-term benefit from early surgical intervention.

SURGICAL TECHNIQUE
Dorsally Located Lesions (Fig. 52-4)

- Preoperative localization is an important part of surgical planning and can be performed using techniques of external skin marking or image guidance with fiducial application.
- Most cavernous malformations can be exposed and resected via posterior approach. Laminectomy or laminoplasty should provide adequate exposure for dorsally located lesions. Laminoplasty has been recommended for cervical or upper thoracic lesions to prevent postsurgical kyphotic deformity.
- Laminoplasty in patients without significant degenerative disease or spinal cord expansion can be performed with a pneumatic drill and a foot plate attachment with laminar cuts on both sides. Ligamentous structures are sharply divided, and the lamina and spinous processes are removed en bloc over the levels of interest. Absolute hemostasis should be obtained before opening the dura.
- The intraoperative microscope is brought into the operative field, and dura mater is incised in the midline with preservation of the underlying arachnoid as described in previous sections. The dural edges are tacked up to the drapes or paraspinous muscles using 4-0 braided nylon sutures.
- The arachnoid is opened sharply in the midline and the edges are secured to the ipsilateral dural leaflet.
- The spinal cord is examined under high magnification, and malformations extending toward the pial surface may be visible at the surface. In other cases blue or red-brown discoloration of the spinal cord caused by hemosiderin deposits will be visible and will point to the location of the malformation. Image guidance or intraoperative ultrasound could be used to localize the lesions that lack any clues to their location.
- The "two-point" method is used to determine the optimal entry point and trajectory through the spinal cord to the

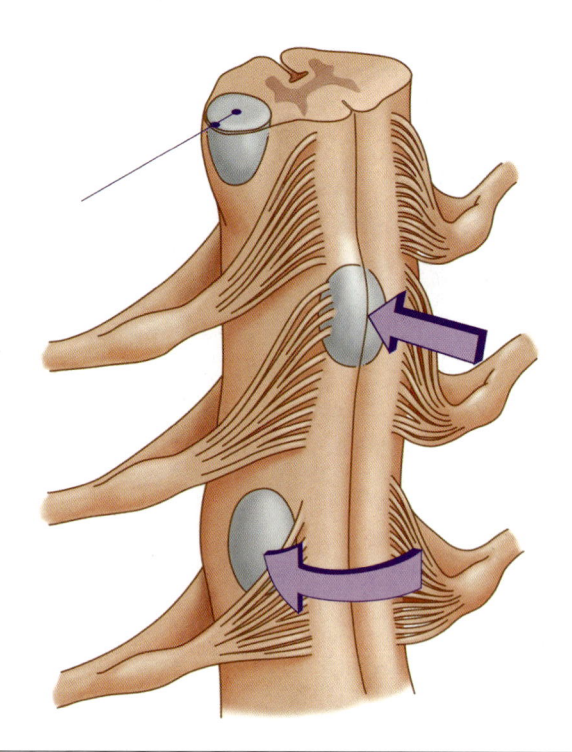

Fig. 52-4 Surgical corridors to the lesions in the spinal cord. *Straight arrow:* Certain lesions in the spinal cord located posteriorly and extending to the pial surface in the midline could be approached safely by performing an incision through the dorsal median septum of the spinal cord. *Curved arrow:* Lesions located paramedially and extending to the pial surface of the spinal cord at the dorsal root entry zone could be approached via dorsolateral sulcus of the spinal cord. *Dotted line:* Two-point method is used to design surgical approach to the lesion of the spinal cord located laterally when anatomic sulci of the spinal cord could not be utilized. First point is placed in the center of the lesion and second point is placed where the lesion comes closest to the pial surface. Line connecting two points will indicate the shortest trajectory to the lesion.

cavernous malformation. A line is drawn through the center of the lesion to the point where it comes closest to the surface. For deeper lesions, this technique is modified in the spinal cord to avoid eloquent tracts and take advantage of better tolerated avenues of approach (see Fig. 52-4).
- For deep-seated lesions, myelotomy is performed under high magnification either through the dorsal median sulcus or along the dorsal root entry zone, whichever offers a better trajectory to the malformation.
- Care must be taken to avoid damaging the adjacent normal spinal cord parenchyma, and sharp dissection with judicious use of bipolar electrocautery is the rule. Myelotomies should be parallel to fiber tracts on the long axis of the spinal cord to minimize damage.
- Resection of the lesion is performed using microcurettes and gentle suction aspiration. Handheld suction devices

with thumb apertures offer controlled suction strength which is critical to avoid damaging surrounding tissues. Typically, lesions will be removed in a piecemeal fashion, although some can be resected en bloc. Although not truly encapsulated, cavernous malformations have a well-defined, gliotic plane separating it from the surrounding spinal cord.
- Bleeding is seldom a problem with cavernous malformations because of their low-flow nature, and hemostasis should be accomplished using hemostatic agents and gentle compression. Bipolar cautery use should be avoided unless absolutely necessary and should be set to a very low power.
- Venous draining anomalies are often associated with cavernous malformations and should be preserved because they may provide venous drainage for adjacent eloquent tissues.
- After hemostasis is obtained, careful inspection of the resection bed under high magnification is imperative to identify and further resect small "tongues" of cavernous malformation that may extend into the adjacent tissue. Incompletely resected lesions can recur and hemorrhage; therefore, every attempt should be made to resect these lesions fully during the first surgery.
- Dura is closed in a watertight fashion as described in previous sections. A multilayer wound closure is performed using standard techniques.

Ventrally Located Lesions (Fig. 52-5)

Lesions involving the anterior and lateral aspect of the spinal cord are much more difficult to approach; however, if the lesion is symptomatic and reaches the anterior or lateral pial surface surgery can be attempted. In these cases surgical morbidity is generally higher owing to the increased spinal cord eloquence and difficulty of the surgical approaches. Generally, only lesions that reach a pial surface are approached from an anterior perspective. Approaches through the dorsal median sulcas and dorsal root entry zone are better tolerated with deep lesions.

Lesions located anteriorly in the cervical spinal cord can be approached via cervical corpectomy, which will require anterior interbody arthrodesis and instrumentation in the conclusion of the surgical procedure. The depth and narrowness of the surgical field in this approach is a challenge. Principles of dural opening, lesion localization and removal, and closure are similar to the posterior technique.

In the thoracic region access to the anterior spinal cord can be obtained via thoracotomy with a corpectomy. Although this approach allows adequate visualization of the anterolateral aspect of the spinal cord, working angle and depth of the field make surgical conditions less ideal. Watertight dural closure is even more crucial in this location because of the potential to develop a cerebrospinal fluid leak into the pleural cavity.

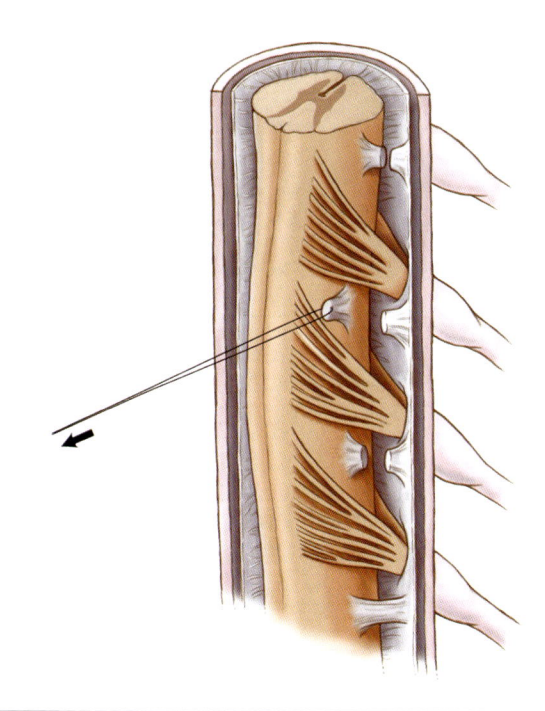

Fig. 52-5 Approach to the lesions of the spinal cord located anteriorly. Lesions extending or located on the anterior surface of the spinal cord are the most challenging for surgical approach. They could be accessed via vertebral corpectomy, or they could be exposed from a posterior approach. Dentate ligament closest to the lesion is cut and 4-0 braided nylon suture is passed through the stump of the ligament. Suture is used to gently rotate the spinal cord, exposing the anteriorly located lesion.

The posterolateral transpedicular approach described by Martin and associates[11] can also be used to access the lesions in the anterolateral thoracic spinal cord. The details of this approach are summarized here:
- Combined posterior midline and transverse incisons are performed over the appropriate levels and the thoracic laminae are exposed on the side from which the lesion will be approached.
- Bony elements of the posterolateral thoracic spine are removed using rongeurs and a high-speed drill.
- The ipsilateral pedicles at the corresponding levels are removed down to their insertion with the vertebral bodies to expose the lateral aspect of thoracic dura.
- Dural opening is performed along the lateral thecal sac in a fashion similar to the one described for the posterior approach.
- The critical part of the approach is to identify and section the dentate ligament several levels above and below the location of cavernous malformation. Stitches are placed in the proximal portion of the ligament to facilitate gentle rotation of the spinal cord and expose the ipsilateral ventral

TABLE 52-1 Classification of Spinal Cord Vascular Malformations

TRADITIONAL CLASSIFICATION*	SPETZLER CLASSIFICATION,† EXTRADURAL AV FISTULAS
I. Arteriovenous (AV) fistulas located in the dura of the nerve root	1. Extradural AV fistulas is a subtype of the AVMs
	2. Intradural dorsal AV fistulas Single feeder (subtype A) Multiple feeders (subtype B)
IV. Intradural arteriovenous fistulas with medullary artery on the pial surface communicating directly with the pial vein without intervening nidus	3. Intradural ventral AV fistulas Type A (small shunt, low flow) Type B (medium shunt, higher flow) Type C (large shunt, highest flow)
III. Juvenile AV malformation (AVM) with abnormal tangle of blood vessels filling the spinal cord at the involved levels and containing neural parenchyma within the nidus of the AVM	4. Extradural-intradural AVM
II. Glomus AVM with localized and tightly coiled intraparenchymal nidus receiving supply from medullary artery and draining via normal venous routes	5. Intramedullary AVM
	6. Conus AVM

*Rosenblum B, Oldfield EH, Doppman JL, et al: Spinal arteriovenous malformations: a comparison of dural arteriovenous fistulas and intradural AVM's in 81 patients. J Neurosurg 1987;67(6):795–802.
†Spetzler RF, Detwiler PW, Riina HA, et al: Modified classification of spinal cord vascular lesions. J Neurosurg Spine 2002;96(2):145–156.

portion of the cord and the cavernous malformation which extends to the pia. Resection of the malformation is then carried out as described in previous sections.
- Limitations of this approach include inadequate visualization of anterior cord surface beyond the anterior midline and anterior spinal artery. Bilateral posterolateral transpedicular approaches may be performed to expose a lesion that crosses the midline. Such aggressive bony resection will likely require stabilization with instrumentation and fusion at the completion of the procedure.

OUTCOMES

Cavernous malformations of the spinal cord can be resected using contemporary microsurgical techniques with overall improvement in patient condition and natural history. Morbidity and recovery after surgical resection usually mimics a bleeding episode and can be justified if the risk of future bleeding is eliminated. If surgical intervention is attempted every possible effort should be made to resect the lesion fully to prevent lesion recurrence, regrowth, and rehemorrhage. MRI immediately after surgery can be ambiguous if blood in the operative bed obscures the presence of residual cavernous malformation. This is particularly the case with T_2-weighted imaging. Patients should undergo MRI surveillance 6 to 12 months after the initial surgery and 2 to 3 years thereafter. If recurrence is suspected clinically and radiographically, reoperation can be considered.

SPINAL CORD ARTERIOVENOUS MALFORMATIONS

CLASSIFICATION

Historical classification schemes for rare spinal cord AVMs were often confusing, but as case numbers and surgical experience grew, more coherent systems of thought were devised. The classification proposed by Rosenblum and associates in 1987 defined four major types of spinal AVMs based on angiographic findings and hemodynamic features (Table 52-1).[12] With later modifications, this system became the most widely accepted. Recent attempts to simplify and offer a more inclusive system of thought for all AVMs affecting the spinal cord led to a new classification by Spetzler and associates.[13] This latter classification system is utilized for subsequent discussion.

EPIDEMIOLOGY AND NATURAL HISTORY
Extradural Arteriovenous Fistulas (Fig. 52-6)

These fistulas are rare lesions. A direct connection between an extradural artery and vein results in venous hypertension, enlargement of the epidural venous complex, mass effect on the spinal cord, and impaired venous outflow. Sometimes these lesions present with acute epidural hemorrhage, which requires urgent surgical intervention.[14] When treated promptly, these patients generally have a very good prognosis.

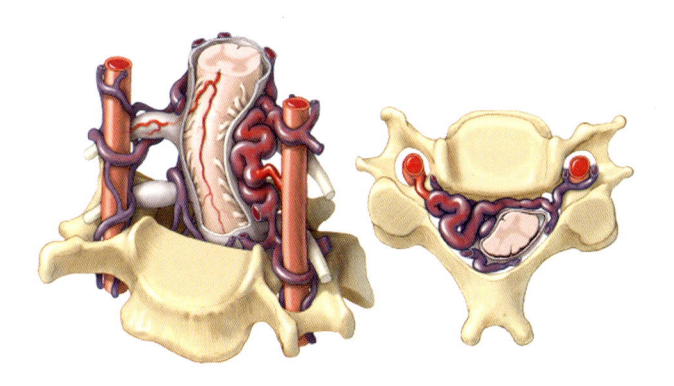

Fig. 52-6 Extradural arteriovenous fistulas. (From Spetzler RF, Meyer FB (eds): Youmans Neurological Surgery, 5th ed., Vol. 2, Section III: Vascular. St. Louis, Elsevier, 2004.)

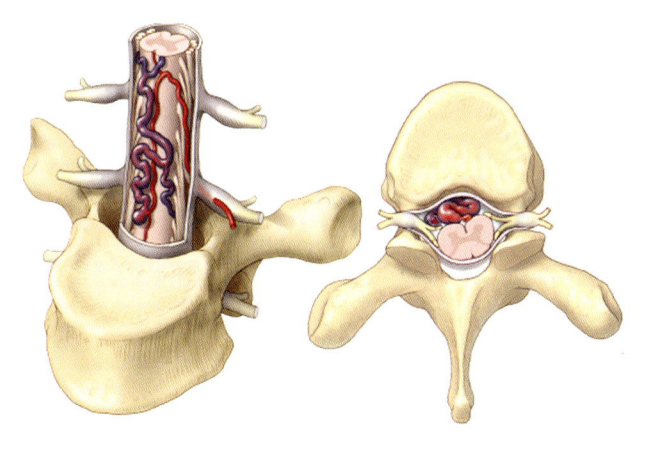

Fig. 52-8 Intradural ventral arteriovenous fistulas. (From Spetzler RF, Meyer FB (eds): Youmans Neurological Surgery, 5th ed., Vol. 2, Section III: Vascular. St. Louis, Elsevier, 2004.)

Intradural Dorsal Arteriovenous Fistulas (Fig. 52-7)

This fistula is the most common type of spinal vascular malformation, responsible for approximately 30% to 80% of spinal vascular malformations. Males are affected approximately three to five times more frequently than females.[11] These lesions predominantly occur in the lower thoracic spinal cord and conus medullaris. They usually consist of a plexiform low-flow shunt from intervertebral (radicular) arterial feeders or less frequently from sacral and hypogastric arteries. The connection to the medullary venous system is within the dural leaflet of the nerve root or immediately adjacent to it. There is no intervening nidus.[14] The shunt produces venous hypertension in the medullary veins, which constitute the sole venous outflow from the coronal venous plexus of the spinal cord. Symptoms are nonspecific and include back pain, weakness, sensory symptoms, and bowel or bladder dysfunction. Hemorrhage is rare and patients rarely present with acute symptoms. Once patients become symptomatic 90% will become disabled within 5 years if treatment is not initiated.

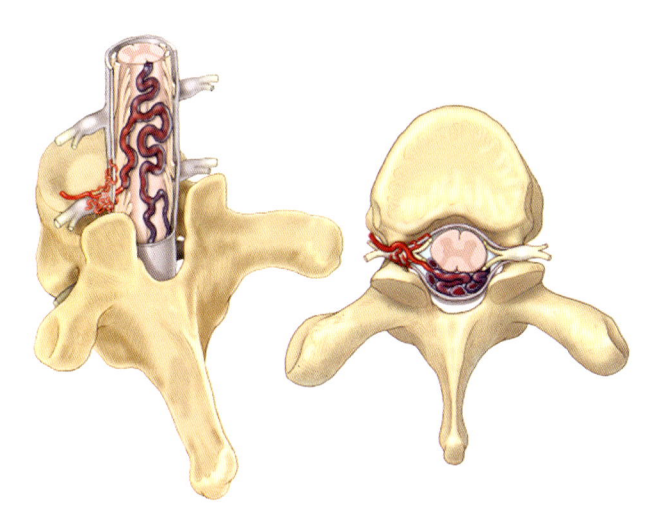

Intradural Ventral Arteriovenous Fistulas (Figs. 52-8 and 52-9)

These malformations account for 15% to 30% of spinal vascular malformations and occur in both males and females with equal frequency. Mean age at presentation is 45 years old. Typical location is thoracolumbar spinal cord and conus medullaris, but they may be found anywhere. These midline lesions derive their blood supply from anterior spinal artery or less frequently from posterior spinal artery with a fistulous component into the superficial venous system of the spinal cord.[15] Patients present with myelopathy, weakness, sensory deficits, pain, or sphincter problems. The incidence of hemorrhage is 10% to 20%. A progressive course is more typical than acute presentation.

Extradural-Intradural Arteriovenous Malformations (Fig. 52-10)

These very rare, large malformations, also known as juvenile AVMs, typically are found in adolescents and young adults in the cervical spinal cord. The vascular supply may arise from anterior and posterior spinal arteries, as well as arteries feeding extradural tissues. They present with hemorrhage, pain, and rapidly progressive neurologic deficit. These AVMs may occupy the entire lumen of the spinal canal and extend into the surrounding tissues and bone.[16] They are felt to arise embryologically from a single metamere. They can have a very aggressive clinical course, are very difficult to treat, and are often considered inoperable. Despite multimodality

Fig. 52-7 Intradural dorsal arteriovenous fistulas. (From Spetzler RF, Meyer FB (eds): Youmans Neurological Surgery, 5th ed., Vol. 2, Section III: Vascular. St. Louis, Elsevier, 2004.)

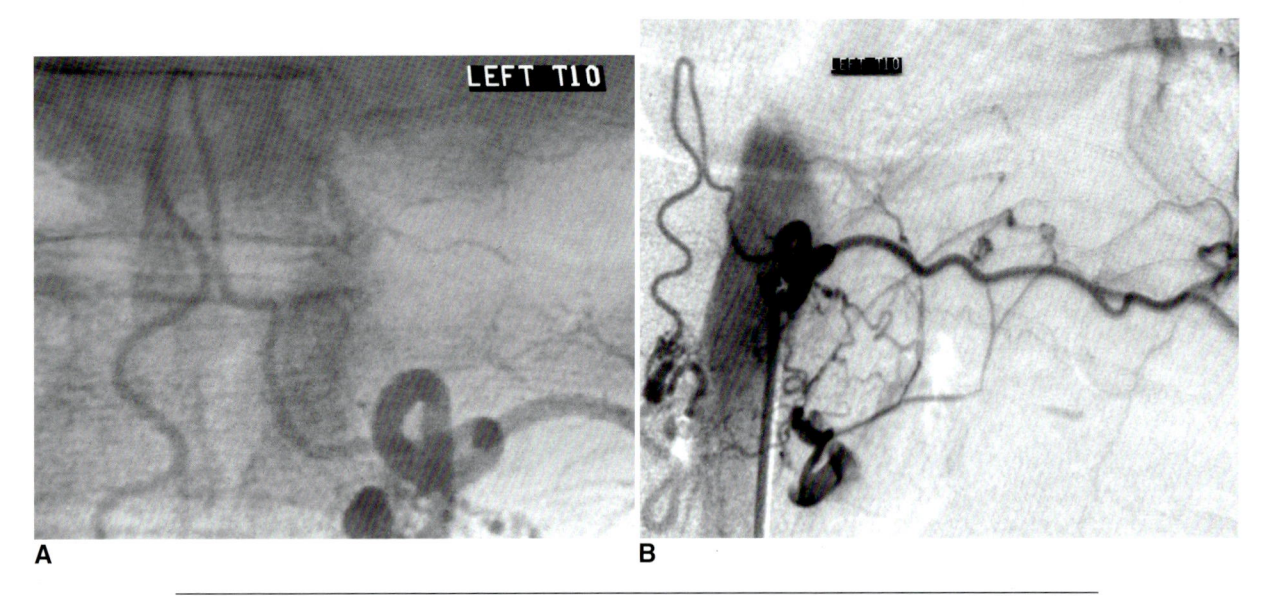

Fig. 52-9 Ventral arteriovenous fistula supplied by Adamkewitz artery. *A,* Non-DSA superselective image of Adamkewitz artery forming arterio-venous fistula. *B,* DSA image of the same patient demonstrating dilated coronal venous plexus of the spinal cord with engorgement of the draining veins.

intervention, prognosis is poor, and "their rarity is perhaps the only favorable aspect."[11]

Intramedullary Arteriovenous Malformations (Figs. 52-11 and 52-12)

A true AVM with a nidal component located within the parenchyma of the spinal cord, this type accounts for 15% to 20% of all spinal cord vascular malformations. There is no gender predilection, and lesions may be located anywhere in the spinal cord. Occasionally, they will extend to a pial surface. The main presenting symptom is acute or progressive myelopathy with or without radiculopathy. These high-flow and high-pressure lesions may harbor aneurysms in

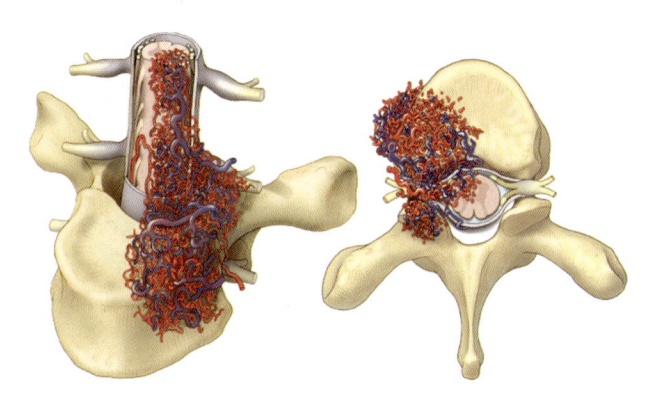

Fig. 52-10 Extradural-intradural arteriovenous malformations. (From Spetzler RF, Meyer FB (eds): Youmans Neurological Surgery, 5th ed., Vol. 2, Section III: Vascular. St. Louis, Elsevier, 2004.)

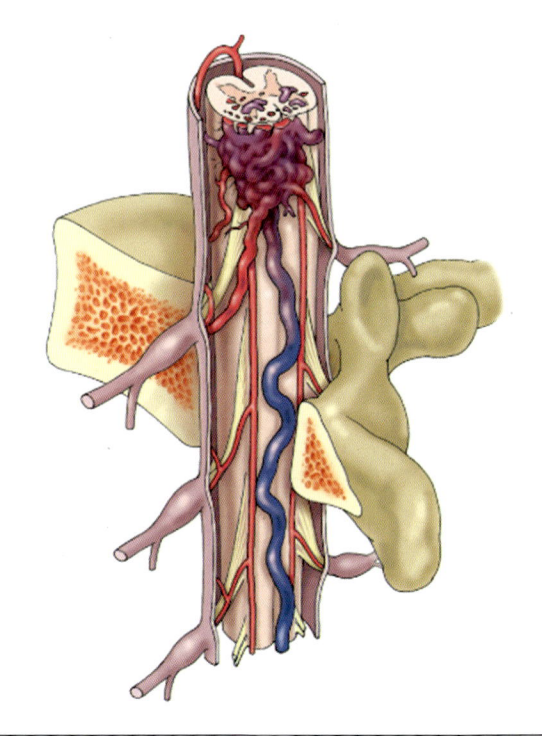

Fig. 52-11 Intramedullary arteriovenous malformations. (From Spetzler RF, Meyer FB (eds): Youmans Neurological Surgery, 5th ed., Vol. 2, Section III: Vascular. St. Louis, Elsevier, 2004.)

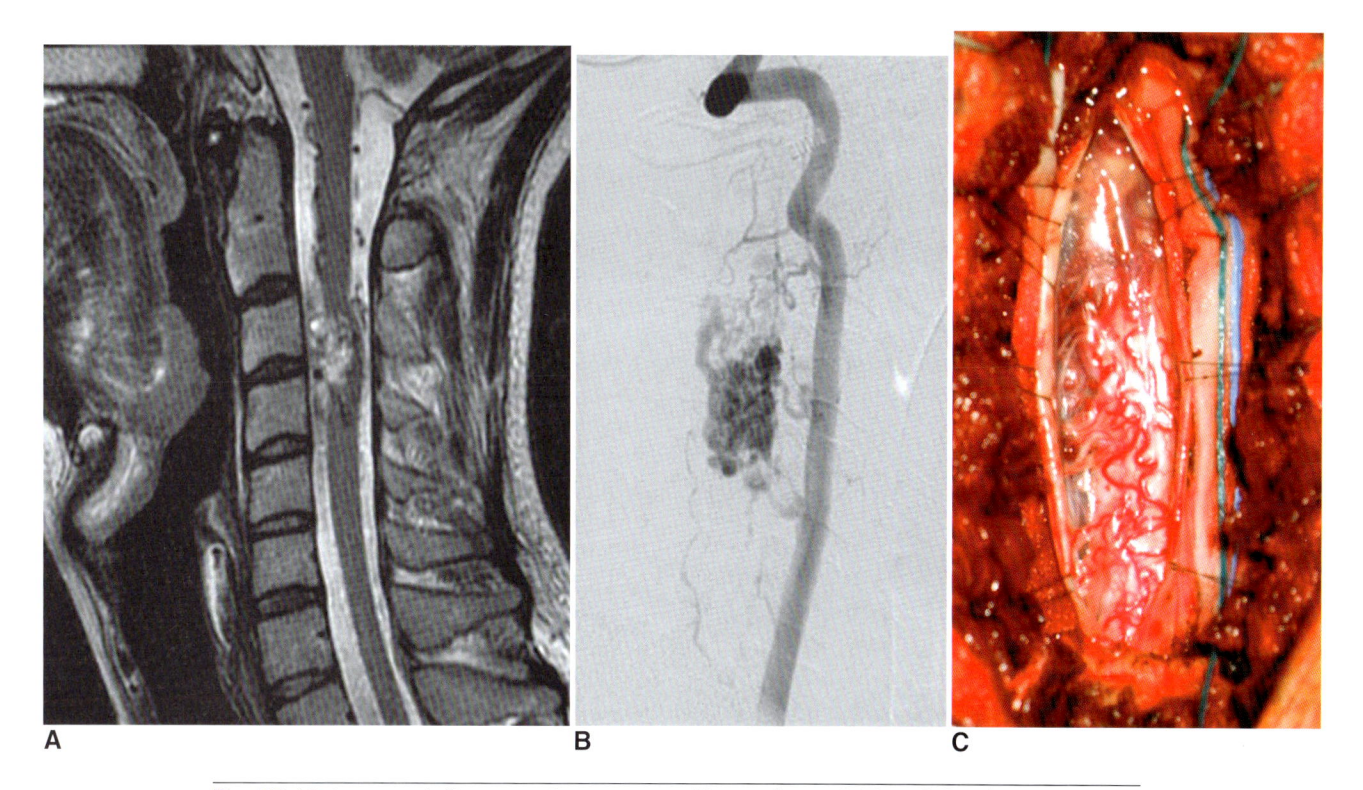

CHAPTER **52** Vascular Lesions of the Spinal Cord   483

A **B** **C**

Fig. 52-12 Intramedullary arteriovenous malformations. *A*, T_2-weighted sagittal magnetic resonance image demonstrating intramedullary arteriovenous malformation at C3-C4 levels with associated hematoma and flow voids from arterialized coronal venous plexus of the spinal cord. *B*, Selective spinal angiogram of the same patient demonstrating intramedullary arteriovenous malformation supplied mainly by the feeders arising from the left vertebral artery. *C*, Intraoperative image of the same patient. The spinal cord at C3-C4 levels was exposed via laminectomy. Note arterialized venous plexus of the spinal cord.

approximately 20% to 50% of cases. This leads to a higher incidence of acute presentation due to subarachnoid or intraparenchymal hemorrhage.

Conus Arteriovenous Malformations (Fig. 52-13)

These location-specific lesions are rare, complex, involving conus medullaris or cauda equina, and consisting of multiple feeders, multiple nidi with complex venous dranage. The arterial supply arises from anterior spinal artery or branches of posterior spinal artery.[13] Presentation is nonspecific and myeloradiculopathy is attributed to mass effect, hemorrhage, or venous hypertension.

PATHOPHYSIOLOGY

By definition, shunting of arterial blood flow into a venous bed without an intervening capillary network is the main feature of any AVM. Histopathologic analysis of recovered specimen will demonstrate vascular tissue with varying degrees of vessel wall breakdown, particularly in the venous elastic lamina. Shunting of arterial flow results in a set of

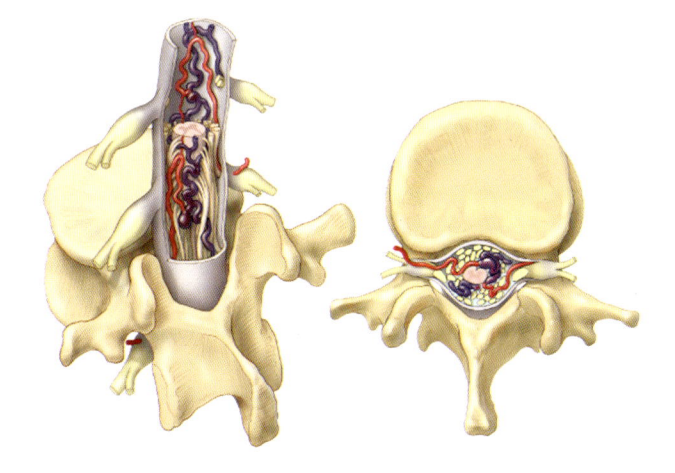

Fig. 52-13 Conus arteriovenous malformations. (From Spetzler RF, Meyer FB (eds): Youmans Neurological Surgery, 5th ed., Vol. 2, Section III: Vascular. St. Louis, Elsevier, 2004.)

pathophysiologic mechanisms responsible for neurologic symptoms. These mechanisms include the following:
- Subarachnoid hemorrhage and intraparenchymal hemorrhage
- Venous hypertension
- Vascular steal
- Arachnoiditis
- Mass effect with compression of the spinal cord or nerve roots

The presence of one or several of these mechanisms varies, depending on the type of the vascular malformation, its location, and the nature of the arterial feeders and venous outflow. A detailed discussion of AVM pathophysiology is beyond the scope of this chapter.

IMAGING

Although conventional myelography and computed tomographic (CT) myelography have been described as an imaging modality of some value in the past, today the patient is most likely to get an MRI of the spine and spinal cord as an initial imaging step. MRI can demonstrate a dilated tortuous venous system with flow-void signals, enlargement of the cord at the level of the nidus, products of blood degradation in case of prior hemorrhage, and changes in the cord attributed to venous hypertension, vascular steal, and previous hemorrhage. Current MRI resolution usually does not demonstrate the nidus or fistula, nor can it clearly delineate the feeding and outflow vascular anatomy precisely; thus, selective and superselective angiography remains the gold standard for evaluation of spinal cord vascular malformations. Endovascular treatment has a role in management of spinal vascular malformations and sometimes is the only treatment option.

SURGICAL CONSIDERATIONS

It is crucial that the vascular anatomy and flow characteristics of these lesions are understood exquisitely before attempting to treat them surgically. Angiography allows precise localization of the nidus or fistula and identification of the vascular supply and venous drainage patterns. It is useful to perform angiography using external markers, which will later serve as a reference for the surgical approach. Intraoperative monitoring of somatosensory evoked potentials has been demonstrated to improve outcomes after endovascular as well as surgical stages of treatment.

The surgical approach is selected based on the location of the lesion. Dorsally located lesions are approached via laminotomy, laminectomy, or hemilaminectony with facetectomy. Intraoperative angiography can be extremely useful both to locate a lesion and to demonstrate its obliteration. The femoral sheath for angiography is usually placed and secured before patient positioning. The patient is generally positioned prone on chest rolls or frame. Careful positioning will avoid abdominal compression, which can increase venous pressure in the venous plexus of the spinal cord. Venous hypertension can make hemostasis problematic. Alternative positions such as sitting and lateral can be considered for appropriate lesions.

The skin incision is planned two levels above and below the level of interest. Laminae are exposed using standard techniques. Skin edges and paraspinous musculature are retracted using self-retaining retractors. Alternatively, fishhooks can be used to retract by securing them to Leila bars on either side of the incision; this will depress the edges of the incision, offer a shallower surgical field, and facilitate surgical technique under the microscope.

Laminotomy is performed en bloc using a high-speed pneumatic drill with pediatric footplate tip. Laminae can be reimplanted at closure and secured with either plates or sutures. The dural opening is performed without violation of the arachnoid membrane and the dural edges are secured to the drapes or paraspinous tissues with 4-0 Neurolon sutures. The microscope is usually brought into the field at this point, although microscopic technique may also facilitate dural opening.

Occasionally, a hemilaminectomy with unilateral facetectomy can be utilized to gain adequate exposure to dorsolateral lesions, such as intradural dorsal arteriovenous fistulas. Stability is usually not an issue after unilateral facetectomy, but a stabilization procedure can be performed at the time of initial surgery or as a second stage after assessment of stability in postoperative period.

The surgical approach to the ventrally located lesions is more difficult. Corpectomy is generally utilized to gain exposure to the ventral dura. The approach for anterior cervical lesions is similar to that used for anterior cervical corpectomies. Thoracic lesions can be approached via thoracotomy, and retroperitoneal approach is used for lumbar lesions. These approaches require a surgical stabilization procedure at the completion of the operation.

SURGICAL TECHNIQUE
Extradural Arteriovenous Fistulas

Surgical treatment of these lesions is focused on interrupting the shunt into the venous plexus of the cord. The lesion is exposed posteriorly using one of the approaches previously described. The feeding vessel is identified and sacrificed using electrocautery and interrupted with microscissors.

Intradural Dorsal Arteriovenous Fistulas

- Goal of the surgical treatment is to eliminate venous hypertension by interrupting communication between the fistula and venous plexus of the spinal cord.
- Rarely, these lesions may be considered for endovascular obliteration, but in general, they are considered surgical cases.

- After the dural opening operative microscope is brought into the operative field.
- The arachnoid is opened with microscissors and the edges are secured to the the dura using small hemoclips or sutures. The underlying veins of coronal venous plexus can be quite dilated and caution should be exercised while opening the arachnoid over them.
- Vascular anatomy should be explored to identify the efferent vein from the fistula. The fistula is generally located in the dural leaflet along the nerve root sleeve. Temporary interruption of the fistula can be accomplished using temporary aneurysm clips
- Coronal venous plexus is observed for decreased venous distention resulting from interruption of the shunt. If this phenomenon does not occur that means that additional vascular contribution to the coronal venous plexus may exist and intraoperative angiography can be utilized to identify it.
- Once the fistula site is confirmed, the fistula itself is cauterized using bipolar cautery and sharply sectioned. Temporary clips are removed and the venous plexus is inspected for resumption of normal venous color and distention.
- The dura is closed in a standard watertight fashion followed by the standard multilayer soft tissue and skin closure.
- General anesthesia is reversed in the end of the case and patient's neurologic function is assessed in the operating room.
- Patients should undergo an intraoperative or postoperative angiogram on the first postoperative day to evaluate the completeness of surgical intervention. If the fistula is not completely obliterated, serious consideration needs to be given to reexploration.

Intradural Ventral Arteriovenous Fistulas

- Goal of the surgery is to interrupt the communication between the arterial feeder (or rarely, feeders) arising most often from the anterior spinal artery and draining veins on the pial surface. These lesions do not have a formal nidus and are superficial.
- Many surgeons agree that type A and some of type B lesions should be approached surgically, not endovascularly, because the fistula is very small and attempting embolization can result in occlusion of the anterior spinal artery with devastating neurologic sequelae.
- The anterior approaches to the spinal cord are described in preceding sections. The dura and arachnoid are opened in the usual manner.
- The ventral surface of the spinal cord is explored using the operative microscope, and the location of the fistulous connection is established. Feeders arising from the posterior spinal arteries must also be interrupted. The veins on the pial surface drain normal tissue and should be preserved during dissection.
- Whenever possible, the fistula should interrupted using clip ligation rather than bipolar electrocautery because of possible current spread and coagulation of the anterior spinal artery with devastating neurologic injury.
- Veins in the ventral surface of the cord are observed for color change and collapse after fistula obliteration. If the veins remain arterialized, additional feeders must be located and ligated.
- Dural closure is performed in a standard watertight fashion. Soft tissues and skin are closed in a multilayer fashion.

Extradural-Intradural Arteriovenous Malformations

- Surgical experience with these lesions is limited owing to their rarity. There are only a few cases of successful treatment of extradural-intradural AVMs in the literature.
- Many surgeons accept these lesions as inoperable, and endovascular treatment predominates in the management of extradural-intradural AVMs. Often, surgical or endovascular treatment is palliative in nature, aimed at reducing shunt flow to ameliorate neurologic symptoms from venous hypertension or mass effect.
- When surgery is an option, it is performed in a staged fashion in combination with preoperative embolization. The surgical techniques employed are described in the sections of this chapter for the other types of vascular malformations.

Intramedullary Arteriovenous Malformations

- Combined endovascular and surgical approach is considered to be most effective for the management of intramedullary AVMs.
- Laminectomy, dural, and arachnoid openings are performed as described earlier.
- Sharp arachnoid opening and dissection are performed because use of bipolar electrocautery may result in current spread to the adjacent dilated veins draining the normal spinal cord.
- Arachnoid dissection should be performed very carefully to avoid damage to the underlying distended veins. Because these AVMs are high-flow and high-pressure lesions hemostasis can be very problematic, and all attempts should be made to avoid violating the integrity of the distended venous vasculature.
- No vessel should be coagulated and interrupted until it has been clearly determined to supply the nidus of the AVM. This can be best ascertained by intraoperative exploration or angiography. As with cerebral AVMs, arterial feeders must be sacrificed before the venous outflow is disconnected; otherwise, a devastating rupture of the nidus could ensue.

- Midline or paramedian myelotomy is performed if nidus of the AVM is deep and does not reach the pial surface. The paramedian myelotomy can be considered if the patient already has fixed sensory deficit.
- A very thin gliotic plane often surrounds the nidus of the AVM. Resection of the nidus is undertaken using bipolar electrocautery within this plane by interruption of the small penetrating vessels. Penetrating vessels should be cauterized and cut with microscissors as close to the nidus as possible because proximal portions of the vessel tends to retract into the cord parenchyma and continue bleeding. Chasing these vessel stumps with electrocautery risks damaging the adjacent spinal cord tissue.
- Many AVMs harbor aneurysms, which can be obliterated using bipolar electrocautery during the early stages of nidus resection. This maneuver gains additional working space for nidus dissection.
- When there is a significant contribution from the anterior spinal artery, hemostasis may become an issue as these feeders may be deep to the nidus. Early identification and interruption of these feeders may decrease the amount of intraoperative bleeding and volume of the nidus. Extreme caution must be used when working near the anterior spinal artery.
- Very meticulous hemostasis and minimal cord manipulation is imperative for successful resection with minimal neurologic deficits.
- Closure is performed in the standard fashion.

Conus Arteriovenous Malformations

Because of their complexity, these lesions often require staged and combined endovascular and neurosurgical approach. Embolization could be used as either a definitive treatment or as an adjunct to surgical resection. Operative technique incorporates approaches and surgical tricks described earlier for intramedullary malformations and intradural fistulas.

SPINAL CORD ANEURYSMS

Spinal cord aneurysms are extremely rare. Only sporadic cases are described in the literature. Spinal cord aneurysms can be classified into two basic groups: (1) aneurysms arising within the abnormal vasculature of preexisting vascular malformations and (2) isolated aneurysms, which form without any associated vascular anomalies. These lesions usually present with subarachnoid hemorrhage or intraparenchymal hemorrhage. Treatment of the aneurysms within the nidus of an AVM is described earlier. Isolated aneurysms can be clipped or treated using endovascular technique. Surgical approaches to specific spinal regions are described in previous sections.

REFERENCES

1. Osborn AG, Maack J: Diagnostic Neuroradiology. St. Louis, Mosby, 1994.
2. Wanebo JE, Lonser RR, Glenn GM, Oldfield EH: The natural history of hemangioblastomas of the central nervous system in patients with von Hippel-Lindau disease. J Neurosurg 2003;98(1): 82–94.
3. Brisman JL, Borges LF, Ogilvy CS: Extramedullary hemangioblastoma of the conus medullaris. Acta Neurochir (Wien) 2000;142(9): 1059–1062.
4. Tibbs RE Jr, Harkey HL, Raila FA: Hemangioblastoma of the filum terminale: Case report. Neurosurgery 1999;44(1):221–223.
5. Escott EJ, Kleinschmidt-DeMasters BK, Brega K, et al: Proximal nerve root spinal hemangioblastomas: Presentation of three cases, MR appearance, and literature review. Surg Neurol 2004;61(3): 262–273.
6. Murota T, Symon L: Surgical management of hemangioblastoma of the spinal cord: A report of 18 cases. Neurosurgery 1989;25(5): 699–707.
7. Minami M, Hanakita J, Suwa H, et al: Cervical hemangioblastoma with a past history of subarachnoid hemorrhage. Surg Neurol 1998;49(3):278–281.
8. Graham DI: Color Atlas and Text of Neuropathology, 3rd ed. St. Louis, Mosby-YearBook, 1996.
9. Fuller GN, Clay J, Goodman MD: Practical Review of Neuropathology. Philadelphia, Lippincott Williams & Wilkins, 2001.
10. Lonser RR, Weil RJ, Wanebo JE, et al: Surgical management of spinal cord hemangioblastomas in patients with von Hippel–Lindau disease. J Neurosurg 2003;98(1):106–116.
11. Martin NA, Khanna RK, Batzdorf U: Posterolateral cervical or thoracic approach with spinal cord rotation for vascular malformations or tumors of the ventrolateral spinal cord. J Neurosurg 1995;83:254–261.
12. Rosenblum B, Oldfield EH, Doppman JL, et al: Spinal arteriovenous malformations: A comparison of dural arteriovenous fistulas and intradural AVMs in 81 patients. J Neurosurg 1987;67(6): 795–802.
13. Spetzler RF, Detwiler PW, Riina HA, et al: Modified classification of spinal cord vascular lesions. J Neurosurg Spine 2002;96(2): 145–156.
14. Riina HA, Spetzler, RA: Classification of vascular lesions affecting the spinal cord. Operative Techniques Neurosurg 2003;6(3): 106–115.
15. Barrow DL, Colohan ART, Dawson R: Intradural perimedullary arteriovenous fistulas (type IV spinal cord arteriovenous malformations). J Neurosurg 1994;81:221–229.
16. Spetzler RF, Zabramski JM, Flom RA: Management of juvenile spinal AVMs by embolization and operative excision: Case report. J Neurosurg 1989;70:628–632.

SECTION

VII

SPINAL INFECTION

CHAPTER 53

MICHAEL J. VIVES
KIAN RAISZADEH

Bacterial, Fungal, and Tuberculosis Diskitis and Osteomyelitis of the Cervical, Thoracic, and Lumbar Spine

INDICATIONS AND CONTRAINDICATIONS FOR SURGICAL MANAGEMENT OF SPINAL INFECTION

INDICATIONS

- Neurologic deficit from spinal cord injury, or progressive root level deficit

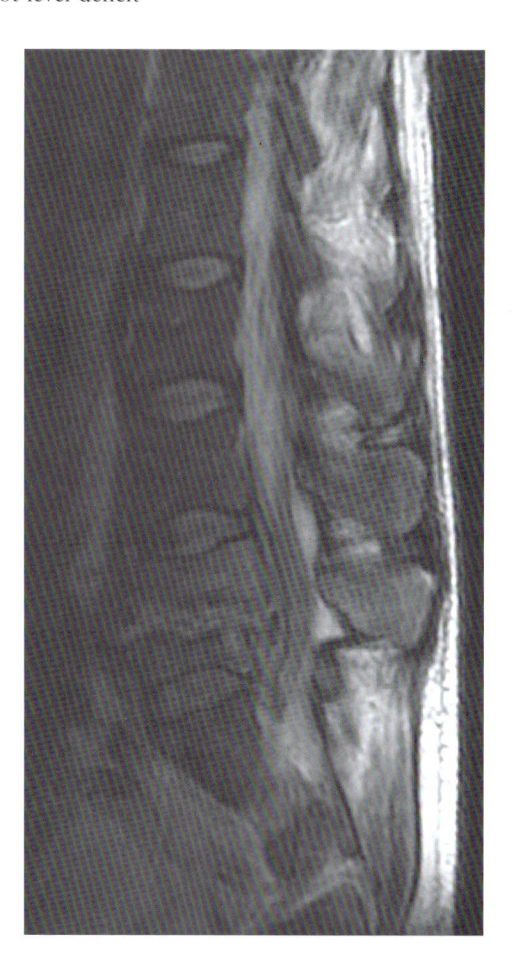

Fig. 53-1 In the setting of diskitis or spinal osteomyelitis, treatment goals can often be achieved without operative intervention.

INTRODUCTION

The management of spinal infections involves several general considerations. The ultimate goals in management are eradication of the infection, preservation of neurologic function, and prevention of sequelae such as progressive deformity or chronic pain. In the setting of diskitis or spinal osteomyelitis (Fig. 53-1), these goals can often be achieved without operative intervention. A presumptive diagnosis is made by the combination of suggestive laboratory findings (elevated erythrocyte sedimentation rate [ESR] and C-reactive protein [CRP]) and advanced imaging studies such as computed tomography (CT) and magnetic resonance (MR) imaging. A definitive tissue diagnosis of the offending pathogen can often be made utilizing percutaneous CT-guided biopsy. After determination of the organism's sensitivity profile, a 6-week course of the appropriate intravenous antibiotic is usually sufficient. Bracing is often prescribed as adjuvant treatment.

- Significant deformity, instability, or bone destruction/pathologic fracture
- Persistent sepsis or abscess formation
- Inability to identify the offending pathogen by closed methods
- Inability to eradicate the infection by medical management alone
- Intractable pain localized to the involved area of the spine

CONTRAINDICATIONS

- Medical comorbidities that make operative intervention prohibitive
- Uncorrected coagulopathies
- Medically stable, immunocompetent patient with early involvement, none of the above indications, and diagnosis made by biopsy

OPERATIVE TECHNIQUE

GENERAL CONSIDERATIONS

When surgical treatment is deemed necessary, several concepts appear to be generally accepted:
- Thorough débridement is a critical step in treatment.
- In most cases, preoperative antibiotics should be held until adequate tissue is obtained (if the microbiologic diagnosis has not been established).
- The location of the lesion is usually anterior; therefore, anterior procedures are usually preferred (with the exception of selective lower lumbar lesions in which the neural elements can be safely manipulated to permit anterior débridement and reconstruction).
- Systemic illness and malnutrition are often present and must be addressed concurrently.

  Conversely, several issues in the surgical management of spinal infections remain controversial.
- Choice of structural graft is controversial. Owing to the attendant morbidity of harvesting large structural autografts, alternative methods of reconstructing the weight-bearing anterior column are increasingly utilized. Despite concerns about the risk of sequestration and delayed healing, recent studies have demonstrated good outcomes (and without the aforementioned complications) utilizing both allograft and titanium cages for spinal reconstruction after débridement of active infection.
- Concerns about the use of instrumentation in the infected spine have led to the common (and effective) practice of performing the anterior reconstruction with a strut graft and instrumenting the spine through a separate, posterior approach. Recent studies, however, have demonstrated successful management of pyogenic and granulomatous infections utilizing anterior instrumentation.
- Same-day anterior-posterior versus staged procedures. Some have advocated staging the posterior placement of hardware to prevent "seeding" of the hardware by bacteremia produced by the anterior débridement. Although this advice is well reasoned, it is unclear if it is necessary. The authors feel that the decision should be made on a case-by-case basis, predicated primarily on the patient's overall physiologic condition on completion of the anterior procedure.
- The techniques for treatment of diskitis and osteomyelitis of the cervical, thoracic, and lumbar spine are generally similar to those utilized for the anterior treatment of degenerative and traumatic conditions. Because these methods have been described in separate, detailed sections, this chapter will review each technique more generally, and highlight important considerations for applying these methods to the management of spinal infections.

CERVICAL DISKITIS AND OSTEOMYELITIS

Positioning

- The patient is positioned supine, with a bump under the buttock if autograft harvesting is planned.
- A roll placed between the shoulder blades may facilitate extension of the neck; taping the shoulders may facilitate visualization of the lower cervical spine.
- Somatosensory and transcranial motor evoked potentials are utilized when patients have preservation of neurologic function.
- If the offending organism has not been previously identified, clear instructions to hold preoperative antibiotics are given to the anesthesia team.

Approach

- A left-sided approach is used by convention. Transverse skin incisions are preferred if three vertebral bodies or less must be visualized. For more extensive procedures, an oblique incision just anterior to the anterior border of the sternocleidomastoid muscle is utilized.
- A standard anterolateral approach to the subaxial cervical spine is performed (Fig. 53-2).
- Localization with fluoroscopy should be performed to clearly identify the levels of interest.
- A self-retaining retractor is used with the blades placed beneath the elevated medial borders of the longus colli.

Débridement and Decompression

- Great care should be taken to maintain orientation with respect to the midline, because the anatomy in the region of the active infection may be distorted. Exposure of an uninvolved level above and below may be helpful.
- Much of the initial débridement can be performed piecemeal using pituitary rongeurs and curettes. Generous sampling of pathologic material should be sent for Gram stain,

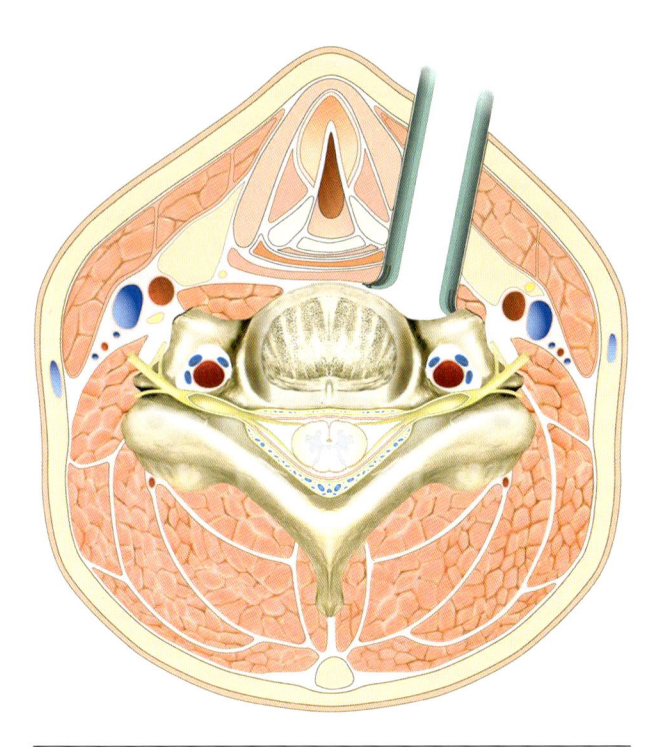

CHAPTER 53   Bacterial, Fungal, and Tuberculosis Diskitis   491

Fig. 53-2 A standard anterolateral approach to the subaxial cervical spine.

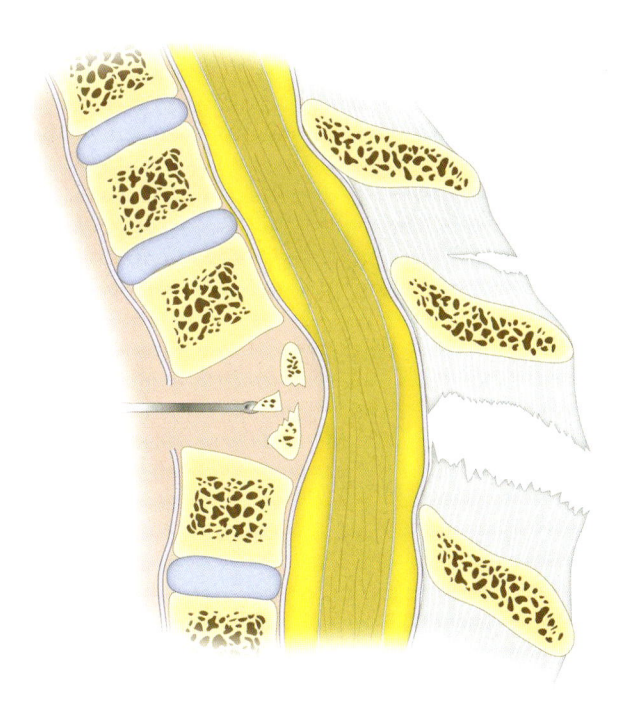

Fig. 53-3 The thin remaining shell of bone is removed with microcurettes.

culture (for aerobic, anaerobic, acid–fast, and fungal organisms), as well as histologic evaluation.
- The remainder of the decompression is accomplished in standard fashion, with a high-speed burr utilized to sequentially thin the bone from anterior to posterior. The thin remaining shell of bone is then removed with microcurettes (Fig. 53-3).

Reconstruction

STRUT GRAFT WITHOUT ANTERIOR INSTRUMENTATION
- To prevent dislodgement, the graft is countersunk into the vertebral bodies above and below.
- A high-speed burr is used to create slots in the bone above and below. The graft is placed in the slot in the superior vertebra first.
- Distraction across the defect using the Caspar distractor or Gardner Wells tongs is helpful for seating.
- With distraction applied, the graft is rotated and tamped into the slot in the inferior vertebra (Fig. 53-4).

STRUT GRAFT WITH ANTERIOR INSTRUMENTATION
If this technique is selected, grafting is done in the manner previously described for cervical corpectomy. Specifics for applying this technique in the infected spine include the following:
- Preservation of end plate integrity by gentle preparation with a high-speed burr.
- Insertion of screws into uninvolved bone. This is done by correlating preoperative imaging with intraoperative findings. Reliance of screw purchase in pathologic bone is not recommended.

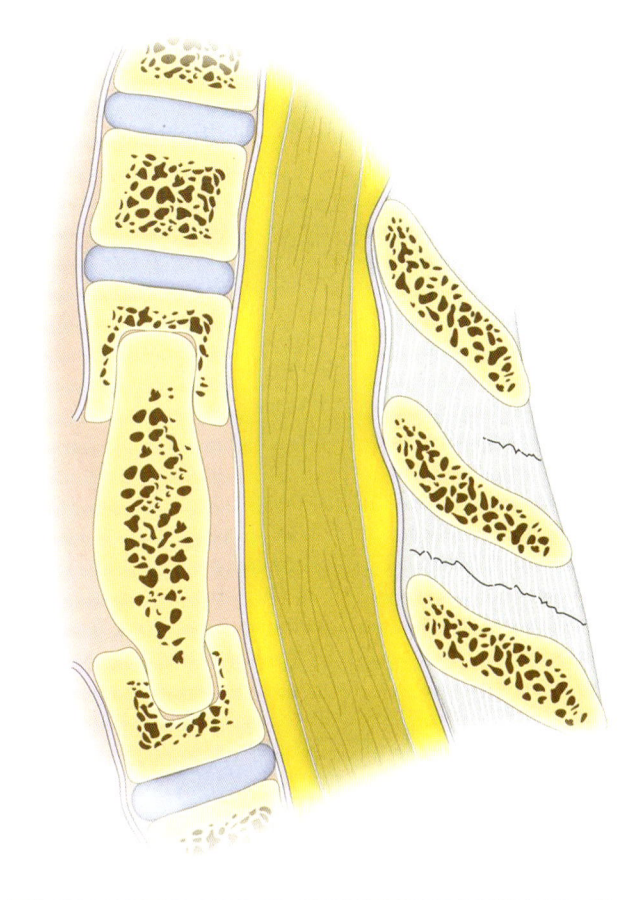

Fig. 53-4 With distraction applied, the graft is rotated and tamped into the slot in the inferior vertebra.

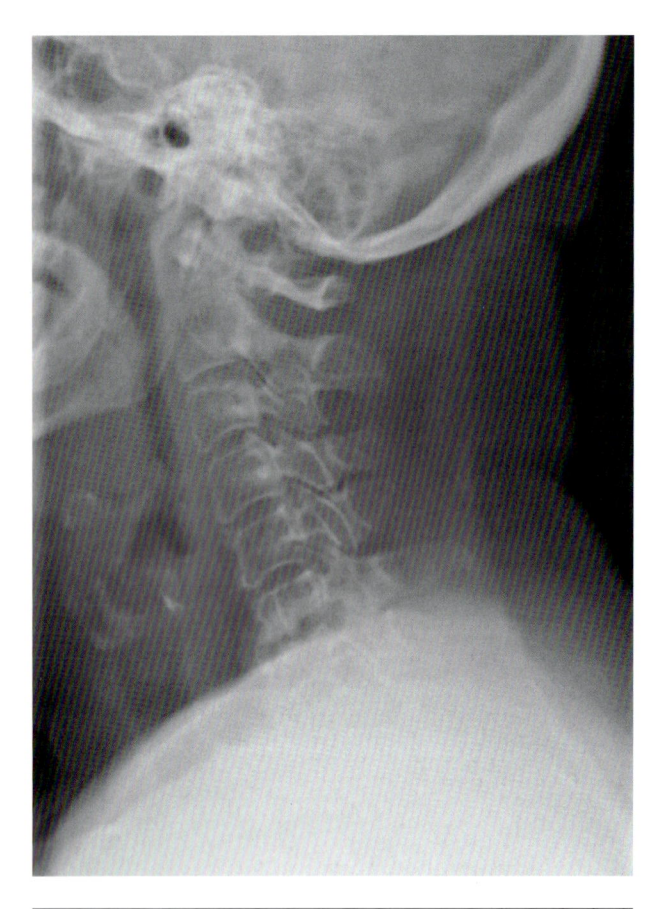

Fig. 53-5 Lateral cervical radiograph of a 42-year-old female (with insulin-dependent diabetes) with cervical diskitis/osteomyelitis.

Posterior Instrumentation

- The authors favor the addition of posterior instrumentation if noninstrumented strut grafting was performed anteriorly, to increase stability of the construct and decrease postoperative immobilization requirements. Posterior instrumentation is also utilized in most cases of three-level corpectomies owing to concerns of inadequate stability with anterior plating.
- Posterior instrumentation is done using standard techniques previously described. Lateral mass screws are generally utilized from C3 to C6. Pedicle screws are used at C7 if at the end of long constructs (anatomy permitting).
- If the posterior procedure is performed under the same anesthesia, a separate set-up table of instruments to be used for the posterior procedure is requested in advance and kept separate from instruments used during the anterior stage.
- Illustrative case:
  - Lateral cervical radiograph of cervical diskitis/osteomyelitis in a 42-year-old female with insulin-dependent diabetes (Fig. 53-5).
  - T_1-weighted sagittal MRI (Fig. 53-6).
  - T_1-weighted gadolinium-enhanced sagittal MRI (Fig. 53-7).

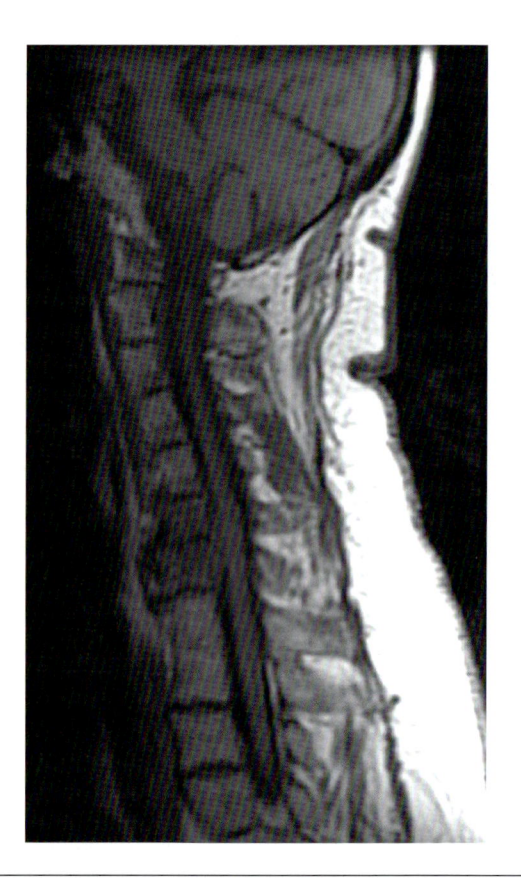

Fig. 53-6 T_1-weighted sagittal MRI.

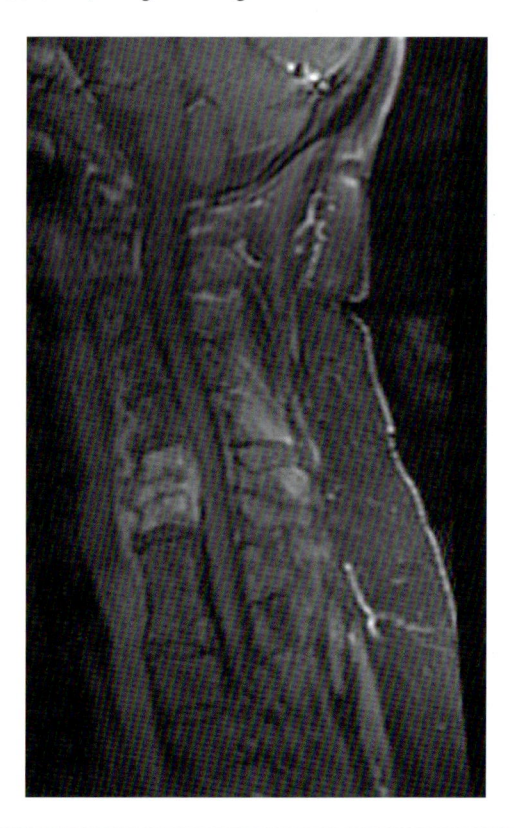

Fig. 53-7 T_1-weighted sagittal gadolinium-enhanced MRI.

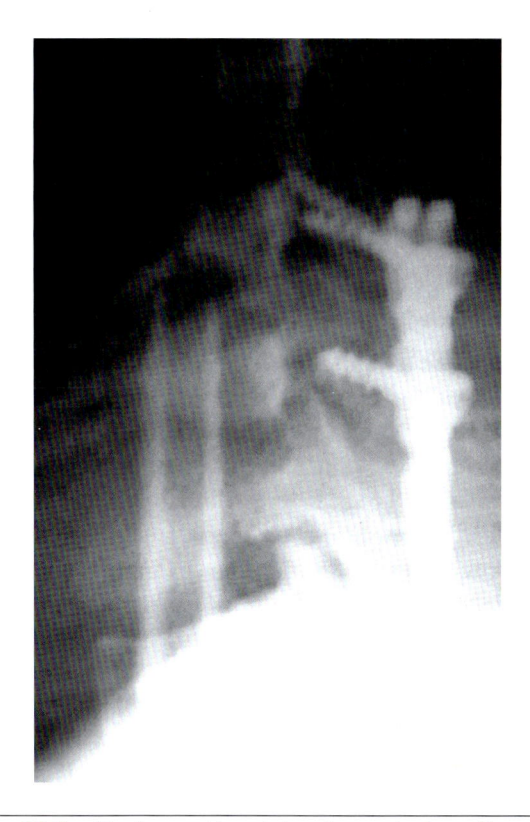

CHAPTER 53 Bacterial, Fungal, and Tuberculosis Diskitis

Fig. 53-8 Postoperative lateral cervical radiograph after anterior débridement and reconstruction with allograft fibula strut and posterior lateral mass fixation.

- Postoperative lateral radiograph after anterior débridement and decompression, allograft fibula strut, and posterior lateral mass fixation (Fig. 53-8).

THORACIC DISKITIS AND OSTEOMYELITIS
Anesthesia
- The thoracolumbar junction can be approached using standard, two-lung ventilation; higher transthoracic approaches may be facilitated by selected intubation and one-lung ventilation with a double-lumen endotracheal tube.
- An arterial line, central venous line, and Foley catheter are typically placed for continuous blood pressure and fluid status monitoring.
- Somatosensory and transcranial motor evoked potentials are utilized when patients have preservation of neurologic function.
- Antibiotics are withheld until specimens are obtained to establish the microbiologic diagnosis.

Patient Positioning
- For anatomic reasons a left-sided approach is favored by many. The thick-walled aorta can be manipulated with less risk than the thin-walled vena cava. In addition, because of the right-sided location of the liver, less caudal access is available to the thoracolumbar junction without a transdiaphragmatic approach. Midthoracic levels can be adequately approached from either side.
- The patient is positioned in a true lateral decubitus position. Care is taken to stabilize the patient at an angle perpendicular to the floor, utilizing padded attachments to the table or a beanbag and tape (Fig. 53-9).
- An axillary roll is placed just below the dependent axilla to protect the neurovascular supply to the arm.

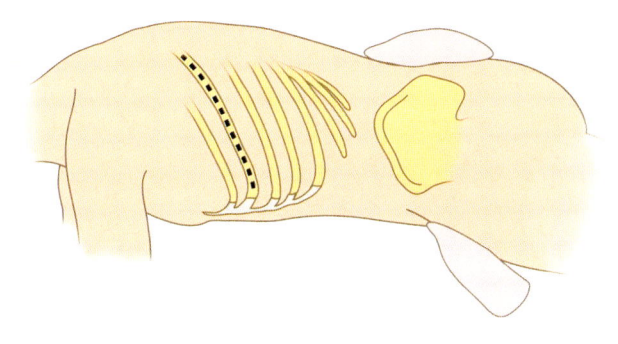

Fig. 53-9 Care is taken to stabilize the patient at an angle perpendicular to the floor, utilizing padded attachments to the table or a beanbag and tape.

Localization
- A high-quality plain radiograph is obtained prior to positioning to correlate the rib with the vertebral body of interest. The ribs are then manually palpated and counted.
- The incision is based over the rib one or two levels above the vertebrae to be resected. This will permit adequate direct access to the cephalad vertebrae if instrumentation is planned.

Surgical Approach
- For access to T4 through T10, a transthoracic-transpleural approach is typically performed through the bed of the resected rib (Fig. 53-10).
- For exposure of the thoracolumbar junction, a transpleural-retroperitoneal thoracoabdominal approach, with detachment of the diaphragm, is commonly employed. (The thoracolumbar junction can also be exposed through an extrapleural-retroperitoneal approach, which avoids incision of the diaphragm and may be associated with less pulmonary related morbidity.)

Decompression and Reconstruction
- After the initial exposure, the lung is gently retracted superomedially away from the spine (Fig. 53-11).
- Confirmation of the involved level is performed by intraoperative imaging. The anatomy of the involved segments may be severely distorted, so careful correlation to the localizing film and preoperative imaging studies is necessary.

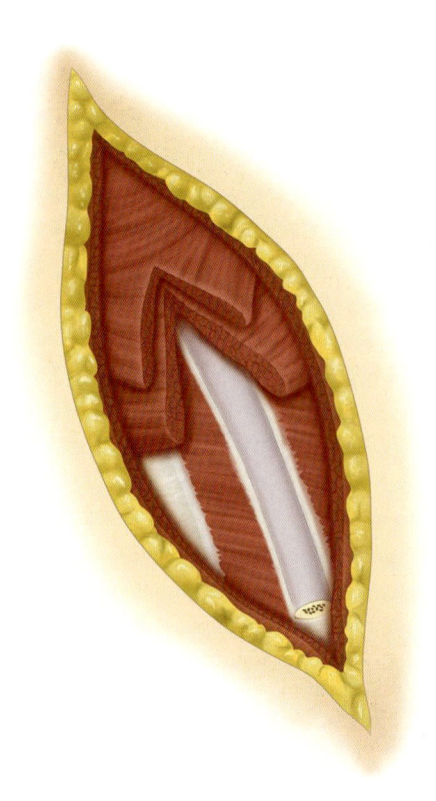

Fig. 53-10 For access to T4 through T10, a transthoracic-transpleural approach is typically performed through the bed of the resected rib.

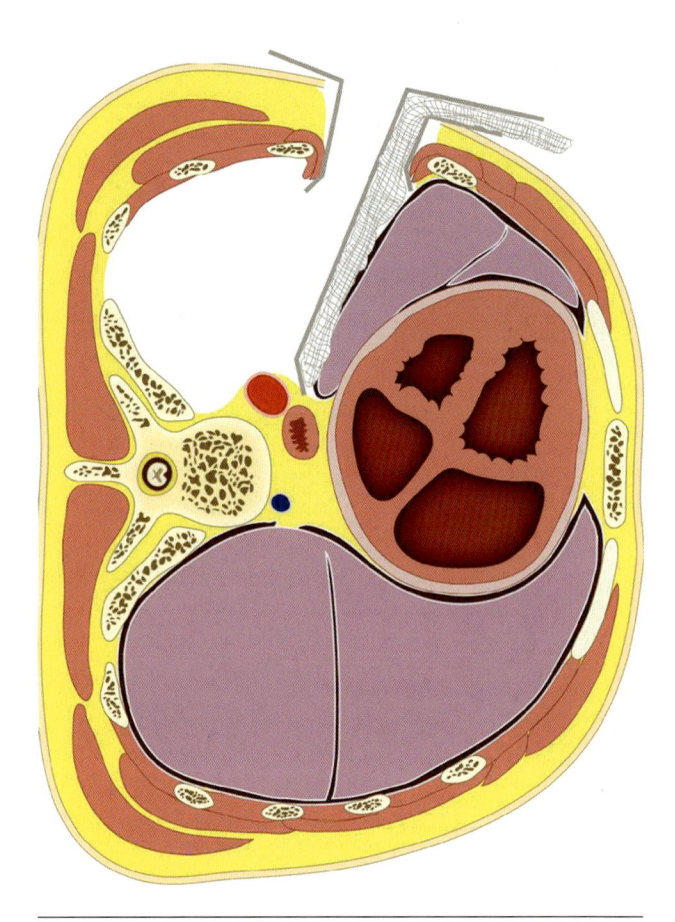

Fig. 53-11 After the initial exposure, the lung is gently retracted superomedially away from the spine.

- Ligation of the segmental vessels overlying the vertebral bodies to be instrumented (as well as the corpectomy level) is generally required (Fig. 53-12).
- Corpectomy of the pathologic vertebrae is then performed, as described in earlier sections, using a combination of osteotomes, rongeurs, punches, and a high-speed burr. Infected and necrotic bone and disk material may be easily removed with rongeurs and curettes and sent for microbiologic analysis.
- If formal neurologic decompression is required, removal of retropulsed bone should continue across the spinal canal until the contralateral pedicle is identified.
- Reconstruction of the anterior weight-bearing column can be performed with structural autograft (typically the iliac crest), structural allograft, or cages packed with morselized autograft or allograft (or combinations of both) (Fig. 53-13).
- If anterior strut grafting without anterior instrumentation is preferred, the graft should be countersunk into the vertebral bodies above and below (Fig. 53-14). If anterior instrumentation is to be utilized, the graft should be fit to span from the inferior end plate of the proximal vertebra to the superior end plate of the inferior vertebra. This will facilitate screw placement into the adjacent vertebral bodies.

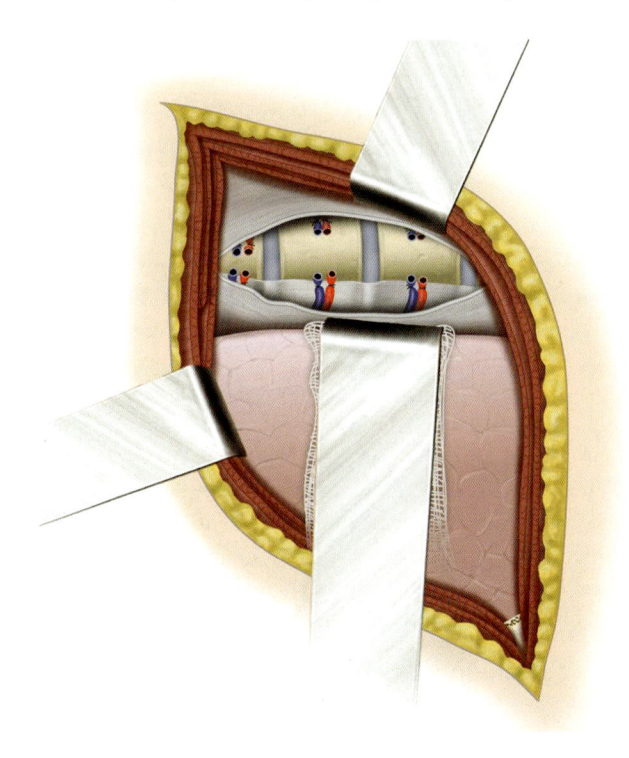

Fig. 53-12 Ligation of the segmental vessels overlying the vertebral bodies to be instrumented (as well as the corpectomy level) is generally required.

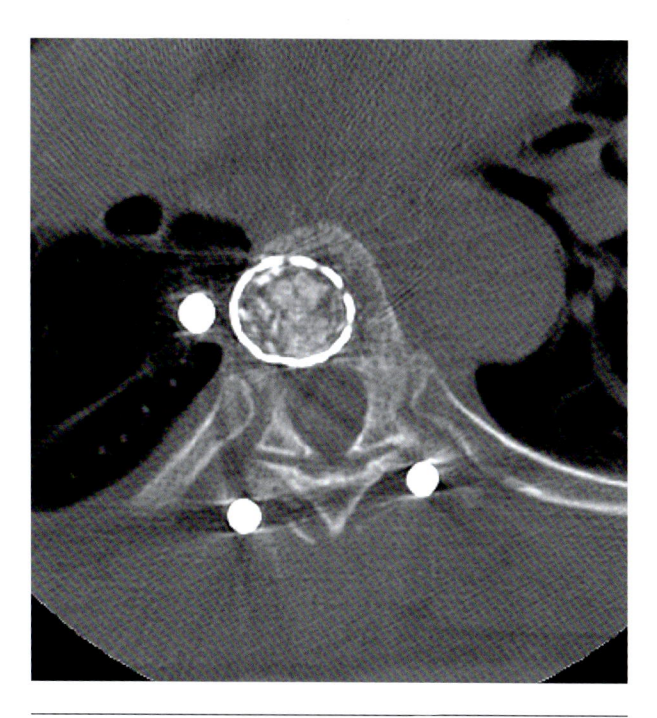

CHAPTER 53 Bacterial, Fungal, and Tuberculosis Diskitis

Fig. 53-13 Reconstruction of the anterior weight-bearing column can be performed with structural autograft (typically the iliac crest), structural allograft, or cages packed with morselized autograft or allograft (or combinations of both).

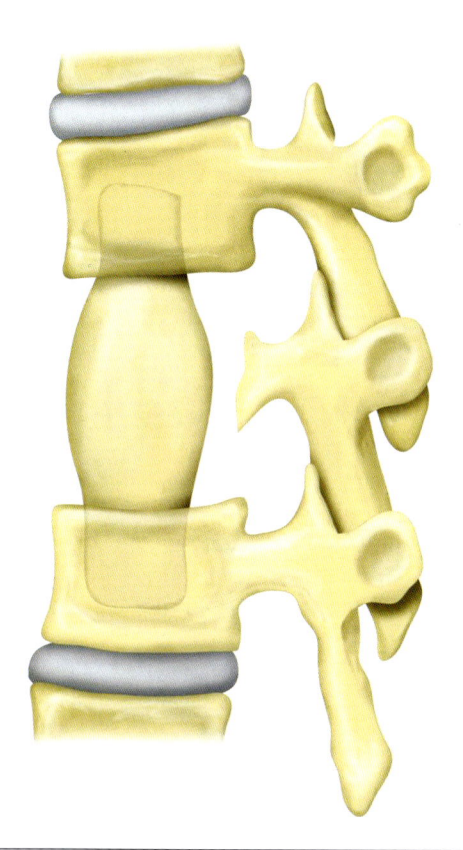

Fig. 53-14 If anterior strut grafting without anterior instrumentation is preferred, the graft should be countersunk into the vertebral bodies above and below.

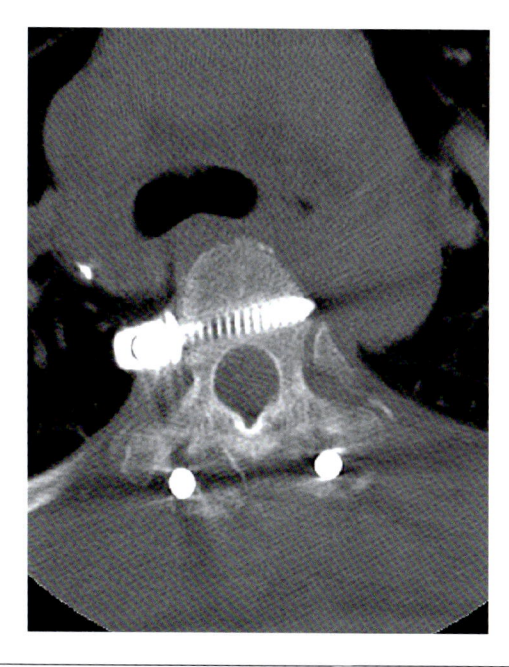

Fig. 53-15 Where possible, bicortical purchase of normal, uninvolved segments is preferable.

Anterior Instrumentation

- If anterior instrumentation is to be utilized, standard techniques for plate or screw-rod devices can be applied. This should be performed after thorough débridement and irrigation of the field.
- Reliance of screw purchase in pathologic bone is not recommended. Where possible, bicortical purchase of normal, uninvolved segments is preferable (Fig. 53-15).
- Illustrative case:
  - A 50-year-old male with history of intravenous drug use presented with thoracic back pain and rapidly progressive cord level neurologic deficit.
  - T_2-weighted sagittal MRI demonstrating T6-T7 diskitis/osteomyelitis with pathologic fracture, epidural extension, and spinal cord compression (Fig. 53-16).
  - Postoperative AP radiograph after anterior débridement and decompression involving T6 and T7 corpectomies, with instrumentation at T5-T8 (Fig. 53-17).
  - The patient had posterior stabilization performed in a staged fashion.

POSTERIOR INSTRUMENTATION

- Posterior stabilization is generally recommended after non-instrumented anterior strut grafting. Standard techniques as described in earlier sections are applicable. Segmental fixation with hook or pedicle screw constructs are favored by the authors.
- In selected cases involving multilevel anterior corpectomies, the authors utilize the addition of posterior instrumentation to achieve greater initial stability, increase fusion

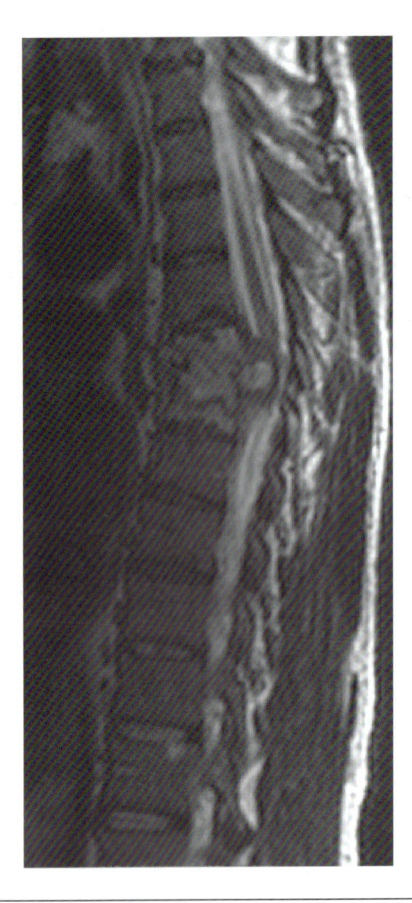

Fig. 53-16 T_2-weighted sagittal MRI demonstrating T6-T7 diskitis/osteomyelitis with pathologic fracture, epidural extension, and spinal cord compression.

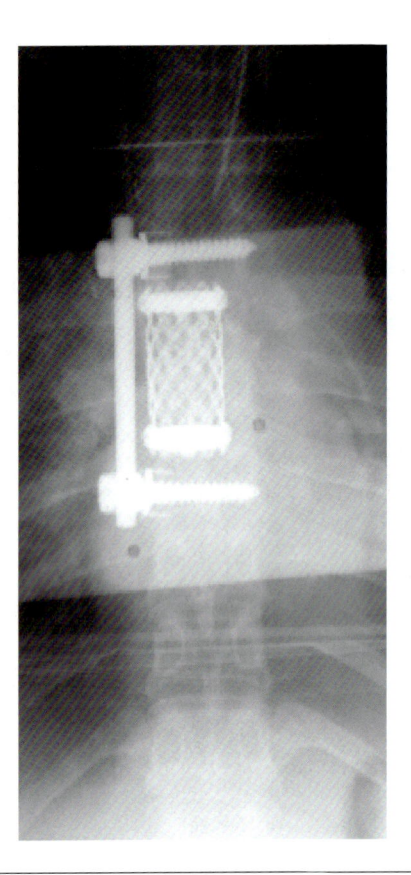

Fig. 53-17 Postoperative anteroposterolateral radiograph after anterior débridement and decompression involving T6 and T7 corpectomies with instrumentation at T5-T8.

rate, and decrease postoperative bracing requirements. In most cases, more limited posterior constructs appear sufficient when combined with anterior plate or screw-rod devices.
- Illustrative case:
  - Postoperative lateral radiograph after addition of posterior instrumentation to the patient presented in Figures 53-16 and 53-17 (Fig. 53-18).
  - Axial CT scan demonstrating appropriate position of the pedicle screws selected for the posterior construct (Fig. 53-19).

LUMBAR DISKITIS AND OSTEOMYELITIS
Positioning and Anesthesia
- For approaches involving levels proximal to L4, a retroperitoneal flank approach is utilized. The patient is placed in a lazy right lateral decubitus position with a bump under the left side (Fig. 53-20).
- To approach the lumbosacral junction, the retroperitoneal approach is performed through a midline vertical incision. The patient is placed supine. A roll may be placed beneath the lumbar spine to maintain lordosis. The legs are slightly flexed and abducted to relax the iliopsoas.
- Antibiotics are withheld until specimens are obtained (if the organism has not been identified).

Exposure
- Standard retroperitoneal approach to the lumbar spine is performed. The flank approach involves division of the external oblique, internal oblique, and transversus abdominis muscles (Fig. 53-21). The vertical midline approach involves splitting the rectus abdominis muscle in the midline linea alba.
- The retroperitoneal space is entered laterally by identification of the retroperitoneal fat. Blunt finger dissection along the anterior surface of the left psoas muscle should lead to the great vessels.
- After ligation and division of the segmentals, the great vessels can be gently retracted the right, with the psoas mobilized toward the left, exposing the spine (Fig. 53-22). The local anatomy may be distorted by the infection. The vessels may be difficult to mobilize secondary to inflammation. Blunt dissection with peanuts and firm, controlled pressure on the surface of the disks and vertebral bodies is most effective.
- The L5-S1 level is exposed through the bifurcation of the great vessels after ligation and division of the middle sacral vessels.

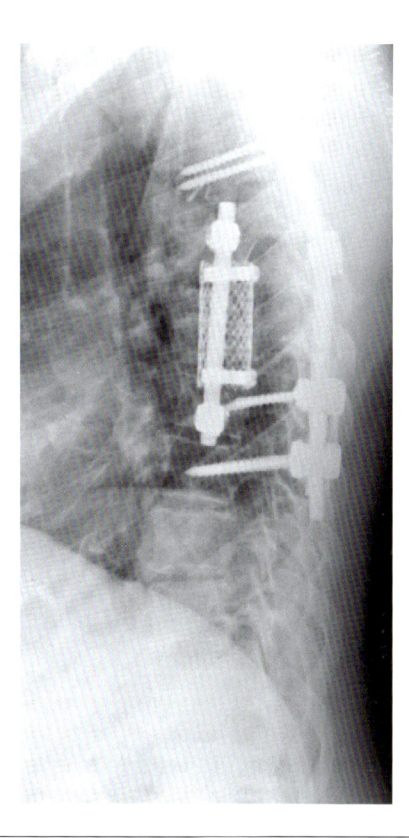

CHAPTER 53 Bacterial, Fungal, and Tuberculosis Diskitis   497

Fig. 53-18 Postoperative lateral radiograph after addition of posterior instrumentation to the patient presented in Figures 53-16 and 53-17.

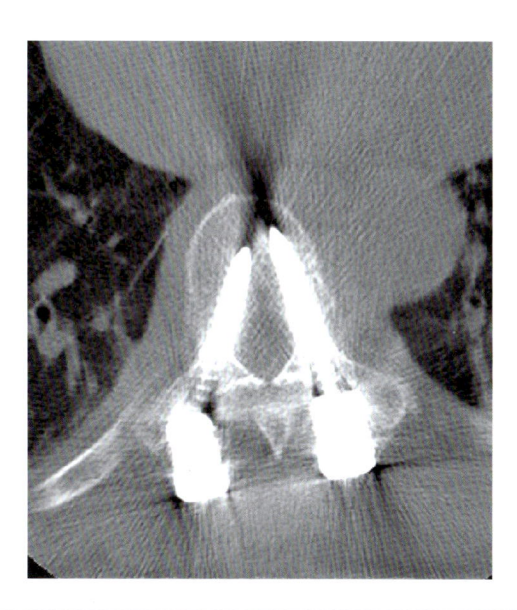

Fig. 53-19 Axial CT scan demonstrating appropriate position of the pedicle screws selected for the posterior construct.

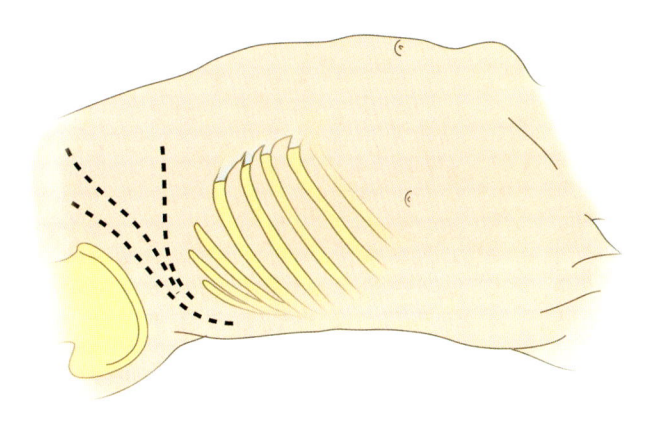

Fig. 53-20 The patient is placed in a lazy right lateral decubitus position with a bump under the left side.

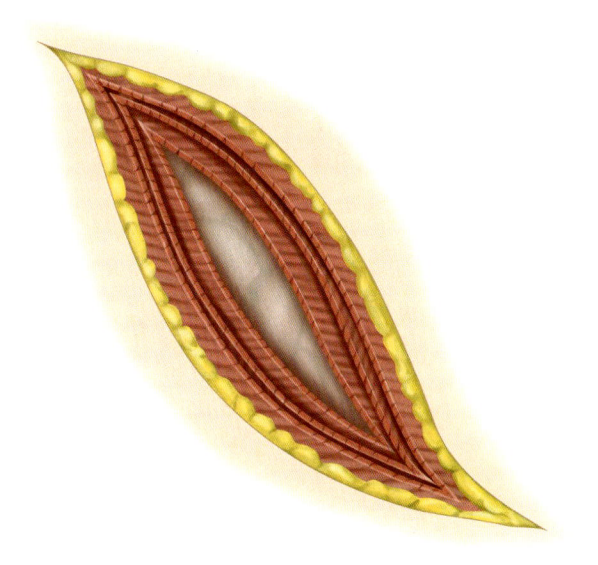

Fig. 53-21 The flank approach involves division of the external oblique, internal oblique, and transversus abdominis muscles.

- A spinal needle is inserted into the appropriate disk and an intraoperative image is obtained to verify the local anatomy.

Débridement and Decompression
- Removal of severely affected bone and disk is readily performed using rongeurs and curettes.
- Generous amounts of tissue should be sent for analysis in order to increase yield. After adequate specimens have been obtained, empiric antibiotic coverage should be started.
- The remainder of the decompression is performed in routine fashion as described in previous sections. All gross purulence and necrotic bone should be removed, back to a margin of healthy, bleeding tissue.

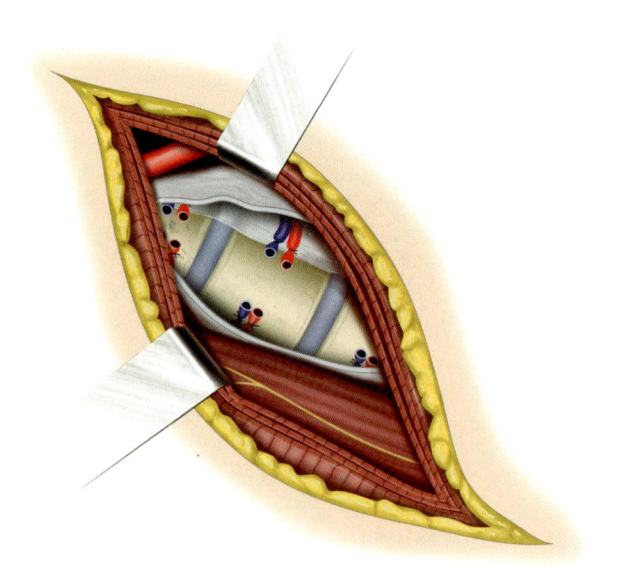

Fig. 53-22 After ligation and division of the segmentals, the great vessels can be gently retracted on the right, with the psoas mobilized toward the left, exposing the spine.

- If an epidural abscess is present anterior to the dural sac, a formal decompression is performed from pedicle to pedicle. The abscess can be gently débrided with a Penfield dissector, and careful suction/irrigation is performed.

Anterior Reconstruction

- Owing to the orientation of the great vessels in the lower lumbar spine, stabilizing anterior plates or screw-rod constructs are rarely used.
- Strut grafting to achieve stability after corpectomy can be performed using iliac crest autograft (Fig. 53-23) or allograft. The graft should be countersunk from the upper end plate above and lower end plate below.
- Illustrative case:
  - A 68-year-old man developed severe unrelenting back pain several months after experiencing bacteremia from a chronic lower extremity infection.
  - Sagittal T_1-weighted MRI demonstrated diskitis and osteomyelitis involving L4-L5 (Fig. 53-24). Sagittal T_2-weighted MRI demonstrated the bony involvement with pathologic fracture of L4 (Fig. 53-25).
  - The patient was treated with intravenous antibiotics after CT-guided biopsy but experienced increasing pain and evidence of further bone loss.
  - Sagittal reconstruction of CT scan performed after anterior débridement, decompression, and reconstruction with an iliac crest strut graft. Posterior stabilization was performed under a separate anesthesia (Fig. 53-26).

Posterior Stabilization

- The authors routinely perform supplemental posterior fusion after noninstrumented decompression and strut

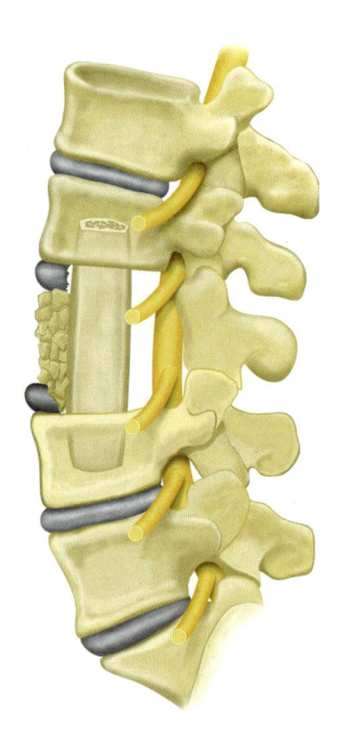

Fig. 53-23 Strut grafting to achieve stability after corpectomy can be performed using iliac crest autograft or allograft.

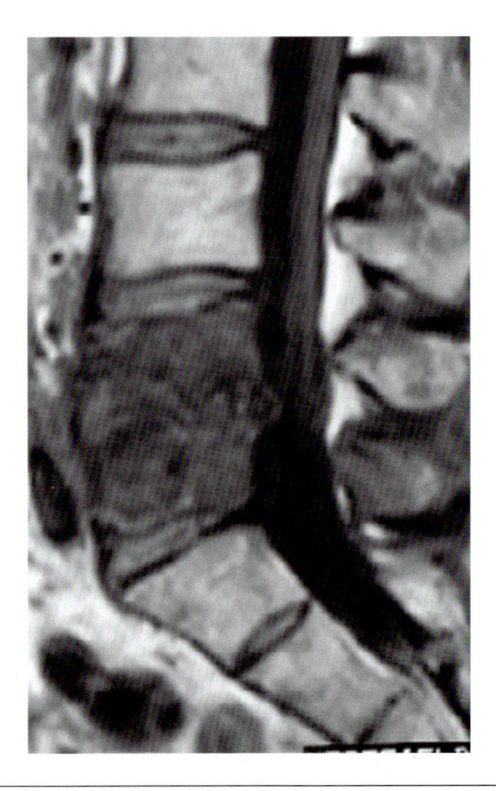

Fig. 53-24 A 68-year-old man developed severe unrelenting back pain several months after experiencing bacteremia from a chronic lower extremity infection. Sagittal T_1-weighted magnetic resonance image demonstrating diskitis and osteomyelitis involving L4-L5.

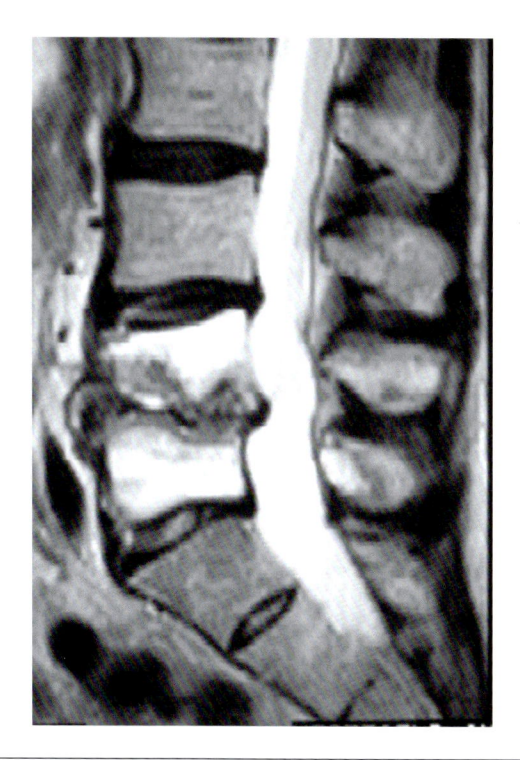

CHAPTER 53 Bacterial, Fungal, and Tuberculosis Diskitis

Fig. 53-25 Sagittal T$_2$-weighted MRI demonstrating the bony involvement with pathologic fracture of L4.

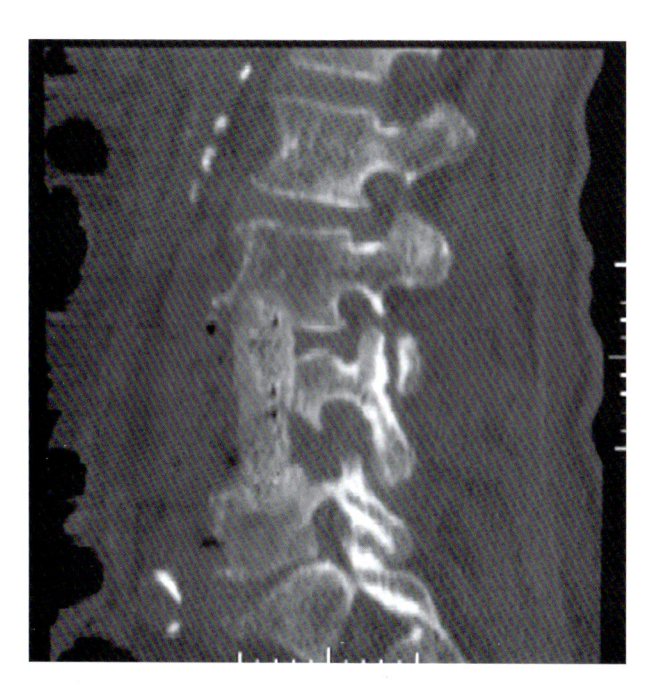

Fig. 53-26 Sagittal reconstruction of CT scan performed after anterior débridement, decompression, and reconstruction with an iliac crest strut graft. Posterior stabilization was performed under a separate anesthesia.

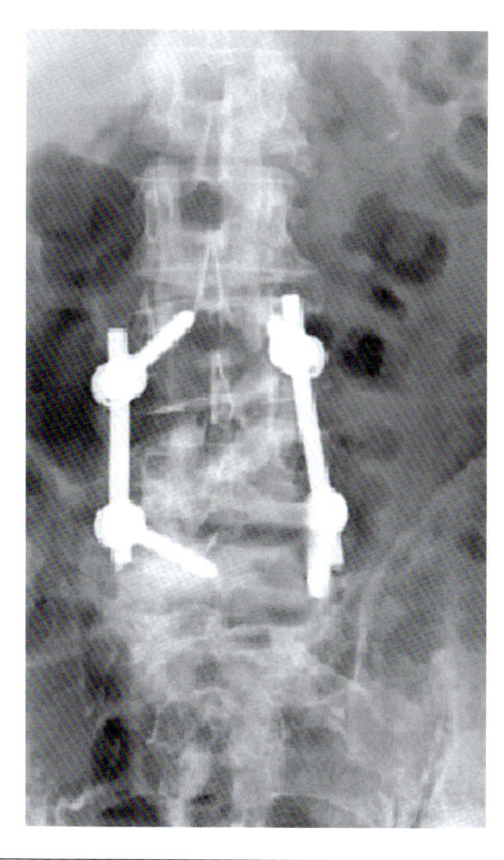

Fig. 53-27 Pedicle screw constructs can be applied in routine fashion as described in earlier sections.

grafting in the lower lumbar spine. Such an approach allows early mobilization with minimal bracing requirements and promotes fusion.
- Pedicle screw constructs can be applied in routine fashion as described in earlier sections. Postoperative AP radiograph after supplemental posterior fusion was performed in the patient discussed in Figures 53-24 to 53-26 (Fig. 53-27).
- The decision to perform both procedures under the same anesthesia (versus in a staged manner) should be made on a case-by case basis.
- In selected cases, posterior techniques may be utilized in the lower lumbar spine to treat diskitis/osteomyelitis. Posterior lumbar interbody fusion (PLIF) or transforaminal lumbar interbody fusion (TLIF) may be applicable as described elsewhere. Cases with more limited bony involvement (with infection confined mostly to the disk space and end plate interface) are better suited to this approach. More extensive bony débridement and reconstruction are more readily performed with the anterior-posterior approach.

Tuberculosis and Fungal Infections of the Spine
- Fungal infections of the spine are managed in similar fashion to pyogenic infections. Antimicrobial therapy must be adjusted based on the culture results.

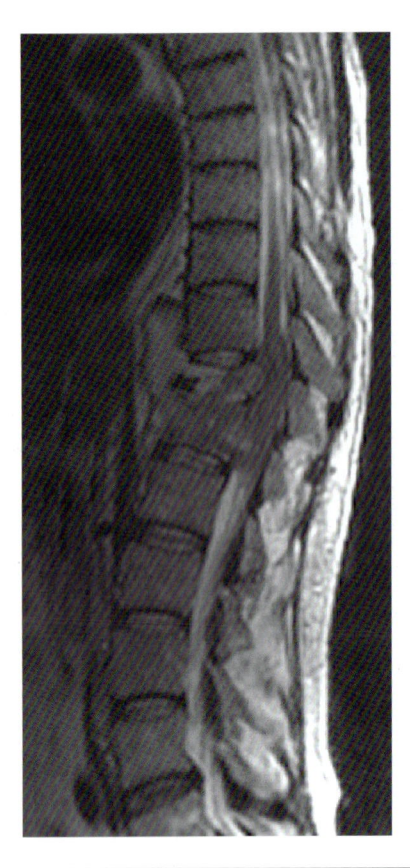

Fig. 53-28 Sagittal T$_2$-weighted MRI demonstrating presumed Pott's disease with anterior soft-tissue abscess, two-level involvement (including pathologic fracture), and preservation of the intervening disc.

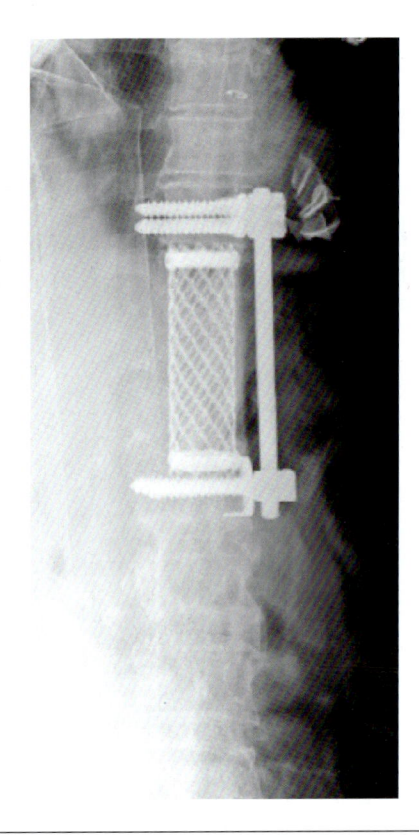

Fig. 53-29 This patient underwent anterior débridement and reconstruction involving two-level corpectomies, cage placement, and anterior instrumentation.

- Patients experiencing fungal infections of the spine are commonly immunocompromised and malnourished. Consultation with medical and nutritional specialists is recommended.
- Tuberculosis (TB) infections of the spine commonly respond well to medical treatment. The diagnosis must be confirmed by biopsy. New testing methods utilizing polymerase chain reaction (PCR) can decrease the amount of time required to definitively establish the diagnosis.
- Surgical indications are similar to those for pyogenic infections, although medical treatment appears effective even in the presence of large soft tissue abscesses associated with TB.
- Operative techniques for management of TB spinal infections are similar to those utilized for pyogenic infections. As with pyogenic infections, recent studies have demonstrated the safety and efficacy of anterior instrumentation for treatment of TB infections, although this continues to be an area of controversy.
- Illustrative case:
  - A 49-year-old male presented with back pain and new onset lower extremity paralysis.
  - Sagittal T$_2$-weighted MR demonstrating presumed Pott's disease with anterior soft tissue abscess, two-level involvement (including pathologic fracture), and preservation of the intervening disk (Fig. 53-28).
  - The patient underwent anterior débridement and reconstruction involving two-level corpectomies, cage placement, and anterior instrumentation (Fig. 53-29). In a staged fashion, posterior stabilization was performed to increase the probability of fusion and decrease postoperative bracing needs (Fig. 53-30).

POSTOPERATIVE CARE

- Postoperative management is similar to that prescribed after performance of these procedures for degenerative or traumatic conditions.
- Empiric antibiotic coverage should continue until culture/sensitivity information is available.
- Appropriate antibiotic treatment should continue for approximately 6 weeks in pyogenic infections, 6 months to 1 year for TB. Infectious disease consultation is recommended to help manage antibiotic selection, dosing, and scheduling.
- Effectiveness of treatment should be monitored by serial evaluation of the ESR. Postoperative radiographs and CT scans to monitor for evidence of hardware failure,

pseudarthrosis, or recurrent abscesses may be helpful. The roles of MRI and nuclear studies to assess the postoperative progress are unclear.

COMPLICATIONS

- Complications of the surgical treatment of spinal infections are similar to those complications reported after the use of these techniques for degenerative and traumatic conditions.
- Failure to eradicate the infection may be due to inadequate débridement or improper antibiotic selection, dosing, or duration.
- Graft dislodgement may occur secondary to improper technique or failure to achieve adequate stability.
- Malnutrition may contribute to delayed wound healing and postoperative wound infections and dehiscence.

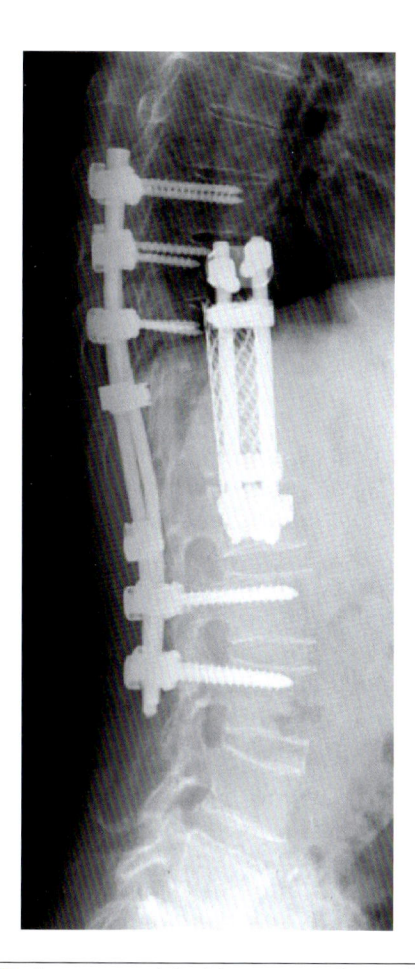

Fig. 53-30 In a staged fashion, posterior stabilization was performed to increase the probability of fusion and decrease postoperative bracing needs.

SECTION

VIII

MISCELLANEOUS

CHAPTER 54

JEFFREY S. HENN
CURTIS A. DICKMAN

Bone Graft Harvesting Techniques

INTRODUCTION

The success of many spinal procedures is determined by successful bone graft fusion. Although instrumentation can provide immediate rigid fixation, ultimately, bone fusion must occur to prevent long-term failure. Whether the person's own bone is harvested (autograft) or cadaveric allograft is used, the goal is the formation of a living, bony arthrodesis.

SELECTING A BONE GRAFT

The type of bone graft used depends on the surgical procedure, the surgeon's preference, and occasionally the patient's preference. Autograft may be either cortical, cancellous, or mixed cortical and cancellous. Cortical bone is the strongest form of autograft and is typically used when strong structural support is required, such as fusion after anterior corpectomies.[1] Compared with cancellous bone, cortical bone has fewer living cells and less surface area. Autologous cancellous bone provides only 60% of the compressive strength of cortical bone but has very high rates of fusion in appropriate cases.[2] Cancellous bone provides the ideal combination of osteogenic, osteoinductive, and osteoconductive properties based on its composition of living cells, bone matrix proteins, and inherent architecture.[1] Typically, pure cancellous bone is used for posterior spinal fusions, which do not require the graft to withstand compressive forces.[1] Cortical-cancellous autografts are composed of both cortical and cancellous bone and offer the advantages of each. The grafts are stronger than cancellous bone and they retain many of its advantages. A common example of cortical-cancellous bone is a tricortical iliac crest graft.

Although autograft remains the gold standard for successful formation of long-term arthrodesis, there are associated drawbacks. Complications associated with graft harvest can range from additional postoperative pain to more significant problems. The quality and quantity of autograft are sometimes inadequate. One alternative is cadaveric allograft. Unlike autograft, which is live, nonreactive, and genetically identical to the host, allograft is nonliving bone. Compared with autograft, allograft becomes vascularized more slowly. The rate of bone fusion is also slower, and the risk of bone resorption, rejection, or infection is higher. However, the distinct advantage of allograft over autograft is the lack of complications associated with harvesting. Similarly, a relatively new category of bone-graft extenders may lead to successful fusion, despite not relying primarily on autograft or allograft.

TECHNIQUES OF BONE GRAFT HARVEST

Regardless of the type of bone graft, the chances of successful arthrodesis can be improved with meticulous surgical technique and adequate preparation of the bone graft and surfaces for spinal fusion.[3] Combining this care and preparation with rigid internal fixation optimizes the likelihood of long-term fusion. In general, local trauma to tissue should be minimized to assure maximum vascularity of the fusion site. Avoiding monopolar coagulation and use of copious irrigation during drilling can minimize the risk of thermal injury to the bone. Periosteum and other soft tissue, which can lead to a fibrous interface and nonunion, should be meticulously removed from the bone graft and fusion bed. Typically, the fusion site should be decorticated to improve the chances of successful fusion. The bone graft should be shaped to fit precisely into the fusion site to maximize the surface area of bone-to-bone contact. In addition, space within the fusion bed should be eliminated. All anti-inflammatory medications should be avoided during the peri- and postoperative period.

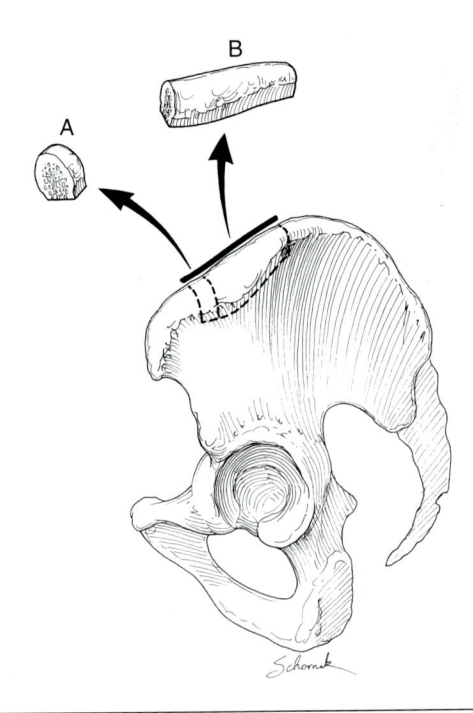

Fig. 54-1 Bone graft harvested from the anterolateral ilium should remain 2 to 3 cm behind the anterior superior iliac spine to avoid an avulsion fracture. Tricortical bone grafts can be harvested for single level interbody fusions (A) or for multisegment vertebral body reconstruction (B).

ANTERIOR ILIAC CREST GRAFTS

Historically, bone graft harvested from the anterior iliac crest was commonly used for anterior cervical spinal procedures requiring cortical-cancellous bone. This particular indication is less common since the recognition that fusion rates are high with allograft. However, there may still be a role for anterior iliac crest bone in anterior cervical fusions in select patients at high risk for nonfusion. Anterior iliac crest bone is still used with some frequency for anterior lumbar fusion procedures.

Anterior iliac crest bone is obtained through a linear incision made parallel to the iliac crest and directly over the harvest site. The bone should be harvested from at least 3 cm behind the anterosuperior iliac spine to avoid disrupting the ilioinguinal ligament or creating an avulsion fracture (Fig. 54-1). A sandbag can be placed under the ipsilateral buttocks to assist with access to the anterolateral iliac spine.

Dissection proceeds through the subcutaneous tissue to the fascial layer. After retractors have been placed, the fascia is opened directly over the iliac crest and subperiosteal dissection is performed. A fascial cuff and periosteum are left intact for secure closure. To expose a tricortical graft, medial and lateral subperiosteal dissection continues with a periosteal elevator until adequate bone has been exposed. Dissection along the medial iliac crest must be done with great care. The dissection must remain subperiosteal to avoid inadvertent peritoneal entry or injury to the iliohypogastric, ilioinguinal, or lateral femoral cutaneous nerves (Fig. 54-2).[4] Cauterization should be used sparingly to prevent the possibility of nerve injury.

After the retractors have been deepened to provide excellent exposure to the tricortical graft, the bone may be harvested using either oscillating saws or osteotomes. If the graft will serve a weight-bearing function, oscillating saws are preferred because osteotomes can cause microfractures that can weaken the graft. Some surgeons temporarily pack the medial and lateral exposure to avoid injury to the muscle or peritoneal cavity.

After the graft has been harvested, bleeding is controlled with bone wax or Gelfoam soaked in thrombin. Drains are rarely needed. The wound is closed in multiple layers; the periosteal layers and fascial layers are closed with interrupted sutures.

POSTERIOR ILIAC GRAFTS

The posterior iliac region can be used to obtain tricortical grafts, cortical matchstick grafts, cortical-cancellous plates, or cancellous bone strips (Fig. 54-3). Bone can be obtained from the iliac crest or in a subcrestal fashion. When a posterior iliac crest tricortical graft is planned, the graft is harvested from the posterior superior iliac spine (PSIS), or lateral to the PSIS to avoid the sacroiliac joint and sciatic notch.[4-6] However, the graft should not be taken more than 8 cm from the iliac spine to avoid the risk of injury to the superior cluneal nerves, which can cause buttock numbness or painful neuromas (Fig. 54-4).

Several variations of incision are used. Some surgeons prefer a vertical incision directly over the PSIS. Others prefer a curved skin incision beginning at the PSIS and extending superolaterally. Dissection proceeds through the subcutaneous tissue, and the fascia is opened directly over the iliac crest. Dissection continues medially and laterally in a subperiosteal fashion to avoid injury to the gluteal artery branches that can cause brisk bleeding. Great care should also be used to avoid dissection in the region of the sciatic notch, where the main trunk of the superior gluteal artery, sciatic nerve, or ureter can be injured. Medial dissection involves stripping off part of the iliacus muscle. Care must be exerted to remain subperiosteal to avoid injury to the ilioinguinal nerve or pelvic contents. Subperiosteal dissection also avoids injury to the ureter, which lies within the retroperitoneal fat pad.

Grafts are obtained using a combination of oscillating saw, osteotomes, or bone gouges/curettes. Hemostasis is obtained with bone wax or Gelfoam soaked in thrombin. Drainage is rarely necessary. The wound is closed in layers; interrupted sutures are used to approximate the periosteal and fascial layers. A layered closure is critical to avoid herniation of the abdominal contents.

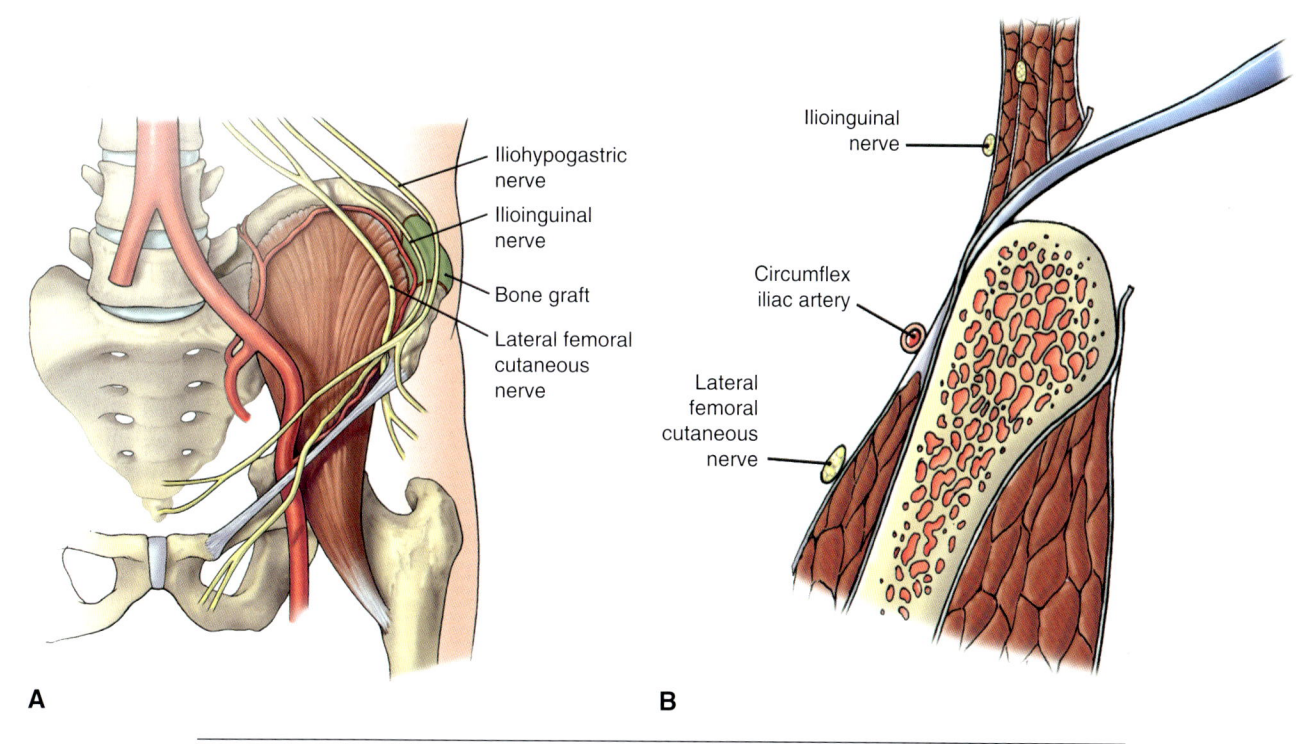

CHAPTER 54 Bone Graft Harvesting Techniques   507

Fig. 54-2 *A,* Fascial and periosteal incisions used for exposure of bone over the anterolateral iliac crest. *B,* The dissection should remain in a subperiosteal plane and cautery should be avoided to prevent injury to the ilioinguinal, iliohypogastric, and lateral femoral cutaneous nerves.

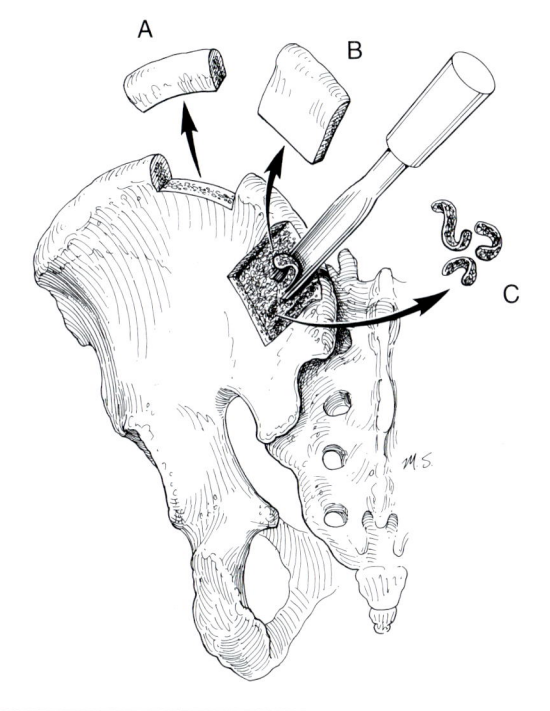

Fig. 54-3 A variety of bone graft can be harvested from the posterior ilium: tricortical strut graft (*A*), cortical cancellous plate (*B*), and cancellous bone strips (*C*).

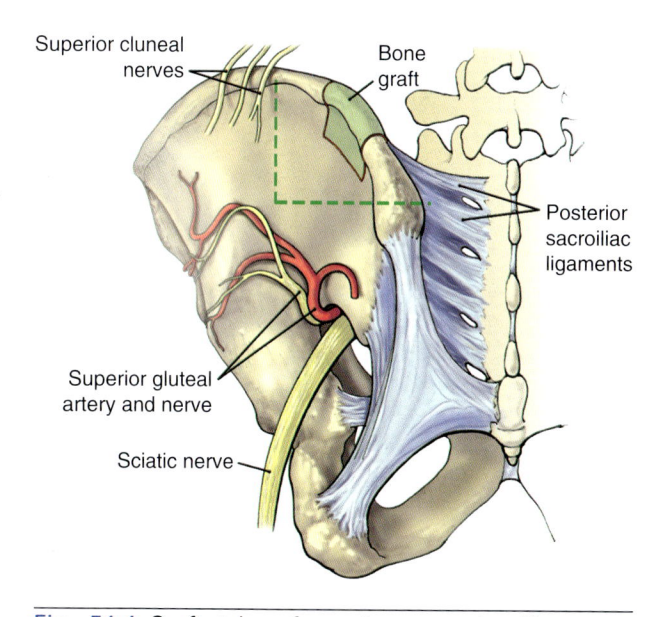

Fig. 54-4 Graft taken from the posterior iliac crest should be kept above the line intersecting the posterior superior iliac spine. Care is taken to protect the sacral iliac ligaments (medially), the sciatic nerve (caudally), the gluteal vessels (caudally and submuscularly), the superior cluneal nerves (laterally), and the ureter (anteriorly).

If tricortical bone is unnecessary, an alternative technique known as the subcrestal exposure can be used to harvest unicortical and cancellous bone. In this case, an incision is centered just lateral to the posterior iliac spine. Dissection proceeds along the posterior surface with the gluteal fascia being detached lateral to the posterior superior iliac spine so that an adequate cuff of connective tissue is left for closure. The dissection avoids the sciatic notch, which can easily be palpated. When dissection is adequate, a Taylor retractor can be used to assist with exposure. A window of cortical bone can be removed using straight osteotomes. If additional cancellous bone is required, it can be obtained easily using bone gouges. The inner cortical table should not be breached. Cancellous bone and cortical-cancellous matchsticks are ideal for occipitocervical posterior fusions. After hemostasis has been obtained using bone wax or Gelfoam, the gluteal fascia must be reapproximated to the periosteum to avoid gait disturbances. Again, the wound is closed in layers with meticulous closure of the periosteum and fascial layer to prevent abdominal herniation.

ALTERNATIVE AUTOLOGOUS SITES

In most cases, the iliac crest is the preferred site for autologous bone graft, but bone can also be harvested from rib, fibula, and the calvarium. Ribs have a relatively thin cortex, are mechanically weak in resisting compressive loads, and provide a relatively small volume of bone. However, they are sometimes a useful alternative if other sites cannot be used.[7-9]

Because of their limited mechanical strength, rib grafts should not be used to reconstruct major spinal deformities without the application of a rigid internal fixation device.

To harvest a rib graft, a linear incision is made in the skin directly over the rib's surface (Fig. 54-5). The outer surface of the rib is exposed by incising the overlying muscles and periosteum. Blunt dissection with a Doyen rib dissector is used to detach the intercostal muscles and parietal pleura from the undersurface. Care is taken to avoid injury to the neurovascular bundle, which lies just along the inferior surface of each rib. The ends of the rib grafts are dissected sharply using a rib cutter or oscillating saw. In most cases, we prefer the oscillating saw because the rib cutter can crush, splinter, and weaken the ends of the ribs. The remaining bone edges are smooth and waxed to prevent pleural puncture and to avoid pneumothorax. After hemostasis is obtained and the wound is closed in multiple layers, a routine postoperative chest radiograph is obtained to rule out pneumothorax.

Fibular grafts are obtained from the middle third of the fibular shafts (Fig. 54-6) to avoid injury to the peroneal nerve at the proximal fibular head and to preserve ankle function distally.[9-13] Overall, functional consequences are avoided. The incision parallels the fibula over the lateral surface of the middle leg. In most cases, a nonvascularized graft is obtained by performing a subperiosteal dissection circumferentially around the desired segment. Fibular graft provides strong, dense cortical bone that is ideal for reconstruction in areas under large loads or stress. However, because there is little cancellous bone, fusion may be relatively slow. Occasionally,

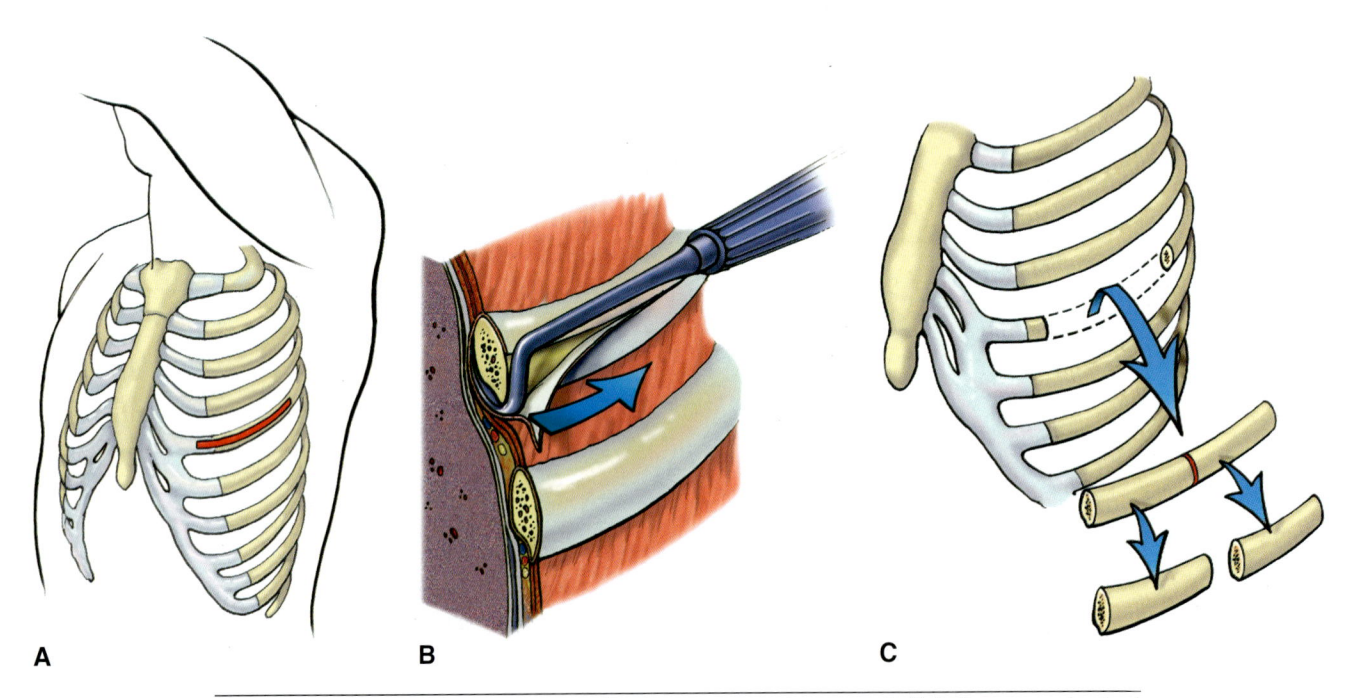

Fig. 54-5 *A*, The incision exposes a rib along a curved segment. *B*, A Doyen periosteal elevator is used to dissect the neurovascular bundle and muscle attachment from the rib, remaining extrapleural. *C*, The rib is cut sharply with a cutting tool.

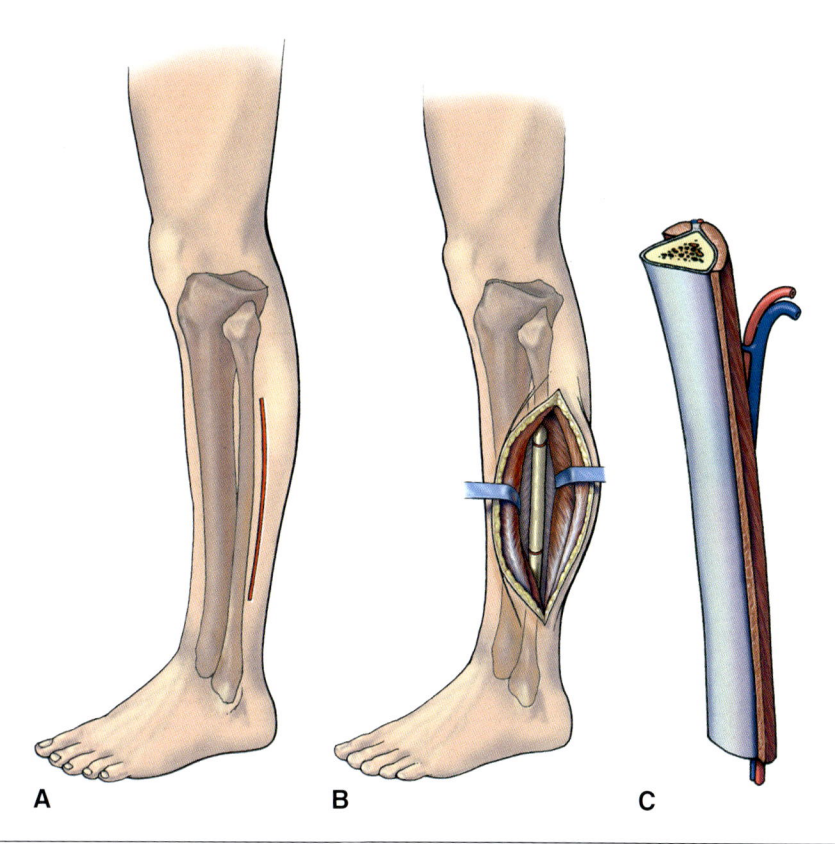

Fig. 54-6 *A,* Incision to obtain a fibular strut graft. The incision is made parallel to the fibular to expose the middle third segment. *B,* A nonvascularized graft can be obtained by performing a subperiosteal dissection circumferentially around the desired segment. *C,* A vascularized graft may be obtained by preserving a muscular cuff around the fibular graft along with the nutrient vessels.

a vascularized graft is preferred, in which case a muscular cuff is preserved around the fibular graft along with nutrient vessels. The muscles and fascia are dissected from the ends of the fibular surface, and a vascular vessel of the peroneal artery and vein is preserved. The bone is transected proximally and distally to the measured length with a Gigli saw or oscillating saw. After hemostasis is obtained, the wound is closed in routine fashion using multiple layers. In the case of vascularized grafts placed in the anterior cervical region, the vessels are usually anastomosed with the superior thyroid artery and vein or other accessible vessels. Posteriorly, the graft can be anastomosed to the occipital artery. Vascularized grafts have the advantage of being living tissue and hence are incorporated rapidly. However, more surgical time and technical expertise is needed for harvesting and placement.

Calvarial bone grafts are used for fusions in young children because the iliac crest and fibula remain nonossified.[9,14–17] Alternatives include a full-thickness graft, which can be obtained from the midline occipital bone, or split-thickness grafts, which can be obtained from the parietal bones (Fig. 54-7). In the case of a suboccipital graft, a linear incision is used to expose the suboccipital skull. One or two burr holes are used to expose the dura, and the atlanto-occipital membrane is dissected along the edge of the foramen magnum. The bone is removed in standard fashion using a high-speed drill. In the case of split-thickness grafts, a bicoronal or C-shaped incision is made at the vertex to expose a paramedian craniotomy. Midline bone is left intact over the superior sagittal sinus if bilateral craniectomies are needed. A reciprocating saw is used to split the diploic layers of the bone longitudinally. The top half of each of the grafts is reattached to the skull with miniplates. The split-thickness graft can then be contoured to the desired shape for fusion.

ALLOGRAFT AND FUSION SUPPLEMENTS

Although autograft remains the gold standard for arthrodesis, many procedures are performed using cadaveric allograft. For example, fibular allografts are routinely used for anterior cervical arthrodesis.[18] Occasionally, fibular, tibial, or femoral strut grafts are used in the thoracolumbar spine. In the case of single-level diskectomies of the cervical spine, autografts and allografts have similar rates of fusion. For multilevel fusions or in patients who have a history of smoking, autografts have a slightly higher rate of fusion than allografts.[19,20]

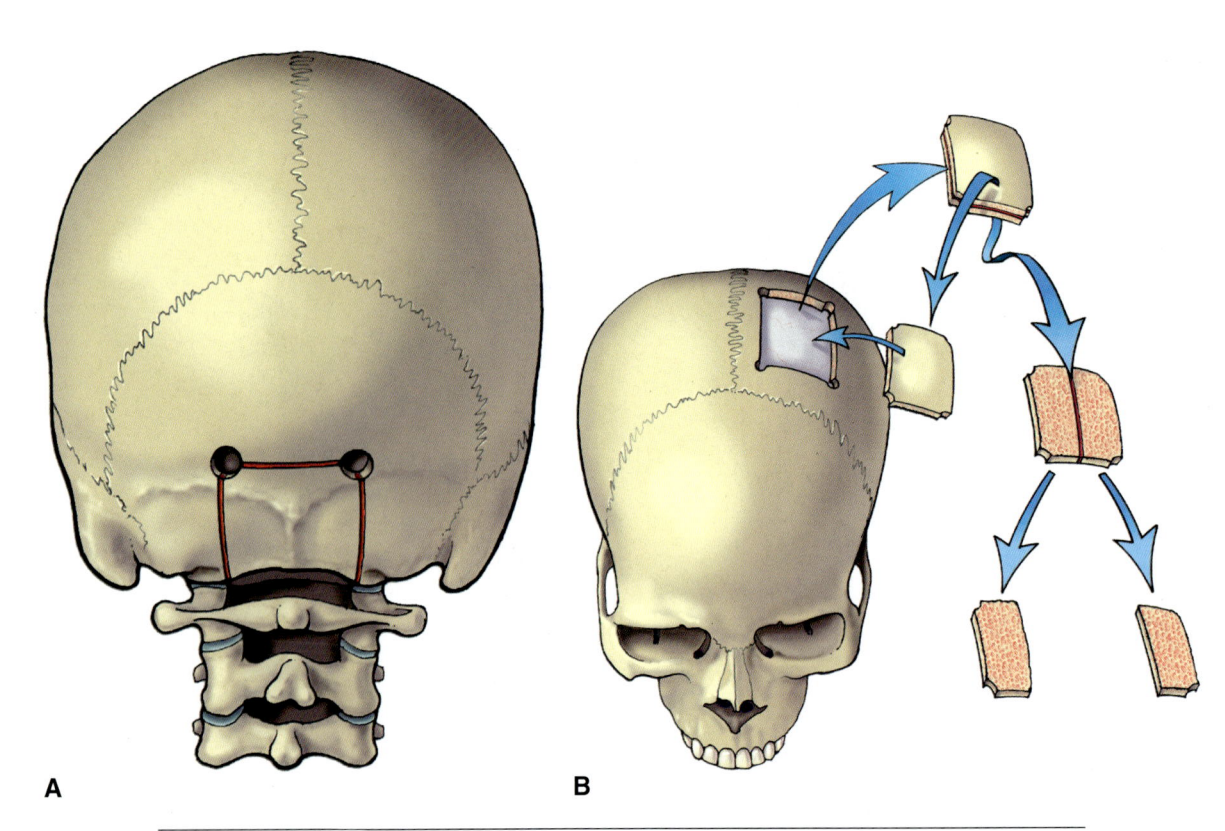

Fig. 54-7 Calvarial bone grafts. *A,* A suboccipital, full-thickness rectangular bone graft is harvested. *B,* A split-thickness parietal calvarial graft is obtained. A full-thickness bone flap is removed and then divided with a reciprocating saw. The upper layer of the calvarial flap is reattached with miniplates.

Allografts are procured by bone banks using established standards. Typically, they are harvested in a sterile fashion, processed, and then freeze-dried or processed in a fresh-frozen manner. Routinely, the donors are screened and undergo serologic tests to minimize the risk of infection. The risk of contracting the human immunodeficiency virus (HIV) through allograft transplantation has been estimated at less than 1 in 1 million.[21] To minimize the risk of immunogenetic reaction, allografts are treated with ethylene oxide, freezing, or freeze-drying.[21] This bone must then be reconstituted in sterile saline before being shaped or cut. To optimize the chance of successful fusion, the hollow center of allograft may be packed with autograft bone, which is obtained during the surgical decompression.

Occasionally, methylmethacrylate is used in place of bone grafts or spinal fusion. Methylmethacrylate, however, does not lead to bone fusion because it is neither osteoconductive, osteoinductive, nor osteogenetic. It does provide strength to resist compression, but it routinely fails under tension and must be anchored to the bone. It can also elicit a foreign-body reaction. Consequently, methylmethacrylate is reserved for patients who are expected to place only minimal mechanical stress on their construct or in those whose life expectancy is short.

Several developments have improved the rate of bone fusion. Numerous studies have shown that pulsed electrical or electromagnetic fields promote fusion, especially in long bones.[22] Although fewer studies have evaluated the effects of electrical and electromagnetic stimulation in spinal fusion, such stimulation appears to increase fusion rates in the spine also.[22] The technology, however, is expensive and patient selection is critical because overall fusion rates are already relatively good.

Other contemporary techniques to improve the rates of bone fusion rely on advances in molecular biology. The degree and strength of fusion are enhanced by a variety of osteoconductive proteins known as bone morphogenic proteins (BMPs). BMPs can lead to higher rates of fusion with allograft, and potentially, combinations of allograft and BMP may obviate the need for autologous bone graft.[23-27] In fact, recent experience shows excellent fusion rates even in cases when BMP is used without autograft or allograft.

CONCLUSION

Successful bone fusion is essential in cases of spinal fixation. The odds of having a successful fusion can be improved by handling the tissue gently, preparing the bone graft and fusion bed meticulously, and avoiding all anti-inflammatory medication perioperatively and postoperatively. Autograft tends to be associated with a higher rate of fusion than allograft, but the benefits and risks of obtaining autograft must be considered. When it is necessary to harvest autograft, the risk of complications can be minimized by meticulous surgical technique and a thorough understanding of the regional anatomy. New developments in molecular biology are providing additional alternatives.

REFERENCES

1. Yonemura KS: Bone grafts: Types of harvesting and their complications. In Menezes AH, Sonntag VKH (eds): Principles of Spinal Surgery. New York, McGraw-Hill, 1996, pp 151–156.
2. Brantigan JW, Cunningham BW, Warden K, et al: Compression strength of donor bone for posterior lumbar interbody fusion. Spine 1993;18:1213–1221.
3. Dickman CA: Techniques of bone graft harvesting and spinal fusion. In Dickman CA, Spetzler RF, Sonntag VKH (eds): Surgery of the Craniovertebral Junction. New York, Thieme, 1996, pp 699–710.
4. Kurz LT, Garfin SR, Booth RE Jr: Harvesting autologous iliac bone grafts: A review of complications and techniques. Spine 1989;14:1324–1331.
5. Coventry MB, Tapper EM: Pelvic instability: A consequence of removing iliac bone for grafting. J Bone Joint Surg Am 1972;54:83–101.
6. Lichtblau S: Dislocation of the sacro-iliac joint: A complication of bone-grafting. J Bone Joint Surg Am 1962;44:193–198.
7. Habal MB: Different forms of bone grafts. In Habal MB, Reddi AH (eds): Bone Grafts and Bone Substitutes. Philadelphia, WB Saunders, 1992, pp 6–8.
8. Prolo DJ, Rodrigo JJ: Contemporary bone graft physiology and surgery. Clin Orthop 1985;200:322–342.
9. Sullivan JA: Bone grafting: Sources and methods. In Weinstein SL (ed): The Pediatric Spine: Principles and Practice. New York, Raven, 1994, pp 1299–1310.
10. Conley FK, Britt RH, Hanberry JW, et al: Anterior fibular strut graft in neoplastic disease of the cervical spine. J Neurosurg 1979;51:677–684.
11. Freidberg SR, Gumley GJ, Pfeifer BA, et al: Vascularized fibular graft to replace resected cervical vertebral bodies: Case report. J Neurosurg 1989;71:283–286.
12. Rossier AB, Hussey RW, Kenzora JE: Anterior fibular interbody fusion in the treatment of cervical spinal cord injuries. Surg Neurol 1977;7:55–60.
13. Whitecloud TS, LaRocca H: Fibular strut graft in reconstructive surgery of the cervical spine. Spine 1976;1:33–43.
14. Chadduck WM, Boop FA: Use of full-thickness calvarial bone grafts for cervical spinal fusions in pediatric patients. Pediatr Neurosurg 1994;20:107–112.
15. Duong DH, Chadduck WM: Reconstruction of the hypoplastic posterior arch of the atlas with calvarial bone grafts for posterior atlantoaxial fusion: Technical report. Neurosurgery 1994;35:1168–1170.
16. Sagher O, Malik JM, Lee JH, et al: Fusion with occipital bone for atlantoaxial instability: Technical note. Neurosurgery 1993;33:926–929.
17. Tanaka T, Ninchoji T, Uemura K, et al: Multilevel anterior cervical fusion using skull bone grafts: Case reports. J Neurosurg 1992;76:298–302.
18. Cloward RB: Gas-sterilized cadaver bone grafts for spinal fusion operations—A simplified bone bank. Spine 1980;5:4–10.
19. Holmes R, Mooney V, Bucholz R, et al: A coralline hydroxyapatite bone graft substitute—Preliminary report. Clin Orthop 1984;188:252–262.
20. Rish BL, McFadden JT, Penix JO: Anterior cervical fusion using homologous bone grafts: A comparative study. Surg Neurol 1976;5:119–121.
21. Elder WJ, Adams M, Dickman CA: Bone harvest techniques, supplementation and alternatives. In Batjer HH, Loftus CM, Ondra SL (eds): Textbook of Neurological Surgery. Philadelphia, Lippincott Williams & Wilkins, 2001.
22. Oishi M, Onesti ST: Electrical bone graft stimulation for spinal fusion: A review. Neurosurgery 2000;47:1041–1055.
23. Sandhu HS, Kanim LEA, Toth JM, et al: Experimental spinal fusion with recombinant human bone morphogenetic protein-2 without decortication of osseous elements. Spine 1997;22:1171–1180.
24. Sheehan JP, Kallmes DF, Sheehan JM, et al: Molecular methods of enhancing lumbar spine fusion. Neurosurgery 1996;39:548–554.
25. Urist MR: Bone transplants and implants. In Urist MR (ed): Fundamentals and Clinical Bone Physiology. Philadelphia, J.B. Lippincott, 1980, pp 331–368.
26. Urist MR, Dawson E: Intertransverse process fusion with the aid of chemosterilized autolyzed antigen-extracted allogeneic (AAA) bone. Clin Orthop 1981;154:97–113.
27. Urist MR, Mikulski A, Lietze A: Solubilized and insolubilized bone morphogenetic protein. Proc Natl Acad Sci U S A 1979;76:1828–1832.

Index

Note: Page numbers followed by "f" indicate an illustration; page numbers followed by "t" indicate a table.

Abdominal wall, anatomy of, 113–115, 114f, 115f
Abscess, psoas, in tuberculosis, 90
Achondroplasia, cervical spine instability in, posterior approaches to, 33
Adamkiewicz, artery of
 anatomy of, in anterolateral approach, 103
 arteriovenous malformation of, 482f
Adams forward bend test, in thoracolumbar scoliosis, 393, 394f
Adolescent idiopathic scoliosis. *See* Scoliosis, idiopathic.
Affinity cage, for anterior cervical fusion, 161–162
Alexander-Farabeuf periosteotome, for thoracic metastasis resection, 452, 453f
Allografts, bone, 505, 509–510
American Spinal Injury Association classification, of thoracolumbar fractures, 356
Aneurysm(s), spinal cord, 486
Aneurysmal bone cysts, 445
Angiography
 in arteriovenous malformations, 484
 in hemangioblastomas, 475
Ankylosing spondylitis, 305–314
 osteotomy for
  contraindications for, 306
  indications for, 305–306
  pedicle subtraction, 311–314, 312f–313f
  posterior cervical, 305f, 306–307, 307f–311f, 310
Ansa cervicalis, anatomy of, 49f, 50f, 51f, 53f, 60f
Ansa hypoglossi, anatomy of, in high cervical retropharyngeal approach, 23
Ant-Cer Dynamic Plate, for anterior cervical fusion, 159
Anterior approaches
 to cavernous malformations, 479–480, 479f
 to cervical facet dislocation reduction and stabilization, 340, 342, 342f, 343f
 to cervical metastasis, 461–462
 to cervical stenosis laminotomy and laminectomy, 175
 to cervicothoracic junction, 65–70
  anatomy of, 65–67, 66f
  low cervical, 67
  supraclavicular, 67
  transmanubrial-transclavicular, 67, 68f, 69f
  trans-sternal-transthoracic, 67, 69f, 70, 70f
 to lumbar metastasis, 458–459, 459f–460f
 to lumbar scoliosis correction, 392–405, 394f–403f
 to lumbar spine fractures, 370–371, 371f
 to midcervical spine, 45–56, 46f–55f

Anterior approaches *(Continued)*
 anatomy of, 45–52, 46f–52f
 lateral, 54, 54f, 55f, 56
 medial (ventral), 52–54, 53f, 54f
 to Scheuermann's kyphosis, 432
 to thoracic metastasis, 452–457, 452f–456f
 to thoracic scoliosis, 379–391, 380f–389f
 to thoracic spine infections, 494–495, 495f, 496f
 to thoracolumbar fractures, 359–362, 359f–362f
 to thoracolumbar scoliosis, 392–405, 394f–403f
Anterior atlantoaxial facet screw fixation, 328, 328f
Anterior cervical corpectomy and fusion, 169–173, 170f–172f
 for ossified posterior longitudinal ligament, 193–194, 194f
Anterior cervical diskectomy and fusion, 141–149, 141f–148f
 instrumentation for, 157–163, 158f–163f
Anterior cervical microforaminotomy, 150–156, 151f–156f
Anterior interbody lumbar fusion, 263–271, 264f–270f
 for spondylolisthesis reduction, 284, 284f
Anterior longitudinal ligament, anatomy of, 45, 47f
Anterior retroperitoneal approach, to lumbar spine, 126–132
Anterior video-assisted thoracoscopic approach, to diskectomy, 208–211, 209f–211f
Anterolateral approaches
 to cervical spine infections, 490–491, 491f
 to cervicothoracic junction, 71–77
  anatomy of, 71–73, 72f
  transaxillary, 73, 73f, 76–77, 77f
  transpleural transthoracic third rib resection, 73–74, 74f–76f, 76
Anterolateral open thoracotomy, for diskectomy, 205–208, 206f, 207f
Anterolateral retroperitoneal approach, to lumbar spine, 101–105, 102f, 105f
Aorta
 anatomy of
  in anterior lumbar interbody fusion, 265, 266f, 268f
  in anterior thoracic scoliosis correction, 381, 382f
  in anterolateral approach, 101, 102f–104f, 103–105
  in anterolateral transthoracic approach, 73
  in lateral lumbar interbody fusion, 273, 274f

Aorta *(Continued)*
 in posterior thoracolumbar approach, 108f
 in posterolateral transthoracic approach, 84, 85f
 in thoracoabdominal approach, 89, 90f
 in transperitoneal approaches, 114–115, 115f
 injury of, in transperitoneal approach, 124
Aortic arch, anatomy of, 66, 73
Arcuate ligaments, anatomy of
 in anterolateral approach, 102f
 in thoracoabdominal approach, 89–91
Arterial thrombosis, in transperitoneal approach, 124
Arteriovenous malformations, spinal cord, 474–486, 480t, 481f–483f
 classification of, 480, 480t
 conus, 480t, 483, 483f, 486
 epidemiology of, 480–483, 481f–483f
 extradural, 480, 480t, 481f, 484
 extradural-intradural, 480t, 481–482, 482f, 485
 imaging of, 484
 intradural dorsal, 480t, 481, 481f, 484–485
 intradural ventral, 480t, 481, 481f, 482f, 485
 intramedullary, 480t, 482–483, 482f, 483f, 485f
 pathophysiology of, 483–484
 surgical treatment of, 484–486
Artery of Adamkiewicz
 anatomy of, in anterolateral approach, 103
 arteriovenous malformation of, 482f
Arthrodesis
 in cervical laminoplasty, 187
 in thoracic diskectomy, 207
Asterion, anatomy of, in far-lateral approach, 42
Astrocytomas, intradural, 462
Atlantis plating system, for anterior cervical fusion, 159
Atlantoaxial subluxation, in rheumatoid arthritis, decompression for, 297–304, 298f, 300f–303f
Atlantoaxial transarticular fixation, for fractures, 321, 321f
Atlanto-occipital junction fractures. *See* Craniocervical junction fractures and dislocations.
Atlanto-occipital ligament, exposure of, in cervicomedullary decompression, 300–301, 301f
Atlanto-occipital membrane, anatomy of, in posterior approaches, 34, 35f, 36

513

Atlas
  anatomy of, in posterior approaches, 34
  exposure of, in cervicomedullary decompression, 301–302, 301f
  transoral approaches to, 3–13, 5f–11f, 14f–15f
Auricular nerve, anatomy of, 38f, 58f, 60f
  in high cervical retropharyngeal approach, 29, 30f
  in lateral approach, 38f
  in lateral retropharyngeal approach, 41
Autograft, bone. See Bone graft, harvesting of.
Awl-staple combination, in anterior scoliosis correction, 387f
Axial compression fractures, thoracolumbar, 353, 353f
Axilla, cervicothoracic junction approach through, 73, 73f, 76–77, 77f
Axis, transoral approaches to, 3–13, 5f–11f, 14f–15f

BAL/D cage, for anterior cervical fusion, 161–162
Basilar artery, anatomy of, in transmaxillary approach, 18, 19f
Basilar invagination, transoral approach to, 3–13, 5f–11f, 14f–15f
Basiocciput, approaches to, lateral retropharyngeal, 41
BendMeister device, for Steinmann pin bending, 318
Bengal cages, for anterior cervical fusion, 161–163, 163f
Bicortical screws, in Caspar plate system, for anterior cervical fusion, 159, 159f
Bilateral apical vertebral derotation maneuver, in scoliosis correction, 415, 416f
Bioabsorbable plating systems, for anterior cervical fusion, 159–160
Biopsy
  in chondrosarcomas, 443
  in metastasis, 451
Bladder
  anatomy of, in transperitoneal approaches, 114
  injury of, in transperitoneal approaches, 124
Bone banks, for grafting, 509–510
Bone graft
  allograft, 505, 509–510
  cancellous, 505
  cortical, 505
  for anterior cervical corpectomy and fusion, 172
  for anterior cervical diskectomy and fusion, 147–148
  for anterior lumbar interbody fusion, 269
  for cervical fractures, 335, 335f
  for cervical laminoplasty, 184–185, 185f, 186f, 194f, 196f, 197
  for cervical spine fixation, 61, 63f
  for cervical spine infections, 491, 491f
  for cervicomedullary decompression, 302, 302f
  for craniocervical junction fractures, 318, 319f, 324–325, 326f, 327, 327f
  for infections, 490–491, 491f, 494, 495f, 498–499, 498f, 499f

Bone graft (Continued)
  for lateral lumbar interbody fusion, 275f, 276–279, 276f
  for lumbar spine fractures, 370–371, 371f
  for lumbar spine infections, 498–499, 498f, 499f
  for lumbosacral junction, 117f, 123, 123f
  for ossified posterior longitudinal ligament, 194f, 196f, 197
  for pedicle screw fixation, 243, 244f
  for posterior cervical osteotomy, 310, 311f
  for posterior lumbar interbody fusion, 248, 248f, 249f, 252, 253f
  for sacral fractures, 374
  for Scheuermann's kyphosis correction, 435
  for Smith-Petersen osteotomy, 424
  for thoracic diskectomy, 204, 204f
  for thoracic metastasis resection, 456, 456f
  for thoracic scoliosis correction, 385
  for thoracic spine infections, 494, 495f
  for thoracolumbar fractures, 358, 360, 361f
  for thoracolumbar scoliosis, 401
  for transforaminal lumbar interbody fusion, 259, 260f, 261, 261f
  harvesting of, 505–511
    complications of, 505
    from calvarium, 509, 510f
    from fibula, 508–509, 509f
    from iliac crest, 123, 124f, 147–148, 248, 248f, 504, 506f, 507f, 508
    from rib, 508, 508f
    techniques for, 505–509, 506f–510f
  selection of, 505
  tricortical, 506, 507f, 508
  types of, 505
  unicortical, 508
  vascularized, 508–509, 509f
Bone morphogenic proteins, for bone fusion, 510
Bone scan
  in metastasis, 451
  in osteosarcomas, 442
Bone tamps, for pedicle subtraction osteotomy, 313, 313f
Brachial plexus, anatomy of, 48
Brachiocephalic artery, anatomy of, 66
Brachiocephalic veins, anatomy of, 66
Brattström technique, for occipitocervical wire fixation, 327, 327f, 328f
Breast cancer, metastasis from, 451
Brooks fusion, for craniocervical junction fractures, 325, 326f
Buccopharyngeal (transoral) approach, to craniocervical junction, 3–13, 5f–11f, 14f–15f
Burrs
  for laminoplasty, 196, 196f
  Midas, 194f
Burst fractures
  cervical spine, 331–336, 332f–335f
  cervicothoracic junction, 345
  lumbar spine, 365

C1-C2, high cervical retropharyngeal approaches to, 22–32, 23f–31f
C2-C3 disk space, transoral approaches to, 3–13, 5f–11f, 14f–15f

Cable fixation
  for cervical facet dislocation, 339
  for cervical spine, 61, 63f
  for cervicothoracic junction fractures, 350f
  for craniocervical junction fractures, 318, 319f, 320f, 324–325, 325f, 326f
Cages
  for anterior cervical fusion, 161–163, 162f, 163f
  for anterior lumbar interbody fusion, 269, 270f
  for cervicothoracic junction fractures, 348f
  for lateral extracavitary approach, 109f
  for lateral lumbar interbody fusion, 276, 277f, 278f
  for lumbar metastasis reconstruction, 459, 460f
  for lumbosacral fusion, 123, 123f
  for posterior lumbar interbody fusion, 248–252, 249f–253f
  for thoracic metastasis resection, 456, 456f
  for thoracolumbar fractures, 360, 360f
  for thoracolumbar scoliosis correction, 399, 399f, 403f, 404
  for transforaminal lumbar interbody fusion, 259, 261f
Calcification, of posterior longitudinal ligament. See Posterior longitudinal ligament, ossification of.
Calvarium, bone graft harvesting from, 509, 510f
Cancellous bone, for grafts, 505
Cancer, 441–442, 443f, 444f
Carbon dioxide insufflation, for laparoscopic surgery, 120
Cardiopulmonary plexi, anatomy of, 66
Carotid artery(ies)
  anatomy of, 50, 50f, 52f, 66
    in cross-sectional view, 58f
    in high cervical retropharyngeal approach, 24, 26, 26f, 27, 28f, 29, 31f
    in transmaxillary approach, 18, 18f
    in transoral approach, 6
  injury of, in cervicomedullary decompression, 303–304
Carotid sheath, anatomy of, 50
  at cervicothoracic junction, 65–66
  in high cervical retropharyngeal approach, 27, 29–30, 30f, 31f
  in lateral approach, 54, 55f
  in medial approach, 52, 53
Carotid triangles, anatomy of, 22, 23f
Caspar distractors
  for anterior cervical corpectomy and fusion, 169, 170f
  for anterior cervical diskectomy and fusion, 145, 145f
Caspar plate, for anterior cervical fusion, 159, 159f
Caspar retractors
  for anterior cervical diskectomy and fusion, 145, 145f
  for anterior cervical microforaminotomy, 152, 152f
Caspar screws, for anterior cervical corpectomy and fusion, 169, 170f
Cauda equina, injury of, in transperitoneal approach, 124

Index

Cauterization, in lumbar microdiskectomy, 215
Cavernous malformations, spinal cord, 476–480, 477f–479f
Cavitron, for tumor removal, 39
Cement
　as bone graft substitute, 510
　for thoracic metastasis reconstruction, 458
Center sacral vertical line, in Lenke curve patterns, 406, 409f
Central disk herniation, definition of, 61f
Cerebellar arteries, anatomy of, in transmaxillary approach, 18, 19f
Cerebrospinal fluid, leakage of
　in lateral extracavitary approach, 111–112
　in transoral approach, 3–4
Cervical corpectomy and fusion, anterior, 169–173, 170f–172f
　for ossified posterior longitudinal ligament, 193–194, 194f
Cervical disk herniation
　anterior cervical diskectomy and fusion for, 141
　anterior microforaminotomy for, 150
　decompression of, nomenclature for, 61f
　posterior approaches to, 33
　posterior keyhole foraminotomy for, 164–167, 165f–167f
　with facet dislocation, 339
Cervical diskectomy, anterior, 141–149, 141f–148f
　instrumentation for, 157–163, 158f–163f
Cervical fascia, anatomy of, 48–49, 49f
Cervical foraminotomy, posterior keyhole, 164–167, 165f–167f
Cervical fusion
　anterior, 141–149, 141f–148f
　　in corpectomy, 169–173, 170f–172f, 193–194, 194f
　　instrumentation for, 157–163, 158f–163f
　with laminectomy, for ossified posterior longitudinal ligament, 193
Cervical ganglion, anatomy of, in lateral approach, 55f
Cervical laminoplasty, 180–190, 181f–189f
Cervical microforaminotomy, anterior, 150–156, 151f–156f
Cervical nerve, anatomy of, in posterior approaches, 36
Cervical osteotomy, posterior, for ankylosing spondylitis, 305f, 306–307, 307f–311f, 310
Cervical plexus, anatomy of, 49, 50f
Cervical spinal cord
　arteriovenous malformations of, 481–482, 484
　cavernous malformations of, 479
Cervical spine
　anatomy of
　　cross-sectional view of, 58f
　　disks, 46, 47f
　　ligaments, 46, 47f
　　neurovascular structures, 49–50, 50f–52f, 52
　　osseous, 45, 46f
　approaches to
　　anterior, 45–56, 46f–55f
　　midregion. See Midcervical spine.
　　posterior, 57–64, 58f–63f

Cervical spine (Continued)
　　transmaxillary, 13–21, 14f–20f
　　transoral, 3–13, 5f–11f, 14f–15f
　facet dislocations of, 337–343, 337f–342f
　fractures of. See Craniocervical junction fractures and dislocations; Fractures, cervical spine.
　intervertebral disks of, anatomy of, 45, 47f
　intradural tumors of, 462–463, 463f, 469f
　metastasis to, 460–461
　osteomyelitis of, 490–493, 491f–493f
　pedicle screw fixation of, 61, 63f
　spondylosis of
　　posterior approaches to, 33
　　posterior keyhole foraminotomy for, 164–167, 165f–167f
　stenosis of. See Cervical stenosis.
　traction on, for cervicomedullary decompression, 299
　trauma to, posterior approaches to, 33
　tumors of, lateral approach to, 37
Cervical spine locking plate, constrained type, for anterior cervical fusion, 159
Cervical stenosis
　anterior cervical corpectomy and fusion for, 169–173, 170f–172f, 193–194, 194f
　clinical evaluation of, 174, 175t
　in posterior longitudinal ligament ossification, 191–199, 192f–198f
　laminoplasty for, 180–190, 181f–187f
　laminotomy or laminectomy for, 174–179, 175f–178f
　natural history of, 175
　pathophysiology of, 174
Cervical sympathetic trunk, anatomy of, 50
Cervical-brachial pain syndromes, anterior cervical diskectomy and fusion for, 141
Cervicocranial junction. See Craniocervical junction.
Cervicomedullary decompression, in rheumatoid arthritis, transoral approach to, 298–304, 298f–303f
Cervicomedullary junction, approach to, 27
Cervicothoracic junction
　anterior approaches to, 65–70
　　anatomy of, 65–67, 66f
　　low cervical, 67
　　supraclavicular, 67
　　transmanubrial-transclavicular, 67, 68f, 69f
　　trans-sternal-transthoracic, 67, 69f, 70, 70f
　anterolateral approaches to, 71–77
　　anatomy of, 71–73, 72f
　　transaxillary, 73, 73f, 76–77, 77f
　　transpleural transthoracic third rib resection, 73–74, 74f–76f, 76
　fractures of, 344–351
　　anatomic considerations in, 346
　　classification of, 344–345, 345f
　　surgical treatment of, 346–351, 347f–351f
　pedicle screw fixation for, 61, 63f
　posterolateral approaches to, 78–88
　　anatomy of, 78–81, 79f–81f
　　costotransversectomy, 82–84, 83f–86f, 86
　　laminectomy, 81, 81f, 82, 83f

Cervicothoracic junction (Continued)
　　lateral extracavitary, 82, 83f, 86–87, 86f–88f
　　parascapular extrapleural, 82, 83f
　　transpedicular, 82–84, 83f
Chance fractures, thoracolumbar, 353, 353f
Chemotherapy
　for chondrosarcomas, 443
　for Ewing's sarcoma, 442
　for giant cell tumors, 446
　for multiple myeloma, 443
　for osteosarcomas, 442
　for plasmacytomas, 443
Chest tube, for thoracoabdominal approach, 98–99, 98f
Chest wall, arterial supply of, 80
Chin, incision through, in transmandibular approach, 3, 4, 6, 11f, 12
Chin-brow angle, in ankylosing spondylitis, 307, 307f
Chondrosarcomas, 442–443
Chordomas, 441
Clamps
　Halifax, 324, 324f
　laminar, for cervical facet dislocation, 339
Claudication, in lumbar stenosis, 227, 231
Clavicle, anatomy of, in high cervical retropharyngeal approach, 22
Clipping, of arteriovenous malformations, 485
Clivus
　approaches to
　　high cervical retropharyngeal, 22–32, 23f–31f
　　transmaxillary, 13–21, 14f–20f
　　transoral, 3–13, 5f–11f, 14f–15f
　exposure of, in cervicomedullary decompression, 301–302, 301f
Cloward procedure
　for anterior cervical diskectomy and fusion, 141, 141f
　for posterior lumbar interbody fusion, 247–248, 247f–249f
Cobb angles, in scoliosis, 393, 394f, 406, 407t, 408f
Cobb elevators
　for posterior approaches, to craniocervical junction, 34
　for sacral fracture fixation, 373
　for thoracolumbar scoliosis correction, 397–398, 397f–399f
Colon
　anatomy of, in transperitoneal approaches, 114, 118, 120, 121, 121f
　cancer of, metastasis from, 451
　injury of, in transperitoneal approach, 125
Compression
　in Scheuermann's kyphosis correction, 434–435, 434f–436f
　in thoracic scoliosis correction, 383, 385, 386f
　in thoracolumbar scoliosis correction, 400, 400f
Compression fractures
　anterior cervical diskectomy and fusion for, 141
　cervicothoracic junction, 344, 345f
　　burst, 345, 345f
　　flexion, 344, 345f
　thoracolumbar, 353, 353f

Computed tomography
  in aneurysmal bone cyst, 445
  in cervical facet dislocation, 337–338
  in cervical spine infections, 497f
  in cervicothoracic junction fractures, 345f
  in chondrosarcomas, 442
  in chordomas, 441
  in craniocervical junction lesions, 37
  in Ewing's sarcoma, 442
  in giant cell tumors, 445
  in metastasis, 451–452
  in multiple myeloma, 443
  in ossified posterior longitudinal ligament, 192, 192f
  in osteoid osteomas, 443
  in osteosarcomas, 442
  in rheumatoid arthritis, 297
  in thoracic pedicle screw fixation, 348f
  in thoracolumbar fractures, 354f, 355f, 356
Computed tomography myelography, in arteriovenous malformations, 484
Constrictor muscles of pharynx, anatomy of, in high cervical retropharyngeal approach, 26, 27, 27f, 28f
Conus arteriovenous malformations, 480t, 483, 483f, 486
Cornerstone HSR cage, for anterior cervical fusion, 161
Coronal venous plexus, arteriovenous malformations of, 485
Corpectomy
  in arteriovenous malformation resection, 484
  in cervical procedures, 169–173, 170f–172f
    fracture treatment, 332, 334f, 335
    instrumentation for, 157–163, 158f–163f
    metastasis resection, 461
    ossified posterior longitudinal ligament treatment, 193–194, 194f
  in infections, 494
  in intradural tumor resection, 470
  in lumbar metastasis resection, 459–460, 460f
  in thoracic metastasis resection, 455, 455f, 457–458, 458f
  in thoracolumbar fractures, 360, 360f
Cortical bone, for grafts, 505
Cortical burring, in scoliosis correction, 412f, 413
Costotransverse ligaments, anatomy of, 80, 80f
Costotransversectomy, 82–84, 83f–86f, 86
  for intradural tumors, 463–467, 465f–467f
  for thoracic diskectomy, 201f–204f, 202–205
Costovertebral ligaments, anatomy of, 80, 80f
Cotrel-Dubousset rod-screw plate, for craniocervical junction fractures, 318, 319f
Cranial nerves, anatomy of, in transmaxillary approach, 18, 19f
Craniectomy, suboccipital
  in cervical Steinmann pin fixation, 318, 319f
  in far-lateral approach, 41, 42, 42f
Craniocervical junction
  far-lateral approach to, 41–43, 42f
  high cervical retropharyngeal approach to, 22–32, 23f–31f

Craniocervical junction (Continued)
  instability of, 33
  lateral approach to, 37, 37f–40f, 39
  lateral retropharyngeal approach to, 39, 41
  posterior approaches to, 33–36, 34f–36f
  transmaxillary approaches to, 13–21, 14f–20f
  transoral approaches to, 3–13, 5f–11f, 14f–15f
Craniocervical junction fractures and dislocations, fixation of, 317–318, 319f
  anterior approaches to, 328, 329f
  atlantoaxial transarticular, 321, 321f
  Halifax clamp for, 324, 324f
  indications for, 327–328
  lateral mass-pars articularis screws for, 318, 320f
  plate, 322, 322f
  rod systems for, 321, 321f
  screw, 318, 320f
  threaded Steinmann pin for, 318, 319f
  wire, 324–325, 325f–328f, 327
Crankshaft phenomenon, in scoliosis, 379, 385, 392
Cricoid cartilage, anatomy of
  in lateral approach, 37, 37f
  in medial approach, 53, 53f
Cricothyroid muscle, anatomy of, 48f
Crura, anatomy of
  in anterolateral approach, 102
  in thoracoabdominal approach, 89
Cubic cages, for anterior cervical fusion, 161–163, 163f
Culture
  in infection management, 489
  oropharyngeal, in cervicomedullary decompression, 299
Curettes
  for anterior cervical microforaminotomy, 151, 151f
  for tumor removal, 39
Cutter, rib, in thoracoabdominal approach, 93, 93f
Cylindrical cages, for anterior cervical fusion, 161–162
Cysts
  aneurysmal bone, 445
  with hemangiomas, 476

Débridement
  in infections
    cervical spine, 490–491, 491f
    lumbar spine, 497–498
    thoracic spine, 494
    tubercular, 500, 500f
  in lateral lumbar interbody fusion, 272
Decompression
  nerve root, in spondylolisthesis reduction, 281–282, 282f, 283f
  spinal cord
    anterior cervical corpectomy and fusion for, 169, 193–194, 194f
    cervical laminoplasty for, 180
    cervical laminotomy or laminectomy for, 174
    cervicomedullary, in rheumatoid arthritis, 298–304, 298f–303f

Decompression (Continued)
  for infections, 489–491, 491f, 493–494, 494f, 495f, 497–498
  for lumbar spine fractures, 370
  for ossified posterior longitudinal ligament, 193–197, 194f–198f
  for thoracic metastasis, 456
  for thoracolumbar fractures, 358–360, 359f
  lateral extracavitary approach to, 108
  lateral lumbar interbody fusion for, 278
  lumbar foraminotomy for, 230, 230f
  lumbar hemilaminectomy for, 230, 230f
  lumbar laminectomy for, 227–229, 228f, 229f
  lumbar laminotomy for, 229, 230f
  posterior midcervical approach to, 60, 61f
  thoracic diskectomy for, 203–204, 204f
Deep cervical fascia, anatomy of, 48–49, 49f
Deformities. See also Flatback syndrome; Kyphosis; Scoliosis.
  lateral lumbar interbody fusion for, 272
Degenerative disease
  cervical
    anterior diskectomy and fusion for, 141–149, 141f–148f, 157–163, 158f–163f
    anterior microforaminotomy for, 150–156, 151f–156f
    stenosis in. See Cervical stenosis.
  lumbar
    microdiskectomy for, 213–218, 214f, 216f, 217f
    percutaneous and endoscopic diskectomy for, 219–225, 220f–224f, 220t
    transpedicular screw fixation for, 239
  thoracic, diskectomy for, 201–211, 201f–211f
Dehiscence, after cervical laminoplasty, 188
Denis classification, of fractures
  lumbar spine, 366, 366f, 367f
  sacral, 366, 366f, 367f
  thoracolumbar spine, 353
Dentate ligament, identification of, in cavernous malformation resection, 479–480
Derotation maneuver, in scoliosis correction, 415, 416f
Diaphragm
  anatomy of
    in anterolateral approach, 101–102, 102f
    in thoracoabdominal approach, 89–90, 90f
  approach through, to thoracolumbar junction, 92–95, 93f–96f
  closure of, in thoracoabdominal approach, 98, 98f
  complications with, in thoracoabdominal approach, 99
  dissection of, in thoracoabdominal approach, 93, 94f–97f, 95–97
  identification of, in thoracolumbar scoliosis correction, 396, 396f, 397f
  splitting of, in thoracolumbar junction metastasis resection, 457

Digastric muscle and tendon, anatomy of, 47, 48f
　in far-lateral approach, 42
　in high cervical retropharyngeal approach, 23, 25f–28f, 26, 29, 31f
Dilators, muscle
　for lumbar decompression, 232, 232f–235f, 234–235
　for percutaneous and endoscopic lumbar diskectomy, 221–222, 222f–224f, 224
Dingman retractor, for cervicomedullary decompression, 299, 300f
Dingman self-retraining mouth retractor, 4
Disk(s)
　anatomy of
　　cervical, 45, 47f
　　lumbar, 213, 214f
　excision of. See Diskectomy.
　herniation of
　　cervical. See Cervical disk herniation.
　　lumbar. See Lumbar disk herniation.
　　thoracic, diskectomy for, 201–211, 202f–211f
　types of, 61f
　infections of. See Diskitis.
Diskectomy
　cervical
　　anterior, 141–149, 141f–148f, 157–163, 158f–163f
　　in fractures, 332, 332f
　lumbar
　　in anterior interbody fusion, 268, 268f
　　in lateral interbody fusion, 274–275, 275f
　　in posterior interbody fusion, 247, 247f, 250, 250f
　　in spondyloptosis reduction, 285
　　micro-, 213–218, 214f, 216f, 217f
　　percutaneous and endoscopic, 219–225, 220f–224f, 220t
　　transmuscular far lateral, 215, 217f, 218
　　unilateral approach to, 257, 258f
　lumbosacral, in transperitoneal approaches, 122–123
　open standard, 214–215, 216f
　thoracic, 201–211, 201f–211f
　　in anterior scoliosis correction, 383
　　in metastasis, 455
　thoracolumbar, in scoliosis correction, 397–398, 397f–399f
Diskitis
　diagnosis of, 489
　surgical management of, 489–501
　　cervical, 490–493, 491f–493f
　　complications of, 501
　　contraindications to, 490
　　fungal, 499–500
　　goals of, 489, 489f
　　indications for, 489–490
　　lumbar, 496–499, 497f–499f
　　postoperative care in, 500–501
　　technique for, 490
　　thoracic, 493–496, 493f–497f
　　tubercular, 500, 500f, 501f
Dislocations
　cervical spine, 337–343, 337f–342f
　cervicothoracic junction, 344, 345f
　craniocervical junction. See Craniocervical junction fractures and dislocations.

Distraction, as injury mechanism
　in cervicothoracic junction region, 344, 345f
　in thoracolumbar region, 353, 354f
Distraction pins
　for anterior cervical diskectomy and fusion, 145, 145f
　for cervical facet reduction, 340, 342, 342f, 343f
　for posterior lumbar interbody fusion, 250–251, 250f–252f
Distraction screws
　for anterior cervical corpectomy and fusion, 169, 170f
　for cervical fracture treatment, 332, 332f–334f
DOC plating system, for anterior cervical fusion, 159
Dorsal root ganglion, anatomy of, 59, 59f
Doyen dissector
　for thoracic metastasis resection, 452, 453f
　for thoracoabdominal approach, 93, 93f
Drilling
　in anterior cervical corpectomy, 169, 171, 171f, 172
　in atlantoaxial wiring, 324, 325f
　in atlanto-occipital fixation, 323, 323f
　in cervical fusion, 160
　in cervical interspinous wiring, 61, 63f
　in cervical laminectomy, 178, 178f
　in cervical laminotomy, 177, 177f
　in cervical microforaminotomy, 152, 154f
　in cervical Steinmann pin fixation, 318, 319f
　in cervicomedullary decompression, 302, 302f
　in intradural tumor resection, 472f
　in lumbar diskectomy, 222
　in lumbar laminectomy, 228, 229f
　in lumbar laminotomy, 235–236
　in ossified posterior longitudinal ligament treatment, 196, 196f
　in pars interarticularis screw insertion, 318, 320f, 321f
　in pedicle screw fixation, 241, 242, 242f
　in posterior keyhole cervical foraminotomy, 166, 166f
　in posterior lumbar interbody fusion, 251, 252f
　in scoliosis correction, 412f, 413
　in thoracic diskectomy, 206–207, 210
　in thoracic metastasis resection, 455
　in transforaminal lumbar interbody fusion, 257, 257f
Ducker classification, of cervicothoracic junction fractures, 345f, 346–347
Dura
　excision of, in hemangioblastoma resection, 476
　incision in, in lateral approach, to craniocervical junction, 39, 40f
　patching of, in transoral approach, 12
　tears of
　　in cervicomedullary decompression, 303
　　in lumbar decompression, 237
　tumors within. See Intradural tumors.
Dwyer instrumentation, for scoliosis, 401
Dynamic plating systems, for anterior cervical fusion, 159

"Eggshell" procedure, in pedicle substraction osteotomy, 313f
Electrical fields, for bone fusion, 510
Electrocauterization
　for arteriovenous malformations, 484
　for hemangioblastoma resection, 476
　for intradural tumors, 462
Electromagnetic fields, for bone fusion, 510
Electromyography, in screw placement, in scoliosis correction, 413, 414f
Elevators
　for posterior approaches, to craniocervical junction, 34, 35f
　for sacral fracture fixation, 373
　for thoracolumbar scoliosis correction, 397–398, 397f–399f
Embolization, preoperative
　for aneurysmal bone cyst resection, 445
　for metastasis treatment, 451–452
Endoscopic procedures
　anterior video-assisted thoracoscopic diskectomy, 208–211, 209f–211f
　lumbar diskectomy, 219–225, 220f–224f, 220t
Endotracheal intubation, for transthoracic approaches, 73
Ependymomas, intradural, 462
Epigastric vessels, anatomy of, in transperitoneal approaches, 114, 114f
Erector spinae muscles, anatomy of
　in cervicothoracic junction approaches, 79–80
　in lateral extracavitary approach, 110, 111
　in posterior thoracolumbar approaches, 106
　in posterior transthoracic approaches, 86, 87f
Esophagus, anatomy of
　in anterolateral transthoracic approach, 73
　in high cervical retropharyngeal approach, 24
Eustachian tube, anatomy of, in transmaxillary approach, 18, 18f
Ewing's sarcomas, 442
Extension injury
　cervicothoracic junction, 345
　thoracolumbar, 355
Extracavitary approach, lateral, to thoracic diskectomy, 201f–204f, 202–205
Extradural tumors, arteriovenous malformations as, 480, 480t, 481f, 484
Extradural-intradural arteriovenous malformations, 480t, 481–482, 482f, 485
Extramedullary intradural tumors, 468, 468f

Facet(s). See also Facetectomy.
　anatomy of
　　cervical, 45, 46f, 57, 59
　　in posterior midcervical approach, 60, 61f
　　in posterior thoracolumbar approaches, 106
　dislocations of, cervical, 337–343, 337f–342f
　fractures of, cervical, posterior approaches to, 33
　hypertrophy of, retractor placement and, 222, 222f

Facet(s) (Continued)
  screw fixation of, in craniocervical junction fractures, 328, 328f
  subluxation of, cervicothoracic junction, 344, 345f
  wiring of, 339
Facetectomy
  definition of, 61f
  in arteriovenous malformation resection, 484
  in posterior cervical keyhole foraminotomy, 165–166, 166f
  in scoliosis correction, 410, 411f
  in Smith-Petersen osteotomy, 424
  in transforaminal lumbar interbody fusion, 257, 258f
Facial artery, anatomy of, 50f
  in high cervical retropharyngeal approach, 25, 27f, 28f
  in medial approach, 53, 54f
Facial nerve, anatomy of, 25, 25f
Facial vein, anatomy of, 25, 27, 27f
Fang and Ong transoral approach, to craniocervical junction, 3
Far-lateral approach, to craniocervical junction, 41–43, 42f
Fascial sling, anatomy of, 26
Fat, retropleural, anatomy of, 80, 81f
Feeding tube
  for transmaxillary approach, 21
  for transoral approach, 6
Femoral cutaneous nerve, protection of, in iliac crest graft harvesting, 123
Ferguson-Allen classification, of thoracolumbar fractures, 352–353, 353f–355f, 356
Fibula, bone graft harvesting from, 508–509, 509f
Finochietto rib spreader, for thoracic metastasis resection, 453, 454f
Fish-hook retractors, 202, 203f, 463, 464f, 467f
Fistulas. See Arteriovenous malformations.
Fixed sagittal imbalance. See Flatback syndrome.
Flatback syndrome, 421–430
  clinical presentation of, 421, 422f
  pedicle subtraction osteotomy for, 425–430, 438f, 439f
  Smith-Petersen osteotomy for, 422–425, 423f, 425f, 427f
Flexion compression injury, of cervicothoracic junction, 344, 345f
Flexion dislocation, of cervicothoracic junction, 344, 345f
Flexion-compression fractures, thoracolumbar, 353
"Floating segment" approach, anterior, to ossified posterior longitudinal ligament, 194, 194f
Fluid shifts, in posterior cervical osteotomy, 310–311
Fluoroscopy
  in lumbar decompression, 234, 235, 235f
  in lumbar diskectomy, 220–221, 220f
  in ossified posterior longitudinal ligament treatment, 196
  in pedicle screw fixation, 240, 241f

Fluoroscopy (Continued)
  in posterior keyhole cervical foraminotomy, 165, 165f
  in thoracic diskectomy, 202
Foramen magnum
  anatomy of, in posterior approaches, 34
  far-lateral approach to, 41–43, 42f
  transmaxillary approaches to, 13–21, 14f–20f
  transoral approach to, 3–13, 5f–11f, 14f–15f
Foraminal disk herniation, definition of, 61f
Foraminotomy
  cervical
    in laminoplasty, 185, 187, 187f
    in stenosis, 177, 177f
    posterior keyhole, 164–167, 165f–167f
    small keyhole, 150–156, 151f–156f
  definition of, 61f
  lumbar
    in laminectomy, 228–229, 229f
    in stenosis, 230, 230f
Forceps, jeweler pick-up, in intradural tumor resection, 466
Four-poster frame, for kyphosis correction, 312, 312f
Fractures
  burst
    cervical spine, 331–336, 332f–335f
    cervicothoracic junction, 345
    lumbar spine, 365
    thoracolumbar, 353, 353f
  C1-C2
    anterior approaches to, 328, 329f
    Halifax clamp for, 324, 324f
    indications for fixation of, 327–328
    lateral mass-pars articularis screw fixation for, 318, 320f
    plate fixation for, 321, 322f, 323
    rod fixation for, 320f, 321, 322f, 323
    screw fixation for, 318, 320f, 321, 321f, 323f, 327–328, 329f
    threaded Steinmann pin fixation for, 318, 319f
    wire fixation for, 318, 319f, 323–327, 325f, 328f
  cervical spine. See also Fractures, C1-C2.
    anterior diskectomy and fusion for, 141, 157
    at cervicothoracic junction, 337–343, 337f–342f
    burst, 331–336, 332f–335f
    posterior approaches to, 33
  cervicothoracic junction, 344–351, 345f–351f
  compression, anterior cervical diskectomy and fusion for, 141, 157
  craniocervical junction. See Craniocervical junction fractures and dislocations.
  lumbar spine
    in thoracolumbar region, 352–353, 353f–354f
    transpedicular screw fixation for, 239
  thoracic spine, 352–353, 353f–354f
    at cervicothoracic junction, 344–351, 345f–351f
    at thoracolumbar junction, 352–353, 353f–354f

Fractures (Continued)
  thoracolumbar, 353, 353f
  vertebral, thoracoabdominal approach to, 91
Free hand pedicle screw fixation, in scoliosis correction, 410, 411f, 412f, 413–414
French door laminoplasty, cervical, 180f, 181
Fungal infections, 499–500
Fusion
  cervical. See Cervical fusion.
  for craniocervical junction fractures, wiring techniques for, 324–325, 325f–328f, 327
  for thoracic scoliosis, 379–391, 380f–389f
  for thoracolumbar fractures, 358
  for thoracolumbar scoliosis, 393, 394f, 395f, 396
  lumbar. See Lumbar fusion.

Gait abnormalities, in cervical stenosis, 174, 175
Gallie fusion, for craniocervical junction fractures, 324–325, 326f
Ganglion retractor, for posterior lumbar interbody fusion, 250, 251f
Gearshift probing, in scoliosis correction, 412f, 413
Genetic factors, in ossified posterior longitudinal ligament, 191
Geniohyoid muscle, anatomy of, 47, 48f
Genitofemoral nerve, anatomy of, in thoracoabdominal approach, 91
Giant cell tumors, 445–446
Glomus (intramedullary) arteriovenous malformations, 480t, 482–483, 482f, 483f
Glossopharyngeal nerve, anatomy of, in high cervical retropharyngeal approach, 23, 27
Glossotomy, in transmandibular approach, 3, 4, 6, 11f, 12
Gluteal nerve, injury of, in sacral approach, 138
Gluteus maximus muscle, anatomy of, 137
Graft, bone. See Bone graft.
Gray rami, cervical, anatomy of, 49, 50f
Grob "Y" plate, for craniocervical fracture fixation, 322f
Guidewires, in thoracic scoliosis correction, 385, 387f

Halifax clamps, for craniocervical junction stabilization, 324, 324f
Halo stabilization
  for cervical facet dislocation, 338
  for posterior cervical osteotomy, 307, 309, 309f
Hard palate, approach through, to craniocervical junction, 3, 4, 7f–10f
Harrington distraction instrumentation, flatback syndrome after, 421
Hartshill rectangle, for craniocervical junction fractures, 318, 319f
Hattori laminoplasty, 195f
Hemangioblastomas
  intradural, 462
  spinal cord, 476–480, 477f–479f

Index

Hemilaminectomy
  definition of, 61f
  in arteriovenous malformation resection, 484
  in intradural tumor resection, 465, 466f
  in lumbar stenosis, 230, 230f
Hemilaminotomy, in lumbar microdiskectomy, 215, 216f, 223, 224
Hemorrhage, in cavernous malformations, 476–477
Hemosiderin, in cavernous malformations, 477
Henry lateral approach, to cervical spine, 54
Herniation
  cervical disk. *See* Cervical disk herniation.
  lumbar disk. *See* Lumbar disk herniation.
  thoracic disk, diskectomy for, 201–211, 201f–211f
High cervical retropharyngeal approach, to craniocervical junction, 22–32, 23f–31f
Hirabayashi classification, of ossified posterior longitudinal ligament, 191, 192f
Hirabayashi laminoplasty, 180, 180f, 195f
Hittori Z-plasty, in cervical laminoplasty, 180, 180f
Hockey-stick incision
  for high cervical retropharyngeal approach, 22, 27, 30f
  for transmanubrial-transclavicular approach, 67, 68f
Hodgson lateral approach, to cervical spine, 54, 54f, 56
Holdsworth classifications, of thoracolumbar fractures, 352–353, 353f–355f, 355
Hook(s)
  for cervicothoracic junction fractures, 346, 347f–350f, 348, 351
  for Scheuermann's kyphosis correction, 434, 434f, 435f
Hook-claw construct, for Scheuermann's kyphosis correction, 434, 434f, 435f
Horseshoe incision, in far-lateral approach, 41
Horsley rongeur, for pedicle subtraction osteotomy, 313
Hyoid bone, anatomy of, 48f, 50f
  in high cervical retropharyngeal approach, 26–27, 26f
  in medial approach, 53, 53f
Hypogastric plexus
  anatomy of
    in anterolateral approach, 101, 104–105, 104f, 105f
    in transperitoneal approaches, 115, 115f, 122
  injury of, in transperitoneal approach, 125
  protection of, in anterior interbody fusion, 268, 268f–269f
Hypoglossal canal, anatomy of, 42
Hypoglossal nerve, anatomy of, 50f, 52f
  in high cervical retropharyngeal approach, 23, 26, 26f, 27, 28f
  in medial approach, 53, 54f
Hypoglossus muscle, anatomy of, 26
Hypothyroid muscle, anatomy of, 48f

Iliac artery, anatomy of
  in anterolateral approach, 103, 103f
  in retroperitoneal approaches, 130, 131f

Iliac artery, anatomy of *(Continued)*
  in transperitoneal approaches, 114–115, 114f
Iliac crest, graft harvesting from, 123, 124f, 147–148, 248, 248f, 506, 506f, 507f, 508
Iliac fixation with four screw foundation, for sacral fractures, 374–376, 374f–376f
Iliac vein
  anatomy of
    in retroperitoneal approaches, 130, 131f
    in transperitoneal approaches, 114, 114f, 115f
  injury of, in transperitoneal approach, 124
Iliocostalis muscles, anatomy of
  in cervicothoracic junction approaches, 79–80
  in posterior approaches, 57, 58f
Iliolumbar veins
  anatomy of, in anterolateral approach, 103, 103f
  ligation of, in anterior lumbar interbody fusion, 266, 266f
Iliosacral screw fixation, for sacral fractures, 372, 372f
Implants, for anterior cervical fusion, 161–163, 163f
Infections. *See also* Diskitis; Osteomyelitis.
  after cervical laminoplasty, 188
  lateral lumbar interbody fusion for, 272
Inflammatory disease
  ankylosing spondylitis as, 305–314, 305f–313f
  rheumatoid arthritis as, 297–304, 298f, 300f–303f
Infrahyoid muscle, anatomy of, 49f
Infraorbital nerve, anatomy of, 17f, 18
Inion, anatomy of, 42
Instrumentation. *See also* Rod systems; Screw fixation.
  for infection reconstruction, 490
    cervical spine, 491–493
    lumbar spine, 498, 498f, 499f
    thoracic spine, 495–496, 495f–497f
    tubercular, 500, 500f, 501f
  for thoracolumbar spine, 108, 109f–110f
Intercostal arteries, anatomy of, 81
  in anterolateral transthoracic approach, 73, 76, 76f
  in lateral extracavitary approach, 111
  in thoracoabdominal approach, 89
Intercostal muscles, anatomy of, 111f
Intercostal nerves, anatomy of, 81
Intercostal neurovascular bundle, preservation of, in thoracoabdominal approach, 93, 93f
Intercostal veins, anatomy of, 66
  in anterolateral transthoracic approach, 73, 76, 76f
  in lateral extracavitary approach, 111
Intercostobrachial nerve, sacrifice of, in transaxillary approach, 76
Interfacet distances, in cervical spine, 45
Interspinal ligaments, anatomy of, 34
Interspinal muscles, anatomy of, 35f
Interspinous fusion technique
  for cervical facet dislocation, 339
  for craniocervical junction fractures, 324, 325f

Interspinous ligament, anatomy of, 47f, 57, 58f
Interspinous wire fixation, for cervical spine, 61, 63f
Intertransverse ligament, in transmuscular far lateral diskectomy, 215, 217f
Intervertebral cages. *See* Cages.
Intervertebral disks. *See* Disk(s).
Intradural tumors, 462–473
  arteriovenous malformations as
    dorsal, 480t, 481, 481f, 484–485
    ventral, 480t, 481, 481f, 482f, 485
  extramedullary, 468, 468f
  posterior approach to, 462–463, 462f, 463f
  posterolateral approach to, 463–473
    costotransversectomy in, 463–467, 465f–467f
    intramedullary, 467–470, 467f–469f
    thoracotomy in, 470, 470f–473f
  types of, 462
Intramedullary tumors
  arteriovenous malformations as, 480t, 482–483, 482f, 483f, 485f
  cavernous malformations as, 477
  hemangioblastomas as, 476–480, 477f–479f
  intradural, posterolateral approach to, 467–470, 467f–469f
ISOLA instrumentation, for sacral fractures, 375
Itoh laminoplasty, 195f

Jackson lordosing table, for kyphosis correction, 312
Jho anterior cervical microforaminotomy, 150–156, 151f–156f
Joints of Luschka, anatomy of, 45, 46f
Jugular bulb, anatomy of, 42, 43
Jugular vein, anatomy of
  external, 29, 30f, 31f, 49f
    in lateral approach, 39
  internal, 50, 51f, 52f
    in far-lateral approach, 43
    in high cervical retropharyngeal approach, 27, 31f
Juvenile arteriovenous malformations (extradural-intradural), 480t, 481–482, 482f

Kaneda device, for thoracolumbar fractures, 361, 362f
Kaneda system, for thoracolumbar scoliosis, 401
Kerrison punches
  for cervical laminoplasty, 183, 184f
  for cervical laminotomy, 177, 177f, 178
  for lumbar laminectomy, 228, 229f
  for pedicle subtraction osteotomy, 313
Kerrison rongeurs
  for anterior cervical microforaminotomy, 155, 155f
  for cervical laminotomy, 177, 178
  for cervical Steinmann pin fixation, 318, 319f
  for lumbar microdiskectomy, 215, 216f
Keyhole foraminotomy, posterior cervical, 164–167, 165f–167f
Kidney cancer, metastasis from, 451
Kittner sponges, for transperitoneal approaches, 122, 122f

Koyama laminoplasty, 195f
Kurokawa French door laminoplasty, cervical, 180f, 181
K-wires
  for craniocervical fracture fixation, 323, 323f
  for scoliosis correction, 413
  for SpheRx pedicle screw system, 291–292, 291f–293f
Kyphoplasty, for compression fractures, 356, 357f
Kyphosis
  cervical laminotomy or laminectomy in, 175, 175f
  in ankylosing spondylitis
    pedicle subtraction osteotomy for, 311–314, 312f–313f
    posterior cervical osteotomy for, 305f, 306–307, 307f–311f, 310
  laminoplasty for, 181
  modifiers for, in Lenke curve patterns, 406, 409f
  Scheuermann's, 432–437, 433f–436f
  Smith-Petersen osteotomy for, 422
  thoracoabdominal approach to, 91
  transforaminal interbody fusion for, 255

Labioglossomandibular approach, to craniocervical junction, 3, 4, 6, 11f, 12
Labiomandibular approach, to craniocervical junction, 3, 4, 6, 11f
Laminar clamps, for cervical facet dislocation, 339
Laminar hooks, for cervicothoracic junction fractures, 346, 347f–350f, 348, 351
Laminectomy
  definition of, 61f
  in arteriovenous malformation resection, 484
  in cavernous malformation resection, 478
  in cervical stenosis correction
    anterior approach, 175
    posterior approach, 175, 175f, 176f
    technique for, 177–178, 177f, 178f
  in cervicothoracic junction region, 81, 81f, 82, 83f
  in intradural tumor resection, 463, 463f
  in lumbar posterior interbody fusion, 247, 247f, 250, 250f
  in lumbar spine fracture fixation, 369
  in lumbar stenosis correction, 227–229, 228f, 229f
  in posterior cervical keyhole foraminotomy, 165–166, 166f
  in posterior cervical osteotomy, 310, 310f
  in sacral fracture fixation, 373
  in transpedicular approach, 106
Laminoplasty
  cervical, 180–190
    advantages of, 181
    arthrodesis in, 187
    bone graft for, 184–185, 185f, 186f
    closure of, 188
    complications of, 188
    contraindications for, 181
    disadvantages of, 181
    equipment for, 181
    evaluation for, 181

Laminoplasty (Continued)
    foraminotomy in, 185, 187, 187f
    Hirabayashi, 180, 180f
    in ossified posterior longitudinal ligament excision, 194–197, 195f–198f
    incision for, 182–183, 183f, 184f
    indications for, 181
    Kurokawa French Door, 180–181, 180f
    open door, 180, 180f
    open hinged, 182–183, 183f, 184f
    positioning for, 181–182, 182f
    postoperative care in, 188
    preparation for, 182
    types of, 180, 180f
    Z-plasty, 180, 180f
  in cavernous malformation resection, 478
  in intradural tumor resection, 462
  open door, for ossified posterior longitudinal ligament, 195–197, 196f–198f
Laminotomy
  in arteriovenous malformation resection, 484
  in cervical stenosis
    anterior approach, 175
    posterior approach, 175, 175f, 176f
    technique for, 176–177, 177f
  in intradural tumor excision, 463, 464f
  in lumbar stenosis, 229, 230f
  in transpedicular approach, 106
Laparoscopic surgery, for lumbosacral junction, 113, 118–122, 119f, 122f
Laryngeal artery, anatomy of, 28f, 52f
Laryngeal nerves
  anatomy of, 50, 50f–52f
  in cervicothoracic approach, 66–67
  in high cervical retropharyngeal approach, 23, 27, 28f
  in medial approach, 53–54
  in trans-sternal-transthoracic approach, 70, 70f
  protection of, in anterior cervical diskectomy and fusion, 143, 143f
Larynx, strap muscles of, anatomy of, 47, 48f
Lateral approaches
  to cavernous malformations, 479–480, 479f
  to craniocervical junction, 37, 37f–40f, 39
Lateral disk herniation, definition of, 61f
Lateral extracavitary approach
  to thoracic diskectomy, 201f–204f, 202–205
  to thoracolumbar region, 108–112, 109f–111f
Lateral extracavitary posterolateral approach, to cervicothoracic junction, 82, 83f, 86–87, 86f–88f
Lateral lumbar interbody fusion, 272–279, 273f–279f
Lateral mass plate fixation, of cervical spine, 60–61, 61f–63f
Lateral retropharyngeal approach, to craniocervical junction, 39, 41
Latissimus dorsi muscle, anatomy of
  in anterolateral transthoracic approaches, 71, 72f
  in cervicothoracic junction approaches, 79
Le Fort I osteotomy, in transmaxillary approach, 13, 16f, 18, 19f, 20f, 21

Leksell rongeur, for pedicle subtraction osteotomy, 313
Lenke curve patterns, in scoliosis, 380, 380f, 381f, 406, 407f–410f, 407t
  modifiers in, 406, 407f, 409f–410f
  type 1 (main thoracic curves), 406, 407f, 407t, 408, 416, 417f
  type 2 (double thoracic curves), 406, 407f, 407t, 408f, 416
  type 3 (double major curves), 406, 407f, 407t, 408f, 416–417, 418f
  type 4 (triple major curves), 406, 407f, 407t, 408f, 417
  type 5 (thoracolumbar/lumbar curves), 406, 407f, 407t, 408f, 417, 419f, 420
  type 6 (thoracolumbar/lumbar and main thoracic curves), 406, 407f, 407t, 408f, 420
Lenke probes, 412f, 413
Levator scapulae muscle, anatomy of, 47
  in cervicothoracic junction approaches, 78–79, 79f
  in lateral approaches, 39, 39f, 40f
Lexal rongeurs, for cervical laminectomy, 178, 178f
Leyla bar, for intradural tumor resection, 463
Lhermitte's sign, in cervical stenosis, 174
Ligamentum flavum
  anatomy of, 213
    in posterior approaches, 57, 58f
    in posterior thoracolumbar approaches, 106
  removal of
    in lumbar decompression, 236
    in lumbar microdiskectomy, 215, 216f
    in transforaminal lumbar interbody fusion, 257, 258f
Ligamentum nuchae, anatomy of, in posterior approaches, 57, 58f
Lin laminoplasty, 195f
Linea alba, anatomy of, 113
Lingual artery, anatomy of, 50f
  in high cervical retropharyngeal approach, 23, 27
  in medial approach, 53, 54f
Lingual vein, anatomy of, 50f
Lip, incision through, in transmandibular approach, 3, 4, 6, 11f, 12
Load-shearing classification system, of lumbar spine fractures, 365
Longissimus capitis muscle, anatomy of, 57, 58f, 59f
Longissimus cervicis muscle, anatomy of, 57, 58f, 59f
Longissimus muscles, anatomy of
  in cervicothoracic junction approaches, 79–80
  in posterior transthoracic approaches, 86f
Longitudinal ligament, anterior, exposure of, in cervicomedullary decompression, 300–301, 301f
Longus capitis muscle, anatomy of, 47, 48f
  in far-lateral approach, 41–42
  in high cervical retropharyngeal approach, 23, 27, 29, 29f, 31f
  in transmaxillary approach, 18f, 21
  in transoral approach, 4, 9f, 13, 14f–15f

Longus colli muscle
  anatomy of, 47, 48f, 50f
    in high cervical retropharyngeal
      approach, 23, 27, 29, 29f, 31f
    in lateral approach, 54, 55f
    in transmaxillary approach, 18f, 21
    in transoral approach, 4, 9f, 13, 14f–15f
  partial removal of, in anterior cervical
    microforaminotomy, 152, 153f
Lordosis
  cervical laminotomy or laminectomy in,
    175, 175f
  loss of, in flatback syndrome, 421, 422f
Low cervical approach, to cervicothoracic
    junction, 67
Lumbar arteries, anatomy of
  in anterolateral approach, 102
  in thoracoabdominal approach, 89
Lumbar disk herniation
  anatomic considerations in, 213–214, 214f
  anterior interbody fusion for, 263
  extraforaminal, transmuscular far lateral
    diskectomy for, 215, 217f, 218
  foraminal, transmuscular far lateral
    diskectomy for, 215, 217f, 218
  microdiskectomy for, 213–218, 214f, 216f,
    217f
  percutaneous and endoscopic diskectomy
    for, 219–225, 220f–224f, 220t
  posterior lumbar interbody fusion for, 246
  transforaminal interbody fusion for, 255
  transpedicular screw fixation for, 239
Lumbar fusion
  anterior interbody, 263–271, 264f–272f,
    284, 284f
  for spondylolisthesis, 280–286, 280f–284f
  lateral interbody, 272–279, 273f–279f
  minimal access, 287–294, 288f–294f
  posterior interbody, 246–254, 247f–253f,
    255, 284
  transpedicular screw fixations for, 239–245,
    240f–244f, 256, 256f, 261, 261f,
    262f, 289–293, 291f–294f
  unilateral transforaminal interbody,
    255–262, 256f–262f
Lumbar plexus, anatomy of
  in anterolateral approach, 102–103
  in thoracoabdominal approach, 91
Lumbar spine
  anterior retroperitoneal approach to,
    126–132, 127f–131f
  anterolateral retroperitoneal approach to,
    101–105, 102f, 105f
  fractures of
    classification of, 365–366
      in thoracolumbar region, 352–353,
        353f–354f
    treatment of, 366–371, 368f, 369f, 371f
  fusion of. See Lumbar fusion.
  infections of, 496–499, 497f–499f
  intradural tumors of, 462
  Lenke curve patterns in
    type 3 (double major curves), 406, 407f,
      407t, 408f, 416–417, 418f
    type 5 (thoracolumbar/lumbar curves),
      406, 407f, 407t, 408f, 417, 419f, 420
    type 6 (thoracolumbar/lumbar and main
      thoracic curves), 406, 407f, 407t,
      408f, 420

Lumbar spine (Continued)
  metastasis to, surgical treatment of,
    452f–460f, 458–460
  posterior and posterolateral approaches to,
    106–112, 107f–111f
  scoliosis of, anterior treatment for,
    392–405, 394f–403f
  stenosis of. See Lumbar stenosis.
Lumbar spine modifiers, in Lenke curve
    patterns, 406, 407f, 409f–410f
Lumbar stenosis
  anatomic considerations in, 227
  foraminotomy for, 230, 230f
  hemilaminectomy for, 230, 230f
  laminotomy for, 229, 230f
  minimally invasive decompression for,
    231–237, 232f–236f
  radiography in, 231, 231f
  symptoms of, 227, 231
  total laminectomy for, 227–229, 228f, 229f
  transpedicular screw fixation for, 239
Lumbar vein
  anatomy of
    in retroperitoneal approaches, 131f
    in transperitoneal approaches, 114, 115f
  injury of, in transperitoneal approaches,
    124
Lumbosacral fascia, anatomy of, 136f
Lumbosacral junction, transperitoneal
    approaches to, 113–125, 114f–124f
Lung cancer, metastasis from, 451
Luque rods, for cervicothoracic junction
    fractures, 347f
Lymphatic system, anatomy of, in
    cervicothoracic approach, 67

McAfee classification, of lumbar spine
    fractures, 365, 366f
McCormack classification
  of lumbar spine fractures, 365–366
  of thoracolumbar fractures, 356
Magerl classification, of thoracolumbar
    fractures, 355–356
Magerl method
  for craniocervical fracture fixation, 322f
  for pedicle screw fixation, 240, 241f
Magnetic resonance imaging
  in aneurysmal bone cyst, 445
  in arteriovenous malformations, 484
  in cavernous malformations, 477
  in cervical facet dislocation, 338
  in cervical spine infections, 492f, 496f
  in cervicothoracic junction fractures, 345f
  in chondrosarcomas, 442–443
  in chordomas, 441
  in craniocervical junction lesions, 37
  in Ewing's sarcoma, 442
  in giant cell tumors, 445–446
  in hemangioblastomas, 475, 475f
  in infections, 492f, 496f, 499f
  in intradural tumors, 462
  in lumbar spine infections, 499f
  in lumbar stenosis, 231, 231f
  in metastasis, 451
  in multiple myeloma, 443
  in ossified posterior longitudinal ligament,
    192–193, 193f
  in osteoblastomas, 445f
  in osteoid osteomas, 443–444

Magnetic resonance imaging (Continued)
  in osteosarcomas, 442
  in rheumatoid arthritis, 297
  in thoracic scoliosis, 382f
  in thoracolumbar fractures, 356
Mandible, osteotomy of, in craniocervical
    junction approach, 3, 4, 6, 11f, 12
Manubrium, anatomy of, 65, 66f, 67, 69f, 70f
Manubriumectomy, for thoracic metastasis,
    457
Masseter muscle, anatomy of, 17f, 18
Master laminoplasty, 195f
Mastoid, anatomy of, 43
Mastoid process, anatomy of, 37, 37f
MaXcess system, for posterior lumbar fusions,
    289–293, 291f–294f
Maxilla, osteotomy of, in transmaxillary
    approach, 13, 16f, 18, 19f, 20f, 21
Maxillary artery, anatomy of, 17f, 18
Maxillary sinus, anatomy of, 13, 16f, 18
MED (microendoscopic diskectomy system),
    219, 220t
Medial (ventral) anterior approaches, to
    midcervical spine, 52–54, 53f, 54f
Median sternotomy, for thoracic metastasis,
    457
Mediastinum, anatomy of, 65–66, 66f
Medullary arteries, segmental, anatomy of,
    103
Meningiomas
  cervical spine, lateral approach to, 37
  foramen magnum, transoral approach to,
    3–13, 5f–11f, 14f–15f
  intradural, 462
Meningitis
  in cervicomedullary decompression, 303
  in transoral approach, 3–4
Metastasis, 449–461
  biopsy in, 451
  clinical evaluation of, 450–451
  clinical presentation of, 450
  from giant cell tumors, 445
  from osteosarcomas, 441, 442
  incidence of, 450
  radiography in, 450–451
  radiotherapy for, 449
  sources of, 451
  surgical treatment of
    cervical, 462–463
      decision making in, 451
      embolization before, 451–452
      lateral lumbar interbody fusion for, 272
      lumbar, 452–458, 452f–458f
      thoracic, 452–458, 452f–458f
Methylmethacrylate cement
  as bone graft substitute, 510
  for thoracic metastasis reconstruction, 458
METRx Quadrant Retractor System,
    289–293, 291f–294f
METRx (microscopic endoscopic tubular
    retractor) system, 287–289, 288f
  for lumbar diskectomy, 219, 220t
  for lumbar stenosis, 232–236, 232f–236f
Metzenbaum scissors, for thoracic metastasis
    resection, 453, 454f
Microcurettes, for anterior cervical
    microforaminotomy, 151, 151f
Microdiskectomy, lumbar, 213–218, 214f,
    216f, 217f

Microdrill, for lumbar laminectomy, 228, 229f
Microendoscopic diskectomy (MED) system, 219, 220t
Microforaminotomy, cervical, anterior, 150–156, 151f–156f
Microscope
  in cavernous malformation resection, 478
  in intradural tumor resection, 467
Microscopic endoscopic tubular retractor (METRx) system, 287–289, 288f, 289f
  for lumbar diskectomy, 219, 220t
  for lumbar stenosis, 232–236, 232f–236f
Midas diamond burr, 194f, 196, 196f
Midas Rex drill, for cervical laminotomy, 177f, 178
Midcervical spine
  anterior approaches to, 45–56, 46f–55f
    anatomy of, 45–52, 46f–52f
    lateral, 54, 54f, 55f, 56
    medial (ventral), 52–54, 53f, 54f
  posterior approaches to, 57–64
    anatomy of, 57, 58f–60f, 59
    midline, 59–61, 60f–63f
Minimally invasive procedures
  anterior cervical microforaminotomy, 150–156, 151f–156f
  anterior video-assisted thoracoscopic diskectomy, 208–211, 209f–211f
  for lumbar stenosis, 231–237, 231f–236f
  percutaneous lumbar diskectomy, 219–225, 220f–224f, 220t
  posterior lumbar fusions, 287–294
    complications of, 292
    MaXcess system, 289–291, 289f–291f, 293f
    monosegmental (METRx system), 287–289, 288f, 289f
    multisegmental (Sextant Spinal System), 289, 289f, 292–293, 293f
    SpheRx pedicle screw system, 291–292, 291f–293f
Monitoring, in posterior cervical osteotomy, 309
Mouth, craniocervical junction approach through, 3–12, 5f–11f
Multifidus muscle, anatomy of
  in cervicothoracic junction approaches, 80
  in lateral extracavitary approach, 110f
  in posterior approaches, 57, 58f, 59f
  in posterior thoracolumbar approaches, 107f
Multiple myeloma, 109f, 443
Multisegmental spinal access, for posterior lumbar fusions, Sextant Spinal System for, 289, 289f, 292, 293, 293f
Muscle dilators
  for lumbar decompression, 232, 232f–235f, 234–235
  for percutaneous and endoscopic lumbar diskectomy, 221–222, 222f–224f, 224
Myelography
  in arteriovenous malformations, 484
  in hemangioblastomas, 475
  in lumbar stenosis, 231
  in metastasis, 451–452
  in rheumatoid arthritis, 297

Myelomas, multiple, 109f, 443
Myelopathy, cervical
  anterior corpectomy and fusion for, 169, 193–194, 194f
  anterior diskectomy and fusion for, 141, 157
  clinical evaluation of, 174, 175t
  in ossified posterior longitudinal ligament, 191–199, 192f–198f
  laminoplasty for, 180–190, 181f–187f
  laminotomy or laminectomy for, 174–179, 175f–178f
Myeloradiculopathy
  anterior diskectomy and fusion for, 157
  cervical, in ossified posterior longitudinal ligament, 191–199, 192f–198f
Myelotomy
  in cavernous malformation resection planning, 478
  in intradural tumor resection, 467–468, 467f
Mylohyoid muscle, anatomy of, 47

Nakano laminoplasty, 195f
Nasal septum, anatomy of, in transmaxillary approach, 13, 16f, 18
Nasogastric feeding tube
  for transmaxillary approach, 21
  for transoral approach, 6
Neck
  fascial planes of, 48–49, 49f
    approach through, to craniocervical junction, 22–32, 23f–31f
  incision in
    anterior, 52–56, 53f–55f
    far-lateral, 41–43, 42f
    lateral, 37, 37f–40f, 39, 54, 54f, 55f, 56
    medial, 52–54, 53f, 54f
    posterior, 33, 34f
  ligaments of, 45, 47f
  muscles of, 36, 36f, 47–49, 48f, 49f
  neurovascular structures of, 49–50, 50f–52f, 52
  osseous structures of, 45, 46f
Neoplasia. See Tumor(s).
Nerve injury
  in cervical laminoplasty, 188
  in ossified posterior longitudinal ligament treatment, 197
Nerve roots
  anatomy of
    cervical, 49, 50f
    in lateral extracavitary approach, 111
    in midcervical region, 59, 59f, 60f
    in posterior thoracolumbar approaches, 106
    lumbar, 213–214, 214f
  decompression of
    in anterior cervical microforaminotomy, 152, 154f
    in spondylolisthesis reduction, 281–282, 282f, 283f
  injury of
    in cervical facet dislocation, 337
    in cervical laminoplasty, 188
    in sacral approach, 138
  ligation of, in thoracic metastasis resection, 457

Neurofibromas
  cervical spine, lateral approach to, 37
  intradural, 462
Nuchal ligament
  anatomy of, in posterior approaches, 57, 58f
  division of, in posterior approaches, 33, 34
Numbness, in cervical stenosis, 174
Nurick, cervical spondylolytic myelopathic gait classification of, 174, 175t

Oblique capitis muscles, anatomy of, 36, 42
Oblique fascia, anatomy of, 113–114, 114f
Oblique muscles, anatomy of
  in lateral lumbar interbody fusion, 273, 274f
  in retroperitoneal approaches, 129, 129f, 130f
Oblique-vertical incision, for high cervical retropharyngeal approach, 22
O'Brien laminoplasty, 195f
Occipital nerves, anatomy of, 58f, 59, 60f
  in lateral approaches, 38f
  in posterior approaches, 34, 36f
Occipital pain, anterior cervical diskectomy and fusion for, 141
Occipital triangle, anatomy of, in high cervical retropharyngeal approach, 22, 23f
Occipitocervical junction. See Craniocervical junction.
Occipitocervical junction fractures. See Craniocervical junction fractures and dislocations.
Odontoid
  approaches to
    high cervical retropharyngeal, 22–32, 23f–31f
    lateral retropharyngeal, 39, 41
    transoral, 3–13, 5f–11f, 14f–15f
  excision of
    high cervical retropharyngeal approach to, 30
    transoral approach to, 6, 8f, 12
  exposure and shelling-out of, in cervicomedullary decompression, 301–302, 301f
  fractures of
    fixation of, 328, 329f
    posterior approaches to, 33
Omohyoid muscle, anatomy of, 47, 48f, 50f, 51f
  in high cervical retropharyngeal approach, 22, 23f
  in lateral approach, 55f
Open door laminoplasty
  cervical, 180, 180f
  for ossified posterior longitudinal ligament, 195–197, 196f–198f
Open hinged laminoplasty, cervical, 183–184, 184f, 185f
Oral cavity, ventral cervicomedullary decompression approach through, in rheumatoid arthritis, 298–304, 298f–303f
Orthosis
  for Scheuermann's kyphosis correction, 435
  for thoracolumbar fractures, 356, 357f

Ossification, of posterior longitudinal ligament. *See* Posterior longitudinal ligament, ossification of.
Osteoblastomas, 444–445, 444f
Osteoclasis, in posterior cervical osteotomy, 310
Osteoid osteomas, 443–444
Osteomyelitis
　diagnosis of, 489
　surgical management of, 498–501
　　cervical, 490–493, 491f–493f
　　complications of, 501
　　contraindications to, 490
　　fungal, 499–500
　　goals of, 489, 489f
　　indications for, 489–490
　　lateral extracavitary approach to, 108
　　lumbar, 496–499, 497f–499f
　　postoperative care in, 500–501
　　technique for, 490
　　thoracic, 493–496, 493f–497f
　　thoracoabdominal approach to, 91
　　transpedicular screw fixation in, 239
　　tubercular, 500, 500f, 501f
Osteophytectomy
　in anterior cervical diskectomy and fusion, 145–146, 146f, 147f, 160, 160f
　in posterior cervical keyhole foraminotomy, 166–167, 167f
　lumbosacral, in transperitoneal approaches, 122–123
Osteoporosis, thoracolumbar compression fractures in, 356, 357f
Osteosarcomas, 441–442
Osteotomes
　for posterior lumbar interbody fusion, 248, 248f
　for thoracic metastasis resection, 452, 453f
　for transforaminal lumbar interbody fusion, 259, 259f
Osteotomy
　for ankylosing spondylitis
　　pedicle subtraction, 311–314, 312f–313f
　　posterior cervical, 305f, 306–307, 307f–311f, 310
　Le Fort I, in transmaxillary approach, 13, 16f, 18, 19f, 20f, 21
　of mandible, in craniocervical junction approach, 3, 4, 6, 11f, 12
　of maxilla, in transmaxillary approach, 13, 16f, 18, 19f, 20f, 21
　pedicle subtraction
　　for ankylosing spondylitis, 311–314, 312f–313f
　　for flatback syndrome, 425–430, 438f, 439f
　Smith-Petersen, for flatback syndrome, 422–425, 423f, 425f, 427f

Pain
　after cervical laminoplasty, 188
　in aneurysmal bone cyst, 445
　in cavernous malformations, 476–477
　in chordomas, 441
　in Ewing's sarcomas, 442
　in giant cell tumors, 445
　in lumbar stenosis, 227, 231
　in metastasis, 451
　in multiple myelomas, 443

Pain *(Continued)*
　in osteosarcomas, 442
　occipital, anterior cervical diskectomy and fusion for, 141
Palate
　approach through, to craniocervical junction, 3, 4, 7f–10f, 18, 20f
　incision of, in cervicomedullary decompression, 299–300, 300f
Palpation, in scoliosis correction, 412f, 413
Pannus formation, in rheumatoid arthritis, 297–298, 298f, 302, 302f
Parascapular extrapleural (lateral extracavitary posterolateral) approach, to cervicothoracic junction, 82, 83f, 86–87, 86f–88f
Parascapular region, anatomy of, 78–81, 79f–81f
Paravertebral muscle, removal of, in lumbar microdiskectomy, 215, 216f
Parotid gland, anatomy of, 29, 30f, 31f
Pars interarticularis
　anatomy of
　　in posterior thoracolumbar approaches, 106, 107f
　　lumbar, 213, 214f
　screws in, for fractures, 318, 320f
PEAK polyaxial anterior cervical plate, for anterior cervical fusion, 159
Pedicle(s), anatomy of
　cervical spine, 45, 46f
　cervicothoracic spine, 84
　lumbar, 213, 214f
Pedicle blush, 108
Pedicle screw fixation, 239–245, 240f–244f
　for cervicothoracic junction fractures, 346, 347f–349f, 348
　for cervicothoracic junction stabilization, 61, 63f
　for kyphosis correction, 313
　for lumbar spine fractures, 368–370, 368f, 369f
　for sacral fractures, 374–376, 374f–376f
　for Scheuermann's kyphosis correction, 434, 434f
　for scoliosis correction, 410, 411f, 412f, 413–414
　for Smith-Petersen osteotomy, 424, 425f–428f
　for spondylolisthesis reduction, 282–283, 282f
　for thoracic metastasis resection, 457
　for thoracolumbar fractures, 358–359
　for transforaminal lumbar interbody fusion, 256, 256f, 261, 261f, 262f
　minimal access systems for, 289–293, 291f–294f
Pedicle subtraction osteotomy
　for ankylosing spondylitis, 311–314, 312f–313f
　for flatback syndrome, 425–430, 438f, 439f
Pediculectomy, in posterior thoracolumbar approaches, 108
PEEK cage, for anterior cervical fusion, 161, 163
Percutaneous diskectomy, for lumbar disk herniation, 219–225, 220f–224f, 220t
Periosteotomes, for thoracic metastasis resection, 452, 453f

Pfannenstiel incision, for lumbosacral junction, 119, 120f
Pharyngeal artery, anatomy of, 23, 27
Pharynx
　incision in, in transoral approach, 4, 7f, 13, 14f–15f
　space behind, craniocervical junction approach through, 22–32, 23f–31f
Phrenic nerve, anatomy of, 50, 52f, 60f, 89–90
Pial vessels, coagulation of, in hemangioblastoma resection, 476
Pin(s)
　distraction, for cervical facet reduction, 340, 342, 342f, 343f
　Steinmann. *See* Steinmann pins.
Plasmacytomas, 443, 443f, 444f
Plate fixation
　for anterior cervical fusion, 157–161, 158f–161f, 172–173
　for anterior lumbar interbody fusion, 269–270, 270f
　for cervical facet dislocation, 339
　for cervical laminoplasty, 196f, 197, 197f
　for cervical spine, posterior, 60–61, 61f–63f
　for cervical stabilization, in rheumatoid arthritis, 303, 303f
　for cervicothoracic junction fractures, 347f
　for craniocervical junction fractures, 318, 319f, 321, 322f, 323, 323f
　for lateral lumbar interbody fusion, 277, 278f
　for Le Fort I osteotomy, 21
　for mandibular osteotomy, in transoral approach, 12
　for maxillary osteotomy, 21
　for sacral fractures, 372–374, 373f
　for thoracic diskectomy, 210–211, 211f
　for thoracic metastasis resection, 456, 456f
Platysma muscle
　anatomy of, 47
　　in lateral approach, 37
　　in medial approach, 53
　incision in, for high cervical retropharyngeal approach, 24, 24f, 25f, 28f, 29
Pleura
　anatomy of, 72, 89–91, 90f
　approach through, to thoracolumbar junction, 96–98, 96f–98f
　dissection of, in lateral extracavitary approach, 111, 111f
　transpleural transthoracic third rib resection approach through, to cervicothoracic junction, 73–74, 74f–76f, 76
Pneumonia, in thoracoabdominal approach, 99
Portals, for video-assisted thoracoscopic approach, to diskectomy, 208–209, 209f, 210f
Posterior approaches
　to cavernous malformations, 478–479, 478f
　to cervical facet dislocation reduction and stabilization, 339, 340f, 341f
　to cervical metastasis, 461
　to cervical spine infections, 492–493, 493f, 494f
　to craniocervical junction, 33–36, 34f–36f
　to infections, 492–496, 493f–497f

Posterior approaches (Continued)
   to laminotomy or laminectomy, for cervical stenosis, 175–176, 175f
   to lumbar metastasis, 459–460
   to lumbar spine, 106–112, 107f–111f, 368–370, 368f, 369f
   to midcervical spine, 57–64
     anatomy of, 57, 58f–60f, 59
     midline, 59–61, 60f–63f
   to sacrum, 133–138, 134f–137f
   to Scheuermann's kyphosis correction, 432–437, 433f–437f
   to thoracic metastasis, 457–458, 458f
   to thoracic spine, 106–112, 107f–111f, 493–496, 494f–497f
   to thoracolumbar fractures, 358–359, 359f
Posterior cervical osteotomy, for ankylosing spondylitis, 305f, 306–307, 307f–311f, 310
Posterior keyhole cervical foraminotomy, 164–167, 165f–167f
Posterior longitudinal ligament
   anatomy of, 45, 47f
   excision of, in thoracolumbar scoliosis correction, 398
   injury of, in cervical facet dislocation, 337
   ossification of, 191–199
     anterior approaches to, 193–194, 194f
     anterior cervical corpectomy and fusion for, 169, 172, 172f, 193–194, 194f
     classification of, 191, 192f
     clinical features of, 191–192
     combined anterior and posterior approaches to, 194
     continuous, 191, 192f
     epidemiology of, 191
     historical review of, 191
     laminectomy and fusion for, 193
     laminectomy for, 193
     laminoplasty for, 194–197, 195f–198f
     localized, 191, 192f
     mixed, 191, 192f
     natural history of, 192
     pathophysiology of, 191
     segmental, 191, 192f
   removal of, in anterior cervical corpectomy, 171–172, 172f
Posterior lumbar interbody fusion, 246–255, 247f–253f, 284
Posterior transpedicular approach, to thoracic diskectomy, 201
Posterolateral approaches
   to cervicothoracic junction, 78–88
     anatomy of, 78–81, 79f–81f
     costotransversectomy, 82–84, 83f–86f, 86
     laminectomy, 81, 81f, 82, 83f
     lateral extracavity, 82, 83f, 86–87, 86f–88f
     parascapular extrapleural, 82, 83f
     transpedicular, 82–84, 83f
   to lumbar spine, 106–112, 107f–111f
   to thoracic spine, 106–112, 107f–111f
Posterolateral transpedicular approach, for cavernous malformation resection, 479–480
Pott's disease
   lateral extracavity approach to, 108
   of lumbosacral junction, transperitoneal approach to, 113

Premier plating system, for anterior cervical fusion, 159
Presacral plexus, anatomy of, in transperitoneal approaches, 121
Prevertebral cervical fascia, anatomy of, 49, 49f, 53f, 54
Prevertebral muscles, anatomy of, 24
Prostate cancer, metastasis from, 451
Pseudoarthrosis
   after thoracolumbar scoliosis correction, 401, 404
   transforaminal interbody fusion for, 255
Pseudomeningocele, in transoral approach, 3
Psoas muscle
   anatomy of
     in anterolateral approach, 101–103, 102f
     in thoracoabdominal approach, 90–91
   dissection of
     in retroperitoneal approach, 130, 131f
     in thoracoabdominal approach, 97, 97f
Pterygoid muscle, anatomy of, 17f, 18
Pterygopalatine fossa, anatomy of, 17f, 18
Pulmonary function, testing of, in scoliosis correction planning, 380, 396
Pulmonary restriction, in ankylosing spondylitis, 307, 309f
Punches
   for cervical laminoplasty, 183, 184f
   for cervical laminotomy, 177, 177f, 178
   for lumbar laminectomy, 228, 229f
   for pedicle subtraction osteotomy, 313
Pyriform aperture, anatomy of, in transmaxillary approach, 16f

Quadratus muscles, anatomy of, in anterolateral approach, 102

Radiculopathy
   cervical
     anterior cervical diskectomy and fusion for, 141
     anterior cervical microforaminotomy for, 150
     anterior corpectomy and fusion for, 169, 193–194, 194f
     anterior diskectomy and fusion for, 157
     in ossified posterior longitudinal ligament, 191–192
     posterior keyhole foraminotomy for, 164–167, 165f–167f
   in cavernous malformations, 477
   in chordomas, 441
   lumbar, transforaminal interbody fusion for, 256
Radiofrequency ablation, for osteoid osteomas, 444
Radiography
   in aneurysmal bone cyst, 445
   in ankylosing spondylitis, 307, 307f
   in cervical facet dislocation, 337–338
   in cervical spine infections, 492f, 493f
   in chondrosarcomas, 442
   in chordomas, 441
   in Ewing's sarcomas, 442
   in flatback syndrome, 421
   in giant cell tumors, 445
   in lumbar spine infections, 497f
   in metastasis, 451–452
   in multiple myeloma, 443

Radiography (Continued)
   in ossified posterior longitudinal ligament, 192
   in osteoid osteomas, 443
   in osteosarcomas, 442
   in rheumatoid arthritis, 297
   in Scheuermann's kyphosis, 432, 433f
   in scoliosis, 380f, 381f, 388f, 389f, 408f–410f, 413–414, 417f
   in thoracolumbar fractures, 356
   in thoracolumbar scoliosis, 393, 394f–395f, 402f, 403f
Radiotherapy
   for aneurysmal bone cyst, 445
   for chondrosarcomas, 443
   for Ewing's sarcoma, 442
   for giant cell tumors, 446
   for multiple myeloma, 443
   for plasmacytomas, 443
Ransford loop, for craniocervical junction fractures, 318, 319f
Ray threaded fusion cage system, for posterior lumbar interbody fusion, 248–252, 249f–253f
Rectus abdominis muscles, anatomy of
   in retroperitoneal approaches, 128, 129f, 130f
   in transperitoneal approaches, 113–114, 114f
Rectus capitis muscles, anatomy of, 36, 42, 47, 48f
Rectus sheath, anatomy of
   in retroperitoneal approaches, 128–129, 129f
   in transperitoneal approaches, 113, 114f
Reflexes, abnormal, in cervical stenosis, 174
Resorbable plating systems, for anterior cervical fusion, 159–160
Respiratory failure, in thoracoabdominal approach, 99
Retractors
   abdominal, in transperitoneal approaches, 116f
   fish-hook, 202, 203f
   for anterior lumbar interbody fusion, 265, 265f, 267f
   for cervical fracture treatment, 332, 332f–334f
   for cervicomedullary decompression, 299, 300f
   for lumbar decompression, 232–236, 232f–236f
   for percutaneous and endoscopic lumbar diskectomy, 221–222, 222f–224f, 224
   for posterior approaches, to craniocervical junction, 33
   for Scheuermann's kyphosis correction, 433–434
   for transoral approach, 4
   in METRx system, 219, 232–236, 232f–236f
   tang, for posterior lumbar interbody fusion, 250–251, 250f–252f
Retroarcuate space, anatomy of, in thoracoabdominal approach, 90–91, 91f
Retrograde ejaculation, after, in transperitoneal approach, 125

Retromediastinal space, anatomy of, 66–67, 80–81, 81f
Retroperitoneal approaches
　to lumbar fractures, 370, 371f
　to lumbar interbody fusion, 264–266, 265f, 266f, 273–275, 273f, 274f
　to lumbar spine, anterior, 126–132, 127f–131f
　to lumbar spine infections, 496–497, 497f
　to lumbar tumors, 458–459, 458f, 459f
　to thoracolumbar junction, through pleura, 96–98, 96f–98f
　to thoracolumbar scoliosis, 396–397, 396f, 397f
Retroperitoneal fat, dissection of, in thoracoabdominal approach, 97, 97f
Retroperitoneal space, anatomy of, 101, 102f
Retropharyngeal approach, to craniocervical junction, 22–32, 23f–31f
Retropharyngeal space, anatomy of, 66–67
Rheumatoid arthritis
　cervicomedullary decompression in, 297–304, 298f, 300f–303f
　diagnosis of, 297
　of cervical spine, posterior approaches to, 33
Rhomboid muscles, anatomy of
　in anterolateral transthoracic approaches, 71, 72f
　in cervicothoracic junction approaches, 78, 79f
　in lateral extracavitary approach, 110
　in posterior transthoracic approaches, 86, 86f, 87f
Rib(s)
　anatomy of, 80, 80f
　　at diaphragm, 89–90, 90f
　　at pleura, 89–90, 90f
　　in lateral extracavitary approach, 110, 111, 111f
　bone graft harvesting from, 508, 508f
　counting of, in anterolateral transthoracic approach, 71
　in anterior scoliosis correction, 381, 383, 384f, 387f
　in intradural tumor resection, 465f, 466, 470, 472f, 473f
　in thoracic diskectomy, 202–204, 203f, 204f, 206, 206f, 207f, 210, 210f
　in thoracic metastasis treatment, 452–454, 452f, 453f, 455f
　in thoracic spinal infection management, 493
　resection of
　　in thoracoabdominal approach, 92–93, 93f, 96, 96f
　　in transpleural transthoracic third rib resection approach, to cervicothoracic junction, 73–74, 74f–76f, 76
Rod systems
　for cervical stabilization, in rheumatoid arthritis, 303, 303f
　for cervicothoracic junction fractures, 346, 347f, 348f, 351, 351f
　for craniocervical junction fractures, 318, 319f, 321, 322f
　for lateral lumbar interbody fusion, 277, 278f

Rod systems (Continued)
　for pedicle screw fixation, 242–243, 243f, 256, 256f, 261, 261f, 262f
　for sacral fractures, 375, 375f
　for Scheuermann's kyphosis correction, 434–435, 434f–436f
　for scoliosis, 414, 414f
　for Smith-Petersen osteotomy, 424, 427f
　for thoracic metastasis resection, 456, 456f
　for thoracic scoliosis correction, 383, 384f–388f, 385
　for thoracolumbar fractures, 362
　for thoracolumbar scoliosis correction, 398–401, 399f–404f
Rongeurs
　for anterior cervical microforaminotomy, 155, 155f
　for cervical laminotomy, 177, 178
　for cervical Steinmann pin fixation, 318, 319f
　for lumbar microdiskectomy, 215, 216f
　for pedicle subtraction osteotomy, 313
Rotational force, in thoracolumbar fractures, 353, 355
Rotator muscles, anatomy of
　in cervicothoracic junction approaches, 80
　in posterior approaches, 57, 58f
Roy-Camille classification, of sacral fractures, 366, 367f
Roy-Camille method
　for cervical facet dislocation fixation, 339
　for pedicle screw fixation, 240, 240f
Roy-Camille plate, for craniocervical fracture fixation, 322f

Sacral ala, anatomy of, 136–137, 136f
Sacral fixation, in spondylolisthesis reduction, 282–283, 282f, 283f
Sacral hiatus, anatomy of, 136, 136f
Sacral ligament, anatomy of, 137, 137f
Sacral vessels, anatomy of
　in anterolateral approaches, 103
　in retroperitoneal approaches, 131f
　in transperitoneal approaches, 114
Sacrospinalis muscles, anatomy of, in posterior approaches, 57, 58f
Sacrum
　anatomy of, 134f, 135–136, 136f
　fractures of
　　classification of, 366, 366f, 367f
　　treatment of, 371–376, 372f–376f
　posterior approaches to, 133–138, 134f–137f
Sagittal imbalance. See Flatback syndrome.
Sagittal thoracic modifier, in Lenke curve patterns, 406, 409f
Sagittal-vertical angle, in ankylosing spondylitis, 307, 307f
Sanger cable, for cervical facet dislocation, 339
Sarcomas, Ewing's, 442
Scalene muscles, anatomy of, 47–48, 48f, 49f, 52f, 55f, 56
Scapula, anatomy of, 71, 72f, 78–81, 79f–81f
Scheuermann's kyphosis, 422, 432–437, 433f–436f
Schwannomas, intradural, 462
Sciatic foramen, anatomy of, 136, 136f
Scissors, for thoracic metastasis resection, 453, 454f

Scoliosis
　congenital, Smith-Petersen osteotomy for, 422
　idiopathic, surgical treatment of
　　bilateral apical vertebral derotation maneuver in, 414–416, 415f
　　classification and, 406, 407f–410f, 407t
　　deformity correction in, 414, 414f
　　equipment for, 406, 408
　　indications for, 406
　　Lenke type 1 (main thoracic curves), 406, 407f, 407t, 408, 416, 417f
　　Lenke type 2 (double thoracic curves), 406, 407f, 407t, 408f, 416
　　Lenke type 3 (double major curves), 406, 407f, 407t, 408f, 416–417, 418f
　　Lenke type 4 (triple major curves), 406, 407f, 407t, 408f, 417
　　Lenke type 5 (thoracolumbar/lumbar curves), 406, 407f, 407t, 408f, 417, 419f, 420
　　Lenke type 6 (thoracolumbar/lumbar and main thoracic curves), 406, 407f, 407t, 408f, 420
　　pedicle screw placement in, 410, 411f, 412f, 413–414
　　positioning for, 408
　　postoperative management in, 416
　　preparation for, 408, 410
　　rod contouring in, 414
　lumbar, anterior treatment for, 392–405, 394f–403f
　thoracic, anterior release and fusion techniques for, 379–391, 380f–389f
　thoracoabdominal approach to, 91
　thoracolumbar, anterior treatment for, 392–405, 394f–403f
　transpedicular screw fixation for, 239
Screw fixation
　for anterior cervical corpectomy and fusion, 169, 170f
　for anterior cervical fusion, 159, 159f
　for cervical facet dislocation, 339
　for cervical fractures, 41, 335
　for cervicothoracic junction fractures, 346, 347f–350f, 348
　for craniocervical junction fractures, 318, 320f, 321f, 323f, 327–328, 329f
　　atlantoaxial transarticular, 321, 321f
　　lateral mass-pars articularis, 318, 320f
　　wiring techniques with, 324–325, 325f, 328f
　for infections, 495, 495f, 497f, 499, 499f
　for lateral lumbar interbody fusion, 277, 278f
　for lumbar spine fractures, 368–370, 368f, 369f
　for lumbar spine infections, 497f, 499, 499f
　for posterior cervical spine, 60–61, 61f–63f
　for sacral fractures, 372, 372f, 374–376, 374f–376f
　for spondylolisthesis reduction, 282–284, 282f, 284f
　for thoracic metastasis resection, 456–457, 457
　for thoracic scoliosis correction, 383, 384f–388f, 385
　for thoracic spine infections, 495, 495f
　for thoracolumbar fractures, 361–362, 361f

Screw fixation (Continued)
  in scoliosis correction, 410, 411f, 412f, 413–414
  pedicle or transpedicular. See Pedicle screw fixation.
  rod systems with. See Rod systems.
Segmental vessels
  anatomy of
    in anterolateral approach, 103, 103f
    in retroperitoneal approach, 131f
  ligation of
    in lateral lumbar interbody fusion, 274–275, 275f
    in thoracic metastasis resection, 454, 454f
    in thoracolumbar scoliosis correction, 397, 397f
Semiconstrained (dynamic) plating system, for anterior cervical fusion, 159
Semilunar line of Douglas, anatomy of, 114
Semispinalis capitis muscle, anatomy of
  in lateral extracavitary approach, 110, 110f, 111f
  in posterior approaches, 57, 58f, 59f
Semispinalis cervicis muscle, anatomy of
  in cervicothoracic junction approaches, 79f
  in far-lateral approach, 41
  in posterior approaches, 35f, 36f, 57, 58f, 59f
Semispinalis muscle, anatomy of
  in cervicothoracic junction approaches, 79f, 80
  in posterior transthoracic approaches, 86f
Sensory deficits, in cervical stenosis, 174
Serratus anterior muscle, anatomy of
  in anterolateral transthoracic approaches, 71, 72f
  in transthoracic approaches, 74, 74f
Serratus posterior muscle, anatomy of, in cervicothoracic junction approaches, 79, 79f
Sextant Spinal System, for posterior lumbar fusions, 289, 289f, 292, 293, 293f
Shear force, in thoracolumbar fractures, 355, 355f
Shikata laminoplasty, 195f
Sibson's fascia, anatomy of, 65, 67
Sigmoid sinus, anatomy of, in far-lateral approach, 42, 43
Single lung ventilation, in thoracic scoliosis correction, 385
Sinuvertebral nerve, anatomy of, 49
SLIM-LOC plating system, for anterior cervical fusion, 159
Small intestine
  anatomy of, in transperitoneal approaches, 114, 120, 121f
  injury of, in transperitoneal approaches, 125
Smith-Petersen osteotomy, for flatback syndrome, 422–425, 423f, 425f, 427f
Smith-Robinson lateral approach, to cervical spine, 54f
Smith-Robinson low cervical approach, 67

Smith-Robinson procedure, for anterior cervical diskectomy and fusion, 141, 142f
Soft palate, approach through, to craniocervical junction, 3, 4, 7f–9f
Songer cable, for cervicothoracic junction fractures, 350f
Spetzler classification, of arteriovenous malformations, 480, 480t
Spetzler retractor, for cervicomedullary decompression, 299
SpheRx pedicle screw system, 291–292, 291f–293f
Spinal accessory nerve, anatomy of
  in high cervical retropharyngeal approach, 23, 29, 31f
  in lateral approach, 37, 39
  in lateral retropharyngeal approach, 41
Spinal cord
  aneurysms of, 486
  arteriovenous malformations of, 476–480, 477f–479f
  cavernous malformations of, 476–480, 477f–479f
  compression of, in metastasis, 451
  decompression of. See Decompression, spinal cord.
  hemangioblastoma of, 474–476, 474f, 475f
  injury of
    in cavernous malformations, 478
    in cervical facet dislocation, 337
    in Scheuermann's kyphosis correction, 437
    in thoracolumbar fractures, 356
Spinal nerves, anatomy of, in midcervical region, 50f, 59, 59f
Spinalis cervicis muscle, anatomy of, 57, 58f
Spinalis muscles, anatomy of
  in cervicothoracic junction approaches, 79–80
  in posterior transthoracic approaches, 86f
Splenius capitis muscle, anatomy of
  in cervicothoracic junction approaches, 79, 79f
  in far-lateral approach, 41
  in lateral approach, 37, 38f
  in posterior approaches, 36f, 57, 58f, 59f
Splenius cervicis muscle, anatomy of
  in far-lateral approach, 42
  in lateral approach, 39, 40f
  in posterior approaches, 57, 58f
Spondylectomy, for chordomas, 441
Spondylitis. See also Ankylosing spondylitis.
  anterior cervical corpectomy and fusion for, 169
Spondylolisthesis reduction, 280–286, 280f–284f
  posterior lumbar interbody fusion for, 255
  transpedicular screw fixation for, 239
Spondyloptosis, 284–285
Spondylosis, cervical
  anterior corpectomy and fusion for, 169
  posterior approaches to, 33
  posterior keyhole foraminotomy for, 164–167, 165f–167f
Sponges, Kittner, for transperitoneal approaches, 122, 122f

Staple fixation
  for thoracolumbar fractures, 361–362, 361f
  for thoracolumbar scoliosis correction, 398, 399f
Steinmann pins
  for craniocervical junction fixation, 318, 319f
  for endoscopic diskectomy, 220–221, 220f, 221f
  for endoscopic lumbar decompression, 233f
  for lumbar spine fracture fixation, 368, 369f
  for pedicle screw fixation, 240, 241f
  for thoracic metastasis resection, 458
Stellate ganglion, anatomy of, 51f
Stenosis. See Cervical stenosis; Lumbar stenosis.
Sternal angle, anatomy of, 65, 66f
Sternocleidomastoid muscle, anatomy of, 47, 48f, 49f
  in cervicothoracic junction approaches, 65
  in far-lateral approach, 41
  in high cervical retropharyngeal approach, 22, 23f, 24, 27, 28f, 29, 30f, 31f
  in lateral approach, 37, 38f, 54, 55f
  in lateral retropharyngeal approach, 41
  in medial approach, 52–53
  in transmanubrial-transclavicular approach, 67, 68f, 69f
Sternohyoid muscle, anatomy of, 47, 48f, 65
Sternothyroid muscle, anatomy of, 47, 65
Sternotomy
  for trans-sternal-transthoracic approach, 67, 69f, 70, 70f
  median, for thoracic metastasis, 457
Strange-Vognsen classification, of sacral fractures, 367f
Strap muscles of larynx, anatomy of, 47, 48f
Styloglossus muscle, anatomy of, 23
Stylohyoid ligament, anatomy of, 23
Stylohyoid muscle, anatomy of, 23, 25f, 26, 47
Stylopharyngeus muscle, anatomy of, 23
Subclavian artery, anatomy of, 48, 50, 66
Subclavian vein, anatomy of, 50
Sublaminar wire fixation, for cervicothoracic junction fractures, 350f
Submandibular gland, dissection of, in high cervical retropharyngeal approach, 25–26, 25f, 28f
Submandibular triangle, anatomy of, 22, 23f
Submental triangle, anatomy of, 22, 23f
Suboccipital craniectomy, in far-lateral approach, 41, 42, 42f
Suboccipital triangle, anatomy of, 42
Subscapular space, anatomy of, 71–72, 75f
Suction, for cavernous malformation resection, 478–479
Supraclavicular approach, to cervicothoracic junction, 67
Supraclavicular nerve, anatomy of, 60f
Supraclavicular triangle, anatomy of, in high cervical retropharyngeal approach, 22, 23f
Suprahyoid muscles, anatomy of, 47

Index

Supraspinous ligament, anatomy of, 47f
Suprasternal notch, anatomy of, 65, 66f
Sutures, tagged, for diaphragm reattachment, 95, 95f
Sympathetic chain, anatomy of
  in anterolateral approach, 101, 103–104, 104f
  in anterolateral transthoracic approach, 73
Sympathetic nervous system, cervical, 50–51
Sympathetic plexus, injury of, in transperitoneal approach, 124–125
Sympathetic trunk, anatomy of
  cervical, 50, 50f, 54
  in posterior thoracolumbar approaches, 108f
  in retroperitoneal approach, 131f
  in thoracic diskectomy, 207f
Syrinx, with hemangioblastoma, 474

Tang retractor, for posterior lumbar interbody fusion, 250–251, 250f–252f
Teardrop flexion fractures, cervicothoracic junction, 344, 345f
Teeth, guards for, in transoral approach, 4
Temporal vein, anatomy of, in high cervical retropharyngeal approach, 28f
Temporomandibular joint, evaluation of, in cervicomedullary decompression, 299
Tension bands
  for cervicothoracic junction fractures, 346
  for sacral fractures, 376f
Texas Scottish Rite Hospital instrumentation, for scoliosis, 401, 402f
Thoracic cage, posterior, anatomy of, 80, 80f
Thoracic disk herniation, 201–211, 202f–211f
Thoracic diskectomy, 201–211
  anterior video-assisted thoracoscopic approach to, 208–211, 209f–211f
  anterolateral open thoracotomy approach to, 205–208, 206f–207f
  approaches to, 201, 201f
  costotransversectomy approach to, 201f–204f, 202–205
  indications for, 201
  lateral extracavitary approach to, 201f–204f, 202–205
Thoracic duct
  anatomy of, 50, 51f, 52f
  identification of, in anterior thoracic scoliosis correction, 381
Thoracic inlet, anatomy of, 65, 66f
Thoracic nerves, anatomy of, 81
Thoracic spinal cord
  arteriovenous malformations of, 484
  cavernous malformations of, 479
Thoracic spine
  fractures of, 352–353, 353f–354f
    at cervicothoracic junction, 344–351, 345f–351f
    at thoracolumbar junction, 352–353, 353f–354f
  infections of, 493–496, 493f–497f
  intradural tumors of, posterolateral approach to, 463–470, 465f–473f
  Lenke curve patterns in

Thoracic spine (Continued)
    type 1 (main thoracic curves), 406, 407f, 407t, 408f, 416, 417f
    type 2 (double thoracic curves), 406, 407f, 407t, 408f, 416
    type 3 (double major curves), 406, 407f, 407t, 408f, 416–417, 418f
    type 6 (thoracolumbar/lumbar and main thoracic curves), 406, 407f, 407t, 408f, 420
  metastasis to, surgical treatment of, 452–458, 452f–458f
  posterior and posterolateral approaches to, 106–112, 107f–111f
  scoliosis of, anterior release and fusion techniques for, 379–391, 380f–389f
Thoracic spine modifiers, in Lenke curve patterns, 406, 407f, 409f–410f
Thoracoabdominal approach, to thoracolumbar junction, 89–100
  anatomy of, 89–91, 90f, 91f
  complications of, 98–99
  contraindications for, 91
  indications for, 91
  positioning for, 91, 92f
  transpleural-retroperitoneal, 96–98, 96f–98f
  transthoracic-transdiaphragmatic, 92–95, 93f–96f
Thoracodorsal fascia, anatomy of, in posterior thoracolumbar approaches, 106
Thoracodorsal nerve, anatomy of, in transaxillary approach, 77
Thoracolumbar fractures, 352–363
  anatomic considerations in, 352
  classification of, 352–355, 353f–355f
  mechanism of injury of, 352–353, 353f–355f, 356
  neurologic status in, 356
  radiography in, 356
  treatment of, 356–362
Thoracolumbar junction
  metastasis at, 457
  thoracoabdominal approach to, 89–100, 90f–98f
Thoracolumbar scoliosis
  anterior treatment for, 392–405, 394f–403f
  Lenke curve patterns in
    type 5 (thoracolumbar/lumbar curves), 406, 407f, 407t, 408f, 417, 419f, 420
    type 6 (thoracolumbar/lumbar and main thoracic curves), 406, 407f, 407t, 408f, 420
Thoracolumbar spine
  fractures of. See Thoracolumbar fractures.
  scoliosis of. See Thoracolumbar scoliosis.
Thoracoscopy
  in scoliosis correction, 380–381, 382f–384f, 383, 385, 387f
  video-assisted, in diskectomy, 208–211, 209f–211f
Thoracotomy
  anterolateral open, for diskectomy, 205–208, 206f, 207f
  for anterior thoracic scoliosis correction, 381

Thoracotomy (Continued)
  for intradural tumors, 470, 471f–473f
  for thoracic metastasis
    anterior, 452–457, 452f–456f
    high posterolateral, 457
"Three-column" concept, of thoracolumbar fractures, 352
Thrombosis, in transperitoneal approach, 124
Thyrohyoid muscle, anatomy of, 47, 48f, 50f
Thyroid cartilage, anatomy of, 53, 53f
Thyroid vein, anatomy of, 53, 53f, 54f
Thyroidal arteries, anatomy of, 50, 50f, 51f, 52f
  in high cervical retropharyngeal approach, 23, 27, 28f
  in lateral approach, 55f
  in medial approach, 53, 54f
Tomita laminoplasty, 195f
Tongue
  incision through, in transmandibular approach, 3, 4, 6, 11f, 12
  swelling of, in transoral approach, 6
Trachea, anatomy of, in anterolateral transthoracic approach, 73
Tracheostomy
  for cervicomedullary decompression, 299
  for high cervical retropharyngeal approach, 22–24
  for transmandibular approach, 6
  for transmaxillary approach, 21
Traction, cervical
  for cervicomedullary decompression, 299
  for posterior cervical osteotomy, 309, 309f
Transaxillary approach, to cervicothoracic junction, 73, 73f, 76–77, 77f
Transcervical (high cervical retropharyngeal) approach, to craniocervical junction, 22–32, 23f–31f
Transcondylar approach, to craniocervical junction, 41–43, 42f
Transforaminal lumbar interbody fusion, 255–262, 256f–262f
Transiliac screws, for sacral fractures, 376f
Transmandibular approach, to craniocervical junction, 3, 4, 6, 11f
Transmanubrial-transclavicular approach, to cervicothoracic junction, 67, 68f, 69f
Transmaxillary approach, to craniocervical junction, 13–21, 14f–20f
Transmuscular far lateral lumbar diskectomy, 215, 217f, 218
Transoral approach
  to craniocervical junction, 3–13, 5f–11f, 14f–15f
  to ventral cervicomedullary decompression, in rheumatoid arthritis, 298–304, 298f–303f
Transpalatine approach, to craniocervical junction, 3, 4, 7f–10f
Transpedicular approach
  to cervicothoracic junction, 82–84, 83f
  to thoracic diskectomy, 201
  to thoracolumbar region, 106, 108

Transpedicular screw fixation. *See* Pedicle screw fixation.
Transperitoneal approaches, to lumbosacral junction, 113–125, 114f–124f
  anatomy of, 113–115, 114f, 115f
  complications of, 124–125
  contraindications for, 116
  indications for, 116
  laparoscopic, 113, 118–122, 119f, 122f
  technique for, 116–124, 117f–124f
Transpleural transthoracic third rib resection approach, to cervicothoracic junction, 73–74, 74f–76f, 76
Transpleural-retroperitoneal approach, to thoracolumbar junction, 96–98, 96f–98f
Trans-sternal-transthoracic approach, to cervicothoracic junction, 67, 69f, 70, 70f
Transthoracic-transdiaphragmatic approach, to thoracolumbar junction, 92–95, 93f–96f
Transversalis fascia, anatomy of, 114, 114f, 121f
Transverse colli nerve, anatomy of, 60f
Transverse foramen, anatomy of, 45
Transverse incision, for high cervical retropharyngeal approach, 22
Transverse sinus, anatomy of
  in far-lateral approach, 42
  in posterior approaches, 34
Transversospinalis muscles, anatomy of
  in cervicothoracic junction approaches, 80
  in posterior approaches, 57, 58f
  in posterior transthoracic approaches, 87, 87f
Transversus abdominis muscle, anatomy of
  in posterior thoracolumbar approaches, 106
  in retroperitoneal approach, 129, 129f, 130f
Transversus fascia, anatomy of, in retroperitoneal approach, 130, 130f
Trapezius muscle, anatomy of, 49f
  in anterolateral transthoracic approaches, 71, 72f
  in cervicothoracic junction approaches, 78, 79f
  in far-lateral approach, 41
  in high cervical retropharyngeal approach, 22, 23f
  in lateral extracavitary approach, 110, 110f, 111f
  in posterior approaches, 34, 36, 36f, 57, 58f, 59f
  in posterior transthoracic approaches, 86, 86f, 87f
Trauma. *See also* Dislocations; Fractures.
  cervical spine, posterior approaches to, 33
  craniocervical
    transmaxillary approach to, 3–12, 5f–11f
    transoral approach to, 3–13, 5f–11f, 14f–15f
  transpedicular screw fixation for, 239
Tricortical bone graft, 506, 507f, 508
Trigeminal nerve, anatomy of, in transmaxillary approach, 17f, 18
Triple-wire technique, for cervical spine fixation, 61, 63f

T-shaped incision, for high cervical retropharyngeal approach, 22, 23, 24f
Tube(s), chest, for thoracoabdominal approach, 98–99, 98f
Tuberculosis, 500, 500f, 501f
  lateral extracavitary approach to, 108
  of lumbosacral junction, transperitoneal approach to, 113
  psoas abscess in, 90
Tubular retractors
  for lumbar decompression, 232–236, 232f–236f, 288, 288f
  for METRx system, 232–236, 232f–236f, 287–289, 288f, 289f
  for percutaneous and endoscopic lumbar diskectomy, 221–222, 222f–224f, 224
Tumor(s)
  benign, 443–446, 444f, 445f
  intradural, 462–473, 462f–473f
  lateral lumbar interbody fusion for, 272
  malignant
    primary, 441–443, 443f, 444f
    secondary. *See* Metastasis.
  of cervical spine, posterior approaches to, 33
  of craniocervical junction
    far-lateral approach to, 41–43, 42f
    lateral approach to, 37, 37f–40f, 39
    transmaxillary approach to, 3–12, 5f–11f
    transoral approach to, 3–13, 5f–11f, 14f–15f
  of spinal cord, 475f–483f, 474–486
  of vertebrae, thoracoabdominal approach to, 91
  transpedicular screw fixation for, 239
"Two-column" concept, of thoracolumbar fractures, 353
"Two-point" method, for cavernous malformation resection planning, 478, 478f

Uncinate process, drilling of, in anterior cervical microforaminotomy, 152, 154f
Uncovertebral joint, anatomy of, 45, 46f, 55f
Uncovertebral junction, exposure of, in anterior cervical microforaminotomy, 151, 152f
Unicortical bone graft, 508
Unicortical screws, in cervical spine locking plate, for anterior cervical fusion, 159
Unilateral transforaminal lumbar interbody fusion, 255–262, 256f–262f
Ureter
  anatomy of
    in anterolateral approach, 101, 102f
    in lateral lumbar interbody fusion, 274
    in thoracoabdominal approach, 91
    in transperitoneal approaches, 114–115, 115f, 121
  injury of, in transperitoneal approach, 124
Uvula, retraction of, in cervicomedullary decompression, 299–300, 300f

Vagus nerve, anatomy of, 28f, 50, 50f, 51f
Vantage anterior thoracolumbar plate, for metastasis, 456–457
Vascular lesions, of spinal cord, 474–486

Vena cava, anatomy of
  in anterior lumbar interbody fusion, 265–266, 266f, 267f
  in anterolateral approach, 103, 103f, 104f, 105
  in lateral lumbar interbody fusion, 273, 274f
  in transperitoneal approaches, 115f
Venous sinus, anatomy of, in posterior approaches, 34
Venous thrombosis, in transperitoneal approach, 124
Ventral (medial) anterior approaches, to midcervical spine, 52–54, 53f, 54f
Verbiest lateral approach, to cervical spine, 54, 54f
Vertebrae
  anatomy of
    cervical, 45, 46f
    lumbar, 213, 214f
  resection of. *See* Vertebrectomy.
  rib attachment to, 80, 80f
Vertebral arches, anatomy of, in posterior approaches, 34, 35f
Vertebral artery
  anatomy of, 49–50, 52f
    in cross-sectional view, 58f
    in far-lateral approach, 41–43, 42f
    in lateral approach, 38f, 39, 40f, 54, 55f, 56
    in lateral retropharyngeal approach, 41
    in midcervical spine, 45
    in posterior approaches, 34, 36
    in transmaxillary approach, 18, 19f
    in transoral approach, 6
  injury of
    in cervicomedullary decompression, 303–304
    in cervicothoracic junction surgery, 346
  lesions of, lateral approach to, 37
Vertebral fractures, thoracoabdominal approach to, 91
Vertebral plexi, anatomy of, in posterior thoracolumbar approaches, 108f
Vertebral veins, anatomy of, 58f, 66
Vertebrectomy
  in anterior cervical corpectomy and fusion, 169, 171, 171f
  in anterior transthoracic approach, 76, 76f
  in lateral lumbar interbody fusion, 275–277, 276f, 277f
  in pedicle subtraction osteotomy, 428–429
  in spondyloptosis reduction, 282, 285
  lumbosacral, in transperitoneal approaches, 122–123
Vertebrobasilar junction, transoral approach to, 3–13, 5f–11f, 14f–15f
Vertebroplasty, for compression fractures, 357
Video-assisted thoracoscopic approach, anterior, to diskectomy, 208–211, 209f–211f
Visceral cervical fascia, anatomy of, 49
Viscerocarotid space, anatomy of, 65–66, 66f
von Hippel-Lindau syndrome, hemangioblastoma in, 474

"Wanding" technique
  in endoscopic lumbar decompression, 234, 234f

"Wanding" technique *(Continued)*
  in endoscopic lumbar diskectomy, 224, 224f
Weakness, in cervical stenosis, 174
Weber-Ferguson incision, in transmaxillary approach, 13, 17f
Wedge compression injury, cervicothoracic junction, 344, 345f
Wertheim-Bohlman technique, for occipitocervical wire fixation, 327, 327f

Wire fixation
  for cervical facet dislocation, 339
  for cervical spine, 61, 63f
  for cervicothoracic junction fractures, 346, 347f, 351
  for craniocervical junction fractures, 318, 319f, 324–325, 325f–328f, 327

"Y" plate (Grob), for craniocervical fracture fixation, 322f

Yellow ligaments, anatomy of, 34, 35f
Yoshida laminoplasty, 195f

Zielke instrumentation, for scoliosis, 401
Z-plasty, in cervical laminoplasty, 180, 180f
Zygapophyseal joints, anatomy of, 34